Medical Management of the Surgical Patient

A Textbook of Perioperative Medicine

Fifth Edition

Medical Management of the Surgical Patient

A Textbook of Perioperative Medicine

Fifth Edition

Editor-in-Chief
Michael F. Lubin MD
Professor of Medicine, Emory University School of Medicine, Atlanta, GA, USA

Associate Editors
Thomas F. Dodson MD
Professor of Surgery and Chief, Division of Vascular and Endovascular Surgery,
Emory University School of Medicine, Atlanta, GA, USA

Neil H. Winawer MD
Associate Professor of Medicine, Emory University School of Medicine, Atlanta, GA, USA and
Director of the Hospital Medicine Service at Grady Memorial Hospital, Atlanta, GA, USA

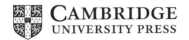

CAMBRIDGE
UNIVERSITY PRESS

CAMBRIDGE
UNIVERSITY PRESS

University Printing House, Cambridge CB2 8BS, United Kingdom

Published in the United States of America by Cambridge University Press, New York

Cambridge University Press is part of the University of Cambridge.

It furthers the University's mission by disseminating knowledge in the pursuit of education, learning and research at the highest international levels of excellence.

www.cambridge.org
Information on this title: www.cambridge.org/9781107009165

First published 2013

Printed in United Kingdom by TJ International Ltd. Padstow Cornwall

A catalogue record for this publication is available from the British Library

Library of Congress Cataloguing in Publication data
Medical management of the surgical patient : a textbook of perioperative medicine / [edited by] Michael F. Lubin, Thomas F. Dodson, Neil H. Winawer. – 5th ed.
        p. ; cm.
Includes bibliographical references.
ISBN 978-1-107-00916-5 (Hardback)
I. Lubin, Michael F., 1947– II. Dodson, Thomas. III. Winawer, Neil H.
[DNLM: 1. Perioperative Care. 2. Intraoperative Complications–prevention & control. 3. Postoperative Complications–prevention & control. 4. Risk Assessment. WO 178]
617.9′1–dc23   2012016725

ISBN 978-1-107-00916-5 Hardback

Michael F. Lubin MD

I would like to dedicate this book to
J. Willis Hurst – my teacher
H. Kenneth Walker – my mentor and co-editor
Robert Smith – my colleague and co-editor

Their contributions to this book are unseen but were critical to its successful completion

Thomas F. Dodson MD

I would like to dedicate this book to my wife, Jan, and my children, Thomas, Michael, and Amy. Their patience has been remarkable and their love and support have been graciously given.

Neil H. Winawer MD

I would like to dedicate this book to my wife Tamara, and my son Matthew for bearing with me during completion of this project and always. You are my everything.

Contents

Contents

Contents

Contributors

Raja-Elie E. Abdulnour
Pulmonary and Critical Care Medicine, Department of Internal Medicine, Brigham and Women's Hospital and Harvard Medical School, Harvard Institutes of Medicine, Boston, MA, USA

Kumari N. Adams
Emory University School of Medicine, Atlanta, GA, USA

Dheera Ananthakrishnan
Emory University School of Medicine, Atlanta, GA, USA

Jordan Angell
Emory University School of Medicine, Atlanta, GA, USA

H. Michael Baddour, Jr.
Emory University School of Medicine, Department of Otolaryngology Head and Neck Surgery, Atlanta, GA, USA

Remzi Bag
Emory University School of Medicine, Atlanta, GA, USA

Daniel L. Barrow
Emory University School of Medicine, Atlanta, GA, USA

Eric E. Berg
Emory University School of Medicine, Department of Otolaryngology Head and Neck Surgery, Atlanta, GA, USA

James C. Black
Emory University School of Medicine, Atlanta, GA, USA

Maxwell Boakye
Stanford University School of Medicine, CA, USA

Duncan Borland
Vancouver, WA, Canada

Bryon J. Boulton
Emory University School of Medicine, Atlanta, GA, USA

Andrew Boxer
Manhattan Veteran's Hospital and Division of Gastroenterology, New York University School of Medicine, New York, NY, USA

Thomas Bradbury
Emory University School of Medicine, Atlanta, GA, USA

Luke P. Brewster
Emory University School of Medicine, Atlanta, GA, USA

Jennifer Brown
Division of Infectious Diseases, UC Davis Medical Center, Sacramento, CA, USA

Grant W. Carlson
Emory University School of Medicine, Atlanta, GA, USA

C. Michael Cawley
Emory University School of Medicine, Atlanta, GA, USA

Kristina Chacko
Manhattan Veteran's Hospital and Division of Gastroenterology, New York University School of Medicine, New York, NY, USA

Amy Y. Chen
Professor, Department of Otolaryngology Head and Neck Surgery, Emory University School of Medicine, Atlanta, GA, USA

Edward P. Chen
Emory University School of Medicine, Atlanta, GA, USA

Andrew I. Chin
University of California Davis, Sacramento, CA and Department of Veterans Affairs Northern California Health Care System, Mather, CA, USA

Jayer Chung
Division of Vascular Surgery, University of Texas Southwestern, Dallas, TX, USA

Carter G. Co
Division of Pulmonary, Critical Care, Allergy, and Sleep Medicine, Department of Medicine, Emory University School of Medicine, Atlanta, GA, USA

Rebecca L. Coefield
Emory University School of Medicine, Atlanta, GA, USA

Stuart H. Cohen
Division of Infectious Diseases, UC Davis Medical Center, Sacramento, CA, USA

Candice C. Colby
Emory University School of Medicine, Atlanta, GA, USA

Michelle V. Conde
University of Texas Health Science Center at San Antonio; San Antonio, TX, USA

William A. Cooper
Emory University School of Medicine, Atlanta, GA, USA

Matthew A. Corriere
Emory University School of Medicine, Atlanta, GA, USA

Anastasios P. Costarides
Emory University School of Medicine, Atlanta, GA, USA

Natario L. Couser
Emory University School of Medicine, Atlanta, GA, USA

Francis X. Creighton
Emory University School of Medicine, Atlanta, GA, USA

John H. Culbertson
Emory University School of Medicine, Atlanta, GA, USA

Vladimir Dadashev
Emory University School of Medicine, Atlanta, GA, USA

Mark J. Dannenbaum
Emory University School of Medicine, Atlanta, GA, USA

S. Scott Davis, Jr.
Emory University School of Medicine, Atlanta, GA, USA

Samuel M. Davis
Emory University School of Medicine, Atlanta, GA, USA

John J. De Caro
Emory University School of Medicine, Atlanta, GA, USA

John M. DelGaudio
Emory University School of Medicine, Department of Otolaryngology Head and Neck Surgery, Atlanta, GA, USA

Sanjay Singh Dhall
Emory University School of Medicine, Atlanta, GA, USA

Thomas F. Dodson
Emory University School of Medicine, Atlanta, GA, USA

Burl R. Don
University of California Davis, Sacramento, CA, USA

Erica C. Dun
Emory University School of Medicine, Atlanta, GA, USA

Mrinal Dutia
Division of Hematology Oncology, UC Davis School of Medicine, Sacramento, CA, USA

James R. Eckman
Emory University School of Medicine, Atlanta, GA, USA

Niels Engberding
Emory University, Grady Memorial Hospital, Atlanta, GA, USA

Greg Erens
Emory University School of Medicine, Atlanta, GA, USA

Annette Esper
Division of Pulmonary, Allergy and Critical Care, Emory University, Atlanta, GA, USA

Christine Doss Esper
Emory University School of Medicine, Atlanta, GA, USA

David V. Feliciano
Emory University School of Medicine, Atlanta, GA, USA

Felix G. Fernandez
Emory University School of Medicine, Atlanta, GA, USA

Lamar L. Fleming
Emory University School of Medicine, Atlanta, GA, USA

Seth D. Force
Emory University School of Medicine, Atlanta, GA, USA

Michael Frankel
Emory University School of Medicine, Atlanta, GA, USA

Taki Galanis
Jefferson Vascular Center, Jefferson Medical College, Thomas Jefferson University Hospitals, Philadelphia, PA, USA

Niall T. M. Galloway
Emory University School of Medicine, Atlanta, GA, USA

Frederick Gandolfo
Manhattan Veteran's Hospital and Division of Gastroenterology, New York University School of Medicine, New York, NY, USA

Leda Gattoc
Emory University School of Medicine, Atlanta, GA, USA

Bonnie B. Germain
Emory University School of Medicine, Atlanta, GA, USA

Steven M. Gorbatkin
Renal Section, Atlanta Veterans Affairs Medical Center and Emory University School of Medicine, Atlanta, GA, USA

Michael B. Gottschalk
Emory University School of Medicine, Atlanta, GA, USA

William J. Grist
Emory University School of Medicine, Atlanta, GA, USA

Robert E. Gross
Emory University School of Medicine, Atlanta, GA, USA

Naren Gupta
VA Boston Health System and Brigham and Women's Hospital, Harvard Medical School, Boston, MA, USA

Regis W. Haid, Jr.
Atlanta Brain and Spine, Inc., Atlanta, GA, USA

Garrett Harper
Emory Division of Plastic and Reconstructive Surgery, Emory University School of Medicine, Atlanta, GA, USA

Katherine L. Hayes
Emory University School of Medicine, Atlanta, GA, USA

John G. Heller
Emory University School of Medicine, Atlanta, GA, USA

Stacy Higgins
Emory University School of Medicine, Atlanta, GA, USA

Kenneth L. Hill, Jr.
Emory University School of Medicine, Atlanta, GA, USA

Christopher D. Hillyer
New York Blood Center, New York, NY, USA

Eric G. Honig
Division of Pulmonary, Critical Care, Allergy, and Sleep Medicine, Department of Medicine, Emory University School of Medicine, Atlanta, GA, USA

Ira R. Horowitz
Emory University School of Medicine, Atlanta, GA, USA

William C. Horton
Emory University School of Medicine, Atlanta, GA, USA

G. Baker Hubbard
Division of Vitreoretinal Surgery and Disease, Department of Ophthalmology, Emory University, Atlanta, GA, USA

Carl C. Hug, Jr.
Emeritus, Emory University School of Medicine; Emory University Hospital, Emory University, Atlanta, GA, USA

Amy K. Hutchinson
Emory University School of Medicine, Atlanta, GA, USA

Walter Ingram
Emory University School of Medicine, Atlanta, GA, USA

Muta M. Issa
Emory University School of Medicine and Atlanta VA Medical Center, Atlanta, GA, USA

S. Mohammad A. Jafri
Emory University School of Medicine, Atlanta, GA, USA

Michael M. Johns
Emory University School of Medicine, Atlanta, GA, USA

Danielle Jones
Emory University School of Medicine, Atlanta, GA, USA

Wright A. Jones
Emory University School of Medicine, Atlanta, GA, USA

Lilith Judd
Emory University School of Medicine, GA, USA

Jorge L. Juncos
Emory University School of Medicine, Atlanta, GA, USA

Julie Katz Karp
Methodist Hospital, Philadelphia, PA, USA

Osama N. Kashlan
Emory University School of Medicine, Atlanta, GA, USA

Karthikeshwar Kasirajan
Emory University School of Medicine, Atlanta, GA, USA

W. Brent Keeling
Division of Cardiothoracic Surgery, Emory University School of Medicine, Atlanta, GA, USA

Craig R. Keenan
Department of Medicine, UC Davis School of Medicine, Sacramento, CA, USA

Jaffar Khan
Emory University School of Medicine, Lawrenceville, GA, USA

Joung Y. Kim
Division of Cornea and External Disease, Emory University School of Medicine, Atlanta, GA, USA

Kathleen Kinlaw
Center for Ethics, Program Director, Health, Science and Ethics, Emory University, Atlanta, GA, USA

S. Robert Kovac
Emory University School of Medicine, Atlanta, GA, USA

John G. Kral
Department of Surgery, SUNY Downstate Medical Center, Brooklyn, New York, NY, USA

Sameh A. Labib
Emory University School of Medicine, Atlanta, GA, USA

David V. LaBorde
Emory University School of Medicine, Atlanta, GA, USA

James J. Lah
Emory University School of Medicine, Atlanta, GA, USA

Omar M. Lattouf
Emory University School of Medicine, Atlanta, GA, USA

Adrienne M. Laury
Emory University School of Medicine, Atlanta, GA, USA

Valerie A. Lawrence
University of Texas Health Science Center at San Antonio; San Antonio, TX, USA

Sung Bae Lee
Emory University School of Medicine, Atlanta, GA, USA

Jeffrey L. Lennox
Emory University School of Medicine, Atlanta, GA, USA

Jason Lesandrini
Grady Memorial Hospital, Atlanta, GA, USA

Bradley G. Leshnower
Emory University School of Medicine, Atlanta, GA, USA

Allan I. Levey
Emory University School of Medicine, Atlanta, GA, USA

Bruce D. Levy
Pulmonary and Critical Care Medicine, Department of Internal Medicine, Brigham and Women's Hospital and Harvard Medical School, Harvard Institutes of Medicine, Boston, MA, USA

Harrell Lightfoot
Emory University School of Medicine, Atlanta, GA, USA

Edward Lin
Emory University School of Medicine, Atlanta, GA, USA

Albert Losken
Emory University School of Medicine, Atlanta, GA, USA

John Louis-Ugbo
Emory University School of Medicine, Atlanta, GA, USA

Michael F. Lubin
Emory University School of Medicine, Atlanta, GA, USA

C. Ronald MacKenzie
Hospital for Special Surgery, New York Weill Cornell Center, New York, NY, USA

Sharmila Makhija
University of Louisville School of Medicine, Louisville, KY, USA

Kamal A. Mansour
Emory University School of Medicine, Atlanta, GA, USA

Douglas E. Mattox
Emory University School of Medicine, Atlanta, GA, USA

Kevin W. McConnell
Emory University School of Medicine, Atlanta, GA, USA

Gary R. McGillivary
Emory University, Department of Orthopedic Surgery, Atlanta, GA, USA

Yuri McKee
Division of Cornea and External Disease, Emory University School of Medicine, Atlanta, GA, USA

Anne Marie McKenzie-Brown
Emory University School of Medicine, Atlanta, GA, USA

J. Nicolas Mclean
Emory University School of Medicine, Division of Plastic and Reconstructive Surgery, Atlanta, GA, USA

Yelena Melyakova
Emory University School of Medicine, Atlanta, GA, USA

Geno J. Merli
Jefferson Vascular Center and Jefferson Medical College, Thomas Jefferson University Hospitals, Philadelphia, PA, USA

Charles E. Moore
Department of Otolaryngology Head and Neck Surgery, Emory University School of Medicine, Atlanta, GA, USA

Thomas J. Moore
Emory University School of Medicine, Atlanta, GA, USA

Benjamin L. Moosavi
Emory University School of Medicine, Atlanta, GA, USA

Radu F. Neamu
Pulmonary and Critical Care Medicine, Emory University School of Medicine, Atlanta, GA, USA

David C. Neujahr
Emory University School of Medicine, Atlanta, GA, USA

Duc Q. Nguyen
Emory University School of Medicine, Atlanta, GA, USA

Peter T. Nieh
Emory University School of Medicine, Atlanta, GA, USA

Kathleen Nilles
Feinberg School of Medicine, Northwestern University, Chicago, IL, USA

Gina M. Northington
Emory University School of Medicine, Atlanta, GA, USA

Kenneth Ogan
Emory University School of Medicine, Atlanta, GA, USA

Timothy W. Olsen
Division of Vitreoretinal Surgery and Disease, Department of Ophthalmology, Emory University, Atlanta, GA, USA

Jeffrey J. Olson
Emory University School of Medicine, Atlanta, GA, USA

Shervin V. Oskouei
Emory University School of Medicine, Atlanta, GA, USA

Kumiko Owada
Emory University School of Medicine, Atlanta, GA, USA

Nelson Oyesiku
Emory University School of Medicine, Atlanta, GA, USA

Monica W. Parker
Emory University School of Medicine, Atlanta, GA, USA

Ted Parran, Jr.
CWRU School of Medicine, Cleveland, OH, USA

Stephen Pastan
Emory University School of Medicine, Atlanta, GA, USA

L. Reuven Pasternak
Health Systems of Stony Brook University Hospital, Storm Brook, NY, USA

John G. Pattaras
Emory University School of Medicine, Atlanta, GA, USA

John F. Payne
Division of Vitreoretinal Surgery and Disease, Department of Ophthalmology, Emory University, Atlanta, GA, USA

Allan Pickens
Emory University School of Medicine, Atlanta, GA, USA

J. Richard Pittman
Emory University School of Medicine, Atlanta, GA, USA

Michael A. Poles
Manhattan Veteran's Hospital and Division of Gastroenterology, New York University School of Medicine, New York, NY, USA

Pamela T. Prescott
University of California at Davis, Division of Endocrinology, Sacramento, CA, USA

David A. Quintero
Division of Pulmonary, Critical Care, Allergy, and Sleep Medicine, Department of Medicine, Emory University School of Medicine, Atlanta, GA, USA

Hassan T. Rahman
Division of Vitreoretinal Surgery and Disease, Department of Ophthalmology, Emory University, Atlanta, GA, USA

Charles L. Raison
Department of Psychiatry and Behavioral Sciences, Emory University School of Medicine, Atlanta, GA, USA

J. Bradley Randleman
Emory University School of Medicine, Atlanta, GA, USA

Madhuri Rao
Department of Surgery, SUNY Downstate Medical Center, Brooklyn, New York, NY, USA

James G. Reeves
Emory University School of Medicine, Atlanta, GA, USA

William M. Reisman
Assistant Professor of Orthopedic Trauma, Emory University School of Medicine, Atlanta, GA, USA

John M. Rhee
Emory University School of Medicine, Atlanta, GA, USA

Paul J. Riesenman
Emory University School of Medicine, Atlanta, GA, USA

Eva Rimler
Emory University School of Medicine, Atlanta, GA, USA

Chad M. W. Ritenour
Emory University School of Medicine, Atlanta, GA, USA

James Roberson
Emory University School of Medicine, Atlanta, GA, USA

Carla P. Roberts
Emory University School of Medicine, Atlanta, GA, USA

Eve Rodler
Division of Oncology, University of Washington School of Medicine, Seattle, WA, USA

Gerald E. Rodts, Jr.
Emory University School of Medicine, Atlanta, GA, USA

Lorenzo Rossaro
University of California Davis, Sacramento, CA, USA

Adil Sadiq
Emory University School of Medicine, Atlanta, GA, USA

Atef A. Salam
Emory University School of Medicine, Atlanta, GA, USA

Neil D. Saunders
Emory University School of Medicine, Atlanta, GA, USA

Alonzo T. Sexton
Emory University School of Medicine, Atlanta, GA, USA

Nisha N. Shah
Department of Psychiatry and Behavioral Sciences, Emory University School of Medicine, Atlanta, GA, USA

Rupa Shah
Department of Ophthalmology, Case Western Reserve University, Cleveland, OH, USA

Jyotirmay Sharma
Emory University School of Medicine, Atlanta, GA, USA

Beth H. Shaz
Chief Medical Officer, New York Blood Center, New York, NY, USA

Adam B. Shrewsberry
Resident in Urology, Emory University School of Medicine, Atlanta, GA, USA

Kimberly A. Singh
Emory University School of Medicine, Atlanta, GA, USA

Cyril O. Spann
Emory University School of Medicine, Atlanta, GA, USA

Nathan Spell
Emory University School of Medicine, Atlanta, GA, USA

Eric Anthony Sribnick
Emory University School of Medicine, Atlanta, GA, USA

Michael S. Sridhar
Emory University, Department of Orthopedic Surgery, Division of Sports Medicine, Atlanta, GA, USA

Jahnavi K. Srinivasan
Emory University School of Medicine, Atlanta, GA, USA

Melissa M. Statham
Emory University School of Medicine, Department of Otolaryngology Head and Neck Surgery, Atlanta, GA, USA

James P. Steinberg
Emory University School of Medicine, Atlanta, GA, USA

Ram Subramanian
Emory University School of Medicine, Atlanta, GA, USA

John F. Sweeney
Emory University School of Medicine, Atlanta, GA, USA

Sudha Tata
Emory University School of Medicine, Atlanta, GA, USA

Sooraj Tejaswi
University of California Davis, Sacramento, CA, USA

Vinod H. Thourani
Division of Cardiothoracic Surgery, Emory University School of Medicine, Atlanta, GA, USA

N. Wendell Todd
Emory University School of Medicine, Atlanta, GA, USA

Ravi K. Veeraswamy
Emory University School of Medicine, Atlanta, GA, USA

J. David Vega
Emory University School of Medicine, Atlanta, GA, USA

Alvaro Velasquez
Emory University School of Medicine, Atlanta, GA, USA

Giri Venkatraman
Dartmouth Hitchcock Medical Center, Lebanon, NH, USA

J. Trad Wadsworth
Emory University School of Medicine, Atlanta, GA, USA

Mark D. Walsh
Emory University School of Medicine, Atlanta, GA, USA

Howard Weitz
Thomas Jefferson University Hospital, Philadelphia, PA, USA

Jill R. Wells
Division of Ocular Oncology, Department of Ophthalmology, Emory University, Atlanta, GA, USA

Neil H. Winawer
Emory University School of Medicine, Atlanta, GA, USA

Sarah K. Wise
Emory University School of Medicine, Atlanta, GA, USA

Ted Wun
Division of Hematology Oncology, UC Davis School of Medicine and UC Davis Clinical and Translational Sciences Center, Sacramento, CA, USA

John W. Xerogeanes
Emory University, Department of Orthopedic Surgery, Division of Sports Medicine, Atlanta, GA, USA

Seth A. Yellin
Clinical Assistant Professor, Emory University School of Medicine, Atlanta, GA, USA

Jane Y. Yeun
University of California Davis, Sacramento, CA and Department of Veterans Affairs Northern California Health Care System, Mather, CA, USA

Vivian M. Zhao
Department of Pharmaceutical Services, Emory University Hospital, Atlanta, GA, USA

Thomas R. Ziegler
Nutrition and Metabolic Support Service, Department of Medicine, Division of Endocrinology, Metabolism and Lipids, Emory University School of Medicine, Atlanta, GA, USA

Shanta M. Zimmer
University of Pittsburgh School of Medicine, Pittsburgh, PA, USA

Preface

In 1977, Dr. Kenneth Walker called his young colleague, Dr. Michael Lubin, to tell him that there was going to be a new consultation service and he was going to be the first attending. Dr. Lubin replied, "A consult service? That's great! I don't know anything about that stuff." Dr. Walker said, "Don't worry," and hung up the phone.

And now, 35 years later, I and my co-editors are publishing the fifth edition of our textbook on perioperative consultation! The core of knowledge in perioperative care has changed immensely; in 1977 there was no information until Dr. Lee Goldman's seminal paper in the *New England Journal of Medicine* [1]. Since then, there has been an explosion of new information. Many medical people have built their academic careers in this area.

In some specialties, like cardiology, there has been a huge amount of exploration and progress, albeit along with some backtracking. In the previous edition, the latest advance was perioperative beta blockade; today, there is less enthusiasm for this intervention. While in the early days of cardiac evaluation, there was great emphasis placed on invasive testing and interventions, for many surgery patients there has been little benefit found in an aggressive approach to perioperative revascularization. The perioperative management of diabetes has also been the focus of much investigation. Indeed, progress is being made in a multitude of fields.

On the other hand, there are areas where there have been fewer advances. I would be very pleased to find better ways to determine which patients with pulmonary and renal disease are at higher risk for complications and death from surgical intervention.

This fifth edition will update the reader on the latest advances in perioperative care and surgical techniques. We have again gathered together the best people we can find to educate us in the best ways to handle the evaluation and care of patients who may need surgical intervention.

There have been some editorial changes as well. Dr. Robert Smith has retired; Dr. Thomas Dodson, our institution's Associate Chairman of the Department of Surgery and the Chief of the Division of Vascular Surgery, has taken up Dr. Smith's job of handling the surgical part of our book. Dr. Neil H. Winawer, selected as one of the 10 best academic hospitalists by the American College of Physicians, and editor-in-chief of *Journal Watch Hospital Medicine*, has come on board to help me with the medical sections.

As in previous editions, we have added new chapters to fill in perceived gaps. There are new chapters on consultation, transplantation medicine, and pain management. There is a new chapter on asthma management (how could we have missed that for four editions?). New surgical chapters include thoracic aortic disease, lung transplantation, esophagomyotomy, cervical spine surgery, reconstruction after cancer ablation, thyroid malignancies, vasectomy, and inflatable penile prosthesis.

We are firm in our belief that this book is an important part of the medical literature. Our target audience is all physicians who contribute to the care of patients in the perioperative period: anesthesiologists, surgeons, internists, and family physicians. The physician assistants and nurse practitioners who assist in patient care will find information that is valuable to them as well. We have again tried to make *Medical Management of the Surgical Patient* a usable and well-documented reference book. While there are excellent handbooks that address "only the facts," we feel very strongly that there should to be a single-volume source for the background information to support the recommendations we have put forward.

Most of all, we hope that all of our patients receive better medical care because of the efforts of our authors.

We are indebted to Cambridge University Press for publishing this fifth edition. Their editorial assistance and patience are deeply appreciated.

Michael F. Lubin, MD

Reference

1　Goldman L, Caldera DL, Nussbaum SR *et al.* Multifactorial index of cardiac risk in noncardiac surgical procedures. *N Engl J Med* 1977: **297**: 845–50.

Introduction

The interchange between physicians discussing a patient's case has been mentioned in written history since ancient Greece. From the time of Hippocrates, physicians have been encouraged to seek consultation on difficult cases when they were in doubt. They were urged not to be jealous of one another but to realize their own limitations and to use the knowledge of their colleagues to help. "Nor, among physicians, do those who treat by diet envy those who employ surgery, but they even call each other into consultation and commend one another." It is clear, however, that there were disagreements in those days: "Physicians who meet in consultation must never quarrel or jeer at one another." There were also "wretched quarrelsome consultations at the bedside of the patient, with no consultant agreeing with another, fearing he might acknowledge a superior."

Over the next 25 centuries, consultation has had its ups and downs. Much of what was written had to do with the etiquette and ethics of the interaction. In medieval Europe, little changed from ancient times. Physicians were encouraged to ask colleagues for help if needed and to refrain from criticizing each other in front of non-physicians.

In the fourteenth century, patients were warned against consulting large numbers of doctors because there would be "endless disagreements and different suggestions" and "the patients [would] suffer from lack of care." The doctor could call in another physician for consultations, but the treatment should be administered by the one knowing the most about the case. Physicians, curiously enough, were warned about consulting with other physicians. "It is better if he have good excuses that he may refuse their demands. He may feign an injury, or illness, or some other likely excuse. But if he accepts their demands let him make a covenant for his work and make it beforehand .... Clearly advise the other leech that he will give no definite answer in any case until he has seen the sickness and the symptoms of the patient." At least the last is sound advice.

The seventeenth and eighteenth centuries brought out the best and the worst in physicians. In Italy, Julius Caesar Claudinius wrote, "There is no part of a Physician's Office more illustrious than Consultation, because by it alone unlearned physicians are known from the Learned .... And there is nothing that brings greater advantage to the Sick." Contrast this with the following: "On December 28, 1750, Drs. John Williams and Parker Bennett, of Jamaica, having become involved in a wrangle about their respective views on bilious fever, came to blows, and, the next day, proceeded to a desperate hand-to-hand combat with swords and pistols, which ended fatally for both. It is said that Johann Peter Frank was so disgusted with the behavior of doctors in consultation that he advised the calling in of the police on all such occasions." Again, in contrast to the brutish behavior in the British colony, John Gregory wrote that "consultation, when required, is to be conducted in a gentlemanly manner. The chief concern is to be the relief of the patient's suffering and not personal advancement. That is, the duty to one's patients takes precedence over personal and professional differences."

During the eighteenth century, there had been (and would continue to be) a great deal of competition between practitioners. At the turn of the nineteenth century, there was much activity in writing about the ethics of medicine, most of which was aimed at avoiding the harmful effect of this competition. Two men in particular bear mention – Johann Stieglitz and Thomas Percival.

In 1798, Stieglitz addressed the problem of the profession's internal difficulties and the distrust they engendered in the public. Many practitioners were afraid to admit their need for help and thus avoided consultation with more knowledgeable physicians. He encouraged consultation for the good of the patient while exhorting the consultants to treat the consulting physicians as colleagues and with respect that would only improve the public's view of the profession.

In 1803, Percival published *Medical Ethics*, a few years after he had been requested to write on the subject by his fellow physicians. Much of the book was devoted to the etiquette of professional interaction, and consultation was addressed in much the same manner as in centuries past: consultation should be obtained to help the patient; no jealousy, competition, or patient stealing should be tolerated; conflict in front of patients was to be avoided at all costs. It is a tribute to the relative timelessness of Percival's work that much of it was used almost verbatim in the AMA Codes of Ethics in 1847, 1911, and 1912.

In the late 1800s, another problem surfaced in England. A great gap had appeared between the eminent consultants and general practitioners. Although the former, because of superior knowledge and prestige, were able to command high fees from wealthy clients, they apparently continued to see less well-to-do patients for the same fees that were being charged by the general practitioners. This attracted business to the consultants but left the ordinary physicians with much less work and poor incomes. The result, as could have been anticipated, was ill feeling between the groups. The conflict was of such consequence that the *British Medical Journal* in 1872 was moved to comment entirely against the "great consultants," who they believed should charge higher fees. This would decrease the burden of the overworked consultants and distribute the workload and the income in a more reasonable manner.

There was great fear among the general practitioners of sending their patients to consultants, because often these patients remained in the care of the more prestigious men whose care was considered better and whose fees were identical. Thus, the patients had no incentive to return to their practitioners. Therefore, in 1886, the Association of General Practitioners was established to try to regulate the relations between these opponents.

In the USA, meanwhile, another problem was developing. In the mid-1800s, many states repealed their laws regulating medicine, resulting in a large influx of quacks and cults. Because of this, a code of ethics restricting competition among doctors was adopted by the medical profession. This code condemned practitioners who did not have orthodox training, who claimed secret medications, and, importantly for consultants, who offered special abilities. (They may have actually had special abilities.) Although the code did much to discourage unqualified practitioners, as medical practice moved into the twentieth century, it allowed ill feeling to exist between general practitioners and a growing group of medical "specialists."

A number of other negative results surfaced. Because the code forbade consultations with unlicensed physicians, if a patient insisted on a consultation with an outsider, the legitimate physician was forced to withdraw from the case, leaving the patient in the hands of these unqualified people. The rules also provided an opportunity for exclusion of even qualified physicians, and in the late 1800s, women, blacks, and those who were trying to specialize were at times subjected to these consultation bans.

In the twentieth century, laws have again been passed reducing the numbers of unqualified practitioners. The International Code of Ethics encourages consultation in difficult cases. The attainment of equal status by osteopathic physicians is an interesting sidelight to these ancient struggles to protect patients and the profession.

Today, the problem is entirely different. In previous centuries, consultation was requested from a physician who, although similarly trained, was thought to be more knowledgeable overall. Even 60 years ago, in "uncomplicated" cases, consultation was generally considered unnecessary. The doctor who took care of the patient was the doctor who did the surgery, attended to preoperative and postoperative care, and continued to do the "primary care" long after.

For the past few decades, however, as medical knowledge has mushroomed and physicians have specialized and subspecialized, these tasks have been divided and subdivided. This division of labor has helped the great advances in medicine in the USA, but it also has created some special problems.

The proliferation in consultative medicine has allowed patients to have a large number of experts taking care of each separate part of an illness. The internist asks the cardiologist to consult on myocardial infarctions; the cardiologist asks the endocrinologist to consult on patients with diabetes; the surgeon asks the internist for help on patients with hypertension and congestive failure. Although this accumulation of expertise is impressive and would seem to lead to the best care possible, it can, and not infrequently does, lead to conflicting orders, incompatible medications, and conflicts between consulting physicians. Unfortunately, these conflicts are at times perceived by the patients and can cause unnecessary insecurity, fear, and anger.

These kinds of problems are common in the perisurgical patient who has complicating medical problems before surgery or who develops complications afterward. The surgeon frequently needs to have medical support to help with the complicated problems of preoperative and postoperative care. Unfortunately, the internist's knowledge of the surgical procedures, the recovery course, and complications is often scanty. This sets up a situation in which each physician has knowledge that the other needs to take optimal care of the patient.

The advantages of the primary care physician, although they should be obvious, have been lost in the tangle of subspecialization. This physician can be either the internist or the surgeon. The important concept is that the responsibility for the integration of therapies falls to that one physician because he or she is most familiar with all aspects of the patient's case. All other physicians must function as advisors (consultants) to the primary care provider.

The consultant's role can be a difficult one. It is imperative that the primary physician be aware of, and approve of, all therapy, and therefore feel free to accept and reject the advice of the consultant. Rejection is, thankfully, an unusual occurrence. Under ideal circumstances, it is best for the consultant to discuss all recommendations with the primary physician before they are written in the chart. In this way, information can be exchanged, theories can be discussed, and a mutually satisfactory plan of treatment can be formulated. This avoids the confusion, anger, and mistakes that can occur when the consultant must institute therapy without discussion; this should be done only in an emergency situation, when delay would cause harm to the patient.

Another area of potential difficulty for the consultant is in discussing plans and diagnoses with patients who are exquisitely sensitive to any discrepancy, real or perceived, between physicians. This can cause misunderstanding and anxiety for the patient, and can require an immense amount of explanation by the primary physician to reestablish the patient's trust, to help him or her understand what is happening, and to allay his or her fears.

In general, it is best for the consultant to communicate treatment plans through the primary physician. When asked, the consultant can give the patient the broad outline of possibilities to be presented to the primary physician. The consultant should always make it clear that the final decision about what is to be done will be made by the primary physician and the patient.

There seem to be five basic principles behind optimal patient care. The first is the one-patient/one-doctor principle of primary care, or the "final common pathway" to integrate therapies as discussed above. Second, the primary doctor and consultant should trust each other. There needs to be a feeling between them that each one is able to provide something important to the patient's care. Third, communication is indispensable. If the physicians take the time to talk to one another, confusion, irritation, anger, and mistakes can be avoided. The fourth principle is really a corollary of the third, and that is cooperation. It is the natural extension of communication:

if two physicians can talk to each other and each one trusts the other's judgment and knowledge, they will be able to cooperate, even in areas of disagreement, in taking the best care of the patient.

The final principle that ties the others together is etiquette. As in all human interactions, the way people deal with each other may be as important as the content of the interaction. A brilliant consultation, handled in a brusque and rude manner may be no more useful than no consultation at all. Controversial or optimal therapies begun before consultation with the primary physician will make further interaction difficult. Finally, and worst of all, improper therapy instituted erroneously or because of inadequate information not only will harm the physicians' relationship but may harm the patient as well.

The art of consultation is one that involves many aspects of interaction. The primary physician and the patient must feel that the consultant is concerned not only with the hard scientific facts of the patient's care from the specialist's viewpoint but with optimal overall management. The request for consultation is not a carte blanche for management; it is a request for advice in treating some part of the patient's illness. Thus, the consultant should feel like an invited guest in someone's house, not the master of ceremonies.

Part

1

Perioperative Care of the Surgical Patient

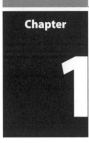

Chapter

Anesthesia management of the surgical patient

L. Reuven Pasternak

Few aspects of healthcare involve as much simultaneous interaction by different physicians as the management of the patient undergoing surgery. At a minimum, the primary care provider, surgeon, and anesthesiologist form a team of physicians, all of whom bring a different perspective and expertise to the care of the patient. As the medical intensity of patients increases, there is also an expanding number of community-based and hospital-based specialty physicians and hospitalists actively involved in this process.

The intersection of the primary care provider and the anesthesiologist first occurs when the surgeon schedules a patient for surgery. At that point the series of events that culminates in medical evaluation, anesthetic assessment, and perioperative management starts. This chapter will begin with that aspect of preparation of the patient for elective surgery. The greatest detail is spent in this area as this is where, by far, the greatest overlap of expertise and communication occurs. The remainder of the chapter will then briefly cover the standard issues involved in perioperative management. These comments are not so much geared to make the primary care provider an expert in the field but are more designed to provide some familiarity with the environment into which the patient is going. It is assumed that detailed information about anesthesia care is provided directly to the patient by the anesthesia provider and/or preoperative systems.

Preoperative evaluation: preparation for surgery

The importance of this phase of clinical management is indicated by its global nature. As the administration of anesthesia may involve a risk for the patient that equals or even exceeds that of the surgery itself, the preoperative evaluation is a crucial first step that may affect the clinical safety and organizational integrity of the entire surgical system. The preoperative assessment of the surgical patient for surgery poses a formidable challenge. While the relative merits of alternative surgical and anesthetic techniques have been extensively studied and reviewed in the literature and other forums, the issue of appropriate preoperative assessment has often remained ambiguous.

Several issues have combined to cause this previously simple process to become more complex.

- While the surgeon has retained the opportunity to examine and assess the patient before the scheduling of surgery, the anesthesiologist often does not have the same access to the patient that had previously existed with routine preoperative admissions.
- The selection of procedures by third-party payers to be done on an outpatient and same-day admission basis is generally determined on the presumed complexity of the procedure and not the patient's other underlying medical problems or potential issues associated with anesthesia. Consequently, the anesthesiologist is often asked to manage patients with complex medical conditions undergoing less complex surgery with little prior information.
- Organized health plans often seek to retain as much of the control of the process as possible, including determining when and where tests and consultations are to be done.
- Many hospitals and surgical units have yet to organize and develop preoperative evaluation units due to the expense of staff and space at a time when financial constraints are increasingly severe.
- There has been no consistent system for risk assessment to determine appropriate preoperative management.
- Multiple professional societies have developed specific and often contradictory guidelines on preoperative evaluation for their members.

To further compound the issues there are multiple strategies and guidelines for assessment of the patient undergoing surgery, often from organizations outside of the anesthesia community and, at times, with little input from anesthesiologists or consideration of anesthesia-related issues.

Medical Management of the Surgical Patient, ed. Michael F. Lubin, Thomas F. Dodson, and Neil H. Winawer. Published by Cambridge University Press. © Cambridge University Press 2013.

Philosophy

The purpose of the preoperative evaluation is to identify and reduce the risks associated with anesthesia and surgery. The preoperative evaluation is that portion of the general process that is designed to address issues related to the perioperative management of the surgical patient by anesthesiologists. All preoperative activities, including evaluation prior to the day of surgery, testing, and consultation, should be undertaken only on the reasonable expectation that they will enhance the safety, comfort, and efficiency of the process for the patient, clinical staff, and overall system. Decisions concerning preoperative management should be associated with a consideration of how any aspect of the evaluation will affect the management and outcome of the perioperative process. Evaluations and interventions that do not have a demonstrated beneficial effect do not have value to the patient, clinician, or manager and should not be undertaken on the basis of custom or convenience.

The preoperative evaluation is therefore a focused assessment to address issues relevant to the safe administration of anesthesia and performance of surgery. The use of this event to perform unrelated general medical screening and intervention should be undertaken only in association with appropriate primary and specialty care support. Only anesthesia staff may determine a patient's fitness for administration of anesthesia and appropriate anesthesia technique. The performance of a history and physical examination by other healthcare providers does not constitute a clearance for administration of anesthesia but provides information to the anesthesia staff to make that determination. Thus, internists and other specialists do not "clear" patients for surgery. Rather, they provide an assessment of the current health status of the patient, including whether the patient is as optimally managed as possible.

When evaluating patients for surgery, it should be remembered that the anesthesiologist has only a temporary but important relationship with the patient. Patients' continuing care, including assessment of new or acute exacerbations of chronic conditions, should be done by their primary care providers and associated consultants with whom they will have long-term relationships. Patients should be apprised of the fact that the preoperative evaluation is not a substitute for regular primary care. Requests by patients for performance of tests not deemed necessary for the performance of surgery or administration of surgery should also be referred to their primary healthcare source.

Risk classification

While the purpose of the preoperative evaluation is to reduce risk, current risk classification systems are ill-equipped to provide assistance with patient classification. The first attempt to quantify risks associated with surgery was undertaken by Meyer Saklad in 1941 at the request of the American Society of Anesthesiology (ASA) [1]. This effort was the first by any medical specialty to stratify risk for its patients. Saklad's system did so based on mortality secondary to the associated preoperative medical condition. Type of anesthesia and nature of surgery were not considerations in this system and the divisions were based on empirical experience rather than on specific sets of data and reflect the techniques and standards of practice as of 50 years ago. Four preoperative risk categories were established ranging from category 1 (least likely to die) to category 4 (highest expectation of mortality).

The current ASA classification system is a modification of this work, adding an additional fifth category for moribund patients undergoing surgery in a desperate attempt to preserve life. Numerous studies have demonstrated an association of mortality with ASA Classification independent of anesthetic technique [2–13]. However, these data have limited application as it relates to mortality as its sole outcome and are based on anesthetic techniques as practiced more than 20 years ago. Apfelbaum [14] and Meridy [15] for example, have noted a lack of correlation between ASA status and cancellations, unplanned admissions, and other perioperative complications in outpatient surgery. In a 2004 review of 564,267 procedures done through the Medicare program, Fleischer et al. [16] found that advanced age, prior admission within the past 6 months, and, most important, invasiveness of procedure were the best predictors of admission.

Thus, while useful as a broad assessment of preoperative medical status, the current ASA classification is limited in its ability to truly establish risk or serve as a basis for formulating clinical guidelines without an associated risk index for the surgical procedure. In addition, while concerning itself with the identification of risk, there is a remarkable lack of data delineating outcomes in ambulatory surgery and anesthesia. When the ASA Task Force on Preoperative Evaluation recently issued its recommendations for all preoperative assessment, it initially tried to do so using an evidence-based approach linking specific tests and interventions with designated outcomes. The literature in this area for all of anesthesia was such that, of over 1,200 articles identified in this area, fewer than 30 fit the criteria for use. Lack of information of sufficient scientific validity mandated that the guideline development had to yield to an advisory that was based on consensus opinion subject to further scientific investigation and validation using evidence-based studies at a future date. For purposes of risk stratification, the ASA advisory adopted a modification of the risk index system for patient medical severity and surgical severity as used by the other most commonly used algorithm for patient preoperative assessment, the AHA/ACC guidelines for preoperative assessment of the cardiac patient for noncardiac surgery [17].

Patient and procedure selection

The nature of patient and procedure selection is a function of medical status, surgical procedure, and availability of appropriate postoperative assistance, ranging from home care to intensive care support. While elective surgical procedures are by definition not emergencies, many are nonetheless relatively urgent in nature. The delay of some procedures, such as biopsies for staging of oncology treatments, may unnecessarily delay and inappropriately compromise the care of the patient. Surgeons and anesthesiologists must make a judgment if delay will truly reduce the risk for the patient or merely postpone the inevitable task of dealing with a potentially difficult challenge in the operating room. Finally, while mandates for early discharge by regulatory and managed care groups are based almost wholly on postoperative physiologic status, patient comfort and availability of appropriate assistance at home should be a major consideration in this process. In these circumstances, it is anticipated that the primary care provider will provide insight about the medical status of the patient and assist with optimal stabilization prior to surgery. Advice as to type of anesthesia technique should be deferred to the anesthesia team, who will tailor their technique to the special needs of the patient.

Time of the evaluation

At the current time, over 60% of surgery performed in the USA is outpatient and another 10–15% is performed on a same-day admission basis. For this 70% of the nearly 40 million surgical procedures performed each year, the challenge of appropriate timing and content of the assessment is important and sometimes difficult. Initially, it was a common assumption that a preoperative visit prior to the day of surgery confers some added measure of safety and comfort for patients. On the basis of this assumption, patients were often asked to take the time and expense required to comply with such requirements while hospitals and anesthesiologists had to staff centers able to handle this demand.

Eventually, the literature called this practice into question. Fischer's study [18] demonstrated for outpatients and inpatients that prior preoperative evaluation by anesthesia staff reduced cancellations, tests, and consultations. This study was thus useful in demonstrating the need for a screening mechanism that allowed for patient assessment prior to the day of surgery. However, the assertion that these benefits could be obtained only in a system where all patients visited a preoperative evaluation center was not demonstrated. Some studies demonstrated that no preoperative evaluation visit prior to the day of surgery was necessary for healthy patients undergoing minor procedures [19,20]. Some of the most comprehensive work in this area has been by Twersky et al. [21] which indicates that patient evaluations on the day of surgery may be performed in a manner that is safe and effective. However, even in these studies, patients were not stratified by medical status or surgical procedure and were not relevant for the larger patient population managed by most anesthesiologists.

In discussions with major academic and private practice medical center directors, it has been observed by this author

that the percentage of patients who required having an onsite visit prior averages about 25–33%. The preoperative assessment must be a balance between patient convenience and the need to have information available in a timely fashion to allow for planning appropriate preoperative and perioperative management. While the ideal system may include a preoperative evaluation prior to the day of surgery for all patients, the logistics of patient schedules and their often otherwise healthy status makes this ideal impractical and, at times, unnecessary. This point is of significant concern to hospital preoperative evaluation staff who believe that resources may be inappropriately committed to patients with little need of those services to the detriment of others with more extensive medical and surgical issues and with waste of resources needed elsewhere.

The algorithm adopted by the ASA for preoperative evaluation [22] recognizes that there are categories of patients (health individuals for low-risk surgical procedures) for whom a preoperative assessment (consisting of information made available prior to the day of surgery for review) is sufficient. Similarly, there are some individuals for whom assessment prior to the day of surgery is mandated by their medical condition and/or planned surgery. It is difficult to provide a standard recommendation for how ambulatory surgical centers should place its patients into these categories; much depends on the ease of availability and validity of data provided prior to the day of surgery. What is uniformly recommended is that appropriate information should be made available to anesthesia staff prior to the day of surgery to allow for review and appropriate action.

It is increasingly recognized that the role of the primary care provider is critical in this process. That individual is most familiar with the health status of the patient. Thus, while they are not in a position to "clear for anesthesia," they are in a position to provide the pertinent medical information prior to the day of surgery that would allow surgical systems staff to determine the need for any additional information or consultation.

Laboratory testing

Laboratory and other diagnostic tests associated with preoperative evaluations represent one of the most costly issues associated with surgery. It is difficult to attach a precise dollar cost on this activity. However, it is conservatively estimated that at least 10% of the over $30 billion spent on laboratory testing each year is for preoperative evaluation. The traditional system of the protocol "battery of tests" evolved from a lack of clear definition of their role in preoperative screening, insufficient information on their utility, and a mistaken belief that voluminous information, no matter how irrelevant, enhanced the safety of care and reduced physician liability for adverse events. Protocol testing relieved physicians and their associates of the responsibility of decision making as an easier, though more costly, alternative to selective tests based on patients' individual health profiles.

At a time when the cost of care and the convenience of patients is a major concern, the role of tests as a screening device is rightfully diminishing. The patient history, physical examination, and judgment of the physician are replacing protocols as the basis for testing. While information about other aspects of the preoperative evaluation may be ambiguous, there is extensive literature and experience to support the selective use of testing which also confirms that the use of broad testing panels has a strong tendency to result in excessive testing. Laboratory testing, like all areas of medical intervention, should be undertaken on a "value-added" basis: a reasonable expectation that a potential issue exists that is relevant to anesthesia.

The utility of the preoperative test is based on several key considerations. The first issue is relevance. While some abnormalities are clearly of concern (e.g., cardiac and respiratory), others may have little or no effect on anesthetic plan and outcome and thus do not warrant thorough investigation in this format. The second issue is the prevalence of the condition in both symptomatic and asymptomatic patients. A low prevalence in asymptomatic patients indicates that screening is of little use. The third issue is that of test sensitivity and specificity. Low sensitivity permits false-negative results and patients at risk undergo anesthesia without appropriate preparation. Low specificity causes a large number of false-positives subjecting patients to additional testing, with coincident inconvenience, costs, and potential morbidity. Testing should therefore be done for conditions that are medically relevant using tests of high sensitivity and specificity. A final consideration is cost. Selection of alternative testing modalities should also take into consideration the financial and non-financial costs of testing with selection of the less costly approach where it does not compromise the quality of the information desired. Testing in the asymptomatic population should only be done in patients for whom the potential condition is significant and of reasonable prevalence with tests of reasonable sensitivity and specificity.

Attaching precise numbers to the above caveats is difficult and is the subject of cost–benefit and cost-effectiveness analysis for each of the tests concerned. While this has not been established for many of the routine diagnostic tests that we employ, it has been established in the medical, surgical, and anesthesia literature that the use of screening tests without specific indication is not appropriate. In a study of 19,980 tests on 1,000 patients, Korvin et al. [23] encountered 2,223 abnormal values of which 993 were initially considered to be unanticipated. Of these, 223 led to further evaluation and new diagnoses and in only one case was the diagnosis unrelated to other known medical issues and resulted in new patient care. This involved elevated liver studies in a male who had received halothane anesthesia and for whom the recommendation was made that this agent be avoided.

Robbins and Mushlin [24] in evaluating preoperative testing from a medical perspective, provide an excellent review of the sensitivity, specificity, and consequent utility of a wide range of tests. Kaplan et al. [25] reviewed the records of 2,000 patients undergoing elective surgery who received a routine battery of complete blood cell count, differential cell count, prothrombin time, partial thromboplastin time, platelet count, glucose level, and six channel chemistries. They found that 60% of these tests would not have been performed had they been done only on the basis of clinical indication and that, of these, only 0.22% revealed abnormalities that might have affected perioperative management. These findings were replicated by Turnbull and Buck [26] in a review of 1,010 otherwise healthy patients undergoing cholecystectomy, who discovered 225 abnormal results in 5,003 tests of which 104 were judged to be important and for whom only four patients might have derived some benefit.

In addition to protocols lacking critical review, another reason for excess testing often relates to a lack of communication between medical colleagues. A retrospective study by Kitz et al. [27] compared the use of chest X-rays, electrocardiograms, and chemistry panels in patients undergoing knee arthroscopy and diagnostic laparoscopy or laparoscopic tubal ligation. The groups were divided into patients electively admitted prior to the day of surgery and those who were outpatients. Both patient groups were healthy ASA I and II with tests ordered in the first group by the admitting surgeon and in the second by the anesthesiologist. Though medically similar, the groups had significantly different rates of testing with the higher test rate by surgeons attributable to their desire to not have cases canceled and lack of information from anesthesia staff about test indications.

Additional studies of specific tests have also confirmed the use of the history and physical as a basis for specific tests. Urinalysis, long a mainstay of testing and still required by law in some states, has been found to be of extremely limited use in patients without a preexisting medical condition or positive physical findings [28]. Their use for prevention of postoperative surgical problems outside the realm of genitourinary surgery was addressed by Lawrence et al. [29]. In a classic application of cost–benefit analysis, it was determined that routine urinalysis for all knee replacement surgery in the USA would cost $1,500,000 per wound prevented and not add to the safety or effectiveness of the surgery. Rucker et al. [30] in a review of 905 routine chest X-rays for elective surgical procedures, determined that 368 had no risk factors by history and physical and that only one had a minor abnormality. Of the remaining 504 patients, 22% (114) had serious abnormalities, virtually all of which would have been anticipated by the history and physical examination. Charpak et al. [31] in a retrospective review of postoperative complications, found no circumstances in which absence of a chest X-ray in patients without prior pulmonary disease would have altered outcome or management, even when the complications were respiratory in nature. In both studies, no correlation was established between age and occurrence of positive chest X-rays in patients independent of coexisting positive history or physical examination. Similar findings are available for hemoglobin determinations [32,33], serum chemistries [34], and pulmonary function testing [35].

In accordance with the philosophy that a test is undertaken because of a realistic possibility of adding valuable information, protocol screening without specific indication is not appropriate. In addition to lack of utility for the physician, such testing may, in fact, do harm to patients through unnecessary and potentially invasive interventions, heightened anxieties, and markedly increased costs that may place the physician in a position of having to explain proceeding with surgery in the face of incomplete or irrelevant data. As observed in the literature, there is little rationale for testing other than on the basis of specific indicators. Testing should be done only on an expectation of a finding that might have reasonable relevance for anesthesia and surgery based on:

- Presence of a positive finding on the history and physical examination.
- Need of the surgeon or other clinician for baseline values in anticipation of significant changes due to surgery or other medical interventions (e.g., chemotherapy).
- Patient's inclusion in a population at higher risk for the presence of a relevant condition even though they may exhibit no individual signs of that condition themselves.

By this standard, patients less than 50 years of age without coexisting medical disease would require no preoperative testing, while patients greater than 50 years of age would require an electrocardiogram as per the anesthesiologist. Further testing is done on an individualized basis as indicated by history, physical, and nature of the surgical procedure. It is estimated conservatively that such testing at our institution could reduce preoperative testing by 70%.

Consultations

Specialty consultations should not be obtained on an automatic basis because of organ-specific problems but because there is a specific issue that remains to be addressed. For example, in some centers it is routine to require all patients with any cardiac risk factor to be seen by a cardiologist prior to surgery. These consultations often provide no new information or insight other than that which can be obtained by a review of existing records and a basic history and physical examination. At worst, these requests for consultation are at times taken as a request for suggestions concerning the perioperative management with recommendations made that are based on erroneous assumptions concerning the risks associated with anesthetic techniques. When indicated, requests for consultations should be specifically and narrowly worded to request the specialist's evaluation of the patient's clinical condition, and not to "clear for anesthesia."

Preparation of the patient on the day of surgery

Preoperative fasting (NPO)

Preoperative fasting is aimed at reducing the risk of aspiration on induction of anesthesia and the risk of postoperative emesis. It had long been assumed that any gastric intake prior to surgery posed a major risk to the patient. This standard assumption, however, has been shown to be misleading. Some recent studies in adults demonstrate reduced and less acidic gastric contents when patients are given 150 mL of clear fluid 2 hours before surgery. Schreiner et al. [36] evaluated this same issue in pediatric patients, comparing those with routine NPO status with those allowed to take clear liquids up to 2 hours before surgery, with the only limitation in volume being the last intake (240 mL). The study group taking oral fluids was found to be less anxious and less irritable at the time of induction, while not having any statistically significant difference in gastric volume or pH. Similarly, Sandhar et al. [37] evaluated oral intake of liquids (5 mL/kg) with and without ranitidine (2 mg/kg) and ranitidine alone up to 2–3 hours before surgery in patients 1–14 years of age. The use of fluids alone did not appear to place patients at risk, and the combination with ranitidine was found to be beneficial.

These findings increasingly suggest that the 8-hour NPO rule for outpatients may be subjecting many low-risk individuals, especially children and the elderly, to unwarranted discomfort and that allowing clear liquids up to 2–3 hours before surgery may be preferable. Current recommendations retain the 8-hour NPO rule for solids, but allow up to 150–200 mL of liquid 2 hours before surgery. From a practical standpoint, however, the ability to convey this in instructions is sometimes difficult for the patient to follow, and it sometimes remains simpler to require a full 8-hour NPO period prior to surgery except for sips of liquids required for medication or for special circumstances on an individualized basis.

Preoperative medication

It is generally recommended that patients take their routine medications prior to, and on the day of, surgery. Exceptions to this recommendation include diuretics, oral hypoglycemic agents, anticoagulants, and insulin. Anticoagulants will usually need to be withheld per instructions of the surgeon. Insulin should be brought by the patient to the hospital or surgical facility on the day of surgery with one-third to one-half of the usual dose administered after testing for blood glucose levels and the start of an IV to prevent hypoglycemia. For this reason, it is strongly recommended that insulin-dependent diabetics be placed as early in the schedule as possible to protect against wide swings in their glucose levels prior to surgery. One area of special interest has been the use of beta-blockers prior to surgery. Early management called for discontinuation of these drugs with deference to management by anesthesiologists on the day of surgery. However, recent analysis by the American Heart Association and the American College of Cardiology [38,39] has determined that the weight of evidence supports continuing administration of beta-blockers prior to and on the day of surgery.

At times, a compassionate primary care physician may prescribe sedation to be taken by the patient prior to arrival for an outpatient or same-day admission procedure. This practice should be discouraged as the patient may not be in an appropriate condition to work with the anesthesiologist who must also then cope with an exogenous agent in determining and obtaining informed consent for an appropriate anesthetic plan.

Perioperative management

As with all other aspects of management, the perioperative care of the ambulatory surgery patient requires scrupulous attention to issues of safety, comfort, convenience, and efficiency. Selection of anesthetic technique must thus ensure a cooperative patient for the surgeon. The anesthesiologist must use a method that ensures rapid induction and emergence from anesthesia, with the patient feeling little discomfort in the recovery period and thus allowing for a reasonably quick discharge. The margin for error is considerably smaller in outpatient procedures, since often little time is available to stabilize a patient during the perioperative period if one discovers excessive or insufficient depth of anesthesia.

As with any procedure, the anesthetic technique is discussed with the patient and a notation made in the record of this fact. This discussion constitutes informed consent and is increasingly being conducted with the same formality as the surgical consent. Just as the surgeon is required to state potential complications and potential unplanned interventions that may occur, patients should be advised of alternative plans that may ensue. These plans are usually in the form of general anesthesia in the event that other techniques are insufficient for the procedure's successful completion. At times, patients for whom general anesthesia is contraindicated may have a procedure performed with sedation or a regional technique. In these circumstances, both surgeon and patient should be fully aware that an attempt to perform the procedure one way does not constitute open clearance to proceed under all circumstances. Also, if the initial effort is unsuccessful, the surgery should be discontinued and performed in a different setting.

On occasion, primary-care providers advise patients, suggest appropriate anesthetic techniques and agents, and at times place these suggestions in the medical record. While done with the best of intention, this practice often prejudices the discussion between the anesthesiologist and the patient and may cause undue confusion and distress on the day of surgery. Accordingly, the primary-care provider is discouraged from this practice. Instead, patient concerns and preferences, if any, should be noted with discussion of technique and agents left to the discussion between the anesthesiologist and patient.

Monitoring and anesthesia equipment

A fully operational anesthesia system includes pulse oximetry, capnography, ECG, blood pressure measurement, and precordial or esophageal stethoscope. The provision of anesthesia services in any location, whether inside or outside of the operating room, requires the availability of these modalities of monitoring as a minimum standard of care. Within the operating room, the ability to monitor inspiratory and expiratory inhalation agents is proving to be of significant value in modifying anesthetic technique to allow for smooth induction and rapid emergence.

Monitored sedation

Monitored sedation, when possible, often provides the safest, most comfortable, and most efficient anesthetic management. It is especially desirable in patients whose medical condition (e.g., major cardiorespiratory disease and difficult airways) makes them relatively more difficult candidates for general anesthesia. Whereas regional and general anesthesia may provide deep anesthesia over a large body area and allow leeway to both anesthesiologist and surgeon, monitored sedation requires scrupulous technique by both. Common procedures using these techniques include carpal tunnel repair; other hand procedures; cataract extraction and lens implanting; significant dermatologic procedures; and some hernia repairs.

Procedures that can often be performed by experienced surgeons in this way include breast biopsies; inguinal hernia repairs; limited superficial procedures on the skin and subcutaneous tissue; ophthalmic procedures such as cataract extraction; and procedures on distal portions of extremities to a local block by the surgeon. Surgery performed with local anesthesia thus requires a technique that is limited, is amenable to local infiltration, is performed rapidly, and does not require excessive doses of either local anesthesia or sedation. Surgical skill is critical; attempts to perform such invasive procedures as tonsillectomy and laparoscopy with sedation and local anesthesia is fraught with potential disaster in the hands of anyone but the most skilled surgeon.

With some surgeons, patient sedation may not be required. In general, however, sedation allows a patient to achieve a more relaxed state and permits a more pleasant and rapid completion of the procedure. A wide array of drugs is employed. The standard technique that has generally worked well involves the use of a benzodiazepine with a short-acting narcotic, replacing the past practice of relying on barbiturates. Midazolam's tendency to cause less postoperative drowsiness than diazepam, combined with its faster onset of action and less vein-irritating nature, has made midazolam the mainstay of current techniques. Contrary to much conventional wisdom, the retrograde amnesia associated with midazolam is minimal and instead is marked by the patient's impaired ability to integrate events into long-term memory after its administration [40–42].

Administration of short-acting narcotics, such as fentanyl (1–2 µg/kg), can supplement the sedative nature of the midazolam, with the anesthesiologist checking closely for any impaired or compromised ventilation. Alfentanil (10–20 µg/kg) is also effective and provides more rapid onset and shorter duration of action than fentanyl. As with all procedures, varying levels of stimulation occur, usually associated with initial and subsequent injections of local anesthetic into the surgical site. Administration of 25–50 mg of a short-acting barbiturate or 10–20 mg of propofol immediately before anesthesia induction may preclude the need for larger doses of longer-acting agents. Frequent need for such medication, however, indicates the need for deeper sedation.

An alternative and increasingly popular approach to sedation involves the intravenous use of propofol, a rapid-onset, short-acting hypnotic. After an initial dose of 1 mg/kg, increments of 0.25 mg/kg up to a total dose of 2.5 mg are used to achieve sedation. A continuous infusion of 20 µg/kg is then used to maintain sedation, adjusting to the patient's level of sedation and vital signs. When using this technique, one must remember that propofol is a hypnotic and not an analgesic. Therefore its success depends even more on appropriate local anesthetic use than with a benzodiazepine or hypnotic, although propofol has the advantage of faster onset and cessation of action.

A critical point to remember is that the surgeon administers the local agent to provide anesthesia. Patient discomfort that persists despite sedation in the unstimulated state may indicate the need for more local anesthetic infiltration or alteration of technique. In some individuals, "light" sedation with local anesthesia may not be satisfactory. While light sedation is designed to provide a calming influence, these individuals may proceed to what is known as "deep" sedation. When used, deep sedation carries many of the risks of general anesthesia and, at times, may be more problematic. Patients receiving deep sedation have a profound alteration of consciousness and may not be able to cooperate with a surgeon's request to remain still, at times becoming agitated. The patient's airway muscles also become relaxed, causing potential airway obstruction and desaturation of blood oxygen content. When this occurs, general anesthesia may be preferred as a means of protecting the airway and providing a situation permitting the surgeon to complete the procedure.

Regional anesthesia

Regional anesthesia offers a potentially major benefit for patients undergoing procedures on the extremities. Although this is especially true for those patients for whom general anesthesia may provide a significant risk, regional anesthesia also provides advantages for the general patient population. The most frequently cited criticisms of regional anesthesia, other than spinal, is the time that is needed to place and establish a block, usually 20 to 30 minutes, and the perceived risk of failure and need to switch to general anesthesia.

In assessing the usefulness of regional anesthesia, one must consider recovery time and the patient's postoperative comfort. In a review of 543 brachial plexus blocks, Davis [43] found a success rate of 93% for anesthesiologists performing such blocks regularly. Bowe et al. [44] and Baysinger et al. [45] demonstrated that brachial plexus anesthesia for carpal tunnel release and upper extremity procedures did not significantly differ from general anesthesia in total OR and recovery room time. However, the incidence of postoperative nausea, emesis, and pain requiring medication was less than half that found in patients who had general anesthesia.

Similar findings have been shown for arthroscopy of the knee with the patient under epidural or spinal anesthesia, and administration of a narcotic by this route for prolonged analgesia [46–48]. As with brachial plexus blockade, the incidence of nausea, emesis, and postoperative pain were significantly less than with general anesthesia. Bach et al. [49] demonstrated a frequency of pain of 20.3% vs 27.0% in patients under regional and general anesthesia, respectively, but found significantly less nausea and emesis (4.1% vs 16.5%, respectively). Bowe et al. [44] found an even greater difference in postoperative pain (27% vs 65% for regional vs general) and nausea with emesis (1.5% vs 25% for regional vs general). In all studies, neither OR nor recovery times were significantly different between these two groups. Of interest is the additional finding of Randel et al. [50] that epidural anesthesia results in a decreased recovery time of 123 minutes, compared with 164 minutes for general anesthesia.

Epidural anesthesia has been found to provide significant benefit and safety for peripheral vascular, urologic, gynecologic, and arthroscopic surgery. Randel et al. [50] showed that the additional time required for placement of the block should be compensated for by reduced time to oral intake, ambulation, voiding, and discharge. Although the incidence of moderate to severe headache was less than with either general or spinal anesthesia, patients undergoing epidural anesthesia did have a higher incidence of moderate to severe backache.

Spinal anesthesia usually offers the benefit of a more rapidly achieved and intense block than that achieved with epidural anesthesia. The risk of spinal headache and subsequent distress used to be a major issue. Three aspects of spinal headache were of concern, especially in the ambulatory setting: (a) its occurrence 2–3 days postoperatively, after routine follow-up has already been accomplished; (b) it incapacitates the patient for several days thereafter; and (c) the potential need for readmission or further intervention with a blood patch. Advocates of spinal anesthesia point out the low incidence of postoperative spinal headache as a justification for its use. Some advocates, such as Mulroy [51] have maintained that alteration in technique and appropriate patient selection can reduce the incidence to well under 1% or less and assert that maintenance of a recumbent position does not help avoid headache [52,53] and may simply delay its onset. The use of 27-gauge needles and use of Greene "pencil point" or Whitacre side-port needles has reduced the incidence of postdural puncture headaches to less than 1%. The decreasing costs and clinical advantages of the 27-gauge Whitacre is increasingly making it the standard for spinal anesthesia.

The use of spinal anesthesia is still relatively contraindicated in patients with preexisting back pain or injury unless it presents a clear advantage in the patient at risk for general anesthesia.

A final but important consideration in this area is the increasing use of regional anesthesia to supplement general anesthesia for postoperative analgesia. This situation usually arises in the administration of caudal anesthetics to pediatric patients undergoing urologic or lower extremity procedures. The most significant of these has been the use of caudal anesthesia in the pediatric population undergoing genitourinary and lower-extremity procedures. It is noteworthy that caudal anesthesia has found widespread favor in alleviating the discomfort associated with inguinal hernia repairs, orchiopexies, and other procedures. Although the delayed discharge associated with caudal anesthesia has been the principal objection to its use, usually by surgeons, the use of 0.125% bupivacaine has diminished the incidence of postoperative urinary retention while maintaining equivalent analgesia to the point that this consideration should no longer prevent its use.

Local infiltration with anesthetics is also useful in diminishing postoperative pain. Placing local anesthetics into the wound is an increasingly popular technique. Casey et al. [54] found that simple instillation of 0.25% bupivacaine was as effective as a more elaborate ilioinguinal or iliohypogastric block with bupivacaine for patients having inguinal hernia repair. Studies have also found a significant reduction in postoperative pain in patients having bilateral tubal ligation, with injection of 5 mL of 1% etidocaine into the banded portion of the tube [55]. Narchi et al. [56] obtained similar results in patients undergoing laparoscopy, with 80 mL of 0.5% lidocaine or 0.5% bupivacaine applied to the right subdiaphragmatic area. Studies are currently evaluating instillation of local anesthetics and narcotics in the knee joint for arthroscopy. Such techniques require close cooperation and communication between the surgeon and anesthesiologist.

General anesthesia

When required, general anesthesia remains a safe and effective manner to achieve the goals of anesthesia. Principal problems associated with the otherwise successful general anesthetic are somnolence, nausea and emesis, postoperative pain, and associated delays in discharge and, in ambulatory surgery, possible admission. As the number of procedures performed with sedation and regional anesthesia increases, general anesthesia may be required less frequently. Nonetheless, it remains a mainstay of anesthetic practice, and considerable progress has been made to reduce the problems just listed.

Before the introduction of propofol, sodium pentothal or thiopental were accepted as the mainstays for induction. Considerable evidence now shows that propofol offers distinct advantages. Sampson et al. [57] in an analysis of the two agents, compared 4 mg/kg of thiopental with 2.5 mg/kg of propofol followed by 100% O_2 for outpatient procedures. The recovery time until patients were comfortable postoperatively was considerably better for the patients receiving propofol than for those receiving thiopental. These findings of reduced recovery time, less nausea, and greater postoperative alertness have also been consistently reported in other studies. Anecdotal information from practitioners also note patient emergence marked by greater satisfaction, at times bordering on a transient pleasant euphoria. Marais et al. [58] and Sung et al. [59] in separate studies indicative of future cost–benefit analyses, also found that propofol, by decreasing patient stay and postoperative symptoms, was also effective in reducing costs. Because of its application on a near-universal basis for sedation and general anesthesia, propofol is the most commonly used anesthetic agent in virtually all parts of the world today.

The availability of newer agents has altered perspectives on optimal maintenance of general anesthesia. Specifically, propofol; the short-acting neuromuscular agents atracurium, vecuronium, mivacurium, and rocuronium; the short-acting narcotics fentanyl, alfentanil, sufentanil, and remifentanil; and newer inhalation agents desflurane and sevoflurane are allowing new approaches to general anesthesia in the outpatient.

Before the availability of these agents, the major issue was whether an inhalation technique or a balanced technique with narcotics and nitrous oxide (N_2O) was optimal. In assessing volatile agents, little has been found to differentiate among them as to postoperative drowsiness, headache, myalgia, or nausea and vomiting [59,60] and perioperative stability. However, the introduction of short-acting hypnotics and narcotics, such as propofol and alfentanil, has assisted in the development of total intravenous anesthesia (TIVA) as a means of providing general anesthesia. In two studies, propofol in a continuous infusion of 12 mg/kg/hour was compared with enflurane [61] and enflurane and isoflurane. In both instances, patients receiving propofol had significantly less nausea and emesis, less recovery time, and less need for intervention for these problems in the recovery room.

Conclusions

The interaction of primary-care providers and anesthesiologists is one of the most critical for the safety, efficiency, and comfort of patients. These individuals bring different perspectives and expertise to the care of the patient undergoing surgical procedures. It is increasingly important for each to have a better understanding of the issues involved in chronic patient care and perioperative management at a time when the healthcare system is placing more demands on physicians and the systems in which they work.

References

1. Saklad M. Grading of patients for surgical procedures. *Anesthesiology* 1941; **2**: 281–4.

2. Brown DL. Anesthetic risk: a historical perspective. In Brown DL, ed. *Risk and Outcome in Anesthesia*. Philadelphia, PA: J. B. Lippincott Co.; 1988.

3. Derrington MC, Smith G. A review of anesthetic risk, morbidity, and mortality. *Br J Anaesth* 1987; **59**: 815–33.

4. Farrow SC, Fowkes FGR, Lunn JN, Robertson IB, Samuel P. Epidemiology in anaesthesia II: factors affecting mortality in hospital. *Br J Anaesth* 1982; **54**: 811–16.

5. Goldstein A, Keats AS. The risk of anesthesia. *Anesthesiology* 1970; **33**: 130–43.

6. Lunn JN., Farrow SC, Fowkes FGR, Robertson IB, Samuel P. Epidemiology in anaesthesia I: anaesthetic practice over 20 years. *Br J Anaesth* 1982; **54**: 803–9.

7. Lunn JN, Hunter AR, Scott DB. Anesthesia-related surgical mortality. *Anaesthesia* 1983; **38**: 1090–6.

8. Vacanti CJ, VanHouten RJ, Hill RC. A statistical analysis of the relationship of physical status to postoperative mortality in 68,388 cases. *Anesth Analg* 1970; **49**: 564–6.

9. Keats AS. Anesthesia mortality in perspective. *Anesth Analg* 1990; **70**: 113–19.

10. Rao TLK, Jacobs KH, El-Etr AA. Reinfarction following anesthesia in patients with myocardial infarction. *Anesthesiology* 1983; **59**: 499–505.

11. Dripps RD, Lamont A, Eckenhoff JE. The role of anesthesia in surgical mortality. *J Am Med Assoc* 1961; **178**: 261–6.

12. Marx GF, Mateo CV, Orkin LR. Computer analysis of postanesthetic deaths. *Anesthesiology* 1973; **39**: 54–8.

13. Carter DC, Campbell D. Evaluation of the risks of surgery. *Br Med Bull* 1988; **44**: 322–40.

14. Apfelbaum JL. Preoperative evaluation, laboratory screening, and selection of adult surgical outpatients in the 1990s. *Anesthesiol Rev* 1990; **17**: 4–12.

15. Meridy HW. Criteria for selection of ambulatory surgical patients and guidelines for anesthetic management:

a retrospective study of 1553 cases. *Anesth Analg* 1982; **61**: 921–6.

16. Fleischer LA, Pasternak LR, Herbert R, Anderson GA. Inpatient hospital admission and death after outpatient surgery in elderly patients. *Arch Surg* 2004; **139**: 67.

17. Fleisher LA. *Applying the New AHA/ACC Perioperative Cardiovascular Evaluation Guidelines to the Elderly Outpatient*. Society for Ambulatory Anesthesia; 2002.

18. Fischer SP. Development and effectiveness of an anesthesia preoperative evaluation clinic in a teaching hospital. *Anesthesiology* 1996; **85**: 196–206.

19. Arellano R, Cruise C, Chung F. Timing of the anesthetist's preoperative outpatient interview. *Anesth Analg* 1989; **68**: 645–8.

20. Rosenblatt MA, Bradford C, Miller R, Zahl K. A preoperative interview by an anesthesiologist does not lower preoperative anxiety in outpatients. *Anesthesiology* 1989; **71**: A926.

21. Twersky RS, Frank D, Lebovits A. Timing of preoperative evaluation for surgical outpatients – does it matter? Part II. *Anesthesiology* 1990; **73**: A1.

22. American Society of Anesthesiologists Task Force on Preoperative Evaluation. Practice Advisory for Preoperative Evaluation. *Anesthesiology* 2002; **96**: 485–96.

23. Korvin CC, Pearce RH, Stanley J. Admissions screening: clinical benefits. *Ann Intern Med* 1975; **83**: 197–203.

24. Robbins JA, Mushlin AI. Preoperative evaluation of the healthy patient. *Med Clin North Am* 1979; **63**: 1145–56.

25. Kaplan EB, Sheiner LB, Boeckman AJ. et al. The usefulness of preoperative laboratory testing. *J Am Med Assoc* 1985; **253**: 3576–81.

26. Turnbull JM, Buck C. The value of preoperative screening investigations in otherwise healthy individuals. *Arch Intern Med* 1987; **147**: 1101–5.

27. Kitz DS, Slusarz-Ladden C, Lecky JH. Hospital resources used for inpatient and ambulatory surgery. *Anesthesiology* 1988; **69**: 383–6.

28. Zilva JF. Is unselective urine biochemical urine testing cost effective? *Br Med J* 1985; **291**: 323–5.

29. Lawrence VA, Gafni A, Gross M. The unproven utility of the preoperative urinalysis: economic evaluation. *J Clin Epidemiol* 1989; **42**: 1185–91.

30. Rucker L, Frye BD, Staten MA. Usefulness of chest roentgenograms in preoperative patients. *J Am Med Assoc* 1983; **250**: 3209–11.

31. Charpak Y, Blery C, Chastang C, Szatan M, Fourgeaux B. Prospective assessment of a protocol for selective ordering of preoperative chest X-rays. *Can J Anaesth* 1988; **35**: 259–64.

32. Hackman T, Steward DJ. What is the value of preoperative hemoglobin determinations in pediatric outpatients? *Anesthesiology* 1989; **71**: A1168.

33. O'Conner ME, Drasner K. Preoperative laboratory testing of children undergoing elective surgery. *Anesth Analg* 1990; **70**: 176–80.

34. Bold AM, Currin B. Use and abuse of clinical chemistry in surgery. *Br Med J* 1965; **2**: 1051–2.

35. Zibrak JD, O'Donnell CR, Marton K. Indications for pulmonary function testing. *Ann. Intern. Med.* 1990; **112**: 763–71.

36. Schreiner MS, Triebwasser A, Keon TP. Ingestion of liquids compared with preoperative fasting in pediatric outpatients. *Anesthesiology* 1990; **72**: 593.

37. Sandhar BK, Goresky GV, Maltby JR, Shaffer EA. Effect of oral liquids and ranitidine on gastric fluid volume and pH in children undergoing outpatient surgery. *Anesthesiology* 1989; **71**: 327.

38. Fleisher LA, Beckman JA, Brown KA et al. ACC/AHA Guidelines on Perioperative Evaluation and Care for Noncardiac Surgery: Executive Summary. *Circulation* 2007; **116**: 1971–96.

39. Fleischman KE, Beckman JA, Buller CE et al. ACCF/AHA focused update on perioperative beta blockade. *Circulation* 2009; **120**: 2123–51.

40. Ghoneim MM, Mewaldt SP. Benzodiazepines and human memory: a review. *Anesthesiology* 1990; **72**: 926.

41. Baughman VL., Becker GL, Ryan CM et al. Effectiveness of triazolam, diazepam, and placebo as preanesthetic medications. *Anesthesiology* 1989; **71**: 196–200.

42. Raybould D, Bradshaw EG. Premedication for day case surgery. *Anaesthesia* 1987; **42**: 591–5.

43. Davis WJ. Outpatient brachial plexus anesthesia. *Anesthesiology* 1990; **73**: A25.

44. Bowe EA, Baysinger CL, Sykes LA, Bowe LS. Subarachnoid blockade versus general anesthesia for knee arthroscopy in outpatients. *Anesthesiology* 1990; **73**: A45.

45. Baysinger CL, Boew EA, Boew LS, Sykes LA. Brachial plexus blockade and general anesthesia for carpal tunnel release in ambulatory patients. *Proceedings of the Fifth Annual SAMBA Conference*, Baltimore, MD, 1990 (abstract).

46. Philip BK. Supplemental medication for ambulatory procedures under regional anesthesia. *Anesth Analg* 1985; **64**: 1117–25.

47. Rice LJ, Pudimat MA, Hannallah RS. Timing of caudal block placement does not affect duration of postoperative analgesia in pediatric ambulatory surgical patients. *Anesthesiology* 1988; **69**: A771.

48. Rice LJ, Binding RR, Vaughn GC, Thompson R, Newman K. Intraoperative and postoperative analgesia in children undergoing inguinal herniorrhaphy: a comparison of caudal bupivacaine 0.125% and 0.25%. *Anesthesiology* 1990; **73**: A3.

49. Bach BR, Parnass SM, McCarthy RJ, Werling W, Hasson S. A prospective evaluation of epidural versus general anesthesia for outpatient arthroscopy. *Arthroscopy* 1991; 7: 311–12.

50. Randel GI, Levy L, Kothary SP, Brousseau M, Pandit SK. Epidural anesthesia is superior to spinal or general for outpatient knee arthroscopy. *Anesthesiology* 1989; **71**: A769.

51. Mulroy MF. Is spinal anesthesia appropriate for outpatients? *SAMBA Newslett* 1989; **4**: 1.

52. Carbaat PA, van Crevel H. Lumbar puncture headache: controlled study on the preventive effect of 24 hours bed rest. *Lancet* 1981; **1**: 1133–5.

53. Thornberry EA, Thomas TA. Posture and post-spinal headache. *Br J Anaesth* 1988; **60**: 195–7.

54. Casey WF, Rice LJ, Hannallah RS *et al.* A comparison between bupivacaine instillation versus ilioinguinal/iliohypogastric nerve block for postoperative analgesia following inguinal herniorrhaphy in children. *Anesthesiology* 1990; **72**: 637–9.

55. Baram D, Smith C, Stinson S. Intraoperative topical etidocaine for reducing postoperative pain after laparoscopic tubal ligation. *J Reprod Med* 1990; **35**: 407–10.

56. Narchi P, Lecoq G, Fernandez H, Benhamou, D. Intraperitoneal local anesthetics and scapular pain following daycase laparoscopy. *Anesthesiology* 1990; **73**: A5.

57. Sampson IH, Plosker H, Cohen M *et al.* Comparison of propofol and thiamylal for induction and maintenance of anaesthesia for outpatient surgery. *Br J Anaesth* 1988; **61**: 707–11.

58. Marais ML, Maher MW, Wetchler BV *et al.* Reduced demands on recovery room resources with propofol (Diprivan) compared with thiopental-isoflurane. *Anesthesiol Rev* 1989; **16**: 29–40.

59. Sung YF, Reiss N, Tillette T. The differential cost of anesthesia and recovery with propofol-nitrous oxide anesthesia versus thiopental-nitrous oxide. *Proceedings of the Fifth Annual SAMBA Conference*, Baltimore, MD; 1990 (abstract).

60. Carter JA, Dye AM, Cooper GM. Recovery after day-case anesthesia: the effect of different inhalational anaesthetic agents. *Anaesthesia* 1985; **40**: 545–8.

61. Pandit SK, Kothary SP, Randel GI, Levy L. Recovery after outpatient anesthesia: propofol versus enflurane. *Anesthesiology* 1988; **69**: A565.

Specialized nutrition support in the surgical patient

Vivian M. Zhao and Thomas R. Ziegler

Introduction

Protein–energy malnutrition (PEM), which includes significant loss of lean body mass and fat stores, and depletion of micronutrients (including essential vitamins and trace elements), is common among hospitalized surgical patients [1–7]. Various studies among total hospital admissions and in intensive care unit (ICU hereafter) settings have reported that varying degrees of malnutrition can occur in 20% to as high as 60% of surgical and medical patients [1–3]. While most patients gradually progress to an oral diet shortly following surgery and require little or no nutritional intervention, major surgery or postoperative complications can delay the progression of an oral diet. The extent of PEM worsens over time in such patients due to the stress of surgery, increased nutritional needs to support wound healing, and increased metabolic rate associated with postoperative recovery, insufficient *ad libitum* dietary intake and repeated catabolic insults [8,9].

Protein–energy malnutrition prior to, and inadequate nutritional intake during, hospitalization are each associated with increased morbidity and mortality, as well as longer hospital stay and cost [9–15]. In 1936, Studley was the first to recognize a direct correlation between preoperative weight loss and operative mortality rate, independent of age, impaired cardio/respiratory function, and types of surgery [16]. Giner *et al.* subsequently confirmed that malnutrition is a major determinant for the development of postoperative complications [3]. In highly catabolic surgical ICU patients, nutritional depletion has been associated with higher incidence of infectious complications, poor wound healing, impaired skeletal muscle strength, and the need for postsurgical mechanical ventilation [4,5,10–15]. Multiple pathophysiologic challenges may compromise nutritional status in patients undergo elective or major surgery (Table 2.1) [17]. Ensuring adequate nutritional intake has been a major focus among surgeons. Nutritional interventions can be safely performed either with enteral nutrition (EN; enteral nutrient supplements and tube feedings) or with complete parenteral nutrition (PN) [18]. Both EN and PN provide fluid, calories (as carbohydrate, protein/ amino acids, and fats) and known essential amino acids, fats, electrolytes, vitamins, and trace elements. The delivery of these interventions is the focus of this chapter.

Nutritional assessment

Comprehensive nutritional assessment involves integration of various factors, as outlined in Table 2.2 [17]. Unfortunately, there is no "gold standard" for nutritional assessment in surgical patients. Conventional blood levels of albumin and pre-albumin might be useful in outpatient or epidemiologic settings; however, they are neither reliable nor practical as nutritional markers after surgery because they may be markedly decreased due to inflammation, infection, decreased hepatic synthesis, and/or increased blood clearance. Plasma levels of these proteins are also susceptible to fluid status (increased with fluid depletion or decreased with fluid overload). Nevertheless, serum albumin is an excellent prognostic indicator of surgical outcomes, with an inverse relationship between postoperative morbidity and mortality compared with preoperative serum albumin level [19]. Blood levels of certain vitamins and trace elements, as well as electrolytes, are useful to follow in certain at-risk patients, but can fluctuate due to fluid status and inter-organ shifts, necessitating serial monitoring to guide repletion strategies. In addition, body weight can also fluctuate dramatically in relation to fluid status in surgical patients.

Subjective global assessment (SGA) is a simple, practical bedside method that has been validated to assess nutritional status and to predict clinical outcomes in stable patients without marked fluid shifts [20,21]. The SGA incorporates multiple components, including weight loss and dietary intake history, functional capacity, gastrointestinal symptoms (diarrhea, nausea, and vomiting), and physical examination evidence (loss of muscle or fat mass, presence of edema/ascite) to classify the severity of malnutrition (e.g., well nourished, mild to moderately malnourished, or severely malnourished [20,21]. A European nutritional risk assessment that is also commonly used involves scoring risk based on whether or not the patient is severely ill, body mass index (BMI), decrease in

Medical Management of the Surgical Patient, ed. Michael F. Lubin, Thomas F. Dodson, and Neil H. Winawer. Published by Cambridge University Press. © Cambridge University Press 2013.

Table 2.1 Major contributing pathophysiologic factors for malnutrition in surgical patients.

- Reduced spontaneous food intake pre- or postoperation (due to anorexia, pain, gastrointestinal symptoms, NPO status)
- Elevated catabolic hormones and cytokines levels (e.g., cortisol, catecholamines, interleukins, tumor necrosis factor-α)
- Decreased anabolic hormones concentrations (e.g., insulin-like growth factor-I, testosterone)
- Resistance to anabolic hormones with subsequent decreased substrate utilization (e.g., insulin resistance)
- Unusual nutrient losses (due to diarrhea, various drainage via tubes, emesis, polyuria, dialysis treatment, wounds)
- Reduced protein synthesis in relation to physical inactivity (due to bed rest, chemical-induced paralysis)
- Drug–nutrient interactions (due to diuretics, vasopressors, corticosteroids)
- Increased caloric, protein and/or specific micronutrient requirements (due to infection, trauma, wound healing, oxidative stress)
- Iatrogenic factors (due to prolonged insufficient enteral or parenteral nutrition provision in relation to metabolic requirements)

NPO, *nil per os* (enteral food restriction due to diagnostic tests or therapeutic procedures).

Table 2.2 Important approaches to assess nutritional status for surgical patients.

- Review past medical and surgical histories, tempo of current illness, underlying condition prompting minor or major surgery, and expected postoperative course
- Review preoperative dietary intake pattern and use of specialized nutrition support
- Obtain body weight and weight history
- Perform physical examination to assess fluid status, organ functions, evidence of malnutrition, signs and symptoms related to vitamin-mineral deficiency, and wound healing
- Evaluate gastrointestinal tract function to select appropriate feeding route (e.g., oral, enteral, and/or parenteral feeding)
- Determine the anticipated duration of inadequate oral intake and the need for intraoperative feeding tube or central venous line placement
- Evaluate ambulatory capacity and mental status
- Measure or assess standard biochemical markers (e.g., electrolytes, organ function indices, pH, triglycerides, selected vitamins/minerals if at risk for deficiencies)
- Estimate caloric and protein requirements

Careful evaluation for malnutrition for the following patients: (1) involuntary body weight loss of > 5–10% of usual body weight within the past several weeks or months; (2) weight < 90% of ideal body weight; (3) body mass index (BMI) < 18.5 kg/m².

percentage of usual dietary intake, change in body weight, and age [22]. Detailed aspects of comprehensive nutritional assessment have been published in a recent review paper [17].

Nutrient intake goals

Major professional societies have recently outlined guidelines for energy (calorie) and protein (amino acid) intake in adult hospital patients [4,5, 23–25]. Specific recommendations for pediatric patients have been recently published [26,27]. Caloric requirements in hospitalized surgical patients, especially those who are critically ill, may vary considerably due to serial changes in clinical conditions over time [4,5, 25]. However, optimal caloric and amino acid needs in surgical patients are unknown because of a lack of current rigorous, randomized, controlled clinical trials [4,5, 28].

Resting energy expenditure (REE) can be determined using indirect calorimetry, but its utilization is limited by cost, availability, and technical issues [4, 29]. Resting energy expenditure can be estimated using traditional predictive equations, such as the commonly used Harris–Benedict equation, which incorporates the patient's age, gender, height, and weight [4, 17]. Unfortunately, predictive equations need to be used with caution as they may over- or underestimate REE in surgical patients secondary to changes in body weight due to fluid status [17, 29]. Recent (2009) American and European clinical practice guidelines suggest 25 kcal/kg/day as an approximate energy goal for most surgical patients, which is approximately equivalent to 1.2 times of the measured or estimated REE. For patient under conditions of severe stress, the estimated daily energy expenditure and requirements may

be closer to 30 kcal/kg, but feeding this level of calories increases the risk for complications (outlined below).

Ongoing randomized controlled trials (RCTs) are designed to better define caloric dosing guidelines in ICU patients, as data are particularly conflicting in this area. Pre-hospital and preoperative body weight should be used when estimating energy requirement because measured body weight in the hospital (especially in the ICU) may reflect fluid status and can be much higher than recent "dry" weight. Ideal body weight (IBW) derived from routine tables or equations can be used as an alternative when recent dry weight is unknown. For obese patients whose body weight is ≥ 20–25% IBW, adjusted body weight to ideal levels should be used to estimate caloric needs [17].

Adequate protein provision is important for tissue maintenance, wound healing, and slowing endogenous protein catabolism, particularly after major surgery. Studies conducted in the 1980s in ICU patients indicate that daily protein loads of > 2.0 g/kg are inefficiently used for protein synthesis and the excess is oxidized and contributes to azotemia [30,31]. The commonly recommended daily amino acid dose is between 1.2–1.5 g/kg for most surgical patients with normal renal and hepatic function (50–100% above the recommended daily allowance (RDA) of 0.8 g/kg/day); although higher doses of 2.0–2.5 g/kg/day have been recommended in specific conditions such as burns, patients with large wounds, and in patients requiring renal replacement therapy [4,5, 17]. Protein requirement may need to be adjusted below recommended range in relation to the extent and progression of renal dysfunction in the absence of dialysis treatment (0.6–0.8 g/kg/day). In patients with evidence of acute hepatic dysfunction with hyperbilirubinemia and altered mental status (who are at risk for amino acid-induced hyperammonia), it may be prudent to provide lower doses of amino acids (0.6–1.2 g/kg/day), based on the severity of hepatic failure.

Timing of nutrition support

Rigorous evidence regarding the efficacy of preoperative nutrition support is limited, but significantly malnourished patients adequately fed for 7–10 days preoperatively and continued into the postoperative period were shown to have improved surgical outcomes in an older trial [32]. Delaying elective surgery for preoperative nutrition support is recommended for patients with preexisting severe malnutrition (e.g., > 10–15% of unintended weight loss from usual body weight within 3–6 months, BMI < 18.5 kg/m^2, or SGA grade C) [9, 24,25].

Although most patients tend to resume oral intake within 2–7 days postoperatively, lack of nutrition for 10–14 days after major surgery is associated with a significant increase in morbidity and mortality [9, 14]. A short period of starvation or inadequate dietary intake was correlated with worse surgical outcome in one study, but the clinical effect of various durations of minimal or no feeding remains an area of uncertainty [33]. Therefore, several clinical practice guidelines recommend starting nutrition support immediately after surgery when patients are expected to not fully meet their caloric requirement within 7–10 days in the postoperative course independently [9, 24,25].

Several studies suggest that postoperative enteral feeding in patients undergoing gastrointestinal (GI) resection and other abdominal operations is safe and well tolerated when started within 12 hours of surgery [34–37]. The timing for initiation of PN (and EN) remains controversial due to a lack of rigorous randomized controlled trials [38]. A large RCT from Belgium (4,640 patients) was recently published on the impact of timing of PN initiation primarily in adult surgical ICU patients receiving inadequate amounts of early enteral feeding (tube feeds in all subjects were begun on day 2 of ICU admission) [39]. In the early initiation group, supplemental PN to meet the caloric goal of 25–30 kcal/kg/day was started on ICU day 2, per 2009 European clinical practice guidelines [5]. In the late initiation group, supplemental PN to meet the caloric goal was started on ICU day 7, per 2009 American clinical practice guidelines [4]. The early initiation of PN was associated with modestly increased ICU and **hospital** length of stay, infectious complications, indices of organ dysfunction, and total hospital costs [39]. However, most patients in this study were not significantly malnourished at entry and those receiving specialized EN or PN on ICU admission were excluded. Nonetheless, this is an important study that provides evidence that PN initiation in the first few days of an ICU admission to supplement inadequate EN should be carefully considered in adults [38].

Current American clinical practice guidelines suggest that: (1) moderately to severely malnourished patients scheduled for major GI surgery should receive 7–14 days of preoperative NS if surgery can be safely postponed; (2) PN should routinely be prescribed in the immediate postoperative period for patients undergoing major GI surgery if adequate EN is not possible; (3) postoperative specialized nutrition support is warranted if inadequate oral nutrition is anticipated for 7–10 days [9].

Enteral nutrition support

Enteral feeding is the preferred route of nutrition support in patients with a functional GI tract. Enteral nutrition in surgical patients should consist of regular foods as tolerated, and oral nutritional supplements as indicated, using the wide variety of commercially available flavored oral liquid formulations or solid nutrient-rich products. Although not evidence-based, it is recommended that most surgical patients receive complete enteral multivitamin-mineral products to cover micronutrient needs when possible [38].

Enteral nutrition is associated with fewer postoperative complications than PN, although direct comparison of EN vs PN in clinically matched patients (including for GI function) has not been rigorously studied [4,9,15,40,41]. Specific indications for EN in children and adults are described in recently published clinical practice guidelines [4,5,15,23–27,42]. Common contraindications to tube feeding are inability to access the GI tract, diffuse peritonitis, ischemic bowel, intractable vomiting, mechanical or paralytic intestinal obstruction, severe diarrhea, paralytic ileus, and hemodynamic instability requiring mid- to high-dose vasopressors [4,5,9,17].

Delivery of EN must be customized for each patient's specific needs. To determine the suitable EN delivery method, GI tract integrity and functional capacity, the presence and extent of malnutrition, underlying comorbidities, and feeding tolerance must be assessed before and after feeding is initiated. Enteral tube feeding is associated with gastrointestinal, mechanical, and metabolic complications; therefore, close monitoring of enterally fed patients is necessary to identify potential complications [42].

Access for enteral feeding

Selection of the appropriate enteral access device and placement technique is a fundamental part of successful enteral tube feeding. Feeding tubes are typically made of polyurethane or silicone with a variety of diameters: small-bore (5–12 French) or large-bore (≥ 14 French) [43]. Feeding tubes are usually based on insertion sites (e.g., nasal, oral, percutaneous) and the location of the tube tip (e.g., stomach, duodenum, proximal small bowel) (Table 2.3).

Nasoenteral (NE) tubes are often inserted blindly at bedside by experienced personnel or with the assistance of endoscopy or fluoroscopy. Endoscopic, fluoroscopic, laparoscopic, and percutaneous tube placement techniques can be used for the placement of gastrostomy and jejunostomy tubes. If patients present with moderate or severe malnutrition and/or are anticipated to have insufficient oral intake for a prolonged period of time

Table 2.3 Advantages and disadvantages of various enteral feeding access routes.

	Indications	Advantages	Disadvantages
Nasoenteric (NE) tube feeding (short term, < 4 weeks)			
Nasogastric (NG)	Normal gastric emptying No esophageal reflux	Easy tube placement Stomach serves as a large reservoir Normal physiologic process of digestion and absorption	Highest aspiration risk Tube displacement
Nasoduodenal (ND) Nasojejunal (NJ)	Delayed gastric emptying Esophageal reflux Gastroparesis As in ND Gastric dysfunction Pancreatitis	Reduced aspiration risk compared with NG As in ND May start feed immediately following operation	Placement may require endoscopy Possible complications: Aspiration GI intolerance (bloating, cramping, diarrhea) Tube displacement
Tube enterostomy (long-term feeding required)			
Gastrostomy Percutaneous* esophagostomy gastrostomy (PEG) Operative laparoscopic** gastrostomy	Refer to NG NE route is not available Persistent dysphasia	Convenient intraoperative tube placement Surgery is not required for PEG PEG is less expensive than surgical gastrostomy Reduced risk of tube occlusion with large bore tube Stomach serves as a large reservoir Normal physiologic process of digestion and absorption	Requires surgery for gastrostomy placement Requires stoma care Possible complications: Aspiration Infection at stoma site Skin excoriation at stoma site Fistula after tube removal
Jejunostomy Percutaneous* endoscopic jejunostomy (PEJ) Needle catheter jejunostomy (NCJ) Operative laparoscopic jejunostomy	As in ND and NJ High aspiration risk Inability to access upper GI tract (esophagus, duodenum, stomach)	Reduced aspiration risk Convenient intraoperative tube placement Surgery is not required for PEJ PEJ is cheaper than surgical jejunostomy May start feed immediately following operation	Requires surgery for jejunostomy placement Requires stoma care Possible complications: GI intolerance Infection at stoma site Skin excoriation at stoma site Fistula after tube removal Tube occlusion risk with small-bore tube or needle catheter

* Percutanous tube placements avoid risks of surgery and general anesthesia; however, may require the assistance of endoscopy, abdominal ultrasound, or radiologic procedure with contrast media. Endoscopy can be challenging in patients with tumor or stricture, altered anatomy, and/or severe obesity.

** Laparoscopic or operative tube placements expose patients to the risks of general anesthesia and surgery; however, patients may be able to return home on the same day following procedure.

following operation, surgeons should consider placing a feeding tube at the time of surgery [43]. Proper placement of a blindly inserted small- or large-bore feeding tube must be verified by radiography prior to the administration of tube feedings and medications [43–46]. If EN is anticipated for short-term (< 4–6 weeks), nasal or oral tubes are generally placed. If EN is expected for long-term (≥ 4 weeks), clinical practice guidelines recommend enterostomies [43–47].

The selection of an appropriate enteral delivery route depends on patient-specific characteristics, including comorbidities and their relation to nutritional requirements, aspiration risk, GI anatomy, gut motility and function, and the anticipated duration of enteral nutrition [42–47]. Gastric feedings require a functional stomach without delayed gastric emptying, fistula, or obstruction. Small bowel feedings are most suitable for patients with esophageal reflux, gastroparesis, gastric outlet obstruction, pancreatitis, and increased aspiration risk (e.g., confusion or other altered mental states, inability to raise head of bed, etc.). Small bowel feedings via nasojejunal (NJ) tube are not required unless patients have gastric feeding intolerance, but they have been associated with a significant reduction in ventilator-associated pneumonia in some, but not all, studies [42]. For patients with impaired gastric motility but with normal intestinal motility and absorption, gastrojejunal tubes are indicated to allow gastric decompression while jejunal feeding is possible [42,46].

Table 2.4 Some commercially available enteral formulations in the USA.

Categories	Potential indications	kcal/mL	Protein (g/L)	Fat (g/L)	Carbohydrate (g/L)	% Water	Osmolality (mOsm/kg H$_2$O)
Standard (e.g., Osmolite®; Isocal®)	Most patients	1.0–1.5	44–63	35–49	144–204	76–84	300–525
Semi-elemental (e.g., Pivot®; Peptamen®)	Malabsorption, pancreatitis	1.0–1.5	40–51	28–39	127–138	83–85	300–585
Fiber-Enriched (e.g., Jevity®; Ultracal®)	Diarrhea	1.0–1.5	44–63	35–49	155–216	76–84	300–525
Diabetic (e.g., Glucerna®)	Diabetes	1.0–1.5	42–82	54–75	95.6–133.1	76–85	355–875
Caloric Dense (e.g., TwoCal HN®)	Fluid restriction, high caloric needs	2.0	84	90	218	70	725
Renal failure (e.g., Nepro®)	On dialysis	1.8	81	96	167	73	600
Renal failure (e.g., Suplena®)	Predialysis	1.8	45	96	202	73	600
Pulmonary (e.g., Oxepa®)	Adult respiratory distress syndrome	1.5	63	94	105	79	535
Immune-enhancing (e.g., Impact Glutamine®; Crucial®)	Immuno-suppressed, critical illness	1.3–1.5	78	43	150	81	630
High protein (e.g., Promote®, Nutren Replete®)	Wound healing	1.0	62	26–28	130–138	84	340–380

This table does not constitute an all-inclusive list. Information provided by manufacturer.

Appropriate selections for tube feeding formula

Selecting an appropriate formula is important prior to starting enteral feeding. Various commercially available enteral formulations can be categorized into the following groups: standardized or polymeric, hydrolyzed, calorically dense, disease-specific, fat-modified, fiber-enriched, and "immune-modulating" (Table 2.4). These formulas differ in terms of caloric density, composition and digestibility of macronutrients, osmolarity, viscosity, and cost. The standardized formulas consist of complex carbohydrates, intact protein, long- and medium-chain triglycerides, vitamins/minerals, and trace elements, and are low in sodium content. Polymeric formulas are lactose- and gluten-free, and are mostly low residue as well as isotonic or slightly hypertonic with a caloric content between 1 to 2 kcal/mL.

The most appropriate product to meet the patient's estimated nutritional needs can be selected by utilizing a systematic comparison of the patient-specific factors and nutrient needs with the specific variables of the available formulas. Patient-specific characteristics include clinical and nutritional status, caloric needs, metabolic abnormalities, organ function, fluid status, absorptive and digestive capacity of the gut, acute underlying conditions, expected outcomes, and availability of possible administration routes.

Most surgical patients can be safely fed with the standardized, inexpensive enteral products (Table 2.4). The standard polymeric formulas are generally tolerated as well as the more expensive hydrolyzed formulas [48–49]. Hydrolyzed formulas, also known as oligomeric, peptide-based, or semi-elemental formulas, were developed for patients with malabsorption and pancreatic insufficiency. Clinical data documenting the advantages of routine use of hydrolyzed formulas are limited; however, one study has shown that patients with acute pancreatitis who received hydrolyzed formulas significantly shortened their length of hospital stay when compared with standard formulas [50]. Soluble fiber-enriched formulations are common in commercial formulas and can be used for management of diarrhea; available data on fiber-supplemented formulas have shown inconsistent benefit, possibly because there are numerous contributing factors for the development of diarrhea in hospital patients [51]. When a high-fiber formula is selected, adequate fluid provision is important to prevent constipation or fecal impaction.

Specialized tube feeding products have been developed for certain conditions and requirements, including diabetes mellitus, immune enhancing, fluid restriction, renal dysfunction, and pulmonary disease (Table 2.4) [52–56]. Diabetes-specific products consist of admixed blends of soluble and insoluble fibers, with lower carbohydrate content and higher fat content (higher amounts of monounsaturated fatty acids compared with polyunsaturated or saturated fatty acids) and have been developed to improve blood glucose control. Some

Table 2.5 Delivery methods for enteral feeding.

Methods	Indications	Advantage	Disadvantage
Continuous	Preferred for initiation of feeding Critical illness Small bowel feeding Intermittent or bolus feeding intolerance	Pump-assisted Better tolerance Lower risk of complications related to high gastric residual, aspiration, and metabolic abnormalities	Ambulatory restriction Requires feeding pump and supplies (more expensive)
Bolus – intermittent	Non-critical illness Home TF Gastric feeding	Simple delivery No pump required Short feeding time Mimics a typical dietary pattern Allows most freedom and mobility	Highest aspiration risk Increased risk of GI intolerance (abdominal pain, diarrhea, nausea, vomiting)
Cyclic – intermittent	Non-critical illness Home TF Small bowel feeding	Flexible schedule Allow for mobility Useful for the transition of TF to oral diet	Delivers high volumes over a short time (8–16 hours) May require caloric/protein dense formula to meet nutritional requirements Increased risk of GI intolerance and aspiration

TF, tube feedings; GI, gastrointestinal.

studies have reported that their use in hospitalized diabetic patients resulted in improved glycemic control and lowered insulin requirements when compared with patients on standard formulas [52–53].

The caloric-dense (concentrated) products are appropriate for patients requiring fluid restriction, such as those with congestive heart failure or renal failure. Because of the smaller volume needed to meet caloric requirements, a caloric-dense product is also appropriate for high calorie requirement, cyclic feeds, or bolus feeds. Renal-specific products are available for patients with different degrees of renal dysfunction with or without dialysis. Formulas with increased amounts of antioxidant nutrients (e.g., vitamins C and E) and anti-inflammatory lipids (e.g., eicosapentanoic acid, gamma-linolenic acid) are also available. Several RCTs suggest that their use improved clinical outcomes compared with standard formulas in patients with acute respiratory distress syndrome (ARDS) [54–55]; however, a recent Phase II study of omega-3 fatty acid-enhanced EN showed no benefit [56].

Enteral nutrition formulas supplemented with one or more of the following ingredients: arginine, glutamine, omega-3 fatty acids, probiotics and/or antioxidants are commercially available [42]. Early EN with immune-enhancing formulation appears promising for general-surgery patients; however, routine use of these formulations remains controversial based on inconsistent results of controlled trials and lack of mortality benefits [57–60].

Tube feeding delivery

Diluting enteral formula is not necessary at the initiation stages of tube feeding. Diluted formulas are more prone to microbial contamination versus standard full-strength

formulas and are associated with increased intolerance [42]. There are limited data to form strong recommendations for the optimal starting infusion rate for enteral tube feeding. Enteral feedings can be delivered as continuous, bolus, or cyclic intermittent, or a combination of these methods (Table 2.5).

Continuous feedings are usually infused at a slow continuous rate over 24 hours via gravity drip or by an electronic feeding pump. Full strength of most commercially available formulas is well tolerated when administered into the stomach or small intestine at 10 to 30 mL/hour. The infusion rate can generally be advanced in increments of 10 to 20 mL/hour every 8–12 hours as tolerated until the goal rate is reached. Hemodynamically stable patients can tolerate a fairly rapid progression of delivery rate and achieve the estimated goal rate within 24 to 48 hours following initiation. There is also evidence to support starting EN at goal rates in stable adult patients [61–62]. Continuous feeding is typically better tolerated with lower incidence of GI intolerance and risk of aspiration than bolus feeding in hospital settings. Patients with post-pyloric feeding tubes require continuous infusion as bolus feeds into the small bowel induce diarrhea.

Bolus and intermittent feedings are the most physiologic feeding methods that mimic a normal dietary lifestyle and allow bowel rest in between feedings (Table 2.5) [42]. They are the simplest to perform and can be infused over a short time via syringes or a feeding container by gravity drip with or without an enteral feeding pump [63]. However, gastric bolus feedings can cause adverse GI effects secondary to the sudden delivery of a large, hyperosmolar formula [42,63].

Regardless of the feeding methods, most enterally fed patients will require supplemental fluid to meet minimum fluid requirements (typically 30–40 mL/kg body weight).

Supplemental fluid, such as sterile water or normal saline, is administered intermittently as flushes daily (e.g., at least 30 mL/ flush every 8 hours). The amount of flush is determined by the amount of free water required to meet the estimated fluid goal. The volume of the additional fluid requirements can be calculated by first determining the patient's total fluid needs, followed by determining the amount of free water provided by the enteral formula by multiplying the percent free water concentration by the total volume of enteral formula to be delivered daily (Table 2.4). Lastly, the volume of the free water supplied by tube feeds is subtracted from the calculated total free water needs to give the remaining required volume of free water, which then is divided into 3 or 4 boluses given as water flushes daily.

Enteral feeding complications

Adverse events of EN include gastrointestinal, mechanical, and metabolic complications (e.g., bronchopulmonary aspiration, feeding tube misplacement and displacement, tube clogging, GI intolerance, and drug–nutrient interactions [42, 64–65]. Table 2.6 reviews some of the potential causes and the management of these complications.

The tolerable ranges for gastric residual volumes (GRVs) at which to lower tube feeding rates have been re-evaluated in recent years, and higher volumes than previously routine practice have been advocated based on available data [66]. For GRVs $\geq$ 250 mL after two consecutive checks, the use of a promotility agent in adult patients has been suggested. Limited evidence to date has verified that elevated GRVs are dependable markers for increased risk of aspiration pneumonia [66]. Gastric residual volumes should be checked more frequently (e.g., every 4–6 hours during the first 48 hours) when gastric feedings are first initiated. Once the desired gastric feeding rate is achieved, gastric residual monitoring can be adjusted to every 6–12 hours in the non-critically ill patients [66]. Pulmonary aspiration of enteral feeding in patients demonstrating intolerance (e.g., emesis, gastric distension) can be minimized by adjustment of patient position, use of post-pyloric continuous feeding, and cautious use of prokinetic agents (e.g., metoclopramide or erythromycin) [67–69].

Clogging of feeding tubes is commonly related to the use of small-bore tubes, inappropriate delivery of medication, and accumulation of formula residue in the lower segment of the tube, especially with a slow infusion of caloric-dense or fiber-enriched formulas [70]. To prevent tube clogging, it is recommended to use cleaning techniques to minimize formula contamination and to adhere to proper tube flushing protocols [42, 70]. Water is preferred for tube flushes, and sterile water should be used for tube flushes in patients who are immunocompromised or critically ill, especially when the safety of tap water cannot be reasonably assumed [70]. If the use of warm water fails to unclog the tube, then a combination use of pancrelipase and sodium bicarbonate solution may dissolve the clog [70].

Enteral nutrition-induced metabolic complications are comparable to PN, but may occur in reduced incidence and severity (see below). Monitoring metabolic parameters before EN was initiated and periodically during enteral feeding should be based on individual institution practice protocols, patient-specific conditions, and duration of therapy. Patients at risk for refeeding syndrome should be recognized, and severe electrolyte abnormalities should be corrected before starting enteral feeding. Prevention of refeeding syndrome and proper monitoring of feeding tolerance in enterally fed patients is essential for the safe delivery of EN [71].

Parenteral nutrition support

Few well-designed, adequately powered intent-to-treat RCTs on PN efficacy in hospital settings have been published [17, 72–73]. Thus, current practices of PN use in hospital patients are largely based on guidelines by professional societies, largely derived from observational studies, expert opinion, and small clinical trials [4–5,9,23–27,38]. Further, many of the earlier trials were conducted with excessive PN caloric doses and liberal blood glucose control strategies compared with current practice today.

Indications for parenteral nutrition

While it would seem intuitive that early nutritional intervention is warranted for most patients, the literature to date suggests that early PN does not improve clinical outcomes [39, 74–79]. Although not evidence-based, PN is generally indicated for malnourished surgical patients when energy requirements were not met after 3–7 days by EN alone. Parenteral nutrition is indicated when EN is either not feasible or tolerable, as in: (1) major upper GI surgery; (2) after extensive small bowel resection with or without colonic resection; (3) with perforated small bowel; (4) with a proximal high-output (> 600 mL) fistula; (4) other conditions resulting in prolonged EN intolerance (e.g., severe diarrhea, persistent emesis, significant abdominal distension, partial or complete bowel obstruction, acute GI bleeding, hemodynamic instability) that preclude sufficient EN provision for > 3–7 days [4,5,17]. Again not evidence-based, PN is generally contraindicated for the following types of patients: (1) those with functional GI tracts and accessibility for EN; (2) fluid-restricted patients who cannot tolerate the intravenous fluid load provided for PN; (3) patients with severe hyperglycemia or electrolyte abnormalities on the day of planned PN initiation; (4) when PN therapy is unlikely to last > 5–7 days; and (5) if placement of a new access line solely for PN causes unnecessary risks [4,5,17].

Parenteral nutrition administration

Parenteral nutrition, as complete solutions, can be infused through a peripheral or central vein. Table 2.7 lists some of the characteristics of peripheral and central vein PN, fluid

Table 2.6 Complications of enteral feeding.

Complications	Possible causes	Possible management
Gastrointestinal		
Diarrhea (> 4 bowel movements per day or large loose stool)	Medications Formula intolerance Bacterial overgrowth Osmotic overload Decreased bulk *Clostridium difficile*	Medication modifications: Discontinue antibiotics, antacids, sorbitol-containing liquid medications when possible Further dilute hypertonic medications Administer medications by intravenous route Use bulking agents (e.g., psyllium), probiotics and/or antidiarrheal agents* Feeding modifications: Consider a low-fat, fiber-enriched, or isotonic formula Reduce administration rate Stool culture for pathogens
Nausea or vomiting	Supine position Delayed gastric emptying GI tract obstruction Hyperglycemia Nutrient intolerances – volume overload	Keep head of bed up 30–45° Position patient on right side to facilitate passage of gastric contents through pylorus Medication modifications: Reduce narcotic use or use narcotic antagonists (e.g., naloxone and alvimopan) Use prokinetic agents (e.g., metoclopramide and erythromycin) and/or anti-emetic Feeding modifications: Reduce total volume or infusion rate Slow progression of delivery rate (e.g., over 12–24 hours) Hold feeding for 2 hours and check residuals Consider low-fat formula
Constipation	Decreased fiber Dehydration GI obstruction	Consider fiber-enriched formula Use bulking agents Use sufficient amount of fluid as flushes to meet hydration needs Hold feeding temporarily
Mechanical		
Aspiration	Impaired gag reflex Reflux Supine position Tube malposition or displacement Delayed gastric emptying	Keep head of bed up 30–45° Use continuous feed or feed through duodenum or jejunum Use a smaller bore feeding tube Correct placement is confirmed via radiography after insertion, severe coughing, vomiting, or a seizure Tape tube in place and mark with indelible ink at exit site as reference point Reconfirmation of tube placement prior to each feeding by checking residuals, ink mark
Clogging	Acid precipitation of formula Insufficient/improper tube flushing Medications	Regular tube flushes (e.g., before and after each medication, residual check, bolus feeding, and every 6–8 hours during continuous feeding, or whenever feeding is stopped) Feed via duodenum or jejunum Do not mix medications with enteral formula Adequately crush and dissolve medications with water; if more than one medication is to be given, flush tube between doses Use liquid medications where possible or administer via different route Avoid using bulk-forming agents via small-bore tube

* Use antidiarrheal agents only when infectious and inflammatory etiologies and fecal impaction have been ruled out and contributing medications have been changed or discontinued.

volume requirements, macronutrient and micronutrient content. Peripheral vein PN (PPN) provides low amounts of dextrose (5%; dextrose = 3.4 kcal/g) and amino acids (≤ 3%; 4 kcal/g) and high caloric content as fat emulsion (≤ 5%; 10 kcal/g; 50–60% of total calories) secondary to the risk of developing phlebitis [9]. Peripheral vein PN generally requires a fluid volume of ≥ 2 liters in order to meet a patient's caloric needs; therefore, it may be contraindicated or not indicated for ICU patients and those require fluid restriction due to cardiac, hepatic, and/or renal dysfunction. Unlike PPN, central venous PN (CPN) is infused through the superior vena cava where concentrated dextrose and amino acids are tolerated. Central

Table 2.7 Composition of typical peripheral and central venous parenteral nutrition formulations

Component	Peripheral vein PN	Central vein PN
Volume (L/day)	2–3	1–1.5
Dextrose (%)	5	10–25
Amino acids (%)	2.5–3.5	3–8
Lipid (%)	3.5–5.0	2.5–5.0
Sodium (mEq/L)	50–150	50–150
Potassium (mEq/L)	20–35	30–50
Phosphorus (mMol/L)	5–10	10–30
Magnesium (mEq/L)	8–10	10–20
Calcium (mEq/L)	2.5–5	2.5–5
Vitamins[1]		
Trace elements/minerals[2]		

[1] Vitamins generally added to PN on a daily basis are composed of commercial mixtures of vitamins A, B_1 (thiamine), B_2 (riboflavin), B_3 (niacinamide), B_6 (pyridoxine), B_{12}, C, D, and E, biotin, folate, pantothenic acid, and with or without vitamin K. Specific vitamins (e.g., vitamin B_1, B_6, B_{12}, K, and folate) are available to be supplemented separately.
[2] Trace elements/minerals typically added to PN on a daily basis consist of commercial mixtures of chromium, copper, manganese, selenium, and zinc. These minerals are available for individualized supplementations.

venous PN is able to meet caloric and protein requirement for the vast majority of patients with just 1–1.5 liters of fluid a day (Table 2.7).

Parenteral nutrition electrolytes are adjusted as indicated to maintain serially measured serum levels within the normal range. With increased and decreased blood levels, dose adjustment of specific electrolytes may be indicated until serum levels are within the normal range. Higher dextrose content in CPN may increase potassium, magnesium, and phosphorus requirements. The relative percentage of sodium and potassium salts as chloride is increased to correct metabolic alkalosis, and the percentage of these salts as acetate is increased to correct metabolic acidosis. Currently clinical practice guidelines recommend tighter glycemic control in ICU and other hospital patients (< 180 mg/dL) [80]. Regular insulin can be added to PN and/or the reduced dextrose load in CPN as needed to achieve these goals. Separate intravenous insulin infusions are commonly required with hyperglycemia in ICU settings [17].

Conventional PN provides all nine essential amino acids and several non-essential amino acids, depending on the commercial amino acid formulation used [28]. Although controversial, European guidelines recommend routine addition of glutamine as a conditionally essential amino acid in ICU patients, given the evidence that this amino acid may become essential in certain catabolic patients [5,28]. The dose of amino acids is adjusted downward or upward in relation to goal amounts as a function of the degree of azotemia or hyperbilirubinemia in patients with acute renal and hepatic failure, respectively. Complete PN provides intravenous lipid emulsions as a source of both energy and essential linoleic and linolenic fatty acids. In the USA, the only commercially available lipid emulsion is soybean oil-based; in Europe and other countries, intravenous soybean oil/medium-chain triglyceride mixtures, fish oil, olive oil/soybean oil mixtures, and combinations of these are approved for use in PN. Lipid is typically mixed with dextrose and amino acids in the same PN infusion bag ("all-in-one" solution) and given with PN over 16–24 hours. Intravenous lipid emulsion may also be infused separately over 10–12 hours. The maximal recommended dose of lipid emulsion infusion is 1.0–1.3 g/kg/day, with monitoring of blood triglyceride levels at baseline and then approximately weekly and as indicated to assess fat clearance [9, 17, 24]. Triglyceride levels should be maintained below 400–500 mg/dL by decreasing the amount of lipid infused to decrease risk of pancreatitis and diminished pulmonary diffusion capacity in patients with severe chronic obstructive lung disease (Table 2.8). In central venous PN, a reasonable initial guideline is to provide 60–70% of non-protein calories as dextrose and 30–40% of non-protein calories as fat emulsion [4,5,17,24].

Specific requirements for intravenous vitamins and minerals have not been rigorously defined in hospital patients [3,5,17,24]. Therefore, therapy is directed at meeting published recommended doses that maintain blood levels in the normal range in most stable patients using standardized intravenous preparations of combined vitamins and minerals (Table 2.7). However, several studies show that a significant proportion of ICU patients receiving conventional nutrition support variously exhibit low zinc, copper, selenium, vitamin C, vitamin E, and vitamin D levels [6,7]. This may be due to pre-ICU depletion, increased ICU requirements (possibly secondary to oxidative stress), and increased excretion and/or tissue redistribution. Depletion of these essential nutrients may impair antioxidant capacity, immunity, wound healing, and other important body functions. Thus, as with electrolytes, therapy is directed at maintaining normal blood levels, with serial measurements in blood as clinically and biochemically indicated.

Parenteral nutrition formulations can be compounded under a sterile hood by trained pharmacists, but "premixes" of the standardized formulations are also available commercially. Parenteral nutrition is administered by an infusion pump to control delivery rates and the infusion catheters incorporate an in-line filter to prevent microbial contamination.

Clinical monitoring of parenteral nutrition

Monitoring of PN therapy in the hospital setting requires daily assessment of the multiple factors outlined in Tables 2.1 and 2.2. Blood glucose should be monitored several times daily and blood electrolytes and renal function tests should generally be determined daily. Blood triglyceride levels should be measured at baseline and then weekly until stable. Although guidelines

Table 2.8 Potential complications of overfeeding and refeeding syndromes in patients receiving parenteral nutrition.

- Intracellular shift of magnesium, phosphorus, and/or potassium (due to excess dextrose content; refeeding hyperinsulinemia)
- Immune cell dysfunction and infection (due to hyperglycemia)
- Cardiac dysfunction or arrhythmias (due to excess fluid, sodium and other electrolytes; refeeding-induced shift of electrolytes)
- Neuromuscular dysfunction (due to thiamine depletion; refeeding-induced shift of electrolytes)
- Azotemia (due to excess amino acid; inadequate caloric provision relative to amino acid dose)
- Edema or fluid retention (due to excess fluid and/or sodium; refeeding hyperinsulinemia)
- Increased liver function tests and/or hepatic steatosis (due to excessive calorie, dextrose, or fat content)
- Elevated blood ammonia concentrations (due to excessive amino acid provision with acute hepatic dysfunction)
- Hypercapnia (due to excessive total caloric provision)
- Respiratory insufficiency (due to refeeding-induced hypophosphatemia; excess fluid, calorie, carbohydrate or fat content)
- Hypertriglyceridemia (due to excessive carbohydrate or fat provision; carnitine-deficiency)

are few, some centers routinely monitor periodic blood levels of copper, selenium, folate, vitamin B_{12}, zinc, thiamine, vitamin B_6, vitamin C, and 25-hydroxyvitamin D [17]. Liver enzymes should be measured at least a few times weekly. pH should generally be monitored daily in ventilated patients when arterial blood gas pH measurements are available. Monitoring of blood glucose, electrolytes, and organ function is routine in the ICU setting.

Adverse effects of parenteral nutrition

Metabolic, infectious, and mechanical complications may occur with PN [24]. Mechanical complications, particularly with insertion and use of central venous catheters, include pneumothorax, hemothorax, thrombosis, and bleeding. Catheter-related bloodstream infections can occur. Proper and safe administration of both peripheral and central vein PN requires strict catheter care protocols, including use of dedicated catheter ports for PN administration and subclavian vein insertion sites for central venous PN [9,24].

Potential metabolic and clinical consequences of overfeeding and refeeding syndrome during central venous PN in critically ill patients are shown in Table 2.8. Risk factors for PN-associated hyperglycemia include: (1) use in obese, diabetic, and/or septic patients; (2) poorly controlled blood glucose at PN initiation; (2) initial use of high dextrose concentrations ($> 10\%$) or dextrose load (> 150 g/day); (3) insufficient insulin administration and/or inadequate monitoring of blood glucose; and (5) concomitant administration of corticosteroids and pressor agents.

Electrolyte administration requires careful monitoring and, in ICU patients, generally day-to-day adjustment in PN to maintain normal blood levels. Overfeeding can induce several metabolic complications of varying degrees of severity affecting several organ systems (Table 2.8). A recent large study found that PN use, overfeeding, and sepsis were the major risk factors for liver dysfunction in critically ill patients [81]. Thus, PN should be advanced carefully to goal rates and the composition adjusted as appropriate based on the results of close metabolic and clinical monitoring performed daily. The calories provided by dextrose in non-PN intravenous fluids, the soybean oil lipid emulsion carrier of propofol, a commonly used ICU sedative, and the nutrients provided in any administered EN must be taken into account in the PN prescription to avoid overfeeding.

Refeeding syndrome is relatively common in at-risk patients (preexisting malnutrition or electrolyte depletion; prolonged periods of intravenous hydration therapy alone) [71,82]. Refeeding syndrome is mediated by administration of excessive intravenous dextrose (> 150–250 g or 1 liter of PN with 15–25% dextrose). This markedly stimulates insulin release, which may rapidly decrease blood potassium, magnesium and especially phosphorus concentrations due to intracellular shift and utilization in metabolic pathways. High doses of carbohydrate increase thiamine utilization and can precipitate symptoms of thiamine deficiency. Hyperinsulinemia may cause sodium and fluid retention by the kidney. This, together with decreased blood electrolytes (which can cause cardiac arrhythmias) can result in heart failure, especially in patients with preexisting heart disease [71,82]. Prevention of refeeding syndrome requires identification of at-risk patients, use of initially low PN dextrose (e.g., 1 liter of PN with 10% dextrose for 1–2 days), empiric provision of higher PN doses of potassium, magnesium, and phosphorus, based on blood levels and renal function, and supplemental PN thiamine (e.g., 100 mg/day for 3–5 days) [17,71,82].

Consultation with an experienced multidisciplinary nutrition support team for recommendations regarding the PN prescription is ideal when such personnel are available. Nutrition support team daily monitoring has been shown to reduce complications, costs and to decrease inappropriate use of PN [83,84].

Future directions

Limited data are available to support a significant impact of nutrition support on surgical patients. The optimal time for EN and PN intervention in surgical patients remains a major area of uncertainty. Few prospective data are available on the clinical effects of minimal or no feeding over time (e.g., > 7 days), and such data are unlikely to be generated. Rigorous RCTs are needed to define optimal caloric and protein dose regimens in subgroups of ICU patients. Some studies show that larger doses of standard soybean oil-based intravenous fat emulsions induce pro-inflammatory and pro-oxidative effects and possibly immune suppression [85]. However, conflicting results of small RCTs comparing soybean oil-based lipid emulsion with other types of lipid emulsion have not clarified optimal use. Available data suggest that glutamine may become a conditionally essential amino acid in ICU patients [28, 86]. Glutamine plays a vital role in nitrogen transport, and serves as an important fuel for immune and gut mucosal cells and has cytoprotective properties, among other potentially beneficial functions. Several clinical trials have shown that glutamine supplementation at 0.2–0.5 g/kg/day as the L-amino acid or as glutamine dipeptides in PN has protein-anabolic effects, enhances indices of immunity, and decreases hospital infections [28, 86]. Thus, some recent expert panels recommend that glutamine be routinely added to PN in ICU patients, if available [5, 23].

Ongoing large, RCTs on glutamine-supplemented PN should provide the needed information. Phase III level double-blind, intent-to-treat RCTs are needed in specific ICU patient subgroups to define clinically optimal calorie, protein/amino acid, and specific vitamin and mineral requirements, as well as the efficacy of supplemental PN combined with EN to achieve caloric and protein/amino acid goals [4–5, 17, 87–88]. In addition, rigorous trials to verify proposed "pharmaconutrition" strategies (e.g., use of high doses of supplemental parenteral and enteral glutamine, vitamin C and other antioxidants, selenium, and/or zinc, etc.) are also needed [88–89]. Fortunately, numerous large, multicenter RCTs in this regard are in progress and will help to define optimal use of these important adjunctive nutritional therapies over the next several years.

References

1. Barker LA, Gout BS, Crowe TC. Hospital malnutrition: prevalence, identification and impact on patients and the healthcare system. *Int J Environ Res Public Health* 2011; **8**: 514–27.

2. De Luis DA, López MR, Gonzalez SM *et al.* Nutritional status in a multicenter study among institutionalized patients in Spain. *Eur Rev Med Pharmacol Sci* 2011; **15**: 259–65.

3. Giner M, Laviano A, Meguid MM *et al.* In 1995 a correlation between malnutrition and poor outcome in critically ill patients still exists. *Nutrition* 1996; **12**: 23–9.

4. McClave SA, Martindale RG, Vanek VW *et al.* Guidelines for the provision and assessment of nutrition support therapy in the adult critically ill patient: Society of Critical Care Medicine and American Society for Parenteral and Enteral Nutrition. *JPEN J Parenter Enteral Nutr* 2009; **33**: 277–316.

5. Singer P, Berger MM, Van den Berghe G *et al.* ESPEN guidelines for parenteral nutrition: intensive care. *Clin Nutr* 2009; **28**: 387–400.

6. Nathens AB, Neff MJ, Jurkovich GJ *et al.* Randomized, prospective trial of antioxidant supplementation in critically ill surgical patients. *Ann Surg* 2002; **236**: 814–22.

7. Luo M, Fernandez-Estivariz C, Jones DP *et al.* Depletion of plasma antioxidants in surgical intensive care unit patients requiring parenteral feeding: effects of parenteral nutrition with or without alanyl-glutamine dipeptide supplementation. *Nutrition* 2008; **24**: 37–44.

8. Villet S, Chiolero RL, Bollmann MD *et al.* Negative impact of hypocaloric feeding and energy balance on clinical outcome in ICU patients. *Clin Nutr* 2005; **24**: 502–9.

9. ASPEN Board of Directors and the Clinical Guidelines Task Force. Guidelines for the use of parenteral and enteral nutrition in adult and pediatric patients. *JPEN J Parenter Enteral Nutr* 2002; **26** (1 Suppl): 1SA–138SA.

10. O'Brien JM Jr, Phillips GS, Ali NA. Body mass index is independently associated with hospital mortality in mechanically ventilated adults with acute lung injury. *Crit Care Med* 2006; **34**: 738–44.

11. Schneider SM, Veyres P, Pivot X *et al.* Malnutrition is an independent factor associated with nosocomial infections. *Br J Nutr* 2004; **92**: 105–11.

12. Bozzetti F, Gianotti L, Braga M *et al.* Postoperative complications in gastrointestinal cancer patients: the joint role of the nutritional status and the nutritional support. *Clin Nutr* 2007; **26**: 698–709.

13. Jagoe RT, Goodship TH, Gibson GJ. The influence of nutritional status on complications after operations for lung cancer. *Ann Thorac Surg* 2001; **71**: 936–43.

14. Sandstrom R, Drott C, Hyltander A *et al.* The effect of postoperative feeding (TPN) on outcome following major surgery evaluated in a randomized study. *Ann Surg* 1993; **217**: 185–95.

15. Chen Y, Liu BL, Shang B *et al.* Nutrition support in surgical patients with colorectal cancer. *World J Gastroenterol* 2011; **17**: 1779–86.

16. Studley HO. Percentage weight loss, a basic indicator of surgical risk in patients with chronic peptic ulcer. *J Am Med Assoc* 1936; **106**: 458–60.

17. Ziegler TR. Parenteral nutrition in the critically ill patient. *N Engl J Med* 2009; **361**: 1088–97.

18. Seike J, Tangoku A, Yuasa Y *et al.* The effect of nutritional support on the immune function in the acute postoperative period after esophageal cancer surgery: total parenteral nutrition versus enteral nutrition. *J Med Invest* 2011; **58**: 75–80.

19. Kudsk KA, Tolley EA, DeWitt RC *et al.* Preoperative albumin and surgical site identify surgical risk for major postoperative complications. *JPEN J Parenter Enteral Nutr* 2003; **27**: 1–9.

20. Detsky AS, McLaughlin JR, Baker JP *et al.* What is subjective global assessment of nutritional status? *JPEN J Parenter Enteral Nutr* 1987; **11**: 8–13.

21. Norman K, Schütz T, Kemps M *et al.* The Subjective Global Assessment reliably identifies malnutrition-related muscle dysfunction. *Clin Nutr* 2005; **24**: 143–50.

22. Rasmussen HH, Holst M, Kondrup J. Measuring nutritional risk in hospitals. *Clin Epidemiol* 2010; **2**: 209–16.

23. Heyland DK, Dhaliwal R, Drover JW *et al.* Canadian clinical practice guidelines for nutrition support in mechanically ventilated, critically ill

adult patients. *JPEN J Parenter Enteral Nutr* 2003; **27**: 355–73.

24. Braga M, Ljungqvist O, Soeters P *et al.* ESPEN guidelines on parenteral nutrition: surgery. *Clin Nutr* 2009; **28**: 378–86.

25. Weimann A, Braga M, Harsanyi L *et al.* ESPEN guidelines on enteral nutrition: surgery including organ transplantation. *Clin Nutr* 2006; **25**: 224–44.

26. Koletzko B, Agostoni C, Ball P *et al.* ESPEN/ESPGHAN Guidelines on paediatric parenteral nutrition. *J Pediatr Gastroenterol Nutr* 2005; **41**: S1–87.

27. Mehta NM, Compher C, A.S.P.E.N. Board of Directors. A.S.P.E.N. Clinical Guidelines: nutrition support of the critically ill child. *JPEN J Parenter Enteral Nutr* 2009; **33**: 260–76.

28. Yarandi SS, Zhao VM, Hebbar G *et al.* Amino acid composition in parenteral nutrition: what is the evidence? *Curr Opin Clin Nutr Metab Care* 2011; **14**: 75–8.

29. Anderegg BA, Worrall C, Barbour E *et al.* Comparison of resting energy expenditure prediction methods with measured resting energy expenditure in obese, hospitalized adults. *JPEN J Parenter Enteral Nutr* 2009; **33**: 168–75.

30. Streat SJ, Beddoe AH, Hill GL. Aggressive nutritional support does not prevent protein loss despite fat gain in septic intensive care patients. *J Trauma* 1987; **27**: 262–6.

31. Shaw JH, Wildbore M, Wolfe RR. Whole body protein kinetics in severely septic patients. The response to glucose infusion and total parenteral nutrition. *Ann Surg* 1987; **205**: 288–94.

32. Veterans Affairs Total Parenteral Nutrition Cooperative Study Group. Perioperative total parenteral nutrition in surgical patients. *N Engl J Med* 1991; **325**: 525–32.

33. Lewis SJ, Egger M, Sylvester PA *et al.* Early enteral feeding versus "nil by mouth" after gastrointestinal surgery: systemic review and meta-analysis of controlled trials. *Br Med J* 2003; **323**: 733–6.

34. Reissman P, Teoh TA, Cohen SM *et al.* Is early oral feeding safe after elective colorectal surgery? A prospective randomized trial. *Ann Surg* 1995; **222**: 73–7.

35. Braga M, Gianotti L, Gentilini S *et al.* Feeding the gut early after digestive surgery: results of a nine-year experience. *Clin Nutr* 2002; **21**: 59–65.

36. Barlow R, Price P, Reid TD *et al.* Prospective multicentre randomized controlled trial of early enteral nutrition for patients undergoing major upper gastrointestinal surgical resection. *Clin Nutr* 2011; **30**: 560–6.

37. Osland E, Yunus RM, Khan S *et al.* Early versus traditional postoperative feeding in patients undergoing resectional gastrointestinal surgery: a meta-analysis. *JEPN J Parenter Enteral Nutr* 2011; **35**: 473–87.

38. Ziegler TR. Nutrition support in critical illness – bridging the evidence gap. *N Engl J Med* 2011; **365**: 562–4.

39. Casaer MP, Mosetten D, Hermans G *et al.* Early versus late parenteral nutrition in critically ill adults. *N Engl J Med* 2011; **365**: 506–17.

40. Beier-Holgersen SR, Boesby S. Influence of postoperative enteral nutrition on post surgical infections. *Gut* 1996; **39**: 833–5.

41. Schroeder D, Gillanders L, Mahr K *et al.* Effects of immediate postoperative enteral nutrition on body composition, muscle function and wound healing. *JEPN J Parenter Enteral Nutr* 1991; **15**: 376–83.

42. A.S.P.E.N. Board of Directors and Enteral Nutrition Practice Recommendations Task Force. Enteral nutrition practice recommendations. *JPEN J Parenter Enteral Nutr* 2009; **33**: 122–67.

43. Minard G. Enteral access. *Nutr Clin Pract* 1994; **9**: 172–82.

44. Baskin WN. Acute complications associated with bedside placement of feeding tubes. *Nutr Clin Pract* 2006; **21**: 40–55.

45. Metheny NA, Meert KL, Clouse RE. Complications related to feeding tube placement. *Curr Opin Gastroenterol* 2007; **23**: 178–82.

46. Metheny NA, Meert KL. Monitoring feeding tube placement. *Nutr Clin Pract* 2004; **19**: 487–95.

47. Heyland DK, Drover JW, Dhaliwal R *et al.* Optimizing the benefits and minimizing the risks of enteral nutrition in the critically ill: role of small bowel feeding. *JPEN J Parenter Enteral Nutr* 2003; **26** (6 Suppl): S51–7.

48. Ford E, Hull S, Jenning L *et al.* Clinical comparison of tolerance to elemental or polymeric enteral feedings in the postoperative patient. *J Am Coll Nutr* 1992; **11**: 11–16.

49. Mowatt-Larssen C, Brown R, Wojtysial S *et al.* Comparison of tolerance and nutritional outcome between a peptide and a standard formula in critically ill, hypoalbuminemic patients. *JPEN J Parenter Enteral Nutr* 1992; **16**: 20–4.

50. Tiengou LE, Gloro R, Pouzoulet J *et al.* Semi-elemental formula or polymeric formula: is there a better choice for enteral nutrition in acute pancreatitis? Randomized comparative study. *JPEN J Parenter Enteral Nutr* 2006; **30**: 1–5.

51. Yang G, Wu XT, Zhou Y *et al.* Application of dietary fiber in clinical enteral nutrition: a meta-analysis of randomized controlled trials. *World J Gastroenterol* 2005; **11**: 3935–8.

52. Elia M, Ceriello A, Laube H *et al.* Enteral nutritional support and use of diabetes-specific formulas for patients with diabetes: a systemic review and meta-analysis. *Diabetes Care* 2005; **28**: 2267–79.

53. Alish CJ, Garvey WT, Maki KC *et al.* A diabetes-specific enteral formula improves glycemic variability in patients with type 2 diabetes. *Diabetes Technol Ther* 2010; **12**: 419–25.

54. Gadek JE, DeMichele SJ, Karlstad MD *et al.* Effect of enteral feeding with eicosapentanoic acid, gamma-linolenic acid and antioxidants in patients with acute respiratory distress syndrome. Enteral Nutrition in ARDS Study Group. *Crit Care Med* 1999; **27**: 1409–20.

55. Singer P, Theilla M, Fisher H *et al.* Benefit of an enteral diet enriched with eicosapentanoic acid and gamma-linolenic acid in ventilated patients with acute lung injury. *Crit Care Med* 2006; **34**: 1033–8.

56. Stapleton RD, Martin TR, Weiss NS *et al.* A phase II randomized placebo-controlled trial of omega-3 fatty acids for the treatment of acute lung injury. *Crit Care Med* 2011; **39**: 1655–62.

57. Marik PE, Zaloga GP. Immunonutrition in critically ill patients: a systematic review and analysis of the literature. *Intensive Care Med* 2008; **34**: 1980–90.

58. Dupertuis YM, Meguid MM, Pichard C. Advancing from immunonutrition to a pharmaconutrition: a gigantic

challenge. *Curr Opin Clin Nutr Metab Care* 2009; **12**: 398–403.

59. Cerantola Y, Hübner M, Grass F *et al.* Immunonutrition in gastrointestinal surgery. *Br J Surg* 2011; **98**: 37–48.

60. Consensus recommendations from the US summit on immune-enhancing enteral therapy. *JPEN J Parenter Enteral Nutr* 2001; **25**: S61–3.

61. Mentec H, Dupont H, Bocchetti M *et al.* Upper digestive intolerance during enteral nutrition in critically ill patients: frequency, risk, factors, and complications. *Crit Care Med* 2001; **29**: 1922–61.

62. Rees RG, Keohane PP, Grimble GK *et al.* Tolerance of elemental diet administered without starter regimen. *Br Med J* 1985; **290**: 1869–70.

63. Lord L, Harrington M. Enteral nutrition implementation and management. In Merritt R, ed. *The ASPEN Nutrition Support Practice Manual.* Silver Spring, MD: American Society for Parenteral and Enteral Nutrition; 2005, pp. 76–89.

64. Gueenter P, Hicks RW, Simmons D *et al.* Enteral feeding misconnections: a consortium position statement. *Jt Comm J Qual Patient Saf* 2008; **34**: 285–92.

65. Malone AM, Seres DS, Lord L. Complications of enteral nutrition. In Gottschlich MM, ed. *The A.S.P.E.N. Nutrition Support Core Curriculum: A Case-Based Approach – The Adult Patient.* Silver Spring, MD: American Society of Parenteral and Enteral Nutrition; 2007, pp. 246–63.

66. Hurt RT, McClave SA. Gastric residual volumes in critical illness: what do they really mean? *Crit Care Clin* 2010; **26**: 481–90.

67. Torres A, Serra-Batlles J, Ros E *et al.* Pulmonary aspiration of gastric contents in patients receiving mechanical ventilation: the effect of the body position. *Ann Intern Med* 1992; **116**: 540–3.

68. Metheny NA, Clouse RE, Chang YH *et al.* Tracheobronchial aspiration of gastric contents in critically ill tube-fed patients: frequency, outcomes, and risk factors. *Crit Care Med* 2006; **34**: 1–9.

69. McClave SA, DeMeo MT, DeLegge MH *et al.* North American Summit on aspiration in the critically ill patient: consensus statement. *JPEN J Parenter Enteral Nutr* 2002; **26** (6 Suppl): S80–5.

70. Lord LM. Restoring and maintaining patency of enteral feeding tubes. *Nutr Clin Pract* 2003; **18**: 422–6.

71. Stanga Z, Brunner A, Leuenberger M *et al.* Nutrition in clinical practice – the refeeding syndrome: illustrative cases and guidelines for prevention and treatment. *Eur J Clin Nutr* 2008; **62**: 687–94.

72. Doig GS, Simpson F, Delaney A. A review of the true methodological quality of nutritional support trials conducted in the critically ill: time for improvement. *Anesth Analg* 2005; **100**: 527–33.

73. Doig GS, Simpson F, Sweetman EA. Evidence-based nutrition support in the intensive care unit: an update on reported trial quality. *Curr Opin Clin Nutr Metab Care* 2009; **12**: 201–6.

74. Heyland DK, Montalvo M, MacDonald S *et al.* Total parenteral nutrition in the surgical patient: a meta-analysis. *Can J Surg* 2001; **44**: 102–11.

75. Heyland DK, MacDonald S, Keefe L *et al.* Total parenteral nutrition in the critically ill patient: a meta-analysis. *J Am Med Assoc* 1998; **280**: 2013–19.

76. Torosia MH. Perioperative nutrition support for patients undergoing gastrointestinal surgery: a critical analysis and recommendations. *World J Surg* 1999; **23**: 565–9.

77. Maxfiled D, Geehan D, Van Way CW. Perioperative nutritional support. *Nutr Clin Pract* 2001; **16**: 69–73.

78. Klein S, Kinney J, Jeejeebhoy K *et al.* Nutrition support in clinical practice: review of published data and recommendations for future research direction. *JPEN J Parenter Enteral Nutr* 1997; **21**: 133–56.

79. Bozzetti F, Gavazzi C, Miceli R *et al.* Perioperative total PN in malnourished gastrointestinal cancer patients: a randomized, clinical trial. *JPEN J Parenter Enteral Nutr* 2000; **24**: 7–14.

80. American Diabetes Association. Standards of medical care in diabetes – 2011. *Diabetes Care* 2011; **34**: S11–61.

81. Grau T, Bonet A, Rubio M *et al.* Liver dysfunction associated with artificial nutrition in critically ill patients. *Crit Care* 2007; **11**: R10.

82. Solomon SM, Kirby DF. The refeeding syndrome: a review. *JPEN J Parenter Enteral Nutr* 1990; **14**: 90–7.

83. Trujillo EB, Young LS, Chertow GM *et al.* Metabolic and monetary costs of avoidable parenteral nutrition use. *JPEN J Parenter Enteral Nutr* 1999; **23**: 109–13.

84. Kennedy JF, Nightingale JM. Cost savings of an adult hospital nutrition support team. *Nutrition* 2005; **21**: 1127–33.

85. Waitzberg DL, Torrinhas RS, Jacintho TM. New parenteral lipid emulsions for clinical use. *JPEN J Parenter Enteral Nutr* 2006; **30**: 351–67.

86. Wischmeyer PE. Glutamine: role in critical illness and ongoing clinical trials. *Curr Opin Gastroenterol* 2008; **24**: 190–7.

87. Cahill NE, Murch L, Jeejeebhoy K *et al.* When early enteral feeding is not possible in critically ill patients: results of a multicenter observational study. *JPEN J Parenter Enteral Nutr* 2011; **35**: 160–8.

88. Wischmeyer PE, Heyland DK. The future of critical care nutrition therapy. *Crit Care Clin* 2010; **26**: 433–41.

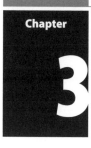

Preoperative testing

Eva Rimler and Danielle Jones

Overview and historical perspective

Preoperative evaluation of patients is a unique opportunity to assess patients who may not have previously been in contact with primary care with the principal goal of intraoperative and postoperative risk reduction. New diagnoses may be identified, or perhaps more frequently, chronic conditions medically optimized in preparation for surgery. In all cases, a meticulous preoperative history and physical exam will be performed. The data gleaned from the history and physical exam, combined with information about the planned procedure, form the basis for selection of medically indicated preoperative tests.

Preoperative evaluation and testing theory has evolved greatly over the last 50 years. Routine preoperative testing for all patients, rather than indicated testing for selected patients, came into vogue with the advent of multiphasic screening in the 1960s. The alluring notion that routine testing would lead to the discovery and treatment of unsuspected abnormalities, thereby decreasing perioperative complications, has not been realized. In a landmark 1985 study, Kaplan *et al.* assessed the value of routine laboratory screening of preoperative patients. In a random sample of 2,000 patients who underwent tests before elective surgery in an academic medical center, Kaplan's group found there was no indication for 60% of the preoperative tests that were performed. Only 3.4% of these tests were abnormal and very few of these tests (0.14%) were potentially significant [1]. Moreover, even though none of these potentially significant results was acted on and no changes in patient care resulted, Kaplan showed that no complications resulted.

Multiple reports echo these findings. A study of routine preoperative testing on patients awaiting cataract surgery found that preoperative testing, including ECG, CBC, electrolytes, BUN, Cr, and glucose, did not alter perioperative morbidity or mortality. This first large, multicenter randomized trial of routine preoperative testing studied 19,557 patients who were randomly assigned to either a testing or no-testing group [2]. The cumulative rates of medical events in the two groups were the same (31.3 events per 1,000 operations). Hypertension and arrhythmia, mostly bradycardia, were the two most common events that

occurred in patients undergoing cataract surgery. Despite the advanced age of the average patient and the likely presence of coexisting illnesses, preoperative testing did not alter perioperative morbidity and mortality.

While cataract surgery is a lower-risk procedure, multiple studies over the past 50 years underscore that there is no appreciable benefit from unfocused batteries of tests. This was again demonstrated in a review done by Narr and colleagues. His group reviewed the charts of 1,044 patients who underwent anesthesia and a surgical procedure without any laboratory work being performed within the preceding 90 days [3]. Despite the absence of preoperative testing these relatively healthy patients underwent their procedures without any deaths or major perioperative morbidity. From this study it was again made clear that large-scale screening tests are not only unnecessary prior to surgery but often lead to the discovery of numerous minor abnormalities with little or no impact on surgical care or recovery. Further, investigation of these abnormal values incur additional cost, potential harm to patients from more invasive testing, and often result in unnecessary surgical delays. The preoperative assessment paradigm has shifted, therefore, from screening labs and studies to focused evaluation and possible intervention when needed.

The healthy perioperative patient

A comprehensive history and physical exam are the most important components of preoperative testing in a healthy patient, especially under the age of 40. A preoperative history should focus on occult or uncontrolled chronic medical problems and exercise capacity. Furthermore, it should evaluate a personal or family history that may contribute to operative risk, such as bleeding disorders, as well as current pulmonary and cardiac risk factors. A physical exam should focus on elements that may signify active cardiovascular or pulmonary disease.

A brief evaluation of self-reported functional status can be very useful in preoperative risk assessment. The Duke (DASI) questionnaire has been found to be a quick and effective means of evaluating functional status. Developed as a way to

Medical Management of the Surgical Patient, ed. Michael F. Lubin, Thomas F. Dodson, and Neil H. Winawer. Published by Cambridge University Press. © Cambridge University Press 2013.

determine functional capacity without performing costly exercise tolerance tests, this simple 12-question self-assessment correlates with peak oxygen uptake and is considered a reasonable surrogate for gauging cardiovascular health [4]. Poor scores on this questionnaire are independent markers for preoperative morbidity, and have been found to correlate with angiographic evidence of heart disease [5]. The most sensitive cut-off for poor performance is the inability to walk more than four blocks or two flights of stairs. The American Heart Association (AHA) together with the American College of Cardiology (ACC) recommends evaluation of a patient's metabolic equivalents (METs). Both these tests are surrogates for maximum tidal volume, and serve as a way to uncover patients at risk of perioperative morbidity and mortality (largely cardiac and pulmonary) without subjecting patients to costly tests. As highlighted by the ACC/AHA there is level B evidence that suggests a patient who can do four METs of activity (e.g., walking up a flight of stairs or do moderate housework) and has no overt cardiopulmonary symptoms should proceed to surgery [6].

In patients younger than 40 years of age with adequate functional status and without concerning history or physical exam findings no testing is needed prior to surgical intervention. Multiple studies have found that there is no combination of labs that effectively identify patients at risk for adverse events [1–3], yet 30 billion dollars is spent on perioperative testing in the United States annually [7]. Even when abnormalities are discovered in healthy patients during preoperative laboratory testing they are of little clinical significance [8]. Moreover, as shown above studies have found that these abnormal tests are often ignored, and their presence leads to neither surgical delay nor adverse surgical outcomes and may even increase medicolegal risk [3]. This may occur because abnormalities that may not affect surgery may herald other health risks if not noted or pursued. Additionally, repeating laboratory work preoperatively that has been completed in the four months before surgery usually does not result in any significant change in the original values [9].

While screening lab tests are unnecessary in otherwise healthy adults, one should always take into consideration the type and risk factors associated with the surgery about to be undertaken. For example, when undergoing an operation where significant blood loss is anticipated, such as some orthopedic procedures, a preoperative hematocrit can be useful even in young healthy patients. In this instance, it helps to anticipate if blood products or a method for autologous transfusions may be necessary. Furthermore, if large fluid shifts are expected or nephrotoxins will be used, a baseline BUN and creatinine may be helpful. Similarly, it is reasonable to check a preoperative platelet or white blood cell count in patients that are on myelosuppressive medications. Notably, although coagulation profiles are commonly ordered, they are generally indicated only when patients have a known or suspected history of liver disease, bleeding diatheses or current use of anticoagulation medication and do not have a role in screening preoperatively

[10]. Selection of laboratory testing in asymptomatic or healthy patients, therefore, depends on existing comorbidities and the surgery involved. For more details and information about cardiac and pulmonary testing, see the section below.

As shown, preoperative testing especially in young, healthy patients hinges on history and physical exam findings. Without a just cause, no further preoperative testing is truly necessary in this patient population and practitioners can adopt a philosophy of "less is more."

Screening in patients with comorbidities
Laboratory testing
Although it has been shown that routine laboratory testing is not indicated in healthy patients, patients with underlying comorbidities often require preoperative laboratory evaluation. Selection of specific tests is largely based on patient comorbidities and occasionally on the potential surgery. For example, patients with underlying renal disease benefit from preoperative electrolytes. Please see Table 3.1 for a more complete listing of indicated testing. Make note that most of these laboratory tests would not be considered screening tests; instead, testing in these cases is conducted to evaluate for known complications of the comorbid conditions present or for abnormalities suspected based on pre-admission history and physical exam.

Cardiac testing
Over the years the appropriate level of cardiac testing prior to surgery has been investigated. As with laboratory examination patients' personal history, physical exam and risk factors determine the necessity for further cardiac testing prior to surgical intervention. Without an appropriate indication preoperative cardiac imaging is costly, potentially invasive, and is not proven to change outcomes.

Electrocardiography
Electrocardiograms (ECGs), much like laboratory work, are not routinely necessary as a preoperative test in healthy patients. It has been hypothesized that ECGs can be used to detect unsuspected cardiac conditions that increase the risk of perioperative cardiac complications. However, preoperative ECGs in a largely healthy outpatient population have not been shown to have useful predictive value [11]. Not only were postoperative adverse cardiac events rare in this population, but abnormal preoperative ECGs were only present half the time in those patients who had an adverse event. Additionally, Ashton *et al.* found routine perioperative ECGs are of little value when the incidence of perioperative infarction is low [12]. Further studies show no difference in the prevalence of perioperative events amongst healthy adults (American Society of Anesthesia grade I and II) with normal ECGs compared with healthy adults with abnormal ECGs undergoing elective ambulatory surgery [13].

Table 3.1 Indications for preoperative laboratory tests.

Preoperative test	Indication
Creatinine/BUN	History of renal disease, diabetes, hypertension, or congestive heart failure, use of diuretics, ACE inhibitors, angiotensin-receptor blockers, NSAIDs, nephrotoxins, age > 40, major surgical procedures
Electrolytes	History of renal disease, diabetes, or endocrinopathy that may lead to electrolyte disorders, use of diuretics, ACE inhibitors, angiotensin receptor blockers, digoxin, steroids, or bowel preparation, age > 40
Glucose	History of diabetes or corticosteroid use
Hemoglobin/hematocrit	History or physical findings of anemia, renal insufficiency, or malignancy, anticoagulant or myelosuppressive therapy, surgery associated with significant blood loss, age > 60
White blood cell count	Signs or symptoms of infection, history of myeloproliferative disorder, high risk of leukopenia from medications or underlying disease
Platelet count	Suspicion of a bleeding diathesis, history of myeloproliferative disease, or recent chemotherapy
PT/PTT	Liver disease, suspicion of or known bleeding diathesis, malignancy, or malnutrition, anticoagulant use
Urinalysis	No indication

PT/PTT, prothrombin time (PT) and partial thromboplastin time (PTT).

Table 3.2 Revised Cardiac Risk Index.

Cardiac risk factor (1 point per risk factor)	Perioperative risk of major cardiovascular event
High-risk surgery	0 Points = 0.4% risk
Ischemic heart disease	1 Point = 0.9% risk
Congestive heart failure	2 Points = 6.6% risk
Creatinine > 2	3 or more points = 11% risk
Insulin-dependent diabetes mellitus	

There is little evidence that a preoperative ECG can predict adverse outcomes; however, many experts recommend an ECG in men over 40 years of age, women over 50 years of age and in patients with cardiovascular risk factors who will undergo intermediate- or high-risk surgeries [14]. It may be reasonable to raise the age threshold for routine preoperative ECGs to 60 years in patients without other cardiovascular risk factors in light of the data reviewed above. Due to the high rate of ECG abnormalities in patients over age 60 years, a "baseline" ECG may be pragmatic, though the value of a baseline has not been studied.

Cardiac imaging

Perioperative cardiac events are a concern for many patients that undergo both cardiac and non-cardiac surgeries. In fact, cardiac complications account for one-third of deaths from non-cardiac procedures [15]. There are certain comorbidities that can be unearthed during a preoperative history and physical that place a patient at greater risk for sustaining a perioperative cardiac event. Largely, these are comorbid conditions

that, in general, lead to cardiovascular disease. Currently the Revised Cardiac Risk Index (RCRI) is commonly, and very effectively, used to determine patients at risk for perioperative cardiovascular mortality [16]. Please see Chapter 9 for a complete discussion of preoperative cardiac risk assessment. Clinicians should consider further cardiac testing in patients who have intermediate- to high-risk cardiac profiles (as determined by the Revised Cardiac Risk Index checklist, Table 3.2).

In general the more cardiac risk factors a patient has the more likely it is that a patient may benefit from cardiovascular evaluation and intervention prior to surgery, especially high-risk surgery. A retrospective cohort study performed by Wijeysundera et al. noted that patients at intermediate (1–2 RCRI points) and high risk (3–6 RCRI points) for cardiovascular disease benefit from further cardiac testing with non-invasive stress testing prior to surgery [17]. The intermediate- and high-risk patients who underwent non-invasive stress testing had improved 1-year survival and decreased length of stay compared with matched counterparts that did not undergo non-invasive stress testing prior to elective surgery. However, this same study found that non-invasive stress testing was associated with harm in low-risk patients (0 RCRI points) [17]. This again suggests that following the "less is more" paradigm in low-risk patients is appropriate, and if patients do not need cardiac evaluation without surgery, they probably do not need cardiac evaluation in order to go for surgery.

The type of cardiac evaluation is key in determining whether preoperative cardiac testing is worthwhile. Studies that have found improvement in patient outcomes are those that have patients with multiple cardiac risk factors who undergo stress testing to evaluate their ischemic burden. However, even in high-risk patients, determination of resting LV function is not useful in determining risk for perioperative events [6]. While echocardiography has been found to be one of the most commonly ordered cardiac tests prior to surgery, there is no evidence that it improves post-surgical outcomes. In fact, a population-based retrospective cohort study with 264,823 patients found that preoperative echocardiography did not decrease mortality or length of hospital stay in patients undergoing major non-cardiac surgery [15].

In select patients with multiple comorbid conditions, preoperative cardiac testing to determine ischemic burden can improve outcomes. As always it is important to gain this information through a focused preoperative history and physical. Preoperative cardiac testing is wrought with complicated decisions that will be discussed in later chapters. It is important to know that the type of testing ordered and the specific patient characteristics are key when determining if further cardiac testing will be of any use in decreasing perioperative cardiac mortality.

Pulmonary testing

Data from the National Surgical Quality Improvement Program show that postoperative pulmonary complications cost more and result in longer lengths of stay than any other cause of major postoperative medical complications (cardiac, infectious, and thromboembolic) [18]. It is generally agreed that both general anesthesia and surgery itself produce physiologic changes in the lungs which can directly lead to postoperative pulmonary complications. Postoperative restrictive reduction of lung volumes, which most commonly occurs with upper abdominal and thoracic procedures, is thought to be one of the largest contributors to these changes [19]. There are a number of factors known to increase the risk of postoperative pulmonary complications, therefore, detailed evaluation of these risks is an important component of any perioperative evaluation (see Chapter [Y] for more details on pulmonary risk assessment). The best tool for evaluating the risk of postoperative pulmonary complications is a detailed history and physical examination [20]. While pulmonary risk reduction should be aggressive, extensive perioperative pulmonary testing is rarely indicated, especially in healthy patients.

Chest radiography

Although there is a paucity of randomized controlled trials investigating the value of preoperative chest radiograph (CXR) in predicting postoperative complications, it remains the most commonly ordered preoperative pulmonary test. A multitude of reviews, meta-analyses, and case series analyses indicate that routine screening CXRs in healthy patients may not be indicated at any age. An extensive review of literature evaluating routine preoperative CXRs by Archer et al. found that abnormalities were common (10%) but in most cases would have been identified based on history and physical exam [21]. Of the 14,390 cases studied, only 1.3% had unsuspected CXR findings and these findings influenced management in 0.1% of patients. Several years later in a review of 46 studies, Munro et al. confirmed very similar rates of abnormal CXR findings (0–2.1%) and concluded that routine preoperative CXR testing should not be recommended [8].

A comprehensive review by Joo et al. of perioperative CXR studies in asymptomatic patients concluded that CXR abnormalities increase with age (markedly over the age of 70) along with pulmonary risk factors but most often these abnormalities are chronic in nature (e.g., COPD) [22]. Importantly, these abnormalities did not appear to correlate with postoperative complications. Thus, the authors concluded that they could not recommend CXRs in asymptomatic patients of any age.

Active pulmonary symptoms indicate significant perioperative risk and if uncovered during routine preoperative history and physical, should be investigated and managed aggressively. Based partly on many of the studies above, the American College of Radiology has also published criteria which state [23]: "given the current evidence, routine preoperative and admission chest radiographs are not recommended except when the following conditions exist:

1. Acute cardiopulmonary disease is suspected on the basis of history and physical examination.
2. There is a history of stable chronic cardiopulmonary disease in an elderly patient (older than age 70) without a recent chest radiograph within the past 6 months."

Despite the data described above, a large gap between current recommendations and practice still exists. Chest radiography remains one of the most commonly ordered preoperative screening tests. As described above reflexive screening CXRs are of little value and a preoperative CXR should only be performed if there is suspicion of an active cardiopulmonary problem uncovered during a preoperative history and physical exam.

Pulmonary function tests

Given the morbidity and cost of postoperative pulmonary complications, many have looked to pulmonary function tests (PFTs) as possible predictors of such complications. While early studies of bedside spirometry suggested FEV1, FVC, and FEV1/FVC ratios could predict increased risk of pulmonary complications postoperatively [24], more recent data suggest PFTs do not predict risk, even in high-risk individuals.

In a study of the effect of chronic obstructive pulmonary disease (COPD) on pulmonary complications after thoracic or major abdominal surgery, Kroenke et al. found that although patients with COPD had higher rates of complications, spirometry was not an independent predictor of pulmonary complications [25]. A case-control study of COPD patients with normal FEV1 compared with abnormal FEV1 (< 40% predicted), found that abnormal spirometry did predict bronchospasm but not postoperative pulmonary complications [26]. Another case control study of all patients undergoing abdominal surgery, again concluded that spirometry did not predict pulmonary complications postoperatively [27].

Despite some early debate, review of the data suggests routine preoperative PFTs are not helpful in most cases. Most abnormalities identified by PFTs confirm what would have likely been predicted by a good history and physical exam, as seen in the case of chest radiography. In their original position paper (1990) on perioperative PFTs, the American College of Physicians (ACP) wrote "Although spirometry clearly assists physicians in making decisions about lung resection, its role in management of other surgical patients remains unclear and needs further investigation" [20].

Table 3.3 Indications for preoperative cardiopulmonary testing.

Chest radiograph	Pulmonary disease, cardiovascular disease, risk of metastatic disease, risk of tuberculosis, acute pulmonary symptoms, age > 70
Pulmonary function tests	For lung resection candidates alone
Electrocardiogram	Known or suspected cardiovascular disease, pulmonary disease, peripheral vascular disease, diabetes, men > 40 years old, women > 55 years old, concern for major electrolyte abnormality
Stress testing	Intermediate or high-risk patients based on RCRI
Echocardiography	Not indicated

RCRI, Revised Cardiac Risk Index.

Updated guidelines from 2006 based upon a systematic review continue to recommend against routine preoperative spirometry for pulmonary risk stratification [28]. The ACP guidelines further state that the most useful tool in predicting postoperative pulmonary complications is a good history and physical exam (Table 3.3). Some experts suggest that in cases where your history and physical exam fails to determine if a patient with lung disease is at his or her baseline, PFTs may be useful to determine if more aggressive preoperative disease management is indicated.

Summary

Since the 1960s preoperative testing practices have shifted dramatically. As a result of large, mostly observational studies, the pendulum has swung from sending batteries of preoperative screening tests to ordering only indicated tests based on a patient's specific risk profile. In fact, there is a small pilot study that questions the efficacy of performing any preoperative testing in ambulatory settings [29]. In truth the goal of preoperative testing is to hone in on the key organ systems that may contribute to perioperative morbidity and mortality. With this focus the practitioner should only perform tests that may help to optimize medical management preoperatively and play a role in surgical planning. This goal is best achieved through a thorough history and physical and rational testing based on these findings.

References

1. Kaplan EB, Sheiner LB, Boeckmann AJ et al. The usefulness of preoperative laboratory screening. *J Am Med Assoc* 1985; **253**: 3576–81.

2. Schein OD, Katz J, Bass EB et al. The value of routine preoperative medical testing before cataract surgery. *N Engl J Med* 2000; **342**: 168–75.

3. Narr BJ, Warner ME, Scroeder DR et al. Outcomes of patients with no laboratory assessment before anesthesia and a surgical procedure. *Mayo Clinic Proc* 1997; **72**: 505–9.

4. Hlatky MA, Boineau RE, Higginbotham MB et al. A brief self-administered questionnaire to determine functional capacity (The Duke Activity Status Index). *Am J Cardiol* 1989; **64**: 651–4.

5. Nelson CL, Herndon JE, Mark DB et al. Relation of clinical and angiographic factors to functional capacity as measured by the Duke Activity Status Index. *Am J Cardiol* 1991; **68**: 973–5.

6. Fleisher LA, Beckman JA, Brown KA et al. ACC/AHA 2007 guidelines on preoperative cardiovascular evaluation and care for noncardiac surgery: a report of the American College of Cardiology/American Heart Association task force on practice guidelines (writing committee to revise the 2002 guidelines on perioperative cardiovascular evaluation for noncardiac surgery). *Circulation* 2007; **116**: e418–500.

7. Marcello PW, Roberts PL. "Routine" preoperative studies. Which studies in which patients? *Surg Clin North Am* 1996; **76**: 11–23.

8. Munro J, Booth A, Nicholl J. Routine preoperative testing: a systematic review of the evidence. *Health Techno Assessm* 1997; **1**(12): 1–62.

9. Macpherson DS, Snow R, Lofgren RP. Preoperative screening: value of previous tests. *Ann Intern Med* 1990; **113**: 969–73.

10. Eckman MH, Erban JK, Singh SK, Kao GS. Screening for the risk for bleeding or thrombosis. *Ann Intern Med* 2003; **138**: W15–24.

11. Gold BS, Young ML, Kinman JL et al. The utility of preoperative electrocardiograms in the ambulatory surgical patient. *Arch Intern Med* 1992; **152**: 301–5.

12. Ashton CM, Tjomas J, Wray NP et al. The frequency and significance of ECG changes after transurethral prostate resection. *J Am Geriat Soc* 1991; **39**: 575–80.

13. Tait AR, Parr HG, Tremper KK. Evaluation of the efficacy of routine preoperative electrocardiograms. *J Cardioth Vasc Anesth* 1997; **11**: 752–5.

14. Goldberger AL, O'Konski M. Utility of the routine electrocardiogram before surgery and on general hospital admission. *Ann Intern Med* 1986; **105**: 552–7.

15. Wijeysundera DM, Beattie WS, Karkouti et al. Association of echocardiography before major elective non cardiac surgery with postoperative survival and length of hospital stay: population based cohort study. *Br Med J* 2011; **342**: d3695.doi:10.1136/bmj.d3695.

16. Lee TH, Marcantonio ER, Mangione CM. Derivation and prospective validation of a simple index for prediction of cardiac risk of major noncardiac surgery. *Circulation* 1999; **100**: 1043–9.

17. Wijeysundera DM, Beattie WS, Austin PC et al. Non-invasive cardiac stress testing before elective non-cardiac surgery: population based cohort study. *Br Med J* 2010; **340**: b5526. doi: 10.1136/bmj.b5526.

18. Dimich JB, Chen SL, Taheri PA et al. Hospital costs associated with surgical complications: a report from the private-sector National Surgical Quality

Improvement Program. *J Am Coll Surg* 2004; **199**: 531–7.

19. Craig DB. Postoperative recovery of pulmonary function. *Anesth Analg* 1981; **60**: 46.

20. American College of Physicians. Position paper: preoperative pulmonary function testing. *Ann Intern Med* 1990; **112**: 793–4.

21. Archer C, Levy AR, McGregor M. Value of routine pre-operative chest X-rays: a meta-analysis. *Can J Anaesth* 1993; **40**: 1022–7.

22. Joo HS, Wong J, Naik VN *et al*. The value of screening preoperative chest x-rays: a systematic review. *Can J Anaesth* 2005; **52**: 568–74.

23. MacMahon H, Khan AR, Mohammed T-L *et al*. Appropriateness criteria: routine admission and preoperative chest radiography. *American College of Radiology* 2000 (Reviewed 2008). www.acr.org/SecondaryMainMenu Categories/quality_safety/app_criteria/ pdf/ExpertPanelonThoracicImaging/ RoutineAdmissionandPreoperative chestradiographyDoc6.aspx

24. Gass GD, Olsen GN. Preoperative pulmonary function testing to predict postoperative morbidity and mortality. *Chest* 1986; **89**: 127.

25. Kroenke K, Lawrence VA, Theroux JF *et al*. Postoperative complications after thoracic and major abdominal surgery in patients with and without obstructive disease. *Chest* 1993; **104**: 1445–51.

26. Warner DO, Warner MA, Offord KP *et al*. Airway obstruction and perioperative complications in smokers undergoing abdominal surgery. *Anesthesiology* 1999; **90**: 372.

27. Brooks-Brunn JA. Predictors of postoperative pulmonary complications following abdominal surgery. *Chest* 1997; **111**: 564.

28. Qaseem A, Snow V, Fitterman N *et al*. Risk assessment for strategies to reduce perioperative pulmonary complications for patients undergoing noncardiothoracic surgery: a guideline from the American College of Physicians. *Ann Intern Med* 2006; **144**: 575–80.

29. Chung F, Yuan H, Yin L *et al*. Eliminating preoperative testing in ambulatory surgery. *Anesth Analg* 2009; **108**: 467–75.

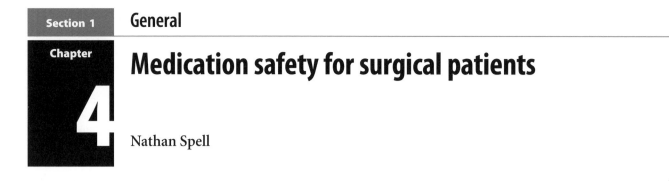

Chapter 4

Medication safety for surgical patients

Nathan Spell

The perioperative period is a dynamic and risky time for patients. After complications related directly to the surgery itself, medication complications are the next most common adverse events in hospitalized patients [1]. This chapter will address patient safety related to medication practices around surgery, excluding anesthesia and intraoperative medication use. A discussion of general principles will be followed by a focus on the more common complications and high-risk medication groups.

General principles
Medication history and reconciliation

Recording a full and accurate medication list is an essential part of a thorough patient history, yet doing so presents a time-consuming challenge in a patient on multiple medications. Reasons for the challenge include the plethora of medications that have been developed and marketed in the last decades that may be unfamiliar to the physician, the difficulty for the patient to remember the full medication list and details of use, and the immature state of electronic health information that does not yet allow universal sharing of data about patients' medical history between multiple health information platforms. As a result, a significant proportion of patients in hospital have incomplete or inaccurate medication histories.

Pippens and colleagues described the occurrence of medication errors in history and reconciliation in two teaching hospitals. In their study medication discrepancies with potential to cause harm occurred on average 1.4 times per patient; most common were discrepancies from the preadmission medication list. Subsequent potential adverse drug events were most often errors of omission originating from the initial medication history [2].

Transitions in inpatient care (entering or leaving the hospital or transferring between levels of care within the hospital) are times when medication orders are often re-evaluated and changed. Purposefully considering the patient's current and prior medications and deciding to stop, resume, change or add is called medication reconciliation. Health care

accreditation organizations such as The Joint Commission expect medication reconciliation to be performed and recorded at transitions of care, with the goal of reducing harm from inadvertent medication errors. While it may seem self-evident that thoughtful decision-making regarding medications at care transitions will reduce adverse drug events, the methods currently used in hospitals for medication reconciliation have shown mixed results [3,4] and may have much to do with the details of how prescribers interact with the medication list and perform reconciliation.

An occasional criticism of the requirement for medication reconciliation is that medications have become so numerous and specialized that a physician cannot be expected to understand all of them. The assertion is then made that medication reconciliation will be fruitless. This is a false argument. The problem is not in medication reconciliation but in the underlying complexity of the medications that may exceed the expertise of any individual physician. The solution, then, is in consultation with other physicians or pharmacists who will have the expertise or focus to assist with managing the medications and the underlying medical conditions.

In addition, the medication history should include specific questions about the use of complementary and alternative therapies, such as herbal medications. Herbal medication use is common in many societies, and patients may not think to include such use with their physicians unless specifically asked. These substances may have direct effects on coagulation or on metabolic pathways common to drugs used in surgery. Ang-Lee and colleagues have published a concise review of several common herbal medications and concur with the recommendations of others that, ideally, herbal medications should be discontinued 2–3 weeks before elective surgery [5]. Interestingly, Beckert and colleagues evaluated the effect of several common herbs on volunteers and did not demonstrate measureable in vivo effects of five common herbs on platelet function assays [6]. Still, without a compelling reason to continue herbal medications, stopping them remains the consensus.

Medical Management of the Surgical Patient, ed. Michael F. Lubin, Thomas F. Dodson, and Neil H. Winawer. Published by Cambridge University Press. © Cambridge University Press 2013.

High-risk drug categories

Some drugs are inherently more risky to use than others – anticoagulants, narcotic analgesics, sedatives, insulin and other glucose-lowering medications, and cardiovascular drugs are examples. Special precautions and monitoring systems can reduce risks from these drugs, and later sections in this chapter will explore options in selected drug categories.

Drug–drug interactions

During the perioperative period new medications are commonly introduced to the patient – anesthetics, paralytics, analgesics, anti-emetics, etc. Each of these medications brings associated side-effects and dangers, and the risk of interaction with other drugs increases exponentially as the number of drugs in a given patient rises. Anticipating and managing all potential drug interactions is beyond the capacity of even the most competent physician. Fortunately, computerized decision support in the form of automated checking for interactions between drugs and between prescribed medication and patients' known drug allergies is capable of handling the huge amount of information available to guard against inadvertent prescribing of drugs with dangerous interactions. Such computerized systems are not yet ubiquitous in clinical settings, however. Where they are in place, their effectiveness may suffer from creation of "alert fatigue" in prescribers, a condition in which the most critical information is lost in a sea of less significant information that is often presented to the prescriber [7].

Inpatient pharmacists can provide a valuable service to physicians and patients by advising on safe and effective medication use and by being members of interdisciplinary teams caring for patients. Pharmacy staffing models differ among hospitals, and having pharmacists integrated into care teams may be uncommon in smaller facilities. Yet, pharmacists are likely to be available for consultations on specific patients in most hospitals in the USA.

Changes in patient physiology that may affect medication safety

Anesthesia and surgery bring about predictable physiological changes in patients. Understanding these changes will help to anticipate and to explain risks from particular medications and guide medication management. The autonomic nervous system, renin–angiotensin–aldosterone (RAA) axis and the hypothalamic–pituitary–adrenal (HPA) axis are all involved within the first hours of surgery. Both general endotracheal and epidural anesthesia result in peripheral vasodilation during surgery that may cause blood pressure to decrease. In response to these effects and to blood loss, RAA activation will work to raise blood pressure and promote volume retention by the kidneys. Sympathetic stimulation from endotracheal intubation and from the stresses of surgery will also tend to raise blood pressure and cardiac output. Production and release of

cortisol begins quickly and peaks within 4–12 hours of starting surgery, tapering off back toward baseline production within 1–2 days if surgery was of average intensity, though it may take about a week to see return of normal diurnal variation [8].

Whether directly related to the surgery or to other events, patients who suffer organ dysfunction, especially kidney, liver, and heart (causing under-perfusion of other organs), will have alterations in metabolism and excretion of most medications. For drugs such as metformin that can have dangerous effects in the setting of renal and hepatic dysfunction, substitutes are available and should be used routinely in the perioperative period for all patients, as the risk–benefit analysis does not support use in the acute surgical period. In patients who develop organ dysfunction, a careful review of medications should be part of the daily evaluation, as drug choices and dosing may need to be changed.

Morbid obesity

Morbidly obese patients have become more common in most developing and advanced societies around the world. For drugs that are dosed based on body weight, dosing by weight may not be appropriate as fat weight increases significantly. As humans gain above ideal body weight, both fat and lean weight increase, with lean mass representing 20–40% of excess weight in most morbidly obese patients. For most drugs, initial volume of distribution and clearance are related to lean body weight (LBW). Dosing by total body weight may result in significant overdosing [9]. Each drug must be individually considered, but LBW is generally the safer weight to use when estimating required dose.

Medications for diabetes and hyperglycemia
Target glucose values for postoperative patients

Uncontrolled hyperglycemia is clearly associated with undesired outcomes among hospitalized patients, both surgical and non-surgical. Mortality, length-of-stay and infection rates are known to be elevated from multiple studies in patients with hyperglycemia [10–12].

The extent to which glycemic control improves these outcomes has been difficult to determine. An influential study of intensive insulin regimens for glycemic control in the critical care setting showed significantly reduced mortality with a target of normoglycemia [13]. For several years hospitals and professional societies recommended tighter glucose control. However, subsequent studies and a systematic review failed to confirm the benefits of tight control and suggested potential for harm from overly aggressive targets [14,15]. More recently, guidelines have begun to recommend against attempts to achieve normoglycemia with intensive insulin therapy, largely because of the dangers of hypoglycemia. Target blood glucose of 7.8–11.1 mmol/L (140–200 mg/dL) is one current recommendation for patients in critical care settings [16]. For patients outside of the critical care unit, there is scant good-quality evidence for the optimal range. The American Association of Clinical Endocrinologists and American Diabetic Association recommend a pre-meal glucose target of < 7.8 mmol/L (140 mg/dL) and that random blood glucose values be kept < 10.0 mmol/dL (180 mg/dL) in most patients [10].

Non-insulin agents for diabetes

For patients admitted for major inpatient surgeries, the best practice is to discontinue oral and other non-insulin agents and to rely on insulin regimens for glycemic control, if therapy is needed [10]. Again, the primary driver of this recommendation is the risk of hypoglycemia from most of these drugs. The harmful effects of hypoglycemia in the postoperative setting include direct neurological injury that profound hypoglycemia can cause and there is reflexive stimulation of the autonomic nervous system that can increase the risk of myocardial ischemia.

Metformin poses unique risks related to its effects on lactic acid metabolism and the altered clearance of the drug if there is renal dysfunction or concomitant administration of intravenous contrast for radiologic imaging [10]. All non-insulin medications for diabetes have the disadvantage that they are not easily titrated to blood glucose values, and the caloric intake of hospitalized patients in the perioperative setting may be significantly below baseline consumption.

For diabetic patients undergoing surgery in an ambulatory setting who will not be hospitalized following surgery, high-quality evidence is lacking to guide recommendations. Non-insulin agents should be held on the day of surgery, with frequent (every 1–2 hour) glucose monitoring and use of rapid-onset insulin formulations to control blood sugar, if needed. Oral agents may be resumed postoperatively when the patient resumes a usual home diet. Patients should have good follow-up with their usual source of diabetes care after surgery in the event that the patient experiences very high or low blood glucose values or side-effects of medications [17].

Insulin

Insulin therapy is the recommended approach in patients with known diabetes or who develop hyperglycemia when hospitalized, whether or not they are having surgery [10]. The goals of therapy are to minimize the complications of hyperglycemia while simultaneously avoiding clinically significant hypoglycemia. In critical-care settings, intravenous (IV) continuous infusion of insulin is the appropriate therapy for most patients, as the short half-life of IV insulin lends itself to rapid adjustment. With clinical stability and resumption of feeding, transition to subcutaneous insulin is made. The first dose of subcutaneous insulin is given at least an hour before stopping IV insulin to avoid hyperglycemia and the potential for ketoacidosis in type 1 diabetics.

A "sliding scale," or corrective, regimen of short-acting insulin has been used traditionally to bring down elevated blood sugar. Without a long-acting "basal" insulin, however, these regimens result in suboptimal control. Addition of a basal insulin (NPH twice daily) or insulin analog (insulin glargine or insulin detemir once daily) results in a greater proportion of time spent in the target range without an increase in significant hypoglycemic episodes. There does not appear to be a difference between the types of long-acting insulin in achieving these outcomes [18], and Umpierrez and colleagues reported that more time in target range for postoperative general surgery patients resulted in improved clinical outcomes for patients on a once-daily glargine plus preprandial glulisine (basal-bolus) regimen compared with a corrective dose alone [19].

Patients who are not eating but are receiving enteral nutrition may require insulin therapy. These patients need to have blood glucose monitored every 4–6 hours [10]. Insulin therapy that includes basal plus corrective insulin achieves better glycemic control than corrective dosing alone without significant hypoglycemic events in a small study of patients on enteral nutrition [20].

Antithrombotic agents

The central challenge of safely managing antithrombotic agents around surgery is to obtain the desired antithrombotic benefits while avoiding clinically significant bleeding. The physician managing these agents must be able to estimate the thrombotic and bleeding risks of the patient's underlying condition and anticipated surgery and understand the mode of action, pharmacodynamics and management of bleeding that may occur with each of these agents. Table 4.1 summarizes this information.

Aspirin

Aspirin acetylates and irreversibly inhibits cyclooxygenase 1 (COX-1) within platelets, reducing production of the platelet-activating substance thromboxane A_2. Because platelets are unable to produce additional COX-1, platelets exposed to aspirin are inhibited for their lifespan of 7–10 days [21]. The effect of aspirin is therefore reversed by replacement of adequate numbers of functional platelets through endogenous production over 5–7 days or through platelet transfusion. The inhibitory effect of aspirin on platelet activity is not complete, however, and many surgeries may proceed despite the patient's use of aspirin unless the surgeon determines the additional risk of bleeding cannot be tolerated.

Thienopyridines

Clopidogrel and related drugs act by permanently blocking surface platelet receptor $P2Y_{12}$ and are more potent inhibitors than aspirin [21]. The risk of bleeding at major surgery is significantly greater than aspirin, and these drugs should be held for 5–7 days preoperatively whenever possible. The patient with recent percutaneous coronary intervention (PCI) is an exception. In combination with aspirin, thienopyridines

Table 4.1 Antithrombotic agents and their mode of action.

Agent	Action	Effect wears off	Reversal agent
Aspirin	Irreversibly inhibits cyclooxygenase	5–7 d	Platelet transfusion
Thienopyridines	Block platelet receptor P2Y$_{12}$	5–7 d	Platelet transfusion
Gp IIb/IIIa inhibitors	Inhibit linking of platelet to fibrinogen	12 h	Platelet transfusion (partial)
Warfarin	Inhibits production of clotting factors	5–6 d	FFP, vitamin K
Unfractionated heparin	Promotes activity of AT to inhibit factor Xa and thrombin	4–6 h	Protamine
Low molecular weight heparins	Promotes activity of AT to inhibit factor Xa	24–36 h	Protamine (partial)
Fondaparinux	Promotes activity of AT to inhibit factor Xa	24–36 h	None
Hirudin, bivalirudin, argatroban	Parenteral direct thrombin inhibitors	4–6 h	None
Dabigatran	Oral direct thrombin inhibitor	24–36 h	None

have proven essential in prevention of thrombosis within the stented portion of the vessel. The risk of stent thrombosis remains significantly elevated until the vascular endothelium has been reestablished. A guideline by the American College of Chest Physicians recommends that a patient requiring surgery within 6 weeks of a bare metal stent or within 12 months of a drug-eluting stent have both aspirin and the thienopyridine continued through surgery [22]. Elective surgery should be postponed until beyond these danger zones when possible, and aspirin should be continued through surgery unless contraindicated. If antithrombotic therapy is interrupted in patients with stents, it should be resumed as soon as the surgeon feels it is safe to do so to reduce risk of thrombosis.

Glycoprotein IIb/IIIa inhibitors

Glycoprotein IIb/IIIa receptors change conformation upon platelet activation and bind to fibrinogen in the formation of a platelet thrombus. Competitive inhibitors to Gp IIb/IIIa (eptifibatide and tirofiban) are short-acting (2 hours). Both are rapid-acting and are used in the management of acute coronary syndromes. The strong inhibitor abciximab (monoclonal antibody) has a longer duration (12 hours). Waiting at least 12 hours after the most recent abciximab dose to operate reduces the risk of bleeding substantially [21].

Warfarin

Warfarin inhibits production of vitamin K-dependent clotting factors. The action of warfarin is slow, both in onset and in reversal, and is measured through the prothrombin time and the International Normalized Ratio. The most common conditions of patients on therapeutic warfarin include venous thromboembolism (treatment of recent events, multiple events, or prophylaxis in patients with thrombophilia) and risks for cardiac sources of emboli (atrial fibrillation,

mechanical heart valves, ventricular thrombus, etc.). Active reversal of the action of warfarin, when needed, is through administration of fresh frozen plasma (FFP) for immediate reversal, or vitamin K (IV or oral) for less urgent reversal over 1–2 days [23]. The anticoagulant effect of warfarin will wane over 5–6 days in most patients when the drug is discontinued.

Patients undergoing minor procedures (for example, cataract surgery, many gastrointestinal procedures such as upper or lower endoscopy with or without biopsy, most dental and dermatological procedures, skin and joint aspirations and injections, and superficial podiatric procedures) may have these procedures done while on warfarin. More significant surgeries will require reversal of warfarin's anticoagulation effect.

For patients at significant risk of thromboembolic events while off warfarin, bridging therapy with a low molecular weight heparin (LMWH) or unfractionated heparin (in some cases) is the recommended approach [22]. Determining and arranging the optimal approach in a given patient may be complex, and consultation with a specialist familiar with anticoagulation management and current recommendations (internist, cardiologist, or hematologist, for example) is advised.

Heparins and fondaparinux

Unfractionated heparin (UFH), LMWH, and fondaparinux share similarities in structure and mechanism of action. Unfractionated heparin is a glycosaminoglycan of complex and variable structure from molecule to molecule. Unfractionated heparin promotes the action of antithrombin III (AT), and AT then inhibits thrombin and factor Xa. The effect of AT on thrombin is dependent upon the size (length) of the heparin molecule in UFH [24], and LMWHs have very little antithrombin activity. The anti-factor Xa activity is mediated through binding of a pentasaccharide in common to UHF and LMWHs to AT. Fondaparinux is a synthetic pentasaccharide that retains this anti-factor Xa activity. Factor Xa activity, therefore, can be used to monitor the effect of all of these agents.

Because of the bleeding risk with these potent anticoagulants, including warfarin, hospitals in the USA that are accredited by The Joint Commission are expected to have written policies and procedures to govern the use and monitoring of anticoagulants. Best practices include scheduled monitoring of the anticoagulant effect through laboratory testing and the use of weight-based dosing protocols for UFH to achieve and maintain a therapeutic level of anticoagulation. LMWH and fondaparinux are weight-based in dosing and are cleared primarily through the kidneys. Dose adjustments are generally not required in mild to moderate renal insufficiency. If creatinine clearance is < 30 mL/min, factor Xa activity should be monitored to adjust LMWH. Other patients in whom monitoring is advised include those who are significantly under- or over-weight and pregnant women on therapeutic LMWH [25]. Fondaparinux is contraindicated at CrCl < 30 mL/min [25]. Heparin-induced thrombocytopenia (HIT) is a known complication of UFH and platelet counts should be monitored. LMWH is significantly less likely to cause HIT than is UFH, and with fondaparinux the risk is extremely small.

Direct thrombin inhibitors

The parenteral direct thrombin inhibitors hirudin, bivalirudin, and argatroban are alternatives to heparins and fondaparinux and may be used to treat HIT. Argatroban is cleared through the liver so is useful especially in patients with renal failure. These drugs have weight-based dosing that is challenging to monitor, and they have no approved antidotes. Fortunately, all have a short half-life, so the effect reverses within several hours of discontinuation [25].

Dabigatran is an oral direct thrombin inhibitor that has shown equivalency to warfarin for stroke prevention in non-valvular atrial fibrillation when dosed twice daily [26]. It does not require monitoring, though it is renally cleared and requires dose adjustment or reconsideration in patients with renal insufficiency. Should a patient taking dabigatran require emergent surgery, FFP will be ineffective in correcting the anticoagulation effect until the drug levels have sufficiently diminished.

Sedatives and analgesics
Preventing withdrawal in chronic benzodiazepine and narcotic users

A general principle of perioperative medication safety is to anticipate and prevent withdrawal effects from discontinuation of a patient's chronic medications. While narcotics are commonly used for analgesia postoperatively, a patient who has opioid dependence and who undergoes prolonged surgery or who has a delay in initiation of narcotic analgesia after surgery may experience withdrawal. Withdrawal increases

physiological stress (accelerated heart rate and blood pressure) and may cause psychological distress or delirium.

It may be more common that a patient taking chronic benzodiazepines will not have these medications routinely prescribed postoperatively and may suffer similar withdrawal effects that may be deleterious to recovery. Anticipation of these effects by the surgeon and anesthesiologist and proper prescribing is the prevention strategy.

Prevention of over-sedation and respiratory depression

Optimal titration of analgesia to achieve adequate pain control while minimizing adverse effects is the goal of postoperative pain management (see Chapter 7 for a full discussion of pain control). Narcotic analgesics can cause respiratory depression, regardless of the route of administration. Strategies to reduce narcotic dosing include use of acetaminophen or non-steroidal anti-inflammatory drugs (NSAIDs) in addition to narcotics and multimodal anesthesia [27]. Short-acting narcotics with rapid onset of action are used to achieve initial pain control through titration of the dose. Long-acting narcotic formulations are now available, such as transdermal fentanyl, that has been shown to be safe and effective in the management of acute postoperative pain in the first days after surgery in a hospital setting [28]. However, reports of deaths and serious adverse events have caused the US Food and Drug Administration (FDA) to issue a safety warning against the use of this product for acute postoperative pain [29].

Prevention of acetaminophen toxicity

A recognized danger of acetaminophen is a toxic threshold not far above that of therapeutic dosing. Because so many commonly prescribed oral analgesic formulations contain acetaminophen in combination with a narcotic, patients may inadvertently ingest larger amounts than the recommended maximum of 4 g per day as the dose of the formulation is titrated upward. Patients may be unaware of the dangers of taking additional non-prescription formulations of acetaminophen. The acetaminophen dose varies among prescription analgesic formulations, increasing the likelihood of prescriber or patient error in dosing. The FDA has asked manufacturers of combination analgesics to limit the dose of acetaminophen to 325 mg per unit so as to improve the safety of the products [30]. A prudent practice in the immediate postoperative setting may be to prescribe a formulation of acetaminophen and a formulation of narcotic separately so as to give clear instructions for each drug.

Cardiac medications
Beta-blockers

Beta-blockers are commonly used to treat ischemic heart disease and systolic heart failure. Withdrawal of beta-blockers removes any protective effect of the drug through surgery and may result in a physiological withdrawal that increases activity of the sympathetic nervous system. Because numerous studies have demonstrated an increased risk of myocardial infarction in the weeks following beta-blocker withdrawal in non-surgical and in surgical patients, beta-blocker therapy should not be discontinued in surgical patients without a clear indication to do so [31].

The recommendations for initiating beta-blocker therapy before surgery have changed over time as research has identified situations in which beta-blocker therapy reduces perioperative risk and where it increases risk. Patients at low risk of cardiac events probably gain no benefit and may be at increased risk of harm from having a beta-blocker added before surgery. Additionally, beta-blockers initiated immediately before surgery and used in high dose without titration to heart rate and blood pressure have been shown to increase the risk of mortality [32]. Therefore, current recommendations are to initiate beta-blocker therapy in patients with indications in advance of surgery such that the dose is titrated to adequate heart rate control without causing bradycardia or hypotension and to continue dose titration through the perioperative period [31]. How far in advance to initiate therapy is not settled, though a randomized study found that patients in whom beta-blockers were started more than 1 week before surgery had better outcomes than those in whom therapy was initiated within a week [33].

Loop diuretics

Based primarily on physiological concerns that patients on diuretics would be more likely to suffer intraoperative hypotension related to intravascular volume depletion, most experts have recommended withholding diuretics on the morning of surgery. Khan and colleagues randomized chronic furosemide users to take furosemide or placebo on the morning of surgery. They found no difference in intraoperative hypotension or postoperative events between the two groups [34]. The traditional recommendation to withhold diuretics may fall to better evidence.

Conclusion

Medications pose a significant risk to patients during surgery and recuperation, and the ever-increasing age of patients and increasing numbers of chronic conditions means that this risk is not diminishing. Careful attention to an adequate medication history and to reconciliation of medications provides a safety net. Following prudent medication practices and consulting colleagues where a physician's expertise is limited may further improve the likelihood of a good outcome for surgical patients.

References

1. Leape LL, Brennan TA, Laird N et al. The nature of adverse events in hospitalized patients. Results of the Harvard Medical Practice Study II. *N Engl J Med* 1991; **324**: 377–84.

2. Pippins JR, Gandhi TK, Hamann C et al. Classifying and predicting errors of inpatient medication reconciliation. *J Gen Intern Med* 2008; **23**: 1414–22.

3. Reckmann MH, Westbrook JI, Koh Y, Lo C, Day, RO. Does computerized provider order entry reduce prescribing errors for hospital inpatients? A systematic review. *J Am Med Inform Assoc* 2009; **16**: 613–23.

4. Schnipper JL, Hamann C, Ndumele CD et al. Effect of an electronic medication reconciliation application and process redesign on potential adverse drug events: a cluster-randomized trial. *Arch Intern Med* 2009; **169**: 771–80.

5. Ang-Lee MK, Moss K, Yuan CS. Herbal medicines and perioperative care. *J Am Med Assoc* 2001; **286**: 208–16.

6. Beckert BW, Concannon MJ, Henry SL, Smith DS, Puckett CL, The effect of herbal medicines on platelet function: an in vivo experiment and review of the literature. *Plast Reconstr Surg* 2007; **120**: 2044–50.

7. Isaac T, Weissman JS, Davis RB et al. Overrides of medication alerts in ambulatory care. *Arch Intern Med* 2009; **169**: 305–11.

8. Udelsman R, Norton JA, Jelenich SE et al. Responses of the hypothalamic-pituitary-adrenal and renin-angiotensin axes and the sympathetic system during controlled surgical and anesthetic stress. *J Clin Endocrinol Metab* 1987; **64**: 986–94.

9. Lemmens HJ. Perioperative pharmacology in morbid obesity. *Curr Opin Anaesthesiol* 2010; **23**: 485–91.

10. Moghissi ES, Korytkowski MT, DiNardo M et al. American Association of Clinical Endocrinologists and American Diabetes Association consensus statement on inpatient glycemic control. *Diabetes Care* 2009; **32**: 1119–31.

11. McAlister FA, Majumdar SR, Blitz S et al. The relation between hyperglycemia and outcomes in 2,471 patients admitted to the hospital with community-acquired pneumonia. *Diabetes Care* 2005; **28**: 810–15.

12. Frisch A, Chandra P, Smiley D et al. Prevalence and clinical outcome of hyperglycemia in the perioperative period in noncardiac surgery. *Diabetes Care* 2010; **33**: 1783–8.

13. van den Berghe G, Wouters P, Weekers F et al. Intensive insulin therapy in the critically ill patients. *N Engl J Med* 2001; **345**: 1359–67.

14. Finfer S, Chittock DR, Su SY et al. Intensive versus conventional glucose control in critically ill patients. *N Engl J Med* 2009; **360**: 1283–97.

15. Kansagara D, Fu R, Freeman M, Wolf F, Helfand M. Intensive insulin therapy in hospitalized patients: a systematic review. *Ann Intern Med* 2011; **154**: 268–82.

16. Qaseem A, Humphrey LL, Chou R, Snow V, Shekelle P. Use of intensive insulin therapy for the management of glycemic control in hospitalized patients: a clinical practice guideline from the American College of Physicians. *Ann Intern Med* 2011; **154**: 260–7.

17. Vann MA. Perioperative management of ambulatory surgical patients with diabetes mellitus. *Curr Opin Anaesthesiol* 2009; **22**: 718–24.

18. Umpierrez GE, Hor T, Smiley D et al. Comparison of inpatient insulin regimens with detemir plus aspart versus neutral protamine hagedorn plus regular in medical patients with type 2

diabetes. *J Clin Endocrinol Metab* 2009; **94**: 564–9.

19. Umpierrez GE, Smiley D, Jacobs S *et al.* Randomized study of basal-bolus insulin therapy in the inpatient management of patients with type 2 diabetes undergoing general surgery (RABBIT 2 Surgery). *Diabetes Care* 2011; **34**: 256–61.

20. Korytkowski MT, Salata RJ, Koerbel GL *et al.* Insulin therapy and glycemic control in hospitalized patients with diabetes during enteral nutrition therapy: a randomized controlled clinical trial. *Diabetes Care* 2009; **32**: 594–6.

21. O'Riordan JM, Margey RJ, Blake G, O'Connell PR. Antiplatelet agents in the perioperative period. *Arch Surg* 2009; **144**: 69–76; discussion 76.

22. Douketis JD, Berger PB, Dunn AS *et al.* The perioperative management of antithrombotic therapy: American College of Chest Physicians Evidence-Based Clinical Practice Guidelines (8th Edition). *Chest* 2008; **133** (6 Suppl): 299S–339S.

23. Grant PJ, Brotman DJ, Jaffer AK. Perioperative anticoagulant management. *Med Clin North Am* 2009; **93**: 1105–21.

24. Petitou M, Hérault JP, Bernat A *et al.* Synthesis of thrombin-inhibiting heparin mimetics without side effects. *Nature* 1999; **398**(6726): 417–22.

25. Hirsh J, Hérault JP, Bernat A *et al.* Parenteral anticoagulants: American College of Chest Physicians Evidence-Based Clinical Practice Guidelines (8th Edition). *Chest* 2008; **133** (6 Suppl): 141S–59S.

26. Connolly SJ, Ezekowitz MD, Elkelboom YS *et al.* Dabigatran versus warfarin in patients with atrial fibrillation. *N Engl J Med* 2009; **361**: 1139–51.

27. Bader P, Fonteyne V, De Meerleer G, Papaioannou EG, Vranken JH. Post-operative pain management. In *Guidelines on Pain Management.* Arnhem: European Association of Urology; 2009, pp. 62–82.

28. Viscusi ER, Siccardi M, Damaraju CV, Hewitt DJ, Kershaw P. The safety and efficacy of fentanyl iontophoretic transdermal system compared with morphine intravenous patient-controlled analgesia for postoperative pain management: an analysis of pooled data from three randomized, active-controlled clinical studies. *Anesth Analg* 2007; **105**: 1428–36, table of contents.

29. Food and Drug Administration. *FDA issues second safety warning on fentanyl skin patch.* Dec. 17, 2007. http://www.fda.gov/NewsEvents/Newsroom/PressAnnouncements/2007/ucm109046.htm.

30. Food and Drug Administration. *FDA drug safety communication: prescription acetaminophen products to be limited to 325 mg per dosing unit.* Jan. 13, 2011. www.fda.gov/Drugs/DrugSafety/ucm239821.htm.

31. Fleischmann KE, Beckman JA, Buller CE *et al.* 2009 ACCF/AHA focused update on perioperative beta blockade: a report of the American College of Cardiology Foundation/American Heart Association Task Force on Practice Guidelines. *Circulation* 2009; **120**: 2123–51.

32. Devereaux PJ, Yang H, Yusuf H *et al.* Effects of extended-release metoprolol succinate in patients undergoing non-cardiac surgery (POISE trial): a randomised controlled trial. *Lancet* 2008; **371**(9627): 1839–47.

33. Flu WJ, van Kuijk JP, Chonchol M *et al.* Timing of pre-operative Beta-blocker treatment in vascular surgery patients: influence on post-operative outcome. *J Am Coll Cardiol* 2010; **56**: 1922–9.

34. Khan NA, Campbell NR, Frost SD *et al.* Risk of intraoperative hypotension with loop diuretics: a randomized controlled trial. *Am J Med* 2010; **123**: 1059 e1–8.

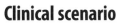

Chapter 5

Informed consent and decision-making capacity

J. Richard Pittman and Jason Lesandrini

Clinical scenario

Ms. P is a 49-year-old-female with obesity and depression who has arrived this morning for her elective cholecystectomy. She initially presented to Surgery Clinic following hospitalization for cholecystitis that was managed medically. Your colleague saw her in clinic and after a discussion of possible options, he scheduled her for the surgery 2 weeks later. His note documents that he discussed "the surgery, the risks, and likely outcomes."

In the preoperative area the patient is notably nervous about surgery, but wants to be rid of her right-upper quadrant pain. Just prior to surgery you approach her with a consent form in hand. You ask, "Do you have any questions about the surgery, prior to signing the consent?" She responds, "No, he said my pain would go away after putting a few holes in my belly." She signs the consent form and you walk back to the operating room.

Introduction

In the high-volume environment of surgical care, the process of informed consent is often the final step before proceeding with surgery. The step may be hurried, poorly timed, and carried out by the least trained member of the team [1]. In so doing, the practical rendering of consent is reduced to a patient's signature on a form they have supposedly read.

Ms. P's case is illustrative of problems frequently encountered in the consent process for surgical procedures. The goal of this chapter is to provide the reader with methods to address these common problems surrounding surgical consent. This chapter will first define informed consent and outline its specific components. Second, several widely accepted exemptions to the informed consent requirement will be reviewed. Finally, practical tips for both systematic use of informed consent and assessing decision-making capacity will be explored.

Shifting the practice of consent

For many decades the ethical principles of beneficence and patient autonomy have been the foundations of doctor–patient interactions [2]. More recently, the ethical literature and court rulings have promoted greater patient involvement by mandating informed consent. Challenges in defining informed consent legally and myths of its intentions have left practitioners ambivalent adherents. Many surgeons view informed consent with skepticism due to limits of patient comprehension, to their ability to persuade patients to assent, and to fears of being reduced to purveyors of medical options without their educated input.

Though doubts of the utility and achievability of true informed consent may remain, most surgeons have complied by using informal scripts – repeated narratives common to a procedure or decision – e.g., "The risks always include infection and bleeding." This script and a request for questions will often yield a signed form and approval for a procedure. These scripted conversations may provide the legal minimum of consent in straightforward situations, but are inadequate in complicated cases, when a patient does not understand or exhibits an inability to make a decision. Furthermore, basic scripted presentations do not constitute "informed" consent nor provide "the basis for a strong and enduring therapeutic alliance between the surgeon and patient, with shared responsibility for decision making" [3].

A shift in the practice of consent to one of shared decision-making through informed consent can be beneficial for both the patient and the surgeon. The American College of Surgeons' Statement of Ethics points out that informed consent "is a standard of ethical surgical practice that enhances the surgeon/patient relationship and that may improve the patient's care and the treatment outcome." Evidence suggests that proper informed consent has a positive impact on the quality of healthcare services [4,5]. In order to live up to their ethical obligations, some surgeons may need to alter their view of obtaining consent, from the exercise of "form signing" to a vital patient encounter of fostering trust and optimizing the principles of beneficence and autonomy.

Returning to the clinical scenario

Ms. P's cholecystectomy that seemed routine and evoked no discussion prior to surgery took an unfortunate turn in the operating room. Her planned laparoscopic surgery had to be

Medical Management of the Surgical Patient, ed. Michael F. Lubin, Thomas F. Dodson, and Neil H. Winawer. Published by Cambridge University Press. © Cambridge University Press 2013.

Table 5.1 Components of informed consent.

A patient possesses decision-making capacity
Surgeon supplies adequate information
Surgeon assesses understanding
Surgeon assesses if voluntary
Surgeon makes a recommendation
Patient responds with clear consent or refusal

Table 5.2 Decision-making capacity.

Cognitive abilities required	Questions to assess abilities
Understand the medical information	What do you understand about your condition now?
Evaluate the risks/benefits	What do you think will happen if you have (or do not have) this procedure?
Employ reason to weigh the decision	How did you reach your decision?
Communicate	Can you explain your decision about the procedure?

converted into an open procedure due to a bile duct injury. During the prolonged surgery, Ms. P developed hypotension and hypoxia that was stabilized with vasopressors and sustained ventilatory support in the ICU. Did Ms. P understand the possible need for a more invasive procedure or the potential complications? Could the use of an informed consent process have better prepared Ms. P for what occurred?

The informed consent process

Informed consent occurs when a patient with decision-making capacity makes a voluntary choice based on an exchange of information with the surgeon.

The informed consent process is ideally a fluid discussion between patient and surgeon about the medical situation at hand. The interaction is not meant to be a monologue by the surgeon prior to handing the patient a paper to sign, nor is it a presentation of a medical menu from which a patient chooses without input from the surgeon. Rather, it is an ongoing dialogue where the patient and surgeon exchange and clarify information until a joint decision is made (Table 5.1).

The process of informed consent highlights the shared burden and decision-making of the patient–surgeon relationship. While the surgeon must provide adequate information (discussed below), patients also have responsibilities. They must provide the surgeon with insight about their values, wishes, and goals relevant to the current situation. Both parties share in the decision-making process and must come to an agreement about what to do. Following this discussion, the surgeon should recommend a treatment plan that is both consistent with the standard of care and best promotes the patient's goals and values.

Decision-making capacity

While no technical starting point to the informed consent process exists, a practical beginning is assessing the patient's decision-making capacity. Decision-making capacity is a clinical term describing a patient's ability to rationally process medical information and make a choice about how to proceed with his or her care. Patients lacking capacity are unable to make informed decisions about their healthcare [6].

Competence and decision-making capacity are often used interchangeably but have technically different meanings. Competence is a legal term describing the global ability to manage

affairs independently. Patients are considered competent unless declared incompetent by a judge. Incompetence is usually a long-term designation for persons who have lost the ability to function independently and require appointment of a guardian [6].

Capacity or decision-making capacity is a clinical term suggesting that a patient has a certain set of cognitive abilities. The set includes the ability to understand the information, to reason, to evaluate the risks and benefits of the options, and to communicate a choice [7]. The difficulty in assessing a patient's capacity is partly due to the lack of an accepted standard of assessment [8,9]. There are formal, time-consuming tools to assess capacity, but a simple, brief questionnaire is all that is needed (see Table 5.2) [10].

Information

As surgeons explain the clinical situation and proposed intervention to the patient they must ensure that "adequate information" is provided. What constitutes adequate information will vary according to legal standards of disclosure in each state. The three main standards require a clinician to provide information as would a (1) "reasonable surgeon", (2) to a "reasonable person", or (3) a "subjective standard" [11]. Which specific standard each state adopts varies, but most have as a minimum requirement for the surgeon to disclose (1) the purpose of the procedure, (2) the risks/benefits, (3) the alternatives, and (4) possible outcomes [12]. The reader should explore different standards via the references and their relevant state statutes. As noted, the statutes above describe the minimum legal standards, but a surgeon fostering shared decision-making would offer additional necessary information needed by the patient to reach a sound decision.

Understanding

Throughout the encounter the surgeon should assess the patient's understanding of the information presented. Depth of knowledge can vary greatly, but at a minimum the patient should appreciate the current situation, treatment options, and likely outcomes [6]. Given the technicality of surgical interventions, patients often struggle to grasp the complex nature of the information exchanged. In addition, the lack of understanding can be compounded by poor medical literacy or education level. This often leaves a patient with vast amounts of information but a lack of clarity about what "the treatment is ultimately meant to do" [13]. What results is that patients often overestimate the benefits of interventions, even when they have acknowledged via "consent forms" that they understand [14]. Providers also often overestimate their patient's understanding. This underscores the importance of focused questions to check a patient's level of comprehension, e.g., "How will this surgery relieve your pain?"

Voluntariness

Voluntariness refers to the ability of the patient to make a choice without undue influence from the surgeon or others through coercion or manipulation. Coercion is a perceived threat to the patient, by a party that has the power to carry out the feared outcome (e.g., the doctor will "fire" me if I don't go through with this procedure) [15]. Manipulation can take many forms, with some more prevalent than others. Framing or presenting information in such a way that inappropriately biases the patient to agree with the recommendation, is a common form of manipulation. In order to avoid manipulation it is important that the surgeon present the information as objectively as possible, being mindful of the temptation to shape or spin the information to strengthen the case [16]. The surgeon should state the facts, provide a medical recommendation, and avoid surreptitiously infusing personal views or opinions unless asked.

Recommendation

A recommendation is a plan of care based on the medical facts and an appreciation of the patient's goals or values. This differs from an attempt to express what the surgeon would do in that patient's situation, i.e., the surgeon's personal opinion. The difficulty in the latter is that in most situations the patient's and surgeon's values contrast significantly enough to yield very different choices. Therefore, by offering an unsolicited opinion the surgeon has the potential to unduly bias his or her patient. However, in cases where this personal opinion is directly sought by a patient, a surgeon may offer it in select situations [17,18].

The ideal consent process for Ms. P would include a recommendation made after assessing her capacity, providing material information, and determining her level of understanding. Given the medical information and an appreciation of her goal of stopping pain, cholecystectomy would be a medically appropriate course of therapy. This is a standard recommendation. If instead, the surgeon suggested no surgery because he or she would not want his or her own body cut to alleviate pain is a personal opinion. This is obviously an exaggeration to show the difference.

Clear consent or refusal

Finally, the patient will need to provide clear consent or refusal for the proposed intervention. The communicated consent can be provided through signature, verbal communication, or other means. Surgeons should adapt the means of a communicated choice to the abilities of the patient. For example, a patient with a stroke and residual dysarthria may still be able to communicate a choice, just through different means. Remember that communication of choice alone does not constitute informed consent; especially communication via a signature on a consent form. A study of 540 informed consent forms from 157 hospitals showed that only 26% included the minimum disclosure requirements. Additionally < 50% of forms provided specific information about risks, and alternatives to the proposed procedure were noted only 57% of the time [19].

Furthermore, consent forms are often poorly written. Even when consent forms are used it is not clear they actually obtain "informed consent." In a study assessing 616 consent forms for readability, the average reading level was 12.6 [20], 7.6 levels above the recommended readability score of 5th grade by the National Work Group on Literacy and Health. Finally, studies often show that patients do not read the consent forms. A 1993 study of 250 patients undergoing intrathoracic, intraperitoneal, or vascular surgery, showed that 69% said they did not read the consent form before signing it [21].

Exceptions to informed consent

While informed consent is held in high regard, surgeons may temporarily defer their obligation to obtain it in three situations. As with all exceptions to the informed consent process inappropriately invoking them must be avoided because it threatens the trust so essential to the therapeutic relationship [7]. The threat is so great that in some situations, disclosure should be sought retroactively in order to protect the patient–surgeon relationship [3].

Emergencies

Surgeons will frequently encounter patients who are in emergent need of an intervention and informed consent cannot be obtained. Under these circumstances, proceeding without the patient's consent can be ethically justified. In a true emergency, it is presumed that the patient would consent if they were able to do so. The challenge is defining an emergency. The definition can vary by state statute but is generally characterized as a situation in which any delay in treatment would put a patient's life in peril. To justly proceed without consent in a true emergency, the patient must lack decision-making capacity, their wishes must be unknown, and there should be no reasonably available authorized decision-maker. What is clear, is that treatment in the emergency room does not alone constitute an emergency, nor that informed consent can be bypassed.

Table 5.3 Scoring the consent of Ms. P against the proposed process.

Decision-making capacity	Neither surgeon documented a capacity assessment
Adequate information	Only a generic statement of disclosure from the clinic without reference to anticipated risks or outcomes No mention of who would be performing the surgery
Understanding	No documentation of her level of understanding from clinic No clarification of her only recorded statement, "No, he said my pain would go away after putting a few holes in my belly" Does this mean she expected a laparoscopic surgery?
Voluntary	Not documented
Recommendation	Not clear how the decision was reached
Clear consent	She signed a consent, but we do not know the extent of her consent

Waiver of consent

Just because a patient can provide informed consent does not mean they must. A patient can consent to waiving the right to make decisions and may delegate that authority to someone else. It is in this decision that the individual exercises autonomy.

Therapeutic privilege

Therapeutic privilege is a less frequent but possible situation in which informed consent may not be obtained prior to a surgical intervention. Under such situations a surgeon decides that informing the patient of their prognosis or diagnosis would be so damaging that it would cause the patient great harm. The use of this exception "is no longer viewed as applicable in any but the most extreme cases (a patient with a history of clinical depression facing terminal diagnosis …). Even then eventual disclosure is considered ethically obligatory" [3].

The case of Ms. P

Contrasting the "consent" of Ms. P with the process explained above reveals numerous opportunities for improvement (Table 5.3). First, the consenting surgeon made no assessment of her decision-making capacity, despite the diagnosis of depression and notable nervousness before surgery. Second, the surgeon made no informational disclosure, relying instead on another surgeon's encounter two weeks prior. A cursory inquiry elicited no questions and an assent was obtained so the case could proceed.

While time constraints exist, Ms. P's surgeons could have improved care by using the outlined process. The clinic surgeon should have concisely documented the elements of consent, with specific attention to likely risks/outcomes and any potential alterations in the procedure. It would also be important to document a plan of decision-making if she lost capacity during the procedure (e.g., who would make decisions.

Practical approach to problems that arise in the informed consent process

Certain challenges or problems will continue to persist during the informed consent process despite our best efforts. An awareness of these challenges will help surgeons anticipate problems and plan accordingly. In this last section we address tips for common challenges during the informed consent process and some unique challenges in the context of Ms. P.

Surgeons should assess capacity for each decision

Decision-making capacity is decision specific such that a patient can have capacity to make one decision and not another [13]. Therefore, to write in a patient's chart that they "do not have decision-making capacity" would imply that the patient lacks the ability to make any decisions for themselves including meals, when to go to the bathroom, take a shower, etc. Rather, when documenting whether a patient lacks decision-making capacity the surgeon should specify the specific decision for which the patient lacks capacity.

In addition, evaluating capacity often varies according to the complexity of the decision. As Chin and Brown point out, "The level of scrutiny applied to the situation depends on the significance of the decision at hand. For minor procedures, capacity may be confirmed with the most cursory of examinations. For refusal of life-saving procedures or consenting to potential risky interventions, more careful consideration must be applied" [22–24]. This seems intuitive, since one would want to be the most confident when the stakes were highest. Furthermore, in helping with assessment of capacity in any setting, the surgeon can look to those who know the patient, e.g., family, friends, loved ones, and ask whether the patient is acting consistently with their past behavior and beliefs.

Psychiatric and/or cognitive disabilities should trigger or create red flags for careful scrutiny in capacity assessments

Healthcare providers often believe that if a patient has a psychiatric diagnosis or decreased cognitive ability that they lack capacity to make decisions. Surgeons should note that neither of these conditions automatically excludes a patient from decision-making [25]. Rather, the conditions should caution the surgeon to be particularly stringent in their capacity assessment. Consulting with psychiatric services may be helpful although not ethically required.

With treatment of the underlying condition a patient can regain capacity during the hospital course

Capacity is likely to wax and wane throughout a patient's hospital stay. Therefore, it is prudent for the surgeon to determine when and if the patient is likely to regain capacity. Some patients are more likely to maintain capacity during certain times of the day due to sleep schedules, e.g., elderly and sundowning situations. The surgeon has a moral obligation to wait until a patient's capacity is restored before proceeding with surgery.

"The concept of decision making is pivotal because as a practical matter assessment of decision-making capacity determines whether patients are empowered to make their own healthcare decisions or whether someone else should be empowered to make decisions for them" [25]. The surgeon should not neglect the views of the patient in situations where others will be empowered to make decisions. Simply because patients have lost the ability to make decisions does not mean we should not treat them with respect and attempt to take what they say into consideration. For example, a patient without decision-making capacity who is refusing amputation of her leg should have her refusal taken into consideration, even if she is not the authorized decision-maker, given the impact the decision will have on her as a human being.

To assess patient's understanding use open-ended questions

The surgeon should use questions that elucidate understanding, rather than adding information until the patient tunes out. "Is this making sense?" is often not an adequate question as it allows the patient to avoid potential embarrassment by nodding. A useful method known as "repeat-back" can be employed to quickly get a sense of understanding [26]. Very simply, you ask, "Can you explain why you need this procedure?" This allows the surgeon to determine whether the information was presented at an appropriate education level.

A surgeon's recommendation should incorporate the medical facts and the patient's values

Often surgeons will arrive at appointments, a patient's bedside or patient meetings with pre-determined plans without hearing the patient's goals of therapeutic interventions. Before surgeons or any healthcare providers can determine whether the intervention is the "best" therapeutic option, they need to determine the patient's values and goals. One easy way to accomplish this is to ask, "Tell me what is important to you?" It is after determining what is important to the patient that a surgeon can then work towards a plan, with the patient, that is medically sound and consistent with the patient's values, goals, and life wishes [27]. After that plan is developed, it may be helpful to clarify with the patient, "Given the medical information we know and the information you have provided me about what is important to you, it sounds like procedure X would fit with your values, wishes, and goals of treatment. What do you think?"

Surgeons should disclose both who will participate in the surgery and each individual's level of training

Depending on the setting and difficulty of the surgical intervention, individuals with a variety of experience will participate in the surgical procedure. The level of experience of these individuals can range from years to months or less. Studies suggest that surgeon volume is related to quality of care, such that surgeons who performed more surgical colorectal resections surgeries had better health outcomes [28]. This also means that if trainees will participate in the surgical procedure the patient should be informed. Withholding this information from the patient would violate the trust the patient has placed in the surgeon to be forthcoming and truthful.

In Ms. P's case an additional challenge presents itself in regard to the informed consent process and who will participate in the surgery. As the case is described, it is not clear that Ms. P was informed that the surgeon from the clinic would not be the surgeon performing the surgery. Again, withholding this information violates the trust she put in the clinic surgeon.

Surgeons should effectively document the informed consent process in the medical record

Adequate documentation is important in recording the interchange between the patient and surgeon. In addition, it allows surgeons who were not present during the informed consent process a partial understanding of what components of the consent process were present or missing. Furthermore, the surgeon can discuss the note with the patient as a means of helping the patient understand what will take place during the surgery. Finally, it also provides the patient with another opportunity to clarify any unresolved issues [29]. Table 5.4 provides a form/checklist to assist the surgeon with completing the informed consent process. While the checklist has not been validated in studies, it may increase completeness of the process and improve patient care. We believe it does provide a simple and clear means of capturing all the components of the informed consent process in one place.

Table 5.4 Checklist for informed consent.

Component	Task to assess	Done	Comments
Decision-making capacity	Does the patient have the ability to understand?	☐	
	Does the patient have the ability to evaluate risks/benefits?	☐	
	Does the patient employ reason to weigh decision?	☐	
	Is the patient able to communicate a choice?	☐	
Provide adequate information	Have you provided the reason for and nature of procedure?	☐	
	Have you explained the risks/benefits of the procedure?	☐	
	Have you provided the alternatives (including no treatment)?	☐	
	Have you explained the possible outcomes?	☐	
Assess for understanding via questions	Why do you need the current procedure?	☐	
	Can you explain the current procedure?	☐	
	What other choices do you have besides this procedure?	☐	
	What are the risks of having this procedure?	☐	
Ensure the patient is acting voluntarily	No threats made	☐	
	No framing of data to encourage acceptance or refusal	☐	
Make a recommendation	Based on medical facts and patients values and goals	☐	
	Have not provided unsolicited personal opinions	☐	
Communicated choice	Patient clearly expressed their decision for or against the recommended intervention	☐	
Contingency for lack or loss of capacity	What should we do if you lose capacity post-surgery?	☐	

Conclusion

In this chapter we have attempted to provide ways for informed consent to be a vital process that builds trust with patients. The informed consent process is about sharing the burden of decision-making with patients. Finally, we provided guidance for the informed consent process and helpful tips to address frequently encountered problems during decision-making.

References

1. Braddock CH 3rd, Fihn SD, Levinson W, Jonsen AR, Pearlman RA. How doctors and patients discuss routine clinical decisions. Informed decision making in the outpatient setting. *J Gen Intern Med* 1997; **12**: 339–45.

2. Emanuel EJ, Emanuel LL. Four models of the physician-patient relationship. *J Am Med Assoc* 1992; **267**: 2221–6.

3. McCullough LB, Jones JW, Brody BA. Informed consent: autonomous decision making of the surgical patient. In McCullough LB, Jones JW, Brody BA, eds. *Surgical Ethics*. New York, NY: Oxford University Press; 1998, pp. 15–37.

4. Beach MC, Sugarman J, Johnson RL et al. Do patients treated with dignity report higher satisfaction, adherence, and receipt of preventive care? *Ann Fam Med* 2005; **3**: 331–8.

5. Beach MC, Keruly J, Moore RD. Is the quality of the patient-provider relationship associated with better adherence and health outcomes for patients with HIV? *J Gen Intern Med* 2006; **21**: 661–5.

6. Lo B. *Decision-making Capacity. Resolving Ethical Dilemmas: A Guide for Clinicians*. 3rd edn. Philadelphia, PA: Lippincott Williams & Wilkins; 2005, pp. 67–74.

7. Post LF, Blustein J, Dubler NN. *Handbook for Health Care Ethics Committees*. Baltimore, MD: Johns Hopkins University Press; 2007.

8. Dunn LB, Nowrangi MA, Palmer BW, Jeste DV, Saks ER. Assessing decisional capacity for clinical research or treatment: a review of instruments. *Am J Psychiatry* 2006; **163**: 1323–34.

9. Vellinga A, Smit JH, van Leeuwen E, van Tilburg W, Jonker C. Instruments to assess decision-making capacity: an overview. *Int Psychogeriatr* 2004; **16**: 397–419.

10. Appelbaum PS. Clinical practice. Assessment of patients' competence to consent to treatment. *N Engl J Med* 2007; **357**: 1834–40.

11. Jonsen AR, Siegler M, Winslade WJ. *Clinical Ethics: A Practical Approach to Ethical Decisions in Clinical Medicine*. 7th edn. New York, NY: McGraw-Hill Medical; 2010.

12. Bernat JL, Peterson LM. Patient-centered informed consent in surgical practice. *Arch Surg* 2006; **141**: 86–92.

13. Meisel A, Kuczewski M. Legal and ethical myths about informed consent. *Arch Intern Med* 1996; **156**: 2521–6.

14. Rothberg MB, Sivalingam SK, Ashraf J et al. Patients' and cardiologists' perceptions of the benefits of percutaneous coronary intervention for stable coronary disease. *Ann Intern Med* 2010; **153**: 307–13.

15. Lo B. *Informed Consent. Resolving Ethical Dilemmas: A Guide for Clinicians.* 4th edn. Philadelphia. PA: Wolters Kluwer Health/ Lippincott Williams & Wilkins; 2009, pp. 18–30.

16. Terry PB. Informed consent in clinical medicine. *Chest* 2007; **131**: 563–8.

17. Kon AA. Answering the question: "Doctor, if this were your child, what would you do?" *Pediatrics* 2006; **118**: 393–7.

18. Ubel PA. "What should I do, doc?": Some psychologic benefits of physician recommendations. *Arch Intern Med* 2002; **162**: 977–80.

19. Bottrell MM, Alpert H, Fischbach RL, Emanuel LL. Hospital informed consent for procedure forms: facilitating quality patient-physician interaction. *Arch Surg* 2000; **135**: 26–33.

20. Hopper KD, TenHave TR, Tully DA, Hall TE. The readability of currently used surgical/procedure consent forms in the United States. *Surgery* 1998; **123**: 496–503.

21. Lavelle-Jones C, Byrne DJ, Rice P, Cuschieri A. Factors affecting quality of informed consent. *Br Med J* 1993; **306** (6882): 885–90.

22. Chin MS, Brown VA. The dilemma of capacity: respecting patient wishes and preferences ≠ decision making ability. *J Hosp Ethics* 2010; **2**(1).

23. Chow GV, Czarny MJ, Hughes MT, Carrese JA. CURVES: a mnemonic for determining medical decision-making capacity and providing emergency treatment in the acute setting. *Chest* 2010; **137**: 421–7.

24. Drane JF. The many faces of competency. *Hastings Cent Rep* 1985; **15**: 17–21.

25. Ganzini L, Volicer L, Nelson WA, Fox E, Derse AR. Ten myths about decision-making capacity. *J Am Med Dir Assoc* 2005; **6** (3 Suppl): S100–4.

26. Fink AS, Prochazka AV, Henderson WG *et al.* Enhancement of surgical informed consent by addition of repeat back: a multicenter, randomized controlled clinical trial. *Ann Surg* 2010; **252**: 27–36.

27. Annas GJ. Informed consent, cancer, and truth in prognosis. *N Engl J Med* 1994; **330**: 223–5.

28. Rogers SO Jr, Wolf RE, Zaslavsky AM, Wright WE, Ayanian JZ. Relation of surgeon and hospital volume to processes and outcomes of colorectal cancer surgery. *Ann Surg* 2006; **244**: 1003–11.

29. Jones JW, McCullough LB, Richman BW. Informed consent: it's not just signing a form. *Thorac Surg Clin* 2005; **15**: 451–60.

Chapter

6

Ethical considerations in the surgical patient

Carl C. Hug, Jr. and Kathleen Kinlaw

In the long tradition of medical ethics, many theories and frameworks for ethical analysis of issues and situations have been developed. The use of primary principles [1] is one such framework that has been identified as relevant for making clinical decisions:

Beneficence	– promoting good; acting in the best interests of the patient.
Non-maleficence	– avoiding or minimizing harm by action or omission.
Autonomy	– respecting patients' rights to make decisions about their healthcare.
	– serves as the foundation for informed consent and informed refusal of diagnostic and therapeutic interventions.
Justice	– fair and equitable treatment that reflects what the patient is due.

These principles can be instrumental in the ethical analysis of clinical situations in which the best option for patient care is not clear. Each is considered "prima facie," a principle that is to be honored unless it is in conflict with an equal or greater principle, in which case, the relative weight of each principle will have to be decided. For example, determining whether aggressive interventions and continuing life-supporting measures are in the best interest of the patient will have to be weighed against the suffering that it engenders and the patient's autonomous expression of their wishes to avoid certain procedures and outcomes. In the USA, high priority has traditionally been placed on patient autonomy in healthcare decisions. Many of the ethical issues covered in this chapter will explore the emphasis on patient autonomy.

Patient autonomy typically refers to the patient's right to make decisions about his or her own health, including the rights to accept or to forego treatments. Information about the state of health and disease, indications for treatment, treatment alternatives with the relative benefits and risks of each, and the consequences of refusing treatment are necessary for the patient to make prudent decisions. From the physician's perspective how one's actions show respect for patient

autonomy is an important ethical commitment and may be specific to the patient/family/cultural context.

Case analysis

Jonsen *et al.* have developed a practical method for analyzing situations for individual patients [2]. They identify four major topics for consideration in any decision about medical interventions. The four-quadrant analysis addresses:

1. What are the *medical indications* for treatment, including the diagnosis and prognosis of the disease with and without treatment, alternative treatments, goals and probabilities of success, balance of benefits and complications for each diagnostic or therapeutic intervention? How is palliation balanced with cure?

2. What do we understand about *patient preferences*, including whether the patient has decision-making capacity, is well informed, and understands information about medical treatment. Central to this quadrant is respect for the patient's values and goals. If the patient is unable to make decisions, is the surrogate using appropriate standards in accordance with previously expressed wishes or advance directives? Within ethical and legal boundaries, is the patient's right to choose being respected?

3. What is the patient's *quality of life*, including the likelihood for returning the patient to a "normal" or usual level of function; physical, mental, and social deficits that are likely if the treatment succeeds or if it fails and the acceptability or unacceptability of such deficits to the patient; conditions that the patient believes would make the patient's continued life undesirable; plans for comfort and palliative care if treatment is foregone?

4. Are there *contextual features* such as family, financial, religious, cultural, or other patient-related issues that might influence the decision? Are there provider, institutional, legal, scientific, or resource allocation issues that could impact the decision? For example, have the

Medical Management of the Surgical Patient, ed. Michael F. Lubin, Thomas F. Dodson, and Neil H. Winawer. Published by Cambridge University Press. © Cambridge University Press 2013.

provider's level of experience, outcomes, and potential conflicts of interest been disclosed? Is the patient willing and able to cooperate with the treatment?

In deciding whether or not an intervention is medically indicated, it is important to keep in mind that at least one of the following goals of medicine mentioned by Jonsen *et al.* [2] should be realistically achievable.

1. Promotion of health and prevention of disease.
2. Relief of symptoms, pain, and suffering.
3. Cure of disease.
4. Prevention of untimely death.
5. Improvement of functional status or maintenance of compromised status.
6. Education and counseling of patients regarding their condition and prognosis.
7. Avoidance of harm to the patient.

*And related to several of Jonsen's goals, we would emphasize: support of humane, dignified and peaceful *death – the last event of natural life.*

The goals of treatment need to be reassessed regularly and continually evaluated against scientific and clinical evidence so that the healthcare team and family reach a consensus on realistic goals for each and every intervention and the overall direction of care.

The importance of providing a realistic prognosis

Presently, medical schools and residency training programs do a very good job in teaching the intricacies of diagnosis and therapy, but there appears to be less emphasis placed on prognostic estimation and communication of those estimates to the patient, especially when the prognosis is poor with or without treatment. An overly optimistic prognosis is dangerous because it may cause a patient and family to be unprepared for disabilities and death, and it makes them reluctant to accept limitations on aggressive treatment that is not medically appropriate. Overly pessimistic prognoses may produce undue anxiety and loss of hope [3]. The physician's challenge is to communicate the facts clearly and accurately, to manage the reactions of the patient and family members to those facts, and to guide them to an appropriate balance of hope with realism.

For a thorough discussion of prognosis, see the book by Nicholas A. Christakis, MD, a physician and sociologist, who has written *Death Foretold*: *Prophecy and Prognosis in Medical Care* [3]. It details the challenges of dealing with uncertainty and offers practical approaches to managing it.

The American Council for Graduate Medical Education (ACGME) and the American Board of Medical Specialties (ABMS) have joined together to assist medical schools and residency training programs in the development of educational protocols designed to achieve six competencies and to implement 13 assessment tools that have been defined by the Outcome Project conducted by the ACGME with the support of the Robert Wood Johnson Foundation. Two of the six competencies, professionalism and communication, relate directly to the professional and ethical obligations of physicians to their patients to provide realistic prognoses and offer reasonable alternatives of curative, restorative, and palliative care [4].

Consent to and refusal of treatment

The right of a patient to be fully informed prior to consenting to medical treatment has been clearly established ethically and legally. Informed consent can be defined as the willing acceptance of a medical intervention by a patient after adequate disclosure and understanding of the nature of the intervention, its risks, benefits, and alternatives. In medical practice the concept of informed consent has evolved from gaining the patient's consent or authorization for the proposed intervention based solely on the physician's recommendation, to informed consent based on adequate disclosure of relevant information, to making sure that the patient understands the information disclosed before providing authorization for the procedure [1].

Fundamental to informed consent is the requirement that the patient has the capacity to make a decision, to understand the medical decision (i.e., the benefits and risks of each proposed diagnostic or therapeutic intervention and their alternatives, including no intervention), and to make his or her own choices free of coercion. Decision-making capacity determinations are typically made by the attending physician, sometimes in consultation with a psychiatrist if capacity is in doubt. Competency, the more global assessment of an individual's ability to manage his or her own life decisions, is a legal concept. As physicians and others interact with patients, they gain insight as to their mental capacity and, barring obvious deficiencies, the patients are presumed to be competent unless legal proceedings determine otherwise.

Assessments of decision-making capacity [5–7] should include:

1. The patient's ability to understand relevant information, including comprehension, recall (verbalization), and retention of information as well as an understanding of causal relationships and probabilities.
2. The patient's ability to appreciate the medical situation and its implications for them, including the alternatives, risks and benefits of each alternative, and the likely consequences.
3. The ability to reason, to deliberate, to reach a conclusion based on the information provided.
4. The ability to express a choice and to recognize one's power to make that choice.

The stress of dealing with pain or other symptoms as well as the influence of medications may impact decision-making capacity. However, medications to relieve pain and other symptoms may actually assist the distressed patient in retaining decision-making capacity. A patient's decision-making capacity should be evaluated regarding the specific medical decision facing the patient. In other words: Can this patient understand and make a choice about the specific intervention under consideration? A patient with limitations in some areas of life (e.g., inability to manage one's fiscal affairs; cognitive limitations or a psychiatric diagnosis; frailty in advanced age) may still have the decision-making capacity needed to make a decision about the medical procedure he or she is facing.

In addition to assessing the patient's capacity to consent, the physician has an ethical obligation to make reasonable efforts to assure that all relevant information has been disclosed and that the patient comprehends that information. There is broad consensus in ethics, law, and medicine confirming the right of the patient to give informed consent to accept or to refuse treatment [8].

Physicians are responsible for:

1. Being knowledgeable and competent in clearly disclosing information relevant to the patient as he or she makes decisions about diagnostic procedures and treatments.
2. Assessing and assuring the patient's understanding of the information.
3. Assuring that the patient's consent is voluntary and free from controlling influences.
4. Obtaining authorization or consent in a way that respects within reason the patient's need for time to make the decision and for reassessing such authorization periodically during longer-term interventions [1].

Physicians may act without the patient or a surrogate's consent in emergencies that are an immediate threat to life and well-being.

Routine utilization of "therapeutic privilege," the ability to withhold information that is felt to be harmful to a patient, needs to be carefully examined and rarely used. Health teams may feel compelled to consider withholding information based on beneficence and non-maleficence. However, physicians should be cautious about making assumptions regarding what information the patient can manage. Alternatively, patients may be asked directly about what type and how much information they wish to receive, e.g., "Mrs. Jones, how would you like us to handle the information we learn from your tests? Do you want us to share all of the information directly with you?" Where limited information is requested, patients may be able to identify a person whom they wish to involve in decision-making.

Right to refuse treatment

Healthcare teams are often troubled when patients do not agree to the recommended course of treatment. Refusal of treatment by an adult, who has decision-making capacity and

is well informed, should be respected, even if that refusal is likely to lead to serious harm to the individual or even ultimately to their death. The right to refuse treatment is ethically based on the principle of autonomy and has been supported in multiple US legal jurisdictions under the constitutional right to privacy. Refusal of treatment by an adult patient with decision-making capacity based on religious beliefs is also generally supported ethically and legally. If no third parties are affected by the refusal of treatment (e.g., a dependent child will be left without a caregiver), religiously based refusals should be honored. (In the case of minors for whom parents or guardians are refusing consent to essential interventions on the basis of their religious beliefs, cultural tradition, etc, a legal intervention should be considered.) Where the physician feels strongly about the compelling reasons for treatment, the physician can certainly continue to discuss the reasons for refusal with the patient and try to persuade the patient to reconsider the decision. Manipulation or coercion are not ethically permissible. A physician who objects on the basis of personal or professional values to the decision not to treat can seek to have the care of the patient transferred to another physician. However, staying with patient and family through discussions of decisions such as refusal of life-sustaining treatments can provide a powerful occasion for developing mutual understanding and respect which will carry over to other healthcare decisions [2].

End-of-life care

In November 2002, the Last Acts organization, funded by the Robert Wood Johnson Foundation, released the report, *Means to a Better End: A Report on Dying in America Today* [9]. The report assessed how well each of the 50 states was doing in providing end-of-life care, utilizing such indicators as the status of advance care planning, where deaths occurred (e.g., home versus acute care settings), time spent in ICUs, pain management, and utilization of hospice services. Addressing the appropriate balance of medical and comfort care, the report concluded "that Americans, at best, have no better than a fair chance of finding good care for their loved ones or for themselves when facing a life-threatening illness."

Despite recent surveys indicating that, on average, more that 70% of Americans wish to die at home, only 25% of Americans actually do so. Approximately 50% of Americans aged 65 and older die in hospitals and 20–25% die in nursing homes [9].

"Do not resuscitate" (DNR) decisions

"Do not resuscitate" decisions include DNR, DNAR (do not attempt to resuscitate), DNI (do not intubate), DNRI (do not attempt resuscitation or intubation), and AND (allow natural death).

From the perspectives of medicine, ethics, and law, a patient suffering pulmonary and/or cardiac arrest is presumed to choose cardiopulmonary resuscitation (CPR), and it should be performed unless and until there is direct evidence that the patient previously has decided to forego CPR (i.e., DNR status). Most states have laws clarifying when and by what process resuscitative procedures may be withheld. Most healthcare organizations have established DNR policies in compliance with state laws and guidelines from the Joint Commission (JC). Many states have laws and protocols for the honoring of "prehospital" DNR orders outside of medical facilities [10].

There are two conceptual justifications for refraining from CPR:

1. The patient has clearly expressed his or her wish that CPR not be performed.
2. It is judged clinically by physicians that CPR would be medically ineffective or inappropriate.

"Do not resuscitate" orders should be written after a careful deliberation with the patient or surrogate and should ideally reflect the patient's preferences or the surrogate's statements about the patient's previously expressed wishes. When the patient's preferences are not known, the surrogate's decision should be based on the patient's best interests. The conversation regarding resuscitation should be clearly documented in the progress notes of the patient's medical record. All members of the healthcare team should be informed and, where applicable, appropriate wristbands and posting on the medical chart cover and elsewhere should occur.

Patients or surrogates may, of course, change their minds at any time regarding DNR orders. Physicians should revisit the decision process if and when improvement in the patient's condition occurs. Some institutions have a policy mandating review of DNR orders on a regular basis.

Many patients and families do not understand either the risks of complications of chest compressions (e.g., trauma to the heart, broken ribs, pneumothorax) or the limited chances of survival until discharge from the hospital, especially in chronically ill patients. Most often TV portrayals of CPR result in successful resuscitation as compared to the published statistics showing much less success.

Meaning of DNR

DNR means that in the case of spontaneous respiration ceasing and/or the heartbeat stopping, measures such as artificial ventilation, chest compressions, electrical defibrillation, and resuscitative doses of epinephrine and other drugs routinely administered according to CPR protocol, will not be employed. DNR may also mean "do not relax" in the sense that all other types of treatment will continue at their current level or may even be increased. This includes both life-supporting measures agreed upon by the patient and physician, and all measures for prevention of pain, anxiety, and other forms of suffering. Other life-supporting measures such as palliative surgery can occur in the presence of an existing DNR status [11].

Managing patients with DNR directives under emergency conditions

Emergency-care providers operate under the rules and laws mandating presumption of a patient's desire to be resuscitated unless and until there is solid evidence to the contrary, such as a living will or communication with a credible healthcare proxy who states that the patient's wishes are not to be resuscitated. Depending on state law and Emergency Medical Service (EMS) standards, a wrist band or other notification worn by the patient may be accepted by emergency medical providers as an indication that the patient does not wish to be resuscitated. Most states require that the band or notification include clear statement of DNR status along with the name(s) and contact number(s) of the person(s) who can verify the patient's wishes. In the presence of a valid DNR order, CPR should not be initiated, or if it is in progress, it should be stopped. Many states allow the honoring of DNR orders outside of the hospital and DNR orders may be "portable," that is, honored by EMS personnel during transport and by the medical and nursing staff at the receiving institution.

Managing patients with DNR directives for elective interventions

If a patient with a DNR order is to undergo anesthesia and surgery, the question of maintenance of the DNR order during the perioperative period arises. The American College of Surgeons issued a statement: recommending "required reconsideration" of prior DNR orders [12]. A new conversation with the patient or surrogate decision-maker should occur, emphasizing that there is added risk for a life-threatening event during the operation, but many such events are transient and correctable. Patients and families need to understand that surgical and anesthetic management of the patient during surgery usually necessitates use of certain procedures (e.g., tracheal intubation, mechanical ventilation, resuscitative drugs) that are components of CPR. Physicians and hospital personnel should work with the patient and family to reconsider the DNR decision during this time, rather than make an assumption either to suspend the DNR order or to maintain the order without the consent of the patient or the surrogate.

The American Society of Anesthesiologists' ethical guidelines suggest four options for managing DNR status or other directives limiting treatment during and immediately after invasive, risky interventions that can lead to cardiopulmonary arrest [13]. These options are discussed below.

Suspension of DNR

This option may be necessary for certain procedures during which it is standard, routine practice to employ multiple life-supporting techniques (e.g., open heart surgery). Generally speaking, the suspension is for the period of time of the procedure per se and continuing through the usual expected time for recovery from medications used to provide anesthesia, analgesia, and sedation. It also includes the usual time required for recovery from the acute insult of the intervention. There may be some concern about how this "time for recovery" is determined and whether there is consistency in implementing suspension timelines.

Some institutions mandate suspension of DNR status for any intervention because there is concern: (a) about the risks of malpractice claims and suits, and (b) the possibility that an anesthesiologist or anesthetist may hold back on the administration of medications for fear of being responsible for the patient's death. Such reluctance to provide drugs creates the risk of patient suffering due to awareness, anxiety, and pain during and after the intervention. For palliative procedures in patients with DNR status who are facing imminent death, we and many others believe that automatic suspension of DNR is inappropriate and contrary to the AMA Code of Ethics and Joint Commission directives.

Maintenance of DNR status

This may be appropriate for some patients who are undergoing palliative interventions for a terminal condition near the end of life. See below.

Modification of DNR status

The patient and/or the proxy for healthcare decisions may choose to negotiate with the physician about whether certain types of resuscitative measures might be suspended during an intervention. For example, if surgery is to be done under general anesthesia when it is routine to assist or support breathing mechanically with or without an endotracheal tube, the DNR order should be suspended. On the other hand, if ventricular fibrillation is not expected or would be rare under the conditions of the intervention, the patient may continue to refuse electrical defibrillation and chest compressions.

Goal-directed CPR

Under this method of management, the patient assents to the judgment of the physicians involved about the specific goals of the intervention. Temporary, easily reversible events (e.g., hypotension, bradycardia) would be treated as long as the specific goals of the intervention are achievable and outcomes unacceptable to the patient are unlikely. Should an outcome that the patient has determined to be unacceptable become apparent after the resuscitative measures are undertaken, continued resuscitative efforts would be discontinued according to the wishes and advance directives of the patient [14]. Many, if not most, anesthesiologists and surgeons would not relish undertaking this responsibility during the operation.

Palliative interventions

In regard to palliative interventions, it should be noted that while the physician accepts responsibility for a complication, there is no obligation to reverse the complication and its consequences, especially when the patient or surrogate has decided to maintain DNR status during a palliative intervention. The occurrence of an iatrogenic complication during a palliative intervention does *not* give the physician the right to override the patient's decision or to perform corrective interventions without the patient's consent [15]. If the physician is unsure about what to do, timely consultation with experienced colleagues and/or an ethics committee team may be helpful.

Most patients receiving end-of-life palliative (comfort) care have accepted the conclusion that they will die of their disease. Though DNR status is not a requirement for admission to hospice care, many patients receiving palliative care near the end of their lives have already decided that they do not want to be resuscitated should their breathing and/or circulation stop. Their DNR preferences may have been communicated through their advance directive or statements to their next of kin or proxy for healthcare decisions. A DNR order needs to be written to effect the patient's preference that resuscitative efforts be withheld.

Advance directives

Advance directives refer to any prior expression by a patient that is intended to guide care, should the patient no longer have decision-making capacity. Directives are a part of the advance care planning process that emphasizes communication about patient preferences with loved ones and healthcare professionals. This concept is founded ethically on the intent to protect the patient's autonomy, the ability of the patient to "govern" or to make decisions prospectively about their own care. Ideally, advance care planning (1) allows the patient to "think through" and communicate their values and preferences to his or her surrogate, family members, and physicians, and (2) it facilitates informed decision making should the patient no longer be able to guide his or her care. Such planning can catalyze family discussion and may minimize dissent at later time when difficult decisions need to be made.

The federal *Patient Self Determination Act of 1990* requires all healthcare facilities receiving Medicare and Medicaid funding to ask all patients whether they have advance directive documents and, if not, whether they wish to receive information about advance planning and to prepare such documents. There are two primary types of legally recognized advance directives:

1. The living will is a document that allows an individual to indicate in writing the interventions she or he would want and those that are not wanted if the individual is no longer able to make decisions. The living will is considered a limited document because in some states the patient's preferences can only be honored if the patient is facing particular medical conditions such as terminal illness or irreversible loss of cognition. The format of some living wills is that of a check-off list which limits the

flexibility of adjusting treatment decisions to the particular circumstances of the patient's condition at a given time.

2. Durable Power of Attorney for Health Care (DPAHC) or medical power of attorney is a more comprehensive document. It allows an individual to appoint another person (usually called an "agent" or "healthcare proxy" or "surrogate") to make any healthcare decisions should the individual lose decision-making capacity.

All 50 states and the District of Columbia have laws that recognize some form of advance directive. Some states have combined the living will and the DPAHC into one advance directive document [9]. Published studies estimate that about 15% of the US population currently has some form of advance directive [9,16]. More recent estimates claim that approximately 25% of US citizens have advance directives.

The utilization of advance directive documents is somewhat controversial and inconsistent in actual practice. Hard copies of the documents must be readily available and family members may not know where they are kept, or even that they exist. Unless the documents are physically present, they cannot be honored. Even when directives are available, they may not contain enough specific information to help surrogates or healthcare professionals make decisions in the immediate context. At the present time, legal directives are often "state specific," meaning that institutions may not be willing to allow a directive to be implemented unless it follows the statutory format recognized in the state where the facility is located. Some state laws allow for forms from other states to be honored. Several groups have worked to create a universal form of advance directive that can easily be recognized and honored across state lines, but such an effort would require changes to the law in many states.

There is some evidence that directives are less likely to be honored if either the treating physician or family disagrees with the patient's preferences expressed in the directive [17]. Communication about the documents, in advance, is essential for surrogates to feel empowered to act on behalf of the patient and for clinicians to understand the patient's wishes. The discussions with physicians and other healthcare professionals that may result from the writing of an advance directive may be more important than the information recorded in the document.

Philosophically, it can be questioned whether any written directive will accurately reflect the preferences of the person when the need to implement the directive actually arises. Patients may change their preferences as a chronic illness progresses or at the point when a medical problem arises. Though imperfect, advance care planning does provide the opportunity to consider one's own values and to communicate them to clinicians and loved ones. Ideally, one's thinking should be revisited regularly and the written and verbal directives revised accordingly.

Therapeutic trials, including surgery and other interventions

Medicine has been described as the science of uncertainty and the art of probability. It is impossible to know with certainty the outcome of any treatment prospectively, whether or not a treatment will be successful, or whether or not complications will occur. There is almost always a statistically based, benefit-to-burden ratio, and the burdens include complications from the intervention or lack of success leading to permanent disabilities or death. Statistical estimates of risks apply to selected groups of patients and cannot be used with certainty to predict the outcome for any individual patient. The teaching point remains: "Never say never or always in medicine."

Faced with these uncertainties, the physician nevertheless has an obligation to provide the patient with a realistic assessment based on group data, statistical estimates, and the physician's personal experience with patients in similar circumstances [3]. The only way to determine whether or not a treatment will be successful or not and whether complications will occur or not, is to do a therapeutic trial. As Sir William Osler said, "Every treatment is an experiment."

In considering such a trial, it is wise for the patient to answer three questions [18,19]:

What are *my* goals for this intervention?

What disabilities & burdens are unacceptable to *me*?

What alternatives exist for *me*?

The intervention should have a realistic chance of achieving the patient's goals, which might range from full restoration of independent function to something as simple as being able to sit in a chair and communicate with grandchildren and other family members and friends.

Most patients do not have realistic and comprehensive appreciation for the impact of disabilities on their quality of everyday life. When patients begin to experience the practical consequences of confinement to a wheelchair or other losses of independence or function, they may find the degree of disability to be unacceptable or they may find sources of support as they adapt to a new phase of life. In addition to changes in physical function, patients may need support in dealing with chronic weakness, fatigue, and/or depression. Along with other members of the health team, the physician has an obligation to help the patient to understand the potential consequences if an intervention is not completely successful.

Ideally, primary care physicians would be compensated for their time in discussing anticipated goals of treatment as well as end-of-life issues with their patients while they retain their decision-making capacity. Healthcare reform proposals under the Obama administration originally proposed to pay physicians for their time spent in such discussions once yearly with each patient, but political claims that this portion of the proposal would create "death panels" resulted in deletion of this item in the final form of the *2010 Patient Protection and Affordable Care Act* later amended as the *Health Care and Education Reconciliation Act of 2010*.

From the physician's point of view, the benefit-to-burden ratio must be high enough to justify offering to provide the treatment. Each physician has to decide what ratio is acceptable for him or herself. It should be noted that, as a group, physicians tend to overestimate the burdens of disabilities compared with patients' estimates [20]. Also, patients often change their opinions about the burdens of disabilities as they experience them and learn to make adjustments to them.

In ethical terms, "the moral burden of proof often should be heavier when the decision is to withhold than when it is to withdraw treatments" [1]. "Only after starting treatments will it be possible in many cases . . . to balance prospective benefits and burdens" [1].

In the case of a surgical trial, the defined benefits must outweigh the potential disabilities in terms of their importance to the patient, but this assessment might not parallel the statistical chance of occurrence. For example, if a patient finds her current state of chronically poor health completely unacceptable, it would be appropriate for the patient to choose a 25% chance of improvement even if the risks of death and disability are considerably higher. The ethical basis of this approach is the principle of double effect in which the improved health condition is intended and the risks of complications and death are recognized and accepted, but not intended [1,19,21]. A therapeutic trial, even with a high risk of death, is not euthanasia or physician-assisted suicide.

In practical terms, a surgical trial includes a period of time after the operation to determine what the likely outcome will be for the patient. In the presence of progressive improvement, continuation of life-supporting measures is indicated. However, the patient, healthcare proxy, family members, and friends in collaboration with the physicians providing care should also discuss the willingness to discontinue futile therapies, including vital function-supporting measures if the patient is unlikely to realize his or her stated goals, deterioration of health status is progressive, and multiple organ systems failure ensues. It has been stated that ". . . trial interventions coupled with hard-nosed clinical realism, may appropriately balance the possibilities for good or ill . . ." [22].

If the physician believes that the benefit-to-burden ratio is not justifiable for an intervention that the patient or family is demanding, the physician must follow his/her own values and judgment and refuse to provide or to participate in the intervention. In maintaining an ongoing therapeutic relationship with the patient, the physician could offer an alternative treatment, refer the patient to another physician, or if the requested treatment is felt to be medically "futile," appeal to an institutional mechanism for dealing with medically non-indicated interventions. (See section on futility below.)

Methods for assessment of the patient's condition and prognosis

Over the years, particularly in the 1980s and 1990s, scoring systems [23,24] have been developed in an attempt to express severity of illness numerically as a means of summarizing and publicizing data, conducting clinical research, measuring and comparing outcomes of treatments, and in the last 10–15 years especially, to provide an objective measure of the benefits of healthcare expenditures. Clinical scoring systems combined with laboratory measures have been correlated individually (univariate analysis) and collectively (multivariate analysis) with outcomes (e.g., benefits of treatment, progression of disease). Such correlations have been expanded into mathematical models intended to assess the risks of morbidity and mortality and to predict short and long-term outcomes for precisely defined groups of patients. For example, a cardiac surgeon considering a cardiac operation for a particular patient can go online to complete the Society of Thoracic Surgeons' questionnaire and obtain a risk score for that patient. Although some of the scoring systems have proven to be quite reliable in predicting outcomes for a particular group of patients with particular characteristics, no system has been able to predict the outcome for any individual patient. There is always residual uncertainty even with the most elaborate mathematical models. But such models may enhance the individual physician's clinical judgment in making treatment or non-treatment decisions for individual patients, and research continues to improve their precision and ease of use at the patient's bedside.

In regard to clinical judgments about critically ill patients in the ICU setting, the effectiveness of prediction models in facilitating decisions about continuing or withdrawing life-supporting measures still remains questionable (e.g., see SUPPORT, Study to Understand Prognosis and Preferences for Outcomes and Risks of Treatments [25]).

One rather simple, easily remembered correlation between the dysfunction of one or more organ systems and in-hospital mortality was elaborated by Knaus and Wagner in 1989 [26]. The basis of their correlations was the precise definition of each organ system's failure (Table 6.1a) and the impact of failure of one or more organ systems on 5,248 patients in 13 US and 27 French hospitals. With the failure of three or more organ systems over a 7-day period, 103 of 105 patients died in hospital (Table 6.1b). This simple correlation has been very useful for an intensive care physician in (1) organizing clinical impressions, (2) documenting the patient's status and likely outcome in the medical record, and (3) communicating prognosis and discussing options with the family members and friends of the patient. The correlation has been particularly useful in supporting the decision of the healthcare proxy and family members when they have chosen to avoid introducing major new interventions, to establish a DNR status, and to withdraw vital function supporting measures.

Table 6.1a Definitions of organ system failure (French definition when different).

If the patient had one or more of the following during a 24-hour period (regardless of values), organ system failure (OSF) existed on that day.

Cardiovascular failure (presence of one or more of the following):
Heart rate ≤ 54/min
Mean arterial blood pressure ≤ 49 mmHg (systolic blood pressure < 60 mmHg)
Occurrence of ventricular tachycardia and/or ventricular fibrillation
Serum pH ≤ 7.24 with a P_aCO_2 of ≤ 49 mmHg

Respiratory failure (presence of one or more of the following):
Respiratory rate ≤ 5/min or ≥ 49/min
P_aCO_2 ≥ 50 mmHg
A_aDO_2 ≥ 350 mmHg; $A_aDO_2 = 713 F_1O_2 - P_aCO_2 - P_2O_2$
Dependent on ventilator or CPAP on the second day of OSF (i.e., not applicable the initial 24 hours of OSF)

Renal failure (presence of one or more of the following):
Urine output ≤ 479 mL/24 hours or ≤ 159 mL/8 hours
Serum BUN ≥100 mg/100 mL (> 36 micromoles/L)
Serum creatinine ≥ 3.5 mg/100 mL (> 310 micromoles/L)

Hematologic failure (presence of one or more of the following):
WBC ≤ 1000 cu mm
Platelets ≤ 20 000 cu mm
Hematocrit ≤ 20%

Neurologic failure
Glasgow Coma Score ≤ 6 (in absence of sedation)

Table 6.1b. Multiple organ dysfunction.

Number of organs	Days	Mortality
1	1	20/40%
1	7	25/50%
> 3	1	80%[a]
> 3	7	~100%[a]

Note: [a] no difference </> 65 years.
Source: (n = 2,843 + 2,405) [26].

The findings of Knaus and Wagner [26] have been replicated and elaborated in multiple publications [23,27], which seek to answer the question: "What can physicians do versus what should physicians do?" [28].

Patient preferences

In US healthcare decision-making there is a strong tradition of respect for the preferences of the patient. This respect for patient autonomy is deeply rooted in an American history noted for liberty interests, civil rights, and an emphasis on consumer rights including patients' rights. In this environment there is a strong presumption of aggressive intervention and continuation of treatment, with patients or families often expecting physicians to comply with treatment requests regardless of their anticipated medical effectiveness.

Surveys indicate that many Americans support limits to aggressive treatment when individuals are dealing with serious illness or end-of-life decisions [9,29]. Many citizens prefer to die peacefully and with dignity at home, avoid pain and suffering, prevent dependence on machines, family members and others, and avoid depleting financial resources of the family and their estates. However, few people prospectively define wishes or formulate advance directives [29]. Death is a feared and taboo subject for discussion among the healthy. As Morrie Schwartz said in *Tuesdays with Morrie*, "Everyone knows they are going to die, but nobody believes it . . . If we did, we would do things differently" [30].

Information about the anticipated course of illness and options for treatment are essential to setting goals with the patient and family. Patients and their family members need to be informed not only about the chances of success and the risks of death of an intervention, but also about the intermediary path the patient will take with or without the intervention, the quality of life, the risks of more or less permanent disabilities, and what sources of support will be available to help the patient along this course.

Withholding and withdrawing life-sustaining treatment

The AMA Council on Ethical and Judicial Affairs defines life-sustaining treatment as "any treatment that serves to prolong life without reversing the underlying medical disease" [31]. Foregoing life-sustaining treatment is ethically, medically, and legally permissible under certain circumstances. Support for the concept comes from multiple medical, nursing, and ethics organizations, as well as from the 1983 President's Commission for the Study of Ethical Problems in Medicine and Biomedical and Behavioral Research [32–35]. One national survey from 1994–1995 indicates that 75% of ICU deaths occurred following a decision to withhold or withdraw some type of life-sustaining treatment [36].

As discussed earlier, respect for patient autonomy requires physicians to respect the patient's own decision to refuse any intervention or to have it withdrawn if the patient has the capacity to decide. If the patient can no longer speak for him or herself, physicians turn first to advance directives and, if those are absent, to surrogate decision-makers. Surrogates are ethically and legally given the right to represent the patient, either through substituted judgment – indicating their knowledge of what the patient would have wanted in the current circumstance – or determining what they believe to be in the best interests of the patient. Surrogate decisions should be honored unless the clinician has valid reason(s) to believe the decision is not what the patient would have wanted or could not "reasonably be judged to be in the patient's best interests."

Many ethicists believe there is no ethically significant difference between withholding and withdrawing treatment from a patient. If important reasons exist to consider withholding an intervention in the first place, but the decision is made to begin treatment, the same rationale would support withdrawing treatment at a later time. Beginning treatment may be permissible and desirable if one anticipates gaining new information about its effectiveness that will clarify future decisions. Removal of a treatment should be considered if the patient's condition indicates that its continuation no longer benefits the patient. In their text, *Clinical Ethics*, ethicists Albert Jonsen, Mark Siegler, and William Winslade state that if we cannot advance the interests of the patient and no goal of medicine is achievable, no duty to treat exists [2,36]. Merely sustaining organic life is not a goal of medicine; often it is only prolonging death.

Futility

Multiple attempts have been made to define the controversial concept of what constitutes a medically futile intervention. Some have attempted a narrow definition such as: "an intervention that has no pathophysiological rationale" [Dr. Bernard Lo] or "an intervention that merely prolongs the dying process." Others like Dr. Laurence Schneiderman attempted a quantitative definition, claiming that a treatment that has been unsuccessful in the last 100 similar cases should be considered "futile." Most professional association guidelines that discuss futile treatment incorporate the concept that these treatments provide no medical benefit to the patient, based on the patient's own values and goals [37].

Yet, there is a sense, even if no consensus definition can be found, that there ought to be limits to treatments that will not meet reasonable medical goals for the patient or will impose unreasonable pain and suffering on the patient. Often the ethical conflict in these cases is between (1) respect for patient autonomy or a surrogate's assessment of what is in the patient's best interest and (2) respect for professional integrity of the clinicians who object to continuing treatment that is perceived to violate professional duty. Communication that identifies the common interests of all involved and focuses on patient goals and values is essential and may lead to resolution.

For situations in which agreement between the patient or surrogate and the physician cannot be reached, the AMA Council on Ethical and Legal Affairs recommends that all healthcare institutions have a medical futility policy that provides for a "fair process" approach to decision-making (Figure 6.1) [31,38].

For an institution, such a process would include a written policy that is published and readily accessible to all parties, a standing committee with public representatives; inclusion of second opinions and external review; support for and inclusion of surrogate decision-makers throughout; and exploration of patient transfer options. If the process ends with a recommendation against continued treatment, "the intervention . . . need not be provided."

An example of such a process exists in the *Guidelines on Medically Inappropriate Interventions*, jointly agreed to by Houston-area hospitals [38]. (In fact the AMA policy draws heavily on the Houston experience.) The Houston guidelines were codified in Texas state law in 1999 under the Texas Health and Safety Code (166.046), which allows for life-sustaining treatment to be withdrawn 10 days after the patient or surrogate receives a written explanation of the decision that treatment is considered "medically inappropriate." Proponents claim that the process, including ethics consultation, has allowed families to accept treatment limitations, many prior to the 10-day notice period [39]. There have been several high-profile cases in recent years that have led to proposed changes in the Texas law. In recent legislative sessions there were attempts to revise the duration of the 10-day notice, require

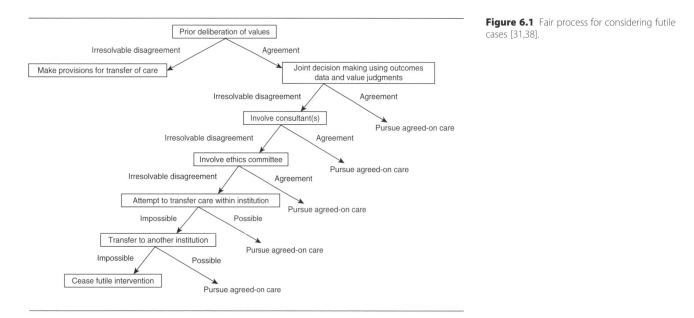

Figure 6.1 Fair process for considering futile cases [31,38].

"treat to transfer" requirements, or limit the ability for withdrawal of treatment against surrogate wishes, but these bills failed.

The state of Virginia also has a state medical futility statute [Virginia Code – Health Decisions Act 54.1–2990] stating that physicians are not required to provide treatment felt to be "medically or ethically inappropriate." There have been two cases to date testing the futility statute in Virginia. One case (Baby K in 1994) supported continued treatment of a child with anencephaly based on the preemption of the futility statute by the federal EMTALA (Emergency Medical Treatment and Active Labor Act). The other case (Bryan vs Rectors and Visitors of the University of Virginia 1996) clarified that EMTALA only required stabilization of the patient in respiratory distress, not continued treatment. Further legal tests in Virginia and Texas are expected in attempts to clarify futility statutes [40].

As of 2008 there were 11 states with laws that provide a process for resolution when there is a conflict between the health team and the patient (or surrogate) about whether to withhold or withdraw treatment [41]. Some of these laws do not utilize the concept of futility explicitly, while other states adopt this language.

The American Medical Association's Council on Ethical and Judicial Affairs: indicates that "Physicians are not ethically obligated to deliver care that, in their best professional judgment, will not have a reasonable chance of benefiting their patients. Patients should not be given treatments simply because they demand them. Denial of treatment should be justified by reliance on openly stated ethical principles and acceptable standards of care . . . not on the concept of 'futility,' which cannot be meaningfully defined" [31].

Comfort care/palliative care and hospice

Diane Meier, Director of the Center to Advance Palliative Care, defines palliative care as "interdisciplinary care that aims to relieve suffering and improve quality of life for patients with advanced illness and their families" [42]. The Joint Commission standard on care at the end-of-life [43] reflects a multidimensional understanding of palliative care, as does the World Health Organization's definition of palliative care, including [44]:

- Provides relief from pain and other symptoms.
- Affirms life and recognizes dying as a normal process and part of life.
- Neither hastens nor postpones death.
- Integrates psychological and spiritual care.
- Supports the patient's living as actively as possible until death.
- Utilizes an interdisciplinary team approach.
- Provides a support system for the family.
- Enhances quality of life if possible.
- Is compatible with life-prolonging therapies.

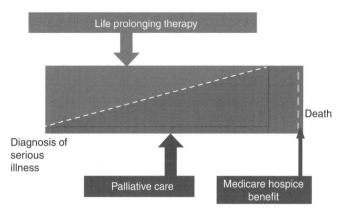

Figure 6.2 Palliative care's place in the course of illness [42].

Palliative care can be "offered *simultaneous with all other appropriate medical treatment*." [42]. Central to this concept is that palliative care can and should be offered early in the course of treatment, rather than be seen as a care alternative that is only offered after curative treatment has been exhausted.

Figure 6.2 demonstrates that palliative care begins at the point of diagnosis with serious illness and is provided along with life-supporting interventions. Through the course of illness, the proportion of interventions of a palliative nature is likely to increase as life-supporting interventions are continued. If restorative interventions are not successful, the patient may reach a point beyond which palliative care alone is provided until the patient dies and bereavement begins.

The good news at present is that resources to provide palliative care support in acute-care settings to patients, families, and healthcare teams is growing rapidly [16,45]. In-hospital hospice units are beginning to emerge. In-service educational programs about pain control in the dying patient have become more prevalent.

When a patient and family are ready to move away from aggressive, restorative therapies and the healthcare team believes that life expectancy is 6 months or less, Medicare patients become eligible for hospice benefits [46]. Hospice care can be provided in the patient's home, a hospice facility, or in a long-term care facility. Hospice benefits may include physicians, nurses, chaplains, and social services; physical and occupational therapy; medical supplies and equipment; respite care; outpatient prescription medications for pain and other symptoms. The number of patients choosing hospice has increased dramatically over the last two decades, with an estimated 41.6% of deaths in the USA in 2009 involving those who were receiving hospice care, according to the National Hospice and Palliative Care Organization. The average length of stay in 2010 was 69 days and several studies now conclude that patients electing hospice care live longer than those not receiving hospice care [47,48].

The multidisciplinary benefits of hospice care cannot be fully realized by the patient and family if referrals are made too close to death. A 2010 study of patients with lung cancer concluded that patients who received palliative care early in their course lived 23.3% longer than patients who started palliative care later [49]. Of course, patients and families require time to make the decision to forego curative interventions. Physician willingness to discuss options for end-of-life care can have a positive influence on patients and families. However, some physicians are reluctant to make referrals possibly because they feel that to do so is signifying treatment failure, patient abandonment, or loss of hope for the patient.

Some physicians do not feel well-informed about end-of-life care options. In a 1993 study of oncologists by Von Roenn *et al.* [50], the findings were:

- 86% of respondents thought that the majority of patients were under-medicated.
- 49% rated pain control in their own practice as fair to very poor.
- 73% evaluated their own training in pain management as fair to very poor.

In a 1998 survey of oncologists by the American Society of Clinical Oncology [51] less than one-third of respondents indicated their training was very helpful in introducing hospice or palliative care, coordinating end-of-life care or communicating with patients near the end of life.

It is not clear that these deficiencies have been fully rectified, but progress is being made in the increased number of palliative care programs and the inclusion of palliative care training in medical schools. Hospice and Palliative Medicine was recognized as an official medical subspecialty by the American Board of Medical Specialties in 2006. Diane Meier, Director of the Center to Advance Palliative Care, has reviewed several palliative care programs utilizing patient/family satisfaction variables and cost-savings factors at Mt. Sinai Hospital in New York City, Kaiser Permanente hospitals, the Ireland Cancer Center, Virginia Commonwealth University, and University of Michigan [52]. The direct discussion of care options, including the option of having the patient's remaining life focused on comfort and time with loved ones rather than on restorative interventions, may be one of the most significant and remembered events in the patient–family–physician relationships. Palliative care in hospitals increases appropriate referrals to hospice care in a hospital's hospice unit, in a nursing home, or in the home of the patient or family, improves continuity of care as the patient is transferred to a new venue, and supports patients and families at a difficult time. Palliative care may also lower expenditures by hospitals and payers by reducing hospital and ICU lengths of stay and direct costs (e.g., laboratory fees, drugs).

Delivering bad news

Bad news comes in a variety of forms: a serious diagnosis with a poor prognosis, treatment complications, less than successful or expected outcomes of interventions, and death itself, especially when it is unanticipated. No one likes to deliver bad news, but

Table 6.2 Delivering bad news.

Compose message – accuracy, consistency

Plan meeting – who, when, setting

Understand your own biases, feelings

Language – concern, empathy, verbal, body

Acknowledge strong reactions, discuss them

Tolerate silence

Achieve common understanding

Follow-up – chart, care team, family

physicians have the obligation to tell the truth and to disclose the facts, as they are known. At the present time, few physicians have been trained in delivering bad news, and they are not comfortable doing so for a number of reasons including their reluctance to give up their view of death as a medical failure, and their lack of preparation for and inability to control the highly variable reactions of patients and family members. Some suggestions for planning and executing the delivery of bad news are shown in Table 6.2 [53]. More detailed discussions of the "do's and dont's" can be found in the literature [52].

Disclosure of medical errors

Beginning with the publication in 2000 of the Institute of Medicine's *To Err is Human*, there has been an increasingly intense focus on medical errors, how to prevent them, and what should be done when they occur [54]. The presumption ethically is that an error should be disclosed to a patient and/or the family; disclosure is based on the principles of respect for patients and truth-telling. However, there is trepidation about disclosure of errors because physicians are concerned about malpractice suits and increasingly larger awards to plaintiffs. Accumulating evidence indicates that attempts to hide errors actually increase the numbers of suits and drive up punitive payouts to injured patients (http://www.med.umich.edu/patientsafetytoolkit/disclosure.htm). Policies supporting full disclosure of errors, the issuing of apologies and, when warranted, prompt financial compensation has been followed by significant reductions in the numbers of malpractice claims and suits as well as a marked decrease in legal costs [55].

An increasing number of institutions are adopting full-disclosure policies based on ethical obligations and mandates to do so from federal and state governments, Joint Commission, and consumer activism [56,57].

It is recognized that the wall of silence that has characterized medical errors undermines trust, ignores patient autonomy, stifles safety advancement, and exacerbates the legal, economic, and public relations problems related to subsequent discovery of non-disclosure. Ignoring or denying culpability is known to increase malpractice risks because many patients and their families sense that something has gone wrong, and the failure to have mistakes disclosed to them by the healthcare

Table 6.3 Serious reportable events.

Surgical: wrong operation, foreign object retained, unexpected death

Products, devices: contamination, unintended use, air embolism

Patient protection: missing, +/− suicide, discharge to wrong person

Care errors: meds, blood reaction, glucose, pressure ulcers (obstetrics, pediatrics)

Environment: restraints, fall, burn, shock

Criminal: assault, abduction, impersonator

providers breaches trust and leads patients and families to seek legal counsel to initiate a claim or suit. The major serious reportable events are listed in Table 6.3.

Several points bear special emphasis. The accurate and complete reporting of facts is required, but speculation about the mechanism of injury and who may be responsible should be avoided. Early in the period after an error, the complete facts are not yet fully known or integrated. Coincidence-in-time is not proof of a cause-and-effect relationship. There are numerous cases in which a complication has been attributed to someone's action when it is ultimately demonstrated beyond doubt that the particular action did not contribute to the injury. Therefore, avoid the "blame game."

It is very important for the physicians, nurses, and others involved in the patient's care to have a common understanding of the facts and to maintain a consistent message. This is often difficult to do, because as the message is passed from one person to another in a series of individuals, the message changes and the original facts of the case may be distorted. Hence, it may be beneficial to have a primary spokesman to lead discussions with the patient and family.

Physicians are human beings, and like everyone else, they can make mistakes of judgment and despite their best efforts, their skills may fail them occasionally. It is ethically both appropriate and laudable for them to accept responsibility for and acknowledge an error or mistake. In many cases, the patient and family members see the concerned and apologetic physician as a human being who is taking responsibility for his or her actions. Families report appreciation for the physician's efforts to minimize the consequences of the mistake, to keep them informed about ongoing investigations, and to implement measures to prevent future repetition of the error. These efforts indicate respect and enhance the physician–patient relationship and often reduce the feelings of anger and abandonment that patients and families experience.

Definition of death

There are two basic definitions of death. Irreversible cessation of circulatory and respiratory function is defined as cardiopulmonary death, and it is the most widely understood and accepted definition of death [58].

However, a second definition is needed because drugs and machines can support circulation and breathing indefinitely, making it impossible to rely on traditional vital signs. Also, concerns about the limited supply of organs for transplantation, and the benefit of harvesting organs during or immediately after cessation of the circulation of oxygenated blood has supported the development of a neurological definition widely referred to as "brain death" [59]. A 1981 Presidential Commission formulated the Uniform Determination of Death Act (UDDA), which incorporates both definitions of death. At least 40 states have adopted the UDDA as a legally acceptable means of determining death, which under this definition is characterized as the "irreversible cessation of all brain functions including the brainstem" [59,60,61]. All states have a judicial or statutory acceptance of brain death [62]. Brain death does not include irreversible coma or a persistent vegetative state.

The neurological definition remains controversial for metaphysical, cultural, legal, and even medical reasons. The basic problem is that the term death typically applies to whole organisms and not to the loss of function in any single organ, even the brain. The neurological definition is not accepted by all cultures, religions, and governments [63]. It leads to questions such as: When is a person really dead? Is brain death a separate type of death that occurs before "real" death? A woman who is brain dead can continue to support fetal growth until successful birth. A brain-dead child continues to grow. All of this creates a suspicion that death is "malleable" and can be adjusted for utilitarian purposes (e.g., organ donation) that contributes to ambivalence among those facing a decision about organ donation [58,59].

There are specific clinical criteria for brain death (Table 6.4), and these criteria must be met through the assessment of two physicians (usually including one neurologist) who complete independent evaluations of the patient separated by some time interval. There are also a number of confirmatory tests for the determination of brain death (Table 6.4) [60,61].

Once brain death has been declared, the common practice today is to inform the patient's family of the fact and to inform the family that aggressive support measures are no longer appropriate. Though the family should not be given the false choice of whether vital function support should be withdrawn, the family should be asked what they would like to happen before withdrawal of vital function support occurs (e.g., time for other family members to arrive, organ donation to be discussed with family, religious traditions observed). Physicians are ethically justified in discontinuing the vital function support at any time as such support is no longer medically appropriate, but it is respectful and compassionate to allow some time (e.g., hours to perhaps days) to accommodate the patient's previously expressed wishes and the family's reasonable requests.

Medical insurance does not cover continuing to support a legally dead patient and the hospital may have a policy about when support should be discontinued. In the case of

Table 6.4 Clinical criteria for brain death.

Absence of:
  Motor responses
  Pupillary responses to light
  Corneal reflexes
  Caloric responses
  Gag reflex
  Coughing during tracheal suctioning
  Respiratory drive at a $P_aCO_2 \geq 60$ mmHg or 20 mmHg
  above patient's baseline
  Pupils at dilation midpoint (4–6 mm)
  Confirmatory tests
  Cerebral angiography
  EEG
  Transcranial Doppler
  Cerebral scintillography

delay required for arranging organ harvesting for transplantation, the United Network for Organ Sharing (UNOS) reimburses the hospital for expenditures after brain death is declared.

Efforts to define brain death continue to raise questions. Biological activity persists for a time after heartbeat and breathing stop; the same is true of the brain which cannot exert its sensing and controlling functions. Should brain death be defined as "total brain necrosis?" Many clinicians believe that permanent unconsciousness negates personhood. Without the potential for thought, the basis of personal identity is lost. Death is a process, a chain of events, before which the patient is fully alive and at the end of which the patient is fully dead. Dying in days or weeks is not the same as "dead." A rigid

definition of death is the irreversible cessation of all integrated functioning of the human *organism* as a whole – mental and physical.

Physicians and other healthcare personnel should be aware of these issues as they address family members and friends of patients who cannot recover independent function and for whom continuing life-support measures appear medically futile. Morrie Schwartz, the subject of the book, *Tuesdays with Morrie*, said to Ted Koppel on *Nightline*, "For me, Ted, living means I can be responsive to the other person. It means I can show my emotions and my feelings. Talk to them. Feel with them . . . When that is gone, Morrie is gone" [30]. Physicians and patients may believe that we should prolong a life that is or can be meaningful, but that it is quite different from prolonging death with its associated suffering. We need to be prepared to discuss these concerns openly with our patients and their families.

Summary

In this chapter, we have attempted to address the most frequently encountered ethical issues that relate directly to the patient facing a surgical operation or other major intervention. Because these interventions entail potential benefits for the patient as well as risks of disability and death, decisions to proceed are often complicated and careful communication with patient and family is vital. Working to establish common goals based on informed understanding and appreciation for values and beliefs will often help everyone involved reach a consensus about how the care of the patient will proceed. Ethical considerations are central to the clinical management of our patients.

References

1. Beauchamp TL, Childress JF. *Principles of Bioethics*. 6th edn. New York, NY: Oxford University Press; 2008.

2. Jonsen AR, Siegler M, Winslade WJ. *Clinical Ethics: A Practical Approach to Ethical Decisions in Clinical Medicine*. 6th edn. New York, NY: McGraw-Hill; 2006.

3. Christakis NA. *Death Foretold; Prophecy and Prognosis in Medical Care*. Chicago, IL: University of Chicago Press; 1999.

4. ACGME Outcomes Project. www.ACGME.org.

5. Appelbaum PS, Grisso T. Assessing patient's capacities to consent to treatment. *N Engl J Med* 1988; **319**: 1635–8.

6. Appelbaum PS, Grisso T. The MacArthur Treatment Competency Study, I: mental illness and competence

to consent to treatment. *Law Hum Behav* 1995; **19**: 105–26.

7. Venesy BA. A clinician's guide to decision making capacity and ethically sound medical decisions. *Am J Phys Med Rehabil* 1994; **73**: 219–26.

8. National Commission for the Protection of Human Subject of Biomedical and Behavioral Research. *The Belmont Report.* (Washington, DC: DHEW Publication 0578–0012; 1978). Salgo v. Stanford University Board of Trustees, 154 Cal. App. 2d560; 1957. Canterburg v. Spence, 464 F.2d 772 (D.C. Cir. 1972).

9. *Last Acts. Means to a Better End: A Report on Dying in America Today.* 2002; www.rwjf.org; http://www.rwjf.org/pr/product.jsp?id=15788pdf

10. Sabatino CP. Survey of State EMS-DNR Laws and Protocols. *J Law Med Ethics* 1999; **27**: 297–315.

11. AMA Council on Ethical and Legal Affairs. Opinion no. 2.22. Do-not-resuscitate orders. In *Code of Medical Ethics, Current Opinions*. Chicago, IL: American Medical Association; 1999, pp. 67–9.

12. Statement of the American College of Surgeons on Advance Directives by Patients. "Do not resuscitate" in the operating room. *Am Coll Surg Bull* 1994; **79**(9): 29.

13. American Society of Anesthesiologists. Ethical guidelines for the anesthesia care of patients with do-not-resuscitate orders or other directives that limit treatment. *ASA Standards, Guidelines and Statements*; www.ASAhq.org.

14. Truog RD, Waisel DB, Burns JP. DNR in the OR: a goal-directed approach. *Anesthesiology* 1999; **90**: 289–95.

15. Casarett D, Ross LF. Overriding a patient's refusal of treatment after an

iatrogenic complication. *N Engl J Med* 1997; **336**: 1908–10.

16. Schwartz CE, Wheeler B, Hammes B *et al*. Early intervention in planning end-of-life care with ambulatory geriatric patients. *Arch Int Med* 2002; **162**: 1611–18.

17. Kinlaw K, Trotochaud K, Thompson N. End of Life Care Practices: A Survey of Organizational Members of the Health Care Ethics Consortium of Georgia. January 2001; 11–12.

18. Hug CC Jr. End-of-life issues and the anesthesiologist. *Int Anesthesiol Clin* 2001; **39**(3): 35–52.

19. Hug CC Jr: Surgical interventions near the end of life: therapeutic trials. In Van Norma GA, ed. *Clinical Ethics in Anesthesiology: A Case-based Textbook.* New York, NY: Cambridge University Press; 2011, pp. 92–6.

20. Leplege A, Hunt S. The problem of quality of life in medicine. *J Am Med Assoc* 1997; **278**: 47–50.

21. Didzinski DM. The principle of double effect in palliative care: euthanasia by another name? In Van Norma GA, ed. *Clinical Ethics in Anesthesiology: A Case-based Textbook.* New York, NY: Cambridge University Press; 2011, pp. 88–91.

22. Ware S, Milch R, Weaver WL *et al*. Care of dying patients. In McCullough L, Jones JW, Brody BA, eds. *Surgical Ethics.* New York, NY: Oxford University Press; 1998, p. 182.

23. Knaus WA, Wagner DP, Draper EA *et al*. (1991). The APACHE III prognostic system. Risk prediction of hospital mortality for critically ill hospitalized adults. *Chest* 1991; **100**: 1619–36.

24. Goldman L, Caldera DL, Nussbaum SR *et al*. Multifactorial index of cardiac risk in non-cardiac surgical procedures. *N Engl J Med* 1977; **297**: 845–50.

25. The SUPPORT Principal Investigators. A controlled trial to improve care for seriously ill hospitalized patients; The Study to Understand Prognoses and Preferences for Outcomes and Risks of Treatment (SUPPORT). *J Am Med Assoc* 1995; **274**: 1591–8.

26. Knaus WA, Wagner DP. Multiple systems organ failure: epidemiology and prognosis. *Crit Care Clinics* 1989; **5**: 221–32.

27. Walter LC, Brand RJ, Counsell SR *et al*. Development and validation of a prognostic index for 1-year mortality in older adults after hospitalization. *J Am Med Assoc* 2001; **285**: 2987–94.

28. Hug CC Jr. Rovenstine lecture: patient values, Hippocrates, science and technology: what we (physicians) can do versus should do for the patient. *Anesthesiology* 2000; **93**: 556–64.

29. Pew Research Center for the People & the Press. January 5, 2006. Survey report. *More Americans Discussing – and Planning – End-of-Life Treatment: Strong Public Support for Right to Die.* http://people-press.org/files/legacy-pdf/266.pdf.

30. Albom M. *Tuesdays with Morrie, An Old Man, A Young Man, and Life's Greatest Lesson.* New York, NY: Doubleday; 1997, pp. 80–81, 162.

31. AMA Council on Ethical and Judicial Affairs. Opinion no. 2.03, Allocation of limited medical resources; Opinion no. 2.035, Futile Care. June 1994; Opinion no. 2.037, Medical futility in end-of-life care; Opinion no. 2.20, Withholding or withdrawing life-sustaining medical treatment. In *Code of Medical Ethics, Current Opinions.* Chicago, IL: AMA; 1998.

32. *Guidelines on Termination of Life-Sustaining Treatment and the Care of the Dying.* Briarcliff Manor, NY: The Hasting Center; 1987.

33. Task Force on Ethics of the Society of Critical Care Medicine. Consensus report on the ethics of foregoing life-sustaining treatments in the critically ill. *Crit Care Med* 1990; **18**: 1435–9.

34. American Nurses Association. Foregoing Nutrition and Hydration (1992), and Promotion of Comfort and Relief of Pain in Dying Patients (1991). Code of ethics for nurses with interpretive statements, Provision 1. (12/14/09). http://www.nursingworld.org/readroom/position/ethics.

35. The President's Commission for the Study of Ethical Problems in Medicine and Biomedical and Behavioral Research Deciding to Forego Life-Sustaining Treatment. Washington, DC: US Government Priority Office; 1983.

36. Prendergrast TJ, Claessens MT, Luce JM. A national survey of end of life care for critically ill patients. *Am J Respir Crit Care Med* 1998; **158**: 1163–7.

37. American College of Emergency Physicians. Nonbeneficial ("Futile") Emergency Medical Interventions. www.acep.org/sitemap/to policy statements.

38. Halevy A, Brody BA. For the Houston City-Wide Task Force on Medical Futility: a multi-institution collaborative policy on medical futility. *J Am Med Assoc* 1996; **276**: 571–4.

39. Fine, R. Tackling medical futility in Texas. *N Engl J Med* 2007; **357**: 1558–9.

40. Futility Court Cases: In re Baby K, 16 F.3d 590 (4th Cir.), *cert. denied*, 115 S. Ct. 91, 1994. Bryan vs. Rectors and Visitors of the University of Virginia, 95 F. 3d 349 (4th Cir.) 1996.

41. Dahm L. Medical futility and the Texas Medical Futility Statute: a model to follow or one to avoid? *The Health Lawyer*, August 2008.

42. Meier D. *Making the case 2010, Power Point presentation available at Center to Advance Palliative Care.* www.capc.org/support-from-capc/capc_presentations/.

43. Joint Commission for the Accreditation of Healthcare Organizations. *Chapter 3, Patients Rights and Organization Ethics*, Standards R1.1.2.8-R1.1.2.9, 2002.

44. World Health Organization. *Definition of Palliative Care.* 1990. Available at www5.who.int/cancer. Accessed 3-19-03.

45. Analysis of US Hospital Palliative Care Programs 2010. Snapshot. *New York Center to Advance Palliative Care*, 2010. www.aha.org/aha/resource-center/bibliography/LIFE.html.

46. General Accounting Office Report GAO/HEHS-00–182. *Medicare: More Beneficiaries use Hospice but for fewer days of Care.* September 2000.

47. NHPCO Facts and Figures Hospice Care in America. 2010 edition. http://www.nhpco.org/files/public/Statistics_Research/Hospice_Facts_Figures_Oct-2010.pdf.

48. Connor SR, Pyenson B, Fitch K, Spence C, Iwasaki K. Comparing hospice and non-hospice patient survival among patients who die within a three year window. *J Pain Symptom Manage* 2007; **33**(3): 238–46.

49. Ternel JS, Greer JA, Muzinkansky A *et al*. Early palliative care for patients

with metastatic non-small-cell lung cancer. *N Engl J Med* 2010; **363**: 733–42.

50. Von Roenn JH, Cleeland CS, Gonin R *et al.* Physician attitudes and practice in cancer pain management. A survey from the Eastern Cooperative Oncology Group. Physician attitudes and practice in cancer pain management. A survey from the Eastern Cooperative Oncology Group. *Ann Intern Med* 1993; **119**(2): 121–6.

51. Foley KM, Gelband H, eds. *National Cancer Policy Board, Institute of Medicine and National Research Council. Improving Palliative Care for Cancer.* Washington, DC: National Academy Press; 2001, p. 289.

52. Lilly CM, DeMeo DL, Sonna LA *et al.* An intensive communication intervention for the critically ill. *Am J Med* 2000; **109**: 469–75.

53. Buckman R. *How to Break Bad News: a Guide for Health Care Professionals.* Baltimore, MD: Johns Hopkins University Press; 1992.

54. Kohn KT, Corrigan JM, Donaldson MS, eds, for the Committee on Quality of Health Care in America, Institute of Medicine. *To Err is Human: Building a Safer Health System.* Washington, DC: National Academy Press; 1999.

55. Kachalia A, Kaufman SR, Boothman R *et al.* Liability claims and costs before and after implementation of a medical error disclosure program. *Ann Intern Med* 2010; **153**: 213–21.

56. Leape LL. Reporting of adverse events. *N Engl J Med* 2002; **37**: 1633–8.

57. Flynn E, Jackson JA, Lindgren K *et al. Shining the Light on Errors: How Open Should We Be?* Oak Brook, IL, University HealthSystem Consortium; 2002.

58. Younger SJ, Arnold RM, Schapiro R, eds. *The Definition of Death: Contemporary Controversies.* Baltimore, MD, Johns Hopkins University Press; 1999.

59. Wijdicks EFM, ed. *Brain Death.* Philadelphia, PA: Lippincott Williams and Wilkins; 2001.

60. Wijdicks EFM. The diagnosis of brain death. *N Engl J Med* 2001; **344**: 1215–21.

61. Wijdicks EFM, Varelas PN, Gronseth GS, Greer DM. Evidence-based guideline update: Determining brain death in adults: Report of the Quality Standards Subcommittee of the American Academy of Neurology. *Neurology* 2010; **74**: 1911–18.

62. Legal Foundations for the Neurological Definition of Death. Abstracted from Burke K for April 2003 Forum, Canadian Council for Donation and Transplantation. http://www.ccdt.ca/english/publications/background-pdfs/Legal-Neurological-Death.pdf.

63. Capron AM. Brain death – well settled yet still unresolved. *N Engl J Med* 2001; **344**: 1244–6.

Perioperative pain management

Anne Marie McKenzie-Brown

Overview: Benefits of postoperative pain control

Acute pain, highlighted by Marks and Sachar's 1973 landmark article on the undertreatment of pain in inpatients, has been discussed in the medical literature for many years [1]. Despite the advances made, the attention given, the development of national guidelines on the evaluation and treatment of acute pain, and adoption of pain as the "fifth vital sign," postoperative pain is still undertreated [2,3]. A 2003 survey of postoperative patients in the USA showed that 82% of patients reported postoperative pain lasting until 2 weeks after discharge; 39% of these described the pain as severe [3].

Both over- and undertreatment of pain can result in negative consequences in the outpatient perioperative setting [4,5]. Untreated pain results in stimulation of the stress response and increased sympathetic activity which can then lead to increased myocardial demand and systemic hypercoagulability [3,5]. Inactivity, inability to take deep breaths and other activities limited by pain may increase the chance of developing postoperative ileus, deep vein thrombosis and atelectasis [3]. Undertreated pain is the most common reason for delayed discharge home following ambulatory surgery and it is often a reason for unanticipated hospital admission [5,6].

There are many techniques available for postoperative pain control. While many studies have alluded to decreased morbidity and mortality due to appropriate treatment of postoperative pain, the evidence is inconclusive [5]. The reason for this is largely due to the overall safety and low incidence of complications associated with surgery. Therefore detecting a significant difference in outcome requires evaluation of a very large patient population [5].

Any discussion involving control of postoperative pain has to address all aspects of the perioperative experience. The treatment of postoperative pain, which often starts in the preoperative holding area (POHA), is continued during surgery then maintained postoperatively until discharge.

Evaluation of the patient

The treatment plan for postoperative pain is best initiated prior to the start of surgery. The approach is similar to the evaluation of other patients; a thorough review of the patient's history and the performance of a directed physical examination are key to successful management of their pain. Preoperative anxiety and a history of "hypervigilance," i.e., enhanced awareness of and prioritization of pain, has been proposed as a predictor of postoperative pain intensity [3]. Preoperative patient reassurance may thus be helpful in decreasing their anticipated postoperative pain.

Options for postoperative analgesia range from oral short-acting opioid analgesics to more complex regional anesthesia techniques. Patient evaluation includes obtaining a history and a review of the pertinent lab tests to determine the medical condition of the patient. Particular attention needs to be paid to liver and kidney function, platelet and coagulation status. Liver dysfunction affects metabolism of some medications; in addition it limits the amount of acetaminophen-containing drugs that a patient may receive. Many of the short-acting opioids prescribed for postoperative pain relief contain acetaminophen. Patients may have either increased or decreased analgesia from drugs metabolized in the liver.

Renal insufficiency similarly affects medications that are excreted by the kidney unchanged and those with active metabolites, e.g., morphine and meperidine. Morphine's metabolite, morphine-6-glucuronide (M6G) accumulates in patients with renal insufficiency [7–9]. M6G, more so than the parent morphine, accumulates in patients with renal failure and is responsible for a lot of the resulting side-effects, particularly sedation and respiratory depression [7–9]. Although M6G and morphine have similar υ (mu) receptor affinity, υ opioid activity of M6G is greater than that of morphine, particularly when given centrally [7–11]. Both have poor bioavailability [12]. A randomized, double-blind study of postoperative knee surgery patients found that, when given via subcutaneous patient-controlled analgesia (PCA), the pain relief over 24 hours was the same whether morphine or M6G was given.

Medical Management of the Surgical Patient, ed. Michael F. Lubin, Thomas F. Dodson, and Neil H. Winawer. Published by Cambridge University Press. © Cambridge University Press 2013.

Meperidine is the least desirable opioid for postoperative analgesia, due to its low potency and high side-effect profile. Its metabolite nor-meperidine has neuroexcitatory activity and has been associated with seizures in patients with renal insufficiency [13,14]. Non-steroidal anti-inflammatory drugs should be used with caution in patients with renal disease or those that will require postoperative venous thrombosis prophylaxis, e.g., low molecular weight heparin.

Underlying diseases are important to note. Patients with sickle cell anemia are at risk for renal insufficiency. Patients with obstructive sleep apnea, particularly those who use home continuous positive airway pressure (CPAP) require increased vigilance for respiratory insufficiency and should get CPAP postoperatively. While patient-controlled analgesia is an acceptable form of postoperative analgesia for patients with sleep apnea, they are not candidates for a basal opioid infusion [15]. Patients with morbid obesity may present technical challenges when performing regional anesthesia techniques.

Pain assessment

In order for the acute postoperative pain to be treated it must be assessed. There are numerous pain assessment tools that are used in practice. Patient self-report is considered the most reliable. Perhaps the most common assessment tool used for postoperative pain is the numerical rating scale (NRS). It is equivalent in sensitivity to the visual analog scale (VAS) [16]. They are best used to assess pain at the moment of questioning [16]. There is also a four-point categorical verbal scale but it does not correlate as well with the NRS and VAS, called the verbal rating scale (VRS). The four measurements of pain on this scale include none, mild (pain rating 1–3/10), moderate (pain rating 4–6/10), and severe (pain rating 7–10/10) [16]. The goal is to keep the pain at a VRS rating of "mild" or below. The VRS is useful only as a course screening tool and should not replace the VAS or NRS in assessing postoperative pain since it tends to overestimate pain at the higher ends of the scale [16].

Post-surgical patients are encouraged to become ambulatory as soon as possible after surgery to decrease the incidence of thromboembolic, gastrointestinal and pulmonary complications associated with remaining sedentary. Thus it is important to assess both pain at rest and pain with movement (dynamic pain) [16]. Pain assessment involves not only numerical scales, it involves obtaining an accurate history of the pain generator, the pain quality, duration and aggravating and alleviating factors, e.g., for some patients the nasogastric tube may be the most painful aspect of the postoperative course. Simply asking a pain score in that situation would not necessarily elicit information that would be used appropriately to produce pain relief.

In patient populations where communication is difficult, e.g., patients with dementia, ventilated patients and children, other forms of assessment may be used [17]. The Pain Assessment in Advanced Dementia (PAINAD) Scale was developed in 2003 to address the need for accurate assessment of pain in non-communicative patients [17]. This scale uses a combination of several observable behaviors to assess pain: quality of breathing, vocalization, facial expression, body language and consolability to determine whether patients with advanced dementia are in pain [17]. The Wong–Baker Scale uses facial expressions to assess pain in children but has been used also in adults with cognitive impairment [18].

Pathophysiology of pain

Pain can be divided into three broad categories: nociceptive, inflammatory, and dysfunctional pain [19,20]. Nociceptive pain can be thought of as protective. It is only activated when the stimulus has reached a certain threshold [19,20]. Inflammatory pain is part of the healing process, e.g., following a surgical incision [19,20]. It can be thought of as protective as well; but the threshold for this type of pain is low and serves to guard against unnecessary contact and aid in the timely healing of the wound [19,20]. Finally there is dysfunctional pain which has no positive attributes [19,20]. It is self-sustaining long after the initial stimulus, through a process called central sensitization [19,20]. This type of pain is pathological and may lead to the development of chronic pain.

Nociception has been described as "the neural processes of encoding and processing noxious stimuli" [20]. It is transmitted via the spinal cord through a series of specialized nerves to the brain where it is perceived as pain. Specialized nerve endings, primary afferent neurons called nociceptors respond to noxious stimuli [21,22]. They may respond to noxious chemical, thermal, or mechanical stimuli [21,22]. The signal that is generated and transmitted by the small Aδ (delta) and C fibers then synapse in the dorsal horn [21,22]. The second-order neurons transmit the pain signal to the thalamus via the spinothalamic tract where third-order neurons project to the central nervous system where the subjective perception of pain occurs. These nociceptors can become activated by prolonged stimuli and result in peripheral and eventually central sensitization which may eventually result in chronic pain states [21].

Preemptive and multimodal analgesia
Preemptive analgesia

There is evidence that blocking nociceptive afferent input to the spinal cord prior to the time of tissue damage may prevent the development of an excitable state known as "wind up" which may mitigate postoperative pain and even prevent the development of chronic pain following surgery [23]. This technique is called preemptive analgesia and it is thought to work best when the nociceptive input is inhibited pre-, intra- and postoperatively [23–25]. Preemptive analgesia may be achieved by giving analgesics preoperatively, e.g., oral opioids and non-steroidals and now more recently the gabapentinoids (gabapentin and pregabalin), or by preoperatively blocking the afferent impulses via regional or neuraxial anesthesia.

Some studies indicate that preoperative gabapentin has an opioid sparing effect and has shown promise in preventing some forms of acute postoperative pain [23,26]. Gabapentin and pregabalin bind to the α2δ-1 subunit of the voltage gated calcium channel [27]. In models of inflammatory or incisional injury gabapentin and pregabalin reduce thermal and mechanical hypersensitivity [28]. There are also data to suggest synergistic effects of these drugs combined with naproxen [28]. In addition, both gabapentin and pregabalin have anxiolytic properties [29,30]. The doses of gabapentin (600–1,200 mg) and pregabalin (150–300 mg) given one hour prior to surgery for preemptive analgesia are much larger than those usually prescribed as an initial single dose for chronic pain [28,29,31]. A single dose of 300 mg pregabalin is enough to produce anti-hyperalgesic levels in the central nervous system [32].

Other medications such as NSAIDs may be given preemptively. In addition, preoperative peripheral nerve blockade may be performed and supplemented with a continuous infusion postoperatively to continue to provide sustained analgesia in the postoperative period.

Increasing attention is being paid to reducing the risk of acute postoperative pain being transitioned to chronic persistent pain after surgery [33]. In theory preemptive analgesia may help to prevent the emergence of chronic pain following surgery. The presence of nerve injury and increased postoperative pain are predisposing characteristics for the development of chronic persistent pain [15]. Thus adequate control of postoperative pain may help to prevent the development of chronic pain after surgery. The distinction between acute and chronic post-surgical pain is defined by the duration of time since the initial insult, generally beginning approximately 3 months after the initial injury. Macrae proposed four criteria for the diagnosis of chronic post-surgical pain: the pain should be (1) post-surgical; (2) at least 2 months duration; (3) other causes should be pursued; and (4) excluded [34].

Some surgeries pose greater risk for the development of chronic post-surgical pain than others. There are many reports of pain post-mastectomy and other breast surgeries. The patient complaints generally involve painful scar, chest wall, arm pain or phantom breast pain [34]. Perhaps the most commonly recognized surgery associated with persistent post-surgical pain is pain after thoracotomy. As many as 50% of patients who have had thoracotomies describe persistent pain one year after surgery which may persist for many years [35,36]. This pain is characterized by dysesthesia, burning and stabbing in the distribution of the intercostal nerves [36]. The use of less-invasive methods to access the thoracic cavity, e.g., video-assisted thoracoscopic surgery, has not resulted in significant decrease in the incidence of persistent post-thoracotomy pain but there may be a decrease in the intensity [35,37]. A thoracic epidural placed preoperatively and continued intra- and postoperatively is the current standard and

may decrease the likelihood of intra-operative peripheral and central sensitization with resulting acute and chronic post-thoracotomy pain [35].

Many of the early preemptive analgesia studies were done on patients who had dental surgery. This type of surgery is also associated with chronic pain, particularly endodontic surgery [34]. The incidence has been reported as 5 to 13% [34,38]. Inguinal hernia repair is also associated with chronic, usually neuropathic pain, particularly when mesh is used [34]. Finally, chronic pain following spine surgery is a frequent reason for visits to pain physicians. The pain may be either axial back or neck pain with or without associated radicular symptoms. The difficulty with assessing the incidence of chronic post-surgical pain in these patients is the high incidence of pre-procedural pain, e.g., sciatic pain that may have been present for weeks or even months prior to surgery.

Multimodal analgesia

The term "multimodal" or "balanced" analgesia was introduced by Kehlet and Dahl in 1993 and describes the use of more than one form of analgesia to provide postoperative pain control [39]. This approach was thought to take advantage of potential additive or even synergistic effects of combining analgesic techniques to provide analgesia at lower doses with fewer side-effects, particularly the side-effects related to opioids [4,39,40].

While this concept has logical appeal, the literature is conflicting. The benefits of reducing opioid-related side-effects include reduced postoperative nausea/vomiting, pruritis, sedation, respiratory insufficiency and the costs (nursing care, medications, prolonged stay, unanticipated admission) associated with treating these side-effects [41]. Seventy-two percent of patients surveyed in one study said they would choose an analgesic other than a narcotic to treat their pain due to the side-effects they experienced with opioids [3].

Oral non-steroidal anti-inflammatory (NSAIDs) medications are a useful adjunct to opioid medications for outpatient surgery. Ketorolac has the advantage of coming in an intravenous formulation but the adverse side-effect profile, particularly GI bleeding and CHF, limits its long-term use [4,42,43]. The dose should be reduced in elderly patients to reduce the risk of side-effects. There are many classes of anti-inflammatory drugs with similar efficacy but slightly different side-effect profiles. There are some surgeries where postoperative NSAID use is controversial, e.g., as an analgesic for spinal fusions and surgery for bone fractures where there is a theoretical concern about healing [44].

Adding acetaminophen may also help to decrease the need for opioids. A systematic review found that the combination of acetaminophen and NSAID provided superior relief to either drug given alone [45]. Intravenous acetaminophen is now available and may be given as supplemental analgesia in the postoperative patient who is *nil per os* (NPO) [46]. Acetaminophen has no anti-inflammatory or antiplatelet effects. Other analgesic methods have been used for multimodal analgesia including local infiltration, regional analgesia, oral and intravenous opioids, peripheral and neuraxial opioids [39].

Analgesic methods of delivery
Oral opioids and other analgesics

Opioids are synthetic or naturally occurring. The naturally occurring opioids are morphine and codeine and there are semi-synthetic derivatives, e.g., hydromorphone, hydrocodone, buprenorphine, etc. [11]. The synthetic opioids include the phenylpiperidines e.g., fentanyl and meperidine, and the pseudo-piperidines, e.g., methadone [11]. The choice of techniques for controlling pain in the perioperative period is affected by the patient's ability to eat and drink. The cheapest and simplest form of postoperative analgesia is oral medication. Most patients remain NPO during the immediate postoperative period and thus oral medications are not practical for the first few days and other methods, often interventional techniques, are employed until the patient is able to take oral medications.

Most postoperative pain following ambulatory procedures can be treated with short-acting oral analgesics. Oral oxycodone or hydrocodone with or without acetaminophen every 4 hours as needed effectively controls the pain following most basic outpatient surgeries. Codeine, only available in oral form, is considered a pro-drug for morphine, although it also occurs naturally along with morphine in the poppy seed [11]. Approximately 10% of codeine is metabolized to morphine via the CYP2D6 enzyme, which is thought to be the clinical analgesia for this drug [11,47]. Thus poor metabolizers result in decreased morphine production and this is thought to be an explanation for poor responders to codeine [11,47]. However most of the codeine is glucuronidated to codeine-6-glucuronide (C6G) via the uridine diphosphate glucuronosyl transferase enzyme, UGT 2B7, leading some to postulate that the C6G, and not morphine, is the main source of codeine's analgesic activity [11]. Codeine is less potent than morphine with weak υ receptor affinity and is often associated with nausea, so is not the first-line oral medication for postoperative pain [11].

Morphine has substantial first-pass metabolism and poor bioavailability [12]. It too is glucuronidated via the UGT 2B7 to M6G as described above [12]. The other conjugate, M3G, does not contribute to analgesia [12]. Oral morphine comes in both an immediate-release and sustained-release formulations. Morphine, hydromorphone, and oxymorphone are glucuronidated by the UGT enzymes [12]. UGT enzymes generally inactivate medications; morphine's metabolite M6G is an exception [12]. Hydrocodone and oxycodone are metabolized by the CYP 2D6 to hydromorphone and oxymorphone respectively [12]. Most postoperative pain decreases over time as the wound heals so short-acting opioids are appropriate as they are more easily titrated to the patient's analgesic requirements. Long-acting opioids are

not indicated for postoperative pain in the majority of patients, particularly those who are opioid naïve.

Transdermal fentanyl has been associated with respiratory depression when used for acute postoperative pain control and has a black box warning against use in acute pain and in opioid naïve patients [48]. Tapentadol is a newer classification of opioid. It is a centrally acting synthetic opioid that is a υ agonist, a norepinephrine and a weak serotonin receptor uptake inhibitor [49]. Its potency is derived from its opioid agonist and norepinephrine reuptake inhibitor properties [49]. Its side-effect profile is similar to other opioids, however it does have the advantage of the additional norepinephrine reuptake inhibition which may decrease the gastrointestinal side-effects associated with other more traditional opioids [49]. For patients who have difficulty swallowing pills but intravenous access is limited, some of the oral analgesics (e.g., oxydocone/acetaminophen, morphine) come in liquid form and may be placed via feeding tube.

Intravenous opioids

Intravenous patient-controlled analgesia (IV-PCA) has largely replaced the intermittent nurse-delivered intramuscular and intravenous opioids for the treatment of acute postoperative pain in patients who are NPO. As needed, intermittent dosing of fixed doses of opioids is inherently inflexible and does not allow for tailoring to the patients needs [50]. The PCA pump can be programmed to deliver small amounts of opioid intravenously on demand. The concept of small intravenous doses of opioids providing adequate postoperative analgesia with fewer side-effects was first described in 1963 by Roe. He felt that repeated evaluation of the postsurgical patient and titration of multiple small doses of opioid could lead to an overall reduction in pain and side-effects [51,52]. Later Austin described large variations in the blood concentration of intramuscular meperidine during the first 2 postoperative days [53]. He used the term "minimum effective analgesic concentration" (MEAC) to describe the lowest serum concentration of a particular drug that would produce adequate analgesia in that particular individual [51,53]. The MEAC varies between drugs and between individuals but is consistent in an individual patient [51,53]. Patients using patient-controlled analgesia are in effect attempting to reach their MEAC by self-administration of small amounts of opioid and titrating to an endpoint of acceptable analgesia with minimal acceptable side-effects. Intramuscular injections of opioid given on an as-needed basis result in serum concentrations above MEAC with increased chance of sedation [51,53,54].

In theory, patients consume less opioid with PCA as they titrate themselves to their required analgesic levels but supporting evidence is mixed [40,54]. A study of patients using PCA for the treatment of pain following total knee replacement titrated themselves, not to the point of complete analgesia, but to steady-state levels of "moderate" pain, trading pain relief for decreased sedation [54]. Patient-controlled analgesia gives patients autonomy to make these decisions, which in itself enhances patient satisfaction [40,47]. In fact the best evidence for improved outcome with PCA is in the area of overall patient satisfaction [40]. Patient-controlled analgesia has many safety features, e.g., secured opioid-filled syringe, small dose, lock-out period, hourly maximal dose; but the most important aspect of PCA is self-administration. As sedation generally precedes respiratory depression, having the patient as the only one administering the opioid provides their own feedback loop and overdosing is avoided.

Basal infusions are not recommended in the opioid naïve patient and have not been shown to improve efficacy or to improve night-time pain [48,51]. In particular, patients with baseline respiratory disorders and sleep apnea are not candidates for basal infusions [48]. Co-administering sedative medications, e.g., benzodiazepines and barbiturates to patients receiving postoperative opioids should be avoided, as it increases the risk of respiratory depression.

A periodic intravenous or intramuscular injection of large doses of opioids every 3 or 4 hours relies on a relative overdose of opioid to provide analgesia for a few hours at a time. This has several disadvantages including inefficient use of nursing time, the potential for feelings of euphoria during the peak effect of the drug and inadequate analgesia during the times of the trough [49]. A variety of opioids have been used for PCA; the most commonly prescribed is morphine. Age, not weight, is the best predictor of postoperative PCA morphine consumption [50]. The typical concentration is 1 mg/mL morphine or its equivalent, and the typical dose is 1 mL. The dose should be small, but enough to provide analgesia without sedation. Hydromorphone (0.2 mg is approximately 1 mg morphine) and fentanyl (10 ʋg fentanyl is approximately equivalent to 1 mg morphine) are other opioids used in PCA. The typical lock-out time is between 6 and 10 minutes. This is the time in between doses when no medication is delivered even if the demand button is pressed several times. Monitoring of the number of times the demand button is pressed during the lock-out period provides valuable information about possible underdosing of the patient. Human error and equipment failure are sources of morbidity and mortality that diminish the effectiveness of PCA [40]. Intubated patients also have analgesic requirements even if they are sedated. There is often a balance between the effort at weaning toward extubation and pain control. Newer medications, e.g., dexmedetomidine, commonly used for sedation in the ICU, are now also used to alleviate pain in intubated patients.

Topical lidocaine

Transdermal lidocaine, which may be applied either as an ointment (generally compounded at a 5% concentration) or as a patch, is a useful adjunct for postoperative pain control [51,52]. Up to three lidocaine patches may be applied topically and removed after 12 hours; absorption is related to the duration of the patch and the amount of patches applied [51]. Clinical data suggest that in adults the patch is safe even when

applied for longer than 12 hours for up to 3 days [51,54]. The patches do not provide enough analgesia to be used as a sole analgesic but is a useful adjunct for postoperative pain control with minimal side-effects [52]. It appears to be most helpful in pain from abdominal surgery [52]. The lidocaine patch must be placed on intact skin [51].

Interventional techniques for the prevention and control of acute postoperative pain

Epidural anesthesia

Epidural analgesia has been associated with a decrease in the surgical stress response and improved pulmonary toilet. There is even evidence from retrospective data to suggest that it may reduce the incidence of tumor recurrence following surgery for certain cancers, e.g., breast and prostate cancer [55,56]. Epidural analgesia for the treatment of postoperative pain carries the benefit of neuraxial placement of a combination of local anesthetic and opioid, decreasing the need for both medication. Thoracotomies and upper abdominal operations are notoriously painful and associated with pulmonary abnormalities [57]. Thoracic epidural analgesia provides superior analgesia to prescribed as needed (prn) intravenous opioids and can avoid the side-effects of decreased respiratory effort due to pain, e.g., splinting, atelectasis, and pneumonia [58,59]. Thoracic epidurals may also be placed for large abdominal and retroperitoneal operations, where patients may be NPO for several days. There is little evidence in the literature to support leaving the epidural in place for longer than 3 days for postoperative pain control but in clinical practice the catheters are often left in for up to 5 days until the patient is able to tolerate clear liquids. After that the patient may be switched to oral analgesics.

Lumbar epidural analgesia has been used postoperatively for years in orthopedic surgery. This technique was limited by the need for postoperative deep vein thrombosis (DVT) prophylaxis in orthopedic patients. Peripheral catheters have removed the concern of epidural hematoma that was associated with epidural analgesia following orthopedic procedures.

Thoracic epidural analgesia is well suited to treat post-thoracotomy pain. Postoperative pain from thoracic surgery, particularly when a thoracotomy is used, impacts not only levels of pain but also pulmonary function due to splinting [58–60]. While epidural local anesthetic and opioid infusions provide superior analgesia to nurse-administered opioid, this technique is more frequently accompanied by systemic hypotension [58]. Due to the large variety of epidural analgesic regimens (epidural opioids with or without local anesthetic, lipophilic vs hydrophilic opioids, continuous infusion vs patient-controlled epidural analgesia) used in studies it may be difficult to make the statement that epidural analgesia is superior, e.g., to patient-controlled intravenous analgesia. The benefit of a combination of epidural local anesthetic and opioid was more pronounced with more lipophilic opioids, e.g., fentanyl than with the more hydrophilic opioids, e.g., morphine and hydromorphone [59,60]. Some aspects of post-thoracotomy pain are less responsive to thoracic epidural analgesia, e.g., post-operative shoulder pain. The shoulder pain associated with thoracic surgery is thought to be related to afferent phrenic activity and may respond to phrenic nerve blocks or adjuvant medications such as NSAIDs [35].

Over the past few years nerve blocks and catheters in the paravertebral and transverses abdominis planes (TAP) have increased in popularity. Both of these approaches were originally described using landmarks and are now being performed routinely under ultrasound guidance. Single shot and continuous paravertebral blocks have the advantage over epidural analgesia of providing equivalent postoperative analgesia without the associated sympathectomy and subsequent hypotension. Paravertebral catheters are a viable option in patients for whom epidural analgesia is not feasible, e.g., severe scoliosis [58]. The paravertebral technique is particularly useful for analgesia following breast cancer surgery, thoracic and abdominal surgery [61]. It can also be an effective analgesic technique for pain following rib fractures. While it does carry a risk of pneumothorax, the incident is mitigated by performance under ultrasound guidance.

Single shot and continuous transversus abdominis plane (TAP) blocks have been used successfully to treat a variety of abdominal post surgical pain. Using this technique blockade of the lower intercostal nerves and upper lumbar nerves can be achieved. A recent systematic review [62] found improved analgesia using this technique for both abdominal laparotomies and laparoscopic procedures. TAP blocks also allow for avoidance of the sympathetic blockade that may be associated with continuous epidural catheters.

Continuous catheters (femoral, brachial plexus, sciatic, lumbar plexus)

Continuous catheters are rapidly replacing epidural analgesia as the interventional analgesic regimen of choice for extremity surgery. Consensus from the 2005 Acute Pain Summit was that "continuous peripheral-analgesic techniques provide superior analgesia, reduce opioid consumption and reduce opioid-related side-effects" [40]. However, significant technical skill is required to successfully perform these techniques and the evidence for reduced hospital stay and reduction in morbidity and mortality is conflicting [40].

Femoral or lumbar plexus catheters have been used with success for total knee replacement surgery. A low concentration of local anesthetic is infused along the plexus for approximately 48 hours providing analgesia with minimal motor blockade. Patients who have had this technique can walk the day after surgery and participate in physical therapy earlier than was possible using epidural analgesia. Continuous sciatic catheters are used for foot and ankle surgery, and brachial plexus catheters for shoulder, arm, and hand surgery. The advantage of using a continuous catheter technique is the ability to isolate a single extremity for analgesia with little to no sedation, greatly reducing the need for any supplemental opioid analgesia. In addition, unlike epidural analgesia, the catheter is generally placed in a location where nearby vessels are compressible in the case of traumatic catheter placement. These catheters may be placed under ultrasound guidance with or without additional nerve stimulation; or simply using nerve stimulation for needle guidance. Ultrasound guidance has the advantage of allowing visualization of the local anesthetic spread, minimizing intraneural or intravascular injection. Continuous catheter techniques are not limited to inpatients but can be utilized in ambulatory surgery where the patients can be instructed on how to withdraw the catheters at home with telephone backup from hospital staff. Peripheral local anesthetic analgesia may also be provided by single injection techniques. Single injection techniques provide several hours of postoperative analgesia until the patient is able to tolerate oral analgesics.

Wound infiltration

With the advent of catheters that can be attached to disposable bulb containers of local anesthetics delivered to the wound at a set rate for 24–48 hours, continuous wound infiltration with local anesthetic has become popular for some types of surgery. These infusion pumps have been attached to intra-articular catheters, placed inside the wound and placed near nerves for analgesia [49]. Continuous local anesthetic infusions have been successfully placed at the median sternotomy site and significantly reduced opioid requirements while increasing patient satisfaction [63].

Special populations
Elderly

Older adults have a disproportionate risk of coming to surgery with preexisting painful conditions, particularly elderly patients with dementia [17,64]. They are more likely to have medical comorbidities and more likely to have negative effects from drug–drug interactions and the effects of polypharmacy must be taken into account when prescribing medications in this population [64]. Inadequate postoperative pain control in the elderly patient may prolong hospital stays [65,66]. Pain assessment can be a challenge in elderly patients as they are more likely to have impaired cognition and depression [66].

This difficulty with assessment, in addition to excessive fears of opioid addiction and increased stoicism in the elderly increases the risk for the under-treatment of their pain [67]. A consensus statement on pain assessment in the elderly recommends preferentially supplementing a patient's self-report with observed pain behaviours [67]. They also recommend using "synonyms for pain (i.e., hurt, aching, discomfort)" that may be easier for elderly patients with cognitive impairment to understand and thus be more likely to self-report pain [67]. In 2009 the American Geriatrics Society revised its clinical practice guidelines on the pharmacological management of persistent pain in older persons [68]. They recommend that NSAIDs and

COX-2 inhibitors be considered only on rare occasions and those patients on aspirin should not also take ibuprofen [68].

Chronic pain patients

Patients who come for surgery with preexisting chronic pain may have been taking opioids chronically and are now tolerant to opioids. Tolerance is not the same as opioid dependence or addiction. When the body becomes tolerant to a drug, the effectiveness decreases and the patient requires an increased dose of the medication to achieve the same effect. If the patient is taking a stable daily dose of opioid that dose should be considered a baseline amount and additional opioid given for the postoperative analgesia [69]. If the patient has been taking a long-acting opioid preoperatively then that should be resumed as soon as is feasible and a short-acting opioid added for the treatment of the acute postoperative pain. This can then be weaned off shortly after discharge. Discharge planning in these patients should include making sure that there is communication with the physician in the community who has been managing the patient's opioids as an outpatient. The patient should be encouraged to resume care with that physician as soon as the immediate postoperative pain is controlled.

History of substance abuse

The risk of addiction in patients who received opioids for the treatment of postoperative pain without risk factors or a history of substance abuse is very low. There are times when postoperative patients may have the added diagnosis of current or past substance abuse. Controlling the pain of postsurgical patients who come to surgery with a history of substance abuse poses a particular challenge. They are more likely to have concomitant medical and psychological illnesses [70]. Many of these patients have been on maintenance programs where they receive once-daily opioid (methadone or buprenorphine). Methadone when given for analgesia is dosed in intervals during the day. Methadone given for maintenance in substance abuse patients is usually given daily, often in large doses. It is important to remember that these patients have been taking these medications chronically prior to surgery so reestablishing their preoperative regimen is key. This dose should not be considered part of the postoperative analgesia, but simply their maintenance medication. The analgesic half life of methadone is shorter than its elimination half life. Thus the once-daily methadone dose should be divided into thrice-daily (tid) dosing for maximal effect. A short-acting opioid should be given to treat the subsequent postoperative pain. The supplemental opioid given in the postoperative period for the treatment of pain does not increase the chances of relapse for this patient population [70]. Withholding postoperative opioids in these patients may paradoxically lead to relapse. They have a strong fear of experiencing pain and of relapse [70].

In 1989 Weissman and Haddox introduced the term "pseudoaddiction" in a case report describing iatrogenic aberrant drug-seeking behavior in a young leukemia patient with no substance abuse history [31]. This behavior was characterized by a combination of inadequate analgesia and aberrant behavior by the patient in an attempt to convince others of the pain severity resulting in mutual mistrust [31]. The difference between addiction in pseudoaddiction is that appropriate treatment of the pain eliminates the behavior in pseudoaddiction [69].

Note that physical and psychological dependence are not interchangeable terms. Physical dependence simply refers to the physical symptoms seen with withdrawal of a medication, in this case an opioid, and has no aberrant behavioral association. A joint statement by the American Academy of Pain Medicine, American Pain Society and American Society of Addiction Medicine defined it as "a state of adaptation that is manifested by a drug class specific withdrawal syndrome that can be produced by abrupt cessation, rapid dose reduction, decreasing blood level of the drug, and/or administration of an antagonist" [69].

Psychological dependence is more closely associated with addiction. The consensus paper defines addiction as "characterized by behaviors that include one or more of the following: impaired control over drug use, compulsive use, continued use despite harm, and craving" [69]. That is not to say that issues may not arise in the postoperative setting related to the patient's substance abuse history and drug-seeking behavior. Appropriate treatment of their postoperative pain includes careful monitoring of their opioid consumption and behavior. Psychiatry consultation may be helpful in difficult cases. More recently ketamine has been added to PCA solutions, particularly in the more complicated patient who may have opioid tolerance or a higher opioid requirement. Tolerance involves decreased response to repeated doses or requiring more medication to achieve the same effect. Hyperalgesia involves exaggerated pain response to a painful stimulus [70]. Both conditions involve the N-methyl-D-aspartate (NMDA) receptor, both conditions may result in the administration of large doses of opioids [15,70]. Ketamine, a non-competitive NMDA receptor antagonist has been shown to inhibit both opioid and nociceptive hyperalgesia in addition to opioid tolerance [15,71]. Ketamine has been added to PCA solutions along with an opioid to provide analgesia in complex patients with elevated opioid requirements or who may not be getting adequate analgesia with PCA opioid alone [15]. Ketamine has promise as an opioid-sparing analgesic that is effective in patients whose pain is traditionally difficult to control [60].

In summary, adequate treatment of postoperative pain is important not only for the comfort of the patient, it may reduce postoperative morbidity [41,52,65]. Utilization of more than one form of analgesia may result in maximizing pain control while minimizing side-effects and is cost effective [41,52,65].

References

1. Marks RM, Sachar EJ. Undertreatment of medical inpatients with narcotic analgesics. *Ann Intern Med* 1973; **78**: 173–81.

2. Carr DB. The development of national guidelines for pain control: synopsis and commentary. *Eur J Pain* 2001; **5**: 91–8.

3. Lautenbacher S, Huber C, Kunz M *et al.* Hypervigilance as predictor of postoperative acute pain: its predictive potency compared with experimental pain sensitivity, cortisol reactivity, and affective state. *Clin J Pain* 2009; **25**: 92–100.

4. Elvir-Lazo OL, White PF. The role of multimodal analgesia in pain management after ambulatory surgery. *Curr Opn Anesthesiol* 2010; **23**: 697–703.

5. Liu SS, Wu CL. Effect of postoperative analgesia on major postoperative complications: a systematic update of the evidence. *Anesth Analg* 2007; **104**: 689–702.

6. Pavlin JD, Chen C, Penaloza A *et al.* Pain as a factor complicating recovery and discharge after ambulatory surgery. *Anesth Analg* 2002; **95**: 627–34.

7. Lagas JS, Wagenaar JFP, Huitema ADR *et al.* Lethal morphine intoxication in a patient with a sickle cell crisis and renal impairment: case report and a review of the literature. *Hum Exp Toxicol* 2011; **30**: 1399–1403.

8. Chauvin M, Sandouk P, Scherrmann JM *et al.* Morphine pharmacokinetics in renal failure. *Anesthesiology* 1987; **66**: 327–31.

9. Mazoit JX, Butscher K, Samii K. Morphine in postoperative patients: pharmacokinetics and pharmacodynamics of metabolites. *Anesth Analg* 2007; **105**: 70–8.

10. Hanna MH, Elliott KM, Fung M. Randomized, double-blind study of the analgesic efficacy of morphine-6-glucuronide versus morphine sulfate for postoperative pain in major surgery. *Anesthesiology* 2005; **102**: 815–21.

11. Armstrong SC, Cozza KL. Pharmacokinetic drug interactions of morphine, codeine and their derivatives: theory and clinical reality, part II. *Psychosomatics* 2003; **44**: 515–20.

12. Armstrong SC, Cozza KL. Pharmacokinetic drug interactions of morphine, codeine and their derivatives: theory and clinical reality, part I. *Psychosomatics* 2003; **44**: 167–71.

13. Hagmeyer KO, Mauro LS, Mauro VF. Meperidine-related seizures associated with patient-controlled analgesia pumps. *Annals Pharmacotherapy* 1993; **27**: 29–32.

14. Szeto HH, Inturrisi CE, Hounde R *et al.* Accumulation of normeperidine, an active metabolite of meperidine, in patients with renal failure of cancer. *Ann Intern Med* 1977; **86**: 738–41.

15. Wilder-Smith QH, Arendt-Nielsen L. Postoperative hyperalgesia. *Anesthesiology* 2006; **104**: 601–7.

16. Breivik H, Borchgrevink PC, Allen SM *et al.* Assessment of pain. *Br J Anaesth* 2008; **101**: 17–24.

17. Warder V, Hurley AC, Volicer L *et al.* Development and Psychometric Evaluation of the Pain Assessment in Advanced Dementia (PAINAD) Scale. *J Am Med Dir Assoc* 2003; **4**: 9–15.

18. Stinson JN, Kavanagh T, Yamada J *et al.* Systematic review of the psychometric properties, interpretability and feasibility of self report pain intensity measures for use in clinical trials in children and adolescents. *Pain* 2006; **125**: 143–57.

19. Woolf CJ. What is this thing called pain? *J Clin Invest* 2010; **120**: 3742–4.

20. Loeser JD, Treede RD. The Kyoto Protocol of IASP Basic Pain Terminology. *Pain* 2008; **137**: 473–7.

21. Willis WD. The somatosensory system, with emphasis on structures important for pain. *Brain Res Rev* 2007; **55**: 297–313.

22. Cross SA. Pathophysiology of pain. *Mayo Clinic Proceed* 1994; **69**: 375–83.

23. Katz J, Sletzer Z. Transition from acute to chronic postsurgical pain: risk factors and protective factors. *Expert Rev Neurother* 2009, **9**: 723–44.

24. Gottschalk A, Smith DS, Jobes DR *et al.* Preemptive epidural analgesia and recovery from radical prostatectomy: a randomized controlled trial. *J Am Med Assoc* 1998; **279**: 1076–82.

25. Bach S, Noreng MF, Tjellden NU. Phantom limb pain in amputees during the first 12 months following limb amputation, after preoperative lumbar epidural blockade. *Pain* 1988; **33**: 297–301.

26. Fassoulaki A, Triga A, Melemeni A *et al.* Multimodal analgesia with gabapentin and local anesthetics prevents acute and chronic pain after breast surgery for cancer. *Anesth Analg* 2005; **101**: 1427–32.

27. Field MF, Cox PJ, Stott E *et al.* Identification of the $\alpha2$-δ-1 subunit of voltage-dependent calcium channels as a molecular target for pain mediating the analgesic actions of pregabalin. *Proc Natl Acad Sci USA* 2006; **103**: 17537–42.

28. Hurley RW, Chatterjea D, Feng MR, Taylor CP *et al.* Gabapentin and pregabalin can interact synergistically with naproxen to produce antihyperalgesia. *Anesthesiology* 2002; **97**: 1263–73.

29. Tiippana EM, Hamunen K, Kontinen VK *et al.* Do surgical patients benefit from perioperative gabapentin/ pregabalin? A systematic review of efficacy and safety. *Anesth Analg* 2007; **104**: 1545–56.

30. Menigaux C, Adam F, Guignanrd B *et al.* Preoperative gabapentin decreases anxiety and improves early functional recovery from knee surgery. *Anesth Analg* 2005; **100**: 1394–9.

31. Weissman DE, Haddox JD. Opioid pseudoaddiction – an iatrogenic syndrome. *Pain* 1989; **36**: 363–6.

32. Buvanendran A, Kroin JS, Kari M *et al.* Can a single dose of 300 mg of pregabalin reach acute antihyperalgesic levels in the central nervous system? *Reg Anesth Pain Med* 2010; **35**: 535–8.

33. Katz J, Seltzer Z. Transition from acute to chronic postsurgical pain: risk factors and protective factors. *Exp Rev Neurother* 2009; **9**: 723–44.

34. Macrae WA. Chronic pain after surgery. *Br J Anaesth* 2001; **87**: 88–98.

35. Gottschalk A, Cohen SP, Yang S *et al.* Preventing and treating pain after thoracic surgery. *Anesthesiology* 2006; **104**: 594–600.

36. Dajczman E, Gordon A, Kresiman H *et al.* Long-term postthoracotomy pain. *Chest* 1991; **99**: 270–4.

37. Bertrand PC, Regnard JF, Spaggiari L *et al.* Immediate and long-term results

after surgical treatment of primary spontaneous pneumothorax by VATS. *Ann Thorac Surg* 1996; **61**: 1641–5.

38. Campbell RL, Parks KW, Dodds RN. Chronic facial pain associated with endodontic therapy. *Oral Surg Oral Med Oral Pathol* 1990; **69**: 287–90.

39. Kehlet H, Dahl J. The value of "multimodal" or "balanced analgesia" in postoperative pain treatment. *Anesth Analg* 1993; **77**: 1048–56.

40. Rathmell JP, Wu CL, Sinatra RS *et al.* Acute post-surgical pain management: a critical appraisal of current practice. *Reg Anesth Pain Med* 2006; **31**: 1–42.

41. Philip BK, Reese PR, Burch SP. The economic impact of opioids on postoperative pain management. *J Clin Anesth* 2002; **14**: 354–64.

42. Goetz CM, Sterchele JA, Harchelroad FP. Anaphylactoid reaction following ketorolac tromethamine administration. *Ann Pharmacother* 1992; **26**: 1237–8.

43. Franceschi F, Buccelletti F, Carroccia A *et al.* Acetaminophen plus codeine compared to ketorolac in polytrauma patients. *Eur Rev Med Pharmacol Sci* 2010; **14**: 629–34.

44. Pradhan BB, Tatsumi RL, Gallina J *et al.* Ketorolac and spinal fusion. *Spine* 2008; **33**: 2079–82.

45. Ong CKS, Seymour RA, Lirk P *et al.* Combining paracetamol (acetaminophen) with nonsteroidal antiinflammatory drugs: a qualitative systematic review of analgesic efficacy for acute postoperative pain. *Anesth Analg* 2010; **110**: 1170–9.

46. Wininger SJ, Miller H, Minkowitz HS *et al.* A randomized, double-blind, placebo-controlled, multicenter, repeat-dose study of two intravenous acetaminophen dosing regimens for the treatment of pain after abdominal laparoscopic surgery. *Clin Ther* 2010; **32**: 2348–69.

47. Kirchheiner J, Schmidt H, Tzvetkov M *et al.* Pharmacokinetics of codeine and its metabolite morphine in ultra-rapid metabolizers due to CYP2D6 duplication. *Pharmacogenomics J* 2007; **7**: 257–65.

48. Bulow HH, Linnemann M, Berg H *et al.* Respiratory changes during treatment of postoperative pain with high dose transdermal fentanyl. *Acta Anaesthesiol Scand* 1995; **39**: 835–9.

49. Frampton JE. Tapentadol immediate release: a review of its use in the treatment of moderate to severe acute pain. *Drugs* 2010; **70**: 1719–43.

50. Macintyre PE, Jarvis DA. Age is the best predictor of postoperative morphine requirements. *Pain* 1995; **64**: 357–64.

51. Grass JA. Patient-controlled analgesia. *Anesth Analg* 2005; **101**: S44–61.

52. Roe BB. Are postoperative narcotics necessary? *Arch Surg* 1963; **87**: 912–15.

53. Austin KL, Stapelton JV, Mather LE. Relationship between blood meperidine concentrations and analgesic response: a preliminary report. *Anesthesiology* 1980: **53**: 460–6.

54. Ferrante FM, Orave EJ, Rocco AG *et al.* A statistical model for pain in patient-controlled analgesia and conventional intramuscular opioid regimens. *Anesth Analg* 1988; **67**: 457–61.

55. Exadaktylos AK, Buggy DJ, Moriarty DC *et al.* Can anesthetic technique for primary breast cancer surgery affect recurrence or metastasis? *Anesthesiology* 2006; **105**: 660–4.

56. Biki B, Mascha E, Moriarty DC *et al.* Anesthetic technique for radical prostatectomy surgery affects cancer recurrence. *Anesthesiology* 2008: **109**: 180–7.

57. Sabanathan S, Eng J, Mearns AL. Alterations in respiratory mechanics following thoracotomy. *JR Coll Surg Edinb* 1990; **35**: 144–50.

58. Davies RG, Myels PS, Graham JM. A comparison of the analgesic efficacy and side-effects of paravertebral vs. epidural blockade for thoracotomy – a systematic review and meta-analysis of randomized trials. *Br J Anaesth* 2006; **9**: 418–26.

59. George KA, Wright PM, Chisakuta A. Continuous thoracic epidural fentanyl for post-thoracotomy pain relief: with or without bupivacaine? *Anaesthesia* 1991; **46**: 732–6.

60. Mahon SV, Berry PD, Jackson M, Russell GN *et al.* Thoracic epidural infusions for post-thoracotomy pain: a comparison of fentanyl-bupivacaine mixtures versus fentanyl alone. *Anaesthesia* 1999; **54**: 641–6.

61. Boezart AP, Raw RM. Continuous thoracic paravertebral block for major breast surgery. *Reg Anesth Pain Med* 2006; **31**: 470–6.

62. Abdallah FW, Chan VW, Brull R. Transversus abdominis plane block: a systematic review. *Reg Anesth Pain Med* 2012; **37**: 193–209.

63. White PF, Rawal S, Latham P *et al.* Use of a continuous local anesthetic infusion for pain management after median sternotomy. *Anesthesiology* 2003; **99**: 918–23.

64. Reisner L. Pharmacological management of persistent pain in older persons. *J Pain* 2011; **12**: S21–9.

65. Morrison RS, Magaziner J, McLaughlin MA *et al.* The impact of post-operative pain on outcomes following hip fracture. *Pain* 2003; **103**: 303–11.

66. Heer K. Pain assessment strategies in older patients. *J Pain* 2011; **12**: S3–13.

67. Hadjistavropoulos T, Heer K, Turk D *et al.* An interdisciplinary expert consensus statement of assessment of pain in older persons. *Clin J Pain* 2007; **23**: S1–43.

68. American Geriatrics Society Panel on the Pharmacological Management of Persistent Pain in Older Persons. Pharmacological management of persistent pain in older persons. *J Am Geriatr Soc* 2009; **57**: 1331–46.

69. Savage S, Covington EC, Heit HA *et al.* Consensus document. Definitions related to the use of opioids for the treatment of pain. The American Academy of Pain Medicine, The American Pain Society, and the American Society of Addiction Medicine, 2002. Available at: www.asam.org/pain/definitions2.pdf.

70. Bekhit MH. Opioid-induced hyperalgesia and tolerance. *Am J Therapeut* 2010; **17**: 498–510.

71. Nesher N, Serovian I, Marouani N, Chazan S, Weinbroum AA. Ketamine spares morphine consumption after transthoracic lung and heart surgery without adverse hemodynamic effects. *Pharmacolog Res* 2008; **58**: 38–44.

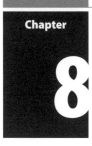

Chapter

8

The medical consult

Michael F. Lubin

As mentioned in the Introduction, consultation has been a topic of discussion at least since the time of Hippocrates; the introduction also discusses a number of the moral, ethical, and interpersonal minefields in the process.

In this chapter, however, my purpose is to discuss the functional process of consultation so that other problems and obstacles can be avoided. The chapter is primarily addressed to clinicians doing consultations for surgical patients, both preoperative evaluations and postoperative management.

Perhaps the most useful and concise recommendations for consultation were developed by Goldman and Rudd in 1983 in a paper entitled "Ten commandments for effective consultation" in the *Archives of Internal Medicine* [1]. These recommendations were: (1) determine the question; (2) establish urgency; (3) look for yourself; (4) be as brief as appropriate; (5) be specific; (6) provide contingency plans; (7) honor thy turf; (8) teach with tact; (9) talk is cheap and effective; (10) follow up. I will address all of these commandments as we proceed.

For the consulting physician: A number of papers have identified one of the common and problematic difficulties in preoperative consultation. Consulting physicians frequently don't identify what problem or problems the consultant is supposed to address. It is crucial for the care of the patient (and for more pragmatic billing purposes) for any problems to be identified. The most common consulting error is the referral for "surgical clearance." Clearance for surgery implies that the consultant can identify which patients will or will not survive surgery, a task that requires more celestial talent than most consultants possess. "Preoperative evaluation" and "risk stratification" imply that there are reasons to think that the patient is at increased risk; if no problem can be identified, then there is no medical (or reimbursable) reason for consultation. Identifiable reasons (e.g., hypertension, diabetes, congestive heart failure) should be the consulting problem or problems.

The timing of surgery is the next area that needs identification. If a patient is having elective surgery, then there is time to get all important information prior to the consult. There may be testing that should be done, e.g., blood tests, chest X-ray, electrocardiogram; these tests can be ordered by the consulting physician. More complicated and or invasive testing is best left to the discretion of the consultant. If the surgery is urgent or emergent, phoning the consultant is often the best method of ensuring a timely consultation.

Timeliness is also very important. Frequently requests for preoperative consultation are submitted within days of the scheduled surgery. If the surgery is urgent or emergent, this obviously can't be avoided. On the other hand, when the contemplated surgery is elective, consultation should be done well before the scheduled date as this will allow time for further testing or optimization of the underlying disease process. Accomplishing these tasks will avoid any unnecessary delays and prevent unhappiness in the patient, the surgeon, and the consultant.

For the consultant: Patients who are having surgery often will not have seen a doctor in some time. The preoperative consult therefore presents an opportunity for the identification of undiagnosed conditions that can improve a patient's long-term care.

Knowing the reason for the consultation is a critically important part of what needs to be done for the patient. If no appropriate request is identified, it is incumbent upon the consultant to call the consulting physician to address the needed questions. Addressing random problems of interest during the consultation will not be helpful if the concern is for something else. If the patient is going to surgery in a few hours, staffing the consult the next day will also not be helpful.

Perhaps the most important task that a preoperative consultant can perform is to "Look for yourself." There is perhaps no more important commandment than this one. The consultant is the most likely person who will take the time to review as much previous information as is available. The consultant should review all old records, looking for information that may have been overlooked that could identify important potential perioperative problems. In particular, this includes the patient's current medications and previous hospitalization. While some of this effort may not be of significance for the surgical procedure, the review can identify other important problems that can result in much improved health status for the patient overall.

Medical Management of the Surgical Patient, ed. Michael F. Lubin, Thomas F. Dodson, and Neil H. Winawer. Published by Cambridge University Press. © Cambridge University Press 2013.

The history of the patient should include a significantly detailed review of previous health problems but also a thorough review of systems. Positive findings such as shortness of breath, chest pain, polyuria, etc. could signal previously unidentified illness. Detecting new or undiagnosed COPD, unstable angina, or diabetes could significantly alter the perioperative treatment plan.

There are several pitfalls during the physical exam worth mentioning. During the assessment of vital signs, many ancillary staff use the wrong cuff in the wrong place, particularly in obese patients, which can be misleading. Pulse should be retaken particularly in patients with significant irregularity since peripheral pulse evaluation can easily miss an important tachycardia. Premature beats often are not transmitted to the peripheral circulation. Detailed examination of the heart and lungs may uncover new congestive heart failure, important valvular disease, or chronic lung disease. Other unexpected findings are also possible, such as lymphadenopathy, thyroid abnormalities, abdominal masses, and focal neurologic findings.

The review of indicated laboratory tests is clearly important. In particular, abnormalities in hemoglobin, white cell count, and platelet count (if indicated) may have been overlooked. Other chemical abnormalities, such as abnormal sodium concentration, metabolic acidosis or alkalosis and renal disease may also be present. Preoperative chest X-ray and electrocardiogram may show important abnormalities as well.

There may be other important tests that need to be individualized prior to surgery. The indications for this testing will be found in the chapters discussing each organ system. Without a good indication, however, it is important to avoid excessive testing as it can be expensive, dangerous, and delays surgery for no good reason.

After having gathered information, the consultant's job is to organize and communicate recommendations. It is important to include only necessary information and exclude the rest. As Voltaire said "The secret of being a bore is to tell everything." There is little that is worse in medicine than having to wade through a lot of information that is never-ending, irrelevant and useless. This also often makes the reader skim the information which may lead to missing important information.

Standardizing the write-up of the consult provides a framework which makes leaving out important parts of the work-up less likely (Box 8.1). It also allows the consulting service to learn how to find the information they are looking for more easily.

The consult should start with a short statement about the patient, the service requesting the consult, the reason(s) for the consult and the procedure to be done, since risk is frequently directly related to the procedure.

This should be followed with a listing of the important medical problems of the patient, those that need to be addressed and any others that should be noted. The listing of an appendectomy in a patient having a lobar pneumonectomy is unnecessary; the recording of COPD in the same patient is quite important.

The positioning of the assessment and plan is personal. While I generally place these most important parts of the note

---

Box 8.1   A brief sample write up of a preoperative consult.

The patient is a 62-year-old man referred by the general surgery service for preoperative evaluation for an inguinal herniorrhaphy.

Problem list
1. Hypertension.
2. Diabetes mellitus.
3. Renal insufficiency.

History
1. The patient has a 30-year history of hypertension. He was not treated for about 10 years but had no complications that he knows of. In the last 20 years he has been treated with a number of agents and is currently on hydrochlorothiazide and lisinopril. He has had no chest pain, shortness of breath, orthopnea, or paroxysmal nocturnal dyspnea. He has had no strokes or kidney disease that he knows of. He takes his medications and has regular follow-up in the geriatric clinic with Dr. Smith.
2. Same kind of history of diabetes as above.
3. The patient is unaware of any kidney disease. He has had recent creatinine of 2.0. He is asymptomatic except for nocturia three times a night. He has no complaints of dysuria, dribbling, difficult starting or stopping his stream, kidney stones, or hematuria.

Review of systems
A review of systems including: head, eyes, ears, nose, and throat (HEENT), endocrine, lymph system, pulmonary, cardiac, GI, liver, hematologic (especially bleeding), neurologic, renal (if there is a listed problem above, these areas should not be repeated).
Past surgical history – s/p appendectomy at age 16.
Family history – often not critical to the surgical problem.
Social history especially drugs, alcohol, and tobacco.
Medications – with doses
atenolol 50 mg daily
metformin 500 mg 2× daily
glipizide 10 mg daily.
Allergies.

Physical examination.
Vital signs (are vital …) 120/80 pulse 80 resp 12 temp 37.

Head, eyes, ears, nose, and throat (HEENT) (including a fundoscopic exam).
Neck.
Pulmonary exam.
Cardiac exam including pulses.
Abdominal exam.
Neurologic exam including reflexes, gait, cerebellar exam, and sometimes a mini mental status exam.
Musculoskeletal exam.
Laboratory review
all needed
creatinine 1.8
glucose 190
Hgb A1C= 7.6

Assessment:
1. Cardiac risk: revised cardiac risk index = 1 No increase in risk.

Box 8.1 *(cont.)*

2. Pulmonary risk: moderate increase in risk secondary to long smoking history and age.
3. Hypertension: well controlled.
4. Diabetes mellitus reasonable control.
5. Renal insufficiency stable.
6. Metformin.
7. DVT risk: moderate risk because of age and longer procedure.

Plan:
1. Routine cardiac monitoring.
2. Pre- and postoperative incentive spirometry.
3. Continue anti-hypertensive medications.
4. Discontinue metformin because of renal insufficiency; continue oral glipizide until day of surgery; suggest sliding scale regular insulin for high sugars (in my institution, we are not asked for details about sugar control; at your hospital, you may be asked to provide detailed instructions in perioperative glucose control).
5. Close attention to volume since his renal insufficiency can result in over- or underhydration since kidney injury affects the ability to concentrate and dilute urine.
6. Low-dose heparin DVT prophylaxis (depending on your institution and consultors, you may or may not need to list exact drugs and doses).

at the end (because I would like the surgeon to look over the body of the consult), it is certainly reasonable and perhaps preferable to put the assessment and plan before the body. This fulfills Goldman's commandment to be appropriately brief.

In doing my assessment, I always write it up in the same way. I number each important piece. I first list cardiac risk with the Revised Cardiac Risk Index (RCRI) score listed. I also list mitigating or worrying factors. Despite the RCRI score, if the patient is having an emergency procedure, a vascular procedure, or a low-risk procedure, that fact will impact the cardiac risk.

I then list the pulmonary risk. While we don't have a really good way to quantitate risk, we can say whether we believe that there is high risk (a pulmonary operation in a patient with a lung cancer resection) moderate risk (an abdominal operation in a patient with hypertension) or low risk (a mastectomy in a patient with hypertension). I again list the factors that increase or decrease the risk.

I then follow this with a listing of the important medical issues (e.g., hypertension, diabetes, stable angina) to be addressed and note whether they are well managed. If a patient is referred for evaluation of chest pain, I make sure that I assess the patient as having non-cardiac chest pain, possible angina, or definite angina, since this will critically affect the management plan.

Following the medical problems to be addressed, I list medications that need to be thought about in the context of surgery. Diuretics, aspirin, anticoagulants, and many other medications should be addressed. Finally I discuss the

indication for venous thrombosis prophylaxis. There are good data for this evaluation and I try to list those that pertain to the patient such as age, procedure, and other risk factors.

The listing of recommendations parallels the assessment so that the numbers coincide. This allows the consultant to identify which recommendations go with each assessed item. Cardiac risk plans such as routine cardiac monitoring (the anesthetists and surgeons know what that consists of); more intensive monitoring such as more frequent electrocardiograms or cardiac enzyme measurement surveillance should be listed. Pulmonary recommendations such as routine care for those with no significant problems, pre- and postoperative incentive spirometry in those with intermediate risk, or chest physical therapy, intensive nebulizer or steroid treatment in those with high risk should be listed.

For the medical problems, perioperative actions should be recorded. In patients with controlled hypertension, continuance of hypertensive medications through surgery should be stated. If the hypertension is not controlled, recommendations for increased medication and delay in the surgery should be stated. This type of notation should be done for every important medical problem.

Medication recommendations should be stated. Holding diuretics on the day of surgery, discontinuing warfarin, withholding non-steroidal anti-inflammatory agents before surgery should be explicit. Deep vein thrombosis prophylaxis has good solid data supporting recommendations. Latitude for the surgeon and anesthesiologist may be important in cases where the indications are soft or non-existent.

When done in this way, I believe that the consultant is "teaching with tact" by listing the indications and ideas behind his or her recommendations.

Honoring one's turf is really important in doing a consult. I have had no training in anesthesia. It would be inappropriate for me and irritating to the anesthesiologist to have any recommendation about anesthetic technique. This is also true about surgical technique for the surgeons. Recommend what you know and can defend. "Talk is cheap and effective" should be obvious. When you need to communicate quickly, talk to your consultants. When there are problems with communication, talk to them; fighting in the chart is a very bad thing to do and often happens because of those problems.

The body of the consult should include a short discussion of each important problem that should be addressed followed by a substantial review of systems to be sure that no other important problems are missed.

Recording the social history is particularly important in identifying tobacco use, and alcohol and drug abuse. Past surgical procedures are important to note along with abnormal bleeding or unusual reactions to anesthesia. A list of medications being taken is of obvious import.

A thorough clinician can do a really good screening examination in less than 15 minutes (Box 8.1) and can identify some important areas that were missed by others. I have found bruits, thyroid nodules, heart murmurs, and abdominal masses that had not been previously identified. While these findings may not be important for the surgical consult, their follow-up may be important or critical for the patient's long-term care. Finally, it is critical that all pertinent data including laboratory findings be documented.

Goldman's final point is follow-up. The necessity or need for follow-up will depend on your own institution and practice. In general, it is a good idea for the consultant to look in on the patient if there are significant preoperative problems. Your involvement can sometimes make a significant difference in those patients who have subtle or complicated postoperative problems.

Reference

1. Goldman L, Lee T, Rudd P. Ten commandments for effective consultation. *Arch Int Med* 1983; **143**: 1753–5.

Chapter

9

Cardiovascular disease

Niels Engberding and Howard Weitz

General overview

The number of non-cardiac surgeries in patients with cardiovascular diseases has been steadily rising. As perioperative myocardial infarctions are the leading cause of death after anesthesia and surgery, it is not surprising that patients with coronary artery disease (CAD) have an increased risk of perioperative morbidity and mortality. Therefore, the determination of cardiac risk generally implies a determination of "coronary risk." Although this is suitable for the vast majority of cases due to the high prevalence of CAD, other cardiac conditions, such as heart failure, arrhythmias, valvular disease, and congenital heart disease, also increase perioperative complications and require distinct perioperative management.

A team approach to patients with cardiovascular disease who undergo non-cardiac surgery is the ideal way to expedite perioperative care. It is essential to assess patients' risk of cardiac complications and to identify those risk factors that may be reversed or ameliorated if time allows before surgery. The most likely cardiovascular problems that patients may encounter in the perioperative period should also be anticipated and an approach to these problems planned in advance. For the patient who undergoes surgery on an emergency basis, preoperative evaluation may be limited to those components that are critical and essential for the surgical procedure. In these circumstances the consultant may well perform a more detailed evaluation in the postoperative period. For many patients the preoperative evaluation is their only opportunity for medical assessment. The consultant should bear this in mind and consider the preoperative evaluation visit as an opportunity for assessment of general cardiovascular risk and development of a plan for cardiac risk reduction.

The physicians who are responsible for preoperative cardiac risk assessment and perioperative care vary according to locale. In many regions, family physicians, general internists, or cardiologists perform these duties. In other areas, these tasks are performed by surgeons or anesthesiologists. The selection of anesthetic agents as well as their means of administration is typically the domain of anesthesiologists; however, it is essential that surgeons and medical consultants understand the basic cardiovascular and hemodynamic effects of anesthesia.

Anesthesia considerations
Physiologic response to anesthesia and surgery

Anesthesia and surgery are accompanied by physiologic stress responses to preserve homeostasis. In the patient with compensated heart disease these adaptive responses may precipitate decompensation by altering myocardial oxygen demand and supply. Catecholamine production increases in response to the stress of surgery, leading to increases in myocardial oxygen demand by increasing afterload and heart rate. In addition, several perioperative factors may decrease myocardial oxygen supply, particularly in the presence of significant coronary obstructive lesions. Hypoventilation and atelectasis may reduce arterial oxygen saturation. Anemia decreases myocardial oxygen delivery. Volume depletion or perioperative hypotension may result in coronary artery hypoperfusion that may provoke myocardial ischemia in the patient with fixed coronary obstructions. Sodium and water retention are increased in response to aldosterone secretion in an effort to maintain intravascular volume. In the patient with impaired ventricular function and/or "fixed" cardiac output (e.g., critical aortic stenosis, severe left ventricular dysfunction), this may result in congestive heart failure. Interestingly, postmortem analysis has shown that many perioperative myocardial infarctions occur in the absence of obstructive coronary disease suggesting plaque rupture and thrombotic occlusion as etiology. Not only do anesthesia and surgery induce a state of systemic inflammation and hyper-coagulability, changes in hemodynamics during surgery may also change shear stress in coronary arteries, which may trigger acute plaque rupture. It is noteworthy, that most unstable plaques cannot be identified by conventional angiography or stress testing, as they usually do not cause hemodynamically significant luminal

Medical Management of the Surgical Patient, ed. Michael F. Lubin, Thomas F. Dodson, and Neil H. Winawer. Published by Cambridge University Press. © Cambridge University Press 2013.

obstruction of a coronary artery. This has important implications for preoperative evaluation and treatment.

Cardiovascular effects of anesthetic agents

Inhalation agents

To achieve a state of general anesthesia, a combination of different agents is usually required. Unconsciousness is induced either by inhalation agents or potent intravenous narcotics, while analgesia is commonly provided by an opioid and muscle relaxation by a neuromuscular blocker. Volatile anesthetics allow for very rapid induction and recovery, which makes them attractive agents for general anesthesia. Aside from nitrous oxide there are five other agents approved for anesthesia, all of which are called halogenated anesthetics. Inhalation agents all produce dose-dependent myocardial depression, which led to theoretical concerns of their use in cardiac patients. However, no randomized trial could be large enough to show a difference in perioperative complications when comparing volatile with intravenous anesthetics. Nitrous oxide is the least depressant and, because its use is associated with an increase in peripheral vascular resistance, systemic blood pressure is maintained. Halothane, rarely used in adults because of idiosyncratic hepatotoxicity, produces the greatest degree of myocardial depression of all the inhaled agents. All inhalational agents cause decreases in blood pressure. For halothane and enflurane it is direct myocardial depression in conjunction with decreased cardiac output and stroke volume that result in the blood pressure decrease. For isoflurane, sevoflurane, and desflurane the associated blood pressure decrease is caused by a reduction in systemic vascular resistance with peripheral vasodilation. This may result in hypotension in the patient who is concurrently receiving vasodilators (angiotensin converting enzyme inhibitors, angiotensin receptor blockers, nitrates, hydralazine, and nifedipine) or is intravascularly volume depleted. Treatment of hypotension in this setting should be with fluid administration. The depressant effects of inhalational anesthetics may be accentuated in patients with abnormal hearts [1]. Desflurane is associated with sympathetic activation and tachycardia and has therefore been considered of limited use in patients with cardiac disease. Using a narcotic in conjunction with desflurane can ameliorate tachycardia. Sevoflurane appears to be similar to isoflurane and safe in the patient with ischemic heart disease. It has been described as having a more stable effect on heart rate than the other inhaled agents. Despite these theoretical differences no clinical trial ever proved a significant impact on patient outcomes depending on the choice of inhalation anesthetic, and their similarities appear greater than their differences. Interestingly, the use of volatile halogenated anesthetics appears to reduce the amount of perioperative ischemia in patients undergoing coronary artery bypass grafting compared with other anesthesia techniques. Volatile anesthetics activate myocardial cellular pathways similar to ischemic preconditioning, which is the proposed mechanism for this observation. A meta-analysis of roughly 2,000 patients undergoing cardiac surgery may even show a reduction in morbidity and mortality by the use of volatile anesthetics [2]. The latest AHA guidelines from 2007 speculate that this effect can likely be generalized to patients with coronary artery disease undergoing non-cardiac surgery [3].

Intravenous agents

Thiopental, a barbiturate, is the prototypical intravenous anesthetic agent. Its cardiac effects during non-cardiac surgery can be significant. It leads to venous dilatation with a reduction in preload as well as myocardial depression. These physiologic responses may result in an increase in heart rate. It should be used with caution therefore in the patient with decreased preload (e.g., hypovolemia) receiving vasodilator medications as well as in the patient in whom increased heart rate would be detrimental, e.g., the patient with ischemia.

Opioids are commonly used in anesthesia to blunt the sympathetic response to intubation and surgical manipulation. Sufentanil and fentanyl are the most commonly used agents of this class. They serve to prevent increases in intraoperative myocardial oxygen demand by maintenance of cardiac output and preventing increases in heart rate [4]. Due to their lack of myocardial depression intravenous opioids have classically been regarded the anesthetics of choice in cardiac anesthesia, however they prolong the need for postoperative ventilation. Newer shorter-acting narcotics may overcome these limitations.

Propofol is commonly used for induction and maintenance of general anesthesia and for sedation during regional anesthesia. It is particularly well suited for use in outpatient surgery because of its short duration of action and anti-emetic properties. Its use may be associated with hypotension, especially after bolus administration [5].

In general, no general anesthesia type is better than another in patients undergoing non-cardiac surgery as long as hemodynamics are tightly controlled. Therefore, it probably is the safest to let the anesthesiologist perform the type of anesthesia that he or she has the most experience with.

Spinal anesthesia

Spinal anesthesia causes sympathetic blockade leading to vasodilation and venous pooling with preload and afterload reduction. Therefore, this type of anesthesia is relatively contraindicated in patients with "fixed" cardiac output (e.g., critical aortic stenosis, severe left ventricular dysfunction) because these patients are unable to augment cardiac output in response to the vasodilation and subsequent hypotension that often accompany this technique. Spinal anesthesia at the lumbar or low thoracic level can also evoke reflex sympathetic activation above the level of block potentially leading to tachycardia and myocardial ischemia.

Regional vs general anesthesia

Several studies have found no difference between the effects of regional and general anesthesia on cardiovascular morbidity or mortality. There are some unique settings in which one modality may be preferable. Regional anesthesia produces less respiratory and cardiac depression than general anesthesia, and its use may be advantageous in the patient with left ventricular dysfunction, congestive heart failure, or pulmonary disease. Some have suggested that, in certain high-risk groups (e.g., those who undergo vascular surgery), epidural analgesia along with general anesthesia is associated with a lower risk of perioperative cardiac complication than general anesthesia alone, but this could not be shown in most randomized trials [6,7]. The use of neuraxial anesthesia has been shown to reduce perioperative cardiac events in patients with CAD undergoing abdominal aortic surgery, when a thoracic epidural approach was used and when epidural analgesia was extended into the postoperative period [8].

A systematic review showed that postoperative epidural analgesia had a significant effect on the incidence of perioperative myocardial infarctions. The results were favorable when the epidural analgesia was performed at the thoracic level but not at the lumbar level [9]. A possible explanation is reflex sympathetic activation above the level of block. For instance, lumbar epidural anesthesia has been found to worsen segmental cardiac wall motion in patients with CAD [10]. Another meta-analysis assessing the impact of epidural vs systemic analgesia on postoperative outcomes reported that the incidence of postoperative myocardial infarction was significantly decreased by epidural analgesia. Although episodes of hypotension were more common with neuraxial anesthesia there was no overall effect on mortality [11]. In terms of specific surgical procedures and non-cardiac outcomes, there is some evidence that peripheral vascular graft patency is enhanced if regional anesthesia is utilized and continued in the immediate postoperative period [12,13]. The sympathetic blockade associated with epidural anesthesia has been credited with improved arterial inflow and venous emptying as well as with reduction in the hypercoagulable state of surgery. Furthermore, return of bowel function is quicker in colonic surgery when epidural anesthesia is used [14]. A Cochrane review comparing regional vs general anesthesia in hip fracture surgery found that there may be a reduction in blood loss, incidence of deep venous thrombosis, and postoperative confusion by regional anesthesia [15]. Complications of regional anesthesia are rare but include the possibility of an epidural hematoma and subsequent paraplegia. In conclusion, the approach to anesthesia in patients with cardiac risk undergoing non-cardiac surgery should be guided by individual preference of the patient and expertise of the anesthesiologist. Pertaining to postoperative analgesia it appears more important that the regimen is effective rather than whether it is applied regionally or systemically, although thoracic epidural analgesia seems to have a slight advantage in preventing myocardial infarctions in patients with CAD.

Assessment of cardiac risk

The main goal of preoperative cardiac risk assessment is to give a reasonable estimate of risk of perioperative cardiac morbidity and mortality to a patient requiring non-cardiac surgery. Once it is clear that a patient's risk is increased, the next question will be if there are any interventions that may reduce the risk.

The rationale for assessing cardiac risk is based on the observation that patients with a history of myocardial infarction or signs and symptoms of cardiac disease have increased risk of perioperative myocardial infarction [16–18]. The mortality of perioperative myocardial infarction is very high [19,20]. Additionally, there was hope that the outcomes of high-risk individuals can be improved by coronary revascularization. This was based on data showing that patients after coronary bypass surgery had an operative mortality for non-cardiac surgery comparable to that of patients without significant coronary disease [21,22]. Subsequently, considerable attention was devoted to the development of cardiac risk indices and algorithms. In 1977 a multifactorial risk factor index was defined by Goldman and associates to identify the high-risk surgical patient preoperatively as well as to delineate cardiovascular risk factors that could be corrected prior to non-cardiac surgery [23]. Nine clinical or historical features, the majority of which were reversible, were found to be associated with an increased incidence of perioperative complications. The factors were assigned "risk points" by multivariate analysis, enabling a preoperative estimate of total cardiac risk and determination of the likelihood of life-threatening complications (e.g., myocardial infarction, pulmonary edema, ventricular tachycardia, and cardiac death). Patients were stratified into four risk classes based on their total accumulated risk points. Risk determined with the original multifactorial cardiac risk index has been integrated with the type of surgery to estimate the probability of cardiac complications in non-cardiac surgery.

The multifactorial risk index has been validated in prospective studies stratifying unselected, consecutive patients who undergo non-cardiac surgery. It has been less reliable when used to risk-stratify selected patient subgroups particularly those with or at high risk for coronary artery disease and those who are to undergo major vascular surgery. This index was derived from relatively small numbers of patients and predated significant change in anesthesia and surgery and has therefore not maintained its clinical relevance [24].

A more recent modification of the multifactorial index has been developed in 1999 by Lee *et al.* for use with stable patients age 50 years and older undergoing major non-cardiac surgery and has been shown to perform well as a tool to predict the probability of major cardiac complications [25]. This index, known as the Revised Cardiac Risk Index (RCRI), uses six readily available clinical factors to place the preoperative patient into one of four risk groups:

- High-risk type of surgery (intraperitoneal, intrathoracic, or suprainguinal vascular).
- History of ischemic heart disease.
- History of congestive heart failure.
- History of cerebrovascular disease.
- Diabetes requiring treatment with insulin prior to surgery.
- Renal insufficiency with preoperative serum creatinine > 2.0 mg/dL.

Rates of major cardiac complication (myocardial infarction, pulmonary edema, ventricular fibrillation or primary cardiac arrest, and complete heart block) with 0, 1, 2, or ≥ 3 of these factors were 0.4%, 0.9%, 7%, and 11%, respectively, but the risk was substantially lower than described in most of the previous risk indices. This was probably due to advances in surgical technique and anesthesia as well as in management of coronary artery disease. Due to its ease of use the RCRI has gained popularity.

To facilitate preoperative risk assessment of patients with cardiovascular disease, a consensus guideline was developed by a panel of the American College of Cardiology and the American Heart Association [3]. The panel acknowledged that the number of evidence-based trials pertaining to perioperative cardiovascular evaluation and therapy was limited and therefore the guidelines are based on a large part from studies not directly derived from non-cardiac surgery and on expert opinion. The guidelines initially published in 1996 and revised in 2002 seek to identify and define those clinical situations in which preoperative testing and intervention may improve patient perioperative outcome. In 2007, these guidelines were updated because new data from randomized controlled trials have emerged that necessitated a practice change. The new guidelines diminished the role for an extensive preoperative coronary work-up and raised questions about the benefit of preoperative revascularization. The overriding theme of the document is that cardiac intervention is rarely necessary to lower the risk of surgery, unless such intervention is indicated regardless of the planned surgery. Based on multifactorial scoring systems such as the Goldman approach the 1996 guidelines initially introduced the concept of clinical risk predictors classified by their importance into major, intermediate, and minor predictors.

The 2007 revision of the guidelines has incorporated the RCRI and abandoned the distinction of major, intermediate, and minor clinical predictors. The general approach to the patient requires assessment of clinical risk factors, functional status, and surgery specific risk. The preoperative history and physical examination should focus on identifying the presence of serious active cardiac conditions and clinical risk factors as well as a history of prior pacemaker or implantable cardioverter defibrillator. A goal of the guideline is the identification of the patient at increased risk who would benefit, in the long term, from medical therapy or coronary artery revascularization.

The major clinical predictors from the 2002 guidelines are now called active cardiac conditions (Table 9.1). In the presence of one of these, the risk of a perioperative complication

Table 9.1 Active cardiac conditions.

Condition
Unstable coronary syndromes Unstable or severe angina[a] (CCS class III or IV)[b] Acute myocardial infarction (within the past 7 days) Recent myocardial infarction (within the past 30 days) with evidence of ischemia by clinical symptoms or non-invasive study[c]
Decompensated heart failure NYHA functional class IV Worsening or new-onset heart failure
Significant arrhythmias Greater than Mobitz II atrioventricular block Symptomatic or uncontrolled (ventricular rate > 100 bpm at rest) tachycardia Symptomatic bradycardia Newly recognized ventricular tachycardia
Severe valvular disease Symptomatic or severe aortic stenosis (mean pressure gradient > 40 mmHg, aortic valve area < 1.0 cm^2) Symptomatic mitral stenosis

CCS, Canadian Cardiovascular Society; NYHA, New York Heart Association.
[a] According to Campeau [16].
[b] May include "stable" angina in patients who are unusually sedentary.
[c] If a recent stress test does not indicate ischemia, the likelihood of perioperative myocardial re-infarction is low, however it is deemed reasonable to wait 4–6 weeks after MI to perform elective surgery.
Reproduced from Fleisher LA, Beckman JA, Brown KA et al. 2009 ACCF/AHA focused update on perioperative beta-blockade incorporated into the ACC/AHA 2007 guidelines on perioperative cardiovascular evaluation and care for noncardiac surgery: a report of the American College of Cardiology Foundation/American Heart Association Task Force on practice guidelines. *Circulation* 2009; **120**: e169–276.

for an elective surgery is unacceptably high and it is recommended to evaluate and stabilize the patient first and cancel or delay elective non-cardiac surgery. The rate of perioperative MI or death is as high as 28% in patients with unstable angina (Figure 9.1) [19]. On the other hand, if a surgery is emergent the benefits of the surgery will probably justify the increased risks. Reducing perioperative mortality under these circumstances has not been well addressed by the current guidelines and evidence is scarce. There are several favorable case reports for using intra-aortic balloon counterpulsation to support the patient during surgery, but trial data are not available [26,27]. Another special situation is the rare case of a patient who presents simultaneously with both a cardiac and a surgical emergency. This is exemplified by a patient with ST-elevation myocardial infarction and significant trauma. In such a case, management must be individualized based on clinical judgment. If the sustained injuries are life-threatening, a life-saving surgery needs to be performed first with supportive cardiovascular care perioperatively, again with potential consideration of intra-aortic balloon counterpulsation. If the injuries do not require immediate surgical correction and antiplatelet therapy is possible it is prudent to proceed with coronary angiography

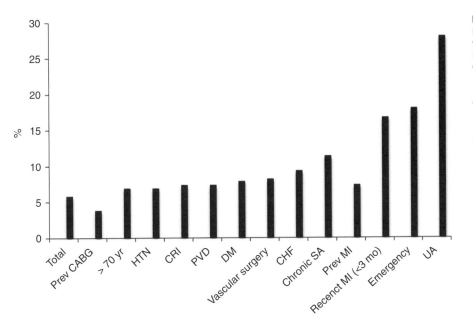

Figure 9.1 Incidence of perioperative myocardial infarction or cardiac death in patients with high cardiovascular risk (patients with known coronary artery disease or age > 70 years). CABG, coronary artery bypass graft surgery; HTN, hypertension; CRI, chronic renal insufficiency; PVD, peripheral vascular disease; DM, diabetes mellitus; CHF, congestive heart failure; SA, stable angina; MI, myocardial infarction; UA, unstable angina.
Reproduced from Shah KB, Kleinman BS, Rao TL, *et al*. Angina and other risk factors in patients with cardiac diseases undergoing noncardiac operations. *Anesth Analg* 1990; **70**: 240–7.

and balloon angioplasty and address surgical issues after an appropriate time interval [28].

The former intermediate clinical predictors have been replaced by clinical risk factors (Table 9.2), which are the same as the risk correlates of the RCRI, with the exclusion of the type of surgery as it is considered elsewhere in the approach to the patient. The consensus committee described the five risk factors as follows: ischemic heart disease (defined as history of myocardial ischemia (MI), history of positive treadmill test, use of nitroglycerine, current complaints of chest pain thought to be secondary to coronary ischemia, or ECG with abnormal Q waves); congestive heart failure (HF) (defined as history of HF, pulmonary edema, paroxysmal nocturnal dyspnea, peripheral edema, bilateral pulmonary rales, presence of a third heart sound, or X-ray with pulmonary vascular redistribution); cerebral vascular disease (history of transient ischemic attack or stroke); preoperative insulin treatment for diabetes mellitus; and preoperative creatinine of greater than 2 mg/dL.

Advanced age (greater than 70 years), abnormal ECG (LV hypertrophy, left bundle branch block, ST-T abnormalities), rhythm other than sinus, and uncontrolled hypertension used to be called minor predictors. However, these minor predictors are no longer incorporated into the algorithm as they have not been proven to increase perioperative risk independently. Nevertheless, they are recognized markers for cardiovascular disease and should raise the suspicion of coronary artery disease when present.

Assessment of functional capacity continues to be a main goal of the general approach to the patient. It has been shown that poor functional capacity is a marker for subsequent cardiac events [29,30]. Formal exercise testing can be used to identify individuals at risk for perioperative complications [31]. Alternatively, the Duke Activity Status Index (DASI) can be obtained

by a simple questionnaire and has been found to be a valid measure of functional capacity as it correlates well with maximum oxygen uptake by exercise treadmill testing [32]. This enables the physician to estimate functional capacity by evaluating the patient's capability to perform common tasks of daily living and expressing that activity in terms of metabolic equivalents (METs). In a series of 600 patients who underwent non-cardiac surgery it has been shown that perioperative MI and cardiovascular events were more common in patients unable to walk four blocks or climb two flights of stairs [33]. Perioperative cardiac risk is increased in patients unable to reach or exceed an aerobic demand of 4 METs during normal activity. Energy expenditures of eating, dressing, walking, and other low-level activities range from 1–4 METs. More vigorous activity, e.g., climbing a flight of stairs, brisk walking, playing golf is equivalent to 4–10 METs. Strenuous activity like tennis and swimming exceeds 10 METs.

Surgery-specific risk is determined by urgency, type of surgery and its associated hemodynamic stress (Table 9.3). Emergent surgeries are generally considered high risk, particularly in the elderly. However, the new preoperative algorithm considers emergent surgeries separately. Major open vascular surgeries represent the highest-risk elective procedures and are therefore considered distinctly in the decision-making process. These procedures have a reported cardiac risk greater than 5%. They include aortic and peripheral vascular surgery. Endovascular procedures are classified as intermediate-risk for perioperative cardiac complications. However, the long-term survival of endovascular interventions appears similar to open vascular surgery strategies [34,35]. Intermediate-risk procedures have variable mortality and morbidity depending on surgical location as well as duration, extent, and associated hemodynamic stress of the procedure. In general, the associated risk is considered less than 5% but greater than 1%. They

Table 9.2 Clinical risk factors for increased perioperative cardiovascular risk.[a]

Ischemic heart disease
Congestive heart failure
Cerebral vascular disease
Insulin-treated diabetes mellitus
Chronic renal insufficiency (serum creatinine > 2 mg/dL)

[a] Major cardiac complications included myocardial infarction, pulmonary edema, ventricular fibrillation or primary cardiac arrest, and complete heart block [25].
Reproduced from Fleisher LA, Beckman JA, Brown KA *et al.* 2009 ACCF/AHA focused update on perioperative beta-blockade incorporated into the ACC/AHA 2007 guidelines on perioperative cardiovascular evaluation and care for noncardiac surgery: a report of the American College of Cardiology Foundation/American Heart Association Task Force on practice guidelines. *Circulation* 2009; **120**: e169–276.

Table 9.3 Cardiac risk stratification for non-cardiac surgical procedures.[a]

Vascular (reported cardiac risk often > 5%)
Aortic and other major vascular surgery
Peripheral vascular surgery
Intermediate (reported cardiac risk < 5%)
Carotid endarterectomy
Head and neck surgery
Intraperitoneal and intrathoracic surgery
Orthopedic surgery
Prostate surgery
Low[b] (reported cardiac risk < 1%)
Endoscopic procedures
Superficial procedures
Cataract surgery
Breast surgery
Ambulatory surgery

[a] Combined incidence of cardiac death and non-fatal myocardial infarction.
[b] Do not generally require further preoperative cardiac testing.
Reproduced from Fleisher LA, Beckman JA, Brown KA *et al.* 2009 ACCF/AHA focused update on perioperative beta-blockade incorporated into the ACC/AHA 2007 guidelines on perioperative cardiovascular evaluation and care for noncardiac surgery: a report of the American College of Cardiology Foundation/American Heart Association Task Force on practice guidelines. *Circulation* 2009; **120**: e169–276.

include carotid endarterectomy, head and neck surgery, intraperitoneal and intrathoracic surgery, orthopedic surgery, and prostate surgery. Low-risk procedures are those associated with a cardiac risk less than 1%. They include endoscopic procedures, superficial procedures, cataract surgery, and breast surgery.

After the patient's clinical risk factors, functional capacity and surgery-specific risk are identified, a five-step algorithm guides decision-making regarding further cardiac testing or proceeding to surgery (Figure 9.2).

1. *Is the surgery an emergency?* If so, the patient should proceed to surgery without delay for further preoperative evaluation. We typically treat patients in this group as if they did have coronary artery disease, if they have coronary artery disease risk factors, or if their functional capacity is poor and coronary disease could be occult (i.e., asymptomatic) due to decreased activity. The patient's cardiac risk profile as well as overall medical state should be assessed in the postoperative period. If the surgery is not an emergency, we then ask:

2. *Does the patient have one of the active cardiac conditions?* In patients being considered for an elective non-cardiac surgery the presence of an active cardiac condition usually leads to cancellation or delay of surgery until the cardiac problem has been clarified and treated. In patients with unstable or severe angina this means referral for coronary angiography to define coronary anatomy and assess further therapeutic options. Depending on the result of the test, it may be appropriate to proceed to surgery after a prespecified time interval. For the patient with severe valvular heart disease, evaluation is performed to assess whether valve repair or replacement is indicated. If the patient needs an urgent surgery balloon valvuloplasty can sometimes be considered as a bridge through non-cardiac surgery, but there are no convincing data for the benefit of this approach. Some data show that non-cardiac surgery can be performed with 11% risk of mortality in patients with severe aortic stenosis who were not able to receive

preoperative aortic valve replacement for various reasons [36]. For the patient with decompensated congestive heart failure or significant arrhythmias, stabilization of these problems should be undertaken before non-emergency non-cardiac surgery is performed. For the patient who has undergone recent coronary angioplasty with placement of a non-drug eluting intracoronary stent, it is recommended that non-cardiac surgery be delayed until the patient's mandatory dual antiplatelet regimen is completed, which is typically 30–45 days following stent implantation. This is to avoid the risk of major hemorrhage if surgery is performed while the patient is receiving aggressive antiplatelet therapy as well as to prevent premature termination of antiplatelet therapy, which would dramatically increase the stent thrombosis risk. For most patients who have undergone coronary stent placement, this approach would delay non-cardiac surgery for at least 4–6 weeks following intracoronary stent placement. By that time, stents are generally endothelialized and the post-stent placement antithrombotic therapy should only consist of a low-dose aspirin [37,38]. In patients with stents it is recommended to continue the daily aspirin perioperatively, but the risks of bleeding from surgery need to be weighed against the risk of stent thrombosis. For the patient who has undergone placement of a drug-eluting stent, the period of dual-antiplatelet therapy after stenting is 365 days and should similarly be completed before non-cardiac surgery is performed to avoid the risk of delayed stent thrombosis. After balloon angioplasty without stenting the recommended treatment time for dual-antiplatelet therapy is 2 weeks, but it takes about 1 week for the effects of a

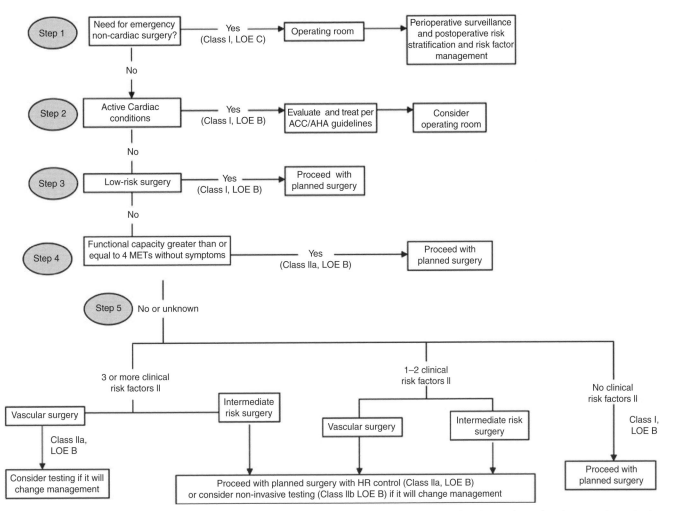

Figure 9.2 Cardiac evaluation and care algorithm. Reproduced from Fleisher LA, Beckman JA, Brown KA *et al.* ACCF/AHA focused update on perioperative beta-blockade incorporated into the ACC/AHA 2007 guidelines on perioperative cardiovascular evaluation and care for noncardiac surgery: a report of the American College of Cardiology Foundation/American Heart Association Task Force on practice guidelines. *Circulation* 2009; **120**: e169–276. With permission.

thienopyridine (e.g., clopidogrel) to subside and thus it is reasonable to wait an extra week. The best time frame for non-cardiac surgery after balloon angioplasty appears to be from 3–4 weeks after angioplasty up to 8 weeks after angioplasty because waiting for more than 8 weeks increases the chance that restenosis has occurred. In patients without stents it is prudent to also stop aspirin preoperatively to reduce the risk of surgical bleeding.

3. *Is the patient undergoing a low-risk surgery?* Low-risk procedures are usually associated with a combined morbidity and mortality rate of less than 1%, even in high-risk patients provided they are stable. Therefore additional cardiac testing is not necessary in this patient group.

4. *Does the patient have a functional capacity greater than or equal to 4 METs without symptoms?* When answering this question we take into consideration the patient's daily activity, realizing that for the patient who is sedentary, progression of coronary artery disease may be occult because their physical activity is not strenuous enough to provoke symptoms of ischemia. Perioperative cardiac risk

has been shown to be increased in patients with poor exercise tolerance, e.g., those who are unable to carry out activity of 4 METs during their daily activities [13]. Cardiac risk is increased even if the inability to perform this degree of activity is due to a non-cardiac cause, i.e., osteoarthritis. As defined by the DASI, activities that utilize 4 METs include performing light work around the house and climbing a flight of stairs [18]. Clinical questionnaires can only estimate functional capacity, thus a standardized exercise test can help determine the patient's functional capacity. For the patient with at least moderate functional capacity, i.e., capability of performing 4 or more METs activity, management will rarely be changed based on the results of any further cardiac testing and it is therefore appropriate to proceed with the planned surgery.

5. *If the patient has poor or unknown functional capacity or is symptomatic at this low level of exertion the presence of clinical risk factors should be determined.* If the patient has one or two clinical risk factors it is reasonable to proceed with the planned surgery. Non-invasive testing can be

considered if it will change management, although the effectiveness of this approach is less well established. In patients with three or more clinical risk factors who are going into vascular surgery, non-invasive testing is favored if it will change management. Other types of surgery have not been well studied in this setting and the decision for preoperative testing should be based on individual clinical judgment. If non-invasive testing reveals high-risk features of active ischemia, coronary angiography is indicated and the non-cardiac surgery will be cancelled or delayed. It is important to keep in mind that the positive predictive value of preoperative stress testing generally is low, ranging from 2–20%, while their negative predictive value is high at approximately 99%. The positive predictive value of myocardial perfusion imaging correlates with the clinical pretest probability of the patient [39]. Therefore, non-invasive testing prior to non-cardiac surgery should only be used selectively in high-risk patients if it will change management. A large retrospective cohort study demonstrated that non-invasive cardiac stress testing reduces 1-year mortality and length of hospital stay in intermediate- and high-risk patients going for intermediate- and high-risk surgery, while this approach actually was harmful in low-risk patients [40].

Risk assessment prior to vascular surgery

Major vascular surgery presents a special challenge for pre-operative assessment, as it is associated with greater cardiac morbidity and mortality than other forms of non-cardiac surgery. Patients with major vascular disease have been demonstrated to have an increased prevalence of CAD. Coronary artery disease exists in up to 70% of patients with peripheral artery disease [41]. If their vascular disease or other comorbid conditions result in physical inactivity, the patient with major vascular disease may have no symptoms of myocardial ischemia despite the presence of significant coronary artery disease because of their limited activity. Additionally, major open vascular surgery may involve substantial fluid shifts during surgery.

Advanced age, a history of diabetes, myocardial infarction, angina, or congestive heart failure have been validated as risk factors for cardiac complication in vascular surgery. The absence of any of these factors was shown by L'Italien et al. to be associated with only a 3% incidence of perioperative cardiac complication, while presence of one or two of these factors was associated with an 8% risk. If three or more risk factors were present, the risk of perioperative cardiac complication or death was 18% [42]. In a database review of vascular surgery patients, Paul et al. found that the presence of these risk markers correlated with the likelihood of underlying coronary artery disease. The absence of any of these risk factors predicted a low likelihood of severe coronary artery disease while the presence of three or more of these factors was linked to a high incidence of left main or triple vessel coronary artery disease [43].

The American College of Cardiology/American Heart Association *Guideline for Perioperative Cardiac Evaluation Prior to Noncardiac Surgery* classifies aortic, major vascular, and peripheral vascular surgery as the highest-risk non-cardiac surgery with a specific risk of cardiac complication greater than 5%. Carotid endarterectomy is classified as an intermediate risk procedure with risk of cardiac complication at less than 5%. The preoperative evaluation of these patients proceeds as it would for non-vascular surgery. The patient who has undergone a recent coronary angiogram or stress test with favorable results is estimated to be at favorable cardiac risk and proceeds to the operating room. For the patient who does not meet these criteria, their functional status potentially supplemented by clinical risk factors aid in the determination of their risk. For the patient with active cardiac conditions, aorta, major vascular, or carotid surgery is delayed until these predictors can be reversed. In this case the patient typically requires coronary angiography with coronary revascularization, if indicated, prior to vascular surgery. For the patient with a critical carotid artery stenosis who requires coronary artery bypass surgery, we often perform simultaneous carotid and coronary artery revascularization to decrease the risk of stroke in the period during coronary artery bypass surgery. Patients with good functional capacity able to perform 4 METs or more activity are deemed to be at low cardiac risk and undergo surgery. The DECREASE-II (Dutch Echocardiographic Cardiac Risk Evaluation Applying Stress Echo II) trial assessed the value of cardiac testing before major vascular surgery in 770 patients with 1–2 cardiac risk factors. The primary endpoint of cardiac death or myocardial infarction at 30 days was no different between those randomized to receive stress testing or no stress testing. As all patients were receiving beta-blockers the authors concluded that cardiac testing can safely be omitted in these patients if beta-blockers are titrated for heart rate control perioperatively [44]. For patients with low functional capacity and three or more cardiac risk factors, the high-risk nature of major vascular and peripheral vascular surgery necessitates non-invasive testing of myocardial perfusion (e.g., dipyridamole thallium imaging) to aid in risk assessment. A high-risk finding on non-invasive testing usually leads to a delay of surgery to allow for coronary angiography with myocardial revascularization if indicated, otherwise the patient proceeds to surgery. It is important to realize that the above approach pertains to the patient undergoing elective aorta repair or major vascular surgery. The guideline suggests that patients who require emergency surgery proceed to surgery without delay and that their cardiac status be closely observed in the perioperative period.

Risk assessment prior to transplant surgery

In many instances transplantation surgery is performed in patients with significant medical comorbidities. The patient who undergoes kidney transplantation usually carries important clinical risk factors aside from chronic renal insufficiency, namely hypertension and diabetes. The prevalence of obstructive CAD in this population ranges from 40–80% [45,46]. As survival of the graft has steadily improved, patients with obesity, old age and CAD are increasingly being accepted for transplantation. Despite the high prevalence of CAD in renal transplant candidates they are oftentimes asymptomatic. Guidelines therefore recommend evaluation of asymptomatic high-risk renal transplant candidates with stress testing or coronary angiography and to perform revascularization in case of significant CAD [47]. A retrospective review of 2,694 patients who underwent renal transplantation identified age > 50 and preexisting heart disease especially in diabetics as risk factors that significantly increased the risk of perioperative cardiac complication [48]. Despite improved long-term survival, the risk of death among renal transplant recipients during the first 2 weeks after transplantation is almost three times higher than that among the patients on the waiting list for renal transplant, which most likely reflects the perioperative risk of transplantation itself [49]. The benefit of pre-transplant cardiac risk assessment in order to identify and treat CAD prior to transplantation is not clear and it has been reported that oftentimes the information gained from preoperative testing is used for estimating the patient's prognosis and potentially restricts access to transplantation [50]. A study in 429 renal transplant recipients compared patients who required pre-transplant coronary revascularization with those who were not revascularized. The post-transplant cardiac prognosis was not improved by coronary revascularization [51]. In 176 patients who underwent kidney or kidney–pancreas transplant the occurrence of postoperative cardiac complications correlated with the presence of reversible myocardial perfusion defects on preoperative dipyridamole thallium imaging [52]. In 126 renal transplant candidates the accuracy of non-invasive testing to detect CAD was limited while clinical risk stratification and coronary angiography predicted freedom from cardiac events [45]. However, contrast-induced nephropathy is a significant concern in this population and therefore coronary angiography is reserved for patients with high-risk findings on non-invasive testing.

In a study in the early 1990s, patients with known CAD have mortality rates as high as 50% during orthotopic liver transplantation [53]. Furthermore, patients with chronic liver disease and cardiac risk factors have a higher prevalence of CAD. While diabetes was the strongest risk factor, patients with chronic liver disease and no cardiac risk factors do not seem to have a higher prevalence of CAD [54]. For the patient who undergoes liver transplantation dobutamine stress echocardiography has been shown to have utility in the prediction of postoperative cardiac complications [53,55].

Elderly patients

In the elderly patient who undergoes surgery the cardiovascular response to surgery may be affected by the presence of preexisting heart disease as well as by normal physiologic changes of the cardiovascular system that accompany aging. Many physiologic changes that occur in response to aging have a significant effect on the cardiovascular response to surgery. The resting heart rate and the heart rate response to stress decrease [56]. Because cardiac output is a function of heart rate and stroke volume, output increases in elderly patients in response to stress primarily by increasing the left ventricular end-diastolic volume [57]. In patients with left ventricular dysfunction, decreased ventricular compliance, or intravascular volume overload, this compensatory response may result in congestive heart failure. Baroreceptor responsiveness decreases with increased age and may cause exaggerated hypotension after intravascular volume loss or with the administration of vasodilators or diuretics. The incidence of sick sinus syndrome and other cardiac conduction disorders is also increased, and occult conduction disorders may be unmasked when beta-blockers or calcium channel antagonists are used in the perioperative period. Other cardiovascular changes that may affect cardiac function in the perioperative period are left ventricular hypertrophy with associated decreased left ventricular compliance, elevated left ventricular end-diastolic pressure, and subsequent interstitial edema. In this situation, which often results from long-standing hypertension, left ventricular hypertrophy may cause diastolic left ventricular dysfunction. Drug metabolism is altered in the elderly. Renal function declines and cardiovascular drugs cleared by the kidney (e.g., digoxin, enalapril) may have increased half-lives. Hepatic blood flow also decreases, leading to delayed metabolism of agents such as lidocaine, propranolol, and verapamil [58].

Age has been demonstrated to be a risk factor for perioperative cardiovascular complication. Patients older than 70 years have been shown to have a higher rate of major perioperative complications and mortality after non-cardiac surgery as well as a longer length of hospital stay. In a study of surgical patients aged 80 or older the overall postoperative mortality rate was 4.6%; 25% of the patients developed one or more adverse postoperative events. Neurological and cardiovascular complications were the leading cause of morbidity. Risk factors for development of a postoperative complication were preoperative history of neurologic disease, particularly preoperative dementia, as well as preoperative history of congestive heart failure and arrhythmia [23,59–61]. In a study of 513 surgical patients aged 70 or older, 386 had at least one abnormality on the preoperative electrocardiogram. The presence of abnormalities on preoperative ECGs, however, was not associated with an increased risk of postoperative cardiac complications (OR = 0.63). Abnormalities on preoperative ECGs are common but are of limited value in predicting postoperative cardiac complications in older patients undergoing non-cardiac surgery. These results suggest that obtaining preoperative ECGs based on an age cut-off alone may be indicated to have a comparative baseline, because ECG abnormalities in older people are prevalent but non-specific and less useful than the presence and severity of comorbidities in predicting postoperative cardiac complications [62].

Prevention of perioperative myocardial ischemia and myocardial infarction

Evidence to support the use of beta-blockers to decrease the incidence of myocardial ischemia and infarction related to non-cardiac surgery is based upon several small studies. Mangano, in a study of 200 patients with coronary artery disease or coronary disease risk factors, found a long-term benefit of atenolol when given prior to, and for several days following, surgery. In this study, myocardial ischemia was reduced by 50% in the atenolol-treated group during the first 48 hours following surgery. There was no difference between groups in terms of non-fatal or fatal myocardial infarction during the first week following surgery; however, during the 2-year follow-up period, the mortality rate was 10% in patients given atenolol and 21% in controls [63]. Raby et al., in a small pilot study of 26 patients with preoperative ischemia on 24-hour Holter monitoring, demonstrated that strict heart rate control with IV esmolol in the immediate postoperative period, when tailored to an individual's ischemic threshold (determined by preoperative continuous ambulatory ischemia monitoring), was associated with a reduction of postoperative myocardial ischemia during the 48 hours following surgery [64].

Recent studies have shed some light on the question of who should receive perioperative prophylactic beta-blockers and how beta-blockers should be administered in the perioperative period. In the DECREASE study, Poldermans et al. reported on 112 patients with stress-induced ischemia who underwent elective vascular surgery [65]. The study was stopped prematurely after it became clear that the treatment group had a dramatic decrease in perioperative cardiac events. Subsequently, Boersma et al. performed a retrospective observational cohort study of all patients screened for the DECREASE study [66]. It was shown that counting clinical risk factors effectively stratifies vascular surgery patients into low-risk (0 risk factors), intermediate-risk (1–2 risk factors), and high-risk (≥ 3 risk factors) categories. Clinical risk factors, as well as quantitation of inducible myocardial ischemia using dobutamine stress echocardiography, were used to risk-stratify patients. Clinical risk factors tabulated for each patient were: age ≥ 70, current angina, prior myocardial infarction, congestive heart failure, prior cerebrovascular event, diabetes mellitus, and renal insufficiency with Cr > 2.0. For patients with fewer than three risk factors, those who received perioperative beta-blockers (bisoprolol 5–10 mg/day beginning at least 1 week prior to surgery and continued for 30 days following surgery with the bisoprolol titrated to heart rate < 80 bpm) had a lower incidence of cardiac complications (0.8%) than those who did not receive beta-blockers (2.3%). Based on their risk classification model, patients with 0–2 clinical risk factors (83% of the patients belonged to this category) who received perioperative beta-blockers had a low estimated cardiac complication rate (< 2%), irrespective of the DSE result. It appears therefore reasonable to omit further preoperative risk stratification in these patients. In patients with three or more risk factors, those whose preoperative dobutamine stress echo revealed no inducible ischemia or ischemia in four or fewer left ventricular segments (of a total of 16 segments), perioperative beta-blockers were effective in decreasing the incidence of cardiac complication, 2.3% vs 10.6%. Patients in the highest risk group, those with three or more risk factors and inducible ischemia involving five or more left ventricular segments were at a considerable cardiac risk (> 6%) and beta-blockers were ineffective in decreasing cardiac complications. The latter result forms the basis of current recommendation that this group of high-risk patients may potentially benefit from coronary angiography and revascularization.

The same investigators subsequently confirmed this retrospective observation with a prospectively randomized controlled trial, DECREASE-II [44]. A large cohort study, evaluating the effect from 663,635 surgical procedures confirmed the benefit of beta-blockers in those with an RCRI of 3 or more. These patients were significantly less likely to die in the hospital. However, this was not true for patients with fewer than three clinical risk factors. In fact, those with an RCRI of 0 were even more likely to die in the hospital if they received a beta-blocker [67]. Also in the POBBLE (Perioperative Beta-Blockade) study, low-risk vascular surgery patients did not benefit from perioperative beta-blockade [68]. The favorable results in high-risk patients were questioned by a meta-analysis of eight randomized clinical trials evaluating a total number of 1,152 patients [69], but it was criticized due to the heterogeneity of methods and study populations in the included trials.

Since publication of the 2007 AHA/ACC guidelines, a large randomized controlled trial with more than 8,000 patients undergoing non-cardiac surgery examined the effect of perioperative beta-blockade. Although a reduction of perioperative myocardial infarction and cardiac death was observed in patients randomized to beta-blockers, this benefit was offset by an increased risk of stroke and total mortality [70]. An explanation for this surprising outcome may lie in the way beta-blockers were administered in this trial. Patients received a fixed higher dose of extended-release metoprolol started on the day of surgery. The two studies by Poldermans and Boersma suggested that beta-blockers should be started days to weeks before elective surgery. Furthermore, it seems more beneficial to titrate the dose of beta-blockers to achieve tight heart rate control rather than the "one size fits all" approach of a single fixed dose daily. The important lesson to learn from these new data is that perioperative beta-blockade is associated with risks. These mainly pertain to perioperative bradycardia and hypotension. Interestingly, there were more patients dying of sepsis in the metoprolol-treated group than in the placebo group in the POISE trial, suggesting that it is important to investigate the cause of tachycardia before initiating beta-blockade [70]. Although data are limited, continuation of beta-blockade throughout the perioperative period in patients already on these medications seems to be important, as abrupt withdrawal of beta-blockers may increase mortality [71].

Based on this evidence, we attempt to utilize perioperative beta-blockers in all patients with inducible ischemia, known cardiovascular disease, or with more than one cardiac risk factor as listed above going for at least intermediate-risk surgery. For patients going into vascular surgery it is reasonable to use perioperative beta-blockers in patients with only one clinical risk factor. We attempt to initiate beta-blockers at least 1 week prior to surgery, realizing that in many patients the realities of surgery lead to identification of these patients at time periods considerably less than 1 week prior to surgery, and continue for at least 30 days following surgery. Many patients whom we identify as requiring these agents in the perioperative period have indications for long-term beta-blocker use. We attempt to titrate the beta-blocker to a heart rate of 60–80 bpm. Particular care must be taken to avoid excessive bradycardia when patients are treated with perioperative beta-blockers. Routine administration of beta-blockers without dose titration is not useful and potentially harmful in patients not currently taking beta-blockers. This may particularly be true if there is not enough run-in time for beta-blockers prior to surgery (less than 1 week).

There is no evidence that intraoperative nitrates are of benefit to prevent intraoperative myocardial ischemia [72]. Prophylactic nitrates may actually be harmful if they lead to excessive preload reduction with subsequent hypotension. There are some data indicating that perioperative diltiazem may reduce cardiac events, however this was not shown for any of the other calcium channel blockers [73]. Both diltiazem and verapamil may be able to protect from supraventricular tachycardias. Given the scarcity of data the guidelines have no specific recommendations for calcium channel blockers.

Alpha-2 adrenoceptor agonists (clonidine, dexmedetomide, mivazerol) have been studied to assess whether reducing central sympathetic activity is effective in decreasing perioperative myocardial ischemia. There is evidence that they reduce myocardial ischemia and/or myocardial infarction following vascular surgery [74]. A randomized controlled trial in 190 patients with or at risk for CAD proved that perioperative clonidine reduces the incidence of perioperative myocardial infarction and death [75]. Recent evidence from a large meta-analysis of 31 trials with 4,578 patients provides encouraging evidence that alpha-2 adrenoceptor agonists may reduce cardiac risk. The strongest data pertained to vascular surgeries [76]. More research is needed for these agents to be able to answer questions such as whether it is safe to combine them with other perioperative interventions like beta-blockers. Pending results of large-scale randomized trials, the available data to date led the guidelines to recommend alpha-2 agonists for perioperative control of hypertension in patients with known CAD or at least one cardiac risk factor.

In a study of 300 patients with known CAD or high risk for CAD who underwent abdominal, thoracic, or vascular surgery, maintenance of perioperative normothermia led to a decreased incidence of perioperative morbid events (unstable angina, cardiac arrest, myocardial infarction) (6.3% morbid events in the hypothermic group vs 1.4% morbid events in the normothermic group) as well as a decrease in episodes of ventricular tachycardia [77].

There are observational data that suggest that perioperative use of statins can reduce cardiac morbidity and mortality. The authors of a recent meta-analysis concluded that statin therapy before non-cardiac surgery reduced the absolute risk of post-procedural myocardial infarction by 4.1% [78]. However questions remain regarding the timing of initiation as well as dose and duration.

Until the publication of the 2007 AHA/ACC guidelines, all of the evidence regarding the value of preoperative coronary revascularization stemmed from cohort studies. These suggested a protective effect of previous coronary artery bypass surgery prior to non-cardiac surgery. Pooled data from studies that used historical control subjects reveal that, of 2,000 patients who underwent non-cardiac surgery, the rate of postoperative infarction was significantly lower in those who underwent previous coronary artery bypass surgery (0–1.2%) than in those who did not (1.1–6%) [79]. In addition to the perioperative benefit, Hertzer noted a late benefit that he attributed to perioperative coronary revascularization. In a group of patients who underwent coronary artery bypass surgery before aortic aneurysm repair, survival 5 years after aneurysm surgery was similar to that of patients with trivial coronary disease [80].

In other studies, the overall benefit of preoperative myocardial revascularization has been less clear. Data from the Coronary Artery Surgery Study (CASS) reveal higher perioperative mortality in non-randomized patients who underwent non-cardiac surgery without preceding coronary surgery (2.4%) than in those who had preceding coronary surgery (0.9%). The operative mortality for coronary artery bypass surgery was 1.4%. Therefore, the combination of coronary surgery followed by non-cardiac surgery was no less risky than was non-cardiac surgery alone in medically treated patients [21]. In a subsequent analysis of the CASS registry database, Eagle et al. found that, in patients with known coronary artery disease, non-cardiac surgery (involving the thorax, abdomen, vasculature, head and neck) was associated with increased risk of perioperative cardiac complication, which was reduced in patients with prior coronary artery bypass grafting (CABG) [81]. It was also demonstrated that the protection afforded by CABG was sustained for at least 6 years following the coronary revascularization procedure. In the first large, randomized trial (CARP) of elective coronary artery revascularization prior to elective vascular surgery, coronary revascularization was found to not be of benefit in reducing overall perioperative mortality in patients with stable coronary artery disease if treated with beta-blockers, aspirin and statins in the absence of left main coronary artery disease, aortic stenosis and severe left ventricular dysfunction (ejection fraction < 20%) [82]. A subsequent analysis of all the patients screened for the CARP trial identified the subgroup of patients with unprotected left main disease as the only subset with improved survival from preoperative coronary revascularization [83].

The American College of Cardiology/American Heart Association consensus-based guidelines for preoperative cardiovascular evaluation prior to non-cardiac surgery recommend that the individual patient's long-term risk be considered when deciding whether or not to perform CABG surgery prior to non-cardiac surgery. They advocate that coronary revascularization to get a patient safely through non-cardiac surgery is appropriate only in a small subset of very high-risk patients who meet established criteria for coronary bypass, i.e., left main coronary stenosis, three-vessel coronary artery disease in conjunction with left ventricular dysfunction, two-vessel coronary disease when one of the vessels is the left anterior descending coronary artery with a severe proximal stenosis, and myocardial ischemia despite a maximal medical regimen. The guidelines highlight that coronary artery bypass grafting should be performed in the above patients prior to vascular or intermediate-risk non-cardiac surgery when long-term outcome would be improved by the coronary surgery.

In the CARP trial, 59% of the patients who received preoperative coronary revascularization had percutaneous coronary interventions (PCI; balloon angioplasty and/ or stents), and 41% had bypass surgery. As these patients were not randomized but rather received their coronary procedure at the discretion of their local physician comparisons between the two groups can only be made with caution. A subsequent analysis found fewer myocardial infarctions in the bypass surgery group compared with the PCI group. These differences were explained by the fact that the bypass group had more complete revascularization [84]. Data from the BARI trial, which examined the impact of PCI versus CABG surgery in patients with multi-vessel coronary disease, indicated that the rate of perioperative cardiac complications is approximately equal in the two groups [85]. To date, there is no convincing data that prophylactic PCI confer any protective benefit prior to non-cardiac surgery. Therefore, PCI before non-cardiac surgery is only indicated in those patients in whom PCI is independently indicated for an acute coronary syndrome.

For the patient who has undergone coronary angioplasty with placement of an intracoronary stent, it is recommended that non-cardiac surgery be delayed until the patient's mandatory antiplatelet regimen is completed, which is typically a 4-week regimen of clopidogrel and aspirin following stent implantation with continued long-term aspirin. This is to avoid the risk of major hemorrhage if surgery is performed while the patient is receiving aggressive antiplatelet therapy as well as to prevent premature termination of antiplatelet therapy which would dramatically increase the stent thrombosis risk [37]. For most patients who have undergone coronary stent placement, this approach would delay non-cardiac surgery for at least 5–6 weeks following intracoronary stent placement. This focused approach serves to reduce the risk of stent thrombosis in those patients whose antiplatelet agents would be prematurely discontinued, and bleeding in those who would undergo surgery while still receiving their antiplatelet regimen [86].

For the patient who has undergone placement of a drug-eluting stent, the period of dual antiplatelet therapy after stenting is 12 months and ideally longer. At least 12 months of dual-antiplatelet therapy needs to be completed before non-cardiac surgery is performed, as these stents have an increased risk of late and very late stent thrombosis compared with bare-metal stents [87]. The cytotoxic agents that are aimed at preventing neo-intimal hyperplasia also prevent or delay the physiologic healing process of endothelialization. This means that the stent struts may be uncovered and exposed to blood. The duration of 1 year of dual antiplatelet regimen after drug-eluting stents has not been established and should depend on the physician's judgment. It seems that late stent thrombosis is a steadily ongoing process at a rate of 0.2% per year with no evidence of diminution up to 3 years of follow-up [87,88].

For patients with chronic stable angina it is important to continue their anti-anginal therapy in the perioperative period. Beta-blockers are continued through the time of surgery. For prolonged effect, a long-acting preparation (i.e., nadolol or atenolol) may be given on the morning of surgery. If patients are unable to resume oral intake 24 hours after surgery, beta-blockers may be given intravenously (e.g., propranolol, 0.5–2 mg every 1–6 hours). Parenteral metoprolol or esmolol may also be used. Oral beta-blocker therapy is resumed as soon as possible after surgery.

Patients who are receiving long-term antianginal treatment with calcium channel antagonists are usually given a long-acting oral preparation on the morning of surgery. If they are unable to resume oral intake 24 hours after surgery, we generally add intravenous or topical nitrates to the regimen. The only calcium channel antagonists available for intravenous use are verapamil and diltiazem. Because their effect is primarily antiarrhythmic when they are given intravenously, we do not use these agents as primary anti-ischemic therapy for patients who are unable to take oral medications.

Management of cardiac medications in the perioperative period

Perioperative continuation of patient's long-term cardiac medications is often challenging. Many oral medications have no parenteral substitutes. The stress of surgery may render patients' long-term cardiac medical regiments inadequate during the perioperative period. Finally, few controlled studies have evaluated the use of cardiac medications during and after non-cardiac surgery. Several guidelines are helpful in attempting to maintain patients' long-term medical therapeutic regimens in the perioperative period.

Beta-adrenergic blockers are used in the treatment of myocardial ischemia, arrhythmias, hypertension, and left ventricular systolic dysfunction. Patients who receive beta-blockers on a long-term basis should be given oral doses on the morning of their surgical procedure. Long-acting agents such as atenolol and sustained-release metoprolol provide beta-blockade for as long as 24 hours. Patients' long-term beta-blocker regimens are then restarted 24 hours after surgery if oral intake has resumed. For patients whose gastrointestinal tracts are not functional at that time, the administration of intravenous beta-blockers (e.g., propranolol, 0.5–2 mg every 4–6 hours) is begun and continued until the usual long-term oral beta-blocker is tolerated. This regimen is often effective for patients who are receiving beta-blockers for coronary artery disease or cardiac arrhythmias but may require alteration in patients who take these drugs for hypertension or congestive heart failure. For the patient with hypertension, labetalol (a test dose of 2.5–5.0 mg intravenously, then an infusion of 20–80 mg) may also be given by intravenous infusion at 2 mg/min until the blood pressure is controlled or until a total of 300 mg has been given. The short-acting intravenous beta-blocker esmolol (at a loading infusion of 500 μg/kg per min for 1 minute followed by a continuous infusion of 50 μg/kg per min) may also be used to control blood pressure in the postoperative period. Patients whose blood pressures are not controlled with these agents may require supplemental antihypertensive agents in addition to intravenous beta-blockers until oral medications are resumed. For patients receiving beta-blockers as treatment for chronic congestive heart failure, we try to avoid discontinuation of beta-blockers in the perioperative period unless the patient develops deterioration of their clinical status as manifest by hypoperfusion or requires intravenous positive inotropic agents. In these cases we temporarily discontinue the beta-blocker but reinstitute it as soon as the patient is stabilized in an effort to reduce the risk of significant deterioration.

Nitrates are commonly used by patients with ischemic heart disease. Patients who are stable and receiving nitrates on a long-term basis typically are given their oral nitrate preparations on the morning of the surgical procedure. Topical nitroglycerine ointment (0.5–2 inches) is then applied every 8 hours until oral nitrates are resumed. This approach helps to maintain a "nitrate-free" period to decrease the risk of development of nitrate vasotolerance. Nitrates may cause excessive preload reduction and hypotension, which may be exacerbated by intravascular volume depletion and by the simultaneous use of other vasodilator medications or anesthetic agents. In some patients, hypotension may occur unpredictably with the initial administration of nitrates. For this reason, we recommend that the initiation of nitrates, given to decrease the likelihood of perioperative myocardial ischemia, be administered well before surgery. Intravenous nitroglycerine should be considered when nitrates are used to treat perioperative myocardial ischemia.

Intravenous nitroprusside is effective in controlling perioperative hypertension but the need for continuous blood pressure monitoring, and the risk of cyanate toxicity, makes its use impractical for more than a few days. Intravenous methyldopa and enalaprilat, given 3–4 times daily, are effective in controlling postoperative hypertension, are well tolerated, and may be used without continuous blood pressure monitoring in stable patients. They are useful adjuncts for controlling hypertension in the perioperative period.

Intravascular volume depletion may occur in patients receiving long-term diuretic therapy and places them at risk of hypotension when anesthetic agents that produce vasodilation are administered. Intravascular volume depletion is suggested by the presence of orthostatic changes in the blood pressure and heart rate and should be corrected with fluid administration, before surgery if possible. Patients who take diuretics may also have hypokalemia or hyperkalemia from potassium-sparing agents. Serum potassium levels should be checked in these patients before surgery. It has been suggested that a chronic serum potassium level of 3 mmol/L or higher is acceptable for anesthesia and surgery, and that chronic asymptomatic hypokalemia as low as 2.5 mmol/L may be adequate in patients who are at low risk for cardiac complications [89]. Hypokalemia has been shown to increase the incidence of cardiac arrhythmias in patients taking digoxin; therefore, perioperative hypokalemia should be corrected in this patient group.

Calcium channel antagonists are used to treat angina, hypertension, and arrhythmias. Sustained release preparations of the calcium channel antagonists that patients have been using may be given on the morning of surgery in an effort to achieve effective drug levels for the next 24 hours. Patients who are capable of oral intake the day after surgery may resume oral calcium channel antagonists. Problems exist, however, in substituting appropriate parenteral formulations for patients who cannot resume oral calcium channel antagonists at this time. The few calcium channel antagonists that are available for parenteral administration often have their primary effect on the cardiac conduction system rather than in treating hypertension or angina. Intravenous verapamil has potent negative chronotropic effects and can induce heart block. Intravenous diltiazem is indicated primarily to control the ventricular response in patients with atrial fibrillation and to convert paroxysmal supraventricular tachycardia to sinus rhythm in patients who have atrioventricular nodal re-entrant tachycardia. There is no parenteral preparation of nifedipine or amlodipine.

In patients who receive calcium channel antagonists for their anti-anginal effects, topical or intravenous nitrates may be substituted until oral intake resumes. In patients who take calcium channel antagonists for hypertension, intravenous alpha methyldopa or enalaprilat is often effective until oral medications are resumed.

Digitalis glycosides may be given orally on the morning of surgery and then intravenously on a daily basis until patients' long-term oral regimens are resumed. The intravenous administration of these agents increases their bioavailability by as much as 20%, and the maintenance parenteral dose may have to be reduced appropriately.

Angiotensin-converting enzyme inhibitors are used to treat hypertension and left ventricular systolic dysfunction. Enalaprilat is the only agent of this class available for parenteral administration and is given intravenously every 6 hours.

The abrupt withdrawal of centrally acting antihypertensive agents, which may occur in the perioperative period, may result in a "discontinuation syndrome" characterized by sympathetic overactivity and rebound hypertension [90]. Symptoms may resemble those of pheochromocytoma. Clonidine is the prototype drug of this class. The discontinuation syndrome may occur 18 to 72 hours after clonidine is withdrawn but rarely occurs in patients who receive less than 1.2 mg of clonidine daily. This syndrome may be aggravated by the simultaneous use of beta-blockers, which may block peripheral vasodilatory beta-receptors, leaving vasoconstrictor alpha receptors unopposed [91]. The syndrome may be terminated by resumption of clonidine therapy. If that is not possible because patients cannot resume oral intake, rebound hypertension may be controlled with intravenous nitroprusside or labetalol. Clonidine withdrawal syndrome may be prevented by slow tapering of clonidine before surgery. For patients in whom this is not feasible, transdermal clonidine may be given in the perioperative period. The transdermal clonidine requires about 48 hours to achieve therapeutic drug levels. Therefore, it should be given well in advance of surgery and, at its initiation, be administered simultaneously with oral clonidine for about 48 hours. The transdermal preparation maintains therapeutic clonidine levels for as long as 7 days.

Clopidogrel is a thienopyridine antiplatelet agent administered along with aspirin typically for 2–4 weeks to patients who have had bare metal coronary stenting or 12 months following placement of a drug-eluting stent depending on the type of stent used. There is evidence that a beneficial effect on the reduction of stent thrombosis may exist with up to 9 months of clopidogrel use post-stent placement [92]. It is also used in the treatment of patients with acute coronary syndromes [93]. Clopidogrel may increase the risk of bleeding during or immediately following major surgery. Because its effect on platelets and bleeding may last for 5 days, many surgeons request at least a 5-day period between the discontinuation of clopidogrel and subsequent major surgery [94]. Dual-antiplatelet therapy with aspirin and clopidogrel increases the risk of major bleeding compared with aspirin alone. In patients in need of dual-platelet inhibition who require urgent surgery with increased risk of bleeding it should be considered to stop the clopidogrel but continue aspirin perioperatively.

Aspirin given for primary prevention should be stopped 5–7 days prior to surgery. Monotherapy with either aspirin or clopidogrel for secondary prevention can be continued throughout most types of surgery, except those procedures where bleeding can cause significant morbidity (e.g., intracranial procedures) [95]. In non-cardiac vascular surgery, preoperative aspirin is routinely used and is associated with improved bypass graft patency.

Perioperative invasive cardiac monitoring

Invasive pulmonary artery pressure monitoring is often used in patients who are at increased risk for myocardial infarction during and after surgery in an effort to diagnose and treat perioperative myocardial ischemia. Indications for perioperative pulmonary monitoring are ill-defined. Myocardial ischemia decreases left ventricular compliance and increases left ventricular end-diastolic pressure, left atrial pressure, pulmonary capillary wedge pressure, and pulmonary artery pressure. If it is extensive, myocardial ischemia may also reduce cardiac output. These hemodynamic consequences may occur before myocardial ischemia is apparent on standard electrocardiographic monitoring or manifest as abnormalities of cardiac hemodynamics.

Although it is attractive in theory, invasive pulmonary artery pressure monitoring has suboptimal sensitivity and specificity for the detection of perioperative myocardial ischemia. Numerous perioperative situations (e.g., intravascular volume overload, increased afterload) may result in increased pulmonary artery capillary wedge pressure without associated myocardial ischemia. Similarly, myocardial ischemia may be present without changes in pulmonary artery capillary pressure. No evidence was found of reduction in complication rates associated with use of perioperative pulmonary artery catheters in an observational study of patients undergoing high-risk non-cardiac surgery. Because of the morbidity and the high costs associated with pulmonary artery catheters, this intervention in perioperative care may only be beneficial in a select group of patients at very high risk for hemodynamic disturbances. The indication for use of pulmonary artery catheters in the perioperative period is thus unclear. A multicenter, randomized, controlled clinical trial comparing perioperative therapy guided by pulmonary artery catheter derived data vs standard care in high risk (American Society of Anesthesiologists (ASA) class III or IV risk) patients 60 years of age or older found no mortality benefit to therapy directed by pulmonary artery catheter [96]. Hemodynamic optimization of critically ill patients without sepsis and overt organ failure may decrease mortality [97]. It has been our approach to assess the need for invasive hemodynamic monitoring on an individual basis. Intuitive indications for invasive hemodynamic monitoring are: anticipation of fluid shifts in the patient with left ventricular dysfunction or fixed cardiac output; major vascular surgery in the patient with left ventricular dysfunction; and surgery in the patient with recent myocardial infarction or unstable angina.

References

1. Park KW. Cardiovascular effects of inhalational anesthetics. *Int Anesthesiol Clin* 2002; **40**: 1–14.

2. Landoni G, Biondi-Zoccai GG, Zangrillo A *et al.* Desflurane and sevoflurane in cardiac surgery: a meta-analysis of randomized clinical trials. *J Cardiothorac Vasc Anesth* 2007; 21: 502–11.

3. Fleisher LA, Beckman JA, Brown KA *et al.* 2009 ACCF/AHA focused update on perioperative beta blockade incorporated into the ACC/AHA 2007 guidelines on perioperative cardiovascular evaluation and care for noncardiac surgery: a report of the American College of Cardiology Foundation/American Heart Association Task Force on practice

guidelines. *Circulation* 2009; **120**: e169–276.

4. Wiklund RA, Rosenbaum SH. Anesthesiology. First of two parts. *N Engl J Med* 1997; **337**: 1132–41.

5. Higgins TL, Yared JP, Estafanous FG *et al*. Propofol versus midazolam for intensive care unit sedation after coronary artery bypass grafting. *Crit Care Med* 1994; **22**: 1415–23.

6. Rigg JR, Jamrozik K, Myles PS *et al*. Epidural anaesthesia and analgesia and outcome of major surgery: a randomised trial. *Lancet* 2002; **359**: 1276–82.

7. Peyton PJ, Myles PS, Silbert BS *et al*. Perioperative epidural analgesia and outcome after major abdominal surgery in high-risk patients. *Anesth Analg* 2003; **96**: 548–54.

8. Park WY, Thompson JS, Lee KK. Effect of epidural anesthesia and analgesia on perioperative outcome: a randomized, controlled Veterans Affairs cooperative study. *Ann Surg* 2001; **234**: 560–9; discussion 9–71.

9. Nishimori M, Ballantyne JC, Low JH. Epidural pain relief versus systemic opioid-based pain relief for abdominal aortic surgery. *Cochrane Database Syst Rev* 2006; **3**: CD005059.

10. Saada M, Duval AM, Bonnet F *et al*. Abnormalities in myocardial segmental wall motion during lumbar epidural anesthesia. *Anesthesiology* 1989; **71**: 26–32.

11. Popping DM, Elia N, Marret E, Remy C, Tramer MR. Protective effects of epidural analgesia on pulmonary complications after abdominal and thoracic surgery: a meta-analysis. *Arch Surg* 2008; **143**: 990–9; discussion 1000.

12. Tuman KJ, McCarthy RJ, March RJ *et al*. Effects of epidural anesthesia and analgesia on coagulation and outcome after major vascular surgery. *Anesth Analg* 1991; **73**: 696–704.

13. Christopherson R, Beattie C, Frank SM *et al*. Perioperative morbidity in patients randomized to epidural or general anesthesia for lower extremity vascular surgery. Perioperative Ischemia Randomized Anesthesia Trial Study Group. *Anesthesiology* 1993; **79**: 422–34.

14. Breen P, Park KW. General anesthesia versus regional anesthesia. *Int Anesthesiol Clin* 2002; **40**: 61–71.

15. Parker MJ, Handoll HH, Griffiths R. Anaesthesia for hip fracture surgery in adults. *Cochrane Database Syst Rev* 2004; CD000521.

16. Campeau L. Letter: Grading of angina pectoris. *Circulation* 1976; **54**: 522–3.

17. Tarhan S, Moffitt EA, Taylor WF, Giuliani ER. Myocardial infarction after general anesthesia. *J Am Med Assoc* 1972; **220**: 1451–4.

18. Rao TL, Jacobs KH, El-Etr AA. Reinfarction following anesthesia in patients with myocardial infarction. *Anesthesiology* 1983; **59**: 499–505.

19. Shah KB, Kleinman BS, Rao TL *et al*. Angina and other risk factors in patients with cardiac diseases undergoing noncardiac operations. *Anesth Analg* 1990; **70**: 240–7.

20. Sprung J, Abdelmalak B, Gottlieb A *et al*. Analysis of risk factors for myocardial infarction and cardiac mortality after major vascular surgery. *Anesthesiology* 2000; **93**: 129–40.

21. Foster ED, Davis KB, Carpenter JA, Abele S, Fray D. Risk of noncardiac operation in patients with defined coronary disease: The Coronary Artery Surgery Study (CASS) registry experience. *Ann Thorac Surg* 1986; **41**: 42–50.

22. Hertzer NR, Beven EG, Young JR *et al*. Coronary artery disease in peripheral vascular patients. A classification of 1000 coronary angiograms and results of surgical management. *Ann Surg* 1984; **199**: 223–33.

23. Goldman L, Caldera DL, Nussbaum SR *et al*. Multifactorial index of cardiac risk in noncardiac surgical procedures. *N Engl J Med* 1977; **297**: 845–50.

24. Detsky AS, Abrams HB, McLaughlin JR *et al*. Predicting cardiac complications in patients undergoing non-cardiac surgery. *J Gen Intern Med* 1986; **1**: 211–19.

25. Lee TH, Marcantonio ER, Mangione CM *et al*. Derivation and prospective validation of a simple index for prediction of cardiac risk of major noncardiac surgery. *Circulation* 1999; **100**: 1043–9.

26. Jafary FH. Preoperative use of intra-aortic balloon counterpulsation in very high-risk patients prior to urgent

noncardiac surgery. *Acta Cardiol* 2005; **60**: 557–60.

27. Khan AL, Flett M, Yalamarthi S *et al*. The role of the intra-aortic balloon pump counterpulsation (IABP) in emergency surgery. *Surgeon* 2003; **1**: 279–82.

28. Pride YB, Frost EJ, Anderson PD, Cutlip DE. Precordial steering wheel: a fortunate accident. *J Emerg Med* 2011; **41**: e83–7. Epub 2008 Nov 20.

29. Nelson CL, Herndon JE, Mark DB *et al*. Relation of clinical and angiographic factors to functional capacity as measured by the Duke Activity Status Index. *Am J Cardiol* 1991; **68**: 973–5.

30. Weiner DA, Ryan TJ, McCabe CH *et al*. Prognostic importance of a clinical profile and exercise test in medically treated patients with coronary artery disease. *J Am Coll Cardiol* 1984; **3**: 772–9.

31. Gerson MC, Hurst JM, Hertzberg VS *et al*. Prediction of cardiac and pulmonary complications related to elective abdominal and noncardiac thoracic surgery in geriatric patients. *Am J Med* 1990; **88**: 101–7.

32. Hlatky MA, Boineau RE, Higginbotham MB *et al*. A brief self-administered questionnaire to determine functional capacity (the Duke Activity Status Index). *Am J Cardiol* 1989; **64**: 651–4.

33. Reilly DF, McNeely MJ, Doerner D *et al*. Self-reported exercise tolerance and the risk of serious perioperative complications. *Arch Intern Med* 1999; **159**: 2185–92.

34. Blankensteijn JD, de Jong SE, Prinssen M *et al*. Two-year outcomes after conventional or endovascular repair of abdominal aortic aneurysms. *N Engl J Med* 2005; **352**: 2398–405.

35. Endovascular aneurysm repair versus open repair in patients with abdominal aortic aneurysm (EVAR trial 1): randomised controlled trial. *Lancet* 2005; **365**: 2179–86.

36. Torsher LC, Shub C, Rettke SR, Brown DL. Risk of patients with severe aortic stenosis undergoing noncardiac surgery. *Am J Cardiol* 1998; **81**: 448–52.

37. Kaluza GL, Joseph J, Lee JR, Raizner ME, Raizner AE. Catastrophic outcomes of noncardiac surgery soon after coronary stenting. *J Am Coll Cardiol* 2000; **35**: 1288–94.

38. Wilson SH, Fasseas P, Orford JL et al. Clinical outcome of patients undergoing non-cardiac surgery in the two months following coronary stenting. *J Am Coll Cardiol* 2003; **42**: 234–40.

39. Shaw LJ, Eagle KA, Gersh BJ, Miller DD. Meta-analysis of intravenous dipyridamole-thallium-201 imaging (1985 to 1994) and dobutamine echocardiography (1991 to 1994) for risk stratification before vascular surgery. *J Am Coll Cardiol* 1996; **27**: 787–98.

40. Wijeysundera DN, Beattie WS, Austin PC, Hux JE, Laupacis A. Non-invasive cardiac stress testing before elective major non-cardiac surgery: population based cohort study. *Br Med J* 2010; **340**: b5526.

41. Hertzer NR. Basic data concerning associated coronary disease in peripheral vascular patients. *Ann Vasc Surg* 1987; **1**: 616–20.

42. L'Italien GJ, Paul SD, Hendel RC et al. Development and validation of a Bayesian model for perioperative cardiac risk assessment in a cohort of 1,081 vascular surgical candidates. *J Am Coll Cardiol* 1996; **27**: 779–86.

43. Paul SD, Eagle KA, Kuntz KM, Young JR, Hertzer NR. Concordance of preoperative clinical risk with angiographic severity of coronary artery disease in patients undergoing vascular surgery. *Circulation* 1996; **94**: 1561–6.

44. Poldermans D, Bax JJ, Schouten O et al. Should major vascular surgery be delayed because of preoperative cardiac testing in intermediate-risk patients receiving beta-blocker therapy with tight heart rate control? *J Am Coll Cardiol* 2006; **48**: 964–9.

45. De Lima JJ, Sabbaga E, Vieira ML et al. Coronary angiography is the best predictor of events in renal transplant candidates compared with noninvasive testing. *Hypertension* 2003; **42**: 263–8.

46. Hickson LJ, Cosio FG, El-Zoghby ZM et al. Survival of patients on the kidney transplant wait list: relationship to cardiac troponin T. *Am J Transpl* 2008; **8**: 2352–9.

47. Kasiske BL, Cangro CB, Hariharan S et al. The evaluation of renal transplantation candidates: clinical practice guidelines. *Am J Transpl* 2001; **1** (Suppl 2): 3–95.

48. Humar A, Kerr SR, Ramcharan T, Gillingham KJ, Matas AJ. Perioperative cardiac morbidity in kidney transplant recipients: incidence and risk factors. *Clin Transpl* 2001; **15**: 154–8.

49. Wolfe RA, Ashby VB, Milford EL et al. Comparison of mortality in all patients on dialysis, patients on dialysis awaiting transplantation, and recipients of a first cadaveric transplant. *N Engl J Med* 1999; **341**: 1725–30.

50. Patel RK, Mark PB, Johnston N et al. Prognostic value of cardiovascular screening in potential renal transplant recipients: a single-center prospective observational study. *Am J Transpl* 2008; **8**: 1673–83.

51. Jeloka TK, Ross H, Smith R et al. Renal transplant outcome in high-cardiovascular risk recipients. *Clin Transpl* 2007; **21**: 609–14.

52. Mistry BM, Bastani B, Solomon H et al. Prognostic value of dipyridamole thallium-201 screening to minimize perioperative cardiac complications in diabetics undergoing kidney or kidney-pancreas transplantation. *Clin Transpl* 1998; **12**: 130–5.

53. Plotkin JS, Scott VL, Pinna A et al. Morbidity and mortality in patients with coronary artery disease undergoing orthotopic liver transplantation. *Liver Transpl Surg* 1996; **2**: 426–30.

54. Carey WD, Dumot JA, Pimentel RR et al. The prevalence of coronary artery disease in liver transplant candidates over age 50. *Transplantation* 1995; **59**: 859–64.

55. Donovan CL, Marcovitz PA, Punch JD et al. Two-dimensional and dobutamine stress echocardiography in the preoperative assessment of patients with end-stage liver disease prior to orthotopic liver transplantation. *Transplantation* 1996; **61**: 1180–8.

56. Roseberg B, Wulff K. Hemodynamics following normovolemic hemodilution in elderly patients. *Acta Anaesthesiol Scand* 1981; **25**: 402–6.

57. Rodeheffer RJ, Gerstenblith G, Becker LC et al. Exercise cardiac output is maintained with advancing age in healthy human subjects: cardiac dilatation and increased stroke volume compensate for a diminished heart rate. *Circulation* 1984; **69**: 203–13.

58. Wenger NK. Cardiovascular disease in the elderly. *Curr Probl Cardiol* 1992; **17**: 609–90.

59. Leung JM, Dzankic S. Relative importance of preoperative health status versus intraoperative factors in predicting postoperative adverse outcomes in geriatric surgical patients. *J Am Geriatr Soc* 2001; **49**: 1080–5.

60. Liu LL, Leung JM. Predicting adverse postoperative outcomes in patients aged 80 years or older. *J Am Geriatr Soc* 2000; **48**: 405–12.

61. Polanczyk CA, Marcantonio E, Goldman L et al. Impact of age on perioperative complications and length of stay in patients undergoing noncardiac surgery. *Ann Intern Med* 2001; **134**: 637–43.

62. Liu LL, Dzankic S, Leung JM. Preoperative electrocardiogram abnormalities do not predict postoperative cardiac complications in geriatric surgical patients. *J Am Geriatr Soc* 2002; **50**: 1186–91.

63. Mangano DT, Layug EL, Wallace A, Tateo I. Effect of atenolol on mortality and cardiovascular morbidity after noncardiac surgery. Multicenter Study of Perioperative Ischemia Research Group. *N Engl J Med* 1996; **335**: 1713–20.

64. Raby KE, Brull SJ, Timimi F et al. The effect of heart rate control on myocardial ischemia among high-risk patients after vascular surgery. *Anesth Analg* 1999; **88**: 477–82.

65. Poldermans D, Boersma E, Bax JJ et al. The effect of bisoprolol on perioperative mortality and myocardial infarction in high-risk patients undergoing vascular surgery. Dutch Echocardiographic Cardiac Risk Evaluation Applying Stress Echocardiography Study Group. *N Engl J Med* 1999; **341**: 1789–94.

66. Boersma E, Poldermans D, Bax JJ et al. Predictors of cardiac events after major vascular surgery: role of clinical characteristics, dobutamine echocardiography, and beta-blocker therapy. *J Am Med Assoc* 2001; **285**: 1865–73.

67. Lindenauer PK, Pekow P, Wang K et al. Perioperative beta-blocker therapy and

mortality after major noncardiac surgery. *N Engl J Med* 2005; **353**: 349–61.

68. Brady AR, Gibbs JS, Greenhalgh RM, Powell JT, Sydes MR. Perioperative beta-blockade (POBBLE) for patients undergoing infrarenal vascular surgery: results of a randomized double-blind controlled trial. *J Vasc Surg* 2005; **41**: 602–9.

69. Devereaux PJ, Beattie WS, Choi PT *et al.* How strong is the evidence for the use of perioperative beta blockers in non-cardiac surgery? Systematic review and meta-analysis of randomised controlled trials. *Br Med J* 2005; **331**: 313–21.

70. Devereaux PJ, Yang H, Yusuf S *et al.* Effects of extended-release metoprolol succinate in patients undergoing non-cardiac surgery (POISE trial): a randomised controlled trial. *Lancet* 2008; **371**: 1839–47.

71. Hoeks SE, Scholte Op Reimer WJ, van Urk H *et al.* Increase of 1-year mortality after perioperative beta-blocker withdrawal in endovascular and vascular surgery patients. *Eur J Vasc Endovasc Surg* 2007; **33**: 13–19.

72. Thomson IR, Mutch WA, Culligan JD. Failure of intravenous nitroglycerin to prevent intraoperative myocardial ischemia during fentanyl-pancuronium anesthesia. *Anesthesiology* 1984; **61**: 385–93.

73. Wijeysundera DN, Beattie WS. Calcium channel blockers for reducing cardiac morbidity after noncardiac surgery: a meta-analysis. *Anesth Analg* 2003; **97**: 634–41.

74. Wijeysundera DN, Naik JS, Beattie WS. Alpha-2 adrenergic agonists to prevent perioperative cardiovascular complications: a meta-analysis. *Am J Med* 2003; **114**: 742–52.

75. Wallace AW, Galindez D, Salahieh A *et al.* Effect of clonidine on cardiovascular morbidity and mortality after noncardiac surgery. *Anesthesiology* 2004; **101**: 284–93.

76. Wijeysundera DN, Bender JS, Beattie WS. Alpha-2 adrenergic agonists for the prevention of cardiac complications among patients undergoing surgery. *Cochrane Database Syst Rev* 2009; CD004126.

77. Frank SM, Fleisher LA, Breslow MJ *et al.* Perioperative maintenance of normothermia reduces the incidence of morbid cardiac events. A randomized clinical trial. *J Am Med Assoc* 1997; **277**: 1127–34.

78. Winchester DE, Wen X, Xie L, Bavry AA. Evidence of pre-procedural statin therapy: a meta-analysis of randomized trials. *J Am Coll Cardiol* 2010; **56**: 1099–109.

79. Mangano DT. Perioperative cardiac morbidity. *Anesthesiology* 1990; **72**: 153–84.

80. Hertzer NR, Young JR, Beven EG *et al.* Late results of coronary bypass in patients with infrarenal aortic aneurysms. The Cleveland Clinic Study. *Ann Surg* 1987; **205**: 360–7.

81. Eagle KA, Rihal CS, Mickel MC *et al.* Cardiac risk of noncardiac surgery: influence of coronary disease and type of surgery in 3368 operations. CASS Investigators and University of Michigan Heart Care Program. Coronary Artery Surgery Study. *Circulation* 1997; **96**: 1882–7.

82. McFalls EO, Ward HB, Moritz TE *et al.* Coronary-artery revascularization before elective major vascular surgery. *N Engl J Med* 2004; **351**: 2795–804.

83. Garcia S, Moritz TE, Ward HB *et al.* Usefulness of revascularization of patients with multivessel coronary artery disease before elective vascular surgery for abdominal aortic and peripheral occlusive disease. *Am J Cardiol* 2008; **102**: 809–13.

84. Ward HB, Kelly RF, Thottapurathu L *et al.* Coronary artery bypass grafting is superior to percutaneous coronary intervention in prevention of perioperative myocardial infarctions during subsequent vascular surgery. *Ann Thorac Surg* 2006; **82**: 795–800; discussion –1.

85. Hassan SA, Hlatky MA, Boothroyd DB *et al.* Outcomes of noncardiac surgery after coronary bypass surgery or coronary angioplasty in the Bypass Angioplasty Revascularization Investigation (BARI). *Am J Med* 2001; **110**: 260–6.

86. Weitz HH. How soon can a patient undergo noncardiac surgery after receiving a drug-eluting stent? *Cleve Clin J Med* 2005; **72**: 818–20.

87. Daemen J, Wenaweser P, Tsuchida K *et al.* Early and late coronary stent thrombosis of sirolimus-eluting and paclitaxel-eluting stents in routine clinical practice: data from a large two-institutional cohort study. *Lancet* 2007; **369**: 667–78.

88. Hodgson JM, Stone GW, Lincoff AM *et al.* Late stent thrombosis: considerations and practical advice for the use of drug-eluting stents: a report from the Society for Cardiovascular Angiography and Interventions Drug-eluting Stent Task Force. *Catheter Cardiovasc Interv* 2007; **69**: 327–33.

89. Restrick LJ, Huddy N, Hoffbrand BI. Diuretic-induced hypokalaemia and surgery: much ado about nothing? *Postgrad Med J* 1992; **68**: 318–20.

90. Houston MC. Abrupt cessation of treatment in hypertension: consideration of clinical features, mechanisms, prevention and management of the discontinuation syndrome. *Am Heart J* 1981; **102**: 415–30.

91. Bailey RR, Neale TJ. Rapid clonidine withdrawal with blood pressure overshoot exaggerated by beta-blockade. *Br Med J* 1976; **1**: 942–3.

92. Mehta SR, Yusuf S, Peters RJ *et al.* Effects of pretreatment with clopidogrel and aspirin followed by long-term therapy in patients undergoing percutaneous coronary intervention: the PCI-CURE study. *Lancet* 2001; **358**: 527–33.

93. Yusuf S, Zhao F, Mehta SR *et al.* Effects of clopidogrel in addition to aspirin in patients with acute coronary syndromes without ST-segment elevation. *N Engl J Med* 2001; **345**: 494–502.

94. Cannon CP, Mehta SR, Aranki SF. Balancing the benefit and risk of oral antiplatelet agents in coronary artery bypass surgery. *Ann Thorac Surg* 2005; **80**: 768–79.

95. Korte W, Cattaneo M, Chassot PG *et al.* Peri-operative management of antiplatelet therapy in patients with coronary artery disease. Joint position paper by members of the working group on Perioperative Haemostasis of the Society on Thrombosis and Haemostasis Research (GTH), the working group on

Perioperative Coagulation of the Austrian Society for Anesthesiology, Resuscitation and Intensive Care (OGARI) and the Working Group Thrombosis of the European Society for Cardiology (ESC). *Thromb Haemost* 2011; **105**: 743–9.

96. Sandham JD, Hull RD, Brant RF *et al.* A randomized, controlled trial of the use of pulmonary-artery catheters in high-risk surgical patients. *N Engl J Med* 2003; **348**: 5–14.

97. Poeze M, Greve JW, Ramsay G. Meta-analysis of hemodynamic optimization: relationship to methodological quality. *Crit Care* 2005; **9**: R771–9.

Arrhythmias and conduction abnormalities

Incidence and clinical significance of perioperative arrhythmias

Cardiac arrhythmias are common in the perioperative period. They are usually clinically insignificant. In one study using continuous electrocardiographic monitoring, 84% of patients were documented to have at least transient arrhythmias during their hospitalization for surgery. Only 5% of these arrhythmias were clinically important [1]. In another study Kuner *et al.* noted a 62% incidence of one or more transient arrhythmias in the perioperative period. The dysrhythmias were primarily supraventricular, most commonly wandering atrial pacemaker, isorhythmic atrioventricular (AV) dissociation, junctional rhythm, and sinus bradycardia. Isorhythmic AV dissociation is more frequently seen in anesthesia with volatile anesthetics, and small doses of IV beta-blockers were described as effective in reverting it back to normal sinus rhythm [2,3]. Ventricular premature contractions were common but paroxysmal ventricular tachycardia was rare [3]. The Multicenter Study of General Anesthesia reported a 70.2% incidence of tachycardia, bradycardia, or dysrhythmia in more than 17,000 patients who underwent a variety of surgical procedures. Adverse outcomes as a result of these dysrhythmias were reported in only 1.6% of the patients [4,5].

In a study of men who underwent non-cardiac surgery and had known coronary artery disease or significant risk factors for coronary artery disease, O'Kelly found that frequent or major ventricular arrhythmias (more than 30 ventricular premature contractions per hour or ventricular tachycardia) occurred in 44% of the patients who were monitored (21% before operation, 16% during operation, and 36% after operation). Preoperative ventricular arrhythmias were associated with the occurrence of intraoperative and postoperative arrhythmias. These arrhythmias were largely benign, and sustained ventricular tachycardia or ventricular fibrillation did not occur [6].

Multifactorial risk indices identified preoperative ventricular premature contractions and rhythms other than sinus rhythm as markers of risk in non-cardiac surgery. We currently believe that ventricular premature contractions and related ventricular ectopy are markers of risk when they occur in the presence of ischemic or structural heart disease. The American College of Cardiology/American Heart Association *Practice Guideline on Perioperative Cardiovascular Evaluation for Noncardiac Surgery* classifies symptomatic ventricular arrhythmias in the presence of underlying heart disease, supraventricular arrhythmias with uncontrolled ventricular rate, and high-grade atrioventricular block in the presence of underlying heart disease as active cardiac conditions that warrant evaluation of the patient and delay of surgery if possible. This guideline classifies preoperative rhythm other than sinus rhythm (e.g., atrial fibrillation) as a minor predictor that should raise suspicion for underlying cardiovascular disease, but it is not an independent risk factor for perioperative myocardial infarction or death [7,8].

We look for evidence of structural or ischemic heart disease, metabolic derangements, and electrolyte abnormalities when arrhythmias or conduction abnormalities are identified prior to surgery. We do not consider preoperative ventricular premature contractions or complex ventricular arrhythmias in the absence of heart disease or metabolic or electrolyte abnormality to be significant risk factors. Patients with atrial premature contractions and supraventricular arrhythmias that occur without the development of hemodynamic instability are also not considered to be at increased risk. While the presence of atrial fibrillation is a minor predictor for possible cardiac disease, a challenge in the perioperative period is adjustment of anticoagulation regimens for those patients who are receiving long-term anticoagulant therapy. Patients with chronic atrial fibrillation may be treated with medications to control the ventricular response or with medications to maintain sinus rhythm. Care is required to maintain these medications or appropriate substitutes in the perioperative period.

Risk factors for, and etiology of, perioperative arrhythmias and conduction abnormalities

In a study of patients who underwent non-cardiac surgery and developed supraventricular arrhythmias in the perioperative period, Polanczyk identified the following preoperative correlates for the development of perioperative arrhythmia: male sex (odds ratio (OR), 1.3; 95% CI, 1.0–1.7), age 70 years or older (OR, 1.3; CI, 1.0–1.7), significant valvular disease (OR, 2.1; CI, 1.2–3.6), history of supraventricular arrhythmia (OR, 3.4; CI, 2.4–4.8) or asthma (OR, 2.0; CI, 1.3–3.1), congestive heart failure (OR, 1.7; CI, 1.1–2.7), premature atrial complexes on preoperative electrocardiography (OR, 2.1; CI, 1.3–3.4), American Society of Anesthesiologists class III or IV (OR, 1.4; CI, 1.1–1.9), and type of procedure: abdominal aortic aneurysm (OR, 3.9; CI, 2.4–6.3) or abdominal (OR, 2.5; CI,

1.7–3.6), vascular (OR, 1.6; CI, 1.1–2.4), and intrathoracic (OR, 9.2; CI, 6.7–13) procedures [9]. Multiple studies have shown that the only consistent independent risk factor for postoperative atrial fibrillation is age ≥ 60 [10,11].

Sinus tachycardia is common in the perioperative period and often results from catecholamine release precipitated by stress, pain, or anxiety. Hypovolemia or anemia may cause sinus tachycardia as a compensatory response to increase cardiac output. Less common but ominous causes of sinus tachycardia are perioperative congestive heart failure and myocardial infarction. The anesthetic agent ketamine may cause sinus tachycardia as a result of central sympathetic stimulation. Hypercarbia and hypoxemia resulting from inadequate ventilation may cause sinus tachycardia as well as ventricular tachycardia.

Bradycardia is seen frequently during hospitalization for surgery and has numerous causes. Narcotics, with the exception of meperidine, may cause bradycardia by producing central vagal stimulation [12]. Anticholinesterases which are administered to antagonize the effect of non-depolarizing neuromuscular blocking agents may result in bradycardia [13]. An imbalance between sympathetic and parasympathetic tone may be produced in patients undergoing spinal or epidural anesthesia if cardiac stimulating sympathetic fibers are anesthetized. This can occur if the spinal cord is anesthetized at the level of the sympathetic ganglia (T-1 to T-4) or if spinal anesthesia is placed 2–6 segments distant from this region because the anesthetic agent may migrate or ascending preganglionic sympathetic fibers in the paravertebral chain may be blocked. Unopposed parasympathetic (vagal) activity may occur and lead to peripheral vasodilation and hypotension in addition to bradycardia [14].

Reflex bradycardia, occasionally associated with heart block and sinus arrest, may occur during surgical procedures (Table 9.4) [15–22]. It is usually caused by a reflex arc whose efferent limb is the vagus nerve. In addition to bradycardia, this vagally mediated reflex may result in peripheral vasodilation and hypotension. Anesthetic agents such as vecuronium, atacurium, halothane, fentanyl, and succinylcholine may predispose to this reflex [15]. It can be prevented by premedication with an anticholinergic agent such as atropine. If reflex bradycardia does occur, it often can be terminated by discontinuing the procedure or administering anticholinergic agents.

In O'Kelly et al.'s study of perioperative ventricular arrhythmias, the presence of preoperative ventricular ectopy was the most significant predictor of intraoperative and postoperative ventricular arrhythmias. Other risk factors were history of congestive heart failure and history of cigarette smoking. Additional causes of perioperative arrhythmias include hypoxia, hypercarbia, and acute hypokalemia [6].

Arrhythmias may be precipitated by medications used specifically during ophthalmic surgery as a result of systemic absorption of eye drops. Ophthalmic atropine has been reported to cause supraventricular tachycardia and atrial fibrillation; timolol and pilocarpine eye drops have been reported to cause bradycardia [23].

Patients with preoperative cardiac arrhythmias

If atrial fibrillation is detected during the initial preoperative evaluation, we often delay non-emergency surgery and evaluate the patient in a manner similar to our approach to that for the patient with newly diagnosed atrial fibrillation not going to surgery. We attempt to identify precipitating causes. An echocardiogram is performed to evaluate for the presence of structural cardiac abnormalities. Electrolytes as well as thyroid function are assessed. Since the AFFIRM Trial found that, in patients with persistent or recurrent atrial fibrillation, rhythm control was not superior in terms of mortality to rate control with antithrombotic therapy, our approach in newly diagnosed atrial fibrillation is to assess the need for restoration of sinus rhythm vs rate control of atrial fibrillation; to evaluate the patient's need for antithrombotic therapy to prevent stroke; and to appropriately control ventricular response of the atrial fibrillation [24,25].

If the patient is unstable (e.g., pulmonary edema, unstable angina) urgent cardioversion may have to be performed. If the patient is stable, our approach is to slow the ventricular rate with A–V nodal blocking agents (e.g., diltiazem, verapamil, esmolol, metoprolol, propranolol). Up to two-thirds of

Table 9.4 Reflex bradycardia during surgery.

Surgical procedure	Afferent reflex pathway	Reference
Abdominal manipulation	Celiac plexus	16
Mesenteric traction	?	17
Liver biopsy	Hepatic, celiac plexus	18
Laparoscopy	Parasympathetic stimulation from peritoneal stimulation	19
Ocular stimulation (Oculocardiac reflex)	Parasympathetic fibers in the ciliary nerves and the ophthalmic nerve run to the trigeminal nerve which is adjacent to the nucleus ambiguous, which is the origin of the vagus	15
Maxilla or zygoma stimulation	Trigeminal nerve	20
Neurosurgery (tentorium stimulation)	Ophthalmic nerve innervates tentorium; reflex similar to oculocardiac reflex	21
Laryngoscopy	Laryngeal stimulation	22
Blepharoplasty	Same as oculocardiac reflex	15

Table 9.5 CHADS2 score for atrial fibrillation.

Risk factor	Point score	Total score	Annual risk of stroke
		0	1.9%
Congestive heart failure	1	1	2.8%
Hypertension	1	2	4.0%
Age > 75 years	1	3	5.9%
Diabetes on insulin	1	4	8.5%
Previous stroke or TIA	2	5	12.5%
Total score	1–6	6	18.2%

CHADS2: Congestive heart failure, Hypertension, Age over 75 years, Diabetes mellitus, Stroke or TIA history.

patients will spontaneously convert to sinus rhythm within 24 hours of the onset of atrial fibrillation [24]. If we are unable to determine the duration of the patient's atrial fibrillation, we initiate warfarin anticoagulation to decrease the likelihood of systemic embolism. When cardioversion is planned, we either perform cardioversion after 3 weeks of therapeutic warfarin therapy or, as an alternate approach, transesophageal echocardiography is performed and cardioversion is attempted if there is no evidence of left atrial thrombi. In both approaches warfarin is continued with maintenance of international normalized ratio (inr) 2.0–3.0 for 3–4 weeks following conversion. We then plan surgery to occur after completion of this warfarin course.

For the patient with chronic atrial fibrillation who receives long-term anticoagulation, there is no clear evidence for the management of anticoagulation in the perioperative period. A consensus recommendation from the latest guidelines for the management of patients with atrial fibrillation states that it is reasonable to interrupt anticoagulation for up to 1 week without substituting heparin for surgical or diagnostic procedures that carry a risk of bleeding in patients with AF who do not have mechanical prosthetic heart valves [26].

Patients with an intermediate risk CHADS2 score (CHADS is a mnemonic for Congestive heart failure, Hypertension, Age over 75 years, Diabetes mellitus, Stroke or TIA history) have an annual stroke risk of 3–5% without treatment (Table 9.5). Thus, if therapy is stopped for 5 days their risk for a thromboembolic event during this time would be 0.04–0.07%. Patients at high risk of thrombosis, defined as those with atrial fibrillation and mechanical heart valve or history of previous thromboembolism or mitral stenosis have an estimated annual stroke risk of 10–30%, and their risk of stroke in 5 days without treatment would be 0.14–0.41% [26,27]. In these patients it is recommended that therapeutic doses of intravenous unfractionated heparin should be started when the INR falls below 2.0 (typically 48 hours before surgery), stopped 4–6 hours before the procedure, restarted as early after surgery as bleeding stability allows, and continued until the INR is again therapeutic with warfarin therapy [26,28]. Alternatively, therapeutic doses of subcutaneous unfractionated heparin

(15,000 U every 12 hours) or low-molecular weight heparin (100 U/kg every 12 hours) may be considered during the period of a subtherapeutic INR. If time does not allow for these protocols the effects of warfarin can be reversed by parenteral vitamin K or fresh frozen plasma. Of note, in patients with mechanical valves who require interruption of warfarin therapy for non-cardiac surgery, high-dose vitamin K should not be given routinely, because this may create a hypercoagulable condition [28].

Patients are commonly found to have asymptomatic ventricular ectopy at the time of preoperative evaluation. When significant ventricular ectopy (e.g., frequent ventricular premature contractions, non-sustained ventricular tachycardia) is identified, we search for a metabolic cause such as hypoxia or hypokalemia. If none is identified, we then search for the presence of underlying structural cardiac disease and perform an echocardiogram to evaluate left ventricular function. We frequently perform an exercise stress test or vasodilator myocardial imaging to investigate the possibility that myocardial ischemia is playing a role, although this is controversial in patients without symptoms of ischemic disease. In the patient with normal left ventricular function and no evidence of inducible myocardial ischemia, asymptomatic ventricular ectopy is usually benign. Patients with severe left ventricular dysfunction or inducible myocardial ischemia as a cause of ventricular ectopy are at increased risk of death. These patients are further evaluated for the reversibility of their cardiac dysfunction by revascularization.

Special consideration must be given to patients who take the antiarrhythmic agent, amiodarone. This drug is used to treat serious ventricular arrhythmias and, in lower doses, to treat supraventricular tachycardia and atrial fibrillation. One side-effect of this drug is chronic pulmonary interstitial disease. Acute life-threatening pulmonary complications such as the adult respiratory distress syndrome have been observed in patients undergoing cardiac, as well as non-cardiac, surgery while receiving amiodarone. Respiratory failure has been reported 16–72 hours after surgery, unrelated to the dose of amiodarone. Amiodarone levels persist in the body for weeks after its use has been discontinued and amiodarone-related postoperative adult respiratory distress syndrome has been observed in patients who stopped taking the drug 6 days before surgery. The cause of this complication is speculative and may be linked to oxidative lung injury induced by high concentrations of inspired oxygen in the perioperative period. Thus acute amiodarone pulmonary toxicity should be kept in mind for the patient receiving amiodarone who develops perioperative adult respiratory distress syndrome.

Identification and treatment of specific disorders of cardiac rate and rhythm

The guiding principle in the treatment of perioperative cardiac arrhythmias is that the cause of the arrhythmia should be treated and reversed if possible. In the setting of an unstable or life-threatening tachyarrhythmia, cardioversion is frequently utilized to restore regular rhythm while the cause of the arrhythmia is being identified and treated.

Common causes of perioperative arrhythmias are catecholamine release; alterations in autonomic tone; electrolyte abnormalities (e.g., acute hypokalemia, hyperkalemia); acid–base disturbances (e.g., acidosis, alkalosis); anemia; and acute volume depletion. Less commonly, myocardial ischemia is the cause of serious cardiac arrhythmias or conduction abnormalities. Indications for the treatment of perioperative arrhythmias include hemodynamic instability, myocardial ischemia, and myocardial infarction, or the suspicion that these deleterious consequences may occur if the arrhythmia persists.

Sinus tachycardia

Sinus tachycardia is the most common perioperative rhythm abnormality and is almost always benign. It is characterized by a heart rate between 100 and 160 beats/min. The electrocardiogram demonstrates a regular rhythm with a normal P wave before each QRS complex. The QRS complex is normal unless patients have myocardial ischemia, aberrant ventricular conduction, or conduction abnormalities. The most common causes of sinus tachycardia are pain, hypovolemia, anemia, hypoxia, fever, and hypercarbia. Treatment is directed at the inciting factor. Patients with coronary artery disease may develop myocardial ischemia as a result of increased heart rate and increased myocardial oxygen demand. Beta-adrenergic blockers may be beneficial in this instance to decrease the heart rate and alleviate myocardial ischemia while the underlying cause of the sinus tachycardia is being treated.

Atrial premature contractions

Atrial premature contractions are of minor clinical significance but may be harbingers of supraventricular tachycardia or atrial fibrillation. They arise in the atria at a site other than the sinus node and therefore are represented on the electrocardiogram by a P wave that has a different configuration and occurs earlier in the cardiac cycle than does a normal P wave. Atrial premature contractions typically produce a normal QRS

complex. If the premature contraction arrives at the ventricular conduction tissue when it is still refractory and has not fully repolarized, it may result in no QRS complex or one that is abnormal as a result of aberrant ventricular conduction. The aberrant QRS complex is usually of right bundle branch block morphology because the refractory period of the right bundle is longer than that of the left bundle.

Atrial flutter and atrial fibrillation

The incidence of atrial fibrillation after cardiac and thoracic surgery is much higher than after non-cardiothoracic surgery. Nevertheless, aside from sinus tachycardia it is the most common arrhythmia after non-cardiac surgery. Its incidence has been reported as high as 2.5% in older data and at less than 1% in more recent studies [29,30]. The American College of Cardiology/American Heart Association/European Society of Cardiology *Guidelines for the Management of Patients with Atrial Fibrillation* provide recommendations for treatment of postoperative atrial fibrillation [26]. These recommendations are adapted in large part from our approach to atrial flutter and atrial fibrillation in the non-surgical setting. We treat perioperative atrial flutter and atrial fibrillation in similar fashion.

Hemodynamic instability and the presence of myocardial ischemia or congestive heart failure dictate the treatment that should be employed for postoperative atrial flutter or atrial fibrillation. If atrial fibrillation causes the patient to be unstable, the immediate goal is to restore sinus rhythm, usually by direct current (DC) cardioversion. DC cardioversion of atrial fibrillation in adults should begin at 200 J for monophasic shock delivery waveforms, while the initial biphasic energy dose is recommended at 120–200 J. If the initial shock does not restore sinus rhythm, shocks at higher energy levels should be administered [31]. If the arrhythmia is well tolerated, the initial plan should be to control the ventricular rate. If patients remain in atrial flutter or fibrillation and are hemodynamically stable, conversion to sinus rhythm may be attempted under elective conditions.

Digoxin has traditionally been the agent of choice for controlling the ventricular rate in either atrial fibrillation or atrial flutter. Unfortunately, it has a slow onset of action and may have significant side-effects [32]. Digoxin's main role is as an adjunct to a beta-blocker or a calcium channel blocker for additional rate control. Digoxin is still the drug of first choice for ventricular rate control in patients in atrial fibrillation with decompensated heart failure because of the drug's positive inotropic effect. Acute rate control is commonly achieved with continuous intravenous infusion of diltiazem. Verapamil and esmolol are also available as continuous infusion agents. Some data suggest that beta-blockers accelerate return to sinus rhythm in patients with postoperative supraventricular tachycardia [33]. It is our preference that, when patients are switched from continuous intravenous medications to oral medications, beta-blockers be used (if it is possible to do so) because of the long-term beneficial effects of beta-blockers in patients with ischemic heart disease.

The treatment of persistent atrial fibrillation after surgery has not been standardized; different centers have different approaches. The basic decision is whether it is best to aggressively pursue rhythm control or whether it is preferable to employ a rate control strategy. One study of cardiac surgery patients with postoperative atrial fibrillation treated with a rate control strategy noted that 90% of their patients were in sinus rhythm at 4 weeks [34]. We prefer that all patients with either frequent paroxysms or persistent atrial fibrillation have systemic anticoagulation for several weeks following surgery if they have a low risk for bleeding. After that period, the patient's risk for recurrent atrial fibrillation is reassessed and a decision about long-term therapy can be made.

For patients at high risk for developing bleeding complications and those in whom ventricular rate control is difficult, a rhythm control approach is frequently undertaken. In such patients, we usually restore sinus rhythm with direct current electrical countershock. Most anti-arrhythmic medications have only moderate efficacy in terminating atrial fibrillation. However, Ibutilide, a Class III antiarrhythmic medication is effective in terminating atrial flutter or atrial fibrillation of recent onset [35,36]. Ibutilide can also be used to raise the atrial defibrillation threshold, an approach that allows a higher success rate for electrical cardioversion [37]. The shorter the duration of the atrial fibrillation, the better is the success rate of cardioversion. However, it should again be noted that new onset atrial fibrillation has a high spontaneous conversion rate to sinus rhythm [38].

Because of the known increased risk of acute thromboembolic complication following cardioversion we do not perform pharmacologic or electrical cardioversion if atrial fibrillation or flutter has persisted for more than 48 hours [39]. If a rhythm control approach is undertaken, antiarrhythmic medications are usually initiated to prevent the recurrence of atrial fibrillation if the patient reverts to sinus rhythm spontaneously. It is our preference to use a class III antiarrhythmic medication, either amiodarone, sotalol, or dofetilide, in patients with structural heart disease. However, we avoid sotalol and dofetilide in patients with significant left ventricular hypertrophy (LV free wall > 14 mm) as these patients are considered to be at higher risk for drug-induced torsade des pointes. Amiodarone and dofetilide are the only antiarrhythmics safe in heart failure patients [40,41]. On occasion, a class I-A agent such as quinidine can be used if bradycardia prevents the use of sotalol or amiodarone [42]. Evidence-based data regarding the use of dofetilide in the management of postoperative atrial fibrillation have not yet been reported, but there are some data that it may be useful in preventing perioperative atrial fibrillation [43]. We do not use class I-C drugs such as propafenone or flecanide in patients with ischemic heart disease; however, we frequently use them in patients without ischemic heart disease [44].

We prefer to discontinue anti-arrhythmic medications 4–8 weeks after surgery unless the patient is at high risk for recurrent atrial fibrillation. No large randomized studies have been performed evaluating the risk–benefit ratio of systemic anticoagulation, or comparing rhythm control to rate control for the management of postoperative atrial fibrillation. Therefore, an individual approach is required in the management of these conditions.

Of all non-cardiac surgical procedures, thoracic surgery is probably most often complicated by the onset of postoperative atrial fibrillation. The peak incidence of atrial fibrillation that accompanies thoracic surgery is between postoperative days 2 and 4. The mechanism for thoracic surgery-induced atrial fibrillation is unclear. The pulmonary veins in non-surgical patients have been found to be a trigger zone for the onset of atrial fibrillation as well as an important factor to sustain atrial fibrillation once it starts [45]. Manipulation of the pulmonary veins may play a role in the occurrence of atrial fibrillation following thoracic surgery. It is important to note that digoxin is particularly ineffective in the control of ventricular response to atrial fibrillation that follows thoracic surgery [46,47].

Paroxysmal supraventricular tachycardia

Paroxysmal supraventricular tachycardia (PSVT) is characterized by the sudden onset of a rapid regular rhythm with rates between 150 and 250 beats/min. The most common mechanism requires two different electrical pathways, one to conduct faster than the other. With atrioventricular nodal re-entrant tachycardia (AVNRT), the most common type of PSVT, a premature atrial complex that is blocked in the fast pathway and redirected through the slow pathway typically triggers the tachycardia. The electrical impulse, after proceeding down the slow pathway, re-enters the fast pathway in retrograde fashion. It then travels back, in antegrade fashion toward the ventricles and again re-enters the fast pathway to travel back to the atria in retrograde fashion. In AVNRT this circuit is found in the AV node. Re-entrant PSVT that utilizes an accessory pathway outside of the AV node (e.g., Wolff–Parkinson–White syndrome) is called atrioventricular re-entrant tachycardia (AVRT). On occasion, an atrial tachycardia or atrial flutter will have the 12-lead ECG pattern of PSVT.

The management of PSVT is identical, regardless of whether the mechanism is AVNRT or AVRT. If patients are unstable hemodynamically, have angina or congestive heart failure because of the tachycardia, immediate synchronized DC cardioversion should be performed. PSVT is usually responsive to DC cardioversion with 50 J monophasic or biphasic shock. If a 50 J shock does not restore sinus rhythm, shocks at higher energy levels should be administered (i.e., 100 J, 200 J) [31]. Most clinicians advocate starting at a high energy output to reduce the need for multiple DC cardioversions. If the QRS complex is wide and the rhythm has not been definitely proven to be supraventricular, it should be treated as ventricular tachycardia. If patients are stable hemodynamically during PSVT, vagal maneuvers or medical therapy may suffice to terminate the arrhythmia. Vagal maneuvers slow conduction through the AV node by increasing parasympathetic tone. These maneuvers terminate the arrhythmia by disrupting the re-entrant circuit that is necessary to sustain the tachycardia. The most effective vagal maneuver is the Valsalva maneuver (54% termination rate) [48]. However, the Valsalva maneuver may be impossible to perform in the perioperative period, either because of the inability of patients to cooperate or because of the high sympathetic tone. Carotid sinus massage has a success rate of 17% using the right carotid and 5% using the left, and may be the easiest vagal maneuver in the perioperative period to perform. It must be performed while using electrocardiographic monitoring; intravenous atropine and other antiarrhythmic drugs should be available in the event that advanced heart block or another arrhythmia occurs. Carotid sinus massage should not be used in elderly patients or in those with carotid bruits or known cerebrovascular disease because of the risk of inducing a stroke. If vagal maneuvers are unsuccessful or contraindicated and patients remain stable hemodynamically, intravenous adenosine should be administered. This agent is the initial drug of choice for the conversion of hemodynamically stable PSVT and is successful in more than 90% of cases. Adenosine should be given as a 6 mg rapid infusion over 1 to 3 seconds. If conversion is not achieved after 1 or 2 minutes, an additional 12 mg rapid infusion should be given. If the rhythm does not convert with the use of adenosine, rate control with diltiazem or beta-blockers is recommended. If patients become hemodynamically unstable during attempts at conversion to sinus rhythm using medical therapy, DC cardioversion should be performed promptly. In one of the few studies of PSVT in the postsurgical patient, adenosine had only a 44% successful conversion rate, and arrhythmia recurrences were common (52% of patients) [49]. The high recurrence rate of PSVT suggests that many patients will require suppressive therapy while they are critically ill.

Multifocal atrial tachycardia

Multifocal atrial tachycardia (MAT) is an automatic arrhythmia characterized by an atrial rate greater than 100 beats/min with organized, discrete, non-sinus P-waves with at least three different forms in the same electrocardiographic lead [50]. It is usually associated with severe pulmonary disease and often accompanies critical illness. When the onset of MAT occurs in the perioperative period, respiratory failure, pneumonia, and congestive heart failure are common causes. Therapy centers on treating the pulmonary, cardiac, or other acute illness that led to the onset of the arrhythmia [51]. When MAT persists despite these maneuvers, additional medical therapy may be indicated if the arrhythmia is hemodynamically significant (i.e., contributing to hypotension, congestive heart failure, or myocardial ischemia). Correction of serum electrolyte levels may be helpful for patients with hypomagnesemia or hypokalemia. Beta-blockers may be effective in

decreasing the ventricular rate but must be used with extreme caution, if at all, in patients with reactive airway disease or severe acute congestive heart failure. For patients with bronchospastic lung disease calcium channel blockers or amiodarone may be used instead of beta-blockers. It serves to decrease the tachycardia rate by decreasing the degree of atrial ectopy. Digitalis preparations are rarely effective in the treatment of MAT. Aminophylline, even at therapeutic levels, may aggravate the tachycardia by increasing the atrial rate and the number of ectopic atrial beats. Multifocal atrial tachycardia is usually resistant to DC cardioversion.

Ventricular premature contractions and non-sustained ventricular tachycardia

No specific medical therapy is indicated for patients who develop asymptomatic, hemodynamically insignificant ventricular premature contractions, or non-sustained ventricular tachycardia in the perioperative period. The cause of these dysrhythmias should be determined and the provoking factors corrected if possible. Common causes of acute ventricular arrhythmias in the perioperative period include acute myocardial ischemia, hypoxia, hypokalemia, and hypomagnesemia. Right heart catheters may cause ventricular irritability and ectopy as a result of trauma to the right ventricular outflow tract in patients who require these devices to aid in hemodynamic monitoring during the perioperative period. This should resolve on repositioning or removal of the monitoring catheter.

No well-studied data are available regarding the treatment of symptomatic or hemodynamically significant non-sustained ventricular tachycardia that develops acutely in the perioperative period. It is our approach to conduct an immediate search for a reversible etiology. We occasionally initiate medical antiarrhythmic therapy with intravenous beta-blockers, amiodarone, lidocaine, or procainamide.

Sustained ventricular tachycardia and ventricular fibrillation

Patients who develop sustained ventricular tachycardia or ventricular fibrillation in the perioperative period should be treated according to the Advanced Cardiac Life Support protocol. Patients who have ventricular fibrillation or hemodynamically unstable ventricular tachycardia should undergo immediate defibrillation or DC cardioversion. For the patient with normal left ventricular function and hemodynamically stable ventricular tachycardia, an alternate approach to electrical therapy is intravenous procainamide or amiodarone. For the patient with left ventricular dysfunction, amiodarone is the antiarrhythmic agent of choice. If these agents are ineffective in restoring normal rhythm, DC cardioversion should be performed. Readers are referred to the *Advanced Cardiac Life Support Guidelines* for further information [52].

Wide-complex tachycardia of unknown type

Supraventricular tachycardia occasionally may be accompanied by aberrant ventricular conduction, resulting in a wide QRS complex. Although criteria have been established to aid in the identification of the arrhythmia, a definite diagnosis is often elusive. A 12-lead ECG should be obtained. If atrial–ventricular dissociation is present (e.g., loss of a 1 : 1 relationship between P wave and QRS complex) the ECG is highly specific for ventricular tachycardia. We treat the patient with perioperative wide-complex tachycardia of unknown type in the manner recommended by *2010 American Heart Association Guidelines* [53]. For the hemodynamically stable patient with preserved left ventricular function we utilize intravenous amiodarone 150 mg over 10 minutes with the dose repeated as needed to a maximum dose of 2.2 g/24 hours. If these agents are ineffective, or if the patient develops hemodynamic instability, synchronized cardioversion should be used.

Perioperative conduction abnormalities

In the perioperative period, sinus bradycardia and a Mobitz I type of second-degree AV block are common. Mobitz I AV block is a progressive prolongation of the PR interval until a P-wave is not conducted to the ventricles. The P-wave that follows is conducted to the ventricles with a PR interval that is shorter than the PR interval that was associated with the last conducted P-wave. These conduction abnormalities usually result from enhanced vagal tone and, if they are hemodynamically significant, they typically respond to 0.5 to 1 mg of intravenous atropine.

A Mobitz II type of second-degree AV block (a fixed PR interval with P-wave conduction to the ventricles blocked on a constant (e.g., 2:1, 3:1, 4:1) or variable basis) is usually caused by diffuse disease of the conduction system distal to the AV node. Many patients with this conduction disturbance are at high risk for progression to complete heart block, and a means of providing temporary-demand cardiac pacing should be quickly available in the event that this occurs. New-onset Mobitz II AV block in the perioperative period should initiate a search for myocardial ischemia or myocardial infarction.

Third-degree AV block occurs when no atrial impulses reach the ventricles. An associated ventricular rate of 40 to 60 beats/min with normal appearing QRS complexes suggests that the escape rhythm is originating at the level of the AV node. This type of heart block may result from enhanced vagal tone; medications that depress AV nodal conduction (e.g., beta-blockers, digitalis) and, less commonly, AV nodal ischemia. It is often reversible and may respond to the administration of intravenous atropine or the discontinuation of offending pharmacologic agents. If complete heart block is associated with a ventricular escape rate of 20 to 40 beats/min and the QRS complex is wide, the escape rhythm is originating from the ventricles. This strongly suggests the presence of extensive conduction system disease and warrants the placement of a cardiac pacemaker.

Table 9.6 Selected indications for implantation of cardiac pacemakers.

Third-degree or advanced second-degree AV block associated with:
    Symptomatic bradycardia
    Documented asystole > 3 seconds or escape rate less than 40 beats/min in an awake symptom-free person

Second-degree AV block, regardless of site or type, with: Symptomatic bradycardia; bifascicular block with intermittent complete heart block with symptomatic bradycardia; symptomatic bifascicular block with intermittent type II second-degree AV block; sinus node dysfunction with documented symptomatic bradycardia

Following acute myocardial infarction:
    Persistent second-degree AV block in the His–Purkinje system with bilateral bundle–branch block or third-degree AV block within or below the His–Purkinje system
    Persistent and symptomatic second- or third-degree AV block

Source: Adapted from Epstein *et al.* (2008) [60].

Chronic bifascicular block (i.e., right bundle–branch block with either left anterior hemiblock or left posterior hemiblock, or left bundle–branch block) rarely progresses to advanced hemodynamically significant heart block in the perioperative period [54–56]. The preoperative insertion of temporary pacemaker therefore, is not indicated, in general, for this patient group. Possible exceptions are patients with preexisting left bundle–branch block who are undergoing perioperative pulmonary artery catheterization. Transient right bundle–branch block, which is well tolerated in normal patients, may occur in as many as 5% of patients who undergo pulmonary artery catheterization [57]. Transient complete heart block has been reported in patients with preexisting left bundle–branch block who have developed acute right bundle–branch block related to this procedure [58,59]. Given the potential for this significant complication, a method for pacing the left ventricle should be available in the event that complete heart block develops in this clinical setting. A temporary pacemaker should be inserted before surgery if patients meet the criteria for permanent pacemaker implantation and if a permanent pacing device has not yet been implanted (Table 9.6) [60].

Long QT syndrome

The long QT syndrome is a heterogeneous group of disorders characterized by a prolonged QT interval when corrected for heart rate, malignant ventricular arrhythmias (classically the torsades de pointes form of ventricular tachycardia), and the risk of sudden death. It is most commonly acquired as a result of a drug or metabolic abnormality (see Table 9.7). It may also occur as a congenital form inherited as a result of either autosomal dominant or recessive genetic mutations. To date, seven different genetic defects which encode for abnormal cardiac ion channels have been identified that may result in long QT syndrome.

Table 9.7 Selected causes of acquired long QT syndrome.

Antiarrhythmic drugs

Type IA agents (e.g., quinidine, procainamide, disopyramide)

Type III agents (Amiodarone, Sotalol)

Non-cardiac drugs

Phenothiazines

Tricyclic antidepressants

Haloperidol

Selective serotonin reuptake inhibitors (SSRIs)

Antibiotics (e.g., erythromycin, azithromycin, clarithromycin, ampicillin, trimethoprin-sulfamethoxazole, ketoconazole, itraconazole)

Metabolic and electrolyte disorders

Hypokalemia

Hypomagnesemia

Nutritional disorders (starvation, liquid protein diets)

Central nervous system disorders

Subarachnoid hemorrhage

Intracerebral hemorrhage

Head trauma

Encephalitis

The approach to patients in the perioperative period depends on whether the long QT is congenital or acquired. Congenital long QT syndrome is adrenergic dependent and ventricular arrhythmias are typically provoked by sympathetic stimulation (i.e., pain, physical exertion). Long-term treatment with beta-blockers, permanent pacing, or left cervicothoracic sympathectomy is frequently effective [61]. ICD implantation is recommended for selected patients in whom syncope, sustained ventricular arrhythmias, or aborted sudden cardiac death has occurred despite this standard therapy. ICD implantation as primary treatment should be considered in the patient in whom aborted sudden cardiac death is the initial presentation of the long QT syndrome and in those patients with long QT who have a strong family history of sudden cardiac death [62].

For patients with congenital long QT syndrome, we provide perioperative beta-blockade to blunt the adrenergic response to the surgery. Beta-blockers also shift the rate-adjusted QT interval to the normal range, which may contribute to their efficacy. We attempt to avoid anesthetics that may prolong the QT interval (e.g., succinylcholine, propofol, enflurane, or halothane) [62]. Although isoflurane has been demonstrated to prolong the QT interval in normals, it shortens the QT interval in those with long QT syndrome and has been proposed as an acceptable anesthetic agent for this patient group [63]. Thiopental has also been reported to prolong the QT interval in normals but has no effect on the QT duration in patients with long QT syndrome [63]. Finally we minimize sympathetic stimulation and provide adequate sedation to blunt the adrenergic response to surgery.

In patients who have acquired long QT syndrome, we discontinue administration of the offending drug or correct the metabolic or electrolyte abnormality before undertaking surgery.

Despite these measures, malignant ventricular arrhythmias may still occur in the patient with long QT in the perioperative period. The treatment for ventricular ectopy is the same for idiopathic and acquired long QT syndrome. Intravenous magnesium sulfate, 2 g given over 1–2 minutes, with a follow-up dose 15 minutes later if required is often effective in restoring regular rhythm. Immediate ventricular pacing should be used if magnesium sulfate is ineffective. Pacing at rates of 70–80 beats/min may shorten the QT interval and decrease the dispersion of refractoriness of the cardiac conduction system. Intravenous isoproterenol may be used cautiously to increase the heart rate and suppress ventricular arrhythmia until temporary ventricular pacing is achieved. If these methods are unsuccessful in restoring the patient's baseline stable rhythm, DC cardioversion should be considered.

Cardiac conduction issues in the patient with a cardiac transplant who requires non-cardiac surgery

Cardiac physiology is altered after cardiac transplantation. Because the transplanted heart is denervated, cardiac reflexes mediated by the autonomic nervous system are blunted or absent. As a result, heart rate abnormalities may be seen in the perioperative period. The resting heart rate is higher than normal but the heart rate response to stress is less than that of an innervated heart. When the heart rate does increase as a result of stress, it does so gradually in response to circulating catecholamines. Reflex tachycardia does not occur in response to vasodilation or volume loss. The effect of certain cardiac drugs on cardiac conduction is altered. Agents that affect the heart indirectly through their action on the autonomic nervous system are generally ineffective. Therefore, the chronotropic effect of atropine is absent, as is the AV nodal inhibitory effect of digoxin. The antiarrhythmic efficacy of beta-blockers and calcium channel antagonists (e.g., verapamil, diltiazem) is unchanged. The transplanted heart becomes overly sensitive to adenosine, and reduced doses (i.e., one-third to one-half lower than those given to patients with intact cardiac innervation) should be used when this drug is administered to control arrhythmias [64,65].

Bradyarrhythmias following acute spinal cord injury

Acute injury to the cervical spinal cord is frequently accompanied by clinically significant bradyarrhythmias and, in some cases, hypotension. Acute autonomic dysfunction is thought to be the cause. Sympathetic nerves exit the spinal cord in preganglionic fibers at the first through fourth thoracic levels. With a complete cervical spinal cord lesion, sympathetic control from higher centers is interrupted. Parasympathetic control, which is mediated by the vagus nerve, is unaffected by spinal cord interruption. The clinical picture therefore is one of unopposed parasympathetic activity in the setting of markedly reduced sympathetic activity. Sympathetic stimulation with low-dose isoproterenol has been used in several patients for the treatment of clinically significant bradyarrhythmias. These cardiovascular abnormalities have been demonstrated to resolve within 14–30 days following acute cervical spinal cord injury. The reason for resolution is not known but may be related to adaptive sympathetic disinhibition (i.e., loss of reflex sympathetic inhibitory control from higher centers or increase in the number and function of adrenergic receptors) [66,67].

Management of permanent cardiac pacemakers

While most pacemakers are implanted as treatment of bradyarrhythmias or conduction system abnormalities, other indications for pacemakers include treatment of heart failure in the patient with severe left ventricular dysfunction and cardiac dyssynchrony (bi-ventricular pacemaker), neurocardiogenic syncope, long QT syndrome, and selected patients with hypertrophic cardiomyopathy. It is important to know the indication that led to implantation of the patient's pacemaker and whether or not they are pacemaker dependent.

There is no industry-wide standard regarding pacemaker programming, estimation of battery reserve, etc. It is therefore important that the type of pacemaker and the name of its manufacturer be identified prior to surgery. If the patients or their physicians are unable to provide this information, it may be identified by chest X-ray, which reveals radio-opaque identification markers on the pacemaker generator. The pacemaker should be tested and its settings recorded.

While pacemaker problems are uncommon in the perioperative period, one series identified a pacemaker abnormality (e.g., inhibition, acceleration, change in pacing mode) in 13% of pacemaker patients [68].

The most significant pacemaker problem in the perioperative period is alteration of pacemaker function inhibition resulting from electrocautery-induced electromagnetic interference (EMI). If the pacemaker interprets EMI as the patient's electrical heart activity, the pacemaker may be inhibited. If the patient has a dual chamber pacemaker and EMI is sensed only by the atrial sensing circuitry, the ventricular pacing channel may pace at the pacemaker upper rate limit. Some pacemakers respond to the "noise" of EMI by pacing in an asynchronous (fixed rate) mode. Some older pacemakers may respond to EMI by reprogramming. The pacemaker response to the electrical interference of electrocautery may be obtained from the pacemaker manufacturer. This alteration of pacemaker function may be prevented by avoiding the application of electrocautery directly over the pacemaker pulse generator and by keeping the electrocautery current path, which is from electrode tip to ground plate, as far away as possible from the pulse generator. The pacemaker should be programmed to the asynchronous (fixed rate mode) so that it does not inhibit in response to EMI. Many pacemakers will operate in an asynchronous mode if a magnet is applied to the skin over the pulse generator and, while that has been a common approach to perioperative pacemaker management, it is important to realize that a number of new pacemakers have a programmable option that prevents this pacemaker response to magnet application.

Since the early 1990s many pacemakers have "rate-adaptive" systems devised to facilitate a change in heart rate response to a change in the desired cardiac output. Various biologic parameters have been used to trigger heart rate responses. The most common include sensation of vibration at the pulse generator site as a manifestation of perceived patient physical activity and respiratory rate as determined by a minute ventilation sensor. The adaptive rate system may therefore sense surgical-induced vibration or shivering, which commonly occurs upon recovery from anesthesia, and inappropriately pace at a high rate. Similarly, intraoperative hyperventilation may also lead to the pacemaker generating a heart rate more rapid than actually desired if the pacemaker adaptive rate sensor is linked to the patient's minute ventilation. For these reasons the rate-responsive feature should be deactivated during surgery.

For patients who require placement of central venous catheters or right heart pulmonary artery catheters, care should be taken to avoid tangling these catheters in the pacemaker leads. Newly placed pacemaker leads are at risk of becoming dislodged by right heart catheter insertion. For the patient who requires external defibrillation, electrical discharge to their pacemaker will be minimized if the defibrillator paddles are placed in an antero-posterior position [69].

It should be noted that many of the new pacemakers have a programmable option that would make magnet application ineffective. For this reason, knowledge of the patient's pacemaker dependency state and programming of the device may be required. Some pacemakers respond to magnet application only with a brief period of asynchronous pacing. Therefore, it is recommended that continuous telemetry be available during the surgical procedure.

There is no industry-wide standard response to either EMI or magnet application. It is therefore important that data regarding the individual pacemaker response to EMI and magnet application be obtained from the pacemaker manufacturer. However, in general the recommendations outlined above will be effective.

Management of automatic implantable cardioverter defibrillators (AICDs)

Automatic implantable cardioverter defibrillators (AICDs) are used for secondary prevention for the patient who has survived sudden cardiac death and are effective in the primary prevention of sudden cardiac death for the patient with prior myocardial infarction and advanced left ventricular dysfunction (ejection fraction ≤ 30%) [70]. The number of AICD implants is expected to increase significantly in this latter group as it is estimated that, in the USA, 3–4 million patients have coronary heart disease and advanced left ventricular dysfunction with 400,000 new cases each year [71,72].

Electrocautery may affect AICDs in the same manner as it does pacemakers; the electromagnetic signal produced by electrocautery may be interpreted as intrinsic cardiac events. This phenomenon can lead to inhibition of pacing. In addition, if the electrocautery-induced electromagnetic interference is interpreted by the AICD as a rapid ventricular rate, the AICD may deliver unnecessary and undesired shocks. While the frequency of such an occurrence is small, the results of AICD shock delivered during a surgical procedure can be devastating. Therefore, it is recommended that AICDs be deactivated before surgery if the use of electrocautery is a possibility. Continuous electrocardiographic monitoring and advanced cardiac life support, including an external defibrillator, should be available during the time that the AICD is deactivated. The AICD should be deactivated by one of two techniques. Either a magnet may be placed over the AICD for the duration of electrocautery, or the device can be deactivated with the use of the programmer. Magnet application over the pulse generator will disable the device from detecting tachyarrhythmias. For most AICDs, magnet application only deactivates the device temporarily, but some AICDs can be permanently deactivated with magnet application. Magnet application will not affect pacing functions of the AICD. Therefore, electrocautery may inhibit pacing from an AICD. It should be remembered that most patients with AICDs have significant left ventricular dysfunction with ischemic heart disease. These patients require close observation during the perioperative period.

References

1. Marchlinski F. Arrhythmias and conduction disturbances in surgical patients. In Goldman D, ed. *Medical Care of the Surgical Patient*. Philadelphia, PA: J. B. Lippincott; 1982, pp. 59–77.

2. Hill RF. Treatment of isorhythmic A-V dissociation during general anesthesia with propranolol. *Anesthesiology* 1989; **70**: 141–4.

3. Kuner J, Enescu V, Utsu F *et al*. Cardiac arrhythmias during anesthesia. *Dis Chest* 1967; **52**: 580–7.

4. Forrest JB, Cahalan MK, Rehder K *et al*. Multicenter study of general anesthesia. II. Results. *Anesthesiology* 1990; **72**: 262–8.

5. Forrest JB, Rehder K, Cahalan MK, Goldsmith CH. Multicenter study of general anesthesia. III. Predictors of severe perioperative adverse outcomes. *Anesthesiology* 1992; **76**: 3–15.

6. O'Kelly B, Browner WS, Massie B *et al*. Ventricular arrhythmias in patients undergoing noncardiac surgery. The Study of Perioperative Ischemia Research Group. *J Am Med Assoc* 1992; **268**: 217–21.

7. Fleisher LA, Beckman JA, Brown KA *et al*. 2009 ACCF/AHA focused update on perioperative beta blockade incorporated into the ACC/AHA 2007 guidelines on perioperative cardiovascular evaluation and care for noncardiac surgery: a report of the American College of Cardiology Foundation/American Heart Association Task Force on Practice Guidelines. *Circulation* 2009; **120**: e169–276.

8. Goldman L, Caldera DL, Nussbaum SR *et al*. Multifactorial index of cardiac risk in noncardiac surgical procedures. *N Engl J Med* 1977; **297**: 845–50.

9. Polanczyk CA, Goldman L, Marcantonio ER, Orav EJ, Lee TH. Supraventricular arrhythmia in patients having noncardiac surgery: clinical correlates and effect on length of stay. *Ann Intern Med* 1998; **129**: 279–85.

10. Amar D, Zhang H, Leung DH, Roistacher N, Kadish AH. Older age is the strongest predictor of postoperative atrial fibrillation. *Anesthesiology* 2002; **96**: 352–6.

11. Sebel PS, Bovill JG. Opioid analgesics in cardiac anesthesia. In Kaplan JA, ed. *Cardiac Anesthesia*. Orlando, FL: Grune & Stratton; 1987, pp. 67–123.

12. Marymount JH, O'Connor BS. Postoperative cardiovascular complications. In Veder JS, Spiess BD, eds. *Post Anesthesia Care*. Philadelphia, PA: W. B. Saunders; 1992, p. 42.

13. Underwood SM, Glynn CJ. Sick sinus syndrome manifest after spinal anaesthesia. *Anaesthesia* 1988; **43**: 307–9.

14. Doyle DJ, Mark PW. Reflex bradycardia during surgery. *Can J Anaesth* 1990; **37**: 219–22.

15. Merli GJ, Weitz H, Martin JH *et al*. Cardiac dysrhythmias associated with ophthalmic atropine. *Arch Intern Med* 1986; **146**: 45–7.

16. Rocco AG, Vandam LD. Changes in circulation consequent to manipulation during abdominal surgery. *J Am Med Assoc* 1957; **164**: 14–18.

17. Seltzer JL, Ritter DE, Starsnic MA, Marr AT. The hemodynamic response to traction on the abdominal mesentery. *Anesthesiology* 1985; **63**: 96–9.

18. Sullivan S, Watson WC. Acute transient hypotension as complication of percutaneous liver biopsy. *Lancet* 1974; **1**: 389–90.

19. Doyle DJ, Mark PW. Laparoscopy and vagal arrest. *Anaesthesia* 1989; **44**: 448.

20. Robideaux V. Oculocardiac reflex caused by midface disimpaction. *Anesthesiology* 1978; **49**: 433.

21. Hopkins CS. Bradycardia during neurosurgery – a new reflex? *Anaesthesia* 1988; **43**: 157–8.

22. Podolakin W, Wells DG. Precipitous bradycardia induced by laryngoscopy in cardiac surgical patients. *Can J Anaesth* 1987; **34**: 618–21.

23. Mishra P, Calvey TN, Williams NE, Murray GR. Intraoperative bradycardia and hypotension associated with timolol and pilocarpine eye drops. *Br J Anaesth* 1983; **55**: 897–9.

24. Falk RH. Atrial fibrillation. *N Engl J Med* 2001; **344**: 1067–78.

25. Wyse DG, Waldo AL, DiMarco JP *et al*. A comparison of rate control and rhythm control in patients with atrial fibrillation. *N Engl J Med* 2002; **347**: 1825–33.

26. Fuster V, Ryden LE, Cannom DS *et al.* ACC/AHA/ESC 2006 Guidelines for the Management of Patients with Atrial Fibrillation: a report of the American College of Cardiology/American Heart Association Task Force on Practice Guidelines and the European Society of Cardiology Committee for Practice Guidelines (Writing Committee to Revise the 2001 Guidelines for the Management of Patients With Atrial Fibrillation): developed in collaboration with the European Heart Rhythm Association and the Heart Rhythm Society. *Circulation* 2006; **114**: e257–354.

27. Cannegieter SC, Rosendaal FR, Wintzen AR *et al.* Optimal oral anticoagulant therapy in patients with mechanical heart valves. *N Engl J Med* 1995; **333**: 11–17.

28. Bonow RO, Carabello BA, Chatterjee K *et al.* 2008 Focused update incorporated into the ACC/AHA 2006 guidelines for the management of patients with valvular heart disease: a report of the American College of Cardiology/American Heart Association Task Force on Practice Guidelines (Writing Committee to Revise the 1998 Guidelines for the Management of Patients With Valvular Heart Disease): endorsed by the Society of Cardiovascular Anesthesiologists, Society for Cardiovascular Angiography and Interventions, and Society of Thoracic Surgeons. *Circulation* **2008**; 118: e523–661.

29. Goldman L. Supraventricular tachyarrhythmias in hospitalized adults after surgery. Clinical correlates in patients over 40 years of age after major noncardiac surgery. *Chest* 1978; **73**: 450–4.

30. Christians KK, Wu B, Quebbeman EJ, Brasel KJ. Postoperative atrial fibrillation in noncardiothoracic surgical patients. *Am J Surg* 2001; **182**: 713–15.

31. Link MS, Atkins DL, Passman RS *et al.* Part 6: Electrical therapies: automated external defibrillators, defibrillation, cardioversion, and pacing: 2010 American Heart Association Guidelines for Cardiopulmonary Resuscitation and Emergency Cardiovascular Care. *Circulation* 2010; **122**: S706–19.

32. Tisdale JE, Padhi ID, Goldberg AD *et al.* A randomized, double-blind comparison of intravenous diltiazem and digoxin for atrial fibrillation after coronary artery bypass surgery. *Am Heart J* 1998; **135**: 739–47.

33. Balser JR, Martinez EA, Winters BD *et al.* Beta-adrenergic blockade accelerates conversion of postoperative supraventricular tachyarrhythmias. *Anesthesiology* 1998; **89**: 1052–9.

34. Myers MG, Alnemri K. Rate control therapy for atrial fibrillation following coronary artery bypass surgery. *Can J Cardiol* 1998; **14**: 1363–6.

35. Stambler BS, Wood MA, Ellenbogen KA *et al.* Efficacy and safety of repeated intravenous doses of ibutilide for rapid conversion of atrial flutter or fibrillation. Ibutilide Repeat Dose Study Investigators. *Circulation* 1996; **94**: 1613–21.

36. Volgman AS, Carberry PA, Stambler B *et al.* Conversion efficacy and safety of intravenous ibutilide compared with intravenous procainamide in patients with atrial flutter or fibrillation. *J Am Coll Cardiol* 1998; **31**: 1414–19.

37. Oral H, Souza JJ, Michaud GF *et al.* Facilitating transthoracic cardioversion of atrial fibrillation with ibutilide pretreatment. *N Engl J Med* 1999; **340**: 1849–54.

38. Danias PG, Caulfield TA, Weigner MJ, Silverman DI, Manning WJ. Likelihood of spontaneous conversion of atrial fibrillation to sinus rhythm. *J Am Coll Cardiol* 1998; **31**: 588–92.

39. Laupacis A, Albers G, Dalen J *et al.* Antithrombotic therapy in atrial fibrillation. *Chest* 1998; **114**: 579S–89S.

40. Doval HC, Nul DR, Grancelli HO *et al.* Randomised trial of low-dose amiodarone in severe congestive heart failure. Grupo de Estudio de la Sobrevida en la Insuficiencia Cardiaca en Argentina (GESICA). *Lancet* 1994; **344**: 493–8.

41. Torp-Pedersen C, Moller M, Bloch-Thomsen PE *et al.* Dofetilide in patients with congestive heart failure and left ventricular dysfunction. Danish Investigations of Arrhythmia and Mortality on Dofetilide Study Group. *N Engl J Med* 1999; **341**: 857–65.

42. Salerno DM. Quinidine. Worse than adverse? *Circulation* 1991; **84**: 2196–8.

43. Serafimovski N, Burke P, Khawaja O, Sekulic M, Machado C. Usefulness of dofetilide for the prevention of atrial tachyarrhythmias (atrial fibrillation or flutter) after coronary artery bypass grafting. *Am J Cardiol* 2008; **101**: 1574–9.

44. Reiffel JA. Drug choices in the treatment of atrial fibrillation. *Am J Cardiol* 2000; **85**: 12D–9D.

45. Haissaguerre M, Jais P, Shah DC *et al.* Spontaneous initiation of atrial fibrillation by ectopic beats originating in the pulmonary veins. *N Engl J Med* 1998; **339**: 659–66.

46. Amar D, Roistacher N, Burt ME *et al.* Effects of diltiazem versus digoxin on dysrhythmias and cardiac function after pneumonectomy. *Ann Thorac Surg* 1997; **63**: 1374–81; discussion 81–2.

47. Ritchie AJ, Whiteside M, Tolan M, McGuigan JA. Cardiac dysrhythmia in total thoracic oesophagectomy. A prospective study. *Eur J Cardiothorac Surg* 1993; **7**: 420–2.

48. Mehta D, Wafa S, Ward DE, Camm AJ. Relative efficacy of various physical manoeuvres in the termination of junctional tachycardia. *Lancet* 1988; **1**: 1181–5.

49. Kirton OC, Windsor J, Wedderburn R *et al.* Management of paroxysmal atrioventricular nodal reentrant tachycardia in the critically ill surgical patient. *Crit Care Med* 1997; **25**: 761–6.

50. Kastor JA. Multifocal atrial tachycardia. *N Engl J Med* 1990; **322**: 1713–17.

51. Scher DL, Arsura EL. Multifocal atrial tachycardia: mechanisms, clinical correlates, and treatment. *Am Heart J* 1989; **118**: 574–80.

52. Field JM, Hazinski MF, Sayre MR *et al.* Part 1: executive summary: 2010 American Heart Association Guidelines for Cardiopulmonary Resuscitation and Emergency Cardiovascular Care. *Circulation* 2010; **122**: S640–56.

53. Cave DM, Gazmuri RJ, Otto CW *et al.* Part 7: CPR techniques and devices: 2010 American Heart Association Guidelines for Cardiopulmonary Resuscitation and Emergency Cardiovascular Care. *Circulation* 2010; **122**: S720–8.

54. Bellocci F, Santarelli P, Di Gennaro M, Ansalone G, Fenici R. The risk of cardiac complications in surgical patients with bifascicular block. A clinical and electrophysiologic study in 98 patients. *Chest* 1980; **77**: 343–8.

55. Berg GR, Kotler MN. The significance of bilateral bundle branch block in the

preoperative patient. A retrospective electrocardiographic and clinical study in 30 patients. *Chest* 1971; **59**: 62–7.

56. Gauss A, Hubner C, Radermacher P, Georgieff M, Schutz W. Perioperative risk of bradyarrhythmias in patients with asymptomatic chronic bifascicular block or left bundle branch block: does an additional first-degree atrioventricular block make any difference? *Anesthesiology* 1998; **88**: 679–87.

57. Sprung CL, Pozen RG, Rozanski JJ *et al.* Advanced ventricular arrhythmias during bedside pulmonary artery catheterization. *Am J Med* 1982; **72**: 203–8.

58. Abernathy WS. Complete heart block caused by the Swan–Ganz catheter. *Chest* 1974; **65**: 349.

59. Thomson IR, Dalton BC, Lappas DG, Lowenstein E. Right bundle-branch block and complete heart block caused by the Swan–Ganz catheter. *Anesthesiology* 1979; **51**: 359–62.

60. Epstein AE, DiMarco JP, Ellenbogen KA *et al.* ACC/AHA/HRS 2008 Guidelines for Device-Based Therapy of Cardiac Rhythm Abnormalities: a report of the American College of Cardiology/American Heart Association Task Force on Practice Guidelines (Writing Committee to Revise the ACC/AHA/NASPE 2002 Guideline Update for Implantation of Cardiac Pacemakers and

Antiarrhythmia Devices) developed in collaboration with the American Association for Thoracic Surgery and Society of Thoracic Surgeons. *J Am Coll Cardiol* 2008; **51**: e1–62.

61. Richardson MG, Roark GL, Helfaer MA. Intraoperative epinephrine-induced torsades de pointes in a child with long QT syndrome. *Anesthesiology* 1992; **76**: 647–9.

62. Medak R, Benumof JL. Perioperative management of the prolonged Q-T interval syndrome. *Br J Anaesth* 1983; **55**: 361–4.

63. Wilton NC, Hantler CB. Congenital long QT syndrome: changes in QT interval during anesthesia with thiopental, vecuronium, fentanyl, and isoflurane. *Anesth Analg* 1987; **66**: 357–60.

64. Ellenbogen KA, Thames MD, DiMarco JP, Sheehan H, Lerman BB. Electrophysiological effects of adenosine in the transplanted human heart. Evidence of supersensitivity. *Circulation* 1990; **81**: 821–8.

65. O'Connell JB, Bourge RC, Costanzo-Nordin MR *et al.* Cardiac transplantation: recipient selection, donor procurement, and medical follow-up. A statement for health professionals from the Committee on Cardiac Transplantation of the Council on Clinical Cardiology, American Heart Association. *Circulation* 1992; **86**: 1061–79.

66. Leaf DA, Bahl RA, Adkins RH. Risk of cardiac dysrhythmias in chronic spinal cord injury patients. *Paraplegia* 1993; **31**: 571–5.

67. Lehmann KG, Lane JG, Piepmeier JM, Batsford WP. Cardiovascular abnormalities accompanying acute spinal cord injury in humans: incidence, time course and severity. *J Am Coll Cardiol* 1987; **10**: 46–52.

68. Trankina MF, Black S, Gibby G. Pacemakers: perioperative evaluation, management, and complications (abstr.). *Anesthesiology* 2000; **93**: 1193.

69. Senthuran S, Toff WD, Vuylsteke A, Solesbury PM, Menon DK. Implanted cardiac pacemakers and defibrillators in anaesthetic practice. *Br J Anaesth* 2002; **88**: 627–31.

70. Moss AJ, Zareba W, Hall WJ *et al.* Prophylactic implantation of a defibrillator in patients with myocardial infarction and reduced ejection fraction. *N Engl J Med* 2002; **346**: 877–83.

71. Cohn JN, Bristow MR, Chien KR *et al.* Report of the National Heart, Lung, and Blood Institute Special Emphasis Panel on Heart Failure Research. *Circulation* 1997; **95**: 766–70.

72. Myerburg RJ. Sudden cardiac death: exploring the limits of our knowledge. *J Cardiovasc Electrophysiol* 2001; **12**: 369–81.

Valvular heart disease

Mitral stenosis

Mitral stenosis in adults is usually a result of rheumatic fever. Rheumatic valvulitis causes scarring of the mitral valve leaflets, with fusion of the commissures as well as subvalvular apparatus. With the reduced incidence of rheumatic fever in developed countries, non-rheumatic causes of mitral valve stenosis should be considered. In the elderly idiopathic calcification of the mitral valve annulus with extension to the mitral valve, leaflets may result in functional mitral stenosis. Rare causes of mitral stenosis are systemic lupus erythematosus, rheumatoid arthritis, and carcinoid syndrome.

In normal adults, the mitral valve area is 4–5 cm^2. Mitral stenosis is critical when the valve area is reduced to 1 cm^2 or less. As mitral valve leaflet fusion progresses, left atrial pressure increases to maintain left ventricular filling, and a diastolic transvalvular pressure gradient exists between the left atrium and ventricle. Increased left atrial pressure leads

to increased pulmonary vascular pressure. Conditions that decrease diastolic filling time (e.g., tachycardia) as well as those that increase cardiac blood flow across the mitral valve (e.g., physical exercise, fever) further increase left atrial and pulmonary vascular pressure. The pressure gradient across the mitral valve is proportional to the square of the transvalvular flow rate. Therefore, modest increases in transvalvular flow result in significant increases in the pressure gradient [1]. The onset of atrial fibrillation with the loss of the atrial contribution to ventricular filling as well as decreased diastolic filling time associated with a rapid heart rate may also lead to increased left atrial pressure. Pulmonary hypertension occurs as mitral stenosis progresses. Although pulmonary venous and arterial hypertension is usually reversible after mechanical correction of mitral stenosis, advanced disease is often associated with mitral regurgitation, hypertrophy of the pulmonary vasculature, and an irreversible component of pulmonary hypertension. Right ventricular pressure overload may occur as a consequence of pulmonary hypertension.

The clinical findings of mitral stenosis result from inability of the left atrium to empty normally and from pulmonary venous and arterial hypertension. Symptoms such as exertional dyspnea may occur when the mitral valve area decreases to less than 2.5 cm^2. Rest symptoms such as orthopnea and paroxysmal nocturnal dyspnea occur when the valve area is less than 1.5 cm^2. Fatigue resulting from decreased cardiac output characterizes late disease. Hoarseness may occur and is caused by compression of the left recurrent laryngeal nerve by the enlarged left atrium and pulmonary artery. Atrial fibrillation commonly accompanies mitral stenosis and is the result of persistently elevated left atrial pressure and left atrial dilatation as well as involvement of the left atrium by rheumatic carditis. Atrial fibrillation with rapid ventricular response may lead to pulmonary edema due to the decreased diastolic filling time that occurs when heart rate increases. Patients with atrial fibrillation are at high risk for intracardiac thrombus formation with subsequent systemic embolization. The risk of embolization increases with increased size of the left atrium and atrial appendage as well as with decreased cardiac output.

Physical findings of mitral stenosis include an accentuated first heart sound that decreases in intensity as stenosis worsens and a high-pitched opening snap heard after the second heart sound that is caused by opening of the stenotic but pliable mitral valve. As mitral stenosis progresses, left atrial pressure rises and the interval between the second heart sound and the opening snap shortens. When valve mobility is lost, the opening snap disappears. A low-pitched diastolic rumble is heard at the apex and its duration correlates with the severity of stenosis. Patients in whom sinus rhythm is preserved may have presystolic accentuation of the murmur.

Transthoracic echocardiography is essential in patient evaluation. It confirms the diagnosis, identifies the etiology (e.g., leaflet fusion of rheumatic mitral valve stenosis, mitral annulus calcification in the elderly), allows for estimation of valve orifice area, and with the use of Doppler techniques facilitates an approximation of the transvalvular pressure gradient. When findings on echocardiography are concordant with the clinical assessment invasive hemodynamic assessment of mitral stenosis is not necessary [2]. Echocardiography may also facilitate identification of mitral regurgitation which coexists in as many as 40% of patients with mitral stenosis, as well as other valve lesions. Though not indicated in every patient with mitral stenosis, transesophageal echocardiography is an effective tool to determine the presence or absence of left atrial thrombi, the presence of which would be a contraindication to restoration of sinus rhythm in the mitral stenosis patient who is in atrial fibrillation.

Therapy is based on the severity of symptoms. Patients with minimal symptoms often respond to diuretics; those with atrial fibrillation respond to control of the ventricular response with digoxin, beta-blockers, or calcium channel antagonists. Survival is decreased when symptoms are more than mild. Therefore, patients with New York Heart Association functional class II symptoms and moderate or severe stenosis

(mitral valve area ≤ 1.5 cm^2 or mean gradient ≥ 5 mmHg) may be considered for mitral balloon valvotomy if they have suitable mitral valve morphology (i.e., valve with minimal calcification, good leaflet mobility, little involvement of the subvalvular apparatus, and minimal or no valve regurgitation). Balloon mitral valvotomy is contraindicated in patients with left atrial thrombi. The prognosis is poor for patients who have New York Heart Association functional class III or IV symptoms and evidence of severe mitral stenosis if left untreated. They should be considered for treatment with either balloon valvotomy or valve replacement [2]. Percutaneous balloon mitral valvuloplasty or mitral valve replacement is only indicated prior to non-cardiac surgery if the patient otherwise meets the indications for interventional treatment of their mitral stenosis irrespective of the non-cardiac surgery [3].

Intravascular volume status and heart rate are key factors that require attention in patients undergoing non-cardiac surgery. Volume overload must be avoided because further increases in left atrial pressure may result in pulmonary edema. Conversely, excessive volume depletion or preload reduction may decrease left ventricular filling pressure and cardiac output. Perioperative tachycardia may impair left ventricular filling and can be treated with beta-blockers, calcium channel antagonists, or digoxin in patients who have atrial fibrillation with rapid ventricular response. Because of the significant hemodynamic alterations that occur with relatively small volume shifts in patients with severe mitral stenosis, invasive hemodynamic monitoring of the pulmonary capillary wedge pressure should be considered if perioperative volume changes are anticipated. Since the most recent update of the ACC/AHA *Guidelines for the Management of Patients With Valvular Heart Disease* infective endocarditis prophylaxis is no longer indicated in patients with isolated mitral stenosis [2].

Mitral stenosis increases the risk of embolism in the patient with atrial fibrillation. Many of these patients are chronically anticoagulated with warfarin. For the patient who undergoes surgery, care should be taken to minimize the time that the patient will be not anticoagulated in the perioperative period. Strategies include performing surgery without stopping anticoagulation in the patient in whom perioperative bleeding is unlikely, e.g., cataract surgery. As mitral stenosis in a patient with atrial fibrillation is a factor associated with the highest risk of stroke, we often stop the warfarin several days prior to surgery and treat with heparin when the INR becomes subtherapeutic. Heparin is discontinued several hours prior to surgery and restarted as soon as possible following surgery. Warfarin is then restarted. Heparin is discontinued when the INR is therapeutic. An alternative approach, though not studied in prospective randomized trials and not approved by the US Food and Drug Administration for this indication, is to use low molecular weight heparin as "bridge" anticoagulation rather than continuous unfractionated heparin. For this purpose enoxaparin can be given at 1 mg/kg subcutaneously every 12 hours after warfarin is withheld and INR decreases below therapeutic range. Low molecular weight heparin should be stopped 12 hours prior to surgery and resumed when hemostasis is stable in the postoperative period. Warfarin is restarted in the postoperative period and low molecular weight heparin discontinued when INR is therapeutic [4].

Mitral regurgitation

Mitral regurgitation may be caused by one or more abnormalities of the structures that comprise the mitral valve apparatus: the anterior and posterior valve leaflets, chordae tendineae, papillary muscles, and mitral valve annulus. Functional mitral regurgitation may result from poor alignment of a structurally normal valve apparatus or from mitral annular dilation, both of which are caused by left ventricular dysfunction or dilatation. Common causes of mitral apparatus dysfunction are myxomatous degeneration of the mitral valve leaflets or chordae, infective endocarditis that may involve the valve leaflets, coronary artery disease with myocardial ischemia resulting in papillary muscle dysfunction, or rheumatic valve disease. Less common but clinically significant causes of mitral regurgitation include mitral annular calcification (usually limited to the elderly) and distortion of the mitral valve apparatus as a result of systolic anterior motion of the mitral valve in the setting of hypertrophic cardiomyopathy. Degeneration of the mitral valve may be seen in patients receiving long-term hemodialysis as well as those with the antiphospholipid antibody syndrome.

The pathophysiology of mitral regurgitation depends on whether the regurgitation occurs on an acute or chronic basis. Acute mitral regurgitation is characterized by sudden increase in left atrial volume and pressure as blood is ejected back into the left atrium during systole. This acute volume overload will also result in decreased cardiac output and acute pulmonary edema. The patient with chronic mitral regurgitation develops ventricular dilatation slowly which helps to accommodate significant increases in blood volume without significant increases in left ventricular end-diastolic pressure. Thus pulmonary congestion is initially prevented. Although patients may be stable for long periods, chronic left ventricular volume overload eventually leads to left ventricular dysfunction with decreased ejection fraction, decreased cardiac output, elevated left ventricular filling pressure, and pulmonary congestion.

The total left ventricular ejection fraction (forward and regurgitant) is increased in patients with preserved left ventricular function and should be greater than normal (55%). A "normal" ejection fraction (50–55%) in the patient with severe mitral regurgitation gives the appearance that ventricular function is preserved but in reality is evidence of significant left ventricular dysfunction.

In otherwise healthy persons, the sudden onset of fulminant heart failure with the presence of an apical holosystolic murmur strongly suggests acute mitral regurgitation resulting from chordal rupture. Congestive heart failure in patients with inferior wall myocardial infarctions indicates the possibility of papillary muscle dysfunction. Sudden respiratory distress after a febrile illness suggests acute mitral regurgitation caused by ruptured chordae or valve leaflet perforation due to infective endocarditis.

In the presence of acute mitral regurgitation, patients usually have sinus tachycardia and a non-displaced hyper-dynamic left ventricular apical impulse. An apical systolic murmur begins with S1 but often ends before S2 as left atrial and left ventricular pressures equalize and valvular regurgitation ceases. In chronic mitral regurgitation, the left ventricular apical impulse is displaced because of left ventricular dilatation. A holosystolic blowing murmur is heard at the apex and radiates to the axilla. A third heart sound is common and does not necessarily indicate the presence of left ventricular dysfunction. It may occur solely as a result of early diastolic filling [5]. A left parasternal lift and accentuated pulmonic component of the second heart sound suggest coexistent pulmonary hypertension and may indicate severe mitral regurgitation.

Echocardiography is an essential diagnostic study for evaluation of the patient with mitral regurgitation. It provides a measure of the degree of regurgitation as well as an estimate of left ventricular chamber size and function. It usually leads to the identification of the component of the mitral valve apparatus that is responsible for the mitral regurgitation. If tricuspid regurgitation is present, echo-doppler techniques can be used to measure the pressure gradient between the right ventricle and the right atrium and enable an estimate of pulmonary artery systolic pressure.

When surgical correction of mitral regurgitation is performed, it is desirable to repair rather than replace the valve. Valve repair is associated with lower perioperative mortality and better preservation of left ventricular function and, if sinus rhythm is maintained, freedom from the use of warfarin, which is necessary in the patient with a mechanical valve prosthesis. Patients with mitral valve calcification and scarring as well as those with severe myxomatous degeneration and destruction of the valve and chordae are usually not candidates for valve repair.

Left ventricular function is a major determinant of postoperative survival. Non-invasive measurements of ventricular function, ejection fraction and ventricular dimension determined by echocardiography guide the timing of operation. In the patient with severe chronic mitral regurgitation normal ejection fraction should be ≥ 60%. An ejection fraction less than 60% is indicative of a reduced long-term survival. For the patient with severe asymptomatic mitral regurgitation, mitral valve surgery should be performed if there is evidence of left ventricular dysfunction, e.g., left ventricular ejection fraction < 60%. Left ventricular end systolic dimension should be < 40 mm in the patient with normal left ventricular function. Therefore, for the patient with asymptomatic severe mitral regurgitation, surgery should be considered when the left ventricular end systolic dimension exceeds this value.

Surgery is considered in the asymptomatic patient with severe mitral regurgitation and preserved left ventricular function if the patient has had recent onset of episodic or chronic atrial fibrillation or has evidence of pulmonary hypertension (pulmonary artery systolic pressure > 50 mmHg at rest or > 60 mmHg with exercise). Surgery can also be considered in asymptomatic patients with severe chronic mitral regurgitation and preserved left ventricular ejection fraction if the likelihood of mitral valve repair without residual mitral regurgitaion is highly likely ($> 90\%$) [2]. In the symptomatic patient with severe mitral regurgitation, surgery should be performed as long as the ejection fraction is greater than 30% and/or left ventricular end-systolic dimension (LVESD) < 55 mm (LVESD > 55 mm in the patient with severe mitral regurgitation is indicative of severe left ventricular dysfunction) [2,6]. When the left ventricular ejection fraction is $< 30\%$ operative, mortality increases significantly. In this high-risk group surgery should only be considered if it is highly likely that mitral valve repair will be performed [7].

The status of left ventricular function is a major determinant of perioperative complications in patients with mitral regurgitation who undergo non-cardiac surgery. We believe that patients with severe chronic mitral regurgitation should undergo non-invasive assessment of left ventricular function before non-cardiac surgery. If the ejection fraction is not greater than normal, as would be expected, we are particularly vigilant regarding fluid administration and volume shifts in an effort to avoid the development of congestive heart failure. Patients with mitral regurgitation tolerate afterload reduction well in the perioperative period. Agents that increase afterload (e.g., vasopressors) increase the amount of regurgitant blood, and their uses should be avoided if possible. Infective endocarditis prophylaxis is not indicated in patients with isolated mitral regurgitation.

Mitral valve prolapse

Mitral valve prolapse (MVP) is a condition in which one or both mitral valve leaflets extend above the mitral annular plane during systole and prolapse into the left atrium. The degree of valve abnormality varies greatly, ranging from relatively normal valves with only intermittent prolapse to markedly abnormal valve structures with valve leaflet thickening, redundancy, and regurgitation. Mitral valve prolapse occurs in about 1–2.5% of the population [8].

Most persons with MVP are asymptomatic. Some have symptoms that are unrelated to the valve abnormality. These symptoms may be associated with autonomic dysfunction and include chest pain, palpitations, dizziness, and symptoms of panic [9,10].

The diagnosis is usually made on hearing the classic midsystolic click and, in patients with mitral regurgitation, a mid to late systolic murmur. Conditions that decrease the size of the left ventricle (i.e., the Valsalva maneuver, dehydration) cause the valve to prolapse earlier, in which case the click is heard closer to S1 and the intensity and duration of the murmur may be increased. The diagnosis is confirmed by transthoracic echocardiography.

Based on case-control studies from the 1980s it is known that infective endocarditis occurs more frequently in patients with mitral valve prolapse when compared with those with a normal mitral valve [11]. The risk of developing endocarditis, in the setting of bacteremia, has been estimated to be 1 in 1,400 in patients who have MVP and mitral regurgitation, 35 times greater than in those who have MVP without valve regurgitation [12]. Therefore, the risk of infective endocarditis has been the greatest concern for patients with MVP who are undergoing non-cardiac surgery. Particularly patients with the characteristic click-murmur of MVP with mitral regurgitation, and those with an isolated click and echocardiographic evidence of MVP with mitral leaflet thickening have been subjected to infective endocarditis prophylaxis for many years [13,14]. The most recent focused update on infective endocarditis does not recommend antibiotic prophylaxis for these patients [15]. The rationale for the drastic changes is that infective endocarditis is more likely to result from frequent exposure to random bacteremia (e.g., daily tooth brushing) than from bacteremia caused by surgical procedures [16]. Therefore, an increased lifetime risk for infective endocarditis is unlikely to be reduced by prophylaxis prior to surgical procedures. In addition, antibiotic use is not risk free and may contribute to increasing antibiotic resistance of bacterial strains worldwide. While infective endocarditis can be devastating for the patient [17], there have also been reports of failure of antibiotic prophylaxis [18]. Due to the drastic change of practice pattern advocated, the guidelines acknowledge that in select circumstances some clinicians and some patients may still feel more comfortable continuing with prophylaxis for infective endocarditis, particularly for those with severe mitral valve prolapse. In those settings, the clinician should determine that the risks associated with antibiotics are low before continuing a prophylaxis regimen. Over time, and with continuing education, there will be increasing acceptance of the new guidelines among both provider and patient communities [15].

It has been suggested that patients with MVP have a slightly higher incidence of cardiac arrhythmias. The etiology is unclear and the risk of serious arrhythmias is low. These arrhythmias often respond to cessation of caffeine, alcohol, or other stimulants. Beta-adrenergic blockers may be used if these maneuvers are not successful [19]. Patients who have dizziness associated with MVP often have decreased blood volume [20]. The onset of this symptom in the perioperative period should prompt an assessment of volume status and the administration of fluids if indicated.

Aortic regurgitation

Aortic regurgitation may be caused by processes that affect the aortic valve leaflets (e.g., rheumatic fever, infective endocarditis, congenital bicuspid aortic valve) or the aortic root and valve-supporting structures (aortic dissection, systemic hypertension, cystic medial necrosis, Marfan's syndrome). Eighty percent of cases that come to medical attention are chronic.

Chronic aortic regurgitation is accompanied by left ventricular dilatation and a gradual, progressive increase in left ventricular end-diastolic volume with only an initial slight increase in left ventricular end-diastolic pressure. The dilated left ventricle facilitates the rapid return of blood back to the ventricle during diastole, resulting in decreased peripheral arterial diastolic pressure. Left ventricular stroke volume, composed of both forward and regurgitant blood flow, is increased. The heart rate usually remains normal. This compensation often permits patients to remain asymptomatic even with severe aortic regurgitation. This combination of increased stroke volume and decreased diastolic blood pressure explains several of the classic physical findings of chronic aortic regurgitation: wide pulse pressure, water-hammer pulse (brisk pulse upstroke with rapid collapse), de Musset's sign (head bobbing during systole related to increased stroke volume), and Quincke's pulse (visible nail bed capillary pulsations).

Acute aortic regurgitation, in contrast, is characterized by the abrupt regurgitation of blood into a normal left ventricle leading to a sudden increase in left ventricular volume and marked elevation of left ventricular end-diastole pressure. Compensatory mechanisms do not occur as in chronic aortic regurgitation. The heart rate increases, cardiac output decreases, and peripheral vasoconstriction occurs. The wide pulse pressure of chronic aortic regurgitation is not present and systolic blood pressure may decrease. Acute heart failure and pulmonary edema are common. Because of the absence of chronic compensation, the classic physical findings of chronic aortic regurgitation are not present.

Acute aortic regurgitation may rapidly progress to intractable heart failure. Therefore, it is an indication for urgent aortic valve replacement. In contrast, chronic aortic regurgitation may be associated with minimal or no symptoms for years.

Aortic valve replacement is indicated for patients with acute severe aortic regurgitation. For the patient with chronic aortic regurgitation the indications for surgery vary based on the presence of symptoms. Surgery is indicated for the patient with New York Heart Association functional class III, IV symptoms, severe aortic regurgitation and normal left ventricular systolic function (ejection fraction ≥ 50%). Patients with New York Heart Association functional class II, III, IV symptoms with mild-to-moderate left ventricular dysfunction (ejection fraction 25–49%) should also undergo aortic valve replacement. The risks of surgery increase markedly when ejection fraction is less than 25%, but the benefit of surgery often outweighs that risk. For patients with asymptomatic severe aortic regurgitation aortic valve replacement is indicated in the setting of left ventricular dysfunction (ejection fraction < 50%). Aortic valve replacement is also suggested for patients with severe left ventricular dilatation (left ventricular end-systolic dimension > 55 mm or left ventricular end-diastolic dimension > 75 mm) even in the absence of symptoms [2].

In non-cardiac surgery operative risk correlates more closely with the status of left ventricular function than with the degree of aortic valve regurgitation. Vasopressors that raise peripheral vascular resistance may increase the degree of regurgitation and when used must be done so with caution. Bradycardia is associated with increased diastolic filling time which raises the magnitude of regurgitant volume by lengthening the period during which regurgitation may occur. In contrast to patients with aortic stenosis, patients with aortic regurgitation typically tolerate vasodilatation well, often with an increase in cardiac output. Caution must be exercised to prevent excessive decreases in already lowered diastolic pressure in an effort to preclude reductions in coronary artery perfusion pressure. Infective endocarditis prophylaxis is not indicated prior to surgical procedures.

Aortic stenosis

In adults, clinically significant aortic stenosis is usually the result of degenerative calcification of otherwise normal tricuspid aortic valves. When aortic stenosis manifests in adults younger that 50 years old, it is usually a result of calcification and fusion of a congenital bicuspid aortic valve. Even when it is severe, aortic stenosis remains clinically silent for many years. The onset of symptoms indicates that patients are at risk for sudden cardiac death. In patients with untreated symptomatic aortic stenosis, the occurrence of angina or syncope indicates a potential survival of only 2–3 years. The onset of congestive heart failure is more ominous and suggests the likelihood of death within 1–2 years. Sudden death is rare in those with asymptomatic, hemodynamically severe aortic stenosis (i.e., aortic gradient greater than 50 mmHg and aortic valve area $\leq 1.0\ cm^2$).

The classic physical findings of significant aortic stenosis are a low-amplitude and slow-rising carotid pulse pressure (pulsus parvus and tardus), a sustained apical impulse, a crescendo–decrescendo harsh systolic murmur heard at the second right intercostal space radiating to the carotids and precordium, an S4, and diminished intensity of the aortic component of the second heart sound. As the degree of aortic obstruction increases, the systolic murmur peaks later in systole and the intensity of the aortic component of the second heart sound decreases and may disappear.

The absence of these classic findings does not rule out the presence of critical aortic stenosis. The intensity of the heart murmur may decrease as the left ventricle fails. The carotid pulse findings may be altered in elderly patients with non-compliant peripheral vasculatures. Transthoracic echocardiography is essential to estimate the degree of aortic stenosis more precisely and to quantitate left ventricular function.

Adults with critical aortic stenosis (e.g., aortic valve area $\leq 1.0\ cm^2$) should undergo aortic valve replacement once they experience symptoms (e.g., angina, presyncope, syncope, congestive heart failure) or manifest evidence of left ventricular dysfunction even without symptoms. Fifty percent of adults with critical aortic stenosis and angina have significant coronary artery disease that may require revascularization at the time of aortic valve replacement. Survival after aortic valve replacement is excellent and patients with left ventricular dysfunction often experience marked improvement in ventricular function following surgery.

Because the risk of aortic valve replacement exceeds the risk of sudden death in patients with asymptomatic critical aortic stenosis with normal left ventricular function, aortic valve replacement is not performed until the patient develops symptoms or left ventricular dysfunction. An exception is for the patient with asymptomatic critical aortic stenosis who requires coronary artery bypass surgery; aortic valve replacement at the time of coronary artery bypass surgery is recommended.

Balloon aortic valvuloplasty has been described as a non-surgical means of decreasing the degree of aortic obstruction in aortic stenosis. The immediate and long-term results of this procedure have been disappointing. Although the aortic valve area following this procedure may be increased up to 60%, many patients with critical aortic stenosis still have significant aortic stenosis after the procedure. Mortality or major morbidity occurs in as many as 13% of patients who undergo balloon aortic valvuloplasty, and aortic valve restenosis occurs in 50% of patients within 6 months. This modality has a limited role in patients with aortic stenosis who require non-cardiac surgery. It may be considered for those clinically unstable patients with critical aortic stenosis and either congestive heart failure or hypotension who require urgent non-cardiac surgery. It may also be considered before non-cardiac surgery in patients with hemodynamic compromise as a result of critical aortic stenosis who are not candidates for aortic valve replacement [21].

Aortic stenosis was the only valvular heart disease abnormality found by Goldman to be associated with an increased risk of perioperative cardiac complication or death [22]. Patients with critical aortic stenosis have a 13% cardiac perioperative mortality, compared with an overall cardiac mortality of 1.9%. Other studies that have examined the multifactorial risk index have confirmed aortic stenosis to be a risk factor for perioperative cardiac complications [23,24]. O'Keefe reported a small series of patients with moderate or critical aortic stenosis who underwent elective non-cardiac surgery. Although no deaths occurred, 10% of the patients had significant perioperative hypotension that was transient in all but one case [25]. Local anesthesia was used in about half the cases and was not associated with any cardiac complications. Subsequent observations of patients with severe aortic stenosis indicate that their adverse event rate in relation to non-cardiac surgery is similar to patients without aortic stenosis. This overall lower than expected complication rate was attributed to effective preoperative identification of aortic stenosis as well as careful perioperative anesthesia monitoring and management [26,27].

One of the hemodynamic consequences of severe aortic stenosis is a "fixed" cardiac output resulting from left ventricular outflow tract obstruction. Patients are unable to increase cardiac output in response to the stress of surgery and there is decreased left ventricular compliance related to left ventricular hypertrophy. Patients become dependent on adequate preload. Hypovolemia and the vasodilatation that may accompany

spinal anesthesia or vasodilators are tolerated poorly and may result in profound hypotension. The onset of atrial fibrillation with loss of the atrial contribution to ventricular filling may lead to severe hemodynamic compromise.

We believe that the perioperative approach to patients with aortic stenosis must be individualized and based on the severity of the aortic stenosis, the patient's symptoms, left ventricular function, and the anticipated hemodynamic demands of the surgical procedure. Patients with aortic stenosis do not need to receive bacterial endocarditis prophylaxis. Patients with asymptomatic critical aortic stenosis who have preserved left ventricular function are monitored closely during the perioperative period. Invasive hemodynamic monitoring is used if the surgical procedure is associated with significant fluid shifts or changes in pre-load or afterload. For patients with asymptomatic AS, it is unclear whether corrective aortic valve surgery prior to non-cardiac surgery is beneficial. In a small study of 30 patients with asymptomatic, severe AS, there was no significant difference in perioperative complications compared with age- and gender-matched controls with mild-to-moderate AS (33% vs 23%, p = n.s.). The difference was mostly driven by episodes of intraoperative hypotension [28]. Patients with symptomatic critical aortic stenosis or aortic stenosis associated with severe left ventricular dysfunction should undergo aortic valve replacement before non-cardiac surgery if possible. If the non-cardiac surgery cannot be delayed or if the patients are not candidates for aortic valve replacement, the risks and benefits of aortic valvuloplasty are considered. If patients are not candidates for aortic balloon valvuloplasty and surgery is absolutely necessary, it is performed under the guidance of invasive hemodynamic monitoring with a mortality of about 10% [27]. The use of vasodilators and anesthetic techniques that may cause vasodilatation are avoided if possible.

A unique clinical association that may result in the need for non-cardiac surgery in the patient with severe aortic stenosis is bleeding from gastrointestinal dysplasia (Heyde's syndrome). In this syndrome bleeding often ceases after aortic valve replacement. While the cause of this relationship is unknown, there have been case reports of deficiency of von Willebrand factor that has normalized after aortic valve replacement [29].

Treatment of patients with prosthetic heart valves

The major concerns for the patient with a prosthetic heart valve who undergoes non-cardiac surgery are the management of anticoagulation for the patient with a mechanical valve and the need for endocarditis prophylaxis.

Few trials describe the rates of prosthetic valve thrombosis in patients who are not receiving anticoagulants. Overall, the risk of valve thrombosis or thromboembolism is higher in patients with valve prostheses in the mitral position. Although data are scant, the incidence of valve thrombosis is probably greater in patients who are not receiving anticoagulants and who have tilting disc valves (e.g., Bjork–Shiley) and are lower in patients with bileaflet valves (e.g., St. Jude, On-X). Guidelines of the American College of Cardiology/American Heart Association recommend that for patients in whom the risk of thromboembolism is high without anticoagulation (e.g., mechanical valve in the mitral or tricuspid position, older-generation valve or multiple valves in any position, or any one of the following risk factors: atrial fibrillation, previous thromboembolism, hypercoagulable condition, and left ventricular ejection fraction less than 30%) that warfarin be withheld prior to surgery and continuous full-dose intravenous heparin be initiated when the international normalized ratio (INR) becomes subtherapeutic. Heparin is discontinued 4–6 hours prior to surgery and then resumed as soon as is feasible following surgery [2]. Warfarin is resumed at the patient's maintenance dose when oral intake is resumed and heparin discontinued when the INR reaches therapeutic range. For patients with a bileaflet mechanical valve in aortic position, who do not have any one of the risk factors mentioned above, the risk of valve thromboembolism is lower and warfarin is usually discontinued 48–72 hours before surgery with the goal of an INR ≤ 1.5 at the time of surgery. It is resumed as soon as possible during the 24 hours following surgery. If the patient is unable to take oral medications at that time, continuous full-dose intravenous heparin is begun and continued until warfarin is restarted. For patients at low risk of bleeding during surgery while anticoagulated (e.g., cataract surgery, superficial procedures) a recommendation of the American College of Cardiology/American Heart Association Guidelines for the management of patients with valvular heart

disease is to continue the anticoagulation regimen [2]. Dental extractions can be safely performed on patients at a therapeutic level of anticoagulation [30]. Bridging with low molecular weight heparin is more convenient and cost effective as it can be initiated on an outpatient basis. Overall, the safety profile appears comparable to unfractionated heparin [31]. Routine monitoring of anti factor-Xa levels is not necessary in nonpregnant patients.

Bacterial endocarditis prophylaxis

Bacterial endocarditis prophylaxis is reasonable for patients with specific cardiac structural abnormalities that puts them at highest risk for adverse outcomes from infective endocarditis (Tables 9.8, 9.9, 9.10). No randomized trial has ever shown that antibiotic prophylaxis of endocarditis is effective. Since bacteremia is common after mechanical disruption of mucosal surfaces colonized with bacteria, and animal studies provided plausible data for a possible connection of bacteremia and infective endocarditis of damaged heart valves, the AHA has made recommendations for antibiotic prophylaxis of infective endocarditis for decades [32]. However, it is estimated that, even if endocarditis prophylaxis was completely effective, less than 10% of cases of bacterial endocarditis could be prevented. Reasons include the fact that the organisms targeted by currently recommended antibiotic regimens, *Streptococcus viridans* and *Enterococcus*, account for only 50% of all cases of endocarditis, and only 25% of patients with *Streptococcus*

Table 9.8 Patients at highest risk from adverse outcome from infective endocarditis.

Endocarditis prophylaxis is reasonable[a]
Patients with prosthetic cardiac valves or prosthetic material used for cardiac valve repair
Patients with previous infective endocarditis
Unrepaired cyanotic congenital heart disease, including palliative shunts and conduits.
Completely repaired congenital heart defect repaired with prosthetic material or device, whether placed by surgery or by catheter intervention, during the first 6 months after the procedure
Repaired CHD with residual defects at the site or adjacent to the site of a prosthetic patch or prosthetic device (both of which inhibit endothelialization)
Cardiac transplant recipients with valve regurgitation due to a structurally abnormal valve

Notes: [a] Clinical judgment may indicate antibiotic use in selected circumstances.
Source: From Nishimura RA, Carabello BA, Faxon DP et al. ACC/AHA 2008 guideline update on valvular heart disease: focused update on infective endocarditis: a report of the American College of Cardiology/American Heart Association Task Force on Practice Guidelines: endorsed by the Society of Cardiovascular Anesthesiologists, Society for Cardiovascular Angiography and Interventions, and Society of Thoracic Surgeons. *Circulation* 2008; **118**: 887–96.

Table 9.9 Procedures and endocarditis prophylaxis.

Endocarditis prophylaxis is reasonable
Dental procedures that involve manipulation of either gingival tissue or periapical region of the teeth, or perforation of oral mucosa
Respiratory tract
Tonsillectomy and/or adenoidectomy
Surgical operations that involve respiratory mucosa
Bronchoscopy with biopsy
Vaginal delivery at the time of membrane rupture
Invasive procedures in patients with active infections of gastrointestinal or genitourinary tract, respiratory tract, or soft tissues

Source: Modified from
Nishimura RA, Carabello BA, Faxon DP et al. ACC/AHA 2008 guideline update on valvular heart disease: focused update on infective endocarditis: a report of the American College of Cardiology/American Heart Association Task Force on Practice Guidelines: endorsed by the Society of Cardiovascular Anesthesiologists, Society for Cardiovascular Angiography and Interventions, and Society of Thoracic Surgeons. *Circulation* 2008; **118**: 887–96.
Warnes CA, Williams RG, Bashore TM et al. ACC/AHA 2008 Guidelines for the Management of Adults with Congenital Heart Disease: a report of the American College of Cardiology/American Heart Association Task Force on Practice Guidelines (writing committee to develop guidelines on the management of adults with congenital heart disease). *Circulation* 2008; **118**: e714–833.

Table 9.10 Prophylactic regimens for dental procedures.

Situation	Agent	Regimen
Standard general prophylaxis	Amoxicillin	Adults: 2.0 g; children: 50 mg/kg orally 1 hour before procedure
Unable to take oral medications	Ampicillin OR Cefazolin or ceftriaxone	Adults: 2.0 g IM or IV; children: 50 mg/kg IM or IV within 30 min before procedure Adults: 1.0 g IM or IV; children: 50 mg/kg IM or IV within 30 min before procedure
Allergic to penicillin – oral	Clindamycin OR Cephalexin[a] or cefadroxil[a] OR Azithromycin or clarithromycin	Adults: 600 mg; children: 20 mg/kg orally 1 hour before procedure Adults: 2.0 g; children; 50 mg/kg orally 1 hour before procedure Adults: 500 mg; children: 15 mg/kg orally 1 hour before procedure
Allergic to penicillin and unable to take oral medications	Clindamycin OR Cefazoline[a] or Ceftriaxone[a]	Adults: 600 mg; children: 20 mg/kg IV within 30 min before procedure Adults: 1.0 g; children: 50 mg/kg IM or IV within 30 min before procedure

IM, intramuscularly; IV, intravenously.
[a] Cephalosporins should not be used in individuals with immediate-type hypersensitivity reaction (urticaria, angioedema, or anaphylaxis) to penicillins.
Source: From Nishimura RA, Carabello BA, Faxon DP *et al.* ACC/AHA 2008 guideline update on valvular heart disease: focused update on infective endocarditis: a report of the American College of Cardiology/American Heart Association Task Force on Practice Guidelines: endorsed by the Society of Cardiovascular Anesthesiologists, Society for Cardiovascular Angiography and Interventions, and Society of Thoracic Surgeons. *Circulation* 2008; **118**: 887–96.

viridans and 40% of those with *Enterococcus endocarditis* develop their infection after procedures for which prophylaxis would have been given. Only half of all patients with endocarditis have a cardiac condition that would have made them candidates for antibiotic prophylaxis.

Antibiotic prophylaxis is recommended for those with certain high-risk cardiac lesions: prosthetic cardiac valves or prosthetic material used for cardiac valve repair, specific congenital cardiac lesions (e.g., unrepaired cyanotic congenital heart lesions, incompletely repaired congenital heart lesions with residual defects adjacent to prosthetic material, completely repaired congenital heart lesions with prosthetic material

during the first 6 months after the procedure), a previous history of bacterial endocarditis even in the absence of structural heart disease, cardiac transplant recipients with valvular regurgitation due to a structurally abnormal valve. Even though endocarditis prophylaxis is not recommended for patients without these high-risk conditions the guideline panel acknowledges that there is room for clinicians to exercise their own clinical judgment in individual cases and special circumstances [15].

The risk of infective endocarditis is considered highest for dental procedures that involve manipulation of gingival tissue, or the periapical region of the teeth or perforation of the oral mucosa (Table 9.9). Procedures that involve incision or biopsy of respiratory tract mucosa, e.g., tonsillectomy, adenoidectomy, bronchoscopy with biopsy are also likely to transiently produce significant bacteremia with a microorganism that has the potential to cause infective endocarditis. There is not sufficient evidence to suggest that genitourinary, gastrointestinal, gynecologic, obstetric, and general surgical procedures cause infective endocarditis in the absence of active infection, and therefore prophylaxis is not indicated prior to these procedures. In general, prophylaxis against infective endocarditis is not recommended for non-dental procedures in the absence of active infection. Prophylactic antibiotic regimens are directed specifically toward the most likely infecting organism, which is *S. viridans* in dental and upper respiratory tract procedures. For patients with active genitourinary or gastrointestinal infection it may be reasonable that the antibiotic regimen includes an agent active against *enterococcus* [32]. In patients with a known enterococcal urinary tract infection or colonization eradication of the organism is recommended prior to an invasive urinary procedure. In patients with an active respiratory tract infection who undergo an invasive procedure of the respiratory tract (even without incision or biopsy of respiratory tract mucosa) endocarditis prophylaxis against S. *viridans* is reasonable. If the respiratory tract infection is known or suspected to be caused by *Staphylococcus aureus*, the regimen should include an agent active against S. *aureus*. In patients with an established infection with a pathogen that could cause bacteremia and infective endocarditis the underlying infection should be treated in the usual fashion but the treatment should include an intravenous agent effective for this microorganism. In case of polymicrobial infections (e.g., soft tissue infections) the antibiotic for endocarditis prophylaxis should be directed against staphylococci and streptococci because only bacteremia due to these pathogens has the potential to cause infective endocarditis. A consensus recommendation from the ACC/AHA 2008 guidelines for the management of adults with congenital heart disease included the following recommendation that deviates from the above: it is reasonable to consider antibiotic prophylaxis against infective endocarditis before vaginal delivery at the time of membrane rupture in selected high-risk patients with prosthetic cardiac valve or prosthetic material used for cardiac valve repair, or unrepaired and palliated cyanotic congenital heart disease, including surgically constructed palliative shunts and conduits [33].

References

1. Gorlin R, Gorlin SG. Hydraulic formula for calculation of the area of the stenotic mitral valve, other cardiac valves, and central circulatory shunts. I. *Am Heart J* 1951; **41**: 1–29.

2. Bonow RO, Carabello BA, Chatterjee K *et al.* 2008 Focused update incorporated into the ACC/AHA 2006 guidelines for the management of patients with valvular heart disease: a report of the American College of Cardiology/American Heart Association Task Force on Practice Guidelines (Writing Committee to Revise the 1998 Guidelines for the Management of Patients With Valvular Heart Disease): endorsed by the Society of Cardiovascular Anesthesiologists, Society for Cardiovascular Angiography and Interventions, and Society of Thoracic Surgeons. *Circulation* 2008; **118**: e523–661.

3. Fleisher LA, Beckman JA, Brown KA *et al.* 2009 ACCF/AHA focused update on perioperative beta blockade incorporated into the ACC/AHA 2007 guidelines on perioperative cardiovascular evaluation and care for noncardiac surgery: a report of the American College of Cardiology Foundation/American Heart Association Task Force on Practice Guidelines. *Circulation* 2009; **120**: e169–276.

4. Spandorfer J. The management of anticoagulation before and after procedures. *Med Clin North Am* 2001; **85**: 1109–16, v.

5. Folland ED, Kriegel BJ, Henderson WG, Hammermeister KE, Sethi GK. Implications of third heart sounds in patients with valvular heart disease. The Veterans Affairs Cooperative Study on Valvular Heart Disease. *N Engl J Med* 1992; **327**: 458–62.

6. Otto CM. Clinical practice. Evaluation and management of chronic mitral regurgitation. *N Engl J Med* 2001; **345**: 740–6.

7. Otto CM. Timing of surgery in mitral regurgitation. *Heart* 2003; **89**: 100–5.

8. Freed LA, Levy D, Levine RA *et al.* Prevalence and clinical outcome of mitral-valve prolapse. *N Engl J Med* 1999; **341**: 1–7.

9. Fontana ME, Sparks EA, Boudoulas H, Wooley CF. Mitral valve prolapse and the mitral valve prolapse syndrome. *Curr Probl Cardiol* 1991; **16**: 309–75.

10. Gaffney FA, Karlsson ES, Campbell W *et al.* Autonomic dysfunction in women with mitral valve prolapse syndrome. *Circulation* 1979; **59**: 894–901.

11. MacMahon SW, Roberts JK, Kramer-Fox R *et al.* Mitral valve prolapse and infective endocarditis. *Am Heart J* 1987; **113**: 1291–8.

12. MacMahon SW, Hickey AJ, Wilcken DE *et al.* Risk of infective endocarditis in mitral valve prolapse with and without precordial systolic murmurs. *Am J Cardiol* 1987; **59**: 105–8.

13. Clemens JD, Horwitz RI, Jaffe CC, Feinstein AR, Stanton BF. A controlled evaluation of the risk of bacterial endocarditis in persons with mitral-valve prolapse. *N Engl J Med* 1982; **307**: 776–81.

14. Marks AR, Choong CY, Sanfilippo AJ, Ferre M, Weyman AE. Identification of high-risk and low-risk subgroups of patients with mitral-valve prolapse. *N Engl J Med* 1989; **320**: 1031–6.

15. Nishimura RA, Carabello BA, Faxon DP *et al.* ACC/AHA 2008 guideline update on valvular heart disease: focused update on infective endocarditis: a report of the American College of Cardiology/American Heart Association Task Force on Practice Guidelines: endorsed by the Society of Cardiovascular Anesthesiologists, Society for Cardiovascular Angiography and Interventions, and Society of Thoracic Surgeons. *Circulation* 2008; **118**: 887–96.

16. Strom BL, Abrutyn E, Berlin JA *et al.* Dental and cardiac risk factors for infective endocarditis. A population-based, case-control study. *Ann Intern Med* 1998; **129**: 761–9.

17. Cunha BA, D'Elia AA, Pawar N, Schoch P. Viridans streptococcal (*Streptococcus intermedius*) mitral valve subacute bacterial endocarditis (SBE) in a patient with mitral valve prolapse after a dental procedure: the importance of antibiotic prophylaxis. *Heart Lung* 2010; **39**: 64–72.

18. Durack DT, Kaplan EL, Bisno AL. Apparent failures of endocarditis prophylaxis. Analysis of 52 cases submitted to a national registry. *J Am Med Assoc* 1983; **250**: 2318–22.

19. Babuty D, Cosnay P, Breuillac JC *et al.* Ventricular arrhythmia factors in mitral valve prolapse. *Pacing Clin Electrophysiol* 1994; **17**: 1090–9.

20. Devereux RB, Kramer-Fox R, Kligfield P. Mitral valve prolapse: causes, clinical manifestations, and management. *Ann Intern Med* 1989; **111**: 305–17.

21. Hayes SN, Holmes DR, Jr., Nishimura RA, Reeder GS. Palliative percutaneous aortic balloon valvuloplasty before noncardiac operations and invasive diagnostic procedures. *Mayo Clin Proc* 1989; **64**: 753–7.

22. Goldman L, Caldera DL, Nussbaum SR *et al.* Multifactorial index of cardiac risk in noncardiac surgical procedures. *N Engl J Med* 1977; **297**: 845–50.

23. Detsky AS, Abrams HB, McLaughlin JR *et al.* Predicting cardiac complications in patients undergoing non-cardiac surgery. *J Gen Intern Med* 1986; **1**: 211–19.

24. Zeldin RA. Assessing cardiac risk in patients who undergo noncardiac surgical procedures. *Can J Surg* 1984; **27**: 402–4.

25. O'Keefe JH, Jr., Shub C, Rettke SR. Risk of noncardiac surgical procedures in patients with aortic stenosis. *Mayo Clin Proc* 1989; **64**: 400–5.

26. Raymer K, Yang H. Patients with aortic stenosis: cardiac complications in non-cardiac surgery. *Can J Anaesth* 1998; **45**: 855–9.

27. Torsher LC, Shub C, Rettke SR, Brown DL. Risk of patients with severe aortic stenosis undergoing noncardiac surgery. *Am J Cardiol* 1998; **81**: 448–52.

28. Calleja AM, Dommaraju S, Gaddam R *et al.* Cardiac risk in patients aged >75 years with asymptomatic, severe aortic stenosis undergoing noncardiac surgery. *Am J Cardiol* 2010; **105**: 1159–63.

29. Warkentin TE, Moore JC, Morgan DG. Gastrointestinal angiodysplasia and aortic stenosis. *N Engl J Med* 2002; **347**: 858–9.

30. McIntyre H. Management, during dental surgery, of patients on anticoagulants. *Lancet* 1966; **2**: 99–100.

31. Spyropoulos AC, Turpie AG, Dunn AS *et al.* Clinical outcomes with unfractionated heparin or low-molecular-weight heparin as bridging therapy in patients on long-term oral anticoagulants: the REGIMEN registry. *J Thromb Haemost* 2006; **4**: 1246–52.

32. Wilson W, Taubert KA, Gewitz M *et al.* Prevention of infective endocarditis: guidelines from the American Heart Association: a guideline from the American Heart Association Rheumatic Fever, Endocarditis, and Kawasaki Disease Committee, Council on Cardiovascular Disease in the Young, and the Council on Clinical Cardiology, Council on Cardiovascular Surgery and Anesthesia, and the Quality of Care and Outcomes Research Interdisciplinary Working Group. *Circulation* 2007; **116**: 1736–54.

33. Warnes CA, Williams RG, Bashore TM *et al.* ACC/AHA 2008 Guidelines for the Management of Adults with Congenital Heart Disease: a report of the American College of Cardiology/ American Heart Association Task Force on Practice Guidelines (writing committee to develop guidelines on the management of adults with congenital heart disease). *Circulation* 2008; **118**: e714–833.

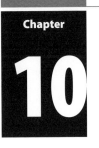

Chapter

10

Postoperative chest pain and shortness of breath

Taki Galanis and Geno J. Merli

Chest pain and shortness of breath are frequently encountered medical problems in the postoperative period. The differential diagnosis for these symptoms ranges from benign causes to medical emergencies necessitating immediate intervention. In order to accurately identify the etiology of these symptoms, the clinician must rely on a thorough history and physical examination in conjunction with the utilization of appropriate diagnostic tests. This chapter will review the differential diagnosis and evaluation of a patient with postoperative cardiopulmonary symptoms.

Evaluation and risk factor assessment

Potential pulmonary complications that may result in postoperative cardiopulmonary complaints include but are not limited to atelectasis, pneumonia, pleural effusion, pulmonary embolism (PE) and bronchospasm. These morbidities have been found to occur as frequently as cardiac complications in the postoperative period and have been identified as predictors of long-term mortality following surgery [1]. Risk factors for these complications are older age, emergency surgery, underlying chronic lung disease, poor nutritional status and advanced American Society of Anesthesiologists (ASA) class. Certain surgeries, such as those closest to the diaphragm as well as head and neck surgeries, incur a higher risk for postoperative pulmonary complications [1–4]. In addition, smoking appears to affect postoperative outcomes [5]. Table 10.1 includes a more comprehensive list of risk factors for pulmonary complications.

Pulmonary embolism is a potential complication that may have devastating consequences. Certain surgical procedures, such as hip or knee arthroplasty as well as trauma surgery, are associated with a higher risk for venous thromboembolism (VTE) than others. In addition, individual patient characteristics such as the presence of an active malignancy or a prior history of a deep vein thrombosis (DVT) or PE increase the potential for a VTE in the postoperative period [6]. Tables 10.2 and 10.3 provide a more detailed list of surgical and patient risk factors that increase the risk for VTE. A lack of appropriate DVT prophylaxis in patients with these risk factors should

raise suspicion for a PE in patients with postoperative cardiopulmonary complaints.

In addition to assessing for pulmonary and VTE risk factors, the clinician must also consider conditions that increase the patient's risk for cardiac complications, which include myocardial infarction (MI), congestive heart failure (CHF) and arrhythmias. Several criteria have been proposed to identify those who are at an increased risk of developing such complications [7–9]. The ACC/AHA 2007 guideline on perioperative cardiovascular evaluation and care for non-cardiac surgery utilizes major cardiac conditions to identify high-risk patients. In addition, it incorporates the Revised Cardiac Risk Index to further stratify a patient's likelihood of developing cardiac complications [10]. Table 10.4 summarizes the major conditions and cardiac risk index that have been incorporated into the ACC/AHA algorithm for the preoperative cardiac evaluation.

The clinician must consider the aforementioned risk factors during the evaluation of a patient with postoperative chest pain and shortness of breath. This entails a bedside assessment that utilizes a focused but thorough history and physical examination. Appropriate adjuvant tests, such as an electrocardiogram (ECG), chest radiography (CXR), and arterial blood gas (ABG) assessment, should then be selected to narrow the differential diagnosis. There is no validated, systematic approach to a patient with postoperative cardiopulmonary symptoms. Figure 10.1 outlines a proposed algorithm

Table 10.1 Risk factors for postoperative pulmonary complications.

Advanced age
General anesthesia
Prolonged surgery
Underlying chronic obstructive lung disease
Emergency surgery
Procedures near the diaphragm
Head, neck, thoracic, aortic surgeries
Poor nutritional status (albumin < 35 g/L)
American Society of Anesthesiologists class > 2
Heart failure
Smoking

Medical Management of the Surgical Patient, ed. Michael F. Lubin, Thomas F. Dodson, and Neil H. Winawer. Published by Cambridge University Press. © Cambridge University Press 2013.

Table 10.2 Classification of the risk of postoperative venous thrombosis and pulmonary embolism.

Level of risk	Approximate DVT risk without prophylaxis
High risk	40–80%
Total hip or knee arthroplasty	
Hip fracture	
Major trauma	
Spinal cord injury	
Moderate risk	10–40%
Most general, open gynecologic, or urologic surgery patients	
Low risk	< 10%
Minor surgery (not listed above) in mobile patients	

Modified from Geerts WH, Bergqvist, Pineo G *et al.* Prevention of venous thromboembolism. *Chest* 2008; **133**: 381S–453S.

Table 10.4 Major cardiac conditions and the Revised Cardiac Risk Index.

Major cardiac conditions

> Unstable coronary syndromes
>> Severe or unstable angina
>> Myocardial infarction within past month

> Decompensated heart failure
>> New-onset symptoms
>> Worsening condition

> Significant arrhythmias
>> High-grade atrioventricular block
>> Supraventricular arrhythmias with uncontrolled heart rates
>> Symptomatic bradycardia
>> New-onset or symptomatic ventricular arrhythmias

> Severe valvular disease
>> Severe aortic stenosis
>> New-onset or worsening symptoms likely of valvular pathology

Revised Cardiac Risk Index

> History of heart disease

> History of compensated or prior heart failure

> History of cerebrovascular disease

> Diabetes mellitus

> Renal insufficiency

Adapted from Fleisher LA, Beckman JA, Brown KA *et al.* ACC/AHA 2007 guidelines on perioperative cardiovascular evaluation and care for noncardiac surgery: Executive summary: A report of the American College of Cardiology/American Heart Association Task Force on Practice Guidelines (writing committee to revise the 2002 guidelines on perioperative cardiovascular evaluation for noncardiac surgery): Developed in collaboration with the American Society of Echocardiography, American Society of Nuclear Cardiology, Heart Rhythm Society, Society of Cardiovascular Anesthesiologists, Society for Cardiovascular Angiography and Interventions, Society for Vascular Medicine and Biology, and Society for Vascular Surgery. *Circulation* 2007; **116**(17): 1971–96.

Table 10.3 Risk factors for venous thromboembolism.

1. Surgery
2. Trauma (major trauma or lower extremity injury)
3. Immobility; lower extremity paresis
4. Cancer (active or occult)
5. Cancer therapy (hormonal, chemotherapy, angiogenesis inhibitors or radiotherapy)
6. Venous compression (tumor, hematoma, arterial abnormality)
7. Previous deep vein thrombosis or pulmonary embolism
8. Increasing age
9. Pregnancy and the postpartum period
10. Estrogen containing oral contraceptives or hormone replacement therapy
11. Selective estrogen receptor modulators
12. Erythropoiesis-stimulating agents
13. Acute medical illness
14. Inflammatory bowel disease
15. Nephrotic syndrome
16. Myeloproliferative disorders
17. Paroxysmal nocturnal hemoglobinuria
18. Obesity
19. Central venous catheter
20. Inherited or acquired thrombophilia

Adapted from Geerts WH, Bergqvist, Pineo G *et al.* Prevention of venous thromboembolism. *Chest* 2008; **133**: 381S–453S.

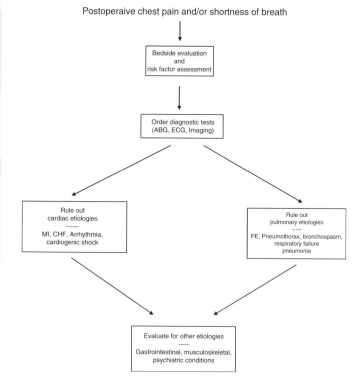

Figure 10.1 Algorithm for the evaluation of postoperative cardiopulmonary complaints. ABG, arterial blood gases; ECG, electrocardiogram; MI, myocardial infarction; CHF, congestive heart failure; PE, pulmonary embolism.

for the evaluation of postoperative chest pain and/or shortness of breath. As delineated in this algorithm, life-threatening conditions such as myocardial infarction and pulmonary embolism must be excluded via a thorough bedside assessment before attributing the symptoms to other potential causes, which include gastrointestinal as well as psychiatric conditions.

Myocardial infarction

Postoperative MI has been associated with an increased risk of death, ranging from 40% to 70% [10]. The reported incidence of this condition has varied depending on the criteria used to define it. In the POISE (PeriOperative Ischemic Evaluation) trial, perioperative MI occurred in 5% of patients with most MIs (74.1%) occurring within 48 hours after surgery [11]. The observation that most MIs occur in the early postoperative period has been observed in other studies but differs from prior reports which noted a peak between postoperative days 3 to 5 [12,13]. Two groups of patients appear to be at greatest risk for postoperative MIs: those with clinically diagnosed coronary artery disease and those with significant peripheral vascular disease [14].

Cardiac-induced angina is classically described as a deep, prolonged, and poorly localized discomfort that is reproduced with physical activity and alleviated with rest or nitroglycerine. However, the clinician must also keep in mind that postoperative MIs may be associated with complaints other than chest pain. In one series, only 40% of patients had chest pain as a presenting complaint [15] while in another only 30% of patients with ECG changes experienced chest discomfort [6]. "Anginal equivalents," which include jaw, neck, shoulder and epigastric pain, isolated dyspnea or a change in mental status, may be the only manifestations of acute coronary syndrome. Also atypical symptoms may still be due to a cardiac etiology. For example, cardiac ischemia has been observed in 22% of patients who presented with sharp pain and 7% of those whose symptoms were reproducible upon palpation of the chest. The resolution of symptoms with GI cocktails also does not exclude acute coronary syndrome [7].

The bedside examination begins with an assessment of the patient's vital signs and general appearance. Evidence of hypoperfusion, such as hypotension and cool extremities, may be suggestive of cardiogenic shock that is associated with a poor prognosis and mandates immediate medical intervention. The presence of rales and/or an S3 gallop, especially in a patient with a normal preoperative examination, suggests cardiac ischemia. In addition to assessing for MI, the cardiovascular examination may point to an alternative cardiac etiology. For example, the presence of a pericardial friction rub is suggestive of pericarditis while the presence of back pain, unequal pulses, and a new aortic regurgitation murmur suggests an aortic dissection [16].

An ECG should be ordered on most patients with postoperative cardiopulmonary complaints. The presence of ECG changes when a patient is symptomatic that resolve when the symptoms subside strongly implies the presence of cardiac ischemia. Several caveats regarding the ECG deserve mention. First, a normal ECG does not exclude cardiac ischemia as 1–6% of such patients are found to have an MI while 4% of such cases are ultimately found to have unstable angina. Conversely, ECG changes do not always indicate cardiac ischemia. ST-segment elevations, for example, can be caused by pericarditis, myocarditis, left ventricular aneurysm or apical ballooning, early repolarization, or Wolff–Parkinson–White syndrome. Intracranial abnormalities and certain medications, such as phenothiazines and tricyclic antidepressants, may cause deep T-wave inversions [16].

Cardiac biomarkers should also be used to complement the bedside evaluation and ECG interpretation. Creatine kinase-MB (CK-MB) was historically the biomarker of choice for diagnosing acute coronary syndrome. However, it is no longer considered a first-line test because of its decreased sensitivity and specificity as compared with the newer biomarkers, the cardiac troponins. CK-MB levels, for instance, can be detected in the blood of healthy volunteers and in situations in which skeletal muscle has been damaged [16,17]. However, CK-MB may still be useful because of its different half-life compared with the troponins. Although both biomarkers can be detected within several hours of myonecrosis, CK-MB levels typically return to normal within 2–3 days whereas troponins may remain elevated for 5–14 days. Thus, CK-MB may be helpful in evaluating patients with recurrent symptoms, especially in the context of persistently elevated troponins. In addition, one must also keep in mind that an elevation of cardiac troponins does not identify the exact cause of myonecrosis. Such elevations can be seen in cardiac or chest trauma (including from procedures), tachyarrhythmia, myocarditis or pericarditis, as well as critical conditions such as sepsis, pulmonary embolism, and neurologic events. Renal insufficiency may also be associated with an elevation of troponins and may be due to metabolic imbalances in addition to myonecrosis [7]. Because of the above caveats, routine measurement of cardiac troponins in the postoperative period is more likely to identify patients without an acute coronary syndrome than with an MI [10]. The bedside evaluation and risk-factor assessment should therefore guide the clinician's decision to order the ECG and cardiac biomarkers.

Pulmonary embolism

Pulmonary embolism (PE) is the most common, preventable cause of death in hospitalized patients. The incidence of VTE varies widely depending on the patient population being studied. Without any form of prophylaxis the incidence of PE is 10–40% in medical and general surgery patients and 40–60% in orthopedic patients [6]. However, patients may still develop a VTE even if they receive prophylaxis because of patient-specific risk factors. In one series, a third of patients who were diagnosed with a PE were receiving appropriate DVT preventative measures [18]. In another trial, approximately one-third of patients in the medical ICU were diagnosed with a VTE despite receiving prophylaxis. However, not all of these patients received prophylaxis continuously [19]. Thus, a careful review of the inpatient medication administration record (MAR) is warranted along with an assessment of VTE risk factors as described above.

The signs and symptoms of a PE are non-specific. Dyspnea, pleuritic chest pain, cough, and hemoptysis may occur [20]. In the postoperative period, tachycardia and hypotension may be its only manifestations [21]. Signs and symptoms of a lower extremity DVT such as edema, pain, and erythema, were common in one series [20]. The physical exam findings are equally non-specific. Auscultation of the heart may reveal an increased component of the second heart sound. A pleural rub may be noted on auscultation over the chest wall where the underlying pulmonary infarction has occurred. In addition, crackles may be heard over the involved lung segments [21].

Because of the non-specific signs and symptoms of a PE, the clinician will often need to supplement the bedside evaluation with diagnostic tests. An ABG is often ordered but the clinical utility of this test has been questioned [22]. Although it may reveal hypoxemia, hypocapnia, and respiratory alkalosis, these findings are neither specific nor sensitive for the diagnosis of PE. Furthermore, these finding are not always present [22,23]. An ECG also appears to have limited diagnostic utility when evaluating patients with a suspected PE. Sinus tachycardia is the most common finding but is non-specific [24]. Right bundle branch block and a "S1Q3T3" pattern have also been observed but are encountered more frequently in patients with large thrombotic burdens [25,26].

If the bedside evaluation suggests a PE, further imaging with either a ventilation-perfusion (V/Q) or a spiral CT scan is warranted. The Prospective Investigation of Pulmonary Embolism Diagnosis (PIOPED) trial illustrated the importance of combining clinical probability with the results of the V/Q scan. Patients with both a high pretest probability of PE and a high probability V/Q scan had a 95% likelihood of having a PE, whereas patients with a low pretest probability of PE combined with a low probability V/Q scan was associated with a 4% likelihood of a PE. Most patients, however, were found to have an intermediate probability of a PE with a wide likelihood range of actually having this condition [27].

The use of a spiral CT scan to evaluate for a PE has increased over the past several years. However, the sensitivity and specificity of this test, especially with the use of the multidetector scans is highly variable, based upon the location of the thromboembolism. In the PIOPED II study, for example, the positive predictive value of the CT scan decreased for the peripheral vessels as follows: 97% in a main or lobar artery, 68% for a segmental vessel, and 25% for a subsegmental branch [28]. Other studies have raised the possibility that such scans may detect perfusion defects of unknown significance [28,29]. Compared with V/Q scanning, another study showed that CT scans detected more pulmonary emboli which were predominantly in the peripheral vessels. However, long-term follow-up of patients evaluated with V/Q scanning did not differ from those evaluated with CT scanning, implying that peripheral perfusion defects may have little clinical significance [29]. More studies are needed to determine whether subsegmental defects merit anticoagulation, especially in the postoperative period where the risk–benefit ratio of anticoagulation may be greater.

Conclusion

The differential diagnosis of postoperative cardiopulmonary symptoms is broad and includes potentially life-threatening conditions. A focused bedside evaluation, coupled with an assessment of a patient's risk factors for pulmonary, cardiac, and VTE complications, is essential. Adjuvant diagnostic tests, while helpful in narrowing the differential diagnosis, must be interpreted in the context of the patient's pretest probability for disease and the characteristics of that particular test.

References

1. Smetana GW, Lawrence VA, Cornell JE, American College of Physicians. Preoperative pulmonary risk stratification for noncardiothoracic surgery: systematic review for the American College of Physicians. *Ann Intern Med* 2006; **144**: 581–95.

2. McAlister FA, Bertsch K, Man J, Bradley J, Jacka M. Incidence of and risk factors for pulmonary complications after nonthoracic surgery. *Am J Respir Crit Care Med* 2005; **171**: 514–17.

3. Pedersen T, Eliasen K, Henriksen E. A prospective study of risk factors and cardiopulmonary complications associated with anaesthesia and surgery: risk indicators of cardiopulmonary morbidity. *Acta Anaesthesiol Scand* 1990; **34**: 144–55.

4. Brooks-Brunn JA. Predictors of postoperative pulmonary complications following abdominal surgery. *Chest* 1997; **111**: 564–71.

5. Turan A, Mascha EJ, Roberman D *et al.* Smoking and perioperative outcomes. *Anesthesiology* 2011; **114**: 837–46.

6. Geerts WH, Bergqvist D, Pineo GF *et al.* Prevention of venous thromboembolism: American College of Chest Physicians evidence-based clinical practice guidelines (8th edition). *Chest* 2008; **133** (6 Suppl): 381S–453S.

7. Younis LT, Miller DD, Chaitman BR. Preoperative strategies to assess cardiac risk before noncardiac surgery. *Clin Cardiol* 1995; **18**: 447–54.

8. Eagle KA, Coley CM, Newell JB *et al.* Combining clinical and thallium data optimizes preoperative assessment of cardiac risk before major vascular surgery. *Ann Intern Med* 1989; **110**: 859–66.

9. Fleisher LA, Eagle KA. Clinical practice. Lowering cardiac risk in noncardiac surgery. *N Engl J Med* 2001; **345**: 1677–82.

10. Fleisher LA, Beckman JA, Brown KA *et al.* ACC/AHA 2007 guidelines on perioperative cardiovascular evaluation and care for noncardiac surgery: Executive summary: A report of the American College of Cardiology/American Heart Association Task Force on Practice Guidelines (writing committee to revise the 2002 guidelines on perioperative cardiovascular evaluation for noncardiac surgery): Developed in collaboration with the American Society of Echocardiography, American Society of Nuclear Cardiology, Heart Rhythm Society, Society of Cardiovascular Anesthesiologists, Society for Cardiovascular Angiography and Interventions, Society for Vascular Medicine and Biology, and Society for Vascular Surgery. *Circulation* 2007; **116**: 1971–96.

11. Devereaux PJ, Xavier D, Pogue J *et al.* Characteristics and short-term prognosis of perioperative myocardial infarction in patients undergoing noncardiac surgery: a cohort study. *Ann Intern Med* 2011; **154**: 523–8.

12. Goldman L, Caldera DL, Nussbaum SR *et al.* Multifactorial index of cardiac risk in noncardiac surgical procedures. *N Engl J Med* 1977; **297**: 845–50.

13. Badner NH, Knill RL, Brown JE, Novick TV, Gelb AW. Myocardial infarction after noncardiac surgery. *Anesthesiology* 1998; **88**: 572–8.

14. Ashton CM, Petersen NJ, Wray NP *et al.* The incidence of perioperative myocardial infarction in men undergoing noncardiac surgery. *Ann Intern Med* 1993; **118**: 504–10.

15. Becker RC, Underwood DA. Myocardial infarction in patients undergoing noncardiac surgery. *Cleve Clin J Med* 1987; **54**: 25–8.

16. Anderson JL, Adams CD, Antman EM *et al.* ACC/AHA 2007 guidelines for the management of patients with unstable angina/non-ST-elevation myocardial infarction: A report of the American College of Cardiology/American Heart Association Task Force on Practice Guidelines (writing committee to revise the 2002 guidelines for the management of patients with unstable angina/non-ST-elevation myocardial infarction) developed in collaboration with the American College of Emergency Physicians, the Society for Cardiovascular Angiography and Interventions, and the Society of Thoracic Surgeons endorsed by the American Association of Cardiovascular and Pulmonary Rehabilitation and the Society for Academic Emergency Medicine. *J Am Coll Cardiol* 2007; **50**: e1–157.

17. Charlson ME, MacKenzie CR, Ales KL *et al.* The post-operative electrocardiogram and creatine kinase: implications for diagnosis of myocardial infarction after non-cardiac surgery. *J Clin Epidemiol* 1989; **42**: 25–34.

18. Goldhaber SZ, Visani L, De Rosa M. Acute pulmonary embolism: clinical outcomes in the international cooperative pulmonary embolism registry (ICOPER). *Lancet* 1999; **353** (9162): 1386–9.

19. Hirsch DR, Ingenito EP, Goldhaber SZ. Prevalence of deep venous thrombosis among patients in medical intensive care. *J Am Med Assoc* 1995; **274**: 335–7.

20. Stein PD, Beemath A, Matta F *et al.* Clinical characteristics of patients with acute pulmonary embolism: data from PIOPED II. *Am J Med* 2007; **120**: 871–9.

21. Desciak MC, Martin DE. Perioperative pulmonary embolism: diagnosis and anesthetic management. *J Clin Anesth* 2011; **23**: 153–65.

22. Rodger MA, Carrier M, Jones GN *et al.* Diagnostic value of arterial blood gas measurement in suspected pulmonary embolism. *Am J Respir Crit Care Med* 2000; **162**: 2105–8.

23. Stein PD, Terrin ML, Hales CA *et al.* Clinical, laboratory, roentgenographic, and electrocardiographic findings in patients with acute pulmonary embolism and no pre-existing cardiac or pulmonary disease. *Chest* 1991; **100**: 598–603.

24. Rodger M, Makropoulos D, Turek M *et al.* Diagnostic value of the electrocardiogram in suspected pulmonary embolism. *Am J Cardiol* 2000; **86**: 807–9, A10.

25. Panos RJ, Barish RA, Whye DW Jr, Groleau G. The electrocardiographic manifestations of pulmonary embolism. *J Emerg Med* 1988; **6**: 301–7.

26. Thames MD, Alpert JS, Dalen JE. Syncope in patients with pulmonary embolism. *J Am Med Assoc* 1977; **238**: 2509–11.

27. PIOPED investigators. Value of the ventilation/perfusion scan in acute pulmonary embolism. results of the prospective investigation of pulmonary embolism diagnosis (PIOPED). *J Am Med Assoc* 1990; **263**: 2753–9.

28. Stein PD, Fowler SE, Goodman LR *et al.* Multidetector computed tomography for acute pulmonary embolism. *N Engl J Med* 2006; **354**: 2317–2327.

29. Anderson DR, Kahn SR, Rodger MA *et al.* Computed tomographic pulmonary angiography vs ventilation-perfusion lung scanning in patients with suspected pulmonary embolism: a randomized controlled trial. *J Am Med Assoc* 2007; **298**: 2743–53.

Preoperative and postoperative hypertension

Craig R. Keenan

Introduction

Hypertension affects an estimated 76 million persons in the USA, including one in three adults and more than 65% of individuals over age 65 years [1]. Thus, it is a very common disorder affecting many surgical patients. Hypertension often causes end-organ damage of the brain, heart, and kidneys, with important implications for surgical risk and perioperative management. Patients with chronic hypertension will often have perioperative episodes of hypertension that will require intervention. In addition, postoperative hypertension is common even without preexisting hypertension, especially in patients undergoing cardiac or carotid surgery. This chapter concentrates on the preoperative risk assessment and management of hypertensive patients and on the perioperative management of hypertension.

Hemodynamic response to anesthesia

A discussion of perioperative hypertension requires a basic understanding of the physiologic responses to anesthesia in normotensive and hypertensive patients. There are four main periods during anesthesia: induction, intubation, maintenance, and recovery periods. During induction, most patients' blood pressure falls. During laryngoscopy and intubation, the sympathetic nervous system is activated and blood pressure and heart rate rise. With deepening anesthesia, a decline in mean arterial pressure and heart rate occur due to the effects of pharmacologic agents, a decrease in sympathetic nervous system activity, and loss of the baroreceptor reflex. During recovery from anesthesia around the time of extubation, blood pressure and heart rate slowly increase in the first 15 minutes, and are accompanied by general arousal.

Patients with untreated hypertension can have exaggerated responses during all phases [2–4]. During induction, blood pressure declines more precipitously. During laryngoscopy and intubation, the blood pressure and heart rate often increase to a much greater degree, due to larger rises in plasma catecholamines as compared with normotensive patients. In maintenance, hypertensive patients are more likely to have blood pressure lability, with episodes of both hypertension and hypotension. During recovery, hypertensive patients can have exaggerated arousal responses with large increases in blood pressure and heart rate.

Preoperative risk assessment of hypertensive patients

Hypertension as a surgical risk factor

In discussing the operative risk of hypertension, the complexity of studying hypertension as an independent risk factor must be recognized. Hypertension causes target-organ diseases, including coronary artery disease (CAD), chronic kidney disease, cerebrovascular disease, left ventricular hypertrophy (LVH), and systolic and diastolic congestive heart failure (CHF) (Figure 11.1). Many patients have hypertension without these conditions, but many others have overt or previously unrecognized target-organ disease. These diseases can all contribute to increased perioperative risk above that of hypertension alone. Thus, the study of perioperative risk in the hypertensive patient entails determining the risks of hypertension itself plus the risks of any concomitant target-organ disease.

In the early 1970s, Prys-Roberts and colleagues studied intraoperative hemodynamics and myocardial ischemia in hypertensive and normal patients [3,4]. These non-randomized, non-blinded studies found that patients with preoperative diastolic blood pressures > 110 mmHg, regardless of pharmacologic treatment, commonly developed arrhythmias and/or severe intraoperative hypotension with associated myocardial ischemia. Patients with better-controlled hypertension behaved similarly to normotensive patients, with no hypotensive or ischemic events.

These small studies were not designed to assess clinical endpoints. But other studies have found that these surrogate endpoints of intraoperative hemodynamic instability and myocardial ischemia are indeed associated with postoperative renal failure, CHF, cerebrovascular events, myocardial infarction (MI), and cardiac death [5–9].

Medical Management of the Surgical Patient, ed. Michael F. Lubin, Thomas F. Dodson, and Neil H. Winawer. Published by Cambridge University Press. © Cambridge University Press 2013.

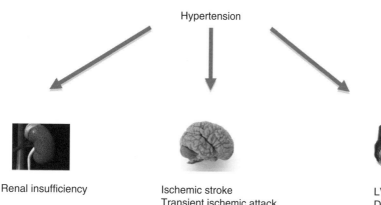

Hypertension

Renal insufficiency

Ischemic stroke
Transient ischemic attack
Hemorrhagic stroke
Retinopathy
Encephalopathy

LVH
Diastolic CHF
Systolic CHF
CAD
PVD

Figure 11.1 Target-organ damage from hypertension, with relatively few pulmonary-specific risk factors. LVH, left ventricular hypertrophy; CHF, congestive heart failure; CAD, coronary artery disease; PVD, peripheral vascular disease.

Despite these concerning findings, Goldman found that preoperative mild to moderate hypertension did not correlate with adverse cardiovascular outcomes [10]. Similarly, multivariate analyses on cohorts of surgical patients have not routinely found preoperative hypertension to be an *independent* risk factor for perioperative cardiac events. In fact, the most widely accepted and validated indices over the past three decades for perioperative cardiac risk assessment for noncardiac surgery do not include hypertension as an independent risk factor [11–13].

Target-organ damage and surgical risk

As discussed above, chronic hypertension can cause damage to the heart, kidney, and brain, termed target-organ damage (TOD). The commonly used Revised Cardiac Risk Index identifies six independent predictors of major cardiac complications, four of which are potentially TOD from hypertension: history of ischemic heart disease, history of CHF, history of cerebrovascular disease, and serum creatinine > 2.0 mg/dL [13]. Hypertensive patients with target-organ damage are likely to have two or more of these predictors and thus are at significantly increased risk for perioperative cardiac events.

Hypertension is a major risk factor for CAD, and CAD definitely increases perioperative cardiac risk. The Perioperative Ischemia Study Group evaluated patients at high risk for CAD or with known CAD *and* concomitant hypertension, and found that this combination is associated with increased in-hospital myocardial ischemia and death for patients undergoing non-cardiac surgery [14]. The same group of patients were monitored for myocardial ischemia with continuous electrocardiograms before, during, and after surgery. A history of hypertension, LVH, diabetes, CAD, and digoxin use were independent predictors of postoperative myocardial ischemia in a multivariate model. In addition postoperative myocardial ischemia was strongly associated with severe cardiovascular complications [8,9].

Hypertension can cause CHF from systolic and/or diastolic dysfunction. The presence of CHF is an independent predictor of major perioperative cardiac complications and of postoperative CHF itself [15,16]. Congestive heart failure is a syndrome, and many of the underlying causes are important surgical risk factors, such as CAD or severe aortic stenosis. Thus, identifying the underlying cause before surgery is very important if at all possible. At a minimum, treatment of those disorders should be optimized prior to surgery.

In a study of 405 patients undergoing major vascular surgery, the presence of LVH on the preoperative ECG, with or without ST segment depression, has an increased risk of perioperative myocardial infarction and cardiac events [17]. As mentioned above, LVH in patients with CAD or at high risk for CAD is an independent predictor of postoperative ischemia [8].

Hypertension is a risk factor for both chronic kidney disease and cerebrovascular disease. A serum creatinine > 3.0 mg/dL was an independent predictor of cardiac risk in Goldman's original cardiac risk study [8]. The Revised Cardiac Risk Index also found that a serum creatinine > 2.0 mg/dL is an independent risk factor for major cardiac complications around non-cardiac surgery [11]. Similarly, a history of transient ischemic attack or stroke was also an independent predictor of major cardiac complications [11].

Summary of perioperative risks

Observational data indicate that hypertension does not independently predict perioperative adverse cardiac events. The studies, however, have small numbers of patients with severe hypertension. Severely hypertensive patients have significant hemodynamic instability and intraoperative myocardial ischemia, factors that are strongly associated with adverse events in other studies. Thus, patients with severe hypertension (> 180/110 mmHg) are felt to have significant perioperative cardiovascular risk. Patients with only mild to moderate hypertension, who are well represented in the cohort studies, have much less hemodynamic instability and ischemia, and do not show the increased risk. Lastly, hypertensive patients often have end-organ damage leading to CAD, CHF, LVH, cerebrovascular disease, and renal insufficiency, all of which independently increase cardiac risk.

Preoperative evaluation of the hypertensive patient

Preoperative assessment

A recommended preoperative evaluation of patients with existing or newly discovered hypertension is outlined in Table 11.1. The first step is to obtain a thorough history, including questioning the patient about diseases associated with hypertension, including CHF, CAD, renal failure, and cerebrovascular disease. Ask specifically about symptoms of these conditions, including chest pain, paroxysmal nocturnal dyspnea, orthopnea, and edema. Recognizing and optimizing these conditions prior to surgery are important goals.

A complete list of allergies and medications, including over-the-counter preparations, is essential. Always ask about prior anesthetic adverse reactions and for symptoms of abnormal bleeding. The physical examination should include careful measurement of the blood pressure, and should focus on the cardiac and pulmonary exams. Look carefully for evidence of LVH or CHF, including a third or fourth heart sound, a displaced or sustained point of maximal impulse, an elevated jugular venous pressure, pulmonary crackles, and peripheral edema. Findings of severe aortic stenosis (e.g., late peaking systolic crescendo-decrescendo murmur, diminished S2, slow rate of rise of carotid pulse) should be sought.

All patients with hypertension should get a preoperative 12-lead ECG to look for evidence of prior MI and LVH, which have implications of increased cardiac risk, as outlined above. This ECG also serves as a baseline tracing for comparison in the event of suspected ischemic events in the perioperative period.

Many patients have undiagnosed CAD, and up to 25% of MIs are unrecognized (or "silent"). Thus, a significant number of hypertensive patients may show evidence of previously unrecognized CAD and MI, as evidenced by pathologic Q waves on the routine preoperative ECG. Patients with unrecognized MI, however, have the same risks of recurrent MI and death as those with known CAD. When silent MI is discovered, at a minimum, patients need careful evaluation of their cardiac risk, as outlined in Chapter 9.

A chest X-ray should be performed if the history or physical examination suggests new or active pulmonary disease. An echocardiogram, if not previously performed, should be done in patients with evidence of CHF or suspected severe valvular dysfunction.

Serum electrolytes, urea nitrogen, and creatinine should be measured prior to surgery to assess baseline renal function and potassium levels. This is particularly important for patients taking antihypertensive medications known to cause

Table 11.1 Recommended preoperative evaluation of hypertensive patients.

History
  Medical conditions: coronary artery disease, congestive heart failure (CHF), cerebrovascular disease, renal disease
  Prior surgeries and complications. History of excessive bleeding
  Social history: functional status, smoking, alcohol and drug intake
  Review of systems: chest pain, shortness of breath, dyspnea, exertional capacity, edema, orthopnea, paroxysmal nocturnal dyspnea, paroxysmal sweating and/or headache

Allergies
  General allergies and prior adverse reactions to anesthetic agents

Medications
  Prescription and over-the-counter agents

Physical exam
  Emphasis on cardiopulmonary exam: evidence of CHF, aortic stenosis

Laboratory and other tests
  Electrolytes, blood urea nitrogen, creatinine
  12-lead electrocardiogram

Other tests, if indicated by history or examination
  Chest radiograph
  Tests for myocardial ischemia
  Exercise electrocardiography or echocardiography, pharmacologic stress nuclear imaging or echocardiography
  Echocardiogram (suspected CHF or severe valvular disease)
  Serum-free normetanephrine and metanephrines (suspected pheochromocytoma)

hypokalemia or hyperkalemia, including thiazide and loop diuretics, potassium-sparing diuretics, angiotensin converting enzyme inhibitors (ACEI), and angiotensin II receptor blockers (ARB). Hypokalemia can contribute to perioperative ileus, potentiate the effect of non-depolarizing muscle relaxants, and may predispose surgical patients to cardiac dysrhythmias. Hyperkalemia can also cause life-threatening arrhythmias. Of note, perioperative use of depolarizing neuromuscular blocking agents can cause acute rises in serum potassium levels of approximately 0.5 meq/L. Thus, both hypokalemia and hyperkalemia need to be identified and corrected prior to surgery.

Lastly, all patients with hypertension need an explicit consideration of perioperative cardiac risk, as outlined in Chapter 9.

Secondary hypertension

Secondary causes of hypertension must be considered when evaluating any patient with elevated blood pressure, including renal artery stenosis, primary hyperaldosteronism, Cushing syndrome, sleep apnea, hypothyroidism, primary hyperparathyroidism, alcohol or other substance abuse, primary renal disease, and pheochromocytoma. Ideally, patients with suspected secondary hypertension should have an evaluation prior to elective surgery, as identification of these conditions may affect perioperative management.

Specifically, patients with alcohol or substance disorders should be watched closely for the development of withdrawal syndromes postoperatively. Uncontrolled Cushing syndrome may potentiate poor wound healing and electrolyte disturbances. Primary hyperaldosteronism and hyperparathyroidism run the risk of hypokalemia and hypercalcemia, respectively.

Sleep apnea is recognized as a risk factor for postoperative complications, including hypoxia, hypercapnea, bronchospasm, delirium, reintubation, and cardiac events [18]. Treatment with positive airway pressure prior to surgery may prevent complications.

Hypothyroid patients undergoing surgery have increased rates of CHF, neuropsychiatric problems, and gastrointestinal hypomotility. These patients are also more susceptible to intraoperative hypotension, delayed recovery from anesthesia, hypoventilation, and increased sensitivity to anesthetic agents [19]. It seems prudent to delay elective procedures to allow treatment to a euthyroid state, especially with severe hypothyroidism.

Surgery in patients with unrecognized or untreated pheochromocytoma is extremely dangerous, due to catecholamine release triggered by perioperative events, with a mortality rate approaching 80% in reported cases [20]. Thus, patients should be asked about symptoms of pheochromocytoma, including the classic triad of episodic headaches, sweating, and tachycardia. Most patients with pheochromocytoma will have two of these symptoms, which unfortunately are present in many patients without the disorder. Half of the patients have classic paroxysmal hypertension and most of the rest have persistent blood pressure elevations. Because pheochromocytoma can be a familial disorder, obtaining a family history can be helpful.

The diagnosis of pheochromocytoma is challenging. Testing for plasma normetanephrine and metanephrine has a sensitivity of 99% [21]. If normal, it essentially excludes pheochromocytoma, making this test a good initial screen for the rare preoperative patient who has signs and symptoms suggestive of pheochromocytoma. The specificity of this test, however, is only 89% and the prevalence of pheochromocytoma is very low (0.5% to 4%), so false-positive tests will be common. Further biochemical testing must be done to distinguish true-positives from false-positives. A diagnosis of pheochromocytoma by biochemical testing is followed by localizing imaging tests and surgical removal of the tumor. In the rare case when a patient has known pheochromocytoma and surgery is emergent, specific interventions, including alphablockade and aggressive fluid management are used to treat patients in the perioperative period.

Management of preoperative hypertension

The exact management of hypertension in surgical patients depends upon the urgency of the planned surgery and the severity of hypertension. The Seventh Report of the Joint National

Table 11.2 Classification of blood pressure severity [22].

Category	Systolic BP (mmHg)	Diastolic BP (mmHg)
Normal	< 120	< 80
Pre-hypertension	120–139	80–89
Hypertension		
Stage 1	140–159	90–99
Stage 2	≥ 160	≥ 100

Committee on High Blood Pressure classifies hypertension severity as outlined in Table 11.2 [22]. This report further classifies hypertensive crises as a blood pressure of > 180/120 mmHg, which include hypertensive emergencies and urgencies.

Rarely, a preoperative patient may have a hypertensive emergency. This is defined as severe blood pressure elevations (> 180/120 mmHg) complicated by evidence of impending or progressive target-organ dysfunction, which would include encephalopathy, intracerebral or subarachnoid hemorrhage, acute stroke, acute aortic dissection, myocardial ischemia, or heart failure. Hypertensive emergencies require immediate treatment with parenteral antihypertensive agents in an intensive care setting to limit target organ damage. The initial goal of therapy is to reduce mean arterial BP within minutes to an hour by no more than 25%, then if stable, to 160/100–110 mmHg within the next 2–6 hours. Excessive blood pressure reductions can precipitate renal, cerebral, or coronary ischemia, and should be avoided. Usually surgery is deferred in patients with hypertensive emergencies, though occasionally a patient must go for emergent surgery for life-threatening conditions and the anesthesiologist is tasked with reducing blood pressure in the operating suite.

Most patients with preoperative severe hypertension, however, have a hypertensive urgency. This is defined as severe elevation in blood pressure without evidence of progressive target-organ damage. Hypertensive urgencies require less rapid reductions in blood pressure over hours to days. As noted above, small studies demonstrated hemodynamic instability, arrhythmia, and myocardial ischemia in patients with severe hypertension.

Based on these observations, experts have advocated postponing surgery to allow antihypertensive therapy to be instituted or adjusted to control the blood pressure prior to surgery, even though no data show that such treatment reduces postoperative complications. Subsequently, uncontrolled preoperative hypertension is the most common reason for cancellation of elective surgery.

As the recommendation to postpone surgery is based upon limited clinical evidence, there is no agreement on the need to postpone surgery in patients with hypertensive urgencies [23]. For truly elective surgeries, it seems prudent to postpone surgery, especially if patients have underlying medical conditions (e.g., renal insufficiency, CHF, CAD) that may be exacerbated by poorly controlled hypertension. In such patients, it is more likely that blood pressure optimization may reduce complications.

The optimal duration of blood pressure control prior to surgery is not known, but the adverse vascular system changes associated with severe hypertension can take 6–8 weeks to reverse even after blood pressure is controlled. Thus, some recommend that control be maintained for several weeks prior to surgery. Weksler and colleagues attempted to determine if a shorter period of control is safe [24]. They randomized 989 patients with previously well-controlled hypertension who had DBP between 110 and 130 mmHg on arrival to the operating room. The control group (400 patients) had the surgery postponed and the patients were hospitalized for blood pressure treatment. Once the DBP was < 110 mmHg for 3 consecutive days, they proceeded to surgery. The treatment group (589 patients) received a single 10 mg dose of intranasal nifedipine, which was effective in getting their DBP < 100 mmHg in all cases. They then proceeded immediately to surgery. There were no differences in postoperative complications over 3 postoperative days. Thus, the immediate blood pressure control seemed safe in these patients with previously well-controlled hypertension, and significantly reduced surgical delays. This may be extrapolated to support the practice of acute preoperative treatment of severe hypertension in cases that are urgent or emergent. Of note, sublingual and intranasal nifedipine is no longer recommended due to the potential for severe adverse events.

For patients with preoperative blood pressures < 180/110 mmHg, delaying surgery will not reduce risk, and patients can proceed to surgery. If time permits, however, getting improved control of mild to moderate hypertension by adjusting a patient's oral antihypertensive regimen is recommended.

Newly diagnosed hypertension

Making a new diagnosis of hypertension during a preoperative evaluation is common. The preoperative risk assessment, evaluation, and initial blood pressure goals are the same as those outlined above. All patients should start lifestyle modifications with low sodium diet, regular exercise, and weight loss if indicated. Patients with severe hypertension (BP > 180/110 mmHg) need pharmacologic therapy for preoperative blood pressure control. All other patients that do not reach their goal blood pressure with lifestyle modifications alone should be started on medication, with most patients requiring two or more agents to achieve their goals [22].

The recommended first-line antihypertensive agents for most patients are thiazide-type diuretics. Meta-analysis has shown that low-dose diuretics prevent stroke, CHF, CAD, and death, while beta-blockers prevent stroke and CHF [25]. Comorbid conditions may dictate using other agents as first-line therapy. Diabetes with proteinuria, non-diabetic renal insufficiency, and systolic CHF are all indications for an ACEI, or an ARB if they cannot tolerate the ACEI. Coronary artery disease with a history of MI is an indication for beta-blocker therapy. Patients with a normal LVEF who are at higher risk for CAD (i.e., with diabetes or peripheral arterial disease plus another cardiac risk factor) have a reduction of mortality, CAD events, and stroke when treated with ACEI [26].

Perioperative management of chronic antihypertensive medications

In the 1960s, blood pressure medications were routinely held for fear of interactions with anesthetic agents. It is now clear that most antihypertensive medications should be continued up until the time of surgery to maintain blood pressure control and avoid adverse events. Specifically, this includes taking the medications on the morning of surgery with small sips of water. Failure to do so can lead to withdrawal syndromes, severe perioperative hypertension, hemodynamic instability, ischemia, and death [27,28]. If possible, it is helpful to change short-acting antihypertensives to longer-acting preparations at least 2–3 days prior to the surgery. Doing this will help avoid postoperative hypertension that may occur on the day of surgery as the medications wear off. Oral agents should be resumed as soon as possible postoperatively. A discussion of specific agents follows.

Beta-blocking agents

Acute cessation of beta-blockers can cause a withdrawal syndrome that can lead to severe hypertension, myocardial ischemia and infarction, and death in surgical and non-surgical patients [28,29]. Beta-blockers have been shown to have benefits in some surgical patients, including reducing myocardial ischemia in normotensive and hypertensive patients, reducing arrhythmias during surgery, and reducing hemodynamic fluctuations associated with recovery from anesthesia, laryngoscopy, and surgical stimuli [30–32]. Thus, there are many compelling reasons to continue beta-blockers perioperatively. But adding beta-blockers in the perioperative period to reduce cardiac events and death has had conflicting results. For a thorough discussion of perioperative beta-blockade, see Chapter 9. For those patients unable to take oral medications postoperatively, intravenous beta-blockers should be substituted to prevent beta-blocker withdrawal.

Clonidine

Clonidine, a central-acting alpha-2 adrenergic agonist, has proven benefits in the perioperative period. In addition to its antihypertensive and sympatholytic properties, it also has sedative and analgesic effects. Multiple trials show that de novo perioperative clonidine administration in non-cardiac surgery decreases the surrogate endpoint of myocardial ischemia [33]. One small randomized controlled trial also showed a mortality reduction [34]. Patients on chronic clonidine therapy may realize some of these benefits as well, though it has not been studied.

Like beta-blockers, oral and transdermal clonidine have a well-recognized withdrawal syndrome, which can lead to hypertensive crisis, perioperative hemodynamic instability, arrhythmias, and myocardial ischemia. This syndrome can start as early as 12 hours after the last dose. Thus, clonidine should be continued up until the time of surgery and resumed in the immediate postoperative period. If it is anticipated that a patient will be unable to take oral medications by 12 hours after surgery, oral clonidine can be converted to a transdermal patch preoperatively. As it can take 48–72 hours to get therapeutic drug levels after placing a patch, the conversion should be started 3 days prior to the surgery, while tapering the oral dose of clonidine to 50% on day 2 and 25% on day 3. The dose relationship between oral and transdermal therapy is not always equivalent, so a 0.1 mg/day patch is used first, except in patients on large oral doses, in which case one may start with a 0.2 mg or 0.3 mg/day patch [35]. Others have successfully used clonidine crushed and suspended in sorbitol or saline for rectal administration in the perioperative period [36].

Angiotensin-converting enzyme inhibitors and angiotensin II receptor blockers

Angiotensin-converting enzyme inhibitors (ACEI) prevent the formation of angiotensin II, a potent vasoconstrictor. Angiotensin receptor blockers (ARB) inhibit the vasoconstrictive action of angiotensin II. Angiotensin-converting enzyme inhibitors and ARB discontinuation do not lead to a withdrawal syndrome, and the long-acting preparations can have hemodynamic effects for 18–24 hours after the last dose. Several small studies have shown that ACEI and ARB therapy administered on the morning of surgery increases the risk of hypotension during anesthetic induction, which in some cases can be severe and refractory to conventional pressor therapy [37–39]. A more recent observational study suggests that this effect is particularly an issue in patients on ACEI/ARB in combination with diuretics [40]. Holding the ACEI/ARB for more than 10 hours before surgery diminishes the incidence of hypotension, without significantly increasing preoperative blood pressure, but may lead to increased postoperative hypertension [37,39,41]. Holding the ACEI/ARB has not been proven to reduce outcomes such as myocardial ischemia or death, but the studies have been small. Thus, there is still no consensus on whether to continue ACEI/ARB on the morning of surgery, or give the last dose on the day prior to surgery. If the ACEI is continued on the day of surgery, the anesthetist must be particularly vigilant for severe hypotension.

Diuretic agents

Diuretics are common and effective antihypertensive agents. Their use in surgical patients carries two major risks. One is the development of potassium imbalance. Hypokalemia (from kaliuretic agents) or hyperkalemia (from potassium-sparing agents) carry risks of arrhythmias and ileus. The other is intravascular volume depletion, which can combine with the systemic vasodilation of anesthetic agents to cause intraoperative hypotension. It is reasonable to withhold diuretics on the morning of surgery to decrease the risk of hypotension, but the clinician must carefully monitor patients' volume status and potassium levels in the perioperative period. Intravenous furosemide can be used in patients unable to resume their oral dosing.

Calcium-channel blockers

Calcium-channel blockers (CCBs) cause vasodilation by inhibiting intracellular transport of calcium through specific calcium channels. With abrupt discontinuation of CCBs, there is no significant rebound hypertension, though some patients on CCBs for angina can infrequently develop coronary vasospasm or recurrent angina. Because CCBs inhibit platelet aggregation, there may be a modest increase in perioperative bleeding, though current guidelines do not recommend discontinuing these agents for this reason. Calcium-channel blockers should be continued in the perioperative period for blood pressure control, as long as there is no hypotension or severe bradycardia.

Given the lack of a significant withdrawal syndrome, other parenteral medications can be used in the place of CCBs for patients unable to take the oral preparations postoperatively. Patients who have been on CCBs for angina pectoris or vasospastic angina should be continued on them or observed very carefully for evidence of worsening angina. Similarly, if patients are on diltiazem or verapamil for rate control of supraventricular arrhythmias, they should be continued in the perioperative period. These agents are available in parenteral form if needed. Nicardipine and clevidipine are available for use in the perioperative period for blood pressure control.

Other agents

Occasionally, patients will be taking older antihypertensive agents. Withdrawal syndromes and adverse outcomes have been associated with methyldopa, guanabenz, reserpine, and hydralazine [27,28]. Thus, these agents should be continued in the perioperative period. If patients are unable to take oral medications postoperatively, hydralazine and methyldopa can be administered parenterally. Reserpine and guanabenz do not have parenteral preparations, and thus tapering off of these medications prior to surgery can be considered. Many other antihypertensive agents with better side-effect and dosing profiles can be used in their place.

Minoxidil is a potent vasodilator that can lead to significant volume retention and reflex tachycardia. Thus, beta-blockers and diuretics are often co-administered with this drug. Rebound hypertension may occur with minoxidil cessation, and patients on this agent usually have underlying severe hypertension. Thus, it should be continued in the perioperative period whenever possible. There is no parenteral preparation of minoxidil.

Management of postoperative hypertension

Postoperative treatment of chronic hypertension

The best strategy for managing postoperative blood pressure in patients with chronic hypertension is to resume their usual antihypertensive medications on their usual dosing schedule. Some patients will have a modest decline in blood pressure after major surgery, and may require less antihypertensive medication (Table 11.3). Blood pressure usually returns to preoperative values within 2–4 weeks of surgery. Thus, close follow-up with a regular provider after surgery is crucial to monitor and adjust medications for optimal treatment. Blood pressure goals for antihypertensive therapy are listed in Table 11.4, and are dependent upon comorbid conditions [22].

A subset of postoperative patients are unable to take oral medications after the surgery, usually due to intra-abdominal surgery, postoperative ileus, or postoperative nausea and vomiting. Until they can resume oral therapy, these patients can be treated with intravenous antihypertensive agents. Medications with a longer half-life, dosed regularly, are effective. Commonly used agents include parenteral hydralazine, labetalol, enalaprilat, or metoprolol. These medications have the benefit of not needing a continuous infusion, and thus can be given outside of intensive care settings with careful monitoring. As discussed, transdermal clonidine may also be useful for these patients, but it must be started preoperatively given the onset of action for the patch is 2–3 days. Once patients are able to take oral agents, they can resume their usual medications.

Acute postoperative hypertension

As patients emerge from anesthesia, many develop mild elevations in blood pressure and heart rate due to generalized arousal. A small subset of patients will have severe elevations in blood pressure (often defined as systolic blood pressure > 20% higher than the preoperative reading), termed acute postoperative hypertension (APH). Acute postoperative hypertension can have significant adverse consequences, including stroke, myocardial ischemia and infarction, heart failure, encephalopathy, hemorrhage and hematoma at the surgical site, disruption of surgical anastamoses, renal failure, arrhythmias, and death. Thus, monitoring for the development of APH and rapid correction when it occurs is important to reduce adverse outcomes.

The onset of APH is usually during the first 10–30 minutes after the end of anesthesia and most episodes resolve within a few hours, although prolonged episodes do occur and present a greater risk for complications. For all patients admitted to the recovery room, the incidence of APH is about 3%, but incidences vary greatly from 3–80% depending upon the population of patients being studied. The incidence is much higher after CABG, aortic valve surgery, carotid endarterectomy, intracranial surgery, abdominal aortic aneurysm resections, and radical neck dissection. Preexisting hypertension is a major risk factor for the development of APH.

Some APH episodes can be avoided by continuing blood pressure medications up until the day of surgery. Many other factors can contribute to APH, including pain, anxiety, hypercarbia, hypoxia, volume overload, hypothermia, and bladder distension. The initial step to treat patients with APH is to look for these factors and correct them. If the hypertension persists, antihypertensive therapy should be instituted.

Since many APH events are of short duration and because hypotension can occur with the use of long-acting medications, the ideal antihypertensive agent for APH has a rapid onset, a short duration of action, an available intravenous preparation, and an easily titratable action. Many different medications can be used for APH and postoperative hypertension, and Table 11.3 summarizes commonly used agents. Medications for APH are the same drugs used for hypertensive emergencies. The usual agents of choice for APH are labetalol, esmolol, nicardipine, and clevidipine; but the choice of drug depends upon characteristics of the patient, the surgical procedure, and the experience of the treating clinicians with specific agents.

Specific medications for APH and postoperative hypertension

Labetalol

Labetalol is a combined alpha- and beta-blocker that is given by either parenteral bolus dosing or continuous infusion. It can be converted easily to pill form when the patient resumes oral intake. It has proven efficacy and safety in APH [42–54]. Major side-effects include postural hypotension, bronchospasm, bradycardia, and exacerbation of heart failure in patients with reduced left ventricular function. Life-threatening hyperkalemia can develop in patients with advanced renal failure, so alternative agents are recommended for such patients [55,56]. Labetalol can be used to replace chronic oral beta-blockers in patients unable to resume oral medications. Labetalol has very little transplacental transfer and so is often used in pregnant women. It is a first-line agent in pregnancy with demonstrated safety and efficacy. It does not increase intracranial pressure, so is a preferred agent after intracranial surgeries.

Esmolol

Esmolol is an ultra-short-acting, cardioselective beta-blocker that can be used effectively in the perioperative period [50,54,57,58]. It requires a continuous infusion in an ICU setting. As with labetalol, esmolol can cause bradycardia, heart block, bronchospasm, and worsening heart failure in patients with left ventricular dysfunction. It is useful in patients with perioperative myocardial ischemia or infarction.

Table 11.3 Intravenous medications for postoperative hypertension.

Agent	Mechanism	Dose	Onset	Duration	Conditions, adverse effects and comments
Labetalol	Beta-blocker and alpha-blocker	20 mg IV over 2 minutes then 10–80 mg IV every 10 minutes to max 300 mg/24 hour; or 0.5–2 mg/min IV infusion	5–10 min	3–6 hours	Useful in pregnancy, myocardial ischemia Can cause bradycardia, heart failure, heart block, bronchospasm, hypotension, nausea, and severe hepatocellular injury. Reduce dose in hepatic insufficiency. Risk of hyperkalemia in patients with advanced renal disease
Esmolol	Beta-blocker	Load 500 µg/kg IV over 1 minute, then 50–300 µg/kg/min IV infusion	1–2 min	10–30 min	Useful in myocardial ischemia Can cause bradycardia, heart block, heart failure, bronchospasm
Nitroprusside	Vasodilator	Start at 0.3–0.5 µg/kg/min IV infusion. Increase in increments of 0.5 µg/kg/min. Max dose 10 µg/kg/min	Seconds	1–10 min	Thiocyanate and cyanide toxicity, with increased risk with renal or hepatic disease. Can cause hypotension, headache, nausea, vomiting, methemoglobinemia, rebound hypertension, coronary steal, elevated intracranial pressure. Can develop tachyphylaxis Doses over 4 µg/kg/min can rapidly lead to toxicity
Nitroglycerin	Vasodilator	5–100 µg/min. Start at 5 µg/min IV infusion. Increase by 5 µg/min every 3–5 min to 20 µg/min. If no response, increase by 10 µg/min every 3–5 min. Max dose 200 µg/min	2–5 min	3–5 min	Useful in myocardial ischemia, pulmonary edema. Can cause headache, hypotension, reflex tachycardia, methemoglobinemia. Can develop tachyphylaxis
Hydralazine	Vasodilator	10–20 mg IV every 4–6 hours. Max dose 40 mg every 4–6 hours.	10–30 min	2–4 hours	Can have unpredictable effect Tachycardia, increased cardiac output, increased sympathetic activity. Avoid in patients with cardiac ischemia, aortic dissection, or increased intracranial pressure
Nicardipine	Calcium channel blocker	Start 5 mg/hour IV infusion, increase by 1–2.5 mg/hour increments every 15 minutes (max 15 mg/hour). Once at goal BP, reduce to 3 mg/hour, titrate as needed. Usual dose 2–15 mg/hour IV	1–5 min	3 hours	Useful in patients with acute ischemic stroke or intracerebral hemorrhage. Can be used in pregnancy Can cause reflex tachycardia, headache, flushing, edema. Reduce dose in hepatic and/or renal insufficiency
Clevidipine	Calcium channel blocker	Start 1–2 mg/hour IV infusion, double every 90 seconds until approach goal. As blood pressure approaches the goal, the dose	2–4 min	5–15 min	Can cause tachycardia. Risk of rebound hypertension when stopped Contraindicated in patients

Table 11.3 (cont.)

Agent	Mechanism	Dose	Onset	Duration	Conditions, adverse effects and comments
		should be increased by less than double, and the time between adjustments should be increased to every 5 to 10 minutes. Usual dose 4–6 mg/hour, max dose 16 mg/hour			with soy or egg allergy and in patients with severe aortic stenosis
Enalaprilat	ACE inhibitor	1.25 mg IV every 6 hours. Max dose 5 mg every 6 hours for up to 36 hours	30 min–4 hours	6 hours	Useful in systolic CHF Can cause renal insufficiency, angioedema, hyperkalemia Response can be variable. Need to lower start dose in renal insufficiency to 0.625 mg every 6 hours Can be converted easily to oral ACEI therapy
Fenoldopam	Dopamine receptor agonist	No bolus. 0.03–1.6 µg/kg/min IV infusion. Adjust at 15 min intervals	5–15 min	10 min–4 hours	Useful in patients with or at risk for renal insufficiency. Can increase GFR and urinary output in patients with renal insufficiency. Can cause reflex tachycardia, headache, nausea, elevated intraocular pressure, flushing Contraindicated in sulfite sensitivity

Table 11.4 Goals of hypertension therapy [22].

Category	Goal (mmHg)
Uncomplicated hypertension	< 140/90
Hypertension in diabetes mellitus	< 130/80
Hypertension in renal disease	< 130/80
Preoperative blood pressure	< 180/110
Ideal	< 140/90
For CEA	< 140/90

Fenoldopam

Fenoldopam is a unique parenteral agent that causes vasodilation by acting on peripheral dopamine-1 receptors. It is given by continuous infusion and is rapidly cleared by the liver. It is effective in treating hypertensive emergencies and APH [59]. It can increase intraocular pressure, and is thus contraindicated in patients with glaucoma. Reflex tachycardia is common, especially at high doses, and should be used with caution in patients with myocardial ischemia. Neither rebound hypertension nor tachyphylaxis has been reported. Fenoldopam increases urine output and glomerular filtration rates, and thus it may improve renal function in severely hypertensive patients with or at risk of impaired renal function [60,61].

Nicardipine, clevidipine, and other CCBs

Nicardipine is a short-acting dihydropyridine CCB that has been effective in treating APH, and has few major side-effects [47,62–67]. It selectively vasodilates the cerebral and coronary vasculature more than the peripheral vasculature, and thus can reduce myocardial and cerebral ischemia. It can cause reflex tachycardia. It has been safely used in pregnant women.

Clevidipine is a new, lipophilic, short-acting dihydropyridine that is approved for the management of acute hypertension. It has been used effectively in patients with hypertensive crises and after cardiac surgery [68]. Clevidipine has a very rapid onset and offset, with a half-life of only 2 minutes. After discontinuation, there is a risk of rebound hypertension, especially if patients have not been transitioned to oral agents after prolonged intravenous use. Thus, patients should be monitored for at least 8 hours after it is discontinued.

The non-dihydropyridine CCBs, diltiazem and verapamil, both have parenteral forms. When used for blood pressure reduction, however, they have a risk of significant arrhythmias and heart block. Thus, they are usually reserved more for the treatment of supraventricular arrhythmias.

Short-acting nifedipine, another dihydropyridine CCB, has been recommended in the past, but sublingual and intranasal administration should not be used given the risk for severe, unpredictable falls in blood pressure which have been linked to serious adverse events, including cerebrovascular ischemia, myocardial ischemia and infarction, conduction disturbances, and death [69].

Nitroprusside

Sodium nitroprusside is a direct arterial and venous vasodilator. It has historically been the prototypical agent for APH and hypertensive crises due to its reliable, immediate onset and easy titration. It is given by continuous infusion and most recommend intra-arterial blood pressure monitoring due to its potency, rapidity of action, and risk of tachyphylaxis. Although very effective, nitroprusside can cause several important adverse effects that require close monitoring.

Nitroprusside can cause cyanide or thiocyanate toxicity, especially in patients with hepatic and renal failure, even at 'safe' infusion rates. Doses over $4\,\mu g/kg/min$ can lead rapidly to cyanide toxicity. Thiocyanate levels and cyanide levels must be monitored closely with prolonged use. Patients on nitroprusside can develop coronary steal and reflex tachycardia, which can be detrimental to patients with CAD. Patients can also develop rebound hypertension when the drug is discontinued. Nitroprusside decreases cerebral blood flow while increasing intracranial pressure, so is avoided in patients after intracranial surgeries. Due to these issues, nitroprusside is no longer the usual first choice, and alternative agents are usually chosen first, especially in patients with CAD, renal failure, or hepatic insufficiency.

Nitroglycerin

Nitroglycerin is a direct vasodilator, particularly of the venous system, though arterial vasodilation occurs at high doses. It is effective but less potent than nitroprusside. Patients can develop reflex tachycardia and tachyphylaxis. Patients on nitroglycerin have improved coronary blood flow and reduced cardiac preload, so it is a good choice in patients with myocardial ischemia and/or pulmonary edema.

Enalaprilat

Enalaprilat is the only available parenteral ACEI. It has been studied extensively in the perioperative period and has been effective [70,71]. It is given by intermittent bolus, so does not require ICU monitoring. Its onset of action can be delayed for up to 6 hours, especially after the first dose. Like other ACEI, it can cause acute renal failure and hyperkalemia. This is especially true in states of diminished renal perfusion, which are common in the perioperative period [70]. Given these issues, it may best be used as an adjunctive agent for APH or hypertensive emergencies. For patients with systolic CHF, it can be used to replace oral ACEI in the perioperative period. It can be converted easily to oral ACEI once a patient resumes oral medications.

Hydralazine

Hydralazine is a direct arteriolar vasodilator. It is commonly used for severe hypertension, but has not been well studied in perioperative hypertension. Hydralazine has a rapid onset of action and a duration of action of 3–8 hours, but its blood pressure lowering can be unpredictable [70]. In addition, it can lead to increased cardiac output, reflex tachycardia, and sympathetic activity and is thus a poor choice in patients with CAD. It should be avoided in patients with cardiac ischemia, elevated intracranial pressure, and aortic dissection. It is not a first-line choice in perioperative blood pressure management. Though previously a preferred agent in pregnancy, a meta-analysis has suggested worse maternal and fetal outcomes than labetalol or CCBs, although the quality of evidence was suboptimal [71]. Thus, labetalol and nicardipine are often recommended as the first-line parenteral agents in pregnancy.

Specific postoperative states

Intracranial surgery

Intraoperative and postoperative hypertension, but not preexisting hypertension, are significant risk factors for intracranial hemorrhage after craniotomy [72]. Thus, perioperative blood pressure control is important. After neurosurgery, patients have disturbed cerebral blood flow autoregulation, and hypertension can cause increases in cerebral blood flow, elevations in intracranial pressure, cerebral edema, and cerebral hemorrhage.

Some antihypertensive agents used to treat APH can cause cerebral vasodilation and subsequent increases in cerebral blood volume, which can cause a rise in intracranial pressure. Drugs that cause cerebral vasodilation (e.g., sodium nitroprusside, nitroglycerin, hydralazine, and calcium channel blockers) can theoretically cause this adverse effect. Esmolol and labetalol do not increase cerebral blood flow. Both have been used to control blood pressure after intracranial surgery, and labetalol has been shown to improve intracranial pressure and cerebral perfusion pressure when added to nitroprusside [50,51,57]. Enalaprilat and clevidipine have also been effective in a small number of patients [73,74]. Another small study that compared adding nicardipine or labetalol to enalaprilat showed that patients in the nicardipine arm had more hypotension, bradycardia, tachycardia, and treatment failures [47]. In general, aggressive management of blood pressure after craniotomy is recommended, and labetalol or esmolol have a theoretic advantage over other agents.

Carotid endarterectomy

Patients after carotid endarterectomy (CEA) have impaired baroreceptor function. This causes significant perioperative hemodynamic instability, including postoperative hypertension and hypotension. Acute postoperative hypertension can affect up to 66% of patients after CEA. Patients who develop APH are more likely to develop both transient and permanent neurologic complications, myocardial ischemia, and wound hematomas (which can potentially obstruct the airway). Patients with preoperative hypertension have a higher incidence of APH, and those with uncontrolled preoperative pressures tend to have more severe episodes. Severe postoperative hypertension is also a risk factor for the development of cerebral hyperperfusion syndrome. This syndrome occurs in about 1% of patients after CEA and characteristic findings are severe headache, neurological deficits, or seizures leading to intracerebral hemorrhage [75].

Given the potential for blood pressure lability, the treatment of APH after CEA requires rapid-acting intravenous agents, and nitroprusside, nicardipine, and labetalol have been shown to be effective in clinical trials [46,76]. Though often used, direct vasodilators (e.g., nitroprusside, nitroglycerin, nicardipine, hydralazine) carry theoretical disadvantages (similar to patients after craniotomy) of cerebral vasodilation in patients who already have increased cerebral blood flow and impaired cerebral autoregulation after the CEA. Thus, labetalol is the first-line agent.

Summary

Hypertension is extremely common in surgical patients. Preoperative assessment requires an assessment of the risks of hypertension itself and the risks of concomitant end-organ diseases. All patients need an explicit assessment of cardiac risk. In general, patients with mild to moderate hypertension can proceed to surgery, while patients with severe hypertension should have elective procedures delayed if possible to allow preoperative control of blood pressure. Postoperative hypertension is common, especially after intracranial surgery, CEA, and CABG. Acute postoperative hypertension can have significant complications and may require intravenous antihypertensive therapy for control and prevention of severe complications. After surgery, close follow-up and control of blood pressure is essential to prevent long-term complications.

References

1. Roger VL, Go AS, Lloyd-Jose DM et al. Heart disease and stroke statistics – 2011 update: a report from the American Heart Association. Circulation 2011; **123**: e18–209.

2. Wolfsthal SD. Is blood pressure control necessary before surgery? Med Clin North Am 1993; **77**: 349–63.

3. Prys-Roberts C, Greene LT, Meloche R et al. Studies of anaesthesia in relation to hypertension. II. Haemodynamic consequences of induction and endotracheal intubation. Br J Anaesth 1971; **43**: 531–47.

4. Prys-Roberts C, Meloche R, Foex P. Studies of anaesthesia in relation to hypertension. I. Cardiovascular responses of treated and untreated patients. Br J Anaesth 1971; **43**: 122–37.

5. Charlson ME, MacKenzie CR, Gold JP et al. The preoperative and intraoperative hemodynamic predictors of postoperative myocardial infarction or ischemia in patients undergoing noncardiac surgery. Ann Surg 1989; **210**: 637–48.

6. Slogoff S, Keats AS. Does perioperative myocardial ischemia lead to postoperative myocardial infarction? Anesthesiology 1985; **62**: 107–14.

7. Raby KE, Barry J, Creager MA et al. Detection and significance of intraoperative and postoperative myocardial ischemia in peripheral vascular surgery. J Am Med Assoc 1992; **268**: 222–7.

8. Hollenberg M, Mangano DT, Browner WS et al. Predictors of postoperative myocardial ischemia in patients undergoing noncardiac surgery. The Study of Perioperative Ischemia Research Group. J Am Med Assoc 1992; **268**: 205–9.

9. Mangano DT, Browner WS, Hollenberg M et al. Association of perioperative myocardial ischemia with cardiac morbidity and mortality in men undergoing noncardiac surgery. The Study of Perioperative Ischemia Research Group. N Engl J Med 1990; **323**: 1781–8.

10. Goldman L, Caldera DL. Risks of general anesthesia and elective operation in the hypertensive patient. Anesthesiology 1979; **50**: 285–92.

11. Goldman L, Caldera DL, Nussbaum SR et al. Multifactorial index of cardiac risk in noncardiac surgical procedures. N Engl J Med 1977; **297**: 845–50.

12. Detsky AS, Abrams HB, McLaughlin JR et al. Predicting cardiac complications in patients undergoing non-cardiac surgery. J Gen Intern Med 1986; **1**: 211–19.

13. Lee TH, Marcantonio ER, Mangione CM et al. Derivation and prospective validation of a simple index for prediction of cardiac risk of major noncardiac surgery. Circulation 1999; **100**: 1043–9.

14. Browner WS, Li J, Mangano DT. In-hospital and long-term mortality in male veterans following noncardiac surgery. The Study of Perioperative Ischemia Research Group. J Am Med Assoc 1992; **268**: 228–32.

15. Goldman L, Caldera DL, Southwick FS et al. Cardiac risk factors and complications in non-cardiac surgery. Medicine (Baltimore) 1978; **57**: 357–70.

16. Charlson ME, MacKenzie CR, Gold JP et al. Risk for postoperative congestive heart failure. Surg Gynecol Obstet 1991; **172**: 95–104.

17. Landesberg G, Einav S, Christopherson R et al. Perioperative ischemia and cardiac complications in major vascular surgery: importance of the preoperative twelve-lead electrocardiogram. J Vasc Surg 1997; **26**: 570–8.

18. Porhomayon J, El-Solh A, Chhangani S et al. The management of surgical patients with obstructive sleep apnea. Lung 2011; **189**(5): 359–67.

19. Edwards R. Thyroid and parathyroid disease. Int Anesth Clin 1997; **35**: 62.

20. Sellevold OF, Raeder J, Stenseth R. Undiagnosed phaeochromocytoma in the perioperative period. Case reports. Acta Anaesthesiol Scand 1985; **29**: 474–9.

21. Chen H, Sippel RS, O'Dorisio et al. The North American Neuroendocrine Tumor Society consensus guideline for the diagnosis and management of neuroendocrine tumors. Pancreas 2010; **39**: 775–83.

22. The Seventh Report of the Joint National Committee on prevention, detection, evaluation, and treatment of high blood pressure. J Am Med Assoc 2003; **289**: 2560–72.

23. Casadei B, Abuzeid H. Is there a strong rationale for deferring elective surgery in patients with poorly controlled hypertension. J Hypertens 2005; **23**: 19–22.

24. Weksler N, Klein M, Szendro G et al. The dilemma of immediate preoperative hypertension: to treat and operate, or to postpone surgery? *J Clinc Anesth* 2003; **15**: 179–83.

25. Psaty BM, Smith NL, Siscovick DS et al. Health outcomes associated with antihypertensive therapies used as first-line agents. A systematic review and meta-analysis. *J Am Med Assoc* 1997; **277**: 739–45.

26. Yusuf S, Sleight P, Pogue J et al. Effects of an angiotensin-converting enzyme inhibitor, ramipril, on cardiovascular events in high-risk patients. *N Engl J Med* 2000; **342**: 145–53.

27. Houston MC. Abrupt cessation of treatment in hypertension: consideration of clinical features, mechanisms, prevention and management of the discontinuation syndrome. *Am Heart J* 1981; **102**: 415–30.

28. Hart GR, Anderson RJ. Withdrawal syndromes and the cessation of antihypertensive therapy. *Arch Intern Med* 1981; **141**: 1125–7.

29. Shammash JB, Trost JC, Gold JM et al. Perioperative beta-blocker withdrawal and mortality in vascular surgical patients. *Am Heart J* 2001; **141**: 148–53.

30. Prys-Roberts C. Interactions of anaesthesia and high preoperative doses of beta-receptor antagonists. *Acta Anaesthesiol Scand Suppl* 1982; **76**: 47–53.

31. Prys-Roberts C, Foex P, Biro GP et al. Studies of anaesthesia in relation to hypertension. V. Adrenergic beta-receptor blockade. *Br J Anaesth* 1973; **45**: 671–81.

32. Pasternack PF, Grossi EA, Baumann FG et al. Beta blockade to decrease silent myocardial ischemia during peripheral vascular surgery. *Am J Surg* 1989; **158**: 113–16.

33. Wallace AW. Clonidine and modification of perioperative outcome. *Curr Opin Anaesthesiol* 2006; **19**: 411–17.

34. Wallace AW, Galindez D, Salahieh A et al. Effect of clonidine on cardiovascular morbidity and mortality after noncardiac surgery. *Anesthesiology* 2004; **101**: 284–93.

35. Bernstein JS. Transdermal clonidine therapy for the perioperative period. *Anesthesiology* 1986; **65**: 451.

36. Johnston RV, Nicholas DA, Lawson NW et al. The use of rectal clonidine in the perioperative period. *Anesthesiology* 1986; **64**: 288–90.

37. Coriat P, Richer C, Douraki T et al. Influence of chronic angiotensin-converting enzyme inhibition on anesthetic induction. *Anesthesiology* 1994; **81**: 299–307.

38. Comfere T, Sprung J, Kumar MM et al. Angiotensin system inhibitors in a general surgical population. *Anesth Analg* 2005; **100**: 636–44.

39. Bertrand M, Godet G, Meersschaert K et al. Should the angiotensin II antagonists be discontinued before surgery? *Anesth Analg* 2001; **92**: 26–30.

40. Kehterpal S, Khodaparast O, Shanks A et al. Chronic angiotensin-converting enzyme inhibitor or angiotensin receptor blocker therapy combined with diuretic therapy is associated with increased episodes of hypotension in noncardiac surgery. *J Cardiothorac Vasc Anesth* 2008; **22**: 180–6.

41. Pigott DW, Nagle C, Allman K et al. Effect of omitting regular ACE inhibitor medication before cardiac surgery on haemodynamic variables and vasoactive drug requirements. *Br J Anaesth* 1999; **83**: 715–20.

42. Chauvin M, Deriaz H, Viars, P. Continuous i.v. infusion of labetalol for postoperative hypertension. Haemodynamic effects and plasma kinetics. *Br J Anaesth* 1987; **59**: 1250–6.

43. Cosentino F, Vidt DG, Orlowski JP et al. The safety of cumulative doses of labetalol in perioperative hypertension. *Cleve Clin J Med* 1989; **56**: 371–6.

44. Cruise CJ, Skrobik Y, Webster RE et al. Intravenous labetalol versus sodium nitroprusside for treatment of hypertension postcoronary bypass surgery. *Anesthesiology* 1989; **71**: 835–9.

45. Dimich I, Lingham R, Gabrielson G et al. Comparative hemodynamic effects of labetalol and hydralazine in the treatment of postoperative hypertension. *J Clin Anesth* 1989; **1**: 201–6.

46. Geniton DJ. A comparison of the hemodynamic effects of labetalol and sodium nitroprusside in patients undergoing carotid endarterectomy. *AANA J* 1990; **58**: 281–7.

47. Kross RA, Ferri E, Leung D et al. A comparative study between a calcium channel blocker (Nicardipine) and a combined alpha-beta-blocker (Labetalol) for the control of emergence hypertension during craniotomy for tumor surgery. *Anesth Analg* 2000; **91**: 904–9.

48. Leslie JB, Kalayjian RW, Sirgo MA et al. Intravenous labetalol for treatment of postoperative hypertension. *Anesthesiology* 1987; **67**: 413–16.

49. Malsch E, Katonah J, Gratz I et al. The effectiveness of labetalol in treating post-operative hypertension. *Nurse Anesth* 1991; **2**: 65–71.

50. Muzzi DA Black S, Losasso TJ et al. Labetalol and esmolol in the control of hypertension after intracranial surgery. *Anesth Analg* 1990; **70**: 68–71.

51. Orlowski JP, Shiesley D, Vidt DG et al. Labetalol to control blood pressure after cerebrovascular surgery. *Crit Care Med* 1988; **16**: 765–8.

52. Orlowski, JP, Vidt DG, Walker S et al. The hemodynamic effects of intravenous labetalol for postoperative hypertension. *Cleve Clin J Med* 1989; **56**: 29–34.

53. Prys-Roberts C, Dagnino J. Continuous i.v. infusion of labetalol for postoperative hypertension. *Br J Anaesth* 1988; **60**: 600.

54. Singh PP, Dimich I, Sampson I et al. A comparison of esmolol and labetalol for the treatment of perioperative hypertension in geriatric ambulatory surgical patients. *Can J Anaesth* 1992; **39**: 559–62.

55. McCauley J, Murray J, Jordan M et al. Labetalol-induced hyperkalemia in renal transplant recipients. *Am J Nephrol* 2002; **22**: 347–51.

56. Hamad A, Salameh M, Zihlif M et al. Life-threatening hyperkalemia after intravenous labetalol injection for hypertensive emergency in a hemodialysis patient. *Am J Nephrol* 2001; **21**: 241–4.

57. Gibson BE, Black S, Maass L et al. Esmolol for the control of hypertension after neurologic surgery. *Clin Pharmacol Ther* 1988; **44**: 650–3.

58. Gray RJ, Bateman TM, Czer LS et al. Comparison of esmolol and nitroprusside for acute post-cardiac surgical hypertension. *Am J Cardiol* 1987; **59**: 887–91.

59. Murphy MB, Murray C, Shorten GD. Fenoldopam: a selective peripheral dopamine-receptor agonist for the treatment of severe hypertension. *N Engl J Med* 2001; **345**: 1548–57.

60. Shusterman NH, Elliott WJ, White WB. Fenoldopam, but not nitroprusside, improves renal function in severely hypertensive patients with impaired renal function. *Am J Med* 1993; **95**: 161–8.

61. Elliott WJ, Weber RR, Nelson KS *et al.* Renal and hemodynamic effects of intravenous fenoldopam versus nitroprusside in severe hypertension. *Circulation* 1990; **81**: 970–7.

62. Goldberg ME, Clark S, Joseph J *et al.* Nicardipine versus placebo for the treatment of postoperative hypertension. *Am Heart J* 1990; **119**: 446–50.

63. IV Nicardipine Study Group. Efficacy and safety of intravenous nicardipine in the control of postoperative hypertension. *Chest* 1991; **99**: 393–8.

64. Halpern NA, Alicea M, Krakoff LR *et al.* Postoperative hypertension: a prospective, placebo-controlled, randomized, double-blind trial, with intravenous nicardipine hydrochloride. *Angiology* 1990; **41**: 992–1004.

65. Halpern NA, Sladen RN, Goldberg JS *et al.* Nicardipine infusion for postoperative hypertension after surgery of the head and neck. *Crit Care Med* 1990; **18**: 950–5.

66. van Wezel, HB, Koolen JJ, Visser CA *et al.* Antihypertensive and anti-ischemic effects of nicardipine and nitroprusside in patients undergoing coronary artery bypass grafting. *Am J Cardiol* 1989; **64**: 22H–27H.

67. Vincent JL, Berlot G, Preiser JC *et al.* Intravenous nicardipine in the treatment of postoperative arterial hypertension. *J Cardiothorac Vasc Anesth* 1997; **11**: 160–4.

68. Nguyen HM, Ma K, Pham DQ. Clevidipine for the treatment of severe hypertension in adults. *Clin Ther* 2010; **32**: 11–23.

69. Grossman E, Messerli FH, Grodzicki T *et al.* Should a moratorium be placed on sublingual nifedipine capsules given for hypertensive emergencies and pseudo-emergencies? *J Am Med Assoc* 1996; **276**: 1328–31.

70. Varon J, Marik PE. Perioperative hypertension management. *Vasc Health Risk Manage* 2008; **4**: 615–27.

71. Magee LA, Cham C, Waterman EJ *et al.* Hydralazine for treatment of severe hypertension in pregnancy: meta-analysis. *Br Med J* 2003; **327**: 955–65.

72. Basali A, Mascha EJ, Kalfas I *et al.* Relation between perioperative hypertension and intracranial hemorrhage after craniotomy. *Anesthesiology* 2000; **93**: 48–54.

73. Tohmo H, Karanko M. Enalaprilat controls postoperative hypertension while maintaining cardiac function and systemic oxygenation after neurosurgery. *Intens Care Med* 1995; **21**: 651–6.

74. Bekker A, Didehvar S, Kim, S *et al.* Efficacy of clevidipine in controlling postoperative hypertension in neurosurgical patients: initial single-center experience. *J Neurosurg Anesth* 2010; **22**: 330–5.

75. Stonham MD, Thompson JP. Arterial pressure management and carotid endarterectomy. *Br J Anaesth* 2009; **102**: 442–52.

76. Dorman T, Thompson DA, Breslow MJ *et al.* Nicardipine versus nitroprusside for breakthrough hypertension following carotid endarterectomy. *J Clin Anesth* 2001; **13**: 281–7.

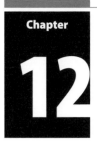

Chapter

12

Perioperative pulmonary risk evaluation and management for non-cardiothoracic surgery

Alvaro Velasquez, Michelle V. Conde, and Valerie A. Lawrence

Introduction

Postoperative pulmonary complications (PPCs) are as common as cardiac complications following non-cardiothoracic surgery and carry significant morbidity and mortality [1]. The incidence of PPCs was higher than cardiac complications (2.7% vs 2.5%) in the cohort of non-cardiac surgical patients used to validate the Revised Cardiac Risk Index [2]. An earlier study of patients undergoing abdominal surgery revealed not only similar results but also longer hospital stays [3]. More recently, Lawrence *et al.* in a large retrospective cohort study of patients undergoing hip repair showed that serious pulmonary and cardiac complications have similar incidence and significant impact on mortality and length of stay [4].

Postoperative pulmonary complications are a marker of poor prognosis. In patients with or without respiratory failure following vascular and general surgical procedures, mortality at 30 days in the respiratory failure group was 26.5% compared with 1.4% in those without it [5]. Similarly, a prospective study of patients age ≥ 70 years examined predictors of mortality up to 3 years following non-cardiac surgery. Postoperative pulmonary complications were independent predictors of decreased long-term survival [6]. These findings confirm the clinical importance of PPCs.

The true incidence of PPCs depends on the criteria used to define them, the population being evaluated, and the type of surgery. The incidence ranges from as low as 5% to as high as 80% for upper abdominal procedures [7,8]. The criteria used to define complications have a significant impact on these estimates. Some authors do not report any criteria for complications and others include clinically unimportant events like microatelectasis [9].

Atelectasis occurs in essentially all patients who undergo general anesthesia. During abdominal surgery, changes of microatelectasis develop routinely and usually do not delay recovery or discharge from the hospital [10]. In high-risk patients, microatelectasis may progress to pneumonia, although atelectasis is not a prerequisite for pneumonia. Microatelectasis may also progress to diffuse, clinically detectable atelectasis that can involve an entire lobe or lung. Pleural effusions are also common after abdominal surgery and develop in about 60–70% of the patients. The majority resolve spontaneously [11,12]. Other pulmonary complications include retained tracheobronchial secretions, bronchospasm, bronchitis, pneumonia, hypercapnia, and respiratory failure.

Respiratory physiology during and after surgery

Over the last 50 years understanding of the physiologic changes during and after general anesthesia has increased. Relevant changes are: (1) monotonous and shallow breathing during moderate anesthesia levels; (2) atelectasis; (3) ventilation/perfusion (V/Q) ratio abnormalities (increased shunt up to 8–10%); (4) reduction of vital capacity (50–60%); (5) attenuation of hypoxic pulmonary vasoconstriction with inhalational anesthetics; and (5) decreased resting lung volume or functional residual capacity (FRC) by 15–30%, which usually occurs during the first few minutes of anesthesia. This reduction in FRC appears to have additional effects on lung compliance and airway resistance and may persist after anesthesia. Some factors implicated in this FRC change are: (1) body positioning (from upright to supine) causing a 4 cm cephalad displacement of the diaphragm; (2) induction of general anesthesia with the associated change in thoracic cage muscle tone; (3) use of paralytic agents; and (4) excessive fluid administration and special surgical positions (i.e., Trendelenburg) [13]. Reduction of FRC also depends on the site of operation. This reduction is most significant and prolonged after upper abdominal surgery.

Atelectasis develops in about 90% of patients under anesthesia and may involve about 15–20% of the lung tissue [14]. Atelectasis can be present during spontaneous or controlled breathing (after muscle paralysis), regardless of the anesthetic used (intravenous or inhaled). The effect of body weight on the extent of atelectasis is supported by the observation that obese patients have more significant atelectasis. Age has no significant impact. Atelectatic areas are associated with the presence of significant shunt and alterations on gas exchange.

Medical Management of the Surgical Patient, ed. Michael F. Lubin, Thomas F. Dodson, and Neil H. Winawer. Published by Cambridge University Press. © Cambridge University Press 2013.

Gas resorption has been implicated in the development of atelectasis during anesthesia by two mechanisms. First, gas uptake in blood continues after airway closure while additional air inflow is prevented. These areas of trapped gas will collapse. The delivery of high concentrations of oxygen (a readily absorbable gas) to those areas during induction and maintenance of anesthesia may accelerate and aggravate this phenomenon. Second, the low V/Q ratios also facilitate movement of gas with high oxygen concentration from alveolar space to blood with the lung unit becoming progressively smaller [15].

Diaphragmatic dysfunction may contribute to further decreases in vital capacity and FRC when incision sites are near the diaphragm. Although not clearly understood, reflex inhibition of diaphragm function during manipulation of viscera close to the diaphragm may result in mechanical failure of the diaphragm [16]. Postoperative pain, splinting, and depression of mucociliary transport also contribute to the development of atelectasis.

Earlier closure of the airways with the increased closing volume (CV) and the reduction in FRC translates into significant reduction of ventilation in dependent lung regions. This leads to hypoxemia and other complications [15,17]. Closing capacity (CC) is the volume at which the dependent airways begin to close. In healthy young subjects, this occurs below functional residual capacity (FRC), which is the volume of air remaining in the lungs after a normal tidal exhalation. In certain circumstances, however, the CV occurs prematurely, FRC is decreased, or both. Because of the increased closing capacity to FRC ratio, airway closure may occur before completion of a normal tidal volume breath, resulting in V/Q mismatch and potential shunting. Non-pulmonary factors contributing to an increased CC/FRC ratio include the supine position, sedative or narcotic drugs, obesity, increased abdominal girth (e.g., ileus), thoracic and abdominal binders, incisional pain, muscle weakness, poor nutrition, immobility, and high and prolonged oxygen concentration. Pulmonary factors contributing to an altered CC/FRC ratio include interstitial edema, loss of surfactant, airway obstruction due to inflammation, bronchoconstriction, and retained secretions. The V/Q mismatch may lead to hypoxemia.

Overview of the preoperative assessment

The most effective preoperative pulmonary evaluation assesses operative risk as a function of the patient's clinical profile and the procedure-related risk. In 2006 the American College of Physicians (ACP) released a guideline on both the risk assessment for PPCs and strategies to reduce PPCs for patients undergoing non-cardiothoracic surgery [18]. These recommendations were based on the first two systematic reviews of the literature during the previous 25 years [1,19]. Odds ratios for different risk factors and interventions were estimated and a letter was assigned to each factor and intervention based on the strength of evidence. Table 12.1 shows the odds ratios and strength of evidence for selected risk factors and Table 12.6 shows the strength of evidence for risk reduction strategies [1].

Table 12.1 Selected risk factors for postoperative pulmonary complications [1].

Factor[a]	Strength of recommendation[b]	Odds ratio[c]
Patient-related risk factor		
Advanced age	A	2.09–3.04
ASA class ≥ II	A	2.55–4.87
CHF	A	2.93
Functional dependence	A	1.65–2.51
COPD	A	1.79
Cigarette use	B	1.26
Alcohol use	B	1.21
Impaired sensorium	B	1.39
Weight loss	B	1.62
Diabetes	C	–
Asthma	D	–
Obesity	D	–
OSA[d]	I	–
Pulmonary hypertension[e]	I	–
Corticosteroid use	I	–
Procedure-related risk factor		
Aortic aneurysm repair	A	6.90
Thoracic surgery	A	4.24
Abdominal surgery	A	3.01
Neurosurgery	A	2.91
Prolonged surgery	A	2.53
Head and neck surgery	A	2.26
Emergency surgery	A	2.21
Vascular surgery	A	2.10
General anesthesia	A	1.83
Hip surgery	D	–
Gynecologic or urologic surgery	D	–

[a] ASA, American Society of Anesthesiologists; CHF, congestive heart failure; COPD, chronic obstructive pulmonary disease; OSA, obstructive sleep apnea.
[b] Recommendation: A, good evidence to support the risk factor; B, at least fair evidence to support the risk factor; C, at least fair evidence to suggest that the factor is not associated with increased risk; D, good evidence to suggest that the factor does not predict risk; I, insufficient evidence to determine whether the particular factor predicts risk; this could be related to lack, poor quality, or conflicting evidence.
[c] Odds ratios are trim-and-fill estimates when available, otherwise pooled estimate.
[d,e] Recent studies indicate that these are probable risk factors.

If the history and physical examination suggest significant pulmonary or cardiac disease, further diagnostic tests may be indicated. Once the risk factors have been identified, the management plan can focus on minimizing risks and preventing complications. Some risk factors are not modifiable prior to surgery while others may provide targets for risk reduction.

Patient-related risk factors
Age

One of the most important patient-related risk factors for PPCs is increasing age. Prior to the 2006 ACP guideline, the influence of age was not well established [1]. In fact, it was considered a minor risk factor. The accumulation of comorbid conditions with age increased the unadjusted risk of complications but the 2006 ACP review concluded that age ≥ 60 years is an important independent predictor of PPCs, even for healthy patients. The odds ratio for PPCs was 2.09 (95% CI, 1.65–2.64) for ages 60–69 and 3.04 (95% CI, 2.11–4.39) for ages 70–79. In a more recent study utilizing the National Surgical Quality Improvement Program (NSQIP) database, the rates of PPCs for patients aged 50–59, 60–69, 70–79, 80–89 and 90–99 years were 6.1%, 8.1%, 11.9%, 14.1%, and 16.7%, respectively [20].

General health status/American Society of Anesthesiologists Class

The American Society of Anesthesiologists (ASA) physical status classification was first published in 1941 and revised in 1963. It provides a general index of overall morbidity and classifies patients preoperatively in one of the following five classes: Class I, a normal healthy patient; Class II, a patient with mild systemic disease; Class III, a patient with systemic disease that is not incapacitating; Class IV, a patient with severe systemic disease that is a constant threat to life; and Class V, a moribund patient who is not expected to survive for 24 hours with or without the operation [21,22]. Class II or higher are associated with increased pulmonary risk [21]. An ASA class III will increase by 2.8 times the risk of respiratory failure while a class IV or V will increase risk by 4.9 times [5]. Another independent predictor that evaluates the patient health status and the presence of medical disorders is the Charlson comorbidity index, which is obtained by evaluating the presence and significance of 19 different medical entities. Summary scores range from 0 to 37. This index was shown to be a good independent risk factor in 2,291 patients undergoing elective abdominal surgery [23]. Each additional point conferred an adjusted odds ratio of 1.6 in the multivariable analysis.

Functional dependence

Total functional dependence is defined as the inability to perform any activities of daily living while partial dependence is the need for equipment or devices and assistance from another person to complete some activities of daily living. The pooled estimates of odds ratios for total and partial dependence were 2.51 (95% CI, 1.99–3.15) and 1.65 (95% CI, 1.36–2.01), respectively in the systematic review [1]. In a separate study of patients undergoing high-risk surgery, patients who were unable to climb two flights of stairs, regardless of etiology, had increased cardiopulmonary complications [24].

Obesity

Obesity is associated with restrictive pulmonary physiology. Combined with anesthesia, obesity may cause further reduction in lung volumes and decrease the ability to take a deep breath postoperatively. Significant V/Q mismatch may ensue [25]. Obesity has been reported as a risk factor for PPCs [26,27]. Several studies that reported obesity as a risk factor, however, did not control for other comorbid conditions [20].

Additionally, the definitions used for PPCs in these studies were broad and included atelectasis [26,27]. Both studies failed to define clinically significant atelectasis and atelectasis comprised the majority of the PPCs. The high prevalence of atelectasis and potentially clinically unimportant atelectasis may have overestimated the strength of obesity as a risk factor. Additional studies have shown no increased PPC risk in obese patients compared with non-obese patients undergoing abdominal surgery [28,29]. In a large cohort of patients undergoing elective non-cardiac surgery, there was no increase in PPCs among patients with BMI ≥ 30 kg/m^2 versus patients with BMI 20 kg/m^2 to 29 kg/m^2 after adjusting for several factors, including smoking history and comorbidities [30]. The absence of a significant increase in PPCs extends to those with severe obesity. A study of 197 morbidly obese patients undergoing gastric bypass surgery found no statistically significant difference in the incidence of PPCs between patients with BMI of ≤ 43 kg/m^2 and those with BMI > 43 kg/m^2 (10% vs 12.3% respectively) [31]. Current evidence suggests that obesity is not an independent risk factor for significant PPCs.

Tobacco use

Cigarette smoking is a well-established risk factor for PPCs [1,4,20,32]. Smoking is associated with an increase in tracheobronchial secretions and depressed mucociliary clearance [33]. In a study of 60 patients undergoing orthopedic surgery under general anesthesia, the phagocytic and microbicidal activities were decreased almost twice as much in smoking (n = 30) as non-smoking (n = 30) patients [34]. In patients undergoing abdominal surgery, smoking is associated with an increased relative risk for PPCs of 1.4–4.3 [20]. The ACP review reported an adjusted odds ratio of 1.26 (95% CI, 1.01–1.56) for cigarette use [1]. Smoking history ≥ 20–40 pack years, even in the absence of chronic bronchitis or airflow limitation, is associated with a higher incidence of PPCs compared with non-smokers [35,36]. The effect of smoking cessation on the development of PPCs was evaluated in a multivariable study of 410 patients undergoing general, orthopedic, urologic as well as cardiovascular surgery [37]. The adjusted odds ratio was 4.2 (95% CI, 1.2–14.8) for development of PPCs in current smokers vs never smokers. Those patients who decreased or discontinued smoking shortly before surgery had an actual increase in the adjusted odds ratio of developing PPCs compared with those who continued usual smoking habits. The adjusted odds ratio was 6.7 (95% CI, 2.6–17.1) [37]. Although selection bias could explain this finding, the transient increase in cough and sputum production may play a significant role. A subsequent study showed that patients with smoking cessation < 2 months before minor surgery had increased intraoperative sputum volume [38].

Impaired sensorium

Three large trials have evaluated the impact of an acutely confused or delirious patient on the development of postoperative pneumonia and respiratory failure after non-cardiac surgery. Two of the trials were included in the 2006 ACP guidelines [1]. The pooled odds ratio estimate for impaired sensorium was 1.39 (95% CI, 1.08–1.79). A subsequent study found that an altered sensorium was an independent predictor of respiratory failure. The odds ratio was 1.49 (95% CI, 1.22–1.83) [5]. This study collected data during a 3-year period from 128 VA hospitals and 14 private-sector academic institutions. Their results provide a more broadly applicable model given the inclusion of female and private sector patients [39].

Preexisting cardiopulmonary disease or symptoms

Clinicians should seek information regarding pulmonary symptoms and previous lung disease, including obstructive lung disease, respiratory infections, occupational lung disease, obstructive sleep apnea (OSA), pulmonary hypertension, and heart failure. Prior chest trauma, thoracic surgery, respiratory difficulty following surgery, and use of cardiopulmonary medications should also be documented. The impact of interstitial lung disease, chest wall abnormalities, and neuromuscular disease in the development of PPCs has not been studied.

Chronic obstructive pulmonary disease (COPD)

Patients with evidence of COPD are unequivocally at increased risk of PPCs. The rate of PPCs in the 2006 ACP review was 18.2% for COPD patients and the estimated odds ratio was 1.79 (95% CI, 1.44–2.22) [1]. Increasing severity of COPD appears to confer a greater risk. A retrospective study evaluated the impact of COPD in patients undergoing thoracic and major abdominal surgery [40]. The rate of serious complications was 23% for those with severe COPD compared with 10% for those with mild to moderate disease and 4% for those with normal spirometry (p = 0.003). A larger and more recent study did not find the severity of COPD by spirometry to be a predictor of PPCs [23].

Preoperative pulmonary symptoms/lung exam findings

Findings during the exam of the chest (e.g., wheezing, rhonchi, rales) are predictors of postoperative pulmonary complications. In a nested case-control study of 2,291 patients undergoing elective abdominal surgery, the presence of abnormal pulmonary findings was the strongest predictor of PPCs (odds ratio, 5.8; 95% CI, 1.04–32.1) [23]. The true magnitude of this effect remains uncertain given the small number of studies. A positive cough test (which is defined by the presence of recurring coughing after a deep breath) was shown to be a risk factor for PPCs (odds ratio 3.8, p = 0.01) [41]. Preoperative sputum production is another risk factor for PPCs [42–44].

Asthma

Given the potential for bronchospasm induced by intravenous agents, it is important to document a history of asthma [45]. Well-controlled bronchial asthma is not a risk factor for

PPCs. Warner *et al.* evaluated PPCs in 706 patients with asthma who underwent surgery at Mayo Clinic [46]. The rate of PPCs was 2%. Most of the complications were minor and did not cause significant morbidity. Increased asthma medication use or visit to the emergency room within 30 days of surgery was associated with a higher rate of complications. The ACP review reported a 3% rate of pulmonary complications in asthma patients, which is comparable to the 3.4% crude adjusted complication rate for all the studies in that review [1].

Obstructive sleep apnea

Obstructive sleep apnea (OSA) is a common disorder with a prevalence that increases with age, in particular after age 65 [47]. The ACP review suggested that the rates of complications were higher for patients with OSA [1]. This conclusion was based on a retrospective case-control study of 101 patients with OSA undergoing joint replacement. Although the study did not measure the rates of pneumonia and respiratory failure after surgery, the overall rate of complications was higher for patients with OSA than among controls (39% vs 18%; p = 0.001) [48]. In 2008 Hwang *et al* reported the results of a retrospective chart review of 172 patients who were scheduled for elective surgery, had features suggestive of OSA, and had completed nocturnal oximetry [49]. They were divided into two groups based on the episodes of oxygen desaturation of 4% or more per hour. Those who had ≥ 5 episodes per hour had a higher rate of PPCs than those with < 5 (15.3% vs 2.7%; p < 0.01). Their adjusted odds ratio was 7.2 (95% CI, 1.5–33.3; p = 0.012) [49].

Two additional studies are now available. Records from the National Inpatient Sample Data between 1998 and 2007 were evaluated for patients who underwent non-cardiac surgery and had a discharge diagnosis of OSA [50]. They were matched to a control group using the propensity scoring method. The frequency of PPCs after orthopedic and general surgery procedures was higher in those with OSA. The need for intubation and mechanical ventilation in OSA patients compared with controls was 10.8% vs 5.94 (odds ratio 1.95; 95% CI, 1.91–1.98) after general surgical procedures. This study is clearly limited by factors inherent to secondary analysis of large administrative databases. Also, no details are provided about OSA severity and the therapy provided after surgery. The relationship between the severity of OSA and the development of PPCs during the first 30 days was evaluated in a group of patients who underwent either open or laparoscopic bariatric surgery at Mayo Clinic [51]. These patients had extensive preoperative evaluation, including polysomnography (PSG). Most patients with OSA (93%) received perioperative positive airway pressure therapy and were closely monitored. The rate of PPCs was higher (p < 0.001) with open procedures, increased BMI and age, but not associated with OSA severity (p = 0.701). These results, however, do not apply to unrecognized and untreated OSA and cannot be extrapolated to non-obese or less intensely monitored populations.

The American Society of Anesthesiologists provided guidelines in 2006 for the management of OSA [52]. The perioperative use of non-invasive positive pressure ventilation, non-supine positioning during extubation, and closer monitoring of patients with established OSA were recommended. The best preoperative evaluation of patients suspecting of having OSA remains to be established.

Pulmonary hypertension

Pulmonary hypertension (PH) has been identified as a risk factor for PPCs. Two studies that evaluated its impact have become recently available. A retrospective cohort study of 145 patients with moderate to severe pulmonary hypertension estimated by echocardiography found a 28% incidence of respiratory failure within 30 days after non-cardiac surgery. A New York Heart Association class $\geq$ II was an independent predictor of short-term morbidity (odds ratio 2.9; 95% CI, 1.2–7.7; p = 0.02) [53]. A more recent prospective case-control study of 124 patients identified the presence of severe pulmonary hypertension (PASP > 70 mmHg) as an important predictor of prolonged endotracheal intubation (21% vs 3%; p = 0.004) [54]. In the same study, the pulmonary artery systolic pressure was an independent predictor of mortality.

These studies highlight the importance of pulmonary hypertension as a risk factor for PPCs. Further studies are needed to clarify the role of preoperative screening for PH.

Congestive heart failure

This condition was identified as a patient-related risk factor by the 2006 ACP guideline and in the updated Respiratory Failure Risk Index [1,5]. In a study of 1,316 patients undergoing laparoscopic colorectal surgery, CHF was found to be a significant risk factor for the development of postoperative medical complications (17.4% vs 7.4%; p < 0.001), with pneumonia as the most common complication [55]. In the 2006 ACP review, the estimated risk associated with CHF was 2.93 (95% CI, 1.02–8.43) [1].

The magnitude of risk due to CHF appears more pronounced in elderly patients. In a study of patients 70 years and older, the relative risk of PPCs after surgery in those with heart failure was 5.7 (95% CI, 2.1–15.5; p = 0.001) [56]. Therefore, CHF should be considered an important risk factor.

Patient-related factors not associated with increased risk of postoperative pulmonary complications

The 2006 ACP review found that diabetes mellitus, HIV infection, and positive oropharyngeal cultures are not significant risk factors for the development of PPCs [1].

Procedure-related risk factors

Surgical site

The surgical site remains the most powerful predictor of PPCs. The closer the surgical incision is to the diaphragm, the higher the risk for PPCs [1,5,20,32,39]. The 2006 ACP review found that open aortic surgery had the highest risk (odds ratio, 6.90; 95% CI, 2.74–17.36) while risk of thoracic (odds ratio, 4.24; 95% CI, 2.89–6.23) and upper abdominal surgery (odds ratio, 2.91; 95% CI, 2.35–3.60) were also high [1]. A cohort study of 355 patients undergoing abdominal aortic aneurysm repair found that the rate of PPCs following endovascular repair (EVAR) vs open surgery was clearly lower (3.2% vs 16.1%; p = 0.001) [57]. Laparoscopic surgery is associated with less pain than open surgery; however, it is not definitive if this translates into fewer clinically important PPCs. Using data from the 2005 Nationwide Inpatient Sample (NIS), a cross-sectional study compared the outcomes of 19,156 patients having open vs laparoscopic bariatric surgery [58]. The rate of PPCs after adjusting for other comorbidities was about two times greater in those undergoing open surgery vs laparoscopic procedure (odds ratio, 1.92; 95% CI, 1.54–2.38; p < 0.001). Cardiovascular events and sepsis were also lower in the laparoscopy group. In contrast, a retrospective cohort study using NSQIP data compared laparoscopic (72%) vs open appendectomy (28%) [59]. Using a propensity-matched cohort, the incidence of major complications, unplanned intubation and pneumonia, was no different between the two groups [59].

The 2006 ACP guidelines, reported that head and neck surgery carried an intermediate risk while hip surgery, gynecologic, and urologic procedures carried a low risk for PPCs. Johnson et al. found that orofacial surgery was an important predictor of respiratory failure (odds ratio, 6.63; 95% CI, 4.78–9.20) [5].

Duration and route of anesthesia

Surgery $\geq$ 2.5 hours is an independent predictor of PPCs [1]. The pooled odds ratio for prolonged surgery was 2.26 (95% CI, 1.47–3.47) in the 2006 ACP review [1]. The authors reported that general anesthesia was an independent predictor of complications and the bias-corrected odds ratio was 1.83 (95% CI, 1.35–2.46) [1].

Emergency surgery

Emergency surgery is an independent predictor of postoperative PPCs (odds ratio, 2.21; 95% CI, 1.57–3.11) [1]. Johnson et al. showed that an emergent procedure was clearly a risk factor for postoperative respiratory failure (odds ratio, 2.41; 95% CI, 2.17–2.69) [5].

Laboratory studies to estimate risk
Pulmonary function testing

The use of spirometry to evaluate for the presence and significance of airflow limitation is well established; however, this clarity does not translate into effective prediction of postoperative pulmonary risk for individual patients undergoing extrathoracic surgery [1]. Since the early systematic review of the predictive value of preoperative spirometry published in 1989 [9], additional studies have failed to provide conclusive data about spirometry as an independent predictor of risk. The results are mixed. Furthermore, those studies comparing spirometric results with clinical data have failed to show an advantage over the history and physical examination. Lawrence *et al.* showed that abnormal results of lung examination predicted PPCs while spirometric results did not [23]. In contrast, Barisione *et al.* showed that pulmonary function testing results were predictive of PPCs; however, a history of mucous hypersecretion, was a stronger predictor [42].

No single spirometric variable consistently correlates with risk and there is no spirometric value that absolutely contraindicates non-cardiothoracic surgery, especially if the procedure will treat a life-threatening condition or may improve long-term survival [60,61].

A retrospective cohort study with controls showed that while patients with severe COPD (FEV1 < 50% predicted) had a higher incidence of PPCs, these occurred only in patients undergoing coronary artery bypass grafting [40]. The subset of patients with severe COPD undergoing non-cardiothoracic surgery had a similar incidence of PPCs compared with patients who had mild to moderate COPD and those without COPD.

No studies have evaluated the predictive value of pulmonary function tests in patients with restrictive physiology.

Finally, an economic analysis concluded that overutilization of routine pulmonary function tests for assessing preoperative pulmonary risk for abdominal surgery was wasteful and that reduced use could generate substantial savings without compromising patients' outcomes [62].

In summary, routine preoperative spirometry, even in the high-risk setting of upper abdominal surgery, rarely contributes additional, useful information to the clinical history and physical exam for predicting PPCs in individual patients. Preoperative spirometry is indicated for further diagnostic evaluation of patients with unexplained dyspnea or chronic cough and for those with obstructive lung disease who have poor control of their disease.

Chest imaging

The common practice of obtaining a chest X-ray as part of the routine preoperative evaluation of healthy patients rarely identifies abnormalities that are new, delays surgery, or changes the perioperative management. Most studies evaluating the value of chest X-rays have focused on the impact during the perioperative management. However, two studies with multivariable analysis found that an abnormal chest X-ray is an independent predictor of PPCs. In one of these studies Lawrence *et al.* evaluated 2,291 patients undergoing abdominal surgery [23]. A total of 82 cases with pulmonary complications were matched with 82 control subjects. An abnormal chest X-ray was found to be an independent predictor of PPCs (odds ratio, 3.2; 95% CI, 1.07–9.4). The

second study was a prospective cohort study of 410 patients scheduled for elective non-cardiac surgery [37]. Although the primary goal of this study was to examine the effect of preoperative smoking behavior on PPCs, the multivariate model found that an abnormal chest radiograph was an independent predictor of pulmonary complications (odds ratio, 6.3; 95% CI, 2.6–15.2) [37].

The impact of an abnormal chest radiograph on the perioperative management has been evaluated in multiple studies. A review by Smetana and Macpherson [63] examined the value of routine preoperative testing. They identified eight studies (n = 14,650), and found that 23% of the preoperative radiographs were abnormal; however, only 3% of these influenced the postoperative management. An earlier meta-analysis of 21 studies (n = 14,390), found abnormalities in 10% of routine preoperative radiographs [64]. The abnormalities were unexpected in only 1.3% of radiographs, and changed perioperative management in only 0.1% of all studies.

One prospective multicenter study identified male gender, age > 60 years, ASA class ≥ III, and presence of respiratory diseases to be significantly related to the probability of a useful preoperative chest radiograph, with utility defined as a positive response by the anesthesiologist regarding a change in the anesthetic management [65].

Clinicians should be able to predict most abnormal chest X-rays from data obtained during the clinical evaluation of the patient. Chest X-rays will rarely provide unexpected information that impacts the preoperative management. The value of chest radiographs as a predictor of PPCs is small.

The current evidence supports the use of chest X-rays for patients with known cardiopulmonary problems and those older than 50 years of age that are undergoing surgery of upper abdomen or thorax as well as abdominal aortic aneurysm repair [1]. Chest radiographs in healthy individuals is a significant waste of healthcare resources.

Arterial blood gases

The value of hypercapnia as a risk factor for PPCs in older studies was confounded by the presence of severe airflow limitation. In a systematic review of blinded studies examining risk factors for PPCs, none of the three studies that evaluated the utility of hypercapnia found it to be an independent predictor [66].

Similarly, old studies that reported hypoxemia to be a risk factor for PPCs were limited by small sample size and lack of added value to the clinical evaluation [67]. Hypoxemia as an independent risk factor for PPCs has not been evaluated in any large series.

In general, arterial blood-gas analyses should not be used to identify patients for whom the risk of surgery is prohibitive as there is no clear threshold that absolutely precludes necessary surgery. In patients with marginal lung function, preoperative arterial blood gas analysis may provide useful baseline information for perioperative management.

Exercise capacity

Cardiopulmonary exercise testing (CPET) has been used as a screening test for patients undergoing cardiothoracic and non-thoracic surgery and found to predict mortality [68]. However, most of these studies have been done to assess patients considered for lung resection due to malignant lung disease or heart, lung, or heart–lung transplantation.

The predictive value of maximum oxygen consumption (VO_{2max}) and anaerobic threshold (AT) obtained during CPET, in calculating perioperative morbidity and mortality during non-cardiothoracic surgery was recently reviewed by Smith *et al.* [69]. They evaluated nine studies and concluded that the VO_{2max} and to lesser extent the AT are valid predictors of perioperative morbidity and mortality. However, the quality of the data in this review had multiple limitations. Further studies should be conducted before CPET is recommended as an independent predictor of PPCs before non-cardiopulmonary surgery and to define the impact of CPET on the postoperative management.

More simple measurements of exercise capacity are the stair-climbing capacity and the 6-minute walking test. These are easy to perform tests that have shown good accuracy and concordance when compared with the VO_{2max} [70]. A prospective study by Girish *et al.* of 83 patients undergoing thoracotomy, sternotomy, or upper laparotomy showed a postoperative cardiopulmonary complication rate of 89% for patients unable to climb one flight of stairs. Those capable of climbing 7 flights did not have complications [24].

Serum measures of renal function

The two groundbreaking studies by Arozullah *et al.* [32,39] identified a serum blood urea nitrogen level of 21 mg/dL or greater as a significant predictor of PPCs. Increasing levels of blood urea nitrogen increased the risk. Johnson *et al.* showed that a preoperative creatinine of ≥ 1.5 mg/dL was associated with an increased risk of postoperative respiratory failure (odds ratio, 1.65; 95% CI, 1.493–1.826) [5].

Serum albumin measurement

The 2006 ACP guidelines [1] confirmed the importance of a low albumin level as a predictor of PPCs. An albumin level < 30 g/L had an adjusted odds ratio of 2.53 (95% CI, 2.28–2.80). A low serum albumin level was also the most important predictor of 30-day perioperative morbidity and mortality in the NSQIP report [71]. The updated risk index for the prediction of respiratory failure also found that a low serum albumin level was an independent predictor of respiratory complications [5]. A serum albumin level ≤ 3.5 g/dL vs > 3.5 g/dL was associated with a higher rate of respiratory failure (odds ratio, 1.485; 95% CI, 1.344–1.641) [5].

Miscellaneous risk factors

Additional risk factors, specifically for respiratory failure, include: preoperative sepsis (odds ratio, 1.999; 95% CI, 1.707–2.341), ascites (odds ratio, 1.846; 95% CI, 1.496–2.278) and hypernatremia (odds ratio, 1.564; 95% CI, 1.205–2.030) [5].

Pulmonary risk indices

The Goldman Cardiac Risk Index and Lee's Revised Cardiac Risk Index have facilitated the preoperative cardiac evaluation of patients undergoing non-cardiac surgery [72,73]. However, early risk indices developed for predicting PPCs were limited by small sample sizes, selected surgical procedures, and conflicting results in validation cohorts. In 2000 and 2001, Arozullah *et al.* published separate multifactorial risk indices for prediction of postoperative respiratory failure and pneumonia [32,39]. They were developed utilizing data from a large surgical cohort. A total of 81,719 male veterans undergoing major non-cardiac surgery were included to develop the respiratory failure index. The pneumonia risk index was derived from data of 160,805 patients from 100 VA hospitals. Both indices were validated on separate cohorts similar in size to the original development cohorts. These risk indices included risk factors related to the patient's general health/nutritional, respiratory, neurological, fluid, and immune status as well as risk factors related to type of anesthesia and the operation per se. Many risk factors were consistent between the two indices and most were not modifiable.

Consistent with previous studies, the most powerful predictor in these risk indices was the surgical site, with abdominal aortic aneurysm repair, thoracic surgery, and upper abdominal surgery conferring the highest risks [20]. These risk indices confirmed other previously established risk factors, including tobacco use, functional status, and COPD. General anesthesia was associated with increased risk of complications compared with spinal or other anesthesia techniques. Additional risk factors identified included: high or very low blood urea nitrogen, preoperative blood transfusion of > 4 units, steroid use, and increased alcohol intake.

Each decade above age ≥ 50 was associated with increasing risk for postoperative respiratory failure and pneumonia.

In both studies, point values were assigned to particular risk factors based on the strength of their association with PPCs in multivariate analysis. Table 12.2 shows the independent preoperative risk factors for pneumonia along with the point value assigned. Table 12.3 shows the probability of postoperative pneumonia in the development cohort according to the risk class.

An updated multivariable risk index for the prediction of respiratory failure after general and vascular surgery was published in 2007 [5]. Respiratory failure was defined as postoperative mechanical ventilation for more than 48 hours or unplanned reintubation. The authors studied a more diverse population. They collected data from 128 Veterans Affairs Medical Centers and 14 academic hospitals for a total of 180,359 patients being evaluated. Twenty-eight of 45 potential risk factors evaluated were found to be significant predictors of respiratory failure. The odds ratios for these factors ranged from 1.114 to 6.635 and they were assigned a point value on

Table 12.2 Postoperative pneumonia risk index (adapted from [32]).

Preoperative risk factor	Point value
Type of surgery	
Abdominal aortic aneurysm repair	15
Thoracic	14
Upper abdominal	10
Neck	8
Neurosurgery	8
Vascular surgery	3
Age	
≥ 80 years	17
70–79 years	13
60–69 years	9
50–59 years	4
Functional status	
Totally dependent	10
Partially dependent	6
Weight loss > 10% in past 6 months	7
History of chronic obstructive pulmonary disease	5
General anesthesia	4
Impaired sensorium	4
History of cerebrovascular accident	4
Blood urea nitrogen level	
< 2.86 mmol/L (< 8 mg/dL)	4
7.85–10.7 mmol/L (22–30 mg/dL)	2
≥ 10.7 mmol/L (≥ 30 mg/dL)	3
Transfusion > 4 units	3
Emergency surgery	3
Steroid use for chronic condition	3
Current smoker within 1 year	3
Alcohol intake > 2 drinks/day in the past 2 weeks	2

Table 12.3 Risk class assignment by postoperative pneumonia risk index score (adapted from [32]).

Risk class	Postoperative pneumonia risk index (point total)	Predicted probability of pneumonia[a]
1	0–15	0.2%
2	16–25	1.2%
3	26–40	4.0%
4	41–55	9.4%
5	> 55	15.3%

[a] Data provided for the development cohort.

Table 12.4 Risk factors for postoperative respiratory failure and the point value (score) assigned (adapted from [5]).

Risk factor	Point value
Orofacial surgery	7
ASA class IV or V	5
Work RVU > 17	4
ASA class III, Thoracic surgery	3
Emergency surgery, work RVU 10–17, cardiac surgery, gastric and bowel surgery, endocrine surgery, preoperative sepsis, preoperative creatinine ≥ 1.5, history of severe COPD, ascites, age > 40 years, preoperative sodium > 145, preoperative acute renal failure	2
Preoperative albumin ≤ 3.5, integumentary surgery, dyspnea, impaired sensorium, preoperative bilirubin > 1.0, more than 2 alcoholic drinks/day in 2 weeks before admission, bleeding disorders, preoperative white blood cell count < 2.5K or > 10K, weight loss > 10%, male gender, CHF < 30 days before surgery, smoker, preoperative platelet count ≤ 150K, CVA, preoperative SGOT > 40, clean/contaminated, contaminated or infected wound, and preoperative hematocrit ≤ 38	1

ASA, American Society of Anesthesiologists; RVU, relative value unit; COPD, chronic obstructive pulmonary disease; CHF, congestive heart failure; CVA, cerebrovascular accident; SGOT, serum glutamic-oxalacetic transaminase.

a scale from 1 to 7. The total number of points determined the risk level in the respiratory risk index. Table 12.4 shows the risk factors (independent predictors) for respiratory failure with the point value assigned. Table 12.5 shows the rates of respiratory failure for the different risk levels in the development cohort.

Most of the risk factors are similar in magnitude to the risk factors identified in the 2006 ACP review. However, this study assigned less risk to low serum albumin level, functional dependence, and congestive heart failure but higher risk to orofacial surgery. New independent risk factors were reported, including high complexity surgery, sepsis, ascites, and hypernatremia. Body mass index and spirometry as potential risk factors for respiratory failure or pneumonia were not evaluated during the development of these indices. This updated RF index is more generalizable since it includes women and patients outside the VA system, as well as VA hospitals.

Strategies to reduce postoperative pulmonary complications

After careful preoperative evaluation, the prevention and treatment of PPCs involve both preoperative and postoperative care. Lung-specific strategies include preoperative smoking cessation, lung expansion techniques, optimizing airflow limitation, and therapy of respiratory infections. Anesthesia, postoperative analgesia, surgical techniques, and

Table 12.5 Rates of postoperative respiratory failure for the different risk levels in the development cohort (adapted from [5]).

Risk level	Postoperative respiratory failure risk index (point total)	Predicted probability of respiratory failure[a]
Low	0–8	0.2%
Medium	8–12	1.0%
High	> 12	6.5%

[a] Data from the development cohort.

Table 12.6 Strategies to reduce the risk of PPCs and the current strength of evidence (adapted from [19]).

Risk reduction strategy	Strength of evidence[a]
Lung expansion maneuvers	A
Postoperative epidural analgesia[b]	A
Selective nasogastric decompression	B
Short-acting neuromuscular blocking agent	B
Laparoscopic vs open surgery[c]	B
Inspiratory muscle training	B
Intraoperative neuraxial blockade	I
Smoking cessation	I
Pulmonary artery catheterization	D
Routine total parenteral or enteral nutrition	D

[a] A, Supported by good evidence; B, Supported by fair evidence; I, At least fair evidence that strategy does not reduce risk or harm outweighs benefit; D, Insufficient or conflicting data to support intervention.
[b] Recent data provide good evidence to support this strategy.
[c] Recent data provide fair evidence to support this strategy (for some surgical procedures).

other perioperative interventions, including pulmonary artery catheterization, nutritional support, and selective nasogastric tube decompression, were also evaluated in the 2006 ACP guidelines and may have significant impact on PPCs. Table 12.6 shows a list of selected interventions that reduce PPCs along with the strength of evidence supporting each strategy.

Lung-specific strategies

Cessation of cigarette smoking

Abstinence from smoking may result in gradual improvement in mucociliary function and decreased upper-airway hypersensitivity [74]. However the effect of preoperative smoking cessation on the rates of PPCs remains controversial. A paradoxical increase in PPCs was presented by earlier reports of patients who quit smoking shortly before surgery [37,38,75]. Although this could be explained by an increase in cough and sputum production during the first few weeks after patients quit smoking, it may be related to methodological flaws in those studies.

Two randomized trials have studied the impact of perioperative smoking intervention programs. The first study evaluated 120 patients scheduled for hip and knee arthroplasty [76]. They were randomized 6–8 weeks before surgery to an intervention of counseling and nicotine replacement vs standard care (control group) [76]. Intervention group patients had an overall complication rate of 18% vs 52% in the control group (p = 0.0003). The most significant effect of intervention was seen for wound-related complications. Postoperative pulmonary complications were low (2%) and identical in both groups. In the second study, 117 patients undergoing hernia repair, laparoscopic cholecystectomy, or arthroplasty of the hip or knee were enrolled [77]. Patients were randomized 4 weeks before surgery to smoking cessation intervention vs standard care. The overall complication rate in the intervention group was 21% vs 41% (p = 0.03). Again, the rate of PPCs was very low for both groups with no statistical difference. These small studies primarily included patients undergoing low-risk procedures and were underpowered to show a difference in PPCs.

Physicians can use the preoperative examination to counsel patients on the overall benefits of long-term smoking cessation, realizing that the maximum benefit most likely occurs with at least 2 months of smoking abstinence before surgery.

Lung expansion techniques

The 2006 ACP guidelines supports the role of lung expansion maneuvers after abdominal surgery [1]. A subsequent qualitative systematic review of lung expansion modalities questioned their beneficial routine use during abdominal surgery [78]. This review identified 35 randomized controlled trials. Thirteen trials had a "no intervention" control group; nine (n = 883) of these 13 trials did not report differences, while four studies (n = 528) did. These conflicting results can be explained by methodological differences between the two systematic reviews: in particular, the inclusion of small studies with few subjects per arm and studies with no explicit definition of PPCs or whose outcomes were physiologic perturbations rather than clinical events. Inclusion of these studies may have biased the results and weakened the conclusions of the latter review.

The overall higher quality data of the systematic review for the ACP guidelines supports the value of lung expansion techniques to decrease the rate of PPCs after abdominal surgery. No particular technique has been identified as the procedure of choice and combined modalities do not provide additional risk reduction.

The optimal duration and frequency of deep breathing exercises or incentive spirometry is unclear. There are different regimens. One utilizes 10 breaths over 15 minutes with an incentive spirometer four times a day [79]. Choosing techniques is probably not as important as is motivating and educating the patients about the desired goals. The presence of experienced personnel to encourage and supervise the patients during the postoperative period is important.

Continuous positive airway pressure (CPAP) may be superior in patients with difficulty performing deep breathing exercises or using an incentive spirometer. A recent meta-analysis of nine randomized controlled trials (n = 654) evaluated the benefit of CPAP vs standard therapy in patients undergoing abdominal surgery [80]. The use of CPAP provided a significant risk reduction in the overall rate of PPCs (odds ratio, 0.66; 95% CI, 0.52–0.85), pneumonia (odds ratio, 0.33; 95% CI, 0.14–0.75) and atelectasis (odds ratio, 0.75; 95% CI, 0.58–0.97).

Inspiratory muscle training

Inspiratory muscle training (IMT) is a fairly novel technique that combines different lung expansion maneuvers including incentive spirometry, education in active cycle of breathing techniques, and forced exhalation maneuver. A single-blind randomized controlled trial evaluated this technique preoperatively in a high-risk group of patients (n = 279) scheduled for coronary artery bypass surgery [81]. The intervention group (IMT) trained 20 minutes every day, 7 days a week, and for a minimum of 2 weeks. Postoperative pulmonary complications developed in 25/139 (18%) patients in the IMT groups vs 48/137 (35%) in the usual group (odds ratio, 0.52; 95% CI, 0.30–0.92). Pneumonia occurred in 9 (6.5%) patients in the MIT group vs 22 (16.1%) in the usual care group (odds ratio, 0.40; 95% CI, 0.19–0.84). Hospital length of stay was shorter in the IMT group as well. A smaller randomized controlled pilot study was conducted in a group of patients (n = 20) undergoing elective abdominal aortic aneurysm repair [82]. Ten patients were assigned to each group. The frequency of atelectasis and mean duration of atelectasis was higher in the control group compared with the IMT set of patients. No adverse events were reported. Larger trials in patients having other types of surgery and evaluating other outcomes are needed to better define the role of this intervention [83].

Optimizing airflow limitation

Patients with COPD are at increased risk for PPCs, while those with well-controlled asthma are not [1]. Exacerbations of COPD or asthma should be treated before elective surgery according to established guidelines [84]. The preoperative use of systemic corticosteroids in asthmatics does not increase the rate of wound complications or respiratory infections. Favorable results were reported by a small prospective study of 60 patients with COPD undergoing coronary artery bypass graft surgery who received a parenteral long-acting corticosteroid vs placebo injection [85]. A third group of 30 patients without COPD was used as control. Although a similar rate of PPCs was reported in the corticosteroid and placebo groups (20%), ICU stay > 48 hours (p = 0.03) and hospital stay (p = 0.013) were longer in COPD patients treated with placebo. This and

other small studies support the safe use of preoperative corticosteroids.

Silvanus *et al.* reported fewer episodes of bronchospasm during intubation in patients with untreated airway hyper-reactivity who were pretreated daily for 5 days with albuterol and methylprednisolone [86].

In patients with moderate or severe COPD, combining bronchodilators with different mechanisms, such as a beta-2-agonist and anticholinergic agents, may provide synergistic effects and a more sustained improvement in FEV1. A subset of these patients may benefit from inhaled glucocorticoid therapy [84].

The weak bronchodilator effect and narrow therapeutic index of theophylline precludes a recommendation for its use during the perioperative period unless significant benefit is anticipated. The potential benefit in diaphragm contractility has not been studied in the preoperative setting.

Finally, cardioselective beta-blockers in patients with COPD are not associated with significant changes in FEV1 or respiratory symptoms, even in those with severe COPD [87].

Respiratory infection

The risk of PPCs in healthy adults with an acute, uncomplicated viral upper respiratory infection (URI) is unknown. Although the issue has been evaluated in the pediatric population, the results are controversial. A prospective cohort study evaluated the rates of perioperative respiratory adverse events in a group of children (n = 9,297) [88]. The risk of bronchospasm, laryngospasm, and desaturation were associated with an upper respiratory tract infection only if symptoms were present or occurred within the last 2 weeks before surgery. Clinical prudence supports the traditional recommendation of postponing elective surgery during URI. Bacterial respiratory infections should be treated before elective surgery. There is no role for prophylactic antibiotics in high-risk patients without acute bacterial infection.

Anesthesia, analgesia, and surgical technique-related strategies

Laparoscopy vs open surgery

The lower rate of PPCs seen after laparoscopic bariatric surgery compared with the open procedure, suggests that this approach could be extended to other abdominal or pelvic interventions [58]. However, similar results were not obtained in a retrospective cohort study that compared laparoscopic appendectomy vs open surgery [59]. Laparoscopy may be another strategy that helps to reduce PPCs in some specific situations.

Postoperative analgesia

Splinting and significant decrease in chest and diaphragmatic excursion due to postoperative pain is a frequent problem after abdominal, thoracic, and aortic procedures. Different strategies for pain control and their impact on the development of PPCs have been evaluated during the past two decades. A 2007 systematic review of the impact of post-operative analgesia on major PPCs supports the use of epidural analgesia over systemic analgesia [89]. In this study only randomized controlled trials of 200 patients or larger were included. A meta-analysis published in 1998 and included in this review, reported that epidural opioids compared with systemic opioids decreased the risk of atelectasis (relative risk, 0.53; 95% CI, 0.33–0.85) and epidural local anesthetics reduced the risk of pulmonary infection (odds ratio, 0.36; 95% CI, 0.21–0.65) and all PPCs (relative risk, 0.58; 0.42–0.80) [90]. A 2000 meta-analysis also included in this study reported lower rates of pneumonia in those receiving epidural analgesia compared with systemic analgesics (odds ratio, 0.61; 95% CI, 0.48–0.81) [91]. A recent meta-analysis by Popping et al. confirmed the above findings but indicated that the relative benefit has decreased due to improvement in the management of systemic analgesia [92]. Based on this volume of information, it is appropriate to conclude that thoracic epidural analgesia reduces the risk of PPCs, particularly during high-risk surgeries. The level of evidence to support the use of patient-controlled analgesia (PCA) and its impact on the rate of PPCs is not sufficient to provide a recommendation about the routine use.

Neuromuscular blocking agents

The use of long acting agents, in particular pancuronium, is not recommended given the higher rate of residual neuromuscular blockade seen with this medication and the increased rate of PPCs compared with intermediate-acting agents like atracurium or vecuronium [93].

Other perioperative interventions
Selective nasogastric tube decompression

Nasogastric tube placement impairs the cough reflex and provides a more direct pathway for oro-pharyngeal bacteria to the lungs, thus potentially increasing respiratory tract infections. The routine placement of a nasogastric tube after abdominal surgery until bowel function returns was questioned during the 2006 ACP guidelines. Selective use refers to placement after surgery only if the patient develops nausea,

vomiting, distension, or ileus. A systematic review reported that the routine use compared with selective use was associated with a significant increase in PPCs, in particular atelectasis and pneumonia (odds ratio, 1.45; 95% CI, 1.08–1.93) [94]. Based on the current level of evidence our recommendation is the selective placement of nasogastric tubes after abdominal surgery.

Nutritional support

Malnutrition and low albumin are risk factors for PPCs. A meta-analysis of randomized controlled trials evaluated perioperative enteral nutrition vs no nutrition treatment, volitional nutrition (scheduled liquid oral diet) vs no nutritional therapy and enteral nutrition vs parenteral nutrition [95]. Enteral nutrition and volitional nutrition were associated with lower infectious complications but no clear decrease in the rate of postoperative pneumonia. Routine perioperative parenteral nutrition was clearly ineffective.

Pulmonary artery catheterization

The potential benefit of pulmonary artery catheters was evaluated in a high-risk group of patients age $\geq$ 60 (n = 1,994) scheduled for urgent or elective surgery [96]. This randomized controlled trial did not show a decrease in the hospital mortality rate and the postoperative pneumonia rates for the pulmonary artery catheter group.

Conclusions

There are numerous risk factors for PPCs. Although many of these risk factors may not be modifiable prior to surgery others may provide a good target for risk reduction. Some of the strategies to reduce risk remained not well defined, as is the case with the optimal duration of smoking cessation. Additionally, current recommendations remain generic, including lung expansion maneuvers, selective use of nasogastric tubes during abdominal surgery, and the use of epidural thoracic analgesia in high-risk interventions. Novel techniques as IMT before CABG may extend its benefit to other types of surgery. Future trials may provide additional evidence-based information that will help to further reduce the rate of complications, Effective communication among the various specialists and an interdisciplinary approach is very important to reduce the PPC risk.

References

1. Smetana GW, Lawrence VA, Cornell JE. Pre-operative pulmonary risk stratification for noncardiothoracic surgery: systematic review for the American College of Physicians. *Ann Intern Med* 2006; **144**: 581–95.

2. Fleischmann KE, Goldman L, Young B et al. Association between cardiac and noncardiac complications in patients undergoing noncardiac surgery:

outcomes and effects on length of stay. *Am J Med* 2003; **115**: 515–20.

3. Lawrence VA, Hilsenbeck SG, Mulrow CD et al. Incidence and hospital stay for cardiac and pulmonary complications after abdominal surgery. *J Gen Intern Med* 1995; **10**: 671–8.

4. Lawrence VA, Hilsenbeck SG, Noveck H et al. Medical complications and outcomes after hip fracture repair. *Arch Intern Med* 2002; **162**: 2053–7.

5. Johnson RG, Arozullah AM, Neumayer L et al. Predictors of postoperative respiratory failure after general and vascular surgery: results from the patient safety in surgery study. *J Am Coll Surg* 2007; **204**: 1188–98.

6. Manku K, Bachetti P, Leung JM. Prognostic significance of postoperative in-hospital complications in elderly patients. I. Long-term survival. *Anesth Analg* 2003; **96**: 583–9.

7. Latimer RG, Dickman M, Day WC *et al.* Ventilatory patterns and pulmonary complications after upper abdominal surgery determined by preoperative and postoperative computerized spirometry and blood gas analysis. *Am J Surg* 1971; **122**: 622–32.

8. Pontoppidan H. Mechanical aids to lung expansion in non-intubated surgical patients. *Am Rev Resp Dis* 1980; **122**: 109–19.

9. Lawrence VA, Page CP, Harris GD. Preoperative spirometry before abdominal operations. A critical appraisal of its predictive value. *Arch Intern Med* 1989; **149**: 280–5.

10. Platell C, Hall JC. Atelectasis after abdominal surgery. *J Am Coll Surg* 1997; **185**: 584–92.

11. Light RW, George RB. Incidence and significance of pleural effusion after abdominal surgery. *Chest* 1976; **69**: 621–5.

12. Nielsen PH, Jepsen SB, Olsen AD. Postoperative pleural effusion following upper abdominal surgery. *Chest* 1989; **96**: 1133–5.

13. Hedenstierna G, Edmark L. The effects of anesthesia and muscle paralysis on the respiratory system. *Intensive Care Med* 2005; **31**: 1327–35.

14. Brismar B, Hedenstierna G, Lundquist H *et al.* Pulmonary densities during anesthesia with muscular relaxation: a proposal of atelectasis. *Anesthesiology* 1985; **62**: 422–8.

15. Wahba RM. Airway closure and intraoperative hypoxaemia: twenty-five years later. *Can J Anaesth* 1996; **43**: 1144–9.

16. Trayner E Jr, Celli BR. Postoperative pulmonary complications. *Med Clin N Am* 2001; **85**: 1129–39.

17. Rothen HU, Sporre B, Engberg G *et al.* Influence of gas composition on recurrence of atelectasis after a reexpansion maneuver during general anesthesia. *Anesthesiology* 1995; **82**: 832–42.

18. Qaseenm A, Snow V, Fitterman N *et al.* Risk assessment for and strategies to reduce perioperative pulmonary complications for patients undergoing noncardiothoracic surgery: a guideline from the American College of Physicians. *Ann Intern Med* 2006; **144**: 575–80.

19. Lawrence VA, Cornell JE, Smetana GW. Strategies to reduce postoperative pulmonary complications after noncardiothoracic surgery: systematic review for the American College of Physicians. *Ann Intern Med* 2006; **144**: 596–608.

20. Turrentine FE, Wang H, Simpson VB *et al.* Surgical risk factors, morbidity and mortality in elderly patients. *J Am Coll Surg* 2006; **203**: 865–77.

21. Smetana GW. Preoperative pulmonary evaluation. *N Engl J Med* 1999; **340**: 937–44.

22. Cohen MM, Duncan PG, Tate RB. Does anesthesia contribute to operative mortality? *J Am Med Assoc* 1988; **260**: 2859–63.

23. Lawrence VA, Dhanda R, Hilsenbeck SG, Page CP. Risk of pulmonary complications after elective abdominal surgery. *Chest* 1996; **110**: 744–50.

24. Girish M, Trayner E Jr, Dammann O *et al.* Symptom-limited stair climbing as a predictor of postoperative cardiopulmonary complications after high-risk surgery. *Chest* 2001; **120**: 1147–51.

25. Ray CS, Sue DY, Bray G *et al.* Effects of obesity on respiratory function. *Am Rev Resp Dis* 1983; **128**: 501–6.

26. Hall JC, Tarala RA, Hall JL, Mander J. A multivariate analysis of the risk of pulmonary complications after laparotomy. *Chest* 1991; **99**: 923–7.

27. Brooks-Brunn JA. Predictors of postoperative pulmonary complications following abdominal surgery. *Chest* 1997; **111**: 564–71.

28. Angrisani L, Lorenzo M, De Palma G *et al.* Laparoscopic cholecystectomy in obese patients compared with nonobese patients. *Surg Laparosc Endosc Percutan Tech* 1995; **5**: 197–201.

29. Pasulka PS, Bistrian BR, Benotti PN, Blackburn GL. The risks of surgery in obese patients. *Ann Intern Med* 1986; **104**: 540–6.

30. Thomas EJ, Goldman L, Mangione CM *et al.* Body mass index as a correlate of postoperative complications and resource utilization. *Am J Med* 1997; **102**: 277–83.

31. Blouw EL, Rudolph AD, Narr BJ, Sarr MG. The frequency of respiratory failure with morbid obesity undergoing gastric bypass. *AANA J* 2003; **71**: 45–50.

32. Arozullah AM, Khuri SF, Henderson WG, Daley J; Participants in the National Veterans Affairs Surgical Quality Improvement Program. Development and validation of a multifactorial risk index for predicting postoperative pneumonia after major noncardiac surgery. *Ann Intern Med* 2001; **135**: 847–57.

33. Kotani N, Hashimoto H, Sessler DI *et al.* Smoking decreases alveolar macrophage function during anesthesia and surgery. *Anesthesiology* 2000; **92**: 1268–77.

34. Dilworth JP, White RJ. Postoperative chest infection after upper abdominal surgery: an important problem for smokers. *Resp Med* 1992; **86**: 205–10.

35. McAlister FA, Khan NA, Straus SE *et al.* Accuracy of the preoperative assessment in predicting pulmonary risk after nonthoracic surgery. *Am J Resp Crit Care Med* 2003; **167**: 741–4.

36. Turan A, Mascha EJ, Roberman D *et al.* Smoking and perioperative outcomes. *Anesthesiology* 2011; **11**: 837–47.

37. Bluman LG, Mosca L, Newman N, Simon DG. Preoperative smoking habits and postoperative pulmonary complications. *Chest* 1998; **113**: 883–9.

38. Yamashita S, Yamaguchi H, Sakaguchi M *et al.* Effect of smoking on intraoperative sputum and postoperative pulmonary complication in minor surgical patients. *Respir Med* 2004; **98**: 760–6.

39. Arozullah A, Daley J, Henderson W, Khuri S. Multifactorial risk index for predicting postoperative respiratory failure in men after noncardiac surgery. *Ann Surg* 2000; **232**: 243–53.

40. Kroenke K, Lawrence VA, Theroux JF *et al.* Postoperative complications after thoracic and major abdominal surgery in patients with and without obstructive lung disease. *Chest* 1993; **104**: 1445–51.

41. McAlister FA, Bertsch K, Man J *et al.* Incidence of and risk factors for pulmonary complications after nonthoracic surgery. *Am J Respir Crit Care Med* 2005; **171**: 514–17.

42. Barisione G, Rovida S, Gazzaniga GM, Fontana L. Upper abdominal surgery: does a lung function test exist to predict early severe postoperative respiratory

complication? *Europ Resp J* 1997; **10**: 1301–8.

43. Mitchell CK, Smoger SH, Pfeifer MP *et al.* Multivariate analysis of factors associated with postoperative pulmonary complications following general elective surgery. *Arch Surg* 1998; **133**: 194–8.

44. Gracey DR, Divertie MB, Didier EP. Preoperative pulmonary preparation of patients with chronic obstructive pulmonary disease: a prospective study. *Chest* 1979; **76**: 123–9.

45. Pizov R, Brown RH, Weiss YS *et al.* Wheezing during induction of general anesthesia in patients with and without asthma. A randomized, blinded trial. *Anesthesiology* 1995; **82**: 1111–16.

46. Warner DO, Warner MA, Barnes RD *et al.* Perioperative respiratory complications in patients with asthma. *Anesthesiology* 1996; **85**: 460–7.

47. Young T, Skatrud J, Peppard PE. Risk factors for obstructive sleep apnea in adults. *J Am Med Assoc* 2004; **291**: 2013–16.

48. Gupta RM, Parvizi J, Hanssen AD, Gay PC. Postoperative complications in patients with obstructive sleep apnea syndrome undergoing hip or knee replacement: a case-control study. *Mayo Clin Proc* 2001; **76**: 897–905.

49. Hwang D, Shakir N, Limann B *et al.* Association of sleep-disordered breathing with postoperative complications. *Chest* 2008; **133**: 1128–34.

50. Memtsoudis S, Liu SS, Ma Y *et al.* Perioperative pulmonary outcomes in patients with sleep apnea after noncardiac surgery. *Anesth Analg* 2011; **112**: 113–21.

51. Weingarten TN, Flores AS, Mackenzie JA *et al.* Obstructive sleep apnoea and perioperative complications in bariatric patients. *Br J Anaesth* 2011; **106**: 131–9.

52. Gross JB, Bachenberg KL, Benumof JL *et al.* Practice guidelines for the perioperative management of patients with obstructive sleep apnea: a report by the American Society of Anesthesiologists Task Force on Perioperative Management of patients with obstructive sleep apnea. *Anesthesiology* 2006; **104**: 1081–93.

53. Ramakrishna G, Sprung J, Barugur SR *et al.* Impact of pulmonary hypertension on the outcomes of noncardiac surgery. *J Am Coll Cardiol* 2005; **45**: 1691–9.

54. Lai HC, Lai HC, Wang KY *et al.* Severe pulmonary hypertension complicates postoperative outcome of non-cardiac surgery. *Br J Anaesth* 2007; **99**: 184–90.

55. Kirchoff P, Selim D, Buchmann P. A multivariate analysis of potential risk factors for intra- and postoperative complications in 1316 elective laparoscopic colorectal procedures. *Ann Surg* 2008; **248**: 259–65.

56. Leung JM, Dzankic S. Relative importance of preoperative health status versus intraoperative factors in predicting postoperative adverse outcomes in geriatric surgical patients. *J Am Geriatr Soc* 2001; **49**: 1080–5.

57. Elkouri S, Gloviczki P, McKusick MA *et al.* Perioperative complications and early outcome after endovascular and open surgical repair of abdominal aortic aneurysms. *J Vasc Surg* 2004; **39**: 497–505.

58. Weller WE, Rosati C. Comparing outcomes of laparoscopic versus open bariatric surgery. *Ann Surg* 2008; **248**: 10–15.

59. Hemmila MR, Birkmeyer NJ, Arbabi S *et al.* Introduction to propensity score: a case study on the comparative effectiveness of laparoscopic vs. open appendectomy. *Arch Surg* 2010; **145**: 939–45.

60. Kroenke K, Lawrence VA, Theroux LF, Tuley MR. Operative risk in patients with severe obstructive pulmonary disease. *Arch Intern Med* 1992; **152**: 967–71.

61. Smetana GW. A 68 year old man with COPD contemplating colon cancer surgery. *J Am Med Assoc* 2007; **297**: 2121–30.

62. De Nino LA, Lawrence VA, Averyt EC *et al.* Preoperative spirometry and laparotomy: blowing away dollars. *Chest* 1997; **111**: 1536–41.

63. Smetana GW, Macpherson DS. The case against routine preoperative laboratory testing. *Med Clin North Am* 2003; **87**: 7–40.

64. Archer C, Levy AR, McGregor M. Value of routine preoperative chest X-rays: a meta-analysis. *Can J Anaesth* 1993; **40**: 1022–7.

65. Silvestri L, Maffessanti M, Gregori D *et al.* Usefulness of routine preoperative chest radiography for anaesthetic management: a prospective multicenter pilot study. *Europ J Anaesth* 1999; **16**: 749–60.

66. Fisher BW, Majumdar SR, McAlister FA. Predicting pulmonary complications after nonthoracic surgery: a systematic review of blinded studies. *Am J Med* 2002; **112**: 219–25.

67. Rao MK, Reilly TE, Schuller DE, Young DC. Analysis of risk factors for postoperative pulmonary complications in head and neck surgery. *Laryngoscope* 1992; **102**: 45–7.

68. American Thoracic Society; American College of Chest Physicians. ATS/ACCP statement on cardiopulmonary exercise testing. *Am J Respir Crit Care Med* 2003; **167**: 211–77.

69. Smith TB, Stonell C, Purkayastha S, Paraskevas P. Cardiopulmonary exercise testing as a risk assessment method in non cardio-pulmonary surgery: a systematic review. *Anaesthesia* 2009; **64**: 883–93.

70. Cataneo DC, Kobayasi S, Carvalho LR *et al.* Accuracy of six minute walk test, stair test and spirometry using maximal oxygen uptake as gold standard. *Acta Cir Bras* 2010; **25**: 194–200.

71. Gibbs J, Cull W, Henderson W *et al.* Preoperative serum albumin level as a predictor of operative mortality and morbidity: results from the National VA Surgical Risk Study. *Arch Surg* 1999; **134**: 36–42.

72. Goldman L, Caldera DL, Nussbaum SR *et al.* Multifactorial index of cardiac risk in noncardiac surgical procedures. *N Engl J Med* 1977; **297**: 845–50.

73. Lee T, Marcantonio E, Mangione C *et al.* Derivation and prospective validation of a simple index for prediction of cardiac risk of major noncardiac surgery. *Circulation* 1999; **100**: 1043–9.

74. Buist AS, Sexton GJ, Nagy JM, Ross BB. The effect of smoking cessation and modification on lung function. *Am Rev Respir Dis* 1976; **114**: 115–22.

75. Nakagawa M, Tanaka H, Tsukuma H, Kishi Y. Relationship between the duration of the preoperative smoke-free period and the incidence of postoperative pulmonary complications after pulmonary surgery. *Chest* 2001; **120**: 705–10.

76. Myers K, Hajek P, Hinds C *et al.* Stopping smoking shortly before surgery and postoperative complications. A systematic review and meta-analysis. *Arch Intern Med* 2011; **171**: 983–9.

77. Moller AM, Villebro N, Pedersen P, Tonnesen H. Effect of preoperative smoking intervention on postoperative complications: a randomized clinical trial. *Lancet* 2002; **359**: 114–17.

78. Pasquina P, Tramer MR, Granier J-M, Walder B. Respiratory physiotherapy to prevent pulmonary complications after abdominal surgery: a systematic review. *Chest* 2006; **130**: 1887–9.

79. Celli BR, Rodriguez KS, Snider GL. A controlled trial of intermittent positive pressure breathing, incentive spirometry, and deep breathing exercises in preventing pulmonary complications after abdominal surgery. *Am Rev Respir Dis* 1984; **130**: 12–15.

80. Ferreyra GP, Baussano I, Squadrone V *et al.* Continuous positive airway pressure for treatment of respiratory complications after abdominal surgery: a systematic review and meta-analysis. *Ann Surg* 2008; **247**: 617–26.

81. Hulzebos EH, Helders PJM, Favié NJ *et al.* Preoperative intensive inspiratory muscle training to prevent postoperative pulmonary complications in high-risk patients undergoing CABG surgery: a randomized clinical trial. *J Am Med Assoc* 2006; **296**: 1851–7.

82. Dronker J, Veldman A, Hoberg E, van der Waal C. Prevention of pulmonary complications after upper abdominal surgery by preoperative intensive inspiratory muscle training: a randomized controlled pilot study. *Clin Rehabil* 2008; **22**: 134–42.

83. Valkenet K, van de Port IGL, Dronkers JJ *et al.* The effects of preoperative exercise therapy on postoperative outcome: a systematic review. *Clin Rehabil* 2011; **25**: 99–111.

84. Pauwels RA, Buist AS, Calverley PM *et al.* The Global strategy for the diagnosis, management, and prevention of chronic obstructive pulmonary disease. NHLBI/WHO Global Initiative for Chronic Obstructive Lung Disease (GOLD) Workshop summary. *Am J Respir Crit Care Med* 2001; **163**: 1256–76.

85. Starobin D, Kramer MR, Garty M, Shitirt D. Morbidity associated with systemic corticosteroid preparation for coronary artery bypass grafting in patients with chronic obstructive pulmonary disease: a case control study. *J Cardiothorac Surg* 2007; **2**: 25.

86. Silvanus MT, Groeben H, Peters J. Corticosteroids and inhaled salbutamol in patients with reversible airway obstruction markedly decrease the incidence of bronchospasm after tracheal intubation. *Anesthesiology* 2004; **100**: 1052–7.

87. Salpeter SR, Ormiston T, Salpeter EE. Cardioselective beta-blockers for chronic obstructive pulmonary disease. *Cochrane Database Syst Rev* 2005; **4**: CD003566.

88. Von Ungem-Sternberg BS, Boda K, Chambers NA *et al.* Risk assessment for respiratory complications in paediatric anaesthesia: a prospective cohort study. *Lancet* 2010; **376**: 773–83.

89. Liu SS, Wu CL. Effect of postoperative analgesia on major postoperative complications: a systematic update of the evidence. *Anesth Analg* 2007; **104**: 689–702.

90. Ballantyne JC, Carr DB, deFerranti S *et al.* The comparative effects of postoperative analgesic therapies on pulmonary outcome: Cumulative meta-analyses of randomized, controlled trials. *Anesth Analg* 1998; **86**: 598–612.

91. Rodgers A, Walker N, Schug S *et al.* Reduction of postoperative mortality and morbidity with epidural or spinal anaesthesia: results from overview of randomized trials. *Br Med J* 2000; **321**: 1–12.

92. Popping DM, Elia N, Marret E *et al.* Protective effects of epidural analgesia on pulmonary complications after abdominal and thoracic surgery. *Arch Surg* 2008; **143**: 990–9.

93. Berg H, Viby-Mogensen J, Roed J *et al.* Residual neuromuscular block is a risk factor for postoperative pulmonary complications. A prospective, randomized, and blinded study of postoperative pulmonary complications after atracurium, vecuronium and pancuronium. *Acta Anaesth Scand* 1997; **41**: 1095–2003.

94. Nelson R, Edwards S, Tse B. Prophylactic nasogastric decompression after abdominal surgery. *Cochrane Database Syst Rev* 2007; **3**: CD004929.

95. Koretz RL, Avenell A, Lipman TO *et al.* Does enteral nutrition affect clinical outcome? A systematic review of the randomized trials. *Am J Gastroenterol* 2007; **102**: 412–29.

96. Sandham JD, Hull RD, Brant RF *et al.* A randomized, controlled trial of the use of pulmonary artery catheters in high-risk surgical patients. *N Engl J Med* 2003; **348**: 5–14.

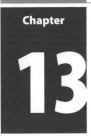

Perioperative management of the asthma patient

Annette Esper

Overview of asthma

Asthma is a common disease, with a worldwide prevalence of about 7–10% [1], and a prevalence in the USA of about 6.7% [2]. Although the incidence of asthma is increasing, morbidity and mortality have decreased [3]. This improvement in morbidity and mortality may be due to changes in management guidelines.

Asthma is diagnosed using a combination of clinical symptoms and physiologic abnormalities. The Global Initiative for Asthma (GINA) defines asthma as a chronic inflammatory disorder of the airways, involving cellular inflammatory responses, and resulting in airway hyperresponsiveness, which may cause symptoms such as wheezing, chest tightness, shortness of breath and coughing [4]. Patient symptoms, lung function, and the number of exacerbations requiring steroids per year typically determine asthma severity. Previous GINA guidelines divided asthma by severity based on level of symptoms, airflow limitation and lung function variability into four categories: intermittent, mild persistent, moderate persistent, and severe persistent. However, asthma severity involves not only severity of underlying disease, which may change over time, but its responsiveness to treatment [5]. Therefore, the current thinking is that assessment of control is more useful [6]. Asthma severity now by consensus is classified on the basis of the intensity of treatment required to achieve good asthma control [5,7]. In 2006, GINA revised their guidelines to emphasize asthma management based on clinical control rather than classification by severity [4]. The goal is for asthma patients to experience infrequent exacerbations, have no or minimal symptoms (including at night), have no limitations on activities, have no or minimal requirement for rescue medications, and have near-normal lung function.

The pathophysiology of asthma is characterized by airway obstruction, inflammation, and airway hyperreactivity in response to various stimuli [8,9] (see Table 13.1). These stimuli result in contraction of the bronchial smooth muscle, leading to bronchoconstriction. Both vagal and sympathetic factors can affect airway tone. The bronchoconstriction that occurs can have cardiopulmonary effects, including increased work of breathing, decreased airflow, air trapping, ventilation-perfusion mismatch, increased pulmonary vascular resistance and right ventricular overload, and decreased FEV1 (forced expiratory volume in 1 second) [8]. The increased airway resistance in asthma is also a product of the inflammatory response to stimuli, which involves lymphocytes, eosinophils, IgE, neutrophils, mast cells, leukotrienes, and cytokines. This inflammatory response results in edema and mucus plugging, which further exacerbates airflow limitation [10]. In chronic asthmatics with poorly controlled disease, airway remodeling, thickening, and injury to airway epithelium occur, promoting resistance to corticosteroid therapy. Multiple factors, including environmental factors and drugs, may trigger bronchoconstriction. Furthermore, tobacco is associated with accelerated decrease in lung function in people with asthma, and increased asthma severity that may not be responsive to steroids [4].

Asthma management is multifaceted and it is important for both patients and healthcare providers to take an active role in the process. The components of management include

Table 13.1 Airway changes seen in asthma. Adapted from the GINA guidelines [4].

Structural changes in asthma
Subepithelial fibrosis
Increase in airway smooth muscle
Blood vessel proliferation
Mucus hypersecretion

Airway narrowing in asthma
Airway smooth muscle contraction
Airway edema
Airway thickening
Mucus hypersecretion

Mechanisms of airway hyperresponsiveness
Excessive contraction of airway smooth muscle
Uncoupling of airway contraction
Thickening of airway wall
Sensitized sensory nerves

Medical Management of the Surgical Patient, ed. Michael F. Lubin, Thomas F. Dodson, and Neil H. Winawer. Published by Cambridge University Press. © Cambridge University Press 2013.

Table 13.2 Classification of asthma control (adapted from GINA guidelines [4]). ACQ, Asthma control questionnaire; ACT, Asthma Control Test; ATAQ, Asthma Therapy Assessment Questionnaire.

Components of control	Classification of asthma control		
	Well-controlled	Not well-controlled	Very poorly controlled
Symptoms	≤ 2 d/wk	> 2 d/wk	Throughout the day
Night-time awakenings	≤ 2 times/mo	1–3 times/wk	≥4 times/wk
Restriction of normal activity	None	Some limitation	Extreme limitation
Short acting beta agonist use	≤ 2 d/wk	> 2 d/wk	Several times a day
FEV1 or peak flow	> 80% of predicted/personal best	60–80% of predicted/personal best	< 60% of predicted/personal best
Validated questionnaires	0	1–2	3–4
ATAQ	≤ 0.75	≥ 1.5	N/A
ACQ	≥ 20	16–19	≤ 15
ACT			

Features associated with increased risk of adverse events in the future: poor clinical control, frequent exacerbations in the past year, admission to a critical care unit for asthma, low FEV1, smoking exposure and high-dose medications.

Table 13.3 Stepwise management of asthma adapted from the EPR-3 and GINA guidelines [4,11]. Each step should involve patient education, control of environmental triggers, and management of comorbid conditions.

	Stepwise approach for asthma management		Step up if needed ⬆
	Preferred therapy	Alternative therapy	
Step 1	SABA as needed		
Step 2	Low-dose ICS	Cromolyn, LTRA, nedocromil, or theophylline	
Step 3	Low-dose ICS+LABA OR medium-dose ICS	Low-dose ICS+LTRA, theophylline, or zileuton	**ASSESS Control**
Step 4	Medium-dose ICS+LABA	Medium-dose ICS+LTRA, theophylline or zileuton	Step down if possible ⬇
Step 5	High-dose ICS+LABA AND consider omalizumab for patients with allergies		
Step 6	High-dose ICS+LABA+oral corticosteroid AND consider omalizumab for patients with allergies		

SABA, short-acting beta agonist; ICS, inhaled corticosteroid; LABA, long-acting beta agonist; LTRA, leukotriene receptor antagonist.

routine monitoring of symptoms and lung function, patient education, control of triggers, and pharmacologic therapy. The goals of asthma therapy are to reduce impairment and reduce risk of adverse outcomes. According to the GINA guidelines, patients should be asked to demonstrate their inhaler device technique at every visit [4]. The most effective and efficient delivery is by a metered-dose inhaler (MDI) and a spacer device. Physicians should assess asthma control at every visit (see Table 13.2). In addition, identifying environmental triggers and comorbid diseases that impact therapy should be addressed. A stepwise approach to pharmacologic therapy as recommended by the National Asthma Education and Prevention Program (NAEPP) Expert Panel report [11], is the mainstay of treatment (see Table 13.3). The guidelines recommend increasing medications until control is established, followed by de-escalation of therapy to minimize side-effects. Prior to stepping up therapy, it is important to check medication compliance, proper inhaler technique, and control of environmental triggers. If asthma is well controlled for at least 3 months, the recommendation is to step down therapy. Studies show that guideline-based management significantly improves quality of life. Table 13.3 lists the common medications used to treat asthma in the acute and chronic setting [8,12].

Perioperative complications

It is known that the incidence of postoperative pulmonary complications is increased in patients with underlying lung disease. Although the frequency of complications that occur in asthmatics undergoing surgery and general anesthesia are low, some complications can be life threatening. The risk of complications depends on the type of surgery performed, the severity of asthma at the time of surgery, and the type of anesthesia used. It is well accepted that well-controlled asthma is not a risk factor for postoperative pulmonary complications [13,14]; however, poorly controlled asthma is a risk factor [11,15].

Therefore, the goal of managing the asthmatic patient undergoing surgery is to achieve good control of the disease in order to reduce the occurrence of operative and postoperative complications. According to one study, about 6.5% of asymptomatic asthmatics develop bronchospasm during surgery [16]. Furthermore, the incidence of operative and postoperative complications has been reported to be 24% in an asthmatic population [15]. Warner and colleagues performed a retrospective study in asthmatics undergoing surgery and observed the frequency of bronchospasm in the perioperative period to be 1.7% [17]. Characteristics associated with complications included recent use of anti-asthmatic drugs, recent asthma symptoms, older age, and recent therapy in a medical facility for asthma. Potential complications in asthmatics that may contribute to an increased risk of postoperative pulmonary complications, and need to be addressed when considering surgery include (1) bronchospasm, which may be precipitated by instrumentation, drugs, infection, aspiration, trauma, and emergence from anesthesia; (2) pain; (3) fluid shifts; and (4) delayed mobilization. Specifically, exacerbations of obstructive symptoms are common after the infusion of general anesthetics [18]. This risk of postoperative complications can be increased even more with concurrent active smoking or COPD. Reduction of these complications can occur with careful preoperative assessment and perioperative management. Perioperative management of asthma involves the following: (1) adequate control of airway hyper-responsiveness; (2) detection of infection before surgery; (3) control of anesthesia; and (4) aggressive treatment of acute attacks. The NAEPP consensus statement recommends that patients with asthma undergo preoperative evaluation to determine asthma control [11].

Preoperative evaluation

The goal of preoperative evaluation of the asthmatic undergoing surgery is to assess their risk of developing intraoperative and postoperative pulmonary complications. Preoperative evaluation should begin with a detailed history and physical exam. It is important to evaluate activities of daily living and physical status; presence of symptoms consistent with infection; presence of allergies; factors known to trigger attacks; use of medications; presence of asthma symptoms; previous history of surgery and anesthesia; and any coexisting disorders [10,19].

It is crucial to distinguish between an asymptomatic asthmatic and one with active disease prior to surgery. Patients with active disease may require more detailed preoperative evaluation to determine precipitating factors and the degree of physiologic impairment. It is important to ascertain whether the patient has other conditions that are potential triggers during the stress of a surgery. Recognition of precipitating factors is essential in asthma management; therefore, physicians should focus on obtaining a history pertaining to infection, allergic factors, irritants, emotional triggers, weather changes, and physical exertion. Elective surgery should not be performed if active bronchospasm is present, and should be postponed until the patient is well controlled and back to baseline status. Assessing control during the preoperative evaluation is necessary, as factors that have been shown to correlate with perioperative bronchospasm include use of anti-bronchospastic medications, recent exacerbations, and recent visit to a medical facility for asthma treatment [19].

Physical exam should focus on detecting signs of acute bronchospasm, active infection, chronic lung disease and right heart failure. A prolonged expiratory phase can be assessed by performing a forced expiratory time (FET) test, which involves listening over the trachea while the patient exhales forcibly. An FET > 6 seconds correlates with a lowered FEV1/FVC and should prompt further investigation [8].

In addition to a history and physical exam, preoperative evaluation may include laboratory studies and other tests, the necessity of which should be determined on a case-by-case basis. Some controversy exists about the utility of pulmonary function tests (PFTs) in the preoperative evaluation. The 2006 American College of Physicians guidelines recommend that clinicians not use preoperative PFTs routinely for predicting the risk for postoperative pulmonary complications [20].

Pulmonary function tests are recommended in asthma patients if clinical evaluation cannot determine if the patients are at their best baseline and that airflow obstruction is optimally reduced. Pulmonary function tests may identify patients who would benefit from more aggressive preoperative management; however, they should not be used as the primary factor to deny surgery. All candidates for lung resection should undergo preoperative PFTs, and such testing should be performed selectively in patients undergoing other procedures [14,21]. Arterial blood gases are also not routinely needed as part of the preoperative evaluation. In severe cases of asthma, ABGs and PFTs may be indicated [19]; however, there are no data suggesting that hypercapnea identifies high-risk patients who would not otherwise have been identified [22].

Once asthma control is assessed, the goal before surgery is to make sure patients are free of wheezing, with a peak flow greater than 80% of predicted [14]. Step-up in asthma therapy is recommended for those patients who are not well controlled [4,11]. If necessary, patients should receive steroids to achieve this control. Studies show that corticosteroid-dependent asthmatics can undergo surgery with minimal complications, provided that they have optimal preoperative clinical evaluation and receive a hydrocortisone regimen prior to surgery [13,23]. In these studies, there was a low risk of postoperative bronchospasm, infections, adrenal insufficiency, and death associated with steroid use.

Preoperative management

The preoperative period should focus on avoidance of triggering factors, pulmonary physiotherapy, control of respiratory infection, and fluid and electrolyte correction [10]. According to Enright [24], preoperative management should include the following:

1. Treatment of bronchospasm with a beta agonist.
2. If at risk for complications, preoperative treatment with 40–60 mg prednisone/day is suggested.
3. Treat any infections.
4. Correct any fluid or electrolyte abnormalities.
5. Prophylactic cromolyn treatment to prevent degranulation of mast cells and release of mediators should be continued.
6. Chest physiotherapy.
7. Treat other comorbid conditions.
8. Smoking cessation.

Recommendations for asthma-related drug therapy prior to surgery include continuation of beta agonist therapy, and inhaled and systemic steroids. An inhaled short-acting beta agonist is recommended 30 minutes prior to intubation, and can be continued in the perioperative and postoperative period. Theophylline should be discontinued the evening before surgery. The leukotriene inhibitors help maintain asthma control, but have no benefit in the acute setting [25]. Their effects continue for up to 3 weeks after cessation of treatment. The recommendation is that the drug be given the morning of surgery and resumed once the patient is taking oral medications.

The decision to administer systemic corticosteroids in the preoperative period will depend on the patient. Woods and colleagues showed that oral methylprednisolone, 40 mg for 5 days before surgery decreased post-intubation wheezing in newly diagnosed or poorly compliant asthmatics [8]. Mitsuta and colleagues concluded that corticosteroid treatment reduces airway hyperresponsiveness and prevents perioperative asthma attacks by suppressing the production of inflammatory cytokines [26]. Other studies have shown that combined treatment with corticosteroids and a beta-2 adrenergic agonist can improve preoperative lung function and decrease the incidence of wheezing following endotracheal intubation [19]. There is evidence that asthmatics treated with steroids can undergo surgical procedures with a low risk of complications [13,23].

Some authors recommend routine administration of 1–2 doses of systemic steroids in the 12 hours prior to surgery to prevent bronchoconstriction at that time of intubation [13,23]. The recommendation is to reserve preoperative systemic steroids to patients with a history of poorly controlled, severe or steroid-dependent asthma. Steroid-induced immunosuppression is unlikely, unless the patient has been on systemic steroids for > 3 weeks within the last 6 months and is undergoing major surgery or stress. Patients who have taken steroids for less than 3 weeks are unlikely to have adrenal insufficiency and should continue usual doses of steroids perioperatively. Patients taking prednisone at a dose greater than 20 mg/day for 3 weeks or more should be assumed to have HPA axis suppression and may need an increased dose of steroids perioperatively [19]. Stress dose steroids (hydrocortisone 100 mg IV Q8 hours) with tapering after 24 hours are recommended.

Intraoperative management

Management of asthma in the intraoperative period includes airway management, appropriate choice of anesthetic, minimizing potential triggers of bronchospasm and treatment of acute bronchospasm. Patients with asthma can present a challenge, and therefore consideration of proper technique and drugs to be utilized is key to avoiding bronchospasm. This is less of a concern in patients who are well controlled. Bronchial hyperreactivity is an important risk factor for potential perioperative bronchospasm. During anesthesia, with or without tracheal intubation, there is a reduction of tone in either the palatal or pharyngeal muscles accompanied by a lung volume reduction and an increase in the layer of liquid on the airway wall. These factors predispose to airway resistance and airflow limitation. Instrumentation of the airway causes reflex bronchoconstriction via the parasympathetic nervous system.

Therefore, the goal during anesthesia is to minimize factors that trigger bronchospasm. Groeben demonstrated a decrease in lung function due to endotracheal intubation, even in symptom-free asthmatics [27]. Therefore, if possible, regional anesthesia is preferred to decrease the risk of bronchospasm. If general anesthesia is required, then prophylactic bronchodilator therapy, volatile anesthetics, propofol, opioids, and muscle relaxants may minimize the risk. The decision whether to intubate the trachea, provide anesthesia by mask, or use a laryngeal mask airway (LMA) is a clinical decision. There is evidence that tracheal intubation causes reversible increases in airway resistance not seen with placement of an LMA. In the perioperative period, bronchospasm can be triggered by laryngoscopy, tracheal intubation, airway suctioning, cold inspired gases, and tracheal extubation, and onset of bronchospasm during general anesthesia typically occurs at induction [8].

Stress is also known to be a trigger for bronchospasm in asthma, so in the setting of preoperative anxiety in a mild asthmatic, the use of sedatives may be useful [10]. The increased airway resistance seen with tracheal intubation can be minimized or prevented, with the use of bronchodilators, steroids, and lidocaine prior to intubation [10]. In addition, studies reveal that the combination of intravenous lidocaine and salbutamol in patients with hyperreactivity may be more effective than either agent alone [27,28].

The choice of anesthetics to be administered during surgery is an important decision to be made by the anesthesiologist. Table 13.4 lists some of the common anesthetics used in asthmatics. Perioperative medications can have

Table 13.4 Common medications used in the management of asthma (adapted from [8] and [12]).

Asthma drug therapy	
Drug	**Mechanism of action**
Acute therapy	
Inhaled short-acting beta-adrenergic agonist	Beta agonist
Inhaled anticholinergic	Muscarinic anti-inflammatory effects (monotherapy not recommended; can be added to beta-agonist therapy for longer-lasting bronchodilator effect)
Parenteral corticosteroids	Anti-inflammatory effects
Volatile anesthetic	Smooth muscle dilation, vagal block, anti-inflammatory actions
Ketamine	Sympathomimetic and endothelin pathway
Magnesium sulfate	Smooth muscle relaxation
Maintenance therapy	
Long-acting beta agonist	Beta agonist
Inhaled corticosteroids	Anti-inflammatory effects
Leukotriene modifiers	Inhibit leukotriene pathway
Anti-IgE therapy	Binds IgE and reduces circulating levels

bronchodilator effects [10], but some can induce bronchospasm via histamine release, muscarinic activity, or by provoking allergic reactions. Inhalational anesthetics possess bronchodilatory effects, decrease airway responsiveness, and decrease histamine-induced bronchospasm [29]. Therefore volatile anesthetic agents are useful in patients with obstructive airway disease [8]. Inhalational anesthetics, such as sevoflurane and isoflurane, have bronchodilator properties, and are appropriate for use in patients with asthma. These agents, at times, are used to treat status asthmaticus that is resistant to medical therapy [30]. These bronchodilator effects are more prominent in the peripheral airways than in the central airways. Desflurane, however, may cause increased secretions, coughing, laryngospasm, and bronchospasm [31,32], and is not recommended for use in asthmatics.

Certain intravenous anesthetics also have properties that may be beneficial for preventing bronchospasm. In general, intravenous (IV) induction agents are safe for use in asthmatics [8]. Intravenous agents such as ketamine and propofol are both useful to prevent increased airway resistance during tracheal intubation. Ketamine is an IV general anesthetic that has excellent induction characteristics, in addition to

sympathomimetic bronchodilatory properties, and has been shown to be effective in treating wheezing in asthmatics who require anesthesia and intubation [19]. Ketamine relaxes the bronchodilator musculature and prevents the bronchoconstriction induced by histamine. These effects result from direct action on bronchial muscle and potentiation of catecholamines. However, it is usually administered with an anticholinergic because it increases bronchial secretions.

Propofol, a widely used short-acting IV anesthetic, has been associated with less bronchoconstriction during induction than other anesthetic agents [33], and is considered safe to use in patients with asthma. In vitro data suggest that propofol has a direct airway smooth muscle relaxant action [34]. The airway smooth muscle relaxation may also occur through vagally mediated mechanisms. Lidocaine intravenously can also prevent bronchospasm by attenuating sensory responses to airway instrumentation or irritation; however, inhalation of lidocaine can be irritating and aggravate bronchospasm [35]. Opioids are also useful during the intraoperative period. They can be administered to suppress the cough reflex and to achieve deep anesthesia [36]; however, attention needs to be paid to making sure these effects are not prolonged in the postoperative period. Opioids have some histamine-releasing effects, but fentanyl and analogous agents can be used safely in patients with obstructive lung disease.

Neuromuscular blocking agents (NMBAs) may be utilized in the intraoperative period as well, and are typically selected based on their affinity for M2 and M3 receptors; histamine-releasing effects; and duration of action. Neuromuscular blocking agents are the most common medications to cause allergic reactions. Those NMBAs with more affinity for M3 receptors, such as vecuronium, rocuronium, and pancuronium, can be used safely [24]. Atracurium and mivacurium have dose-dependent histamine-releasing effects and can cause bronchoconstriction [36], whereas cisatracurium does not cause histamine release or bronchospasm. Rocuronium is a reasonable choice for the asthmatic that requires rapid sequence intubation [37]. Although there are many anesthetics that are safe to use in asthmatics and that may minimize the risk of bronchospasm, it is important to keep in mind that inadequate anesthesia during surgery can precipitate bronchospasm (Table 13.5).

There are no specific guidelines for mechanical ventilation methods in asthmatics; however, it is important to prevent dynamic hyperinflation or auto-PEEP, which can easily occur in patients with obstructive disease and result in hemodynamic instability. The development of auto-PEEP is usually due to inadequate or short expiratory times. This can be corrected by using higher inspiratory flow rates, smaller tidal volumes and by decreasing the respiratory rate. Attention to volume status during the operative period is also necessary in order to prevent volume overload and pulmonary edema, which can precipitate bronchospasm.

Despite precautions to minimize perioperative complications in the asthmatic undergoing surgery, intraoperative bronchospasm may still occur. Intraoperative bronchospasm

Table 13.5 Common anesthetic agents that can be utilized in asthmatics.

Anesthetics safe to use in asthmatics	
Drug	**Comments**
Local Lidocaine	Inhaled lidocaine may cause airway irritation

Inhalational
  Sevflurane
  Isoflurane
  Halothane
	Can be useful in status asthmaticus

Intravenous
  Ketamine
  Propofol
  NMBAs
 	
  Opioids
	Ketamine may cause increased airway secretions
	
	Atracurium and mivacurium have bronchoconstrictive properties

NMBAs, neuromuscular blocking agents.

may be diagnosed by ventilatory abnormalities such as increased peak airway pressures, which indicate increased airway resistance and expiratory wheezing. The treatment of intraoperative bronchospasm should focus on attempting to determine the etiology while treating the patient. The differential diagnosis for intraoperative bronchospasm includes obstruction of the tracheal tube, endobronchial intubation, aspiration, pulmonary embolus, pulmonary edema, pneumothorax, anaphylaxis, adrenal axis and heart failure. Initial treatment involves preventing hypoxemia, and deepening the level of anesthesia, which may be helpful in reducing bronchospasm [8]. This can be done via IV or inhalational route. In patients with status asthmaticus, therapy with inhalational anesthetic agents has been shown to be successful [30]. Next, a rapid acting beta-2 agonist should be administered via a nebulizer or MDI. In the acute setting, consider high-dose steroids, although the effect will take 4–6 hours [38]. If refractory bronchospasm occurs, IV epinephrine can be administered if necessary, although it is not routinely recommended [11]. In patients with severe, acute asthma, who have received maximal inhaled bronchodilator therapy and systemic glucocorticoids and who have not responded adequately, a single dose of magnesium sulfate (2 g IV) is recommended (due to efficacy, low cost, and safety) [4]. Leukotriene receptor antagonists and mast cell inhibitors have no role in the treatment of acute bronchospasm, and

methylxanthines, such as aminophylline, are no longer recommended in the acute setting [11,19].

Postoperative management

The postoperative period is an important part of the management of asthmatics undergoing surgery, and measures should be taken to decrease complications in this period. The GINA guidelines recommend criteria for extubation that may assist the physician [4]. The emergence phase from anesthesia is important to consider in the asthmatic patient, with a slow emergence from anesthesia minimizing the risk of bronchospasm [8]. Aspiration is a risk in the postoperative period; therefore caution must be taken when extubation is being considered. Prior to extubation, respiratory mechanics should be assessed to evaluate for any factors that may result in extubation failure and other postoperative complications. Certain asthmatics may require postoperative mechanical ventilation for a brief period of time, especially in the setting of significant bronchospasm intraoperatively.

To minimize the risk of postoperative complications, the following interventions are key: adequate analgesia, good bronchodilator therapy, incentive spirometry, and early mobilization [8]. The use of epidural anesthesia with local anesthetics increases tidal volume and vital capacity and preserves diaphragmatic function during thoracotomy or laparotomy [10]. Furthermore, studies have shown that epidural anesthesia decreases postoperative atelectasis [39]. There is no consensus to recommend systemic opioid versus epidural drug administration. In patients that have ventilatory difficulty postextubation, non-invasive positive pressure ventilation can be considered [40].

The treatment of asthma, once the patient is out of surgery, is the same as the care of any patient with asthma as shown in Table 13.3.

Conclusion

Although obstructive lung disease may present a challenge in the perioperative period, well-controlled asthma decreases the risk of developing complications. The key in management of the asthmatic in the perioperative period is to establish a sense of disease control, and optimize therapy prior to surgery. Decreasing the risk of complications includes proper management in the preoperative, intraoperative, and postoperative period.

References

1. Lazarus SC. Clinical practice. Emergency treatment of asthma. *N Engl J Med* 2010; **363**: 755–64.

2. The state of asthma in America. Two Landmark Surveys. 2009. http://www.asthmainamerica.com.

3. American Lung Association. *Trends in Asthma Morbidity and Mortality*. 2010. www.lungusa.org.

4. Global Initiative for Asthma (GINA). *Global Strategy for Asthma Management and Prevention*. 2008. www.ginasthma.org.

5. Cockcroft DW, Swystun VA. Asthma control versus asthma severity. *J Allergy*

Clin Immunol 1996; **98** (6 Pt 1): 1016–18.

6. Chen H, Gould MK, Blanc PD *et al.* Asthma control, severity, and quality of life: quantifying the effect of uncontrolled disease. *J Allergy Clin Immunol* 2007; **120**: 396–402.

7. Taylor DR, Bateman ED, Boulet LP *et al.* A new perspective on concepts of

asthma severity and control. *Eur Respir J* 2008; **32**: 545–54.

8. Woods BD, Sladen RN. Perioperative considerations for the patient with asthma and bronchospasm. *Br J Anaesth* 2009; **103** (Suppl 1): i57–i65.

9. Lawal I, Bakari AG. Reactive airway and anaesthesia: challenge to the anaesthetist and the way forward. *Afr Health Sci* 2009; **9**: 167–9.

10. Yamakage M, Iwasaki S, Namiki A. Guideline-oriented perioperative management of patients with bronchial asthma and chronic obstructive pulmonary disease. *J Anesth* 2008; **22**: 412–28.

11. National Asthma Education and Prevention Program. Expert Panel Report 3. Guidelines for the diagnosis and management of asthma. *National Heart, Lung, and Blood Institute*; 2007. www nhlbi nih gov/guidelines/asthma/ 2011.

12. Fanta CH. Asthma. *N Engl J Med* 2009; **360**: 1002–14.

13. Kabalin CS, Yarnold PR, Grammer LC. Low complication rate of corticosteroid-treated asthmatics undergoing surgical procedures. *Arch Intern Med* 1995; **155**: 1379–84.

14. Smetana GW. Postoperative pulmonary complications: an update on risk assessment and reduction. *Cleve Clin J Med* 2009; **76** (Suppl 4): S60–5.

15. Gold MI, Helrich M. A study of complications related to anesthesia in asthmatic patients. *Anesth Analg* 1963; **42**: 238–93.

16. Shnider SM, Papper EM. Anesthesia for the asthmatic patient. *Anesthesiology* 1961; **22**: 886–92.

17. Warner DO, Warner MA, Barnes RD *et al.* Perioperative respiratory complications in patients with asthma. *Anesthesiology* 1996; **85**: 460–7.

18. Liccardi G, Lobefalo G, Di FE *et al.* Strategies for the prevention of asthmatic, anaphylactic and anaphylactoid reactions during the administration of anesthetics and/or contrast media. *J Investig Allergol Clin Immunol* 2008; **18**: 1–11.

19. Burburan SM, Xisto DG, Rocco PR. Anaesthetic management in asthma. *Minerva Anesthesiol* 2007; **73**: 357–65.

20. Qaseem A, Snow V, Fitterman N *et al.* Risk assessment for and strategies to reduce perioperative pulmonary complications for patients undergoing noncardiothoracic surgery: a guideline from the American College of Physicians. *Ann Intern Med* 2006; **144**: 575–80.

21. Smetana GW. Preoperative pulmonary evaluation. *N Engl J Med* 1999; **340**: 937–44.

22. Fisher BW, Majumdar SR, McAlister FA. Predicting pulmonary complications after nonthoracic surgery: a systematic review of blinded studies. *Am J Med* 2002; **112**: 219–25.

23. Pien LC, Grammer LC, Patterson R. Minimal complications in a surgical population with severe asthma receiving prophylactic corticosteroids. *J Allergy Clin Immunol* 1988; **82**: 696–700.

24. Enright A. Bronchospastic disease and emergency surgery. *Middle East J Anesthesiol* 2004; **17**: 927–38.

25. Reiss TF, Chervinsky P, Dockhorn RJ *et al.* Montelukast, a once-daily leukotriene receptor antagonist, in the treatment of chronic asthma: a multicenter, randomized, double-blind trial. Montelukast Clinical Research Study Group. *Arch Intern Med* 1998; **158**: 1213–20.

26. Mitsuta K, Shimoda T, Fukushima C *et al.* Preoperative steroid therapy inhibits cytokine production in the lung parenchyma in asthmatic patients. *Chest* 2001; **120**: 1175–83.

27. Groeben H, Schlicht M, Stieglitz S, Pavlakovic G, Peters J. Both local anesthetics and salbutamol pretreatment affect reflex bronchoconstriction in volunteers with asthma undergoing awake fiberoptic intubation. *Anesthesiology* 2002; **97**: 1445–50.

28. Silvanus MT, Groeben H, Peters J. Corticosteroids and inhaled salbutamol in patients with reversible airway obstruction markedly decrease the incidence of bronchospasm after tracheal intubation. *Anesthesiology* 2004; **100**: 1052–7.

29. Corssen G, Gutierrez J, Reves JG, Huber FC, Jr. Ketamine in the anesthetic management of asthmatic patients. *Anesth Analg* 1972; **51**: 588–96.

30. Jagoda A, Shepherd SM, Spevitz A, Joseph MM. Refractory asthma, Part 1: Epidemiology, pathophysiology, pharmacologic interventions. *Ann Emerg Med* 1997; **29**: 262–74.

31. Klock PA Jr, Czeslick EG, Klafta JM, Ovassapian A, Moss J. The effect of sevoflurane and desflurane on upper airway reactivity. *Anesthesiology* 2001; **94**: 963–7.

32. Goff MJ, Arain SR, Ficke DJ, Uhrich TD, Ebert TJ. Absence of bronchodilation during desflurane anesthesia: a comparison to sevoflurane and thiopental. *Anesthesiology* 2000; **93**: 404–8.

33. Wu RS, Wu KC, Sum DC, Bishop MJ. Comparative effects of thiopentone and propofol on respiratory resistance after tracheal intubation. *Br J Anaesth* 1996; **77**: 735–8.

34. Ouedraogo N, Roux E, Forestier F *et al.* Effects of intravenous anesthetics on normal and passively sensitized human isolated airway smooth muscle. *Anesthesiology* 1998; **88**: 317–26.

35. Groeben H, Silvanus MT, Beste M, Peters J. Combined lidocaine and salbutamol inhalation for airway anesthesia markedly protects against reflex bronchoconstriction. *Chest* 2000; **118**: 509–15.

36. Groeben H. Strategies in the patient with compromised respiratory function. *Best Pract Res Clin Anaesthesiol* 2004; **18**: 579–94.

37. Sparr HJ, Beaufort TM, Fuchs-Buder T. Newer neuromuscular blocking agents: how do they compare with established agents? *Drugs* 2001; **61**: 919–42.

38. Jagoda A, Shepherd SM, Spevitz A, Joseph MM. Refractory asthma, Part 2: Airway interventions and management. *Ann Emerg Med* 1997; **29**: 275–81.

39. Ballantyne JC, Carr DB, deFerranti S *et al.* The comparative effects of postoperative analgesic therapies on pulmonary outcome: cumulative meta-analyses of randomized, controlled trials. *Anesth Analg* 1998; **86**: 598–612.

40. Nowak R, Corbridge T, Brenner B. Noninvasive ventilation. *J Allergy Clin Immunol* 2009; **124** (2 Suppl): S15–18.

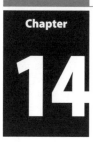

Chapter 14
Acute lung injury and the acute respiratory distress syndrome

Raja-Elie E. Abdulnour and Bruce D. Levy

Introduction and definitions

The acute respiratory distress syndrome (ARDS) is a devastating disorder caused by many underlying medical and surgical diseases. In 1967, Ashbaugh and colleagues first described some key features of ARDS, including: (a) respiratory distress and tachypnea; (b) severe hypoxemia; (c) diffuse alveolar infiltrates on chest radiography; and (d) decreased lung compliance, all occurring in the setting of an acute medical or surgical illness [1]. While this descriptive definition lacks specificity, it encompasses the fundamental concept that ARDS is diffuse lung injury caused either by a direct (e.g., aspiration of gastric contents) or an indirect (e.g., sepsis) pulmonary insult.

In hopes of standardizing clinical care and research studies, attempts have been made to apply more strict criteria to the definition of ARDS. Murray and colleagues in 1988 proposed a comprehensive definition of ARDS, including details on: the severity of lung injury, the mechanism of lung injury, and the presence of non-pulmonary organ dysfunction [2]. Lung injury was quantified based on the severity of four parameters and termed the Lung Injury Score (LIS); it includes: (a) the ratio of the partial pressure of arterial oxygen to the fraction of inspired oxygen (P_aO_2/F_iO_2), (b) the level of positive end-expiratory pressure (PEEP) applied during mechanical ventilation, (c) the static lung compliance, and (d) the extent of alveolar infiltrates on chest radiographs. While the presence of non-pulmonary organ dysfunction and the mechanism of lung injury have important clinical consequences (see below), surprisingly, the extent of lung injury has little predictive value for the clinical course of ALI [3–6]. Thus, in 1994 the American–European Consensus Conference Committee recommended simpler definitions for both ALI and ARDS, requiring only four diagnostic criteria: an acute onset, a $PaO_2/FIO_2 < 300$, bilateral infiltrates and absence of left atrial hypertension [1]. These definitions had the advantages of being applied easily to both clinical work and research protocols [3].

However, the definition of "acute lung injury" (PaO_2/FIO_2 300) was too inclusive and could not be used to risk-stratify patients with ARDS. Therefore, a task force of experts convened in Berlin to update the definition [7]. The most notable change from the AECC definition is elimination of acute lung injury (ALI) as a category and creation of three categories of ARDS based on severity of hypoxemia (as defined by PaO_2/FlO_2 ratio: mild, 200–300; moderate, 101–199; severe, 100). Four ancillary variables were also considered for the definition: radiographic severity, respiratory system compliance, positive end-expiratory pressure, and corrected expired volume per minute. Retrospective application of the definition to preexisting data revealed that the ancillary variables (radiographic severity, respiratory system compliance, positive end expiratory pressure, and expiratory volume) did not contribute to mortality prediction, so these were not included in the definition. Mild, moderate, and sever ARDS were associated with increased mortality rates (27%, 32%, and 45%, respectively) and increased median duration of mechanical ventilation in survivors. Compared with the AECC definition, the Berlin definition of ARDS better predicted mortality and is now the standard definition (Table 14.1).

Although the new definition should be used in future clinical care and research on ARDS, prior literature, including most of the citations in this chapter, refer to the previous AECCC definition [8]. In general, the old definition of acute lung injury (ALI) refers to patients with what is now termed "mild ARDS" and the prior definition of ARDS now encompasses patients with both "moderate" and "severe" ARDS.

Incidence

Until recently, retrospective analyses had reported an annual incidence of ARDS between 1.5 and 70 cases/100,000 [4,9,10]. A recent evaluation of all cases of ALI and ARDS over a 1-year period managed in all the adult ICUs of King County, Washington, reported the results of the first large prospective study of the incidence of, and mortality associated with, ALI and ARDS in the USA [11]. The King County Lung Injury Project (KCLIP) generated national estimates of 86 ALI cases per 100,000, or almost 200,000 cases per year. The incidence of these two syndromes seems considerably higher than previously thought and much higher than that reported from other countries [4].

Medical Management of the Surgical Patient, ed. Michael F. Lubin, Thomas F. Dodson, and Neil H. Winawer. Published by Cambridge University Press. © Cambridge University Press 2013.

Table 14.1 The Berlin Definition of Acute Respiratory Distress Syndrome [1].

Timing	Within 1 week of a known clinical insult or new or worsening respiratory symptoms
Chest imaging (Chest X-ray or computed tomography scan)	Bilateral opacities – not fully explained by effusions, lobar/lung collapse, or nodules
Origin of edema	Respiratory failure not fully explained by cardiac failure or fluid overload Need objective assessment (e.g., echocardiography) to exclude hydrostatic edema if no risk factory present
Oxygenation 　Mild 　Moderate 　Severe	 200 mm Hg $<$ PaO_2/FIO_2 $\leq$ 300 mm Hg with PEEP or CPAP $\geq$ 5 cm H_2O^a 100 mm Hg $<$ PaO_2/FIO_2 $\leq$ 200 mm Hg with PEEP $\geq$ 5 cm H_2O PaO_2/FIO_2 $\leq$ 100 mm Hg with PEEP $\geq$ 5 cm H_2O

a Supplemental oxygen may be delivered noninvasively in mild acute respiratory distress syndrome
1. Modified from Ranieri, V.M., et al., *Acute respiratory distress syndrome: the Berlin Definition*. JAMA, 2012. **307**(23): p. 2526-33.

The incidence of ALI and ARDS increases with age. The lowest age-specific incidence was in those 15–19 years of age (16 cases per 100,000 person-years) whereas the incidence increased with age to a peak of 306 cases per 100,000 person-years in persons 75–84 years of age. With the expansion of the elderly population of the USA, the incidence of ALI and ARDS is expected to grow rapidly with a dramatic impact on the national burden of disease. From a more practical perspective, 11% of all ICU admissions (including community and tertiary care centers) suffer from acute respiratory failure, with ~20% of these patients meeting criteria for ALI [4]. Thus, approximately one out of every 50 patients admitted to ICUs will suffer from ALI or ARDS.

Associated clinical disorders and risk factors

Most cases of ARDS ($>$ 80%) are caused by a relatively few number of clinical disorders (Table 14.2). The majority of ARDS cases (~45%) are seen in medical patients suffering from severe sepsis syndrome and/or bacterial pneumonia [4,6,12,13]. The recent KCLIP study found that ALI was caused by severe sepsis in almost 80% of cases, with a pulmonary source seen in 46% [11]. In contrast, primary surgical illnesses are identified as the cause in 8–35% of ARDS cases [4,12,13]. Pulmonary contusion, multiple bone fractures ($>$ two long bones or unstable pelvic fracture), and chest wall trauma are the most frequently reported surgical conditions in ARDS, whereas head trauma, near-drowning, toxic inhalation, and burns are rare causes (Table 14.3) [4,12]. Less frequent, but important, additional conditions associated with ARDS include multiple transfusions ($>$ 10–15 units in 24 hours), aspiration of gastric contents, drug overdose, and severe pancreatitis.

Certain predisposing conditions carry especially high risk. Sepsis is the at-risk diagnosis most frequently associated with the development of ARDS, with some series reporting ALI/ARDS in up to 40% of sepsis cases [6,12]. In contrast, only 25% of at-risk surgical and trauma patients (including abdominal trauma, multiple fractures, pulmonary contusion, near-

Table 14.2 The most common causes of direct and indirect lung injury with their estimated frequency of association with ARDS [4,12].

Direct lung injury	Frequency (% of total ARDS cases)	Indirect lung injury	Frequency (% of total ARDS cases)
Pneumonia	33–46^a	Sepsis	42^b
Aspiration of gastric contents	10–12	Severe trauma	8.1–35
Pulmonary contusion	5–9	Multiple bone fractures	5.3–12
Near-drowning	0.5–1.5	Flail chest	3
		Head trauma	3–9.1
		Burns	1.5
		Multiple transfusions	2.3–20
		Drug overdose	1.5–11
		Pancreatitis	3.6

^{a} Overlap in cases involving pneumonia-induced sepsis.

drowning, and requirement for hypertransfusion) develop ARDS [12]. The ARDS risk of specific surgical diagnoses varies widely. For example, multiple fractures are complicated by ARDS in 11% of cases; whereas near-drowning and trauma requiring multiple transfusions are associated with increased ARDS risks of ~30% and ~40%, respectively (Table 14.3) [6,12,13]. In addition, ARDS risk is markedly increased in patients suffering from more than one predisposing medical or surgical diagnosis; for example, the incidence of ARDS increases from 25% in patients with trauma to 56% in patients

Table 14.3 The estimated incidence of acute respiratory distress syndrome (ARDS) in several conditions associated with surgery and trauma [12,13]. Note the additive risk of ARDS when a surgical condition is complicated by the need for hypertransfusion.

Clinical condition	Incidence of ARDS (%)
Pulmonary contusion	21–25
Multiple fractures ($\geq$ 2 long bones or unstable pelvic fracture)	$\geq$11
Abdominal trauma (penetrating abdominal trauma index > 15)	18
Hypertransfusion (> 15 units in 24 hours)	21–35
Trauma or surgery complicated by hypertransfusion	50
Near-drowning	30

with trauma and sepsis [6,12]. Similar increased ARDS risk is observed in patients with multiple trauma risk factors [12].

In addition to the underlying clinical disorder, several other clinical variables are predictive for the development of ARDS. Older age is one clear and reproducible risk factor [11]. In a series of 271 trauma patients from Seattle, the incidence of ARDS in patients < 30 years of age was 18% and in patients older than 60 years of age, 33% [12]. Chronic alcohol abuse is also an independent risk factor. In a series of 350 medical and surgical patients, ARDS developed in 20% of septic patients with no alcohol abuse history and in 52% with an alcohol abuse history; similarly, the ARDS incidence in trauma patients with and without a chronic alcohol abuse history was 34% and 22%, respectively [13]. While the mechanism(s) involved in this association are unknown, a contribution from occult liver dysfunction is plausible, especially given the role of the liver in several host-defense mechanisms [14] and the clear association between chronic liver disease and ARDS mortality (see below) [13].

Increased severity of critical illness is also associated with progression to ARDS. A study of 175 trauma patients by Moss and colleagues revealed a 2.5-fold increase in the relative risk of developing ARDS in patients with an acute physiology and chronic health evaluation (APACHE) II score of 16 or greater compared with those patients with scores less than 16 [13]. Similarly, Hudson and colleagues reported ARDS incidences in trauma patients of 13% and 41% in patients with APACHE II scores of $\leq$ 9 and > 20, respectively [12]. The correlation between severity of illness and development of ARDS is further established in trauma patients using the trauma-specific injury severity score (ISS). Acute respiratory distress syndrome developed in no trauma patients with an ISS of $\leq$ 9 and in 25% of patients with an ISS > 20 [12]. Finally, severe metabolic acidosis and acidemia are also risk factors for developing ARDS. For example, in 259 drug overdose and aspiration patients, ARDS was threefold more likely to develop in those patients presenting with a serum pH less than 7.25. Similarly, a serum

bicarbonate lower than 20 meq/L was an independent risk factor for ARDS in trauma patients [12]. Surprisingly, despite the number of non-pulmonary risk factors predictive for the development of ARDS, no pulmonary predictor has been identified, including a history of chronic lung disease [4,12].

Early assessment of risk for ARDS

With the absence of proven and effective therapies aimed at already established ALI, strategies focusing on ALI prevention could have substantial impact on outcomes. Integrating predisposing conditions and risk factors for ALI into a scoring system could provide a clinical prediction tool for early detection of patients at risk for developing ALI during a hospital admission. Identifying high-risk patients creates opportunities for preventive interventions.

A recent single-center observational study developed and internally validated an ALI prediction model, the Lung Injury Prediction Score (LIPS), incorporating the risk factors and risk modifiers present at the time of hospital admission, before ALI onset [15]. The LIPS was subsequently refined and externally validated in a prospective multicenter observational cohort study [16]. After screening patients on admission for ALI risk factors and risk modifiers, the incidence of ALI during the hospital stay was measured. The relative importance of these factors in the development of ALI was calculated using multivariate logistic regression analysis and expressed as LIPS weighting points. For example, the presence of sepsis or a history of alcohol abuse both contributed one point to the overall LIPS. Unsurprisingly, the investigators found that a higher LIPS on admission was associated with increased incidence of ALI during that hospitalization. Optimal sensitivity and specificity occurred at LIPS > 4. At that cutoff point, the negative predictive value was excellent (0.97), but the positive predictive value was more modest (0.18). The latter may still be clinically useful if low-cost and low-risk preventive interventions can be instituted, such as the prevention of second-hit exposures like high tidal volume ventilation or blood transfusions.

Mortality

Mortality in ARDS patients has historically been greater than 50% [17–19], leading to significant frustration for critical care physicians and to marked suffering for patients and their families. While several published reports since 1990 indicate significant improvement in ARDS mortality [3–5, 18,20,21], enthusiasm must be tempered given the wide variability in these data [3,6]. Most encouraging is a report by Milberg and colleagues on a cohort of 900 patients with ARDS followed over 11 years at a single medical center (thereby minimizing variability); overall ARDS mortality from 1983 to 1989 was 67%, decreasing to 41% from 1990 to 1993 [18]. Moreover, three additional reports since 1992, including over 600 ARDS patients, revealed mortality rates ranging from 41% to 47% [4,20,21]. Lastly, the KCLIP study, the most recent and largest prospective cohort of ALI patients in the USA, helped identify

Table 14.4 Non-pulmonary and pulmonary risk factors for mortality in acute respiratory distress syndrome (ARDS). Note the relatively few pulmonary-specific risk factors.

Non-pulmonary	Pulmonary
Advanced age	Increased pulmonary dead space
Sepsis	
Non-pulmonary organ failure	Decreased pulmonary static compliance
Preexisting liver disease or cirrhosis	
Chronic alcohol abuse	
Elevated ISS and APACHE II score	
Immunocompromise	

in-hospital mortality of 38.5% adding further credence to the improving ARDS mortality [11]. If ARDS mortality is improving, then what are the possible reasons? Most deaths in ARDS patients are due to non-pulmonary causes, with sepsis and non-pulmonary organ failure accounting for greater than 80% of deaths [17,19,21]. Thus, improvement in ARDS survival may be attributable to advances in the care of septic/infected patients (e.g., improved antimicrobials) and in supporting patients through multiple organ failure. In partial support of this notion is Milberg and colleagues' observation that ARDS mortality from 1983 to 1993 was most significantly decreased in young septic patients, decreasing from 58% to 26% [18].

More important than knowing overall mortality is understanding the risk factors for mortality in ARDS patients, as risk factor presence can help guide prognosis in individuals and identify ARDS subpopulations that may benefit from new or specialized therapies. Similar to the risk factors for developing ARDS, the predominant risk factors for ARDS mortality are non-pulmonary, with only a few primary pulmonary risk factors recently identified (Table 14.4) [20].

The foremost risk factor for ARDS mortality is advanced age [4,11,18,20]. The KCLIP study showed that mortality increased from a minimum of 24% among those 15–19 years old to 60% among those 85 years of age or older (p < 0.001 for trend) [11]. Several prior studies support this relationship. Luhr and colleagues reported only an 18% mortality in ARDS patients younger than 45 years old compared with 60% in patients older than 75 years of age [4]. Milberg and colleagues reported a threefold higher mortality in ARDS patients with sepsis over the age of 60 compared with patients younger than 60 years old [18]. As with the risk for developing ARDS, different medical conditions predisposing to ARDS are associated with varied risks for mortality. Sepsis remains the diagnosis associated with the highest ARDS mortality [3,11,21]. Doyle and colleagues, for example, demonstrated a mortality odds ratio of 2.8 for ALI/ARDS patients presenting with sepsis [3]. In contrast, surgical and trauma ARDS patients, especially

those without direct lung injury, have a markedly better survival rate than other ARDS patients [13,18]. Milberg and colleagues, for example, reported a 40% mortality for all ARDS patients, but only a 28% mortality in trauma patients with ARDS; moreover, this improved survival was observed over the entire 11-year study period [18]. Similarly, the KCLIP study revealed a 24.1% mortality among ARDS patients with severe trauma, whereas mortality among patients with severe sepsis with a suspected pulmonary source or among patients with witnessed aspiration was above 40% [11].

While perhaps intuitive, the presence and severity of non-pulmonary organ failure in the course of ARDS patients are strong predictors of mortality [13,17,19,21]. In several studies including over 400 ARDS patients, non-survivors had an average of twice the number of organs failing compared with survivors [17,19]. Doyle and colleagues found that the presence of any non-pulmonary organ failure in 123 ALI/ARDS patients was most predictive of mortality, with an odds ratio of 8 [3]. Similarly, increased measures of overall systemic illness also correlate with mortality in ARDS. For example, Luhr and colleagues reported a proportional increase between ARDS mortality and the APACHE II score; APACHE II scores of 10 and 40 were associated with 90-day mortalities of 10% and 90%, respectively [4]. Thus, given the *systemic* inflammatory etiology and sequelae of lung injury (see below) [22,23], non-pulmonary organ dysfunction is likely a marker of the severity of systemic injury and thus a good predictor of mortality.

In addition to acquired organ failure, preexisting organ dysfunction in ARDS patients is also a risk factor for increased mortality. In particular, chronic liver disease and cirrhosis is highly associated with poor outcomes [3–5]. Doyle and colleagues observed an odds ratio for mortality in cirrhotic ARDS patients of 5.2 [3]. Moreover, Monchi and colleagues found in over 200 ARDS patients that cirrhosis was associated with a mortality odds ratio of 27; fivefold greater than any other risk factor [5]. The importance of normal liver function for ARDS recovery is further supported by the observation of Moss and colleagues that ARDS mortality is 1.5-fold greater in patients with a history of chronic alcohol abuse [13]. The hepatic mechanism(s) involved in protection and recovery from ARDS are unknown [13]; however, animal models of sepsis demonstrate a clear increase in inflammatory alveolar infiltrates and alveolar damage in the presence of liver injury [14]. Finally, other chronic diseases have been linked to increased ARDS mortality; most notably, chronic immunosuppression and chronic renal disease [4].

Acute lung injury and ARDS are distinguished by the severity of hypoxemia (Table 14.1) [1]. The degree of hypoxemia present early in the course of ALI and ARDS patients has limited prognostic value [3–5,20,21]. The findings of Luhr and colleagues, in a study of 1,200 patients with acute respiratory failure, illustrate this point, revealing equal mortality (~40%) in patients with acute respiratory failure, ALI, and ARDS [4]. Doyle *et al.* also found no mortality difference between two groups of lung injury patients with markedly different oxygenation, patients with a P_aO_2/F_iO_2 from 150–299 had equal mortality (~58%) to patients with a $P_aO_2/F_iO_2 < 150$ [3]. Moreover, additional measures of lung injury and hypoxemia, including the level of PEEP used in mechanical ventilation, the respiratory compliance, the extent of alveolar infiltrates on chest radiography, and the lung injury score (a composite of all these variables) are of little value in predicting mortality from ARDS [3–5]. On the other hand, further analysis of the KCLIP data revealed that mortality in patients who presented with ARDS (41.1%) or who progressed to ARDS after presenting with ALI (41.0%) was higher than that of patients who presented with ALI without progression (28.6%) [11]. This information therefore conveys that it is most important for the clinician not to judge the severity and prognosis of lung injury patients based on initial respiratory parameters but, instead, to rely more on the non-pulmonary risk factors for disease progression and death discussed above and on the progression of hypoxemia over time which seems to have some prognostic value.

Although respiratory parameters are, in general, of little benefit in risk-stratifying ARDS patients, increased pulmonary dead space and decreased pulmonary compliance may be useful independent predictors of mortality [20]. Pulmonary dead space is that volume of ventilated lung that does not participate in gas exchange with the pulmonary arterial circulation; or, in physiologic terms, it is that area of lung with an infinite ventilation to perfusion ratio. Thus, increased dead space leads to hypoventilation and an increase in the partial pressure of arterial carbon dioxide (P_aCO_2). Increased pulmonary dead space is a well-recognized feature of ARDS and likely occurs as a result of diffuse pulmonary vascular injury and microthrombosis [24,25]. Nuckton and colleagues were the first to study the relationship between pulmonary dead space and ARDS mortality. In their study of 179 ARDS patients, early elevated dead space was associated with increased mortality, with dead space being 18% higher in non-survivors compared with survivors [20]. Low pulmonary compliance indicates "stiff" lungs and is decreased in ARDS as a result of pulmonary edema and loss of surfactant [24,26]. In their study on dead space, Nuckton *et al.* also measured static compliance at uniform tidal volumes and reported a small, but significant, association between decreased lung compliance and increased ARDS mortality [20]. Surprisingly, no prior studies have demonstrated such a relationship; however, this may have been due to varying techniques in measuring respiratory compliance [5]. While further studies are needed to confirm these observations, it is exciting to speculate about the clinical utility of these and other, yet identified, pulmonary-specific predictors of ARDS outcome.

Impact of 2009 H1N1 influenza A pandemic

In the spring of 2009, a previously unrecognized strain of influenza A virus emerged and quickly spread around the world. This ultimately evolved into the H1N1 influenza A pandemic, which was characterized by increased incidence of ARDS and death in young previously healthy adults,

immunocompromised patients, and pregnant women [27,28]. Because of the fulminant nature of the H1N1-initiated ALI/ARDS, extreme measures were implemented to manage refractory hypoxemia, such as extracorporeal membrane oxygenation (ECMO) and high-frequency oscillatory ventilation (HFOV), subsequently allowing for further evaluation of these therapies (discussed later in this chapter).

Clinical course and pathogenesis
Early or exudative phase

The natural history of ARDS usually consists of three phases, each with characteristic clinical and pathologic features [24,29,30]. The first, named the early or exudative phase, generally encompasses the first 7 days of illness [24,29,31]. Clinically, this period represents the onset of respiratory symptoms after exposure to an ARDS risk factor. Although the onset of symptoms is usually rapid, 12–36 hours after the initial underlying insult, symptoms can be delayed by 5–7 days [12]. Symptoms are non-specific, including dyspnea, tachypnea, and ultimately respiratory fatigue. Laboratory values are generally not helpful, but an arterial blood gas will confirm that the P_aO_2/F_iO_2 ratio is less than 300 mmHg in ALI and 200 mmHg in ARDS. Plain chest radiographs usually reveal multi-lobar, "fluffy" alveolar and interstitial opacities (Figure 14.1). While these radiographic findings are characteristic, they are not specific for ARDS and are often indistinguishable from other common conditions, especially cardiogenic pulmonary edema [32]. Because the early presenting features of ARDS are non-specific, alternative pulmonary diagnoses should be considered early in the course of illness. Some common alternative disorders include: congestive heart failure, diffuse infectious pneumonia, toxin injury (e.g., crack cocaine, heroin, radiation pneumonitis), and diffuse alveolar hemorrhage. Other important, but less common, alternative pulmonary disorders include: acute interstitial lung diseases (e.g., acute eosinophilic pneumonia, acute interstitial pneumonitis, cryptogenic organizing pneumonia), acute immunologic injury (e.g., lupus pneumonitis, hypersensitivity pneumonitis, Goodpasture's syndrome), and neurogenic pulmonary edema.

Histologically, the exudative phase is marked by diffuse alveolar damage. Features include degeneration of both alveolar capillary endothelial cells and alveolar epithelial cells (type I pneumocytes), leading to loss of the normally tight alveolar barrier to fluid and macromolecules [24,29]. As a result, protein-rich edema accumulates, containing several pro-inflammatory mediators including interleukin-1, interleukin-8, and tumor necrosis factor [22]. In addition, condensed plasma proteins aggregate with cellular debris and dysfunctional pulmonary surfactant to form hyaline membrane whorls in alveolar septae. As demonstrated by computed tomography (CT) scans of ARDS patients (Figure 14.2), this alveolar edema predominantly involves dependent portions of the lung, leading to marked consolidation and atelectasis [30,33]. The major

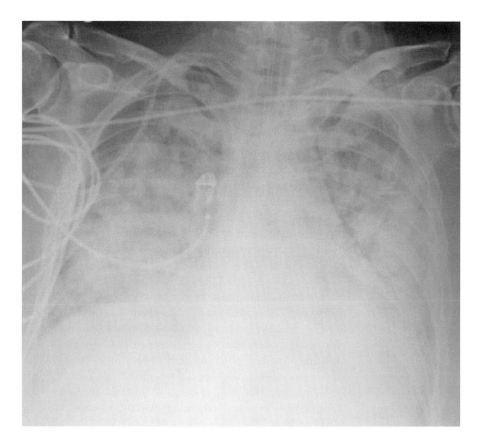

Figure 14.1 Chest radiograph from an acute respiratory distress syndrome (ARDS) patient. This anteroposterior (AP) chest X-ray demonstrates the multilobar and symmetric air space opacities characteristic of the early or exudative phase of ARDS.

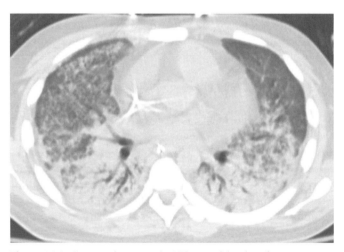

Figure 14.2 Computed tomography (CT) scan of the chest from an acute respiratory distress syndrome (ARDS) patient. This chest CT scan image demonstrates the predominance of dependent alveolar edema and atelectasis in the early or exudative phase of ARDS.

physiologic effect of this pathobiology is a marked decrease in lung compliance, increased intrapulmonary shunt, and hypoxemia [30]. Acute respiratory distress syndrome can be initiated by injury to alveolar epithelial and/or endothelial cells. It remains unknown how a diverse set of clinical disorders can cause such extensive lung injury.

In addition to alveolar injury, pulmonary vascular injury occurs early in ARDS and includes vascular obliteration by both microthrombi and fibrocellular proliferation [25]. These vascular injuries account for the moderate to severe pulmonary hypertension observed in ARDS. Moreover, loss of pulmonary arterial blood flow to ventilated portions of lung increases pulmonary dead space, explaining, in part, why even early ARDS patients can become hypercapneic [20,30].

Intermediate or proliferative phase

The intermediate or proliferative phase of ARDS generally spans from day 7 to approximately day 21 of the disease [24,29]. Histologically, it marks the beginning of lung repair with organization of alveolar exudates and a change from neutrophil to lymphocyte-predominant infiltrates. In addition, type II pneumocytes proliferate along the alveolar basement membrane where they synthesize new surfactant and differentiate into new type I pneumocytes [29]. The proliferative phase is also the clinical point where patients may begin to recover rapidly. Unfortunately, some patients continue to have progressive lung injury and, ultimately, develop pulmonary fibrosis [29,34]. The mechanisms determining progression to fibrosis are unknown, yet the presence of type III procollagen peptide, a marker of pulmonary fibrosis, in alveoli at early stages of ARDS is associated with a protracted clinical course and increased mortality [35].

Late or fibrotic phase

While most ARDS patients have excellent recovery of pulmonary function (see below) [36,37], the few with minimal recovery by 3–4 weeks enter the fibrotic phase of the disease [24]. This late phase is characterized by a transition from alveolar exudates and inflammation to extensive ductal and interstitial fibrosis. These fibrotic changes alter acinar architecture, leading to emphysema-like lesions and large bullae formation [24,29]. In addition, the pulmonary vascular bed undergoes intimal fibroproliferation leading to vascular occlusion and pulmonary hypertension [25]. The physiologic consequences of these pathologic changes include an increased risk for pneumothorax, altered lung compliance, and increased pulmonary dead space [30]. During this phase, patients often require long-term supplemental oxygen and/or ventilatory support. Given the morbidity in this group, it is not surprising that the presence of early pulmonary fibrosis is associated with increased mortality [35,38].

Treatment

General principles

It is important to realize that all medical therapies aimed specifically at lung injury are either unproven or have been unsuccessful. Therefore, the principal goal of ARDS treatment is to support the patient through their disease and allow the lung injury to resolve. This entails optimal general care of critically ill patients, which should include fastidious attention to: (a) recognition and treatment of the underlying at-risk diagnosis for ARDS (e.g., sepsis, pneumonia, trauma); (b) addressing ongoing fevers and infection; (c) minimizing procedures and their complications; (d) maintaining adequate nutrition; and (e) proper prophylaxis against: thromboembolism, gastrointestinal bleeding and injury, and central venous catheter infections. The next step is to ensure the use of lung-protective ventilation strategies with low-tidal volume ventilation, while choosing a restrictive fluid management approach when not in shock. And when faced with refractory hypoxemia, the intensivist needs to identify the treatment option most appropriate to the case at hand. The urgent need for effective management of refractory hypoxemia in ARDS during the H1N1 influenza A pandemic has led to increased awareness and scientific evaluation of the different tools and strategies available. This section will focus on these management principles, offer perspective and insight on several new and promising ARDS-specific therapies and review several treatments of, as yet, unproven benefit.

Management of mechanical ventilation

Ventilator-induced lung injury

While mechanical ventilation can clearly prevent acute hypoxemic death, its potential to aggravate lung injury is well-established [39]. Nearly 30 years ago, Webb and Tierney demonstrated the potential harmful effects of high tidal volume (V_t) mechanical ventilation, observing marked alveolar edema and cellular damage in rats ventilated with high airway pressures and high tidal volumes [40]. Subsequently, Dreyfuss and colleagues, using torso-banding devices in rats to increase airway pressure but limit chest wall excursion and tidal volume, elegantly demonstrated that alveolar damage results from high tidal volume and *not* from high airway pressure [41]. Surprisingly, the alveolar edema and injury induced by high tidal volume ventilation can be completely prevented by applying positive end expiratory pressure (PEEP) [40,41], a maneuver that prevents alveolar collapse at end-expiration. Thus, at least in several animal models, ventilator-induced lung injury appears to require two processes: repeated alveolar over-distension and repeated alveolar collapse.

As described above, ARDS is a heterogeneous process, sparing areas of lung and leaving them with relatively normal compliance. Thus, the impact of ventilator-induced lung injury may be especially prominent in ARDS, where "normal" areas of lung are preferentially over-distended and injured. In fact, in animal models of acute lung injury, high tidal volume ventilation causes additional, synergistic alveolar damage [42]. As a result of these findings in animals, two important theories have emerged regarding mechanical ventilation in ARDS patients. The first is that ventilating ARDS patients with lower tidal volumes may result in less ventilator-induced lung injury and, in turn, improve clinical outcomes, the so-called "lung-protective" ventilation strategy. The second is that prevention of alveolar collapse at end-expiration by addition of PEEP may also reduce ventilator-induced lung injury, the so-called "open-lung" theory [43].

Low tidal volume/lung-protective ventilation

While low-tidal volume ventilation has the theoretical benefit of reducing further lung injury, the principal risks associated with this strategy are respiratory acidosis and lower mean airway pressures, leading to possible alveolar collapse ("de-recruitment" of alveoli) and hypoxemia. Several clinical trials have examined the efficacy of low tidal volume ventilation in ARDS patients [43–46]. Both Stewart *et al.* and Brochard *et al.* randomized over 230 patients with ALI/ARDS to receive either high (formerly conventional) tidal volumes (~12 cm^3/kg predicted body weight) or low tidal volumes (~8 cm^3/kg predicted body weight). In both studies, mortality was equivalent in patients receiving high and low tidal volume ventilation. Moreover, there were no differences in the duration of mechanical ventilation and length of ICU stay between the two groups [39,40]. Importantly, patients in both studies assigned to low-tidal volume ventilation, compared with those assigned to conventional tidal volumes, had significantly higher P_aCO_2 values (so-called "permissive hypercapnia") and lower pH values. Although these data had cast early doubt on the validity of lung-protective ventilation, subsequent studies have yielded more promising results.

Table 14.5 Improved outcomes in acute respiratory distress syndrome (ARDS) with low tidal volume ventilation.[a]

Clinical variable	Low tidal volume (6 cm³/kg)	High tidal volume (12 cm³/kg)
Mortality	31%	40%
Off mechanical ventilation at hospital Day 28	66%	55%

[a] Mechanical ventilation of ARDS patients with a low tidal volume strategy markedly decreases ARDS mortality and leads to more rapid weaning from mechanical ventilation [8]. These findings support the use of tidal volumes of ~6 cm³/kg ideal body weight in ARDS patients.

In 2000, the National Institutes of Health acute respiratory distress syndrome network (ARDS Net) published a large-scale, randomized control trial comparing low-tidal volume (6 cm³/kg predicted body weight) ventilation with high tidal volume (12 cm³/kg predicted body weight) ventilation in over 800 ALI/ARDS patients [44]. High tidal volume patients had their tidal volumes reduced only if the end-inspiratory plateau pressure exceeded 50 cm H_2O; in contrast, low tidal volume patients were permitted to reduce their tidal volumes to as low as 4 cm³/kg if the end-inspiratory plateau pressure exceeded 30 cm H_2O. Remarkably, mortality was significantly lower in the low-tidal volume patients compared with the conventional tidal volume patients, 31% and 40%, respectively. In addition, patients ventilated with low-tidal volumes spent significantly fewer days ventilator-dependent (Table 14.5). A strength of this study was its careful control for other respiratory variables. For example, all study patients were ventilated on volume-cycled assist control mode; and, there were no differences between the two groups in PEEP level, the P_aO_2/F_iO_2 ratio, or the absolute P_aO_2. In addition, respiratory acidosis in the low-tidal volume group was more aggressively treated than in prior studies. In fact, the mean serum pH in the low tidal volume and high tidal volume groups were not significantly different at 7.40 and 7.41, respectively; this was achieved by allowing the respiratory rate to increase to 35 breaths per minute in the low-tidal volume group and by initiating intravenous bicarbonate therapy for a serum pH < 7.30. While further studies would be helpful to confirm the value of low-tidal volume ventilation, several attributes of the ARDS Net study strengthen its findings, including: the large size of the study (it included more patients than all prior studies combined), the "low-tidal volume" group achieved a lower mean tidal volume (~6 cm³/kg) compared with this group in other studies (~8 cm³/kg), and respiratory acidosis was better controlled than in prior studies.

Prevention of alveolar collapse with PEEP

In ARDS, the presence of alveolar and interstitial fluid and the loss of surfactant can markedly decrease lung compliance [30]. Thus, unless end-expiratory pressure is increased, significant alveolar collapse can occur at end-expiration and impair oxygenation by increasing intrapulmonary shunting. The proportion of non-aerated lung responsible for the shunt may be reduced (i.e., recruited) by applying higher levels of PEEP than traditionally used (e.g., 5–12 cm H_2O) in the management of patients with ARDS. Repeated alveolar collapse may also contribute to ventilator-induced lung injury, a phenomenon called atelectrauma [40,41]. However, high PEEP may have serious deleterious effects on other aspects of the patient. First, high levels of PEEP can cause alveolar pressure to exceed pulmonary capillary pressure, creating dead space and potentially increasing pulmonary blood flow through areas of shunt; this may cause both hypoxemia and hypercapnia. Second, excessive alveolar distending pressures may exacerbate ventilator-induced lung injury. And, finally, increased intrathoracic pressures will decrease cardiac pre-load which can decrease systemic blood pressure and critical organ perfusion.

To help assess the overall impact of high PEEP on mortality, three randomized controlled trials have evaluated higher PEEP in patients already receiving pressure and volume-limited ventilation [47–49]. In all three studies, there were no significant differences in mortality, ventilator-free days, length of ICU stay, or extent of organ failure between the low and high PEEP groups. However, in a patient level meta-analysis of these three clinical trials, higher PEEP was associated with improved survival (adjusted RR, 0.90; 95% CI, 0.81–1.00) among the subset of patients with ARDS (P_aO_2/F_iO_2 ratio < 200) [50]. Thus, an open-lung ventilation strategy with high-PEEP could benefit patients with more severe lung injury, but potentially harm patients with P_aO_2/F_iO_2 ratios above 200.

Optimal PEEP

Alveolar distension is determined by the pressure gradient between the alveolus and the space that immediately surrounds it, the pleural space. At end-exhalation, alveoli will collapse if pleural pressure is higher than alveolar pressure, the latter being equal to PEEP. Therefore, optimal PEEP can be considered as the lowest amount of PEEP needed to overcome pleural pressure. Practically speaking, optimal PEEP is 1–2 cm of H_2O higher than pleural pressure.

Pleural pressure is difficult to predict in critical illness due to pleural effusion, elevated abdominal pressure, or variations in the elasticity of the chest wall. For example, a large pleural effusion may raise pleural pressure, thereby reducing transpulmonary pressure at any given PEEP. Unfortunately, direct measurements of pleural pressure in the ICU are rarely possible, and can therefore be estimated only from esophageal pressure. Many assumptions must be made in order to accept that pressure in the esophagus dynamically and accurately reflects pleural pressure. For instance, we must assume that the balloon pressure reflects the esophageal pressure, that the transmural pressure in the esophagus is 0 cm of water, that the esophagus is not compressed by intrathoracic structures such as the heart, that the pressures in the periesophageal area are the same as the pleural pressure, and that pleural pressure is relatively uniform throughout the thorax [51].

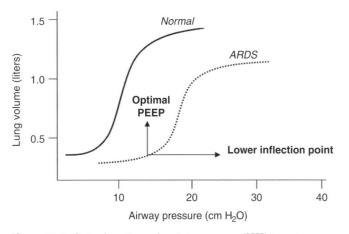

Figure 14.3 Optimal positive end-expiratory pressure (PEEP) in acute respiratory distress syndrome (ARDS) to prevent alveolar collapse at end-exhalation. Schematic static pressure–volume curves for the lung in a normal patient (solid line) and an ARDS patient (dashed line). The arrows mark the lower inflection point, where alveolar opening begins and, therefore, the pressure where PEEP is optimal to prevent alveolar collapse at end-exhalation.

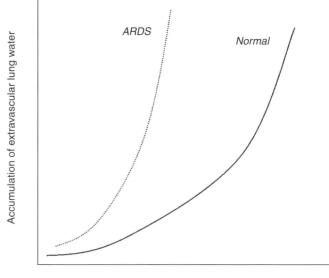

Figure 14.4 Relationship between left atrial pressure and the accumulation of extravascular lung water. Schematic depicting the more rapid accumulation of extravascular lung water with increasing left atrial pressures in an acute respiratory distress syndrome (ARDS) patient (dashed line) compared with a normal patient (solid line).

In most clinical settings, pleural pressure does not need to be measured. The amount of PEEP used is empirically set to minimize F_iO_2 and maximize P_aO_2 [44], with no assurance that the level of PEEP is adequate to prevent significant alveolar collapse at end-expiration. Fortunately, on most modern mechanical ventilators it is possible to construct a pressure–volume curve for the respiratory system. The lower inflection point on the curve represents alveolar opening (or "recruitment"); the pressure at this point is "optimal PEEP" for alveolar recruitment (Figure 14.3) [39,43]. Therefore, titration of the PEEP to the lower inflection point on the static pressure–volume curve might improve oxygenation and minimize lung injury. Again, this theory is referred to as the "open-lung" hypothesis. In our experience, the lower inflection point on the static pressure–volume curve in ARDS is usually from 12–15 cm H_2O.

An alternative method would be to directly estimate pleural pressure. A randomized trial assessed a mechanical-ventilation strategy in which PEEP was adjusted according to end-expiratory transpulmonary pressures [52]. Transpulmonary pressure was measured as the difference between the airway opening pressure and the pleural pressure; pleural pressure was estimated from esophageal pressure. A small catheter with a balloon covering the holes at its end was used to measure pneumatic pressure in the esophagus. PEEP was then adjusted to produce an estimated transpulmonary pressure at end expiration of 0–10 cm of water, according to P_aO_2/F_iO_2 ratio. The esophageal-pressure guided group showed improved oxygenation and respiratory-system compliance at all follow-up time points. The trial was not powered to detect clinically relevant outcomes such as mortality and ventilation-free days. With that in mind, optimal-PEEP ventilation guided by esophageal pressure measurement is a reasonable tool to optimize oxygenation in patients with severe hypoxemia and poor chest wall compliance, such as patients with obesity, elevated abdominal pressures, or pleural effusions.

Fluid management

Increased pulmonary vascular permeability and protein-rich alveolar edema are central features of ARDS [22,24]. Impaired vascular integrity augments the normal increase in extravascular lung water that occurs with increasing left atrial pressure (Figure 14.4). Therefore, maintaining a normal or low left atrial filling pressure should minimize pulmonary edema and improve arterial oxygenation and lung compliance. In several small studies of ARDS patients, aggressive fluid restriction and diuresis reduced extravascular lung water, improved pulmonary mechanics, and in one study improved mortality [53–55]. This ultimately prompted investigators of the ARDS Clinical Trials Network to design a randomized clinical trial aimed at comparing a restrictive and liberal strategy of fluid management [56]. One thousand patients with early ARDS were randomized to the two groups. Attempts at diuresis began 12 hours after resolution of shock (defined as discontinuation of vasopressor use and no intravenous fluid bolus administration). Based on CVP measurements, urine output, and assessments of effective circulation, patients were administered IV furosemide. For example, patients with effective circulation and urine output > 0.5 mL/kg/min received furosemide until CVP fell below 4 in the restrictive group, or below 10 in the liberal group. Although there was no significant difference in mortality at 60 days between the two treatment groups, patients in the group treated according to a restrictive strategy of fluid management had significantly improved lung and central nervous system function and a decreased need for sedation, mechanical ventilation, and intensive care. These salutary effects were achieved without an increase in the frequency of non-pulmonary organ failure or shock. Thus, if there are no hemodynamic or renal contraindications, aggressive attempts at reducing left atrial filling pressures are an important aspect of caring for ARDS patients.

Neuromuscular blockade

Ventilation of ARDS patients with low tidal volumes and permissive hypercapnia is poorly tolerated in the absence of heavy sedation because of the increased drive to breathe. Not infrequently, sedation is either unsuccessful at achieving synchrony between the patient and the ventilator, or causes dose-limiting hypotension. Neuromuscular blockade has been frequently used in such settings. Other theoretical benefits to paralysis include decreased oxygen consumption, stable PEEP requirement thus minimizing atelectrauma, and decreased ventilator-induced lung injury from more accurate tidal volume delivery [57].

A recent randomized controlled trial compared the use of cisatracurium to placebo during the first 48 hours of mechanical ventilation in patients with ARDS [58]. The use of a neuromuscular blockade agent improved the adjusted 90-day survival rate, increased the number of ventilator-free days, and decreased ICU days and the incidence of barotrauma during the first 90 days. Neuromuscular blockade did not significantly improve the overall 90-day mortality, although the study was underpowered for this endpoint. While confirmatory studies are needed, these promising data suggest a therapeutic advantage for the use of neuromuscular blockade early in patients with ARDS who cannot tolerate heavy sedation and permissive hypercapnia.

Treatment of refractory hypoxemia

Recruitment maneuvers

Pulmonary shunting resulting from the perfusion of non-aerated alveoli contributes significantly to hypoxemia, and so ARDS patients may benefit from alveolar recruitment by using higher amounts of PEEP during low volume ventilation. Notably, not all diseased alveoli, in particular some areas in the dependent portions of the lungs, can be recruited by safe PEEP levels. Recruitment maneuvers (RMs), defined as the use of very high levels of PEEP for short periods of time, attempt to recruit these "hard to get" areas while avoiding the potentially adverse consequences of using such high levels for prolonged periods of time.

A variety of techniques have been used in studies evaluating the efficacy and safety of RMs. These include periodic sighs (breaths twice the tidal volume delivered every 25–30 s), one sustained inflation (e.g., PEEP of 35–50 cm H_2O for 30 s), and controlled ventilation at high airway pressures (APRV or

PCIRV). A recent meta-analysis reviewed 40 studies of RMs in close to 1,200 patients with ARDS [59]. It was found that the use of RMs was associated with significant but transient improvement in oxygenation. However, RMs did not improve mortality. In addition, there were no clinically significant changes in short-term hemodynamic or ventilatory variables during RMs, but transient hypotension and desaturation were common. There were few RM-related serious adverse events (e.g., barotrauma or arrhythmias), and only an extremely small number of RMs were terminated early due to adverse events. The authors concluded that while RMs should not be performed on all patients with ARDS, they should be considered on an individualized basis in patients with ALI and life-threatening refractory hypoxemia.

Mechanical ventilation in the prone position

In 1974, Bryan speculated that placing mechanically ventilated ARDS patients into the prone position would improve dependent atelectasis, augment blood flow to ventral lung fields and, thereby, improve ventilation and perfusion matching [60]. Shortly after, several small case series demonstrated impressive improvements in arterial oxygenation after proning; the P_aO_2 in nearly 80% of patients rises 50–60 mmHg within 2 hours of proning [61–64]. While the P_aO_2 will again fall when the patient is supine, re-proning resulted in reproducible gains in arterial oxygenation. While several potential mechanisms have been studied, it still remains unclear how prone positioning improves oxygenation. The following physiologic responses to proning likely contribute to improved arterial oxygenation: (a) decreased intrapulmonary shunt by opening of dependent, atelectatic lung [65]; (b) increased postural drainage of airway secretions; and (c) decreased hydrostatic pressure in dependent and injured lung with subsequent decreased interstitial edema [64]. Although several studies have verified the positive effects of proning on oxygenation [62,63,65,66], until recently, no study has addressed the efficacy of prone positioning on important clinical outcomes.

In 2001, Gattinoni and colleagues randomized over 300 ALI/ARDS patients to supine or intermittent prone mechanical ventilation. While the P_aO_2/F_iO_2 ratio increased by ~50 points in the prone position, both in-hospital and 6-month mortality was equivalent in the supine and proned groups. However, in a post-hoc analysis the sickest quartile of patients (those with a P_aO_2/F_iO_2 ratio < 88, simplified acute physiology (SAP) II score > 49, or a tidal volume >12 cm^3/kg) had a lower 10-day mortality when prone (20%) relative to supine positioning (40%) [67]. This encouraging subgroup analysis led the investigators to organize a second trial in 2009 [68]. More than 300 patients were randomized to supine ventilation or more than 20 hours/day of prone ventilation for 10 days. Patients were then stratified according to severity of hypoxemia; moderate hypoxemia if the P_aO_2/F_iO_2 ratio was between 100 and 200, and severe hypoxemia if the ratio was < 100. Similar to the trial done 8 years earlier, there was no difference in any of the primary and secondary outcomes, including ICU,

28-day and 6-month mortality. Of note, the rate of complications in the proning group of this trial, attended by staff experienced in turning intubated patients, was unacceptably high. The authors of the study followed with a meta-analysis of trials of proning in ARDS patients with severe hypoxemia [69]. A significant improvement in survival among the subset of patients with severe hypoxemia was demonstrated (RR, 0.84; 95% CI, 0.74–0.96) despite an increase in complications including chest tube dislodgement, endotracheal tube obstruction, and facial edema [70]. Therefore, the use of prone positioning should only be considered a rescue strategy in patients with ARDS and severe refractory hypoxemia, and should be limited to centers with specialized equipment and experience.

Inhaled vasodilators

Pulmonary hypertension and right ventricular failure secondary to hypoxic pulmonary vasoconstriction and thromboembolic occlusion of the pulmonary microcirculation are common in ARDS, and may be partially responsible for the high mortality seen in this disease [71]. To address this problem, inhaled pulmonary arterial vasodilators can help curtail right ventricular failure and ventilation/perfusion mismatch caused by refractory hypoxic pulmonary vasoconstriction. Some inhaled vasodilators such as prostacyclin (PGI_2) display additional potential benefits including inhibition of platelet aggregation and anti-inflammatory properties [72]. Commonly used inhaled vasodilators are nitric oxide (NO) and epoprostenol (PGI_2 analog), with similar physiologic effects (improved P_aO_2, reduced pulmonary artery pressure) in ARDS.

Inhaled NO acts locally as a pulmonary arterial vasodilator to selectively increase perfusion to ventilated lung, thereby reducing shunt and improving arterial oxygenation [73]. In 1993, Rossaint and colleagues first tested NO in ARDS patients; administration of 5–20 parts per million (ppm) of NO decreased pulmonary shunt and increased the P_aO_2/F_iO_2 ratio [74]. These positive preliminary findings led to several follow-up randomized clinical trials of NO in ARDS. Although NO reproducibly improves arterial oxygenation, it does not improve mortality or successful ventilator weaning in ARDS patients [75–78]. Of note, pulmonary arterial vasodilation is not always safe. For example, in patients with left-sided heart disease, increased pulmonary arterial blood flow can cause increased left ventricular preload and precipitate acute congestive heart failure. Alternative agents such as inhaled PGI_2 analog lead to similar physiologic improvements with reduced cost [79]. In summary, inhaled vasodilators can be considered for patients with severe refractory hypoxemia, but are not part of the routine care of ARDS patients.

High-frequency oscillatory ventilation (HFOV)

By ventilating at extremely high respiratory rates (5–20 cycles per second), tidal volumes in HFOV can be as low as 1–2 cm^3/kg and high mean airway pressures can be maintained, preventing alveolar collapse while providing lung protective ventilation [80–82].

Early trials of HFOV in adult ARDS patients revealed improved gas exchange but no obvious improvement in mortality [81]. When subjected to a recent meta-analysis that included eight randomized trials (419 patients) uncovered significant reductions in mortality (RR, 0.77; 95% CI, 0.61–0.98) and treatment failure (RR, 0.67; 95% CI, 0.46–0.99) were uncovered, including refractory hypoxemia, among patients receiving HFOV [83]. In contrast, two recent multicenter, randomized trials showed that HFOV was no different from [84] or even inferior [85] to conventional ventilation strategies aimed at targeting low tidal volumes. One of the trials was terminated early because of increased mortality in the HFOV group [85]. Therefore, HFOV should not be applied routinely in patients with ARDS.

Extracorporeal membrane oxygenation (ECMO)

Similar to HFOV, ECMO [86] is another uncommon therapy for refractory hypoxemia that requires a high-level of expertise. Extracorporeal membrane oxygenation provides a clear survival benefit in neonatal ARDS [87,88], but has not proven to result in a survival benefit in adult ARDS [89,90]. To date, ECMO studies have enrolled several hundred adult ARDS patients who otherwise had an expected mortality in excess of 80% [86]. Despite the large number of enrolled subjects, studies have revealed no significant survival benefit for ARDS patients when compared with internal or historical controls [89,90].

Recently however, in the setting of the H1N1 pandemic, a case series of 61 patients from Australia and New Zealand treated with ECMO for severe influenza-associated ARDS reported a survival rate of 79% [91]. In addition, the Conventional Ventilatory Support vs Extracorporeal Membrane Oxygenation for Severe Adult Respiratory Failure (CESAR) trial randomized patients with severe respiratory failure to either consideration for ECMO (with transportation to a single ECMO center) or continued therapy with the best standard practice (i.e. conventional pressure- and volume-limited mechanical ventilation) [92]. Although only 75% of the patients randomized to consideration for treatment by ECMO actually received this therapy, the trial demonstrated a significantly greater survival at 6 months without disability in those patients who were randomized to consideration for ECMO (RR, 0.69; 95% CI, 0.05–0.97). However, it is difficult to separate the effect of ECMO alone compared with the differences in overall care upon transfer to a specialized center for patients randomized to consideration for ECMO. Thus, providing ECMO to patients with life-threatening ARDS may yet prove to be life-saving, but may require transfer to a specialized facility.

Medical therapy in ARDS

All the therapies mentioned above are aimed at supporting the patient with ARDS while the injured lungs recover from the initial injury. To this day, no specific medical therapy to shorten the duration or severity of ALI/ARDS has been identified. Some agents have been studied more extensively than others, and those will be discussed here. Several new potential therapeutic approaches are on the horizon, including the use of pro-resolution molecules [93].

Glucocorticoids

Increased levels of inflammatory cytokines and abundant neutrophils and macrophages are typical features of ARDS [22,24]. Thus, in an attempt to blunt inflammatory lung injury, several research groups and an untold number of individual clinicians have attempted to treat both early and late ARDS with glucocorticoids [94–96]. The most recent attempt at studying corticosteroids in early ARDS is a randomized controlled trial by Meduri et al. in 2007, where patients with ARDS were randomized early to receive long courses (2 weeks at maximal doses, followed by a 2-week taper) of low-dose systemic steroids (1 mg/kg/day of methylprednisolone) [97]. The results were quite impressive, as they demonstrated significant improvement in ICU mortality, duration of mechanical ventilation, and length-of-stay in the ICU, with a trend towards improved in-hospital survival. The study was limited by its small number of patients.

Meduri and colleagues have also reported on several studies demonstrating efficacy of glucocorticoids in treating the later, fibroproliferative stages of ARDS [98–100]. To address their potential role in the treatment of ARDS, the ARDS Network subsequently conducted a multicenter randomized-controlled trial of corticosteroids in late ARDS [101]. Disappointingly, there was no statistically significant improvement in mortality when steroids were started between 1 and 2 weeks after onset of ARDS. Moreover, mortality was worse in the steroid group when the drug was started 2 weeks after disease onset. Together, these data suggest that steroids should not be used for late ARDS, but may be considered for the early phase of ARDS, although this cannot be uniformly recommended in the absence of a more definitive trial [102].

Surfactant replacement therapy

Pulmonary surfactant is a lipid–protein complex secreted by type II pneumocytes that coats the surface of alveoli. It is composed primarily of phosphatidylcholine and has three surfactant-specific proteins. Surfactant reduces alveolar surface tension, thereby helping to prevent alveolar collapse at end-expiration. In addition, surfactant has antibacterial and immuno-regulatory activities [26,103]. The absence of pulmonary surfactant in neonates can lead to severe respiratory failure, named the respiratory distress syndrome (RDS) [26,103]. Unlike RDS, adults with ARDS have pulmonary surfactant but it contains abnormal phospholipid and protein, altering its surface tension-reducing properties [104]. Replacement therapy with exogenous surfactant has markedly reduced neonatal mortality in RDS [103]. To determine the efficacy of this therapy in ARDS, Anzueto et al. randomized over 700 ARDS patients to receive nebulized synthetic surfactant or placebo. Both mortality and arterial oxygenation were equivalent in the surfactant and placebo groups [105]. While these results are disappointing, the surfactant preparation in this study contained only lipid. In addition, the actual quantity of surfactant delivered to the lower airways was likely very small. New investigations are underway testing more native surfactant preparations and efficient surfactant delivery systems.

Other therapies

Inflammatory injury in ARDS is likely mediated, in part, by arachidonic acid metabolites such as thromboxane A_2 (TxA_2), a potent platelet activator [106,107]. Moreover, progression to more severe lung injury may be blunted in some patients by endogenous anti-inflammatory eicosanoids, including prostaglandin E_2 (PGE_2), and lipoxin A_4 [108,109]. In addition to glucocorticoids, several other anti-inflammatory therapies targeted specifically at these arachidonic acid pathways have been tested in ARDS patients [106]. Unfortunately, ketoconazole (a thromboxane synthetase inhibitor) [110–112], cyclooxygenase inhibitors [113] and PGE_1 [108] did not improve clinical outcomes in ARDS. Lipoxins are a distinct class of mediators that hold promise as a novel target for pharmacologic mimetics, as these compounds display potent anti-inflammatory and pro-resolving actions that promote resolution of experimental pulmonary inflammation and ALI [93]. Of interest, statins and aspirin can trigger the formation of 15-epimer-lipoxins [114], and in retrospective analyses pre-exposure to these medications decrease the risk of severe sepsis, ALI/ARDS, and death [115,116]. A more detailed understanding of lipoxins and other pro-resolving lipid mediators will hopefully elucidate mechanisms for restitution of lung homeostasis and provide new therapies for ARDS.

Recommendations

The large number and varied clinical efficacy of ARDS therapies can make it difficult for clinicians to select a rational treatment plan for patients. In addition, the critical illness of ARDS patients can lead practitioners to try unproven, and potentially harmful, therapies. Thus, while applying results of clinical trials to individual patients can be difficult, we advocate an ARDS treatment plan supported by clinical evidence. Table 14.6 lists the therapies discussed in this chapter and contains our summary recommendations regarding their use in ARDS.

Until future studies confirm the efficacy of "adjunctive" ventilator therapies (e.g., high PEEP, prone positioning, HFOV, and ECMO), we recommend the following evidence-based approach to mechanical ventilation in ARDS patients [44]:

- Calculate predicted body weight (PBW) in kilograms (kg)

For men:	PBW (kg) = 50 + 2.3(height (inches) − 60)
For women:	PBW (kg) = 45.5 + 2.3(height (inches) − 60)

Table 14.6 Evidence-based recommendations for acute respiratory distress syndrome (ARDS) therapies.[a]

Treatment	Recommendation
Mechanical ventilation:	
Low-tidal volume	A
High-PEEP or "open-lung"	C
Prone position	C
High frequency ventilation	C
ECMO	C
Minimize left atrial filling pressures	B
Glucocorticoids	C
Surfactant replacement	D
Inhaled nitric oxide	D
Other anti-inflammatory therapy (e.g., ketoconazole, PGE$_1$, NSAIDs)	D

[a] Based on current clinical evidence, several ARDS therapies have been assigned one of the following recommendation scores:
A = Good supportive clinical evidence: Recommended therapy.
B = Supportive evidence, but limited clinical data: Recommended therapy.
C = Indeterminate evidence: Recommended only as alternative therapy.
D = Good evidence against efficacy of therapy: Not recommended.
PEEP, positive end expiratory pressure; ECMO, extracorporeal membrane oxygenation; NSAIDs, non-steroidal anti-inflammatory drugs.

- Ventilator mode.

Volume cycle, assist control.

- Tidal volume (V_t).

Initial V_t 8 cm^3/kg PBW. Reduce to 6 cm^3/kg over 2–4 hours if ventilation adequate (see below).

Goal inspiratory plateau pressures < 30 cm H$_2$O; reduce V_t to as low as 4 cm^3/kg as needed (and permitted by ventilation) to achieve this goal.

- P$_a$O$_2$ goal = 55–80 mmHg or pulse oximetry oxygen saturation 88–95%.
- Follow the F$_i$O$_2$ and PEEP applications used in the ARDS Network study group [44], namely:

F$_i$O$_2$	0.3	0.4	0.4	0.5	0.5	0.6	0.7	0.7	0.7	0.8	0.9	0.9	0.9	1.0
PEEP	5	5	8	8	10	10	10	12	14	14	14	16	18	20–24

- In select patients, consider pleural pressure estimation with an esophageal balloon. Set PEEP to be 0–10 cm H$_2$O higher than pleural pressure.
- Respiratory rate and acidosis management.

Goal arterial pH = 7.30–7.45.

If pH < 7.30, increase respiratory rate up to 35 breaths/minute.

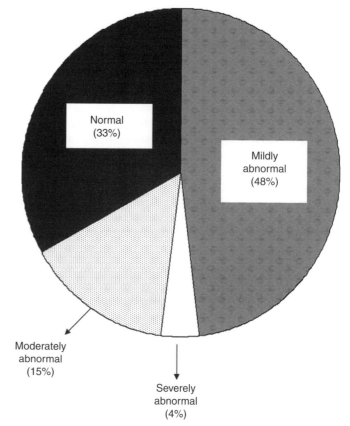

Figure 14.5 Pulmonary function in acute respiratory distress syndrome (ARDS) survivors 1 year after recovery. Pulmonary function was tested using spirometry (measuring the forced expiratory volume at 1 second (FEV1) and the forced vital capacity (FVC)) and by measuring the diffusion capacity for carbon monoxide (DL$_{CO}$). If the FEV1, FVC, and DL$_{CO}$ were all ≥ 80% of predicted values, pulmonary function was considered normal (black). If any of the three values were: 60–79% predicted, 41–59% predicted, or < 40% predicted, then pulmonary function was considered mildly abnormal (gray), moderately abnormal (stippled), or severely abnormal (white), respectively [36].

If pH < 7.30 and the respiratory rate = 35, consider starting intravenous bicarbonate (or equivalent buffer).

If the above strategy fails and the patient is suffering from life-threatening persistent hypoxemic respiratory failure, consider the following:

- Neuromuscular blocking agents (if not already in use).
- Recruitment maneuvers.
- Prone position ventilation.
- HFOV or ECMO as part of a clinical research trial or in selected individuals.

Functional recovery in ARDS survivors

With improving ARDS survival, the functional recovery of ARDS survivors is an increasingly important issue for both patients and the healthcare system. Although ARDS patients can suffer profound and prolonged respiratory failure, it is encouraging that the majority of patients recover nearly normal lung function [36,37]. For example, Ghio et al. reported complete normalization of spirometry values and carbon monoxide diffusion capacities (DL_{CO}) in over a third of ARDS survivors 1 year after endotracheal extubation; most of the remaining patients were left with only mild abnormalities in their pulmonary function tests (Figure 14.5) [36]. Patients recover most of their lung function by 6 months after lung injury [37]. Unlike mortality from ARDS, recovery of lung function is strongly associated with the extent of lung injury early in the disease. For example, McHugh et al. observed 30% lower FVC, DL_{CO}, and total lung capacity (TLC) values at 1 year of recovery in ARDS patients with an initial LIS > 25 (severe) compared with those with a score < 25 (limited) [37].

A recent report on 64 ARDS survivors evaluated 5 years post discharge confirms that lung function returns to near-normal levels at 1 year and remains so at 5 years, suggesting that near-complete recovery of lung function can be expected relatively early in the average ARDS survivor, with no evidence of subsequent deterioration [117,118]. Similarly, quality-of-life assessments appeared to approach near-normal; however, in sharp contrast, physical component scores plateaued at the 2-year mark and never reached the levels seen in a normal population. Six-minute walk tests were substandard and remained so throughout the 5 years of follow-up. In spite of these persistent physical limitations, 78% of these patients were able to return to work by 1 year after ICU discharge; this percentage rose to 94% by the 5-year mark. From the perspective of caring for surgical patients, it is encouraging that survivors from trauma-induced ARDS have nearly 30% greater clinical functional recovery compared with patients surviving sepsis-induced ARDS [119]. Overall clinical recovery from ARDS is a complex process, involving important interactions between physical and psychosocial factors. A better understanding of mechanisms involved in resolution is essential to guide future therapies aimed at reducing long-term ARDS morbidity.

Concluding comments

The Berlin definition of ARDS identifies lung injury as a common clinical disorder in critically ill surgical patients. With general advances in critical care and the discovery of ARDS-supportive therapies, mortality from this disease has decreased. Ongoing basic and clinical research is focused on providing new therapies aimed at both prevention and lung repair, so that future patients will have less severe illness and improved survival and long-term recovery from ARDS.

Acknowledgments

Supported in part by US National Institutes of Health grants HL068669 and HL090927 (BDL).

Disclosures

BDL is a co-inventor on patents on the use of lipoxins in lung disease that are assigned to Brigham and Women's Hospital and have been licensed for clinical development.

References

1. Ashbaugh DG, Bigelow DB, Petty TL, Levine BE. Acute respiratory distress in adults. Lancet 1967; 2(7511): 319–23.

2. Murray JF, Matthay MA, Luce JM, Flick MR. An expanded definition of the adult respiratory distress syndrome. Am Rev Respir Dis 1988; 138: 720–3.

3. Doyle RL, Szaflarski N, Modin GW, Wiener-Kronish JP, Matthay MA. Identification of patients with acute lung injury. Predictors of mortality. Am J Respir Crit Care Med 1995; 152: 1818–24.

4. Luhr OR, Antonsen K, Karlsson M et al. Incidence and mortality after acute respiratory failure and acute respiratory distress syndrome in Sweden, Denmark, and Iceland. The ARF Study Group. Am J Respir Crit Care Med 1999; 159: 1849–61.

5. Monchi M, Bellenfant F, Cariou A et al. Early predictive factors of survival in the acute respiratory distress syndrome. A multivariate analysis. Am J Respir Crit Care Med 1998; 158: 1076–81.

6. Pepe PE, Potkin RT, Reus DH, Hudson LD, Carrico CJ. Clinical predictors of the adult respiratory distress syndrome. Am J Surg 1982; 144: 124–30.

7. Ranieri VM et al. Acute respiratory distress syndrome: the Berlin Definition. JAMA 2012; 307(23): 2526–33.

8. Bernard GR, Artigas A, Brigham KL et al. The American–European Consensus Conference on ARDS. Definitions, mechanisms, relevant outcomes, and clinical trial coordination. Am J Respir Crit Care Med 1994; 149: 818–24.

9. Thomsen GE, Morris AH. Incidence of the adult respiratory distress syndrome in the state of Utah. Am J Respir Crit Care Med 1995; 152: 965–71.

10. Villar J, Slutsky AS. The incidence of the adult respiratory distress syndrome. Am Rev Respir Dis 1989; 140: 814–16.

11. Rubenfeld GD, Caldwell E, Peabody E et al. Incidence and outcomes of acute lung injury. N Engl J Med 2005; 353: 1685–93.

12. Hudson LD, Milberg JA, Anardi D, Maunder RJ. Clinical risks for development of the acute respiratory distress syndrome. Am J Respir Crit Care Med 1995; 151: 293–301.

13. Moss M, Bucher B, Moore FA, Moore EE, Parsons PE. The role of chronic alcohol abuse in the development of acute respiratory distress syndrome in adults. J Am Med Assoc 1996; 275: 50–4.

14. Matuschak GM, Pinsky MR, Klein EC, Van Thiel DH, Rinaldo JE. Effects of D-galactosamine-induced acute liver injury on mortality and pulmonary responses to Escherichia coli lipopolysaccharide. Modulation by arachidonic acid metabolites.

Am Rev Respir Dis 1990; **141**: 1296–306.

15. Trillo-Alvarez C, Cartin-Ceba R, Kor DJ *et al*. Acute lung injury prediction score: derivation and validation in a population-based sample. *Eur Respir J* 2011; **37**: 604–9.

16. Gajic O, Dabbagh O, Park PK *et al*. Early identification of patients at risk of acute lung injury: evaluation of lung injury prediction score in a multicenter cohort study. *Am J Respir Crit Care Med* 2011; **183**: 462–70.

17. Bell RC, Coalson JJ, Smith JD, Johanson WG Jr. Multiple organ system failure and infection in adult respiratory distress syndrome. *Ann Intern Med* 1983; **99**: 293–8.

18. Milberg JA, Davis DR, Steinberg KP, Hudson LD. Improved survival of patients with acute respiratory distress syndrome (ARDS): 1983–1993. *J Am Med Assoc* 1995; **273**: 306–9.

19. Montgomery AB, Stager MA, Carrico CJ, Hudson LD. Causes of mortality in patients with the adult respiratory distress syndrome. *Am Rev Respir Dis* 1985; **132**: 485–9.

20. Nuckton TJ, Alonso JA, Kallet RH *et al*. Pulmonary dead-space fraction as a risk factor for death in the acute respiratory distress syndrome. *N Engl J Med* 2002; **346**: 1281–6.

21. Suchyta MR, Clemmer TP, Elliott CG, Orme JF Jr, Weaver LK. The adult respiratory distress syndrome. A report of survival and modifying factors. *Chest* 1992; **101**: 1074–9.

22. Pugin J, Verghese G, Widmer MC, Matthay MA. The alveolar space is the site of intense inflammatory and profibrotic reactions in the early phase of acute respiratory distress syndrome. *Crit Care Med* 1999; **27**: 304–12.

23. Slutsky AS, Tremblay LN. Multiple system organ failure. Is mechanical ventilation a contributing factor? *Am J Respir Crit Care Med* 1998; **157**: 1721–5.

24. Tomashefski JF Jr, Davies P, Boggis C *et al*. The pulmonary vascular lesions of the adult respiratory distress syndrome. *Am J Pathol* 1983; **112**: 112–26.

25. Tomashefski JF Jr. Pulmonary pathology of acute respiratory distress syndrome. *Clin Chest Med* 2000; **21**: 435–66.

26. Lewis JF, Jobe AH. Surfactant and the adult respiratory distress syndrome. *Am Rev Respir Dis*. 1993; **147**: 218–33.

27. Jain S, Kamimoto L, Bramley AM *et al*. Hospitalized patients with 2009 H1N1 influenza in the United States, April–June 2009. *N Engl J Med* 2009; **361**: 1935–44.

28. Webb SA, Pettila V, Seppelt I *et al*. Critical care services and 2009 H1N1 influenza in Australia and New Zealand. *N Engl J Med* 2009; **361**: 1925–34.

29. Anderson WR, Thielen K. Correlative study of adult respiratory distress syndrome by light, scanning, and transmission electron microscopy. *Ultrastruct Pathol* 1992; **16**: 615–28.

30. Gattinoni L, Bombino M, Pelosi P *et al*. Lung structure and function in different stages of severe adult respiratory distress syndrome. *J Am Med Assoc* 1994; **271**: 1772–9.

31. Ware LB, Matthay MA. The acute respiratory distress syndrome. *N Engl J Med* 2000; **342**: 1334–49.

32. Goodman PC. Radiographic findings in patients with acute respiratory distress syndrome. *Clin Chest Med* 2000; **21**: 419–33, vii.

33. Puybasset L, Cluzel P, Chao N *et al*. A computed tomography scan assessment of regional lung volume in acute lung injury. The CT Scan ARDS Study Group. *Am J Respir Crit Care Med* 1998; **158**: 1644–55.

34. Zapol WM, Trelstad RL, Coffey JW, Tsai I, Salvador RA. Pulmonary fibrosis in severe acute respiratory failure. *Am Rev Respir Dis* 1979; **119**: 547–54.

35. Chesnutt AN, Matthay MA, Tibayan FA, Clark JG. Early detection of type III procollagen peptide in acute lung injury. Pathogenetic and prognostic significance. *Am J Respir Crit Care Med* 1997; **156**: 840–5.

36. Ghio AJ, Elliott CG, Crapo RO, Berlin SL, Jensen RL. Impairment after adult respiratory distress syndrome. An evaluation based on American Thoracic Society recommendations. *Am Rev Respir Dis* 1989; **139**: 1158–62.

37. McHugh LG, Milberg JA, Whitcomb ME *et al*. Recovery of function in survivors of the acute respiratory distress syndrome. *Am J Respir Crit Care Med* 1994; **150**: 90–4.

38. Martin C, Papazian L, Payan MJ, Saux P, Gouin F. Pulmonary fibrosis correlates with outcome in adult respiratory distress syndrome. A study in mechanically ventilated patients. *Chest* 1995; **107**: 196–200.

39. Tobin MJ. Advances in mechanical ventilation. *N Engl J Med* 2001; **344**: 1986–96.

40. Webb HH, Tierney DF. Experimental pulmonary edema due to intermittent positive pressure ventilation with high inflation pressures. Protection by positive end-expiratory pressure. *Am Rev Respir Dis* 1974; **110**: 556–65.

41. Dreyfuss D, Soler P, Basset G, Saumon G. High inflation pressure pulmonary edema. Respective effects of high airway pressure, high tidal volume, and positive end-expiratory pressure. *Am Rev Respir Dis* 1988; **137**: 1159–64.

42. Dreyfuss D, Soler P, Saumon G. Mechanical ventilation-induced pulmonary edema. Interaction with previous lung alterations. *Am J Respir Crit Care Med* 1995; **151**: 1568–75.

43. Amato MB, Barbas CS, Medeiros DM *et al*. Effect of a protective-ventilation strategy on mortality in the acute respiratory distress syndrome. *N Engl J Med* 1998; **338**: 347–54.

44. The Acute Respiratory Distress Syndrome Network. Ventilation with lower tidal volumes as compared with traditional tidal volumes for acute lung injury and the acute respiratory distress syndrome. *N Engl J Med* 2000; **342**: 1301–8.

45. Brochard L, Roudot-Thoraval F, Roupie E *et al*. Tidal volume reduction for prevention of ventilator-induced lung injury in acute respiratory distress syndrome. The Multicenter Trail Group on Tidal Volume reduction in ARDS. *Am J Respir Crit Care Med* 1998; **158**: 1831–8.

46. Stewart TE, Meade MO, Cook DJ *et al*. Evaluation of a ventilation strategy to prevent barotrauma in patients at high risk for acute respiratory distress syndrome. Pressure- and Volume-Limited Ventilation Strategy Group. *N Engl J Med* 1998; **338**: 355–61.

47. Brower RG, Lanken PN, MacIntyre N et al. Higher versus lower positive end-expiratory pressures in patients with the acute respiratory distress syndrome. N Engl J Med 2004; 351: 327–36.

48. Meade MO, Cook DJ, Guyatt GH et al. Ventilation strategy using low tidal volumes, recruitment maneuvers, and high positive end-expiratory pressure for acute lung injury and acute respiratory distress syndrome: a randomized controlled trial. J Am Med Assoc 2008; 299: 637–45.

49. Mercat A, Richard JC, Vielle B et al. Positive end-expiratory pressure setting in adults with acute lung injury and acute respiratory distress syndrome: a randomized controlled trial. J Am Med Assoc 2008; 299: 646–55.

50. Briel M, Meade M, Mercat A et al. Higher vs lower positive end-expiratory pressure in patients with acute lung injury and acute respiratory distress syndrome: systematic review and meta-analysis. J Am Med Assoc 2010; 303: 865–73.

51. Bernard GR. PEEP guided by esophageal pressure – any added value? N Engl J Med 2008; 359: 2166–8.

52. Talmor D, Sarge T, Malhotra A et al. Mechanical ventilation guided by esophageal pressure in acute lung injury. N Engl J Med 2008; 359: 2095–104.

53. Bone RC. Treatment of adult respiratory distress syndrome with diuretics, dialysis, and positive end-expiratory pressure. Crit Care Med 1978; 6: 136–9.

54. Humphrey H, Hall J, Sznajder I, Silverstein M, Wood L. Improved survival in ARDS patients associated with a reduction in pulmonary capillary wedge pressure. Chest 1990; 97: 1176–80.

55. Mitchell JP, Schuller D, Calandrino FS, Schuster DP. Improved outcome based on fluid management in critically ill patients requiring pulmonary artery catheterization. Am Rev Respir Dis 1992; 145: 990–8.

56. Wiedemann HP, Wheeler AP, Bernard GR et al. Comparison of two fluid-management strategies in acute lung injury. N Engl J Med 2006; 354: 2564–75.

57. Slutsky AS. Neuromuscular blocking agents in ARDS. N Engl J Med 2010; 363: 1176–80.

58. Papazian L, Forel JM, Gacouin A et al. Neuromuscular blockers in early acute respiratory distress syndrome. N Engl J Med 2010; 363: 1107–16.

59. Fan E, Wilcox ME, Brower RG et al. Recruitment maneuvers for acute lung injury: a systematic review. Am J Respir Crit Care Med 2008; 178: 1156–63.

60. Bryan AC. Conference on the scientific basis of respiratory therapy. Pulmonary physiotherapy in the pediatric age group. Comments of a devil's advocate. Am Rev Respir Dis 1974; 110: 143–4.

61. Douglas WW, Rehder K, Beynen FM, Sessler AD, Marsh HM. Improved oxygenation in patients with acute respiratory failure: the prone position. Am Rev Respir Dis 1977; 115: 559–66.

62. Langer M, Mascheroni D, Marcolin R, Gattinoni L. The prone position in ARDS patients. A clinical study. Chest 1988; 94: 103–7.

63. Pappert D, Rossaint R, Slama K, Gruning T, Falke KJ. Influence of positioning on ventilation-perfusion relationships in severe adult respiratory distress syndrome. Chest 1994; 106: 1511–16.

64. Piehl MA, Brown RS. Use of extreme position changes in acute respiratory failure. Crit Care Med 1976; 4: 13–14.

65. Albert RK. Prone ventilation. Clin Chest Med 2000; 21: 511–17.

66. Pelosi P, Tubiolo D, Mascheroni D et al. Effects of the prone position on respiratory mechanics and gas exchange during acute lung injury. Am J Respir Crit Care Med 1998; 157: 387–93.

67. Gattinoni L, Tognoni G, Pesenti A et al. Effect of prone positioning on the survival of patients with acute respiratory failure. N Engl J Med 2001; 345: 568–73.

68. Taccone P, Pesenti A, Latini R et al. Prone positioning in patients with moderate and severe acute respiratory distress syndrome: a randomized controlled trial. J Am Med Assoc 2009; 302: 1977–84.

69. Sud S, Friedrich JO, Taccone P et al. Prone ventilation reduces mortality in patients with acute respiratory failure and severe hypoxemia: systematic review and meta-analysis. Intensive Care Med 2010; 36: 585–99.

70. Messerole E, Peine P, Wittkopp S, Marini JJ, Albert RK. The pragmatics of prone positioning. Am J Respir Crit Care Med 2002; 165: 1359–63.

71. Villar J, Blazquez MA, Lubillo S, Quintana J, Manzano JL. Pulmonary hypertension in acute respiratory failure. Crit Care Med 1989; 17: 523–6.

72. Siobal MS, Hess DR. Are inhaled vasodilators useful in acute lung injury and acute respiratory distress syndrome? Respir Care 2010; 55(2): 144–57; discussion 57–61.

73. Payen DM. Inhaled nitric oxide and acute lung injury. Clin Chest Med 2000; 21: 519–29, ix.

74. Rossaint R, Falke KJ, Lopez F et al. Inhaled nitric oxide for the adult respiratory distress syndrome. N Engl J Med 1993; 328: 399–405.

75. Dellinger RP, Zimmerman JL, Taylor RW et al. Effects of inhaled nitric oxide in patients with acute respiratory distress syndrome: results of a randomized phase II trial. Inhaled nitric oxide in ARDS Study Group. Crit Care Med 1998; 26: 15–23.

76. Lundin S, Mang H, Smithies M, Stenqvist O, Frostell C. Inhalation of nitric oxide in acute lung injury: results of a European multicentre study. The European Study Group of Inhaled Nitric Oxide. Intensive Care Med 1999; 25: 911–19.

77. Taylor RW, Zimmerman JL, Dellinger RP et al. Low-dose inhaled nitric oxide in patients with acute lung injury: a randomized controlled trial. J Am Med Assoc 2004; 291: 1603–9.

78. Troncy E, Collet JP, Shapiro S et al. Inhaled nitric oxide in acute respiratory distress syndrome: a pilot randomized controlled study. Am J Respir Crit Care Med 1998; 157: 1483–8.

79. Walmrath D, Schneider T, Schermuly R et al. Direct comparison of inhaled nitric oxide and aerosolized prostacyclin in acute respiratory distress syndrome. Am J Respir Crit Care Med 1996; 153: 991–6.

80. Derdak S, Mehta S, Stewart TE et al. High-frequency oscillatory ventilation for acute respiratory distress syndrome in adults: a randomized, controlled trial. Am J Respir Crit Care Med 2002; 166: 801–8.

81. Fort P, Farmer C, Westerman J et al. High-frequency oscillatory ventilation for adult respiratory distress syndrome – a pilot study. Crit Care Med 1997; 25: 937–47.

82. Slutsky AS, Drazen JM. Ventilation with small tidal volumes. N Engl J Med 2002; 347: 630–1.

83. Sud S, Sud M, Friedrich JO et al. High frequency oscillation in patients with acute lung injury and acute respiratory distress syndrome (ARDS): systematic review and meta-analysis. Br Med J 2010; 340: c2327.

84. Young D et al. High-frequency oscillation for acute respiratory distress syndrome. N Engl J Med 2013; 368(9): 806–13.

85. Ferguson ND et al. High-frequency oscillation in early acute respiratory distress syndrome. N Engl J Med 2013; 368(9): 795–805.

86. Bartlett RH. Extracorporeal life support in the management of severe respiratory failure. Clin Chest Med 2000; 21: 555–61.

87. Bartlett RH, Roloff DW, Cornell RG et al. Extracorporeal circulation in neonatal respiratory failure: a prospective randomized study. Pediatrics 1985; 76: 479–87.

88. O'Rourke PP, Crone RK, Vacanti JP et al. Extracorporeal membrane oxygenation and conventional medical therapy in neonates with persistent pulmonary hypertension of the newborn: a prospective randomized study. Pediatrics 1989; 84: 957–63.

89. Gattinoni L, Pesenti A, Mascheroni D et al. Low-frequency positive-pressure ventilation with extracorporeal CO2 removal in severe acute respiratory failure. J Am Med Assoc 1986; 256: 881–6.

90. Morris AH, Wallace CJ, Menlove RL et al. Randomized clinical trial of pressure-controlled inverse ratio ventilation and extracorporeal CO_2 removal for adult respiratory distress syndrome. Am J Respir Crit Care Med 1994; 149: 295–305.

91. Davies A, Jones D, Bailey M et al. Extracorporeal membrane oxygenation for 2009 influenza A (H1N1) acute respiratory distress syndrome. J Am Med Assoc 2009; 302: 1888–95.

92. Peek GJ, Mugford M, Tiruvoipati R et al. Efficacy and economic assessment of conventional ventilatory support versus extracorporeal membrane oxygenation for severe adult respiratory failure (CESAR): a multicentre randomised controlled trial. Lancet 2009; 374: 1351–63.

93. Levy BD, De Sanctis GT, Devchand PR et al. Multi-pronged inhibition of airway hyper-responsiveness and inflammation by lipoxin A(4). Nat Med 2002; 8: 1018–23.

94. Bernard GR, Luce JM, Sprung CL et al. High-dose corticosteroids in patients with the adult respiratory distress syndrome. N Engl J Med 1987; 317: 1565–70.

95. Luce JM. Corticosteroids in ARDS. An evidence-based review. Crit Care Clin 2002; 18: 79–89, vii.

96. Weigelt JA, Norcross JF, Borman KR, Snyder WH 3rd. Early steroid therapy for respiratory failure. Arch Surg 1985; 120: 536–40.

97. Meduri GU, Golden E, Freire AX et al. Methylprednisolone infusion in early severe ARDS: results of a randomized controlled trial. Chest 2007; 131: 954–63.

98. Meduri GU, Belenchia JM, Estes RJ et al. Fibroproliferative phase of ARDS. Clinical findings and effects of corticosteroids. Chest 1991; 100: 943–52.

99. Meduri GU, Chinn AJ, Leeper KV et al. Corticosteroid rescue treatment of progressive fibroproliferation in late ARDS. Patterns of response and predictors of outcome. Chest 1994; 105: 1516–27.

100. Meduri GU, Headley AS, Golden E et al. Effect of prolonged methylprednisolone therapy in unresolving acute respiratory distress syndrome: a randomized controlled trial. J Am Med Assoc 1998; 280: 159–65.

101. Steinberg KP, Hudson LD, Goodman RB et al. Efficacy and safety of corticosteroids for persistent acute respiratory distress syndrome. N Engl J Med 2006; 354: 1671–84.

102. Tang BM, Craig JC, Eslick GD, Seppelt I, McLean AS. Use of corticosteroids in acute lung injury and acute respiratory distress syndrome: a systematic review and meta-analysis. Crit Care Med 2009; 37: 1594–603.

103. Long W, Thompson T, Sundell H et al. Effects of two rescue doses of a synthetic surfactant on mortality rate and survival without bronchopulmonary dysplasia in 700- to 1350-gram infants with respiratory distress syndrome. The American Exosurf Neonatal Study Group I. J Pediatr 1991; 118: 595–605.

104. Gregory TJ, Longmore WJ, Moxley MA et al. Surfactant chemical composition and biophysical activity in acute respiratory distress syndrome. J Clin Invest 1991; 88: 1976–81.

105. Anzueto A, Baughman RP, Guntupalli KK et al. Aerosolized surfactant in adults with sepsis-induced acute respiratory distress syndrome. Exosurf Acute Respiratory Distress Syndrome Sepsis Study Group. N Engl J Med 1996; 334: 1417–21.

106. Conner BD, Bernard GR. Acute respiratory distress syndrome. Potential pharmacologic interventions. Clin Chest Med 2000; 21: 563–87.

107. Winn R, Harlan J, Nadir B, Harker L, Hildebrandt J. Thromboxane A2 mediates lung vasoconstriction but not permeability after endotoxin. J Clin Invest 1983; 72: 911–18.

108. Abraham E, Baughman R, Fletcher E et al. Liposomal prostaglandin E1 (TLC C-53) in acute respiratory distress syndrome: a controlled, randomized, double-blind, multicenter clinical trial. TLC C-53 ARDS Study Group. Crit Care Med 1999; 27: 1478–85.

109. Fukunaga K, Kohli P, Bonnans C, Fredenburgh LE, Levy BD. Cyclooxygenase 2 plays a pivotal role in the resolution of acute lung injury. J Immunol 2005; 174: 5033–9.

110. The ARDS Network. Ketoconazole for early treatment of acute lung injury and acute respiratory distress syndrome: a randomized controlled trial. J Am Med Assoc 2000; 283: 1995–2002.

111. Slotman GJ, Burchard KW, D'Arezzo A, Gann DS. Ketoconazole prevents acute respiratory failure in critically ill surgical patients. J Trauma 1988; 28: 648–54.

112. Yu M, Tomasa G. A double-blind, prospective, randomized trial of ketoconazole, a thromboxane synthetase inhibitor, in the prophylaxis of the adult respiratory distress syndrome. Crit Care Med 1993; 21: 1635–42.

113. Rinaldo JE, Pennock B. Effects of ibuprofen on endotoxin-induced alveolitis: biphasic dose response and dissociation between inflammation and hypoxemia. *Am J Med Sci* 1986; **291**: 29–38.

114. Levy BD. Resolvins and protectins: natural pharmacophores for resolution biology. *Prostaglandins Leukot Essent Fatty Acids* 2010; **82**: 327–32.

115. Erlich JM, Talmor DS, Cartin-Ceba R, Gajic O, Kor DJ. Prehospitalization antiplatelet therapy is associated with a reduced incidence of acute lung injury: a population-based cohort study. *Chest* 2011; **139**: 289–95.

116. O'Neal HR Jr, Koyama T, Koehler EA *et al*. Prehospital statin and aspirin use and the prevalence of severe sepsis and acute lung injury/acute respiratory distress syndrome. *Crit Care Med* 2011; **39**: 1343–50.

117. Herridge MS, Cheung AM, Tansey CM *et al*. One-year outcomes in survivors of the acute respiratory distress syndrome. *N Engl J Med* 2003; **348**: 683–93.

118. Herridge MS, Tansey CM, Matté A *et al*. Functional disability 5 years after acute respiratory distress syndrome. *N Engl J Med* 2011; **364**: 1293–304.

119. Davidson TA, Caldwell ES, Curtis JR, Hudson LD, Steinberg KP. Reduced quality of life in survivors of acute respiratory distress syndrome compared with critically ill control patients. *J Am Med Assoc* 1999; **281**: 354–60.

Postoperative pulmonary complications

Carter G. Co, David A. Quintero, and Eric G. Honig

Introduction

Postoperative pulmonary complications are defined as pulmonary abnormalities occurring in the postoperative period that produce clinically significant identifiable disease or dysfunction that adversely affects the clinical course [1]. The definition includes pneumonia, atelectasis, respiratory failure, pulmonary embolism, pleural effusion, pneumothorax, pulmonary edema, and hypoxemia. These problems complicate approximately 2–3% of all surgeries varying with the invasiveness of the procedure and the presence of patient-related risk factors [2]. Pulmonary complications are described in 19–59% of thoracic procedures, 16–17% of upper abdominal surgeries, but only 0–5% of lower abdominal procedures [1]. They are most commonly seen in the first week after surgery, especially in the first 24–72 postoperative hours and can be particularly problematic because attention may be relaxed after transfer from a post-anesthesia care unit.

Taken together, they are the most expensive form of postoperative complication, are more common than postoperative cardiac complications, lead to longer hospital stays, and increase the relative risk of death to 14.9 (95% confidence limits 4.76–26.9) particularly from pneumonia [3]. They may cause as much as 84% of postoperative thoracotomy deaths [1].

Surgical factors such as the site of the incision, the type and duration of anesthesia, and postoperative analgesic and sedative care are probably more important determinants of postoperative pulmonary complications than patient-related factors. Among the latter, obstructive airway diseases and smoking, advanced age, obesity, sleep apnea, and pulmonary hypertension pose significant added risks [2]. Patients should be evaluated preoperatively to identify these factors and efforts made to improve risk status. Preoperative respiratory assessment and management are discussed in Chapter 12.

Pathogenesis

The pathogenesis of postoperative pulmonary complications begins in the operating room. Hypoventilation and reduced lung volumes from anesthesia and surgery combine to produce atelectasis and predispose to respiratory tract infection. Immobility leads to higher risk of thromboembolic disease. Respiratory muscle dysfunction is common, especially following cardiac, chest, or upper abdominal procedures. Cardiac surgeries are associated with a 10–85% incidence of phrenic nerve dysfunction due to phrenic-nerve injury, either from cold injury or via direct operative damage. Bilateral phrenic injury is seen in 2% of cases and can lead to ventilator dependence in patients with limited pulmonary reserve, especially during REM sleep. Dysfunction may last from 30 days up to 2 years. Thoracotomies with intercostal incisions and transdiaphragmatic procedures lead to direct muscle injury and may manifest as decreased respiratory muscle pressures for up to a month after surgery. Upper abdominal operations are associated with reflex inhibition of the phrenic nerve for 48 hours to 7 days after surgery. Patients shift to a rib cage-accessory muscle pattern of breathing with consequent basilar atelectasis. Reflex reduction in central phrenic nerve output secondary to vagal, splanchnic, or sympathetic afferent receptors frequently causes diaphragmatic dysfunction. The decline in lung volumes is not as dramatic after laparoscopic abdominal surgery. There is some evidence to suggest that this diaphragm dysfunction may be ameliorated by administration of theophylline [4] or by systemic, regional or local analgesia [5].

All of these mechanisms contribute to postoperative hypoxemia and can progress to respiratory failure in patients with limited respiratory reserve. Most physiological changes regress over 1–2 weeks after surgery [6]. Even with optimal preoperative and perioperative care, some patients will develop significant postoperative pulmonary problems. Intraoperative and post-anesthesia issues remain the province of the surgeon and anesthesiologist.

Medical Management of the Surgical Patient, ed. Michael F. Lubin, Thomas F. Dodson, and Neil H. Winawer. Published by Cambridge University Press. © Cambridge University Press 2013.

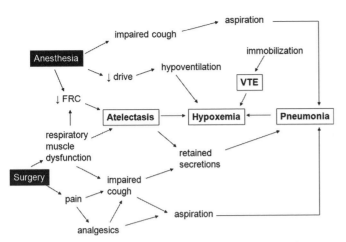

Figure 15.1 Pathogenesis of major postoperative pulmonary complications. VTE, venous thromboembolism; FRC, functional residual capacity.

In this chapter, we will discuss the diagnosis and management of those postoperative pulmonary problems likely to be encountered after transfer back from a post-anesthesia care unit.

Hypoxemia
Epidemiology

Postoperative hypoxemia may occur in up to 30–50% of general surgical cases and is most commonly seen in the first 24–48 hours postoperatively [7]. In a sample of postoperative patients, 60% exhibited desaturations to less than 80% for up to 7 hours after a dose of intravenous morphine. These desaturations were usually associated with apneas and with a decrease in functional residual capacity (FRC) [8]. Patients undergoing bariatric surgery are especially prone to postoperative hypoxemia and desaturation events. In a study using continuous pulse oximetry in postoperative bariatric surgeries, patients spent an average of 165 minutes with oxygen saturation below 90%, and had a mean of 112 desaturation events lasting up to 21 minutes each with an average saturation nadir of 75%. These events were associated with a normal PCO_2, and were unrecognized clinically in every case [9]. Postoperative hypoxemia is not without adverse clinical consequences including cardiac complications, delirium, memory changes, and decreased tissue oxygenation leading to impaired wound healing [10].

Classification

Postoperative hypoxemia can be categorized as constant or episodic.

Constant

Constant hypoxemia is defined as an oxygen saturation less than 90% for more than 3 minutes [8]. It is most closely related to perioperative changes in respiratory mechanics. Each of the common mechanisms of clinical hypoxemia may contribute to postoperative hypoxemia. Shunt is associated with atelectasis, as well as with pneumonia, pulmonary edema, and ARDS. Restrictive lung volume changes, thought to reflect the effects of general anesthesia and muscle relaxants in the supine patient, include anesthetic-induced ventilation-perfusion mismatching and shunt, absorption atelectasis due to high intraoperative F_iO_2 (see below), airway tissue edema, secretions, and upper airway obstruction from excessive relaxation of the tongue. Total lung capacity (TLC) and each of its subdivisions decrease following thoracic and abdominal surgery but not after operations on an extremity. Diminished TLC will impair cough effectiveness. There is a decline of 25–50% in vital capacity (VC), FRC, tidal volume (VT) and in expiratory flow rates, such as forced expiratory volume in 1 second (FEV1). The decline in lung volumes begins during surgery and persists for up to 4 days postoperatively, but it may still take more than 2 weeks for lung volumes to return to baseline. Rapid shallow breathing, impaired cough, mechanical ventilatory inefficiency due to incisional pain or restrictive bandages, and airway closure may further contribute to and complicate postoperative hypoxemia [11]. Dependent atelectasis and loss of FRC are sometimes caused by postoperative diaphragm dysfunction and can be diagnosed at the bedside by ultrasound imaging of diaphragmatic excursion [12]. V/Q mismatching, which generally causes milder and more oxygen responsive hypoxemia may be seen with airways disease or encountered in pulmonary embolism. Constant hypoxemia will be seen in most of the postoperative pulmonary complications discussed below.

Episodic

Episodic hypoxemia is defined as oxygen saturation less than 85% for at least 1 minute at least 10 times a night and is associated with disorders of respiratory control [10]. This may reflect the effects of narcotic and analgesic drugs or postoperative sleep disturbances, but they are particularly associated with sleep apnea. Narcotic analgesics and sedative agents all have the potential to reduce ventilatory drive, blunt arousal responses, decrease upper airway tone to a greater degree than diaphragmatic activation, and to reduce respiratory muscle tone, leading to central apneas, obstructive apneas, and decreased FRC and atelectasis. Surgical stress causes a loss of REM sleep that may persist for up to 7 days. This is followed by a rebound increase in REM sleep which produces further reductions in intercostal and upper airway muscle tone, further exacerbating any tendency towards hypoventilation, atelectasis and apneas [13].

Sleep apnea

Obstructive sleep apnea is a medical condition defined by recurrent cessation of airflow or by partial upper airway obstruction despite respiratory effort during sleep. Arousals from sleep temporarily restore upper airway patency only to be followed by a repetitive cycle of airway collapse and arousal [14]. Obstructive sleep apnea is common in the general population; 4% of men and 2% of women are overtly symptomatic. Among patients referred to a sleep laboratory, the prevalence is 24% and 9% respectively. It is estimated that 70% of bariatric surgery patients have sleep apnea [15]. In one study of 28 postoperative laparotomies, 53% of patients had more than five apnea or hypopnea events per hour on at least one study night; 23% of the hypopneas and 7% of the apneas were associated with desaturations. These events occurred more on the second and third postoperative nights than on the first, possibly reflecting REM rebound [16]. Because postoperative tissue edema precludes immediate benefit, patients undergoing upper airway surgery for the treatment of known sleep apnea are also at increased risk for postoperative pulmonary complications, with rates as high as 25%.

Eighty to ninety percent of sleep apnea in the surgical population is undiagnosed on admission, and may come to attention only because of postoperative hypoventilation, hypoxemia, or apneas [17]. Sleep apnea has been linked to perioperative hypoxemia, arrhythmia, stroke, elevated intracranial pressure, increased risk for ICU transfer, and sudden death. The presence of sleep apnea is predictive of a difficult airway [18]. An apnea index > 5 carries a relative risk for postoperative myocardial infarction of 23 [13]. Sleep apnea patients are especially vulnerable in the perioperative period because of a disproportionate sensitivity to anesthetics and narcotics [19]. The problem can be exacerbated by postoperative REM rebound.

A high clinical index of suspicion is necessary. Sleep apnea should be clinically suspected in patients with a BMI greater than 30, large neck circumference, snoring, excessive daytime somnolence, hypertension, or inability to visualize the tonsils on oral examination. Patients with suspected sleep apnea should be screened carefully preoperatively by a clinical screen such as the Berlin questionnaire or STOP-Bang [19]. Patients with high clinical probability of sleep apnea should undergo formal polysomnographic assessment if possible. Absent a full sleep study, overnight pulse oximetry may be useful. An oxygen desaturation index of $\geq$ 15 events per hour is suggestive of sleep apnea and may warrant positive pressure therapy [20]. The use of oximetry is controversial, however, with issues of standardization and uniformity of interpretation yet to be resolved [21]. Positive results may identify a patient at high risk for postoperative problems and the risks and benefits of the planned surgery should be explicitly reviewed. In the absence of formal confirmation, patients with suspected sleep apnea should be treated presumptively as if they in fact have moderate to severe obstructive sleep apnea. Once again, it is preferable to determine the appropriate level of CPAP with a formal sleep study titrating to a level of CPAP that eliminates apneas, respiratory arousals, and snoring. If a sleep study cannot be obtained, setting CPAP with an auto-titrating apparatus is a reasonable alternative. When possible, CPAP should be provided for several weeks preoperatively, but the optimal duration of treatment is not known. If this is not possible, CPAP or non-invasive ventilation should be instituted as early as the post-anesthesia

recovery unit. Sleep apnea patients should be followed in a monitored (pulse oximetry plus telemetry) bed. Extubation should be delayed until the patient is fully awake. The use of narcotic analgesics should be minimized or eliminated entirely; spinal and epidural anesthesia and NSAIDs are preferred. For patient-controlled analgesia (PCA), the basal dose of narcotic should be eliminated. Supplemental oxygen should be given as needed, targeting a saturation of 94–95% for uncomplicated sleep apnea and 90–92% for patients with the obesity hypoventilation syndrome. The supine posture should be avoided wherever possible in favor of semi Fowler or lateral decubitus. A standardized institutional protocol for the perioperative management of sleep apnea patients is advisable [22].

Platypnea

Platypnea-orthodeoxia is defined as dyspnea or desaturation that is worse in an upright posture compared with supine. This unusual entity may be encountered after liver transplantation for end-stage liver disease, in severe pulmonary hypertension, after major pulmonary resections, and in patients with significant congenital or valvular heart disease, often in association with a patent foramen ovale that may require closure. Bubble echocardiographic studies are frequently diagnostic.

Treatment

Hypoxemia can usually be treated with supplemental oxygen, continuous positive airway pressure (CPAP), or non-invasive ventilation (NIV) without resorting to invasive mechanical ventilation.

Oxygen

Supplemental oxygen can be delivered by nasal cannula, simple face mask, partial non-rebreather mask, or a high flow non-rebreather system [23]. Nasal cannulas at flows of 1–5 L/min are capable of delivering 25–40% oxygen. F_iO_2 increases approximately 4%/L/min flow varying with respiratory rate, tidal volume, and the degree to which the patient mouth breathes. Characteristics of these systems are further summarized in Table 15.1.

Non-invasive ventilation

Indications

Non-invasive ventilation is useful for the prevention and treatment of postoperative hypoxemia and is indicated for the patient in need of respiratory assistance but not in need of immediate intubation and invasive ventilation, specifically patients with a respiratory rate greater than 25 breaths per minute, PCO_2 greater than 45, pH less than 7.35, or P_aO_2/F_iO_2 < 250 [24]. It is an effective treatment modality for patients with sleep apnea and obesity hypoventilation. It has been found to decrease atelectasis and the incidence of pneumonia after abdominal and bariatric surgery better than physical therapy or expansion maneuvers. Non-invasive ventilation has been recommended for preventive use a week before and

Table 15.1 Modes of therapeutic oxygen delivery [23].

Modality	F_iO_2 range	L/min	F_iO_2 control	Comment
Nasal cannula	24–40%	1–5	Poor	Flows > 5 L/min irritating to nose
Simple face mask			Poor	Keep flow > 5 L/min to avoid rebreathing
Venturi mask	35–50%	6–10	Good	
Partial rebreather	50–60%	10–12	Poor	Flow sufficient to keep reservoir bag from collapsing
Non-rebreather	Up to 95%	10–15	Poor	

a week after thoracic, cardiac, and aortic surgery and after lung resection. Non-invasive ventilation is not appropriate for patients who are not sufficiently awake, unable to cooperate, or unable to protect their airways. It should not be used for patients who are hemodynamically unstable, those with a Glasgow coma score (GCS) < 8, minute ventilation greater than 15 L/min, P_aO_2/F_iO_2 < 120, agitated, with swallowing impairment, cannot manage secretions, or have multiple organ failure. Non-invasive ventilation is not suitable in the setting of cardiac or respiratory arrest, recent facial surgery or trauma, or significant deformity. It should be used with caution in patients with upper gastrointestinal tract surgery. Non-invasive ventilation should be provided in a monitored setting where adequate backup (e.g., conventional invasive ventilation) is available. This usually implies an ICU or a stepdown setting but NIV has been successfully applied on well-staffed and experienced general care areas.

Delivery

Non-invasive ventilation can be delivered through full face masks, nasal masks, nasal pillows, mouthpieces or via a fitted helmet. Full face masks are generally used, require less patient cooperation, allow mouth breathing, and lead to fewer problems with air leaks. They do interfere, however, with communication and oral intake. Nasal interfaces require open nasal passages, and will not be effective if the patient is a mouth breather. Gas leaks can be especially problematic. Patients tend to prefer nasal masks over full face masks. Helmets require even less cooperation, but are extremely noisy and are prone to CO_2 rebreathing.

Apparatus

Standard ICU ventilators and dedicated NIV machines are equally capable of providing non-invasive ventilation. The modes employed are similar to those used for invasive ventilation. Continuous positive airway pressure maintains the airway at any preset pressure and helps maintain oxygenation, increases FRC, decreases work of breathing, and decreases left ventricular afterload. The number needed to benefit (NNTB) from CPAP for all postoperative pulmonary complications is 14.2 [7], but the benefit for atelectasis and for pneumonia has been called into question [25]. When minute volume support is needed in addition to defense of FRC, bi-level modes of non-invasive ventilation are used. Pressure support is generally preferred by patients, but is subject to problems with asynchrony in the presence of significant mask leaks. Time cycle ventilation (pressure control) may perform better in this circumstance. Volume control settings are prone to mask leaks, gastric distension, pressure sores, and skin necrosis. The choice of mode is often determined by patient comfort and local expertise. Controlled modes are preferred for more severe disease.

Settings

Necessary settings for non-invasive ventilation include F_iO_2, inspiratory pressure (IPAP), expiratory pressure (EPAP), and rate. F_iO_2 should be titrated to SpO_2 targets of 92–95% as discussed above. Expiratory pressure is analogous to PEEP in conventional mechanical ventilation and is used to maintain FRC and to enhance oxygenation. Expiratory pressure is set to at least 5 cm H_2O, and higher as needed for sleep apnea, atelectasis, or morbid obesity, and in conjunction with F_iO_2 for control of hypoxemia. Eight to 12 cm H_2O will generally suffice. The difference between IPAP and EPAP is analogous to pressure support in conventional ventilation and is used in NIV to provide tidal volume support. Minimal levels of pressure support usually begin at 3–5 cm H_2O, so an average initial IPAP should be 8–10 cm H_2O. The pressure support should be titrated to produce an exhaled tidal volume of 6–10 cc/kg ideal body weight [26]. Bi-level NIV can be provided continuously or on a cyclic basis; 30–45 minutes Q2–4 hours for prophylactic use, and 60–90 minutes Q2–3 hours for curative intent [24]. Inspiratory pressure should generally not exceed 20 cm H_2O so as not to overcome lower esophageal sphincter pressure and produce gastric distension. Current evidence indicates that conventional levels of IPAP are well-tolerated, even in gastric bypass patients. Some authors suggest that for patient comfort, NIV should be initiated with EPAP only, adding IPAP at minimal increments and titrating upwards as needed to meet tidal volume goals. This strategy should be subject to clinical urgency.

Management

Non-invasive ventilation patients should be monitored along with conventional vital signs for mask comfort, tolerance, respiratory distress, respiratory rate, respiratory muscle usage, air leak, adequacy of pressure support, and adequacy of delivered tidal volume, synchrony, and gas exchange (arterial blood gases, pulse oximetry). The best predictor of success of NIV is the clinical response in the first 2 hours. Non-invasive ventilation is successful in 50–80% of cases [27]. Adverse effects of NIV, besides clinical failure, include nasal bridge erosion, pressure necrosis, and facial trauma. Skin injuries can be managed with Duoderm.

As the patient improves, NIV can be weaned either by progressively increasing time off ventilation as tolerated or, analogous to a pressure support wean in conventional ventilation, by decreasing IPAP in steps of 2–4 cm H_2O once or twice daily as tolerated.

Atelectasis
Epidemiology

Atelectasis is the collapse of a group of alveoli, a small lobule, a segment of a lobe, or rarely, a whole lung. It is one of the most common pulmonary complications in the postoperative patient. It is seen in about 90% of all patients who receive general anesthesia [28]. Typically, about 15–20% of the lung is collapsed at the bases during routine anesthesia prior to surgical intervention [29]. Atelectasis formation appears to correlate with the high inspired fractions of oxygen provided during anesthesia, particularly during induction. Providing pre-oxygenation and ventilation with 30% instead of 100% oxygen may prevent atelectasis formation during induction and subsequent anesthesia [30]. In addition, recruitment maneuvers aiming to re-open collapsed lung units during induction of anesthesia may be considered.

Clinically significant atelectasis occurs in 20% of patients undergoing upper abdominal surgery and 30% of thoracic surgery patients [31]. Atelectasis is clinically important because it can lead to increased work of breathing, impaired gas exchange, reduced lung compliance, increased pulmonary vascular resistance, and a predisposition to infection. Even micro-atelectasis, which is not radiographically visible, can cause hypoxemia.

Diagnosis

The diagnosis of atelectasis is based on physical findings and chest radiographs. Tachypnea, râles, absent, reduced, or bronchial breath sounds and dullness to percussion may be encountered. The association of fever with atelectasis is uncertain [32]. Mild leukocytosis may be present. Plain chest films may show increased density in a local segment, displacement of lobar fissures, elevation of the ipsilateral diaphragm, mediastinal shift towards the side of the collapse, or compensatory hyperinflation of other lung segments. Air bronchograms indicate that the bronchus feeding the atelectatic segment is patent. Frequently, it is difficult to differentiate between atelectasis and pneumonia, especially in the absence of bronchial obstruction.

Treatment

The treatment of postoperative atelectasis is based on two principles. The lungs must be expanded with a transpulmonary pressure sufficient to open collapsed lung units, and stagnant secretions must be cleared. Various therapeutic maneuvers have been used to accomplish these goals including early mobilization, sitting posture rather than supine, incentive spirometry, deep breathing exercises, coughing, chest physiotherapy, and NIV. Before initiating NIV in the postoperative period, surgical complications, e.g., leakage of anastomoses should be corrected and the total inspiratory pressure (PSV +PEEP) should be limited to 20–25 cm H_2O to avoid complications [26]. Intermittent positive pressure breathing has been abandoned because of concerns over barotrauma.

Non-invasive treatment

The use of incentive spirometry (IS) is controversial. Although 95% of hospitals in the USA use IS to treat atelectasis after laparotomy and 71% after coronary artery bypass, meta-analyses and reviews have failed to document a consistent beneficial effect [33]. Postoperative IS combined with chest physiotherapy provides no better results than chest physiotherapy alone [34]. Chest physiotherapy generally consists of deep breathing exercises, chest percussion, and postural drainage where needed. Deep breathing is most effective when 5 sequential breaths are held at TLC for 5–6 seconds and repeated hourly during waking hours. For established atelectasis, positive pressure ventilation, delivered as PEEP, CPAP, or PSV+PEEP (BiPAP) at 10–15 cm H_2O appears to provide satisfactory therapeutic results (see above) [35].

When an area of the lung is not ventilated, mucus secreted from the bronchi draining that area becomes thickened and impacted. This makes re-expansion of alveoli in that segment difficult. Chest physiotherapy and postural drainage can help to loosen and clear the mucus. Adequate hydration, along with the use of bronchodilators and mucolytic agents such as acetylcysteine or guaifenesin, may help to liquefy and mobilize secretions. Tracheal suctioning may be used to remove mucus that cannot be removed by cough or other respiratory maneuvers. Adequate pain relief is crucial so that the patient can cough without discomfort but oversedation with narcotics can depress respiratory drive and cause shallow respirations, exacerbating atelectasis. Patient-controlled analgesia, especially by the epidural route appears to offer the best balance between pain relief and respiratory drive [36].

Invasive treatment

Often, conservative therapy is sufficient to reverse atelectasis in the first 24–48 hours. Occasionally, more invasive methods such as bronchoscopy may be needed to extract mucus plugs, instill mucolytic agents directly into affected areas and lavage the airways. If an air bronchogram is present in the area of atelectasis, indicating patent central airways and suggestive of pneumonia, bronchoscopy is not likely to be helpful [37]. Other methods to treat atelectasis include expansion by selective air insufflation of atelectatic areas by a balloon-tipped catheter introduced into the appropriate bronchus under fluoroscopic or bronchoscopic guidance. In some patients adequate expansion cannot be accomplished with the above

Table 15.2 Risk for nosocomial pneumonia among surgical patients [38].

High risk	Relative risk	Low risk
Abdominal aortic aneurysm	4.29	Ophthalmologic
Thoracotomy	3.94	Otorhinolaryngologic
Upper abdominal	2.68	Lower abdominal
Neck	2.3	GU
Neurosurgical	2.14	Extremity
Vascular	1.29	Peripheral vascular
Emergency	1.33	Spine and back

methods, and endotracheal intubation and invasive mechanical ventilation may be needed.

Pneumonia
Epidemiology

Hospital-acquired pneumonia (HAP) is the second most common hospital-acquired infection in the USA and the leading cause of death from nosocomial infections. Any procedure requiring general anesthesia increases the risk for postoperative pneumonia. Hospital-acquired pneumonia, therefore, is more common in surgical than in medical populations [38]. Postoperative pneumonia occurs in up to 9–40% of patients, the risk depending on the specific surgical procedure as well as demographic risk factors. In the ICU, ventilator associated pneumonia (VAP) occurs in about 10–20% of patients receiving mechanical ventilation for more than 48 hours [39]. The rate of VAP per 1,000 ventilator-days was 2.4 for medical ICUs, 4.9 for surgical ICUs, 8.1 for trauma units, and 10.7 for burns units [40]. Relative risks by surgical procedure are summarized in Table 15.2.

Non-modifiable risk factors include age, male sex, functional status, multiorgan failure, preexisting cardiac, pulmonary, or neurological disease, ethanol intake, tobacco abuse within the year prior to surgery, altered sensorium, head trauma, and malnutrition. Potentially modifiable risks include transfusion of more than 4 units packed red blood cells, duration of mechanical ventilation, stress ulcer prophylaxis, enteral nutrition, and use of paralytic agents, antibiotics, and glucose control [41]. Burn patients, particularly those with inhalation injury are at the highest risk, 50% higher than cardiothoracic or neurosurgery patients, and nearly three times higher than medical patients [42].

Postoperative pneumonia increases healthcare cost and total hospital and ICU length of stay. Furthermore, VAP significantly increases the duration of mechanical ventilation. [43–57]. Ventilator associated pneumonia is associated with 6–21 times higher crude mortality rates, the highest rates

(43%) associated with high-risk organisms such as *Pseudomonas*, *Acinetobacter*, or methicillin-resistant *Staphylococcus aureus* (MRSA). Attributable mortality due to VAP is estimated at 30–50% of the crude mortality [44]. The crude mortality rate of HAP has been estimated to be between 30% and 70%, but actual mortality directly attributable to HAP may be lower (between 33% to 50%) [43].

Pathogenesis

The development of nosocomial pneumonia requires that a pathogenic microorganism gain access to the lower respiratory tract. These pathogens arise from a variety of sources including endogenous flora, other patients, hospital staff, the hospital environment, and surgical wound infection [45]. Common to most however, is colonization of the oropharynx, upper airways, and perhaps upper gastrointestinal tract. Colonization of the upper airway with hospital flora occurs within the first 72–96 hours of hospitalization and within a few hours after intubation. Endotracheal intubation plays a crucial role in the pathogenesis of VAP. Intubation may be complicated by aspiration. Additionally, the endotracheal tube can compromise the cough reflex allowing the accumulation of infected secretions in the supraglottic space [46]. Furthermore, bacterial biofilms, which are implicated in the pathogenesis of nosocomial infections, can develop quickly after intubation on the inner surface of the endotracheal tube. Biofilms can easily be dislodged by suction catheters, leading to inoculation of the lower respiratory tract [47].

Microbiology

Nosocomial pneumonia is polymicrobial in 40–60% of cases. Bacteremia is seen in approximately 10% of cases. Most data focus on the microbiology of patients with VAP. The microbiology of HAP is comparable to VAP, therefore similar empiric antibiotic regimes are used [48]. Postoperative pneumonia differs from the flora described for medical HAP by an excess of *Staphylococcus* and aerobic gram-negative isolates [49]. There is considerable variation in the relative proportions of organisms reported in individual studies. Some of the variability may be attributable to a failure to distinguish among early and late, and antibiotic-naïve and antibiotic-exposed infections. Sufficient variability exists to recommend that each institution establish its own lists of likely pathogens for each specific clinical setting. A large series describing VAP in a mixed ICU population is typical, however (Table 15.3). More recent data showed no major changes in these patterns [50]. The role of non-bacterial pathogens in HAP remains unclear. Recent studies reported that viral pathogens (e.g., HSV, CMV) and *Candida* species may play a role in VAP [51,52].

Prior antibiotic use appears more important than timing in predicting the presence of resistant flora. Anaerobes are not frequently reported although they may be present in up to 20% of cases when specifically looked for. Nevertheless, expert

Table 15.3 Microbial spectrum in ventilator associated pneumonia [53]. Percent isolated are shown in parentheses.

Early onset, no antibiotics	Early onset, prior antibiotics
Enterobacteriaciae[a] (24.4)	Enterobacteriaciae[a] (20)
Hemophilus influenzae (19.5)	*Hemophilus influenzae* (10)
MSSA (14.5)	Streptococcus species (25)
Streptococcus pneumoniae (7.3)	*Neisseria* (10)
Other Streptococcus species (17.1)	*Pseudomonas* (20)
	Acinetobacter (5)
Neisseria/Moraxella (12.2)	MRSA (5)
Late onset, no antibiotics	**Late onset, prior antibiotics**
Enterobacteriaciae[a] (21.9)	*Pseudomonas* (21.7)
Streptococcus species (21.9)	*Acinetobacter* (13.2)
MSSA (21.9)	MRSA (19.7)
Neisseria (12.5)	*Stenotrophomonas* (2)
Hemophilus (3)	*Enterobacter* (15)
Pseudomonas (6.3)	Strep species (9)
Acinetobacter (3.1)	MSSA (5)
MRSA (5)	

MRSA, methicillin-resistant *Staphylococcus aureus*; MSSA, methicillin-sensitive *Staphylococcus aureus*.
[a] Enterobacteriaciae (*Escherichia coli, Enterobacter, Serratia, Proteus, Klebsiella*).

consensus is that anaerobes may be safely ignored in the absence of necrotizing pneumonia or abscess formation [54].

Prevention

Ventilator associated pneumonia is a potentially preventable problem. Evidence-based guidelines for the prevention of VAP have been published [55], as well as comprehensive evidence-based guidelines for the prevention of HAP in general [43]. Strategies in these guidelines include general prophylaxis and aggressive infection control (hand disinfection, isolation gowns), oral cleansing with chlorhexidine, microbiological surveillance, antibiotic stewardship programs, avoidance of nasotracheal intubation, preferential use of non-invasive ventilation, a conservative blood transfusion strategy, and the use of orogastric rather than nasogastric tubes. The risk of aspiration can be minimized by keeping the patient in a semi-erect position and through avoidance of gastric over-distension. Small bore feeding tubes and postpyloric feeding tube placement may also be helpful. Ventilator liberation should be pursued as expeditiously as possible. Oropharyngeal secretions should always be suctioned prior to deflation of an endotracheal tube cuff.

The implementation of a ventilator bundle has been promoted to improve the quality of care provided in ICUs. The ventilator bundle includes elevation of the head of the bed to 30–45°, daily sedation holidays, and peptic ulcer disease (PUD) and deep vein thrombosis prophylaxis. Peptic ulcer disease prophylaxis remains a controversial issue, especially whether gastric pH significantly affects the risk of oropharyngeal colonization and VAP. Although implementation of the

ventilator bundle has been shown to decrease rates of VAP [56], it remains underused in many ICUs across the USA [57].

It may be advantageous to treat ventilator associated tracheobronchitis (VAT) to prevent the progression to VAP. In a recent multicenter, randomized trial, the investigators found a statistically significant reduction in the rate of progression to VAP in the group that received 8 days of antibiotics vs a placebo group [58]. In clinical practice however, the diagnosis of VAT is complicated due to the difficulties in standardizing the interpretation of chest radiographs. There is need for further research in this area.

Diagnosis

Combinations of clinical and microbiological strategies provide the best approach in diagnosing VAP [59]. Various criteria for the diagnosis of nosocomial and VAP are presented in Table 15.4. Pulmonary infiltrates present prior to admission or surgery are not considered as postoperative pneumonia.

Clinical diagnosis of VAP is generally characterized by better sensitivity than specificity. Requiring that all three clinical criteria be met increases specificity, but sensitivity falls below 50%. The utility of clinical scoring systems such as the Clinical Pulmonary Infections Score (CPIS) remains unclear. When the CPIS is used alone, it might underestimate the incidence of VAP. Nevertheless, a recent review concluded that using the CPIS could help to determine which patients may be treated with shorter duration of antibiotics [60].

The chest roentgenogram is also sensitive but non-specific. Most infiltrates in ventilated patients are not VAP; rather pulmonary edema, pulmonary hemorrhage, and focal atelectasis are more common [61]. Radiographic appearance can be influenced by respiratory phase, depth of inspiration and even ventilator mode. High rates of interobserver variability in interpretation are common. Absence of an infiltrate, however, effectively excludes a diagnosis of VAP [62]. As can be seen from Table 15.4, specific microbiological sampling does not improve significantly upon clinical criteria, and is helpful only when a high clinical suspicion and an abnormal chest film are both present.

Clinical practice varies regarding the most appropriate method to obtain culture specimens. Endotracheal suction specimens are evaluated in a manner similar to sputum, based on the number of squamous epithelial cells and neutrophils. Diagnoses based on stains are more sensitive but less specific than those based on semi-quantitative cultures, using a threshold of 10^5 or 10^6 cfu/mL. A negative endotracheal specimen, however, is sufficient to exclude infection. More invasive strategies include bronchoalveolar lavage (BAL) and protected brush specimens (PBS). Bronchoscopic specimens are associated with higher specificity than endotracheal aspirates, but do not improve outcomes. Intracellular organisms on stains of any of the above specimens carry a sensitivity of 37–100% and a specificity of 89–100%.

In the absence of ongoing antibiotic therapy, lower concentrations than specified above or negative cultures are sufficient

Table 15.4 Criteria for the diagnosis of ventilator associated pneumonia.

Source	Clinical	CDC	CPIS	Tracheal suction	PBS	BAL
Criteria	New or progressive infiltrate beginning after intubation plus 2 of 3: Temperature > 38 °C WBC > 10,000/mL Purulent endotracheal secretions	1. Râles or dullness to percussion on physical examination of chest AND any of the following: New onset of purulent sputum or change in character of sputum Isolation of organism from blood culture, transtracheal aspirate, bronchial brushing, or biopsy 2. Chest radiography showing new or progressive infiltrate, consolidation, cavitation, or pleural effusion AND any of the following: New onset of purulent sputum or change in character of sputum Isolation of organism from blood culture Isolation of pathogen from specimen obtained by transtracheal aspirate, bronchial brushing, or biopsy Isolation of virus or detection of viral antigen in respiratory secretions Diagnostic single antibody titer (IgM) or fourfold increase in paired serum samples (IgG) for pathogen Histopathologic evidence of pneumonia	≥ 7 points Temperature °C 36.5–38.4 (0) 38.5–38.9 (1) ≥ 39 or ≤ 36 (2) Blood WBC × 10³/L ≥ 4 and ≤ 11 (0) < 4 or > 11 (1) Bands > 0.5 (1) Daily tracheal secretion volume (0–4) Σ < 14 (0) Σ ≥ 14 (1) Purulence (1) P_aO_2/F_iO_2 ratio (mmHg) > 240 or ARDS (0) ≤ 240 no ARDS (2) Chest roentgenogram No infiltrate (0) Diffuse/patchy (1) Localized infiltrate (2) Semiquantitative culture (pathogens, 0–3+) ≤ 1+ or no growth (0) > 1+ (1) Culture matches Gram's stain (1)	Bacteria present on Gram's stain Culture > 10⁵ cfu/mL	Culture > 10³ cfu/mL	Culture > 10⁴ cfu/mL with < 1% squamous cells 2–25% intracellular organisms
Sensitivity (%)	48–100	68	72	Stain 94–100 Culture 38–82	33–100 (mean 67)	42–93 (mean 73)
Specificity (%)	12–91	97.8	85	Stain 14–38 Culture 67–100	50–100 (mean 95)	45–100 (mean 82)

Modified from Welty-Wolf K. Ventilator-associated pneumonia. In MacIntyre NR, Branson RD, eds. *Mechanical Ventilation*. Philadelphia: W.B. Saunders; 2001, pp. 296–328.

to exclude a clinically significant infection. Interpretation in the presence of antibiotics has not been well-standardized and remains problematic [63]. There is insufficient evidence, however, that quantitative or invasive testing improves outcome or decreases mortality [64]. The best use for invasive specimens is to facilitate the elimination of unnecessary antibiotics after an initial empiric regimen is started.

Treatment

Prompt initiation of appropriate antibiotic treatment of VAP within 12 hours of diagnosis leads to improved survival [44]. Conversely, inappropriate initial antibiotic therapy for HAP is associated with poor outcomes and increased mortality [65]. While Gram stain of an adequate respiratory tract specimen may help refine an initial antibiotic choice, culture results, which are not available for 24–48 hours, do not become available in sufficient time to improve outcome. Nevertheless, an initial antibiotic regimen should be modified once culture results become available. Any redundant or unnecessary antibiotics should be discontinued as soon as possible and all antibiotics should be stopped in the event of negative cultures.

Specific treatment recommendations are addressed elsewhere but are available in recently published treatment guidelines [43]. Improved patient outcomes and decreased antibiotic resistance have been reported when guidelines for the management of HAP are followed [65]. To select an appropriate initial antibiotic regiment, it is vital to determine if risk factors for multidrug resistant (MDR) organisms are present. Multidrug resistant risk factors include antimicrobial therapy or hospitalization in the previous 90 days, current hospitalization >5 days, outpatient hemodialysis or infusion therapy, residence of nursing home or extended care facility, high frequency of antibiotic resistance in the community or hospital unit, or immunosuppression [43].

Clinical settings

Management of postoperative pneumonia is based on clinical context. Time since hospital admission and the prior administration of antibiotics as well as the nature of the patient's surgery are key considerations. For the first 72–96 hours of the hospital stay, the microbial flora in the upper airway consists of common community-acquired organisms. This is true of pneumonias seen both on general wards and ICUs, whether the patient is intubated or not. Early-onset pneumonias are generally responsive to shorter courses of antibiotics and tend to be associated with a relatively lower mortality. The microbial flora seen in early pneumonias in surgical patients is the same as that encountered in community-acquired pneumonia in a medical setting. *Staphylococcus*, however, is frequent in neurosurgical and head-injured patients. When encountered early in the absence of prior antibiotics, it is almost always methicillin-sensitive. Increasing length of hospitalization and prior antibiotic use increase the likelihood of a methicillin-resistant isolate.

Many surgical patients receive antibiotics as part of their initial management, either as part of initial resuscitation, or as preoperative wound prophylaxis. The use of antibiotics decreases the incidence of early-onset pneumonias and virtually eliminates *H. influenzae* and *S. pneumoniae* as pathogens. Unfortunately, prior antibiotic use also increases the frequency of late-onset pneumonias which are associated with a less-responsive and higher-risk bacterial flora. This is especially problematic with broad-spectrum antibiotics, leading to the frequent isolation of resistance-prone organisms (e.g., *Pseudomonas, Acinetobacter baumannii*, methicillin-resistant *Staphylococcus aureus*). Patients with a shorter duration of preoperative hospitalization, such as those with trauma, are more likely to develop early-type pneumonia while laparotomy patients tend to present with a late-onset microbial spectrum.

The most widely recommended approach to VAP is that each institution develops customized guidelines on antibiotic use based on local microbiological data and susceptibility profiles. A locally derived algorithm can lead to correct therapy in as many as 94% of cases [66]. Monotherapy and limited spectrum therapy may be safely used for patients with early pneumonia and no prior antibiotic use [54]. As the probability of MDR organisms rises, combination therapy becomes more important and is strongly recommended for patients with late pneumonia and prior antibiotic use. Broad-spectrum therapy including anti-pseudomonal cephalosporins, penicillins, fluoroquinolones or carbapenems, as well as vancomycin or linezolid to cover Gram-positive pathogens including MRSA should be used as part of an initial therapy for patients at risk for MDR organisms.

Optimal duration of treatment has not been definitively determined. Most patients with HAP show a good response within the first week of treatment. Based on randomized clinical trials published over the last decade [67], most clinicians prescribe shorter duration of antibiotics (6–8 days) rather than longer durations (14–21 days) as previously practiced. Failure to improve after 7 days should call for a reassessment of infections and their treatment. When treating VAP caused by non-fermenting Gram-negative bacilli such as *P. aeruginosa, A. baumannii,* and *S. maltophilia* longer courses of antibiotics (14–21 days) are recommended due to a high risk of relapse [68].

Other strategies under consideration include continuous intravenous and aerosolized antibiotics. However, further research is needed in this area to confirm the efficacy of these approaches.

Aspiration
Epidemiology

Aspiration is defined as the inhalation of oropharyngeal or gastric contents into the larynx and lower respiratory tract, due to passive regurgitation or active vomiting in patients with impaired laryngeal protective reflexes. There are two separate aspiration syndromes, aspiration pneumonitis and aspiration pneumonia; clinicians commonly fail to distinguish the two, using antibiotics unnecessarily. Some of the most common pre- and postoperative risk factors for aspiration include depressed level of consciousness, advanced age, pregnancy, recent ingestion of solid food or fluids, esophageal reflux, delayed gastric emptying, and laryngeal incompetence [69]. The highest frequency of aspiration pneumonia involves patients undergoing tracheostomy procedures, 19.1%, compared with an average of 0.7% in patients undergoing procedures other than tracheostomy [70].

Aspiration occurs most frequently during induction of anesthesia and laryngoscopy. The role of cricoid pressure is controversial. In high-risk patients, awake fiberoptic intubation may be a reasonable option [71]. Recently, in an experimental model application of PEEP during cuff deflation and extubation was protective against aspiration, suggesting that unless contraindications are present, the application of PEEP should be considered when extubating patients [72].

Pneumonitis

Aspiration pneumonitis is chemical injury due to inhalation of sterile gastric contents. Traditionally, the severity of the injury has been associated with critical values of pH and volume of aspiration. For instance, aspiration of gastric contents with pH < 2.5 and volumes > 0.3 mL/kg (20–25 mL) may progress to ARDS; however, this concept has recently been questioned [73]. Aspiration pneumonitis may be clinically silent or may progress rapidly to respiratory failure within 2–5 hours after aspiration [74].

Pneumonia

Aspiration pneumonia is defined as inhalation of oropharyngeal secretions colonized by pathogens and is addressed above in the context of pneumonia. It is important to note that in the absence of severe periodontal disease or radiographic evidence of necrotizing pneumonia, anaerobes are only rarely present [75].

Management

The upper airway should be examined in the event of an aspiration episode and should be suctioned. Patients with depressed consciousness should be intubated. Empiric antibiotics are appropriate only for patients with small bowel obstruction or ileus and for pneumonitis that fails to resolve within 48 hours. The injured respiratory epithelium caused by an acid-related aspiration pneumonitis favors the occurrence of aspiration pneumonia due to bacterial superinfection [76]. Fluoroquinolones, piperacillin/tazobactam, or ceftriaxone provide adequate coverage for most cases. There is no benefit to the addition of systemic steroids [74].

Table 15.5 Prevalence of deep vein thrombosis in hospitalized patients without thromboprophylaxis [80].

Patient type	DVT prevalence %
Medical	10–20
General surgery	15–40
Major urologic surgery	15–40
Major gynecologic surgery	15–40
Neurosurgery	15–40
Stroke	20–50
Orthopedic	40–60
Critical care	10–80
Major trauma	40–80
Spinal cord injury	60–80

Deep vein thrombosis (DVT) prevalence is high (see Table 15.5) and if left untreated, progression with associated morbidity and mortality is significant. In patients with VTE, 30 day mortality ranges from 10–30% with the vast majority of deaths due to pulmonary embolism (PE). About 20–25% of PE presents as sudden death, but with early detection and adequate treatment, mortality from PE decreases to 5–8% [82].

Venous thromboembolism
Epidemiology

The postsurgical state is a major risk factor for development of venous thromboembolism (VTE) due to significant alterations in all three components of Virchow's triad resulting in: stasis/blood flow abnormalities, vascular/endothelial damage, and hypercoagulability. The risk of postoperative VTE, which includes deep venous thrombosis (DVT) and pulmonary embolism (PE) is highest during the first 2–3 weeks and remains elevated for 2–3 months [77].

The prevalence of VTE in the general population is steadily increasing, with 432 estimated cases per 100,000 in 2010. Approximately 70% of cases present with DVT, 24% with PE, and 6% with both DVT and PE. The odds of developing VTE in a postoperative patient are 46.7 times higher than in medical patients [78]. With increasing use of intravascular devices and central lines, the incidence of upper extremity (including subclavian, axillary, jugular veins) disease has also been increasing, accounting for approximately 1–4% of all DVT cases and around 18% of in-hospital DVTs (Table 15.5) [79].

According to the most recent guidelines [80], appropriate thromboprophylaxis for hospitalized patients will prevent most VTE events, however studies show that prophylaxis is still underutilized [81].

Risk factors

Multiple risk factors, both genetic and acquired, contribute to development of VTE (see Table 15.6).

Table 15.6 Risk factors for venous thromboembolism (VTE) [83].

Risk factor	
Acquired	**Genetic**
Advancing age	Family history
Race/ethnicity	Factor V Leiden
Chronic disease (cardiac, respiratory, renal, endocrine, neurologic, hematologic, rheumatologic, inflammatory conditions)	Prothrombin G20210A
Obesity	Protein C deficiency
Hospitalization	Protein S deficiency
Surgery (by ASA class, type and emergent status)	Antithrombin deficiency
Immobility	Sickle cell trait
Trauma	
Cancer (and cancer-related therapy)	
Pregnancy and female gender	
Medications (OCP, HRT)	
Prior VTE or antiphospholipid antibodies	
Intravascular catheters	
Infection and critical illness	
Vascular compression or varicose veins	

ASA, American Society of Anesthesiologists; HRT, hormone replacement therapy; OCP, oral contraceptive pills.

Diagnosis

Venous thromboembolism is often clinically silent, making it difficult to diagnose in the surgical patient. In addition, post-operative hardware, dressings, bandages, splints, and casts limit adequate evaluation. Bedside diagnosis carries a sensitivity of 25% and a specificity of 33% [82], and further confirmatory testing is usually required. Despite low sensitivity and specificity, evaluation should focus on signs and symptoms that help rule out VTE. Clinical probability scoring tools are available to stratify patients into low-, intermediate-, and high-likelihood groups [83]. Most surgical patients at the outset already satisfy criteria for intermediate- and high-likelihood groups.

Venous thrombosis

Venous duplex ultrasonography is now the most widely used initial non-invasive screening modality for evaluating DVT. It has high sensitivity (97%) and specificity (94%), and has replaced contrast venography as the diagnostic test of choice. It is also able to image calf veins in 80–98% of cases with high accuracy. However, limitations arise with morbidly obese, edematous, and orthopedic patients with external hardware,

immobilization devices, and surgical wounds [84]. In these situations, further testing using contrast venography (or CT venography, CTV) or magnetic resonance venography (MRV), both with the advantage of visualizing intra-abdominal and proximal vasculature) may be warranted. In patients with a negative screening duplex scan at high risk for DVT, repeat imaging within a week is recommended.

Pulmonary embolism

Computed tomography pulmonary angiography (CTPA) has replaced V/Q scanning as the test of choice for suspected PE. Sensitivity and specificity is 83% and 96%, with positive predictive values of 97% for main and lobar pulmonary arteries [85]. The sensitivity going peripherally is 68% for segmental and 25% for subsegmental branches. Scanning can be combined with CT venography to evaluate extrathoracic vasculature and extremities for clots, however, the risk for contrast-induced nephropathy increases. In patients with renal failure or allergy to contrast, a V/Q scan or perfusion scan may be utilized. When clinical likelihood is low, a low probability scan is sufficient to exclude PE, but an indeterminate scan in the setting of moderate to high clinical likelihood necessitates further evaluation.

Technically adequate MR pulmonary angiography combined with MRV performed in established centers has a sensitivity of 92% and a specificity of 96% for PE. Given the better diagnostic yield compared with the V/Q scan, MR may be used as second-line imaging, however its cost and availability may be limiting [86].

In patients with suspected PE presenting with hemodynamic instability (massive PE) that precludes transport for imaging, bedside echocardiography should be performed to evaluate for RV dysfunction. Signs of RV dysfunction on echo include McConell's sign showing RV free wall hypokinesis with intact apical contraction, RV dilatation indicating pressure overload, and impaired RV ejection (the 60–60 sign) [77]. The absence of these findings effectively rules out PE as a cause for shock. Occasionally, echo may also demonstrate a clot in transit, dilatation of the pulmonary arteries or IVC, and paradoxical septal motion suggesting PE. Echo evaluation should also involve rapid assessment of the left heart, valves, pericardium, pleura, lung parenchyma, and volume status to search for other causes of respiratory and hemodynamic compromise. Other tests for risk assessment include troponin for evidence of ischemia/infarction and BNP for myocardial strain/heart failure. Negative values coupled with absent signs of RV dysfunction in a normotensive patient indicate a low immediate risk of dying (< 3%) [77]. An ECG may show a RBBB or S1Q3T3 pattern with T-wave inversions on V1–4 (sensitivity 18–20%), though most cases will only show sinus tachycardia.

D-dimer testing has high sensitivity but low specificity (< 50%) as levels are already elevated postoperatively. In addition, underlying infection, critical illness, and malignancy, make interpretation of positive results difficult. The utility of this test lies in its negative predictive value where a low or negative D-dimer may be helpful in ruling out VTE.

Pulmonary angiography was once the gold standard test for PE, but is now considered an adjunctive modality when CT or MR imaging is inconclusive. Its use is limited by the invasiveness of the procedure, need for contrast material, and a mortality risk of 0.2%. It is superior in detecting clots up to the subsegmental arteries which may be 1–2 mm in diameter, but consistent interpretation at this level is compromised by low interobserver agreement. Angiography is useful in surgical intervention (thrombectomy/embolectomy) planning, or when catheter directed thrombolysis along with hemodynamic measurements are needed [87].

Treatment

General considerations

Postoperative VTE treatment requires careful balancing of the risks of bleeding and the risks of untreated thromboembolic disease against the benefits of anticoagulation. The risk of bleeding is highest in the first 24 hours, and may remain elevated up to 10 days after surgery. Postoperative bleeding may be seen in 3–5% of surgeries and causes significant morbidity, increases reoperation rates and resource use. Without immediate therapy, mortality of bleeding is high [88].

Surgeries with high risk for bleeding include CABG or valvular surgery, intracranial or spinal operations, aortic aneurysm repair, peripheral artery bypass, or other major vascular surgery, major orthopedic surgery, i.e., hip or knee replacement, reconstructive plastic surgery, major cancer surgery, and prostate and bladder surgery. In addition, the following procedures also carry significant risk: resection of colonic polyps (> 2 cm sessile polyps), prostate or kidney biopsy, and cardiac pacemaker or defibrillator implantation [88].

Other factors increasing bleeding risk include medications, e.g., antiplatelet agents, anticoagulants, or NSAIDs, coagulopathy due to thrombocytopenia, factor deficiency, liver disease, transfusion washout, or DIC, specific factor inhibitors acquired preoperatively or intraoperatively, or an increased postoperative fibrinolytic state.

In the medical setting, the rate of major bleeding from heparin and low molecular weight heparin (LMWH) is < 3% and the case fatality rate from major bleeding is approximately 3% [89]. Among surgical patients, the risk of postoperative bleeding with heparin increases to 10.5%; and bleeding is usually major.

After perioperative initiation of anticoagulation (LMWH and coumadin), the incidence of bleeding following invasive procedures, minor and major operations was reported to be 0.7%, 0%, and 20% respectively. Thromboembolic events occurred in 1.9% of anticoagulated patients and no deaths were reported [90].

Specific medications

Unfractionated heparin (UFH) remains the initial treatment of choice for VTE. Depending on the clinical setting, treatment can be initiated using either: (1) IV infusion of UFH, (2) subcutaneous (SC) LMWH, (3) high-dose SC fixed UFH or SC UFH with monitoring, or (4) SC fondaparinux [91]. Dosing of UFH is weight-based and should follow a nomogram, while titration should aim at maintaining a therapeutic APTT level with anti-Xa activity between 0.3 to 0.7 IU/mL. Intravenous UFH is preferred for critically ill postoperative patients for ease of administration, titration, reversal (with protamine), short half-life, and is not contraindicated in liver or renal failure. For patients on a general ward, SC preparations may be utilized and continued in the outpatient setting.

Low molecular weight heparins such as enoxaparin, tinzaparin, nadroparin, and dalteparin are options for prophylactic and therapeutic anticoagulation in surgical setting. They have longer half-lives, similar to better efficacy as UFH, and a lesser risk of bleeding. In the setting of malignancy with VTE, LMWH has shown reduction in mortality compared with UFH [92]. For long-term treatment of cancer patients with VTE, LMWH decreases recurrence of VTE compared with warfarin. Low molecular weight heparin (enoxaparin) can be dosed at 1.5 mg/kg daily or 1 mg/kg BID, the former being associated with a non-significant lower risk of bleeding, while the latter is associated with lesser VTE recurrence in patients with malignancy [93]. In obese patients (≥ 190 kg), anti-Xa levels may guide dose adjustment, while in renal failure (CrCl < 30), dosing should be decreased by 50%.

Heparin therapy puts patients at risk for development of heparin induced thrombocytopenia (HIT), defined by a 50% drop in platelet counts within 5–10 days of receiving heparin. It occurs via an antibody-mediated reaction directed against Platelet Factor 4 (PF-4) resulting in rapid consumption of platelets with significantly increased risk of arterial and venous thrombotic events. It is seen in up to 5% of patients given UFH, and 1% with LMWH. Platelet counts should be monitored and once HIT is suspected, therapy should be switched to the synthetic pentasaccharides (e.g., fondaparinux, idraparinux) or direct thrombin inhibitors (DTIs) such as argatroban or lepirudin. Likelihood of HIT may be gauged by platelet count and time course, by history of prior heparin exposure and by the presence or absence of competing diagnoses [93].

Synthetic pentasaccharides fondaparinux and idraparinux work by selectively binding antithrombin III, potentiating Factor Xa neutralization and inhibiting thrombin generation. Studies have shown that fondaparinux is non-inferior to LMWH and IV UFH for treatment of DVTs and PEs respectively [91]. Fondaparinux is dosed on a weight-based scale: 5 mg SC daily for < 50 kg, 10 mg for 50–100 kg, and 10 mg for >100 kg.

Direct thrombin inhibitors, as the name implies, directly inhibit thrombin generation. This class of drugs includes: the parenteral preparations – bivalirudin, lepirudin, argatroban; the subcutaneous – desirudin; and oral – dabigatran. The parenteral agents are used as second- to third-line therapy when heparins are contraindicated (i.e., HIT).

The vitamin K antagonist warfarin is the current standard for long-term management of outpatient anticoagulation. It inhibits synthesis of Factors II, VII, IX, and X as well as Proteins C and S. It is necessary to overlap warfarin intake with heparin therapy until an INR level of 2–3 is maintained for > 24 hours due to transient hypercoagulability from initial loss of Proteins C and S. Coumadin is initially dosed at 5–10 mg/day and adjusted thereafter based on the INR level. Subtherapeutic anticoagulation increases the incidence of long-term VTE complications such as: thrombus extension (20%), recurrent VTEs (47%), and development of post-thrombotic syndrome (20–50%) [91]. Duration of therapy is at least 3–6 months for DVT with a reversible risk factor (i.e., surgery, immobilization). However, those with residual risk factors (i.e., malignancy, thrombophilia), will require long-term therapy. The risk of major bleeding on therapeutic warfarin is 0.3–0.5%/year [89].

Newer oral anticoagulants are now being utilized for DVT treatment. These include DTIs – dabigatran – and direct Factor Xa inhibitors – rivaroxaban, apixaban, and betrixaban. Initial studies are promising showing non-inferiority to warfarin with a similar safety profile, without requiring serial monitoring or dosage adjustment [94]. Longer-term studies are ongoing to establish efficacy and safety before warfarin can be replaced as the treatment standard.

Thrombolysis

In the setting of massive PE with hemodynamic compromise, guidelines recommend rapid stratification of patients followed by thrombolytic therapy provided no bleeding contraindication exists [91]. The thrombolytic of choice is recombinant tissue plasminogen activator (rt-PA) given at a dose of 100 mg over 2 hours through a peripheral vein. Recombinant tissue plasminogen activator converts plasminogen to plasmin, promoting fibrinolysis; this infusion should be given with concurrent IV UFH. Rate of major bleeding after thrombolytic therapy with anticoagulation is 13% while intracranial hemorrhage is 1.8% [77]. Optimal time for thrombolytic therapy is within 48 hours, but may be considered up to 14 days. In the decompensating patient in need of intervention emergently (< 2 hours time required for rt-PA infusion) or the surgical patient whose bleeding risk is high where thrombolysis is too risky (or thrombolysis has failed), catheter embolectomy (or fragmentation) may be utilized, provided adequate procedural expertise is available [91]. Pulmonary embolectomy is another option for these patients with contraindications to, or have failed thrombolytic therapy, for repair of patent foramen ovale and removal of intracardiac thrombi [77]. At this time, thrombolysis or surgical intervention is not recommended in patients with submassive PE who are hemodynamically stable, but have RV dysfunction.

Inferior vena cava filter

Inferior vena cava filters (IVCF) have been used when problems arise from anticoagulation therapy. The specific indications for IVCF placement include: (1) confirmed VTE with contraindications to anticoagulation; (2) bleeding complications during anticoagulation; (3) chronic thromboembolic pulmonary hypertension; (4) extension of known thrombosis or recurrent PE during anticoagulation [91]. Encouraging data show that over time, IVCF reduces risk of PE up to 8 years (RR 0.41) but with increases in DVT (RR 1.3) and local thrombosis in 43% of cases. Prophylactic IVCF placement, though not guideline recommended, is accepted in high-risk situations such as submassive PE [95]. In patients with extensive proximal DVT whose symptom duration is 7–14 days with good functional status, low risk of bleeding, and a life expectancy > 1 year, catheter-directed thrombolysis or venous thrombectomy may be considered [91].

Pulmonary edema

Epidemiology

Pulmonary edema is seen in up to 27% of patients with postoperative respiratory failure and is frequently associated with preexisting cardiac disease [96]. Edema is usually mild to moderate in severity, but may present as acute lung injury or acute respiratory distress syndrome (ARDS).

Pathogenesis

Pulmonary edema occurs via a combination of two or more of the following mechanisms: (1) increased intravascular hydrostatic pressures (and/or decreased colloid osmotic pressure); (2) endothelial cell (and glycocalyx layer), damage resulting in increased capillary permeability or frank disruption of vascular integrity; (3) breakdown of alveolar epithelial barrier function; and (4) impaired lymphatic drainage.

Cardiogenic (or hydrostatic) pulmonary edema is seen in patients with heart failure or myocardial infarction. Noncardiogenic (usually permeability) pulmonary edema may occur following acute inflammatory lung injury, airway obstruction, rapid reexpansion of a collapsed lung, transfusion reaction, pulmonary resection, or ischemia-reperfusion injury.

Surgery itself predisposes to pulmonary edema when fluid administered intraoperatively re-enters the intravascular space 72 hours postoperatively causing increased hydrostatic pressures. The amount of fluid that causes pulmonary edema varies with age, body weight, tissue turgor, cardiopulmonary and renal function, and the size of the interstitial space. Net retention of more than 2.2 L/day or more than 20% body weight increases the likelihood of pulmonary edema [97].

Also during surgery, inflammatory mediators along with substances such as bacterial endotoxin, lysosomal enzymes, microemboli, fat emboli, or platelet aggregates may be released into the systemic circulation and deposit in the pulmonary capillary bed producing endothelial damage and increased vascular permeability. Decreased plasma oncotic pressures occur when protein from the intravascular compartment leaks into the interstitial space, promoting edema. In those with underlying infections, the systemic immune response can be severe enough that acute inflammatory lung injury develops.

Etiologies

Pulmonary edema and/or pulmonary hemorrhage from upper airway obstruction or laryngospasm may occur in 0.05–0.1% of general anesthesia cases after extubation. Cases can be severe or even fatal, and usually occur a few hours after extubation, but may be seen as late as 36 hours postoperatively. Inspiration in the presence of an obstructed upper airway generates extremely negative intrathoracic pressures with increasing pulmonary blood volume and hydrostatic pressures. When sufficiently severe, capillary rupture follows leading to alveolar hemorrhage thereby worsening the underlying edema. Immediate therapy involves reestablishing airway patency, supportive ventilation, sedation and muscle relaxants for spasm, and steroids for airway edema if present. Resolution over 24–48 hours is the usual course [98].

Rapid reexpansion of a collapsed lung may also result in what is termed reexpansion pulmonary edema [99]. Among conditions causing the initial compression/atelectasis are: pleural effusion, pneumothorax, a large extrinsic tumor, or lung entrapment from diseases causing chronic pleural inflammation resulting in formation of a fibrinous peel. It is thought that once the cause for collapse is removed, edema occurs from the rapid reperfusion and re-inflation of the atelectatic lung parenchyma with accompanying influx of inflammatory mediators, immune cells, and reactive oxygen species, resulting in endothelial injury and increased permeability.

Transfusion reactions from blood products may also cause non-cardiogenic pulmonary edema. Transfusion-related acute lung injury, or TRALI, is defined as lung injury occurring within 6 hours of transfusion. Risk for TRALI is 1/260,000 for all blood products and is highest for FFP (1/66,000) [100]. The mechanism is multifactorial with a "two hit hypothesis" involving: (1) a susceptible host with activated granulocytes and/or damaged endothelium; and (2) receiving blood products containing antigens (human neutrophil antigen), antibodies (HLA class I and II), ligands (CD40), and biologically active lipids. Once suspected, transfusion should be stopped and supportive therapy/ventilation started immediately. Transfusion-related acute lung injury should be distinguished from transfusion-associated circulatory overload (TACO); the latter is hydrostatic pulmonary edema without the immune reaction and is managed like CHF [101].

Edema after pulmonary resection (lobectomy, pneumonectomy) and ischemia-reperfusion (after lung transplantation) share similar features of increased hydrostatic pressures (after reversal of hypoxic pulmonary vasoconstriction and redistribution of blood flow), endothelial/vascular damage, surgical disruption of epithelium and lymphatic drainage, and inflammation. The extreme form of reperfusion edema, termed primary graft dysfunction, is seen in about 10–25% of lung transplants, while post-resection edema is seen in 5% of pneumonectomies. These forms of edema increase ventilator dependence, length of stay, and are associated with high mortality, approximately 50% [102,103]. Both are treated supportively.

Diagnosis

The diagnosis of pulmonary edema is based on the clinical exam and roentgenographic picture, with bilateral râles, and imaging showing diffuse fluffy infiltrates. Hydrostatic edema is commonly associated with perihilar opacities in a butterfly-wing pattern, widening of the vascular pedicle, Kerley B lines, and an enlarged cardiac silhouette. Jugular venous distension is common. Permeability edema tends to show patchy opacities with normal cardiac and vascular profiles [104]. Arterial blood gases will show hypoxemia and sometimes hypercarbia.

Treatment

Treating pulmonary edema requires correction of the underlying etiology and minimizing fluid overload. In patients with cardiac disease, functional assessment and surgical planning should start preoperatively and medical therapy optimized. Studies have shown that a "rational" intraoperative fluid strategy [97] with goal-directed fluid replacement [105] to maintain normovolemia minimizes postoperative complications and improves outcomes. Fluid administration should aim to match intraoperative losses from bleeding, drains, and urine output, in addition to insensible losses, between 0.5 to 1 mL/kg/hour [97]. Postoperative fluid status should be monitored by daily review of intake and output, physical exam, and weight. With widespread in-hospital utilization of central venous catheters (CVC), pulmonary artery catheter use has fallen out of favor, as trials have shown decreased ventilator and ICU days in surgical patients with ALI managed with a conservative fluid strategy guided by CVC monitoring [106]. Brain natriuretic peptide (BNP) levels may also be used as a marker for fluid overload and followed to judge effectiveness of diuretic therapy. Echocardiography should be performed to assess cardiac function and structural abnormalities. In patients with pre-existing or progressive renal failure refractory to medical therapy, hemodialysis or hemofiltration should be utilized. In patients with overt heart failure, inotropic therapy should be considered.

In addition to supplemental oxygen for hypoxemia, studies show benefit from the use of non-invasive positive pressure ventilation. Continuous positive airway pressure or Bilevel (BiPAP) therapy reduces cardiac and respiratory workload by decreasing venous return (preload), increasing alveolar recruitment, and improving shunt physiology. Moreover, NIV may be used as a bridge for ventilatory support post-extubation in patients with underlying lung disease [107]. If these measures fail, reintubation with full ventilatory support should be reinstituted with a lung protective strategy [108]. In the setting of refractory hypoxemia and severe lung injury, high frequency oscillatory ventilation or extracorporeal membrane oxygenation (ECMO) may be necessary.

Pleural effusion

Epidemiology

Pleural effusions should be high among differential diagnoses for postoperative respiratory failure, as they are commonly associated with problems seen after surgery. Compared with the medical population where effusions are seen in 5–12%, effusions in the surgical population can be found in 49% following abdominal surgery [109], and may be as high as 87% after coronary artery bypass grafting [110].

Classification

The pleural space normally contains a small amount of lubricating fluid (12–15 mL in adults) with a low protein concentration of 1–2 g/dL [111]. Effusions form when the rate of fluid formation exceeds the rate of drainage. Excessive hydrostatic or decreased oncotic pressures produce increased fluid filtration across capillary walls and result in protein-poor transudates. Breakdown of normal formation-resorption mechanisms because of damage to pleural surfaces or blockage of lymphatics results in protein-rich exudates. Effusions can be broadly classified into transudates or exudates according to Light's criteria [112].

The definition of an exudative pleural fluid is based on the presence of any one of the following features:

- Pleural fluid total protein/serum total protein ratio greater than 0.5.
- Pleural fluid LDH/serum LDH ratio greater than 0.6.
- Pleural fluid LDH is greater than two-thirds upper normal for serum LDH.

All three criteria must be absent to define a transudate. Determining characteristics of the fluid is important as it can suggest the underlying causative process and impact therapeutic decisions.

The differential diagnosis of postoperative pleural effusions is shown in Table 15.7.

Diagnosis and treatment

Determining the clinical context in which the effusion is seen and quantifying the amount of fluid present are first steps in evaluation. Chest X-rays are useful for detecting effusions but quantifying volume requires further imaging. Decubitus films can be obtained and as a general rule, thoracentesis should be performed for layering parapneumonic effusions > 10 mm. Other imaging modalities include CT scan and ultrasonography (USG).

The emergence of pleural USG has significantly improved the diagnosis and management of effusions as it not only helps characterize the type of fluid present, but it also optimizes success of thoracentesis and minimizes complications [113]. Contrast-enhanced CT scans may also play a role in characterizing fluid density and identifying other intrathoracic (pleural, parenchymal, mediastinal) processes that may cause effusions.

Table 15.7 Differential diagnosis of postoperative pleural effusions.

Transudates	Exudates
Congestive heart failure	Pneumonia
Hypervolemia	Pulmonary embolism (usually)
Ascites	Subphrenic abscess
Misplaced central venous catheter	Atelectasis
Pulmonary embolism (rarely)	Post-pericardiotomy syndrome or postcardiac injury syndrome
Atelectasis from diaphragmatic dysfunction (paresis/paralysis)	Diaphragmatic contusion
Trapped lung	Thoracic duct injury
Constrictive pericarditis	Pleural injury from internal mammary harvesting
	Pleural space infection
	Lymphocytic effusion of unknown cause
	Lung entrapment

Simple small effusions, usually transudative in nature, do not require therapeutic drainage unless they cause respiratory compromise. In postoperative patients, these effusions are often due to CHF or volume overload, and usually resolve spontaneously with correction of the underlying disorder or diuresis. Occasionally, a patient may have a recurrent transudative effusion causing respiratory compromise. In these cases, completely draining the fluid through a chest tube and performing pleurodesis may be needed to prevent recurrence.

Etiologies

Pneumonia

Pneumonia is among the most common causes of postoperative exudates, where parapneumonic effusions may be seen in 20–57% of patients [114]. Most resolve with appropriate antibiotic treatment (see below), but in about 40% of cases, bacteria may invade a sterile effusion and produce a complicated effusion or empyema. In significant-sized effusions, drainage and pleural fluid analysis should be done. Testing consists of protein, lactic dehydrogenase, glucose, pH, cell count and differential, Gram's stain, microbiological culture, and cytology. Chest tube drainage is necessary if the fluid is thick pus, or reveals bacteria on Gram's stain, if the pH is < 7.2, or if pleural fluid glucose is < 60 mg/dL [115]. Recent studies demonstrated that small-bore chest tubes (< 15 Fr) placed using the Seldinger technique with USG are as effective as large-bore drainage with better patient tolerance and fewer complications [115]. Large parapneumonic effusions left untreated, develop septations, loculations and organize into a fibrous peel that will require video-assisted thoracoscopic surgery (VATS) open thoracotomy or decortication for resolution.

Coronary bypass

Post-CABG effusions can be classified by the timing of occurrence as: (1) perioperative – within the first week after surgery; (2) early – within 1 month; (3) late – 2 to 12 months;

and (4) persistent – present after 6 months. The time intervals can be further subdivided according to the pathophysiologic processes causing fluid accumulation [110]. Effusions within the perioperative period such as those caused by diaphragmatic dysfunction, atelectasis, or internal mammary artery (IMA) harvesting usually resolve early with lung expansion modalities and indwelling chest tubes after chest closure. During the early period, one should be mindful of the postcardiac injury syndrome as a cause of an exudative effusion. This can represent a forme fruste of Dressler's syndrome where there is an inflammatory response consisting of neutrophilic, followed by lymphocytic infiltration with elevated antimyocardial antibodies in the fluid. Management involves NSAIDs and glucocorticoids for severe cases along with drainage. Less common effusions occurring late post-CABG may be related to constrictive pericarditis, lymphocytic exudative effusions, or lung entrapment. Persistent effusions are usually due to trapped lung.

Subphrenic abscess

Postoperative intra-abdominal infections may lead to the development of subphrenic abscesses which may produce an exudative pleural effusion as late as 1–3 weeks. Pleural fluid WBC counts will be very high ($> 10,000/mm^3$) and predominantly neutrophilic, however, the effusion rarely becomes infected. Management requires identification of the abscess by ultrasound guidance or CT, performing drainage, and starting empiric antimicrobials. Initial antibiotics must cover: gram-negative, enterococci, and anaerobic organisms. Useful antibiotic classes include: (1) carbepenems; (2) extended spectrum beta-lactams; (3) third/fourth generation cephalosporins or fluoroquinolones, with metronidazole. Therapy should be narrowed once organism susceptibilities are available. In critically ill patients, coverage for multidrug resistant organisms (adding aminoglycosides or vancomycin) and/or antifungals should be considered [116].

Hemothorax

Hemothorax is uncommon postoperatively, but is usually seen following pulmonary resection (in approximately 3% post-thoracotomy and 2% post-VATS) [117]. Hemothorax can also occur post-CABG or from complications following tube or CVC placement. It is defined by a pleural fluid hematocrit ≥ 50% of peripheral blood. Coagulopathy or anticoagulation contributes to increased risk and severity. A CT scan is helpful in distinguishing hemothorax from pleural effusion as blood has a higher density and may show septations or loculations. In a decompensating patient with a bloody effusion, one should be mindful of acute hemorrhage or tension hemothorax as potential causes. Management options include large-bore thoracostomy, thoracoscopy, VATS, or surgical re-exploration. Surgical management is reserved for massive acute blood loss (> 1.5 L) or successive hourly drainage of > 200 cc requiring blood transfusions to maintain hemodynamic stability. Long-term risks of unresolved hemothorax include infection, lung entrapment, and fibrothorax. Intrapleural fibrinolytic therapy instilled via tube thoracotomy may be an option for lysing organized blood clots prior to surgery [118].

Pulmonary emboli

Pulmonary emboli have been found to cause mostly small exudative effusions in more recent studies [119]. Pleural fluid analysis is not specific and thoracentesis along with drainage are not usually needed unless infection is suspected or to rule out an enlarging hemothorax. Therapy involves anticoagulation for the pulmonary embolism.

Acknowledgment

This chapter represents a revision of chapters previously written by Dr. V.M. Patel and by Dr. Honig.

References

1. Agostini P, Cieslik H, Rathinam S et al. Postoperative pulmonary complications following thoracic surgery: are there any modifiable risk factors? *Thorax* 2010; **65**: 815–18.

2. Smetana GW, Conde MV. Preoperative pulmonary update. *Clin Geriatr Med.* 2008; **24**: 607–24, vii.

3. Stephan F, Boucheseiche S, Hollande J et al. Pulmonary complications following lung resection: a comprehensive analysis of incidence and possible risk factors. *Chest* 2000; **118**: 1263–70.

4. Siafakas NM, Mitrouska I, Bouros D, Georgopoulos D. Surgery and the respiratory muscles. *Thorax* 1999; **54**: 458–65.

5. Beaussier M, El'ayoubi H, Rollin M et al. Parietal analgesia decreases postoperative diaphragm dysfunction induced by abdominal surgery: a physiologic study. *Reg Anesth Pain Med* 2009; **34**: 393–7.

6. Pelosi P, Gregoretti C. Perioperative management of obese patients. *Best Pract Res Clin Anaesthesiol* 2010; **24**: 211–25.

7. Ferreyra GP, Baussano I, Squadrone V et al. Continuous positive airway pressure for treatment of respiratory complications after abdominal surgery: a systematic review and meta-analysis. *Ann Surg* 2008; **247**: 617–26.

8. Jones JG, Sapsford DJ, Wheatley RG. Postoperative hypoxaemia: mechanisms and time course. *Anaesthesia* 1990; **45**: 566–73.

9. Gallagher SF, Haines KL, Osterlund LG, Mullen M, Downs JB. Postoperative hypoxemia: common, undetected, and unsuspected after bariatric surgery. *J Surg Res* 2010; **159**: 622–6.

10. Siriussawakul A, Mandee S, Thonsontia J et al. Obesity, epidural analgesia, and subcostal incision are risk factors for postoperative desaturation. *Can J Anaesth* 2010; **57**: 415–22.

11. Xue FS, Li BW, Zhang GS et al. The influence of surgical sites on early postoperative hypoxemia in adults undergoing elective surgery. *Anesth Analg* 1999; **88**: 213–19.

12. Kim SH, Na S, Choi J-S, Na SH, Shin S, Koh SO. An evaluation of diaphragmatic movement by M-mode sonography as a predictor of pulmonary dysfunction after upper

abdominal surgery. *Anesth Analg* 2010; **110**: 1349–54.

13. Kaw R, Michota F, Jaffer A *et al.* Unrecognized sleep apnea in the surgical patient: implications for the perioperative setting. *Chest* 2006; **129**: 198–205.

14. Bolden N, Smith CE, Auckley D. Avoiding adverse outcomes in patients with obstructive sleep apnea (OSA): development and implementation of a perioperative OSA protocol. *J Clin Anesth* 2009; **21**: 286–93.

15. Liao P, Yegneswaran B, Vairavanathan S, Zilberman P, Chung F. Postoperative complications in patients with obstructive sleep apnea: a retrospective matched cohort study. *Can J Anaesth* 2009; **56**: 819–28.

16. Rosenberg J, Rasmussen GI, Wojdemann KR *et al.* Ventilatory pattern and associated episodic hypoxaemia in the late postoperative period in the general surgical ward. *Anaesthesia* 1999; **54**: 323–8.

17. Finkel KJ, Searleman AC, Tymkew H *et al.* Prevalence of undiagnosed obstructive sleep apnea among adult surgical patients in an academic medical center. *Sleep Med.* 2009; **10**: 753–8.

18. Jain SS, Dhand R. Perioperative treatment of patients with obstructive sleep apnea. *Curr Opin Pulm Med* 2004; **10**: 482–8.

19. Adesanya AO, Lee W, Greilich NB, Joshi GP. Perioperative management of obstructive sleep apnea. *Chest* 2010; **138**: 1489–98.

20. Netzer N, Eliasson AH, Netzer C, Kristo DA. Overnight pulse oximetry for sleep-disordered breathing in adults: a review. *Chest* 2001; **120**: 625–33.

21. Ramsey R, Mehra R, Strohl KP. Variations in physician interpretation of overnight pulse oximetry monitoring. *Chest* 2007; **132**: 852–9.

22. Gross JB, Bachenberg KL, Benumof JL *et al.* Practice guidelines for the perioperative management of patients with obstructive sleep apnea: a report by the American Society of Anesthesiologists Task Force on Perioperative Management of patients with obstructive sleep apnea. *Anesthesiology* 2006; **104**: 1081–93; quiz 117–18.

23. Marley RA. Postoperative oxygen therapy. *J Perianesth Nurs* 1998; **13**: 394–410; quiz -2.

24. Pelosi P, Jaber S. Noninvasive respiratory support in the perioperative period. *Curr Opin Anaesthesiol* 2010; **23**: 233–8.

25. Zarbock A, Mueller E, Netzer S *et al.* Prophylactic nasal continuous positive airway pressure following cardiac surgery protects from postoperative pulmonary complications: a prospective, randomized, controlled trial in 500 patients. *Chest* 2009; **135**: 1252–9.

26. Jaber S, Michelet P, Chanques G. Role of non-invasive ventilation (NIV) in the perioperative period. *Best Pract Res Clin Anaesthesiol* 2010; **24**: 253–65.

27. Lefebvre A, Lorut C, Alifano M *et al.* Noninvasive ventilation for acute respiratory failure after lung resection: an observational study. *Intensive Care Med* 2009; **35**: 663–70.

28. Gunnarsson L, Tokics L, Gustavsson H, Hedenstierna G. Influence of age on atelectasis formation and gas exchange impairment during general anaesthesia. *Br J Anaesth* 1991; **66**: 423–32.

29. Hedenstierna G, Edmark L. Mechanisms of atelectasis in the perioperative period. *Best Pract Res Clin Anaesthesiol* 2010; **24**: 157–69.

30. Edmark L, Kostova-Aherdan K, Enlund M, Hedenstierna G. Optimal oxygen concentration during induction of general anesthesia. *Anesthesiology* 2003; **98**: 28–33.

31. O'Donohue WJ Jr. National survey of the usage of lung expansion modalities for the prevention and treatment of postoperative atelectasis following abdominal and thoracic surgery. *Chest* 1985; **87**: 76–80.

32. Engoren M. Lack of association between atelectasis and fever. *Chest* 1995; **107**: 81–4.

33. Overend TJ, Anderson CM, Lucy SD *et al.* The effect of incentive spirometry on postoperative pulmonary complications: a systematic review. *Chest* 2001; **120**: 971–8.

34. Gosselink R, Schrever K, Cops P *et al.* Incentive spirometry does not enhance recovery after thoracic surgery. *Crit Care Med.* 2000; **28**: 679–83.

35. Matte P, Jacquet L, Van Dyck M, Goenen M. Effects of conventional physiotherapy, continuous positive airway pressure and non-invasive ventilatory support with bilevel positive airway pressure after coronary artery bypass grafting. *Acta Anaesthesiol Scand* 2000; **44**: 75–81.

36. Gust R, Pecher S, Gust A *et al.* Effect of patient-controlled analgesia on pulmonary complications after coronary artery bypass grafting. *Crit Care Med* 1999; **27**: 2218–23.

37. Marini JJ, Pierson DJ, Hudson LD. Acute lobar atelectasis: a prospective comparison of fiberoptic bronchoscopy and respiratory therapy. *Am Rev Resp Dis* 1979; **119**: 971–8.

38. Arozullah AM, Khuri SF, Henderson WG, Daley J, Participants in the National Veterans Affairs Surgical Quality Improvement P. Development and validation of a multifactorial risk index for predicting postoperative pneumonia after major noncardiac surgery. *Ann Intern Med* 2001; **135**: 847–57.

39. Safdar N, Dezfulian C, Collard HR, Saint S. Clinical and economic consequences of ventilator-associated pneumonia: a systematic review. *Crit Care Med* 2005; **33**: 2184–93.

40. Edwards JR, Peterson KD, Mu Y *et al.* National Healthcare Safety Network (NHSN) report: data summary for 2006 through 2008, issued December 2009. *Am J Infect Control* 2009; **37**: 783–805.

41. Bonten MJ, Kollef MH, Hall JB. Risk factors for ventilator-associated pneumonia: from epidemiology to patient management. *Clin Infect Dis* 2004; **38**: 1141–9.

42. Anonymous. National Nosocomial Infections Surveillance (NNIS) System Report, Data Summary from January 1992–June 2001, issued August 2001. *Am J Infect Control* 2001; **29**: 404–21.

43. Guidelines for the management of adults with hospital-acquired, ventilator-associated, and healthcare-associated pneumonia. *Am J Resp Crit Care Med* 2005; **171**: 388–416.

44. Chastre J, Fagon JY. Ventilator-associated pneumonia. *Am J Resp Crit Care Med* 2002; **165**: 867–903.

45. Craven DE. Epidemiology of ventilator-associated pneumonia. *Chest* 2000; **117**: 186S–7S.

46. Ramirez P, Ferrer M, Torres A. Prevention measures for ventilator-associated pneumonia: a new focus on the endotracheal tube. *Curr Opin Infect Dis* 2007; **20**: 190–7.

47. Pneumatikos IA, Dragoumanis CK, Bouros DE. Ventilator-associated pneumonia or endotracheal tube-associated pneumonia? An approach to the pathogenesis and preventive

strategies emphasizing the importance of endotracheal tube. *Anesthesiology* 2009; **110**: 673–80.

48. Weber DJ, Rutala WA, Sickbert-Bennett EE *et al*. Microbiology of ventilator-associated pneumonia compared with that of hospital-acquired pneumonia. *Infect Control Hosp Epidemiol* 2007; **28**: 825–31.

49. Montravers P, Veber B, Auboyer C *et al*. Diagnostic and therapeutic management of nosocomial pneumonia in surgical patients: results of the Eole study. *Crit Care Med* 2002; **30**: 368–75.

50. Hidron AI, Edwards JR, Patel J *et al*. NHSN annual update: antimicrobial-resistant pathogens associated with healthcare-associated infections: annual summary of data reported to the National Healthcare Safety Network at the Centers for Disease Control and Prevention, 2006–2007. *Infect Control Hosp Epidemiol* 2008; **29**: 996–1011.

51. Delisle MS, Williamson DR, Perreault MM *et al*. The clinical significance of Candida colonization of respiratory tract secretions in critically ill patients. *J Crit Care* 2008; **23**: 11–17.

52. Vincent A, La Scola B, Forel JM *et al*. Clinical significance of a positive serology for mimivirus in patients presenting a suspicion of ventilator-associated pneumonia. *Crit Care Med* 2009; **37**: 111–18.

53. Trouillet JL, Chastre J, Vuagnat A *et al*. Ventilator-associated pneumonia caused by potentially drug-resistant bacteria. *Am J Resp Crit Care Med* 1998; **157**: 531–9.

54. Rello J, Paiva JA, Baraibar J *et al*. International conference for the development of consensus on the diagnosis and treatment of ventilator-associated pneumonia. *Chest* 2001; **120**: 955–70.

55. Coffin SE, Klompas M, Classen D *et al*. Strategies to prevent ventilator-associated pneumonia in acute care hospitals. *Infect Control Hosp Epidemiol* 2008; **29** (Suppl 1): S31–40.

56. Wip C, Napolitano L. Bundles to prevent ventilator-associated pneumonia: how valuable are they? *Curr Opin Infect Dis* 2009; **22**: 159–66.

57. Krein SL, Kowalski CP, Damschroder L *et al*. Preventing ventilator-associated pneumonia in the United States: a multicenter mixed-methods study. *Infect Control Hosp Epidemiol* 2008; **29**: 933–40.

58. Nseir S, Favory R, Jozefowicz E *et al*. Antimicrobial treatment for ventilator-associated tracheobronchitis: a randomized, controlled, multicenter study. *Crit Care* 2008; **12**: R62.

59. Welty-Wolf K. Ventilator-associated pneumonia. In MacIntyre NR, Branson RD, eds. *Mechanical Ventilation*. Philadelphia: W.B. Saunders; 2001, pp. 296–328.

60. Rosbolt MB, Sterling ES, Fahy BG. The utility of the clinical pulmonary infection score. *J Intensive Care Med* 2009; **24**: 26–34.

61. Singh N, Falestiny MN, Rogers P *et al*. Pulmonary infiltrates in the surgical ICU: prospective assessment of predictors of etiology and mortality. *Chest* 1998; **114**: 1129–36.

62. Wunderink RG. Radiologic diagnosis of ventilator-associated pneumonia. *Chest* 2000; **117**: 188S–90S.

63. Campbell GD Jr. Blinded invasive diagnostic procedures in ventilator-associated pneumonia. *Chest* 2000; **117**: 207S–11S.

64. Grossman RF, Fein A. Evidence-based assessment of diagnostic tests for ventilator-associated pneumonia. Executive summary. *Chest* 2000; **117**: 177S–81S.

65. Nachtigall I, Tamarkin A, Tafelski S *et al*. Impact of adherence to standard operating procedures for pneumonia on outcome of intensive care unit patients. *Crit Care Med* 2009; **37**: 159–66.

66. Ibrahim EH, Ward S, Sherman G *et al*. Experience with a clinical guideline for the treatment of ventilator-associated pneumonia. *Crit Care Med* 2001; **29**: 1109–15.

67. Chastre J, Wolff M, Fagon JY *et al*. Comparison of 8 vs 15 days of antibiotic therapy for ventilator-associated pneumonia in adults: a randomized trial. *J Am Med Assoc* 2003; **290**: 2588–98.

68. Nseir S, Deplanque X, Di Pompeo C *et al*. Risk factors for relapse of ventilator-associated pneumonia related to nonfermenting Gram negative bacilli: a case-control study. *J Infect* 2008; **56**: 319–25.

69. Janda M, Scheeren TW, Noldge-Schomburg GF. Management of pulmonary aspiration. *Best Pract Res Clin Anaesthesiol* 2006; **20**: 409–27.

70. Kozlow JH, Berenholtz SM, Garrett E, Dorman T, Pronovost PJ. Epidemiology and impact of aspiration pneumonia in patients undergoing surgery in Maryland, 1999–2000. *Crit Care Med* 2003; **31**: 1930–7.

71. Kalinowski CP, Kirsch JR. Strategies for prophylaxis and treatment for aspiration. *Best Pract Res Clin Anaesthesiol* 2004; **18**: 719–37.

72. Hodd J, Doyle A, Carter J, Albarran J, Young P. Increasing positive end expiratory pressure at extubation reduces subglottic secretion aspiration in a bench-top model. *Nurs Crit Care* 2010; **15**: 257–61.

73. Knight PR, Davidson BA, Nader ND *et al*. Progressive, severe lung injury secondary to the interaction of insults in gastric aspiration. *Exp Lung Res* 2004; **30**: 535–57.

74. Marik PE. Aspiration pneumonitis and aspiration pneumonia. *N Engl J Med* 2001; **344**: 665–71.

75. Marik PE, Careau P. The role of anaerobes in patients with ventilator-associated pneumonia and aspiration pneumonia: a prospective study. *Chest* 1999; **115**: 178–83.

76. van Westerloo DJ, Knapp S, van't Veer C *et al*. Aspiration pneumonitis primes the host for an exaggerated inflammatory response during pneumonia. *Crit Care Med* 2005; **33**: 1770–8.

77. Torbicki A, Perrier A, Konstantinides S *et al*. Guidelines on the diagnosis and management of acute pulmonary embolism: the Task Force for the Diagnosis and Management of Acute Pulmonary Embolism of the European Society of Cardiology (ESC). *Eur Heart J* 2008; **29**: 2276–315.

78. Deitelzweig SB, Johnson BH, Lin J, Schulman KL. Prevalence of clinical venous thromboembolism in the USA: current trends and future projections. *Am J Hematol* 2011; **86**: 217–20.

79. Marshall PS, Cain H. Upper extremity deep vein thrombosis. *Clin Chest Med* 2010; **31**: 783–97.

80. Geerts WH, Bergqvist D, Pineo GF *et al*. Prevention of venous thromboembolism: American College of Chest Physicians evidence-based clinical practice guidelines (8th Edition). *Chest* 2008; **133**: 381S–453S.

81. Cohen AT, Tapson VF, Bergmann JF *et al*. Venous thromboembolism risk and prophylaxis in the acute hospital care setting (ENDORSE study): a multinational cross-sectional study. *Lancet* 2008; **371**: 387–94.

82. Dalen JE. Pulmonary embolism: what have we learned since Virchow? Natural history, pathophysiology, and diagnosis. *Chest* 2002; **122**: 1440–56.

83. Caprini JA. Risk assessment as a guide for the prevention of the many faces of venous thromboembolism. *Am J Surg* 2010; **199**: S3–10.

84. Zierler BK. Ultrasonography and diagnosis of venous thromboembolism. *Circulation* 2004; **109**: I9–14.

85. Stein PD, Fowler SE, Goodman LR *et al*. Multidetector computed tomography for acute pulmonary embolism. *N Engl J Med* 2006; **354**: 2317–27.

86. Stein PD, Chenevert TL, Fowler SE *et al*. Gadolinium-enhanced magnetic resonance angiography for pulmonary embolism: a multicenter prospective study (PIOPED III). *Ann Intern Med* 2010; **152**: 434–43, W142–3.

87. Elliott CG, Lovelace TD, Brown LM, Adams D. Diagnosis: imaging techniques. *Clin Chest Med* 2010; **31**: 641–57.

88. Douketis JD, Berger PB, Dunn AS *et al*. The perioperative management of antithrombotic therapy: American College of Chest Physicians evidence-based clinical practice guidelines (8th Edition). *Chest* 2008; **133**: 299S–339S.

89. Schulman S, Beyth RJ, Kearon C, Levine MN. Hemorrhagic complications of anticoagulant and thrombolytic treatment: American College of Chest Physicians evidence-based clinical practice guidelines (8th Edition). *Chest* 2008; **133**: 257S–98S.

90. Dunn AS, Spyropoulos AC, Turpie AG. Bridging therapy in patients on long-term oral anticoagulants who require surgery: the Prospective Peri-operative Enoxaparin Cohort Trial (PROSPECT). *J Thromb Haemost* 2007; **5**: 2211–18.

91. Kearon C, Kahn SR, Agnelli G *et al*. Antithrombotic therapy for venous thromboembolic disease: American College of Chest Physicians evidence-based clinical practice guidelines (8th Edition). *Chest* 2008; **133**: 454S–545S.

92. Akl EA, Rohilla S, Barba M *et al*. Anticoagulation for the initial treatment of venous thromboembolism in patients with cancer. *Cochrane Database Syst Rev*. 2008; CD006649.

93. Pendleton RC, Rodgers GM, Hull RD. Established venous thromboembolism therapies: heparin, low molecular weight heparins, and vitamin

94. Morris TA. New synthetic antithrombotic agents for venous thromboembolism: pentasaccharides, direct thrombin inhibitors, direct Xa inhibitors. *Clin Chest Med* 2010; **31**: 707–18.

95. Tapson VF. Interventional therapies for venous thromboembolism: vena caval interruption, surgical embolectomy, and catheter-directed interventions. *Clin Chest Med* 2010; **31**: 771–81.

96. Arozullah AM, Daley J, Henderson WG, Khuri SF. Multifactorial risk index for predicting postoperative respiratory failure in men after major noncardiac surgery. The National Veterans Administration Surgical Quality Improvement Program. *Ann Surg* 2000; **232**: 242–53.

97. Chappell D, Jacob M, Hofmann-Kiefer K, Conzen P, Rehm M. A rational approach to perioperative fluid management. *Anesthesiology* 2008; **109**: 723–40.

98. McConkey PP. Postobstructive pulmonary oedema – a case series and review. *Anaesth Intens Care* 2000; **28**: 72–6.

99. Neustein SM. Reexpansion pulmonary edema. *J Cardiothorac Vasc Anesth* 2007; **21**: 887–91.

100. Shaz BH, Stowell SR, Hillyer CD. Transfusion-related acute lung injury: from bedside to bench and back. *Blood* 2011; **117**: 1463–71.

101. Gajic O, Gropper MA, Hubmayr RD. Pulmonary edema after transfusion: how to differentiate transfusion-associated circulatory overload from transfusion-related acute lung injury. *Crit Care Med* 2006; **34**: S109–13.

102. Jordan S, Mitchell JA, Quinlan GJ, Goldstraw P, Evans TW. The pathogenesis of lung injury following pulmonary resection. *Eur Respir J* 2000; **15**: 790–9.

103. Lee JC, Christie JD. Primary graft dysfunction. *Proc Am Thorac Soc* 2009; **6**: 39–46.

104. Ely EW, Haponik EF. Using the chest radiograph to determine intravascular volume status: the role of vascular pedicle width. *Chest* 2002; **121**: 942–50.

105. Lees N, Hamilton M, Rhodes A. Clinical review: goal-directed therapy in high risk surgical patients. *Crit Care* 2009; **13**: 231.

106. Stewart RM, Park PK, Hunt JP *et al*. Less is more: improved outcomes in surgical patients with conservative fluid

administration and central venous catheter monitoring. *J Am Coll Surg* 2009; **208**: 725–37.

107. Nava S, Hill N. Non-invasive ventilation in acute respiratory failure. *Lancet* 2009; **374**: 250–9.

108. The Acute Respiratory Distress Syndrome Network. Ventilation with lower tidal volumes as compared with traditional tidal volumes for acute lung injury and the acute respiratory distress syndrome. *N Engl J Med*. 2000; **342**: 1301–8.

109. Light RW, George RB. Incidence and significance of pleural effusion after abdominal surgery. *Chest* 1976; **69**: 621–5.

110. Heidecker J, Sahn SA. The spectrum of pleural effusions after coronary artery bypass grafting surgery. *Clin Chest Med* 2006; **27**: 267–83.

111. Ahmad Z, Krishnadas R, Froeschle P. Pleural effusion: diagnosis and management. *J Perioper Pract* 2009; **19**: 242–7.

112. Heffner JE. Discriminating between transudates and exudates. *Clin Chest Med* 2006; **27**: 241–52.

113. Hooper C, Lee YC, Maskell N. Investigation of a unilateral pleural effusion in adults: British Thoracic Society pleural disease guideline 2010. *Thorax* 2010; **65** (Suppl 2): ii4–17.

114. Wrightson JM, Davies RJ. The approach to the patient with a parapneumonic effusion. *Semin Respir Crit Care Med*. 2010; **31**: 706–15.

115. Davies HE, Davies RJ, Davies CW. Management of pleural infection in adults: British Thoracic Society pleural disease guideline 2010. *Thorax* 2010; **65** (Suppl 2): ii41–53.

116. Solomkin JS, Mazuski JE, Bradley JS *et al*. Diagnosis and management of complicated intra-abdominal infection in adults and children: guidelines by the Surgical Infection Society and the Infectious Diseases Society of America. *Clin Infect Dis* 2010; **50**: 133–64.

117. Litle VR, Swanson SJ. Postoperative bleeding: coagulopathy, bleeding, hemothorax. *Thorac Surg Clin* 2006; **16**: 203–7, v.

118. Boersma WG, Stigt JA, Smit HJ. Treatment of haemothorax. *Respir Med* 2010; **104**: 1583–7.

119. Light RW. Pleural effusion in pulmonary embolism. *Semin Respir Crit Care Med* 2010; **31**: 716–22.

Chapter

16

Peptic ulcer disease

Frederick Gandolfo and Michael A. Poles

Introduction

Peptic ulcer disease (PUD) refers to a defect in the gastrointestinal mucosa of the stomach or duodenum that penetrates through the muscularis mucosa. Most studies of PUD have defined an ulcer as requiring a minimum diameter of 5 mm, although this size criterion is arbitrary. Ulcers form when there is a mismatch in protective and damaging gastrointestinal factors, with the most common destructive factors being infection with the bacteria *Helicobacter pylori* and use of non-steroidal anti-inflammatory drugs (NSAIDs). Without treatment of the primary cause, PUD is typically a relapsing-remitting chronic condition. Symptoms are variable, are often non-specific, and may even be absent. The mainstay of diagnosis of PUD is upper endoscopy. Since PUD is an acid-related condition, treatment includes acid suppression as well as specific treatment aimed at any causative factors identified.

Epidemiology

The worldwide incidence of PUD is approximately 0.1–0.2% and appears to be decreasing [1]. Furthermore, hospitalization rates, need for surgery, and PUD-related mortality are also all decreasing [2,3]. These improvements are likely due to the decreased prevalence of *H. pylori*, use of increasingly potent acid suppression, and the increased therapeutic role of upper endoscopy. The prevalence of PUD in patients with *H. pylori* infection is 1–6% [4], and is 11% in patients taking low-dose aspirin [5]; in the absence of *H. pylori* infection or NSAID use PUD is uncommon [6].

Pathogenesis

All peptic ulcers are thought to occur from an imbalance between gastrointestinal mucosal defense factors and caustic digestive factors. The gastric and duodenal mucosae are highly adapted to the acid–pepsin milieu, and possess several mucosal defense mechanisms. These can be divided into pre-epithelial factors, epithelial factors and post-epithelial factors. The primary pre-epithelial protective mechanism involves gastric mucosal secretion of an adherent mucus-bicarbonate gel that creates an unstirred layer, trapping bicarbonate at the surface of the epithelial cells, resulting in a neutral pH directly adjacent to the mucosa. Gastric and duodenal bicarbonate secretion is enhanced by prostaglandin E. This forms a physical barrier to acid and pepsin and protects the gastric mucosa from their potentially harmful effects. Several epithelial factors are believed to play a role in maintaining the integrity of the mucosal barrier; specifically Toll-like receptors on gastric epithelial cells and lamina propria immunocytes, secreted trefoil proteins, intracellular hypoxia inducible factor and heat shock proteins. Lastly, the primary post-epithelial defense is the rich vascular bed in the submucosa that acts as a sink for excess protons and toxins that enter the mucosa, while providing oxygen, bicarbonate, and nutrients to the gastric epithelium.

As the acidic gastric contents enter the duodenum, acid-sensing mechanisms and epithelial ion transporters work to counteract the pH drop. Due to the action of carbonic anhydrase, the duodenal mucosa can absorb luminal acid and secrete bicarbonate to maintain the pH in an acceptable range. As acid is absorbed from the lumen through the epithelial cells and across their basolateral membranes vasoactive mediators, including nitric oxide, act to vasodilate mucosal vessels and increase the rate at which acid is carried away from the epithelium. Acidification of the portal vein blood after a meal stimulates further increases in intestinal blood flow and augments post-epithelial defense. Intestinal alkaline phosphatase has also been shown to play a role in maintaining duodenal pH [7]. Perturbation of the normal gastroduodenal defense mechanisms can allow acid and digestive enzymes access to the mucosal surfaces with resultant damage leading to ulcer formation.

Helicobacter pylori is the causative agent in the majority of cases of PUD. Infection is thought to occur in childhood, and the prevalence of *H. pylori* infection is inversely correlated with socio-economic status. In the USA, up to 42% of people are seropositive for *H. pylori* [8], while the worldwide prevalence is highly variable, ranging from 7 to 87% [9]. The prevalence of *H. pylori* is thought to be decreasing worldwide, perhaps due to increasing use of antibiotics or improvement in living

Medical Management of the Surgical Patient, ed. Michael F. Lubin, Thomas F. Dodson, and Neil H. Winawer. Published by Cambridge University Press. © Cambridge University Press 2013.

conditions [8]. Approximately 10% of people infected with *H. pylori* will develop ulcers over their lifetime [10,11].

Helicobacter pylori colonizes the entire gastric mucosa and induces chronic inflammation in all carriers. Among infected individuals, two distinct anatomic patterns of gastritis are seen: antrum-predominant gastritis or body-predominant gastritis. In patients who develop duodenal ulcers, antral-predominant gastritis spares the parietal cell mass of the gastric body and results in acid-hypersecretion. *Helicobacter pylori* has high urease activity, producing ammonia that protects the organism from gastric acid, but also disrupts the feedback of luminal acid on somatostatin, which normally serves as a brake on gastrin, and thus, gastric acid secretion. Furthermore, *H. pylori* disrupts antral-fundic neural pathways that normally function to decrease acid production. The resultant gastric acid hypersecretion promotes gastric metaplasia of the duodenal bulb. The metaplastic duodenal tissue becomes colonized with *H. pylori*, causing inflammation and subsequent ulceration due to the high-acid environment.

When *H. pylori* causes body-predominant gastritis, acid secretion is often decreased due to the effect of chronic inflammation on the parietal cell mass. The chronic inflammatory response upregulates epithelial cytokines such as interleukin-8 and interleukin-1β, recruiting neutrophils and macrophages to the gastric mucosa, and causing damage via reactive oxygen species, lysosomal enzymes, and leukotriene release. This induces further immune activation, causing a defect in the gastric mucosal barrier and eventual ulceration [11].

Non-steroidal anti-inflammatory drugs are among the most commonly used prescription and over-the-counter drugs worldwide. NSAIDs are analgesic, anti-inflammatory, and anti-pyretic drugs, whose major mechanism of action is inhibition of prostaglandin synthesis via inhibition of the enzymes cyclooxygenase-1 (COX-1) and COX-2. Non-steroidal anti-inflammatory drugs, including aspirin, are the sole causative factor in approximately one-quarter of all peptic ulcers [12], and are implicated in greater than 50% of bleeding peptic ulcers [10,13]. The risk of developing NSAID-associated ulcers is proportional to the dose taken [14], and a significantly increased risk is present even with low-dose aspirin taken for primary prevention of cardiovascular events [5]. The relative risk of complicated PUD (bleeding, perforation, obstruction) is increased three- to five-fold by the use of NSAIDs. The patients at greatest risk for NSAID-related ulcer disease are those with a prior history of PUD, and patients of advanced age (> 70 years old) [15]. Selective COX-2 enzyme inhibitors appear to carry less of a risk of ulcer formation, however a small risk still exists, due to lack of complete specificity for the COX-2 isoform [16]. Use of COX-2 inhibitors has been limited due to concerns over significant cardiovascular risk [16].

Non-steroidal anti-inflammatory drugs induce gastrointestinal ulceration in several ways. Direct toxicity, by which the drugs act topically on the gastrointestinal mucosa, leading to an increased permeability of the gastric mucus layer, is thought to play only a minor role [10]. The major effect occurs

through their systemic activity. As weak acids, NSAIDs remain protonated in the acidic gastric lumen, and are readily absorbed and concentrated in the epithelial cells, through a phenomenon called ion-trapping. Once inside these cells, the major ulcerogenic effect of NSAIDs is through inhibition of prostaglandin synthesis. Prostaglandin plays a key role in the maintenance of the mucus-bicarbonate layer, a pre-epithelial defense. Furthermore, maintenance of mucosal integrity depends heavily on adequate mucosal blood flow, a post-epithelial defense, which is compromised by NSAID use. Non-steroidal anti-inflammatory drugs also play roles in the inflammatory response, cell proliferation, and apoptosis, although these effects are not as well understood. In addition to their ulcerogenic effects, NSAIDs increase the risk of bleeding from ulcers that have formed due to platelet inhibition; while this effect is reversible for NSAIDS, aspirin inhibition of platelets is irreversible. Non-steroidal anti-inflammatory drugs also have a deleterious effect on ulcer healing by inhibiting the COX-2 enzyme, which plays a role in angiogenesis and wound repair [13].

Although *H. pylori* and/or NSAIDs account for greater than 90% of all cases of PUD, several less common causes also exist, including hypersecretory states (e.g., Zollinger–Ellison syndrome), malignancy, and Crohn's disease. Ulcers can also form after radiation treatment, at the site of surgical anastomoses, or as the result of critical illness (stress ulcers), mainly through the mechanism of splanchnic hypoperfusion [17]. Certain lifestyle factors may also contribute to ulcer formation. Cigarette smoking is thought to increase the risk of PUD twofold [11]; emotional stress, alcohol, and recreational drug use may also amplify ulcer risk although this has not been well demonstrated [11,18].

Clinical features

The most common symptom of PUD is epigastric pain. Classically the pain of duodenal ulcer is relieved with food intake due to buffering of acid; however, this is only seen in 50% of duodenal ulcer patients and is therefore not clinically useful. Gastric ulcer pain often worsens with food intake, though the clinical utility is again dubious. Ulcer patients may also experience non-specific symptoms of early satiety, fullness, bloating, and nausea. The non-specificity of the symptom complex associated with PUD makes distinguishing ulcer pain from non-ulcer dyspepsia challenging. Furthermore, both chronic peptic ulcers and NSAID-associated ulcers may be asymptomatic [19].

Bleeding is the most common manifestation of complicated PUD, with an incidence of 50–80 cases per 100,000 [20,21]. The mortality associated with a bleeding peptic ulcer is approximately 10%, with most deaths occurring among the elderly who possess other comorbid medical conditions. Among otherwise healthy patients under age 60, the mortality of gastrointestinal hemorrhage from PUD is approximately 0.1% [22].

Less common presentations of PUD include perforation, gastric outlet obstruction, and ulcer penetration. Ulcer perforation occurs in 2–10% of patients with PUD and is accountable for over 70% of ulcer-related deaths. Treatment relies on prompt diagnosis and emergent surgical management [23]. Chronic duodenal or pyloric channel ulcer disease can cause scarring and deformity, and is the most common benign cause of gastric outlet obstruction [24]. Ulcers in the posterior duodenal wall or stomach can perforate and penetrate into the adjacent pancreas, biliary system, or less commonly the liver. Penetrating ulcers are rarely seen in the modern era of acid suppression [25].

Diagnostic techniques

Upper endoscopy (EGD) is the gold-standard test for diagnosis of PUD. Since the clinical presentation of PUD is variable and often non-specific, guidelines exist for selection of appropriate patients for EGD. Patients who should undergo EGD for dyspeptic symptoms include those over age 50 with new-onset dyspepsia, or patients of any age with alarm symptoms (family history of upper gastrointestinal malignancy, weight loss, bleeding, iron-deficiency anemia, dysphagia or odynophagia, vomiting, palpable mass, or lymphadenopathy). Of note, these alarm symptoms are geared more towards ruling out upper gastrointestinal malignancy, and none are sensitive or specific for the presence of ulcers on EGD. In selected young patients without alarm symptoms, a non-invasive work-up for *H. pylori* (test and treat strategy) and withdrawal of NSAIDs may preclude the need for EGD [26,27].

Radiographic procedures may have a role in the diagnosis of PUD and its sequelae. Uncomplicated ulcers can be detected by double-contrast barium radiography approximately 80–90% of the time [28]. Skilled radiologists can detect free air on plan films in up to 91% of perforated ulcer cases [29]. Computerized tomography (CT) scan is the best imaging modality to rule out pneumoperitoneum, and is often useful in demonstrating the site of ulcer perforation or penetration [30]. Although suggestive in many cases, radiology is not the best modality to diagnose or exclude ulcer disease.

In all cases of PUD, a thorough effort must be made to definitively rule out *H. pylori* infection. Acceptable non-invasive methods include the ^{13}C-urea breath test or stool antigen test. Because of low diagnostic accuracy the use of *H. pylori* serology should be avoided, except for cases of active ulcer bleeding if other methods of testing are unavailable [31]. During EGD, biopsies should be taken from the stomach to exclude *H. pylori* infection using rapid urease testing or with histology [30]. However, active upper gastrointestinal bleeding (UGIB) can reduce the sensitivity of biopsy-based methods of *H. pylori* testing and to a lesser extent stool antigen testing [32,33]. Proton pump inhibitor (PPI) use, even in the short-term, also decreases the sensitivity of biopsy-based and stool antigen-based *H. pylori* tests [34,35]. Efforts should therefore be made to test for *H. pylori* as soon as possible

after starting PPI therapy. Furthermore, in the presence of UGIB or PPI use, a negative test for *H. pylori* must be interpreted with caution to avoid acting on a false negative result. In addition, an assiduous history of NSAID use should be taken. Specific preparations should be asked about, including aspirin, as well as "hidden" sources of NSAIDs, such as "Alka-Seltzer." Patients with PUD not related to *H. pylori* or NSAIDs should be referred to a gastroenterologist for further evaluation.

Guidelines for therapy

The two basic principles of therapy for established PUD are acid suppression and treatment of the underlying cause of the ulcer. PPI drugs are the first-line acid suppressing agents of choice in PUD. Although efficacious, histamine-2 receptor antagonists (H2RAs) are less potent acid-suppressing agents and may be used as second-line therapy in selected patients. For most ulcers, 4–8 weeks of acid suppression therapy is adequate to promote healing provided that the underlying cause is identified and treated appropriately [11].

When *H. pylori* is identified in a patient with PUD, it is of paramount importance to eradicate the bacteria. Several triple and quadruple therapies (antibiotics plus PPI, with/without bismuth combinations) are effective in treating *H. pylori* [35]. In uncomplicated PUD, eradication of *H. pylori* is known to promote ulcer healing and prevent recurrence in the vast majority of patients [36,37]. In gastrointestinal hemorrhage due to PUD, eradication of *H. pylori* virtually eliminates the risk of rebleeding [38]. Early studies of the efficacy of *H. pylori* treatment using triple therapy reported eradication rates of approximately 80–90% [39,40]. However, the resistance of *H. pylori* to first-line antibiotics, especially clarithromycin, is increasing [41,42]. Therefore, confirmation of eradication with a stool or breath test should be performed in all patients with *H. pylori*-associated PUD after first-line antibiotic treatment (typically performed after a 4–8 week course of PPI therapy) [10,35,42]. Patients who remain *H. pylori* infected should be retreated [43]. Once *H. pylori* eradication has been confirmed, PPI therapy can be stopped indefinitely [42].

For NSAID-associated PUD, the mainstay of treatment is withdrawal of the offending drug whenever possible. If the patient has a condition that necessitates continued NSAID or aspirin use, then acid suppression with a PPI should be given when the NSAID/aspirin is started and continued indefinitely for prevention of new ulcers. For gastric ulcers, both the synthetic prostaglandin misoprostol, or H2RAs may also be efficacious for this indication, although misoprostol is often poorly tolerated and is contraindicated in women of childbearing age due to the risk of inducing abortion [44,45]. For patients with a history of duodenal ulcers, PPI therapy should be first-line [11]. Proton pump inhibitor therapy is also recommended for primary prophylaxis of NSAID associated ulcers in patients age 70 and over, or who use concomitant aspirin, corticosteroids, or anticoagulants [46].

Most patients with gastric ulcers, regardless of *H. pylori* status or NSAID use, should undergo repeat EGD after 6 weeks of treatment with a PPI to confirm healing and obtain biopsies to rule out malignancy. Duodenal ulcers do not require surveillance endoscopy, as the risk of malignancy in the small bowel is exceedingly low [30].

Considerations in the patient with PUD undergoing non-ulcer related surgery

For the patient with a history of PUD who is preparing for non-ulcer related surgery, no special precautions need to be taken in the perioperative period, provided that there is no evidence of active ulcer disease. There is no need for a preoperative EGD or prophylactic acid-suppressing medication. However, since bleeding or complicated ulcers carry a substantial morbidity and mortality, active ulcer disease should be treated before proceeding to surgery in almost all cases. Management should be individualized, taking into account the benefits of endoscopic hemostasis and treatment with a PPI, weighed against the potential delay in surgery. For emergent procedures, any operative delay may be prohibitive. For less acute surgical indications, endoscopic identification, risk stratification, and treatment of the lesion prior to surgery is ideal. In the case of bleeding ulcers, non-emergent operations should be postponed at least 72 hours after the patient is stabilized and started on a PPI, since the risk of rebleeding is highest during that time [47]. Elective operations should be postponed until several weeks after the identification and treatment of active ulcer disease. Patients with ulcer bleeding or complications that occur in the postoperative period should be treated similar to non-surgical patients, as outlined above.

References

1. Sung JJ, Kuipers EJ, El-Serag HB. Systematic review: the global incidence and prevalence of peptic ulcer disease. *Aliment Pharmacol Ther* 2009; **29**: 938–46.

2. Lewis JD, Bilker WB, Brensinger C *et al*. Hospitalization and mortality rates from peptic ulcer disease and GI bleeding in the 1990s: relationship to sales of nonsteroidal anti-inflammatory drugs and acid suppression medications. *Am J Gastroenterol* 2002; **97**: 2540–9.

3. Wang YR, Richter JE, Dempsey DT. Trends and outcomes of hospitalizations for peptic ulcer disease in the United States, 1993 to 2006. *Ann Surg* 2010; **251**: 51–8.

4. Kuipers EJ, Thijs JC, Festen HP. The prevalence of *Helicobacter pylori* in peptic ulcer disease. *Aliment Pharmacol Ther* 1995; **9**: s59–69.

5. Yeomans ND, Lanas AI, Talley NJ. Prevalence and incidence of gastroduodenal ulcers during treatment with vascular protective doses of aspirin. *Aliment Pharmacol Ther* 2005; **22**: 795–801.

6. Sbrozzi-Vanni A, Zullo A, Di Giulio E *et al*. Low prevalence of idiopathic peptic ulcer disease: an Italian endoscopic survey. *Dig Liver Dis* 2010; **42**: 773–6.

7. deFoneska A, Kaunitz JD. Gastroduodenal mucosal defense. *Curr Opin Gastroenterol* 2010; **26**: 604–10.

8. Everhart JE. Recent developments in the epidemiology of *Helicobacter pylori*. *Gastroenterol Clin North Am* 2000; **29**: 559–78.

9. Ford AC, Axon AT. Epidemiology of *Helicobacter pylori* infection and public health implications. *Helicobacter* 2010; **15**: 1–6.

10. van Leerdam ME, Tytgat GN. Review article: *Helicobacter pylori* infection in peptic ulcer haemorrhage. *Aliment Pharmacol Ther* 2002; **16**: 66–78.

11. Malfertheiner P, Chan FK, McColl KE. Peptic ulcer disease. *Lancet* 2009; **374**: 1449–61.

12. Kurata JH, Nogawa AN. Meta-analysis of risk factors for peptic ulcer: nonsteroidal antiinflammatory drugs, *Helicobacter pylori*, and smoking. *J Clin Gastroenterol* 1997; **24**: 2–17.

13. Ramsoekh D, Van Leerdam ME, Rauws EA *et al*. Outcome of peptic ulcer bleeding, nonsteroidal anti-inflammatory drug use, and *Helicobacter pylori* infection. *Clin Gastroenterol Hepatol* 2005; **3**: 859–864.

14. Hawkey CJ. Nonsteroidal anti-inflammatory drug gastropathy. *Gastroenterology* 2000; **119**: 521–35.

15. Sostres C, Gargallo CJ, Arroyo MT *et al*. Adverse effects of non-steroidal anti-inflammatory drugs (NSAIDs, aspirin, and coxibs) on upper gastrointestinal tract. *Best Pract Res Clin Gastroenterol* 2010; **24**: 121–32.

16. Trelle S, Reichenbach S, Wandel S. Cardiovascular safety of non-steroidal anti-inflammatory drugs: network meta-analysis. *Br Med J* 2011; **342**: c7086.

17. Quenot JP, Thiery N, Barbar S. When should stress ulcer prophylaxis be used in the ICU? *Curr Opin Crit Care* 2009; **15**: 139–43.

18. Friedman GD, Siegelaub AB, Seltzer CC. Cigarettes, alcohol, coffee and peptic ulcer. *N Engl J Med* 1974; **290**: 469–73.

19. Soll AH, Graham DY. Peptic ulcer disease. In Yamada T, ed. *Textbook of Gastroenterology*. 5th edn. Chichester: John Wiley & Sons; 2009.

20. Blatchford O, Davidson LA, Murray WR *et al*. Acute upper gastrointestinal haemorrhage in west of Scotland: case ascertainment study. *Br Med J* 1997; **315**: 510–14.

21. Longstreth GF. Epidemiology of hospitalization for acute upper gastrointestinal hemorrhage: a population-based study. *Am J Gastroenterol* 1995; **90**: 206–10.

22. Rockall TA, Logan RF, Devlin HB *et al*. Incidence of and mortality from acute upper gastrointestinal haemorrhage in the United Kingdom. Steering Committee and members of the national audit of acute upper gastrointestinal haemorrhage. *Br Med J* 1995; **311**: 222–6.

23. Bertleff MJ, Lange JF. Perforated peptic ulcer disease: a review of history and treatment. *Dig Surg* 2010; **27**: 161–9.

24. Gisbert JP, Pajares JM. *Helicobacter pylori* infection and gastric outlet obstruction – prevalence of the

infection and role of antimicrobial treatment. *Aliment Pharmacol Ther* 2002; **16**: 1203–8.

25. Venkatesh KR, Halpern A, Riley LB. Penetrating gastric ulcer presenting as a subcapsular liver abscess. *Am Surg* 2007; **73**: 82–4.

26. Banerjee S, Cash BD, Dominitz JA *et al*. The role of endoscopy in the management of patients with peptic ulcer disease. *Gastrointest Endosc* 2010; **71**: 663–8.

27. Talley NJ, Vakil NB, Moayyedi P. American gastroenterological association technical review on the evaluation of dyspepsia. *Gastroenterology* 2005; **129**: 1756–80.

28. Mercer DW, Robinson EK. Stomach. In Townsend CM, Beauchamp RD, Evers MB *et al*., eds. *Sabiston Textbook of Surgery*. 18th edn. Philadelphia. PA: Saunders; 2008.

29. Chiu YH, Chen JD, Tiu CM *et al*. Reappraisal of radiographic signs of pneumoperitoneum at emergency department. *Am J Emerg Med* 2009; **27**: 320–7.

30. Kaewlai R, Kurup D, Singh A. Imaging of abdomen and pelvis: uncommon acute pathologies. *Semin Roentgenol* 2009; **44**: 228–36.

31. Malfertheiner P, Megraud F, O'Morain C *et al*. Current concepts in the management of *Helicobacter pylori* infection: the Maastricht III consensus report. *Gut* 2007; **56**: 772–81.

32. Gisbert JP, Abraira V. Accuracy of *Helicobacter pylori* diagnostic tests in patients with bleeding peptic ulcer: a systematic review and meta-analysis. *Am J Gastroenterol* 2006; **101**: 848–63.

33. Lin HJ, Lo WC, Perng CL *et al*. *Helicobacter pylori* stool antigen test in patients with bleeding peptic ulcers. *Helicobacter* 2004; **9**: 663–8.

34. Udd M, Miettinen P, Palmu A *et al*. Effect of short-term treatment with regular or high doses of omeprazole on the detection of *Helicobacter pylori* in bleeding peptic ulcer patients. *Scand J Gastroenterol* 2003; **38**: 588–93.

35. Gisbert JP, Pajares JM. Stool antigen test for the diagnosis of *Helicobacter pylori* infection: a systematic review. *Helicobacter* 2004; **9**: 347–68.

36. Hentschel E, Brandstatter G, Dragosics B *et al*. Effect of ranitidine and amoxicillin plus metronidazole on the eradication of *Helicobacter pylori* and the recurrence of duodenal ulcer. *N Engl J Med* 1993; **328**: 308–12.

37. Hopkins RJ, Girardi LS, Turney EA. Relationship between *Helicobacter pylori* eradication and reduced duodenal and gastric ulcer recurrence: a review. *Gastroenterology* 1996; **110**: 1244–52.

38. Gisbert JP, Calvet X, Feu F *et al*. Eradication of *Helicobacter pylori* for the prevention of peptic ulcer rebleeding. *Helicobacter* 2007; **12**: 279–86.

39. Walsh JH, Peterson WL. The treatment of *Helicobacter pylori* infection in the management of peptic ulcer disease. *N Engl J Med* 1995; **333**: 984–91.

40. van der Hulst RW, Keller JJ, Rauws EA *et al*. Treatment of *Helicobacter pylori* infection: a review of the world literature. *Helicobacter* 1996; **1**: 6–19.

41. Megraud F. *H pylori* antibiotic resistance: prevalence, importance, and advances in testing. *Gut* 2004; **53**: 1374–84.

42. Fischbach LA, van Zanten S, Dickason J. Meta-analysis: the efficacy, adverse events, and adherence related to first-line anti-*Helicobacter pylori* quadruple therapies. *Aliment Pharmacol Ther* 2004; **20**: 1071–82.

43. Gisbert JP, Pajares JM. *Helicobacter pylori* "rescue" therapy after failure of two eradication treatments. *Helicobacter* 2005; **10**: 363–72.

44. Goldstein JL, Johanson JF, Hawkey CJ *et al*. Clinical trial: healing of NSAID-associated gastric ulcers in patients continuing NSAID therapy – a randomized study comparing ranitidine with esomeprazole. *Aliment Pharmacol Ther* 2007; **26**: 1101–11.

45. Silverstein FE, Graham DY, Senior JR *et al*. Misoprostol reduces serious gastrointestinal complications in patients with rheumatoid arthritis receiving nonsteroidal anti-inflammatory drugs. A randomized, double-blind, placebo-controlled trial. *Ann Intern Med* 1995; **123**: 241–9.

46. Chan FK, Abraham NS, Scheiman JM *et al*. Management of patients on nonsteroidal anti-inflammatory drugs: a clinical practice recommendation from the first international working party on gastrointestinal and cardiovascular effects of nonsteroidal anti-inflammatory drugs and anti-platelet agents. *Am J Gastroenterol* 2008; **103**: 2908–18.

47. Vakil N. Peptic ulcer disease. In Feldman M, Friedman LS, Sleisenger MH, eds. *Sleisenger and Fordtran's Gastrointestinal and Liver Disease*. 9th edn. Philadelphia, PA: Saunders; 2010.

Liver disease

Kristina Chacko and Michael A. Poles

Introduction

Due to the critical synthetic and metabolic functions of the liver, patients with underlying liver disease are at increased risk of morbidity and mortality during the perioperative period. Previously undiagnosed liver disease is estimated to be present in 1 in 700 otherwise healthy surgical candidates [1,2]. Failure to recognize the presence of underlying liver disease during preoperative evaluation can lead to postoperative morbidity and significantly increased mortality [3]. Identification of these patients prior to surgery will aid in proper risk stratification and management.

Classification of patients with liver disease involves determination of the degree of hepatic damage and the type of abnormality. It is equally important to consider the type of surgery that the patient will undergo. Hepatic complications in the perioperative period may also occur, which are frequently related to use of hepatotoxic medications, development of ischemia, or infection.

Preoperative evaluation

The preoperative evaluation should assess the patient for evidence of acute or chronic liver disease. Special attention should be paid to family history of liver disease as well as risk factors for liver disease such as alcohol abuse, distant receipt of blood transfusions, or illicit drug use. The physical exam should include evaluation for signs of chronic liver disease including spider nevi, temporal and/or muscle wasting, ascites, palmar erythema, and hepatosplenomegaly. Jaundice is rare in the absence of liver pathology (< 1% of patients) and raises concern for more significant liver disease [4]. A careful review of the patient's blood work may reveal abnormalities suggestive of an underlying liver condition. While many blood tests may reflect liver diseases, the most clinically relevant are the liver enzymes aspartate aminotransferase (AST), alanine aminotransferase (ALT), as well as bilirubin, albumin, and coagulation tests (prothrombin time, INR). Elevation of gammaglutamyltranspeptidase (GGT) or alkaline phosphatase may reflect underlying cholestatic liver disease; however, the significance of their abnormalities during the preoperative evaluation is directly proportional to the finding of other evidence of chronic hepatic dysfunction.

Elevations of transaminases

Elevations of AST and ALT reflect hepatocellular damage and may be divided into mild (less than 2–5 times the upper limit of normal), moderate (5–10 times the upper limit of normal), and severe (greater than 10 times the upper limit of normal). Each of these categories has its own differential diagnosis and infers its own degree of operative risk. Intuitively, one would expect surgical risk to correspond with the degree of enzyme elevation and studies support this conclusion.

Mild asymptomatic elevations of the liver enzymes are seen most frequently. Possible conditions include mild hepatotoxicity due to medications, the presence of fatty liver disease (both alcoholic or non-alcoholic), infection with hepatotropic viruses, or the presence of autoimmune liver disease. Elevation of ALT is more specific to intrinsic liver disease, but the presence of an isolated elevated AST level should raise consideration of alcoholic liver disease. Recognition of the possibility of a patient's excessive alcohol use prior to surgery is important, as alcohol dependence may result in alcohol withdrawal during the postoperative period. Still, few data suggest that the detection of transaminase elevations in the absence of signs of diminished liver reserve, such as elevated prothrombin time or hyperbilirubinemia, poses a significant risk to a patient undergoing surgery. While not precluding surgery, detection of mild enzyme abnormalities should prompt investigation into its cause.

Moderate elevations of the ALT and AST suggest a greater degree of liver injury and may portend greater vulnerability in the perioperative period. Common causes include use of hepatotoxic medications, viral hepatitis, vascular injury, autoimmune diseases, or fatty liver disease. A carefully obtained drug history, with particular attention to recently initiated medications, including over-the-counter medications, herbal supplements and other alternative therapies becomes more critical as the degree of enzyme elevation worsens. Patients

Medical Management of the Surgical Patient, ed. Michael F. Lubin, Thomas F. Dodson, and Neil H. Winawer. Published by Cambridge University Press. © Cambridge University Press 2013.

with symptoms of acute hepatitis including abdominal pain, nausea, vomiting, and/or clinical signs such as jaundice should be thoroughly evaluated prior to surgery. While data on surgical mortality in patients with acute hepatitis are variable, surgical risk is increased and elective surgery should be delayed pending clinical and laboratory improvement [5–8]. Patients with treatable causes of hepatitis, such as infection with hepatitis B or autoimmune hepatitis, should be evaluated and, if necessary, started on therapy by a liver specialist. Chronic hepatitis may be exacerbated by the stress of surgery, potentially resulting in an acute decompensation of the patient's liver disease. Anesthetic agents can decrease oxygen delivery to the liver by decreasing splanchnic blood flow, thereby worsening liver injury [9,10]. If the surgery proceeds in a patient with moderate transaminitis careful observation during the postoperative period is necessary.

Patients with severe elevation of the liver enzymes represent a special subset. These patients are typically symptomatic, either directly related to the resultant liver dysfunction or due to the primary underlying disease processes. Severe transaminase elevations raise concern for acute viral hepatitis, vascular events such as ischemic hepatitis or Budd–Chiari syndrome, cardiac failure, acetaminophen overdose, traumatic injury, or malignancy. In one review, an AST elevation of greater than 3,000 IU/L was associated with operative mortality of 55% [11]. Patients with severe acute hepatitis should therefore have surgery postponed until their hepatic condition improves. Ischemic hepatitis has been associated with 75% mortality compared with a mortality rate of 33% for other causes of severe transaminase elevations. This high mortality rate reflects the presence of systemic critical illness and multi-organ failure compared with patients who have isolated liver injury. Patients with evidence of acute liver failure, manifested by encephalopathy and coagulopathy should be referred urgently for liver transplantation.

Cholestatic liver disease is the result of impairment of bile formation and/or bile secretion, and early manifestations may include fatigue, pruritis, and elevations of the alkaline phosphatase and GGT. Those patients found to have alkaline phosphatase greater than 1.5 times the upper limit of normal and/or GGT greater than 3 times the upper limit of normal should undergo further evaluation to determine the etiology of these abnormalities [12]. Cholestasis may be characterized as intrahepatic (secondary to hepatocellular dysfunction or obstruction of the intrahepatic biliary ducts) or extrahepatic, as a result of obstruction of the extrahepatic biliary tree. Initial evaluation should utilize abdominal ultrasound to assess for the presence of liver disease, biliary tree abnormalities including ductal dilatation, or obstructing lesions such as extraductal compression by tumor or intraductal blockage due to choledocholithiasis. The differential diagnosis of cholestatic liver disease is broad and beyond the scope of this chapter. However, special consideration should be given to the complications of cholestasis including the presence of osteoporosis and fat malabsorption. Patients with chronic cholestasis may have fat-soluble vitamin deficiencies and should be supplemented with vitamin K prior to undergoing surgical procedures to reduce the risk of severe bleeding [12].

Cirrhosis

Patients with cirrhosis may be identified during the preoperative evaluation through recognition of the stigmata of chronic liver disease and/or through finding abnormal laboratory values suggesting decreased hepatic synthetic function (low albumin, elevated prothrombin time, and elevated bilirubin concentrations). These patients are at increased surgical risk due to diminished functional liver reserve. Surgical risk of patients with cirrhosis can be stratified according to the Child–Pugh–Turcotte score (Child's score), which incorporates clinical evidence of decompensated liver disease such as presence of ascites and encephalopathy along with objective laboratory data, including the levels of bilirubin, albumin, and INR. Child's Class A cirrhosis is associated with low surgical risk and these patients typically may proceed to surgery without further management. Patients with Child's Class B and C cirrhosis are at higher risk for perioperative complications and should be medically optimized if possible prior to undergoing surgery. The Model for End-Stage Liver Disease (MELD) score is a prospectively validated tool that uses only objective data, including the INR, bilirubin, and creatinine to estimate the 3-month mortality in patients with liver disease. Recent studies have shown that the MELD score has similar predictive value in estimating surgical risk when compared with the Child's score [13]. While offering a continuous scale, the MELD score may be divided into three categories to allow for estimation of risk. Low MELD scores of 6–10 are associated with low surgical risk. Patients with moderately increased MELD scores of 11–16 should be evaluated and medically optimized prior to undergoing any elective surgery. Finally, patients with MELD scores greater than 17 should not be offered elective surgery.

Surgical risk also varies depending on the location and type of surgery to be performed. Emergent surgery in patients with cirrhosis is associated with an increase in surgical complications and mortality compared with elective procedures, with several studies showing a 4–5-fold increase in the mortality rate [14,15]. In cirrhotic patients undergoing abdominal surgery the leading complications are severe bleeding due to coagulopathy and sepsis. Mortality associated with abdominal surgery increases proportionally based on Child's classification; the surgical mortality of patients with Child's Class A cirrhosis is 10%, while for those with Child's B cirrhosis, it increases to 30% and for Child's C patients, mortality rates may be as high as 82% [16].

Cholecystectomy is a common abdominal surgery that carries substantial risk in the cirrhotic patient, and is associated with up to a 25% morbidity rate and a 26% mortality rate [17]. For patients with Child's Class A or B cirrhosis, laparoscopic cholecystectomy may be preferable as it is associated with a lower complication rate (morbidity rate 16%, mortality rate 1%) than open procedures [18]. One retrospective study of patients undergoing laparoscopic cholecystectomy showed that a MELD score of greater than 13 was associated with an increased risk of complications including bleeding and infection, as well as an extended length of hospital stay [19]. Child's Class C cirrhotic patients, and by extension, those with a high MELD score, with acute cholecystitis should be managed conservatively with percutaneous drainage as operative management continues to be associated with high mortality rates. Although there is less substantial data, cardiac surgery also carries markedly elevated mortality rates for patients with Child's Class B or C cirrhosis, with reported rates of 50–100% [20,21]. Given the high mortality rates, elective surgery should be avoided in patients with Child's Class C cirrhosis.

Complications of cirrhosis

Ascites develops in cirrhotic patients as the result of portal hypertension and sodium retention. The development of increased portal pressure leads to the release of local vasodilators, particularly nitric oxide, causing splanchnic vasodilation [22]. The abnormalities in splanchnic and systemic hemodynamics cause activation of the sympathetic nervous system and renin-angiotensin-aldosterone system resulting in sodium retention [23]. The presence of ascites is a predictor of poor outcome in patients undergoing abdominal surgery [16] and may increase the risk of wound dehiscence and abdominal wall herniation after abdominal surgery. Individuals with moderate to large volume ascites often develop umbilical hernias, and suffer recurrence of the hernia after repair unless their ascites is adequately treated. Initial control of ascites is often possible simply by instituting a salt-restricted diet (less than 2 g sodium daily) and, if needed, diuresis with furosemide and spironolactone [25]. Combination therapy is recommended to prevent electrolyte abnormalities, and dosing should start with furosemide 40 mg and spironolactone 100 mg daily and then increased every 3–5 days to effect. Intravenous furosemide should be avoided due to risk of azotemia. While diet and combination medical therapy have been shown to be effective in 90% of patients with ascites, some patients develop refractory ascites due to diuretic resistance or intolerance. In this group of patients, performance of large volume paracentesis may relieve symptoms of tense ascites but rapid reaccumulation makes this an inadequate preoperative solution. Therefore, in those patients with recurrent ascites or complications of abdominal wall hernias, placement of transjugular intrahepatic portosystemic shunt (TIPS) prior to surgery is recommended.

Coagulation abnormalities are common in patients with advanced liver disease. Malnutrition and malabsorption may cause vitamin K deficiency resulting in decreased production of coagulation factors II, VII, X, and XI. Hepatic dysfunction,

itself, results in impaired synthesis of clotting factors, as well as anticoagulant factors such as protein C and protein S. In addition, hepatic dysfunction is associated with fibrinogen abnormalities. The overall result is an imbalance of the coagulation pathway that may result in either excessive bleeding or thrombosis, despite elevations of the INR. Thrombocytopenia is also commonly seen in cirrhosis related to hypersplenism with increased platelet sequestration, reduced hepatic production of thrombopoietin, and immune-mediated destruction from antiplatelet antibodies [26]. Administration of vitamin K subcutaneously for 3 days will correct coagulopathy due to vitamin K deficiency. Transfusion of fresh frozen plasma and platelets can be used in the perioperative setting for temporary normalization of an elevated INR (INR > 1.5) and for thrombocytopenia (platelets < 50,000), respectively. Large transfusion requirements may be observed in some cases and caution is necessary to prevent volume overload. In patients with severe coagulopathy, cryoprecipitate, which contains concentrated factor VIII, fibrinogen, von Willebrand's factor (vWF), fibronectin and factor XIII, may be beneficial as it treats dysfibrinogenemia and disseminated intravascular coagulation (DIC) [27]. Recombinant factor VIIa has been studied for the management of coagulopathy in variceal bleeding and liver transplantation, though data have shown limited efficacy. Given the prohibitive cost ($1 per microgram), its use should be limited to patients with severe coagulopathy who have a contraindication to use of fresh frozen plasma.

Malnutrition in patients with cirrhosis is common, affecting up to 80% of patients and has been associated with a reduced quality of life and higher rates of morbidity and mortality. The presence of severe muscle wasting, cachexia, and weight loss of greater than 10% of body weight prior to surgery are associated with poorer outcomes and higher complication rates [28]. Poor nutritional status may result in increased susceptibility to infection, delayed wound healing, and fluid retention and has been shown to be an independent risk factor for increased hospital length of stay [29]. Decreased food intake may be caused, in part, by increased secretion of cachexia-inducing cytokines such as TNF alpha, early satiety due to ascites, and functional dyspepsia. Malabsorption may also occur in individuals with cholestatic liver disease. In addition to those causes resulting in decreased nutritional intake or decreased nutrient absorption, cirrhosis also results in a hypermetabolic state leading to increased protein breakdown and energy expenditure. Additionally, patients with cirrhosis are frequently deficient in vitamins and minerals, including calcium, vitamin D, vitamin A, folate, thiamine, and vitamin B_{12}. Zinc deficiency is also not uncommon and may result in impaired wound healing. Lastly, medications commonly used in cirrhosis such as lactulose and diuretics may also lead to protein and mineral losses [30].

Assessment of nutritional status in patients with advanced liver disease is complicated; low albumin may reflect decreased synthesis rather than protein-energy malnutrition and body weight often fluctuates due to ascites and edema. However, tools such as the Subjective Global Assessment that collect clinical information such as weight loss, dietary changes, and signs of muscle wasting have been shown to provide a more accurate picture of the cirrhotic patients' nutritional state [31]. Optimization of nutritional status prior to elective surgery is strongly recommended to improve postoperative outcomes.

Hepatic encephalopathy is a neuropsychiatric complication of liver disease that is believed to result from accumulation of toxic metabolites as a consequence of hepatic dysfunction and porto-systemic shunting. Manifestations of encephalopathy range from minimal cognitive deficits and day–night reversal of the sleep–wake cycle to overt confusion, obtundation, and even coma. Encephalopathy is frequently precipitated by infection, gastrointestinal bleeding, electrolyte abnormalities, medications, and renal failure. Triggering factors should be identified and corrected early to avoid further decompensation. Perioperative narcotics and benzodiazepines should be used cautiously as decreased hepatic metabolism results in higher serum levels and excessive and more prolonged effects. Treatment of hepatic encephalopathy is typically initiated with use of non-absorbable disaccharides such as lactulose, which may be given orally, or in the obtunded patient, via nasogastric tube or enema. Lactulose should be titrated to 2–3 soft bowel movements daily, with avoidance of excessive fluid loss through diarrhea. Improvement of encephalopathy in hospitalized patients has also been shown with administration of the non-systemic, gut-selective antibiotic, Rifaximin [32]. Rifaximin may be used in conjunction with lactulose or as monotherapy in patients unable to tolerate lactulose. Given the concern for malnutrition, protein-restricted diets are not recommended for the management of encephalopathy.

Patients with cirrhosis should undergo endoscopic surveillance for gastroesophageal varices, and those individuals with large varices or a past history of variceal bleeding should receive prophylaxis with non-selective beta-blocker therapy or attempted obliteration of the varices with endoscopic band ligation. Currently the use of preoperative TIPS placement in patients with portal hypertension is being investigated, and, in small, uncontrolled studies has been shown to reduce intraoperative bleeding and postoperative complications [33,34]. However, data are limited and at this time, TIPS should only be placed in patients with a currently approved indication.

Operative complications

Patients with cirrhosis are at an increased risk of perioperative complications including the development of hepatic decompensation. Cirrhosis and portal hypertension are associated with significant hemodynamic changes including increased cardiac output and decreased systemic vascular resistance, particularly manifested by splanchnic vasodilation, which leads to diminished hepatic perfusion at baseline. Additionally, the presence of arteriovenous shunting leads to decreased tissue perfusion. These alterations make the cirrhotic liver vulnerable to ischemic injury due to hypoxemia and/or hypotension in the perioperative period. Use of inhaled anesthetic agents such as halothane may further reduce portal blood flow by up to 30–50% [35]. Use of alternate agents such as isoflurane and narcotics result in less hemodynamic disturbance [36]. Surgical stress with increased catecholamine release may also lead to alterations in splanchnic circulation. These effects may be compounded by intraoperative hypotension, hemorrhage, and use of vasoactive drugs [37].

Liver disease is also associated with pulmonary dysfunction and may lead to hypoxemia in the operating room. Hepatopulmonary syndrome (HPS) may be seen in 5–47% of patients with advanced liver disease, and the intrapulmonary arteriovenous shunting associated with this syndrome often results in hypoxemia [38,39]. Portopulmonary hypertension (PPH), with an estimated prevalence of 6% among cirrhotics, is also associated with increased perioperative mortality. Neither HPS nor PPH correlate with the severity of underlying liver disease; therefore, the presence of hypoxia or symptoms of platypnea and orthodeoxyia should prompt an investigation. The presence of HPS or PPH significantly increases the risk of perioperative mortality and elective surgery should be avoided in patients with these conditions [40]. Lastly, the presence of ascites and pleural effusions may result in atelectasis and restrictive lung physiology which can complicate mechanical ventilation [40].

Advanced liver disease results in impaired metabolism of anesthetic agents, resulting in prolongation of their action. The use of sedatives, narcotics, and intravenous induction agents should be avoided in patients with decompensated liver disease due to the risk of precipitating hepatic encephalopathy. Medications such as propofol and inhaled anesthetic agents such as isoflurane, desflurane, and sevoflurane are preferred in patients with advanced cirrhosis given their short half-life and minimal hepatic metabolism [37]. Halothane, which is now rarely used, has been associated with fulminant hepatitis in rare cases. While other inhaled anesthetic agents are linked to fewer reported cases of hepatitis, there is cross-reactivity between all halogenated anesthetics so patients with prior anesthetic exposure are at increased risk of liver injury. Severe hepatitis due to these agents typically presents 2–3 weeks after exposure with the development of fever, jaundice, eosinophilia, and tender hepatomegaly [41].

Postoperative complications

In the immediate postoperative setting, sporadic abnormalities in liver-associated tests are common, and mild degrees of transaminitis or cholestasis are typical. When patients exhibit these laboratory abnormalities, a careful review of the operative report, anesthesia record, and quantity of blood products transfused is warranted. If no clear source is found, consideration must be given to drug-induced liver injury (DILI). Acetaminophen, an antipyretic and analgesic frequently utilized in hospitalized patients, can result in a dose-dependent (or intrinsic) hepatitis. Individuals with alcoholic liver disease have an increased risk of developing significant toxicity at doses as low as 2 g of acetaminophen daily. Acute, severe elevations of the ALT/AST (typically > 5,000) should trigger consideration of acetaminophen toxicity as early diagnosis will permit treatment with N-acetylcysteine, which has been shown to be effective in the prevention of acute liver failure due to acetaminophen overdose. Idiosyncratic DILI is more frequent than intrinsic DILI and while unpredictable, certain risk factors have been identified. Age increases the risk of toxicity from certain medications and cholestatic patterns of liver test abnormalities are more frequently seen in elderly patients. While gender does not increase the risk of DILI, women typically experience a more severe course with poorer outcomes [42]. The role of alcohol and underlying liver disease on the risk of developing DILI is not clearly understood; however, these patients tend to have more complicated disease courses and worse outcomes [43]. Hy's rule, now utilized by the US Food and Drug Administration to evaluate drug hepatotoxicity, posits that the development of jaundice (total bilirubin > 2.5 mg/dL) and severe hepatocellular injury in DILI has been associated with increased mortality rates of 10% [44].

Ischemic hepatitis is typically seen within the first several days of the postoperative period, and is associated with severe elevations of the ALT, AST, and lactate dehydrogenase (LDH). Alkaline phosphatase and bilirubin are usually minimally elevated, although in severe cases, conjugated hyperbilirubinemia develops. Ischemic liver injury is usually associated with hypotension related to cardiogenic, septic, or hemorrhagic shock and improvement is typically seen after correction of the inciting cause. In rare instances, inadvertent ligation of the hepatic artery during cholecystectomy has resulted in hepatic necrosis [41]. The severity of liver injury is dependent on the degree of ischemia and the presence of underlying liver disease; acute liver failure may occur in severe cases.

Onset of jaundice in the immediate postoperative period is uncommon, occurring in < 1% of patients, but is more common in patients with preexisting liver disease. Since breakdown of hemoglobin liberates bilirubin, destruction of transfused red blood cells or resorption of a hematoma may cause jaundice in patients with impaired liver function [45]. Additional causes of unconjugated hyperbilirubinemia include destruction of red blood cells by mechanical heart valves, or underlying hemolytic disorders such as sickle cell anemia or G6PD deficiency. Gilbert's syndrome is a common genetic disorder of bilirubin metabolism, and when exacerbated by stress or fasting, can result in mild elevation of unconjugated or total bilirubin. Benign postoperative cholestasis, a progressive rise in the bilirubin within 2–10 days after surgery, is a common process due to a variety of factors. Infection, hypoxemia, passive hepatic congestion during cardiac surgery, and critical illness are all associated with the development of cholestasis. A number of medications have also been associated with cholestasis, including antibiotics, anti-emetics and total parenteral nutrition (TPN) [41,45,46]. Identification of the underlying cause and supportive care are the mainstay of treatment of cholestasis or jaundice postoperatively.

Extrahepatic cholestasis, and conjugated hyperbilirubinemia, due to biliary obstruction or injury is more frequently seen in patients who have undergone upper abdominal surgery. Evaluation with abdominal ultrasound or CT scan can identify the presence of choledocholithiasis, bile leaks or bilomas, and endoscopic retrograde cholangiopancreatography (ERCP) should be performed in patients with biliary obstruction.

Since patients with cirrhosis have intravascular volume depletion but have total corporeal volume overload, a careful assessment of the patient's volume status each day should be obtained. Dehydration may occur due to decreased oral intake (especially in the setting of being NPO), diuresis, or diarrhea. Renal dysfunction in a cirrhotic patient is particularly ominous, and the development of azotemia should prompt an early investigation into the underlying cause. Acute kidney injury in the hospitalized patient is most commonly due to intrinsic kidney damage from nephrotoxic medications such as non-steroidal anti-inflammatory agents, antibiotics, intravenous contrast dye, as well as ischemia causing acute tubular necrosis or allergic interstitial nephritis [47]. In those patients with pre-renal azotemia, an inadequate response to volume resuscitation with colloid or crystalloid fluids suggests the presence of hepatorenal syndrome (HRS). The hemodynamic alterations (systemic and splanchnic vasodilation, activation of the renin-angiotensin system) that cause ascites ultimately lead to progressive renal vasoconstriction resulting in HRS. While the definitive treatment for HRS is liver transplantation, management with vasoactive medications and intravenous albumin is recommended. Vasoconstrictors such as terlipressin (not currently approved for use in the USA) and noradrenaline are used to counter the vasodilation, and when used with albumin, terlipressin has been shown to reverse HRS [48]. Combination therapy of midodrine and octreotide plus albumin infusion has been shown to improve kidney function by improving effective arterial volume [49].

Conclusion

The preoperative evaluation should identify patients with serious underlying liver disease in order to properly assess and modify risks prior to surgery. Individuals with decompensated cirrhosis are at significantly increased risk of perioperative complications and should be medically and nutritionally optimized prior to undergoing surgery. Patients should be closely monitored for evidence of encephalopathy and renal dysfunction in the postoperative setting. Acute elevation of the liver enzymes is common in the postoperative patient and may be related to drug toxicity, ischemia, or underlying infection.

References

1. Schemel WH. Unexpected hepatic dysfunction found by multiple laboratory screening. *Anesth Analg (Cleveland)* 1976; **55**: 810.

2. Wataneeyawech M, Kelly KA Jr. Hepatic diseases unsuspected before surgery. *NY State J Med* 1975; **75**: 1278.

3. Powell-Jackson P, Greenway B, Williams R. Adverse effects of exploratory laparotomy in patients with unsuspected liver disease. *Br J Surg* 1982; **69**: 449–51.

4. Martinez EJ, Boyer TD. Preoperative and postoperative hepatic dysfunction. In Zakim D, Boyer TD, eds. *Hepatology: A Textbook of Liver Disease*. Orlando, FL: W. B. Saunders; 2002.

5. Harville DD, Summerskill WH. Surgery in acute hepatitis. *J Am Med Assoc* 1963; **184**: 257–61.

6. Hardy KJ, Hughes ESR. Laparotomy in viral hepatitis. *Med J Aust* 1968; **1**: 710.

7. Strauss AA, Strauss SF, Schwartz AH *et al.* Decompression by drainage of the common bile duct in subacute and chronic jaundice: a report of 73 cases with hepatitis or concomitant biliary duct infection as cause. *Am J Surg* 1959; **97**: 137.

8. Bourke JB, Cannon P, Ritchie HD. Laparotomy for jaundice. *Lancet* 1967; **ii**: 521.

9. Ngai SH. Effects of anesthetics on various organs. *N Engl J Med* 1980; **302**: 564.

10. Cooperman LH. Effects of anesthesia on the splanchnic circulation. *Br J Anaesth* 1972; **44**: 967.

11. Johnson RD, O'Connor ML, Kerr RM. Extreme serum elevations of aspartate aminotransferase. *Am J Gastroenterol* 1995; **90**: 1244.

12. EASL Clinical Practice Guidelines: management of cholestatic liver diseases. *J Hepatol* 2009; **51**: 237–67.

13. Farnsworth N, Fagan S, Berger DH, Awad SS. Child–Turcotte–Pugh versus MELD score as a predictor of outcome after elective and emergent surgery in cirrhotic patients. *Am J Surg* 2004; **188**: 580–3.

14. Doberneck RC, Sterling WA, Allison DC. Morbidity and mortality after operation in nonbleeding cirrhotic patients. *Am J Surg* 1983; **146**: 306–9.

15. Garrison RN, Cryer HM, Howard DA, Polk HC. Clarification of factors for abdominal operations in patients with hepatic cirrhosis. *Ann Surg* 1984; **199**: 648–55.

16. Mansour A, Watson W, Shayani V, Pickleman J. Abdominal operations in patients with cirrhosis: still a major surgical challenge. *Surgery* 1997; **122**: 730–6.

17. Bloch RS, Allaben RD, Wait AJ. Cholecystectomy in patients with cirrhosis. *Arch Surg* 1985; **120**: 669.

18. Cobb WS, Heniford BT, Burns JM *et al.* Cirrhosis is not a contraindication to laparoscopic surgery. *Surg Endosc* 2005; **19**: 418–23.

19. Delis S, Bakoyiannis A, Madariaga J *et al.* Laparoscopic cholecystectomy in cirrhotic patients: the value of MELD score and Child–Pugh classification in predicting outcome. *Surg Endosc* 2010; **24**: 407–12.

20. Klemperer JD, Ko W, Krieger KH, Connolly M *et al.* Cardiac operations in patients with cirrhosis. *Ann Thorac Surg* 1998; **65**: 85–7.

21. Hayashida N, Shoujima T, Teshima H *et al.* Clinical outcomes of cardiac operations in patients with cirrhosis. *Ann Thorac Surg* 2004; **77**: 500–5.

22. Runyon BA. Ascites and spontaneous bacterial peritonitis. In Feldman M, Friedman LS, Brandt LJ, eds. *Sleisenger and Fordtran's Gastrointestinal and Liver Disease*, Vol. 2. 9th edn. Philadelphia, PA: Saunders Elsevier; 2010, pp. 1517–42.

23. Arroyo V. Pathophysiology, diagnosis and treatment of ascites in cirrhosis. *Ann Hepatol* 2002; **1**: 72–9.

24. Aranha GV, Greenlee HB. Intra-abdominal surgery in patients with advanced cirrhosis. *Arch Surg* 1986; **121**: 275–7.

25. Runyon BA. Management of adult patients with ascites due to cirrhosis: an update. *Hepatology* 2009; **49**: 2087–107.

26. Trotter JF. Coagulation abnormalities in patients who have liver disease. *Clin Liver Dis* 2006; **10**: 665–78.

27. Blonski W, Siropaides T, Reddy KR. Coagulopathy in liver disease. *Curr Treat Options Gastroenterol* 2007; **10**: 464–73.

28. Merli M, Nicolini G, Angeloni S *et al.* Malnutrition is a risk factor in cirrhotic patients undergoing surgery. *Nutrition* 2002; **18**: 978–86.

29. Merli M, Giusto M, Gentili F *et al.* Nutritional status: its influence on the outcome of patients undergoing liver transplantation. *Liver Int* 2010; **30**: 208–14.

30. Tsiaousi ET, Hatzitolios AI, Trygonis SK, Savopoulos CG. Malnutrition in end stage liver disease: recommendations and nutritional support. *J Gastroenterol Hepatol* 2008; **23**: 527–33.

31. Henkel AS, Buchman AL. Nutritional support in patients with chronic liver disease. *Nat Clin Pract Gastroenterol Hepatol* 2006; **3**: 202–9.

32. Mas A, Rodes J, Sunyer L *et al.* Comparison of rifaximin and lactitol in the treatment of acute hepatic encephalopathy: results of a randomized, double-blind, double-dummy, controlled clinical trial. *J Hepatol* 2003; **38**: 51–8.

33. Schlenker C, Johnson S, Trotter JF. Preoperative transjugular intrahepatic portosystemic shunt (TIPS) for cirrhotic patients undergoing abdominal and pelvic surgeries. *Surg Endosc* 2009; **23**: 1594–8.

34. Gil A, Martinez-Regueira F, Hernandez-Lizoain JL *et al.* The role of transjugular intrahepatic portosystemic shunt prior to abdominal tumoral surgery in cirrhotic patients with portal hypertension. *Eur J Surg Oncol* 2004; **30**: 46–52.

35. Gelman S. General anesthesia and hepatic circulation. *Can J Physiol Pharmacol* 1987; **65**: 1762–79.

36. Gelman S, Dillard E, Bradley EL Jr. Hepatic circulation during surgical stress and anesthesia with halothane, isoflurane or fentanyl. *Anesth Analg* 1987; **10**: 936–43.

37. O'Leary JG, Yachimski PS, Friedman LS. Surgery in the patient with liver disease. *Clin Liver Dis* 2009; **13**: 211–31.

38. Rodriguez-Roisin R, Krowka MJ. Hepatopulmonary syndrome – a liver-induced lung vascular disorder. *N Engl J Med* 2008; **358**: 2378–87.

39. Hopkins WE, Waggoner AD, Barzilai B. Frequency and significance of intrapulmonary right-to-left shunting in end-stage

hepatic disease. *Am J Cardiol* 1992; **70**: 516–19.

40. Patel T. Surgery in the patient with liver disease. *Mayo Clin Proc* 1999; **74**: 593–9.

41. Faust TW, Reddy KR. Postoperative jaundice. *Clin Liver Dis* 2004; **8**: 151–66.

42. Chalasani N, Bjornsson E. Risk factors for idiosyncratic drug-induced liver injury. *Gastroenterology* 2010; **138**: 2249–59.

43. Liss G, Rattan S, Lewis JH. Predicting and preventing acute drug-induced liver injury: what's new in 2010? *Expert*

Opin Drug Metab Toxicol 2010; **6**: 1047–61.

44. Bjornsson E. The natural history of drug-induced liver injury. *Sem Liver Dis* 2009; **29**: 357–63.

45. LaMont JT. Postoperative jaundice. *Surg Clin North Am* 1974; **54**: 637.

46. Schmid M, Hefti ML, Gattiker R *et al.* Benign postoperative intrahepatic cholestasis. *N Engl J Med* 1965; **272**: 545.

47. Garcia-Tsao G, Parikh CR, Viola A. Acute kidney injury in

cirrhosis. *Hepatology* 2008; **48**: 2064–77.

48. Sanyal AJ, Boyer T, Garcia-Tsao G *et al.* A randomized, prospective, double-blind, placebo-controlled trial of terlipressin for type 1 hepatorenal syndrome. *Gastroenterology* 2008; **134**: 1360–8.

49. Angeli P, Volpin R, Gerunda G *et al.* Reversal of type I hepatorenal syndrome with the administration of midodrine and octreotide. *Hepatology* 1999; **29**: 1690–7.

Chapter 18

Inflammatory bowel disease

Lorenzo Rossaro and Sooraj Tejaswi

Introduction

Inflammatory bowel disease is an idiopathic chronic inflammatory condition of the gastrointestinal tract. Crohn's disease and ulcerative colitis are two different forms of the condition. While the exact etiology is unclear, it is thought to be the result of a complex interplay of genetic, environmental, and microbial factors. Diagnosis is based on clinical, radiological, endoscopic, and histopathologic findings. The distinction between ulcerative colitis and Crohn's disease has major implications on indications, timing, type, and outcomes of surgical intervention. [1]. However, the distinction remains unclear in a subgroup of 10–15% of cases termed 'indeterminate colitis' [2].

Crohn's disease

The incidence of Crohn's disease in the USA is around 5.0 cases per 100,000 person-years with a prevalence of about 50 cases per 100,000 persons [3]. There is a bimodal pattern of incidence with the first peak between the 2nd–3rd decades of life, and the second peak in the 6th decade [4]. While any part of the gastrointestinal tract can be involved, the most common site of involvement is the ileo-colonic region (50%), but isolated small bowel (30%) and isolated colonic involvement (20%) can also be seen [5].

Common symptoms include diarrhea, abdominal pain, fever, and weight loss. Extraintestinal symptoms involving joints, skin, liver, and eyes can also occur. Physical exam may reveal pallor, cachexia, fever, abdominal tenderness and/or masses, perianal fissures, fistulae, or abscesses [3,6]. Skip lesions (actively diseased areas separated by areas of normal tissue), transmural involvement of the bowel wall, small bowel involvement, fistulizing and perianal disease, deep linear mucosal ulcers, aphthous ulcers, and non-caseating granulomas on histopathology are specific for Crohn's disease [7–11].

Ulcerative colitis

The incidence of ulcerative colitis in the USA is around 7.6 cases per 100,000 person-years with a prevalence of 229 cases per 100,000 persons [3]. It too has a bimodal incidence pattern.

Unlike Crohn's disease, it is confined to the colon, except in 10–15% of cases of "backwash ileitis" when the ileocecal valve and terminal ileum can be involved [12].

The most common presenting complaint is bloody diarrhea that is frequently nocturnal and small in volume. Abdominal pain, tenesmus, and extraintestinal symptoms can also be seen. Physical exam may reveal pallor, fever, weight loss, aphthous ulcers in the oral cavity [13]. Endoscopic findings include rectal involvement in 95% of cases, contiguous mucosal disease without skip lesions, mucosal friability, edema and erythema, superficial ulcers, strictures, and pseudo polyps. The terminal ileum is characteristically spared except in the case of "backwash ileitis." Histopathologically, inflammation is confined to the mucosa and submucosa in contrast to the transmural nature of Crohn's disease. Crypt distortion, crypt abscesses with mixed acute and chronic inflammatory cells is seen but not granulomas [10,11].

Indications for surgery in Crohn's disease

Nearly 80% of Crohn's disease patients will require surgery during their lifetime [14,15]. However, surgery is rarely curative due to the recurrent nature of the disease. Repeated and extensive small bowel resections may result in short bowel syndrome. So decision to operate must be made after due deliberation [14,15]. Acute indications for surgery include bowel perforation, abscess (not amenable to percutaneous drainage), exsanguinating hemorrhage, toxic megacolon, or bowel obstruction. Elective surgery can be performed for strictures, fistulae, malignancy, medically intractable symptoms, and intolerable medication side-effects.

Indications for surgery in ulcerative colitis

Approximately 30–40% of ulcerative colitis patients require surgery in their lifetime [16]. Unlike Crohn's disease, surgery can be curative in ulcerative colitis. Emergent indications for surgery include intractable hemorrhage, toxic megacolon, fulminant colitis, or perforation. Elective surgery can be performed for medically intractable disease, malnutrition, or dysplasia or malignancy seen on surveillance colonoscopy [17].

Medical Management of the Surgical Patient, ed. Michael F. Lubin, Thomas F. Dodson, and Neil H. Winawer. Published by Cambridge University Press. © Cambridge University Press 2013.

Surgical options in inflammatory bowel disease

The type and extent of surgery depends on several factors, such as Crohn's disease versus ulcerative colitis, elective versus emergent, disease extent and activity, coexistent complications and presence of dysplasia. Surgery may be performed by laparotomy or laparoscopy. Laparoscopic technique is continuously evolving and may become a preferred alternative in future [18].

Since Crohn's can affect any part of the GI tract, and result in fistula, stricture, or abscess formation, the surgical options are also varied. The main goal is to preserve as much bowel as possible in view of the need for possible repeat surgeries over time. Emergent surgeries include partial colectomy with ileostomy, followed by secondary reconstruction of continuity in case of toxic megacolon; limited resection of perforated bowel segment and associated stenotic segment if present in case of perforation; limited resection of the bleeding bowel segment in case of hemorrhage [19]. Elective surgeries include fistulectomy, seton placement (silk string or rubber band), abscess drainage, stricturoplasty, segmental bowel resection, and total proctocolectomy [17,19,20].

Surgery for ulcerative colitis is usually a variant of colectomy. For emergent indications, subtotal colectomy with ileostomy is performed, avoiding complicated pelvic dissection, and leaving a rectal stump in place. Once active disease is controlled, an ileal pouch anal-anastomosis can be performed. For elective indications, total restorative proctocolectomy with ileal pouch anal-anastomosis is the procedure of choice. Two-stage procedure is preferred over single stage operation [17,19,21,22]. In experienced hands, the procedure can be safe and effective [23,24]. However, there is growing evidence regarding potential complications post-procedure [21]. They include early complications such as abscess, fistula, sepsis, and late complications such as revision of ostomy, and need for manipulation or repair of bowel [22]. Further by 1 year up to 30% may require reoperation, and this may increase up to 53% by 10 years postoperatively [25–27]. Pouchitis may occurs in up to 50% patients during long-term follow-up [28]. Fecundity may be reduced up to three-fold and patients may experience sexual dysfunction [21,29]. Contraindications to the ileal-pouch anal anastomosis include Crohn's disease, incompetent anal sphincter, distal rectal cancer, and inability of the pouch to reach the anal canal. Relative contraindications include advanced age, obesity, previous small bowel resection, and indeterminate colitis [10]. An alternative procedure would be to leave an ileostomy in place, such the Brooke ileostomy or the continent Kock pouch ileostomy [30].

Preoperative care

Most surgeries in inflammatory bowel disease are elective or semi-elective, providing adequate time for preoperative evaluation. Disease site and extent should be well established.

A recent colonoscopy with terminal ileal examination provides valuable information in this regard. Radiologic studies such as barium studies, computed tomography, and MRI provide useful information in the evaluation of strictures, fistulae, and abscesses.

The specific type of surgery planned should be discussed with the patient and family. The potential for drains, stoma, short gut, and wound closure complications should be discussed as well. The patient and family should understand the goals of the surgery, and should be prepared for potential outcomes, including disease recurrence.

As with any chronic disease, inflammatory bowel disease patients are at risk for malnutrition. When possible, the nutritional status should be assessed and addressed as indicated with enteral or parenteral nutrition. A detailed history and physical exam and serum albumin are often sufficient for evaluation. Total parenteral nutrition (TPN) has not been shown to decrease mortality in surgical patients in general [31], and the proper use of enteral and parenteral nutrition in inflammatory bowel disease remains controversial. Current data support use of preoperative TPN for 5–14 days only in patients with severe malnutrition. When complete nutritional evaluation is not possible, as with emergent surgeries, evaluation and correction of hemoglobin, and fluid and electrolyte status should be undertaken. Caution must be exercised in feeding and ordering bowel preparations in patients with suspected bowel obstruction from stenosis or strictures. Prior to day of surgery, patients should be NPO for 24 hours with an appropriate bowel preparation given the night before.

Patient's medications should be reviewed preoperatively, to ascertain their utility, and to evaluate for risks they may pose in the surgical setting. Maintenance therapy with 5-ASA compounds should be stopped as they are unnecessary in a patient undergoing surgical therapy. Antibiotics for infectious complications may be continued. Immunomodulator therapy (azathioprine, 6-mercaptopurine, methotrexate, and cyclosporine) and biologic therapy (infliximab, adalimumab, certolizumab), raise the major concerns with septic and wound-healing complications. Available literature does not indicate an increased postoperative infectious risk with the use of azathioprine, 6-mercaptopurine, cyclosporine, and infliximab [32–34]. Perioperative steroid use however has conflicting evidence in the literature with regard to postoperative infectious complications and wound healing. Hence, it is prudent to taper off steroids for elective surgeries if possible [35–39].

Perioperative care

A major consideration in perioperative or intraoperative care of inflammatory bowel disease patients is the need for "stress dose" steroids. Normal daily cortisol production by adrenal glands is 15–20 mg. With major surgery this may increase up to 100 mg/day [40,41]. While patients on steroids for less than 3 weeks are not at high risk for adrenocortical suppression, chronic steroid use has been shown to blunt the response to corticotrophin-releasing hormone stimulation test. Patients taking more than 20 mg of prednisone-equivalent daily for 3 consecutive weeks in the preceding year, or patients with Cushingoid appearance should be assumed to have hypothalamic–pituitary–adrenal axis. These patients are commonly given 100 mg of hydrocortisone intravenously before induction of anesthesia, and 50 mg every 8 hours for 24 hours, followed by taper over the next 48 to 72 hours to previous oral maintenance dose [42].

Postoperative care

The postoperative care of the patient with inflammatory bowel disease should focus upon regaining bowel function, providing adequate nutrition, and reducing the risk of disease recurrence or related complications.

Crohn's disease is a leading risk factor for short bowel syndrome. If 50% or less of the small bowel is removed, patients are usually able to maintain their nutritional status and are not at high risk of electrolyte and fluid loss, malabsorption, and other complications of short bowel syndrome. When more than 75% (approximately 450 cm) of small bowel is removed, care must be taken in the early postoperative period to maintain proper hydration, electrolyte balance, and nutrition. In the immediate postoperative weeks profuse watery diarrhea is common, and it is during this time that intravenous hydration and nutrition are often crucial. Diarrheal fluid losses can be slowed with symptomatic treatment with loperamide, diphenoxylate or other antidiarrheal medications. Once oral intake resumes, isotonic oral rehydrating solutions can prevent dehydration. Enteral feeding should be initiated early to aid in intestinal adaptation [10]. Gastric hypersecretion occurring postoperatively can be treated with proton pump inhibitors or H2-receptor blockers [43]. Long-term sequelae of short bowel syndrome such as vitamin deficiencies, nephrolithiasis, and cholelithiasis should be anticipated early, so that preventive and treatment strategies can be initiated.

Crohn's disease recurs postoperatively in up to 50–60% cases by 10 years. This is usually preceded by endoscopic recurrence that is seen in up to 65–90% cases by the first year after surgery. Risk factors for recurrence include smoking, ileo-colonic disease, penetrating disease, and absence of prophylactic therapy [44–46]. Of the available therapies for Crohn's disease, 5-ASA compounds show modest benefit in preventing recurrence [47]. Immunomodulators may be more efficacious [48,49], but based on limited data infliximab therapy shows the greatest promise in preventing recurrence [50]. Steroids have no role in preventing recurrence. Decision to use medications to prevent recurrence should be made on a case-by-case basis. Patients at high risk for recurrence should be started on medication, while those at low risk can be monitored closely for signs of recurrence. The choice of medication should also be on a case-by-case basis. Smoking cessation should be strongly emphasized.

Due to the increased risk of colon cancer, periodic surveillance endoscopies must be undertaken if there is a remnant colonic and rectal segment postoperatively [51].

Summary

Surgery is a vital part of the arsenal in treating inflammatory bowel disease. Indications for surgery are varied and so are the types of surgeries. Differentiating ulcerative colitis from Crohn's disease is very important in planning the surgery to be performed and the postoperative care. Preoperative work-up should include up-to-date laboratory, radiologic, endoscopic, and clinical examinations to accurately determine disease location and activity. Active medications should be reviewed and reassessed. Need for perioperative steroids should be evaluated. Postoperative nutritional and medication needs of the patient should be addressed. Long-term follow-up includes endoscopic surveillance as required. Coordination of care among the surgeon, gastroenterologist, and patient is essential to achieve therapeutic goals.

References

1. Guindi M, Riddell RH. Indeterminate colitis. *J Clin Pathol* 2004; **57**: 1233–44.

2. Price A. Overlap in the spectrum of non-specific inflammatory bowel disease:colitis indeterminate. *J Clin Pathol* 1978; **31**: 567–77.

3. Loftus EV Jr. Clinical epidemiology of inflammatory bowel disease: incidence, prevalence and environmental influences. *Gastroenterology* 2004; **126**: 1504–17.

4. Andres PG, Friedman LS. Epidemiology and the natural course of inflammatory bowel disease. *Gastroenterol Clin North Am* 1999; **28**: 255–81.

5. Steinhardt HJ, Loeschke K, Kasper H, Holtermuller KH, Schafer H. European Cooperative Crohn's Disease Study (ECCDS): clinical features and natural history. *Digestion* 1985; **31**: 97–108.

6. Podolsky DK. Inflammatory bowel disease. *N Engl J Med* 2002; **347**: 1982–4.

7. Haggitt, R. Differential diagnosis of colitis. In Goldman HAH, Kaufman N, eds. *Gastrointestinal Pathology*. Baltimore, MD: Williams & Wilkins; 1988, pp. 325–55.

8. Chambers TJ, Morson BC. The granuloma in Crohn's disease. *Gut* 1979; **20**: 269–74.

9. Schmitz-Moormann P, Pittner PM, Malchow H, Brandes JW. The granuloma in Crohn's disease. A bioptical study. *Pathology Res Pract* 1984; **178**: 467–76.

10. Yamada T, Alpers D, Kalloo A *et al.*, eds. *Textbook of Gastroenterology*. Hoboken, NJ: Wiley-Blackwell: 2009.

11. Feldman M, Friedman L, Brandt L, eds. *Sleisenger and Fordtran's Gastrointestinal and Liver Disease*. Philadelphia, PA: Saunders; 2010.

12. Saltzstein SL, Rosenberg BF. Ulcerative colitis of the ileum and regional enteritis of the colon, a comparative histopathologic study. *Am J Clin Pathol* 1963; **46**: 336–43.

13. Rao SS, Holdsworth CD, Read NW. Symptoms and stool patterns in patients with ulcerative colitis. *Gut* 1988; **29**: 342–5.

14. Yamamoto T. Factors affecting recurrence after surgery for Crohn's disease. *World J Gastroenterol* 2005; **11**: 3971–9.

15. Williams JG, Wong WD, Rothenberger DA, Goldberg SM. Recurrence of Crohn's disease after resection. *Br J Surg* 1991; **78**: 10–19.

16. Wexner SD, Rosen I, Lowry A *et al.* Practice parameters for the treatment of mucosal ulcerative colitis – supporting documentation. The Standards Practice Task Force. The American Society of Colon and Rectal Surgeons. *Dis Colon Rectum* 1997; **40**: 1277–85.

17. Hancock L, Windsor AC, Mortensen NJ. Inflammatory bowel disease: the view of the surgeon. *Colorectal Dis* 2006; **8** (Suppl 1): 10–14.

18. Marcello PW, Milsom JW, Wong SK *et al.* Laparoscopic restorative proctocolectomy: case-matched comparative study with open restorative proctocolectomy. *Dis Colon Rectum* 2000; **43**: 604–8.

19. Leowardi C, Heuschen G, Kienle P, Heuschen U. Surgical treatment of severe inflammatory bowel disease. *Dig Dis* 2003; **21**: 54–62.

20. Schraut WH. The surgical management of Crohn's disease. *Gastroenterol Clin North Am* 2002; **31**: 255–63.

21. Kornbluth A, Sachar DB. Ulcerative colitis practice guidelines in adults: American College of Gastroenterology, Practice Parameters Committee. *Am J Gastroenterol* 2010; **105**: 501–23.

22. Shen B, Remzi FH, Lavery IC, Lashner BA, Fazio VW. A proposed classification of ileal pouch disorders and associated complications after restorative proctocolectomy. *Clin Gastroenterol Hepatol* 2008; **6**: 145–58.

23. Pemberton JH, Kelly KA, Beart RW *et al.* Ileal pouch-anal anastomosis for chronic ulcerative colitis. Long-term results. *Ann Surg* 1987; **206**: 504–13.

24. Robb B, Pritts T, Gang G *et al.* Quality of life in patients undergoing ileal pouch-anal anastomosis at the University of Cincinnati. *Am J Surg* 2002; **183**(4): 353–60.

25. Loftus EV Jr, Delgado DJ, Friedman HS, Sandborn WJ. Colectomy and the incidence of postsurgical complications among ulcerative colitis patients with private health insurance in the United States. *Am J Gastroenterol* 2008; **103**: 1737–45.

26. Weston-Petrides GK, Lovegrove RE, Tilney HS *et al.* Comparison of outcomes after restorative proctocolectomy with or without defunctioning ileostomy. *Arch Surg* 2008; **143**: 406–12.

27. Dhillon S, Loftus EV Jr, Tremaine WJ *et al.* The natural history of surgery for ulcerative colitis in a population-based cohort from Olmsted County, Minnesota. *Am J Gastroenterol* 2005; **100**: A819.

28. Pardi DS, D'Haens G, Shen B, Campbell S, Gionchetti P. Clinical guidelines for the management of pouchitis. *Inflamm Bowel Dis* 2009; **15**: 1424–31.

29. Waljee A, Waljee J, Morris AM, Higgins PD. Threefold increased risk of infertility: a meta-analysis of infertility after ileal pouch anal anastomosis in ulcerative colitis. *Gut* 2006; **55**: 1575–80.

30. Blumberg D, Beck DE. Surgery for ulcerative colitis. *Gastroenterol Clin North Am* 2002; **31**: 219–35.

31. Heyland DK, Motalvo M, MacDonald S *et al.* Total parenteral nutrition in the surgical patient: a meta-analysis. *Can J Surg* 2001; **44**: 102–11.

32. Hyde GM, Jewell DP, Kettlewell MG, Mortensen NJ. Cyclosporine for severe ulcerative colitis does not increase the rate of perioperative complications. *Dis Colon Rectum* 2001; **44**: 1436–40.

33. Kunitake H, Hodin R, Shellito PC *et al.* Perioperative treatment with infliximab in patients with Crohn's disease and ulcerative colitis is not associated with an increased rate of postoperative complications. *J Gastrointest Surg* 2008; **12**: 1730–7.

34. Subramanian V, Pollok RC, Kang JY, Kumar D. Systematic review of postoperative complications in patients with inflammatory bowel disease treated with immunomodulators. *Br J Surg* 2006; **93**: 793–9.

35. Subramanian V, Saxena S, Kang JY, Pollock RC. Preoperative steroid use and risk of postoperative complications in patients with inflammatory bowel disease undergoing abdominal surgery. *Am J Gastroenterol* 2008; **103**: 2373–81.

36. Miki C, Ohmori Y, Yoshiyama S *et al.* Factors predicting postoperative infectious complications and early induction of inflammatory mediators in ulcerative colitis patients. *World J Surg* 2007; **31**: 522–9.

37. Bruewer M, Utech M, Rijcken EJ *et al.* Preoperative steroid administration: effect on morbidity among patients undergoing intestinal bowel resection for Crohn's disease. *World J Surg* 2003; **27**: 1306–10.

38. Colombel JF, Loftus EV Jr, Tremaine WJ *et al.* Early postoperative complications are not increased in patients with Crohn's disease treated perioperatively with infliximab or immunosuppressive therapy. *Am J Gastroenterol* 2004; **99**: 878–83.

39. Lim M, Sagar P, Abdulgader A, Thekkinkattil D, Burke D. The impact of preoperative immunomodulation on pouch-related septic complications after ileal pouch-anal anastomosis. *Dis Colon Rectum* 2007; **50**: 943–51.

40. Salem M, Tainsh RE Jr, Bromberg J, Loriaux DL, Chernow B. Perioperative glucocorticoid coverage. A reassessment 42 years after emergence of a problem. *Ann Surg* 1994; **219**: 416–25.

41. Lamberts SW, Bruining HA, de Jong FH. Corticosteroid therapy in severe illness. *N Engl J Med* 1997; **337**: 1285–92.

42. Jabbour SA. Steroids and the surgical patient. *Med Clin North Am* 2001; **85**: 1311–17.

43. Buchman AL. The clinical management of short bowel syndrome; steps to avoid parenteral nutrition. *Nutrition* 1997; **13**: 907–13.

44. Van Assche G, Rutgeerts P. Medical management of postoperative recurrence in Crohn's disease. *Gastroenterol Clin North Am* 2004; **33**: 347–60.

45. Renna S, Camma C, Modesto I *et al.* Meta-analysis of the placebo rates of clinical relapse and severe endoscopic

recurrence in postoperative Crohn's disease. *Gastroenterology* 2008; **135**: 1500–9.

46. Cottone M, Rosselli M, Orlando A *et al.* Smoking habits and recurrence in Crohn's disease. *Gastroenterology* 1994; **106**: 643–8.

47. Le'mann M. Review article: Can post-operative recurrence in Crohn's disease be prevented? *Aliment Pharmacol Ther* 2006; **24** (Suppl 3): 22–8.

48. Hanauer SB, Korelitz BL, Rutgeerts P *et al.* Postoperative maintenance of Crohn's disease remission with 6-mercaptopurine, mesalamine, or placebo: a 2-year trial. *Gastroenterology* 2004; **127**: 723–9.

49. D'Haens GR, Vermeire S, Van Assche G *et al.* Therapy of metronidazole with azathioprine to prevent postoperative recurrence of Crohn's disease: a controlled randomized trial.

Gastroenterology 2008; **135**: 1123–9.

50. Regueiro M, Schraut W, Baidoo L *et al.* Infliximab prevents Crohn's disease recurrence after ileal resection. *Gastroenterology* 2009; **136**: 441–50.

51. Bernstein CN, Blanchard JF, Kllewer E, Wajda A. Cancer risk in patients with inflammatory bowel disease: a population-based study. *Cancer* 2001; **91**: 854–62.

Postoperative gastrointestinal complications

Andrew Boxer and Michael A. Poles

Introduction

Gut function is often impacted by surgical interventions, and postoperative gastrointestinal complications are common. Fortunately, most are minor and self-limited, but a number may be severe, and rarely, life threatening. Many of the complications can either be prevented or treated with proper prophylaxis and early recognition. Given the escalating use of bariatric surgery in the treatment of obese patients, this population is faced with unique postoperative issues.

Postoperative gastrointestinal bleeding

Postoperatively, gastrointestinal bleeding is an uncommon but potentially serious complication. Clinically significant bleeding occurs in 0.5–1% of patients in the acute postoperative setting [1,2]. The major causes of acute postoperative bleeding include stress ulceration, bleeding from an intestinal anastamosis, ischemic colitis, and bleeding from preexisting lesions such as gastroduodenal ulcers and diverticular disease. Gastrointestinal hemorrhage temporally remote from surgery occurs less commonly, but may be due to aortoenteric fistulae and recurrent or marginal ulcer disease.

Stress-related mucosal disease

Stress-related mucosal disease (SRMD), or stress-ulceration is the most common cause of postoperative GI bleeding, although its incidence has decreased with increased use of prophylaxis since 1999 [3,4]. Stress ulcers are primarily believed to be due to disturbances in the mucosal microcirculation, with relative local hypoperfusion causing a loss of mucosal integrity, an imbalance between aggressive and protective factors and subsequently development of multiple gastric erosions and ulcerations [5–7]. Suppressing gastric acid secretion is currently the best way to protect against these mucosal events; antisecretory agents have been employed successfully for prophylaxis of SRMD in high-risk patients [8].

Prolonged mechanical ventilation and coagulopathy are the main risk factors for clinically important bleeding from SRMD [9]. In studies that identified these risk factors, coagulopathy was defined as a platelet count less than 50,000 mm, an international normalized ratio (INR) greater than 1.5, or a partial thromboplastin time (PTT) greater than two times control [3]. The frequency of bleeding was 3.7% if either mechanical ventilation or coagulopathy were present, whereas patients without either of these complications had a bleeding risk of 0.1%. Other less important risk factors include perioperative hypotension, sepsis, spinal cord injuries, and severe burns [10]. Stress-related mucosal disease prophylaxis should be considered if one or more of these risk factors are present. The earliest studies of stress ulcer prophylaxis utilized weakly alkaline antacid medications to decrease the risk of GI bleeding in ICU patients [11]. Given their low efficacy, subsequent studies have examined use of more powerful antacids, revealing their superiority. Histamine 2 receptor antagonists (H_2 blockers) have been demonstrated to be effective in SRMD prevention in several studies [11,12]. However, tolerance may develop with prolonged use of H_2 blockers, which may limit their effectiveness [7]. Also these agents have been shown to induce thrombocytopenia as a risk factor. Though the mechanism of action of sucralfate has not been adequately elucidated, they have been evaluated as prophylaxis for SRMD, but were found to be less effective than H_2 blockers [13].

Proton pump inhibitors (PPIs) are currently the standard prophylactic agent in critically ill patients. Proton pump inhibitors have been shown to be both superior and cost effective to H_2 blockers in the prevention of GI bleeding from stress ulceration [14,15]. While PPIs have become the standard of care for SRMD prophylaxis, careful consideration must be given to assess if the patient truly necessitates the need for prophylaxis, since these medications are associated with serious adverse events, especially in hospitalized, critically ill patients, including an increased risk of hospital-acquired pneumonia and *Clostridium difficile* infection [16–18].

Ischemic colitis

The most common vascular complication affecting the GI tract in the postoperative period is ischemic colitis. Colonic ischemia is usually due to hypotension and a low flow state in the

Medical Management of the Surgical Patient, ed. Michael F. Lubin, Thomas F. Dodson, and Neil H. Winawer. Published by Cambridge University Press. © Cambridge University Press 2013.

perioperative setting or due to embolic phenomena [19]. While the incidence of ischemic colitis is relatively low, it carries a significant mortality rate. Ischemic colitis occurs in less than 1% of surgical patients overall, but may complicate up to 7% of elective aortic surgeries and up to 60% of surgeries performed for ruptured aortic aneurysms [20–26]. Mortality rates for ischemic colitis in the postoperative period may be as high as 54%, likely reflecting the presence of significant comorbidities [25]. Risk factors for ischemic colitis include older age, the presence of peripheral vascular disease, operative trauma to the colon, perioperative hypotension and the need for emergent surgery [23,26–28]. Patients with prior partial colectomy may also be at higher risk due to disturbed collateral blood supply.

Ischemic colitis typically presents insidiously in the week following a surgical procedure. Depending on the degree of ischemic injury, symptoms may range from mild nausea, diarrhea, heme-positive stool without abdominal pain, to severe colitis presenting with fever, abdominal pain, hematochezia, and peritoneal signs from transmural necrosis and gangrenous bowel. If the patient recovers from the initial episode, chronic sequelae may occur in up to one-third of patients and may include colonic stricture formation or persistence of segmental colitis that can mimic inflammatory bowel disease [29]. Abdominal CT scanning, performed early in the disease course, may be normal or may reveal non-specific colonic thickening, making prompt recognition challenging. In these instances clinicians need to maintain a high index of suspicion and closely monitor the patient's clinical symptoms. Imaging may also show the characteristic thumbprinting, that is associated with ischemic colitis and is due to submucosal hemorrhage. Colonoscopy is the diagnostic procedure of choice as it not only allows for examination of the colonic mucosa, but also allows for acquisition of biopsies and histopathologic examination. In mild disease, colonoscopy may reveal segments of pale mucosa with areas of petechial hemorrhage. As the injury increases in severity, the mucosa may appear blue or black with mucosal sloughing and ulceration. The rectum is often spared due to collateral circulation from the hemorrhoidal vessels off the internal iliacs, but ischemic proctitis may be occasionally seen [30].

Treatment of mild ischemic colitis is supportive, with intravenous hydration to optimize fluid status and bowel rest. If there are signs of infection, broad-spectrum antibiotics should be used. Follow-up endoscopy may be indicated to document lack of disease progression. Increasing abdominal pain, peritoneal signs, and fever suggests colonic infarction and usually requires prompt exploratory surgery and resection of non-viable colon.

Aortoenteric fistula

Aortoenteric fistula (AEF) is a rare but potentially life-threatening cause of GI bleeding, occurring in approximately 1% of patients with previous abdominal aortic graft surgery [31]. Aortoenteric fistula is usually caused by a direct communication between the proximal aorta and the bowel lumen, most typically in the duodenum. Patients characteristically present months to years after their initial operation with evidence of GI hemorrhage. Patients may be seen initially after a minor episode of bleeding, the so-called sentinel bleed. They may then re-present (in hours or as long as several months) with a massive GI hemorrhage that can result in exsanguination if not rapidly addressed. While this presentation is quite dramatic, approximately 50% of patients with AEF will present less dramatically with evidence of chronic GI blood loss, intermittent bleeding, or heme-positive stool [32]. A less common presentation is seen when the aortic graft erodes into the bowel lumen, resulting in a paraprosthetic–enteric fistula (PEF) [33]. In this instance, the graft is bathed in enteric contents, and the patient may present with fever, abdominal pain, and sepsis. Patients with PEF may also have melena or guaiac-positive stools, but rarely experience massive gastrointestinal bleeding [32].

Diagnosis of AEF requires a high index of suspicion. Only one-third of AEFs are demonstrated prior to surgery [34]. If patients are hemodynamically stable, EGD may be performed to identify the source of bleeding. Although endoscopy lacks specificity for AEF, graft erosion into the bowel lumen may sometimes be seen; endoscopy is also useful to exclude other causes of GI hemorrhage [35]. CT angiography may be helpful if a patient presents with fever and sepsis, but the specificity is low for determining the presence of fistulae [34]. If the clinician has a high suspicion for AEF, the patient should undergo urgent exploratory laparotomy.

Postoperative nausea and vomiting

Nausea and vomiting occur frequently in the early postoperative setting. Patient characteristics predisposing to an increased risk include female gender, obesity, history of gastroparesis, prior history of motion sickness or previous postoperative vomiting [36]. Procedural characteristics that increase the risk of postoperative nausea and vomiting include abdominal surgery, laparoscopic procedures, and increasing procedure duration [36]. The anesthetic agents used may also be associated with depression of gastrointestinal motility, but their role in causing postoperative nausea and vomiting is controversial. Postoperative ileus is especially common after abdominal surgery, but is short-lived, typically resolving over 3–5 days. Certain approaches may be associated with a decreased duration of postoperative ileus, including the use of less invasive surgical techniques, use of opioid-sparing agents, use of thoracic epidural anesthetics rather than use of systemic anesthesia, and early institution of oral nutrition. Placement of nasogastric tubes for the treatment of postoperative nausea and vomiting has not been shown to be effective, may increase the risk of postoperative pulmonary complications, and should generally be discouraged [37].

Nausea and vomiting that persists for greater than a few days after abdominal surgery generally warrants further investigation. Care should be taken to assess for metabolic disturbances, gastroesophageal reflux disease (GERD), obstruction, pancreatitis, infection, and neurologic disturbances that may be causative. The complete list of medications the patient is taking should also be examined, as a great number of medications may induce nausea and vomiting [38].

Gastrectomy may be associated with a number of syndromes that may increase the risk of postoperative nausea and vomiting. Billroth II gastrectomy may be associated with afferent loop syndrome, which may cause postoperative vomiting due to a blockage of the afferent limb of the gastrojejunostomy. Symptoms associated with this complication include postprandial epigastric pain as pressure builds in the blocked limb, followed by bilious emesis, without recently ingested food, when the obstruction is relieved. Rarely, patients with chronic high-grade limb-related obstruction may present with pancreatitis and/or obstructive jaundice due to the effects of back-pressure on pancreaticobiliary secretion. Efferent limb syndrome after Billroth II gastrectomy is caused by partial obstruction of the intestinal segment draining the stomach that will also result in nausea and vomiting. While symptoms are similar to those of afferent loop syndrome, with efferent limb syndrome the emesis usually contains recently ingested food. Both afferent and efferent limb syndromes may be diagnosed via barium studies, and treatment is effectively rendered by surgical revision.

Nausea and vomiting occurring remotely from a surgical intervention may be caused by intestinal obstruction, which is commonly due to formation of adhesions after abdominal surgery. In addition, strictures at the site of an intestinal anastomosis may cause postoperative obstruction in approximately 2% of patients [39]. Strictures may be diagnosed and localized with endoscopic or barium studies. Video capsule endoscopy may be helpful in evaluating more distal anastomoses, although concern for capsule impaction warrants cautious use in potentially obstructed patients. If there is a concern for potential retained capsule, a patency capsule should be used first. A patient will ingest a patency capsule then radiologic images are taken days later to see if the capsule travels past the small bowel. After a period of time the patency capsule disintegrates, in comparison to video capsules. Anastomotic strictures may sometimes be treated with balloon dilation, although many patients with distal or refractory strictures may need surgical revision.

Postoperative diarrhea

Diarrhea is commonly seen in the early postoperative setting. The most common etiology of diarrhea in this setting is medication side-effects, though additional causes include resolving ileus, and colonization with pathogenic bacterial flora. Initial evaluation of early postoperative diarrhea should include a review of recent medications, with attention to antibiotic use, magnesium-containing antacids, elixirs containing sorbitol or mannitol, and other medications including

colchicine, lactulose, misoprostol, as well as other stool softeners and laxatives. Diarrhea associated with *Clostridium difficile* infection may present within the first few weeks of surgery and is usually, although not always, associated with antibiotic use. Enteral feeding often causes diarrhea [40]. Patients with fecal impaction may also present with overflow diarrhea [41].

Persistent or chronic postoperative diarrhea may be related to the type of surgical procedure performed. Gastric surgery is frequently associated with diarrhea through a number of mechanisms. Early dumping syndrome is a significant problem in 14–20% of patients after partial gastrectomy [42]. Dumping is characterized by gastrointestinal and vasomotor symptoms due to rapid emptying of hyperosmolar chyme into the small bowel, as well as abnormal release of gut neuroendocrine factors [43–45]. Symptoms typically begin 10–30 minutes after a meal, with patients complaining of postprandial fullness, pain, and explosive diarrhea, often associated with generalized weakness, flushing, and dizziness. The incidence of early dumping is reduced with highly selective vagotomy. Dietary modification is the mainstay of therapy, with patients instructed to eat smaller meals low in simple carbohydrates and to avoid liquid intake during a meal. Symptoms refractory to diet changes and antidiarrheal agents may improve with subcutaneous octreotide [46,47].

Diarrhea may also be seen after vagotomy in 20–30% of patients, and may be due to rapid gastric emptying or impaired gall bladder function leading to bile acid-related ("cholerrheic") diarrhea [48,49]. Patients typically present with frequent watery stools, often with nocturnal symptoms, that are not associated with meals. Treatment includes dietary modifications similar to those used for the dumping syndrome, antidiarrheal medications, and cholestyramine in severe cases [49]. Patients with refractory postvagotomy diarrhea may occasionally benefit from surgical procedures such as the construction of an antiperistaltic jejunal segment in an attempt to slow intestinal transit, although clinical results have not been uniformly positive [50].

Bacterial overgrowth syndrome may be associated with any procedure that interferes with normal intestinal motility, permitting stasis and allowing bacterial colonization of the small bowel. The hallmarks of bacterial overgrowth include diarrhea, steatorrhea, and malnutrition. Patients develop steatorrhea due to bacterial bile acid deconjugation and subsequent fatty acid malabsorption. In the past the diagnosis of bacterial over-growth was made endoscopically by small bowel aspiration and quantitative culture showing greater than 10^5 organisms/mL. However, studies such as the 14C xylose breath test are a less invasive diagnostic alternative. In cases where the clinical suspicion for bacterial overgrowth is high, empiric treatment with antibiotics may be performed without diagnostic testing. Most treatment regimens include agents with effectiveness against both aerobic and anaerobic bacteria. A short (7–10-day) course of antibiotics is generally given, but rotating antibiotics may be needed if symptoms quickly return or become chronic [51].

Chronic diarrhea is a known complication after cholecystectomy. The frequency of postcholecystectomy diarrhea, however, is a matter of debate. Although postcholecystectomy diarrhea has been found to occur very rarely in some clinical investigations, watery diarrhea was observed in up to 12% of patients in other studies. In one of these studies, up to half of the patients were found to have milder changes of bowel habits after the onset of postcholecystectomy diarrhea, such as loose stools or increased stool frequency. This occurs due to increased fecal bile acid excretion [52].

The short bowel syndrome is characterized by diarrhea, steatorrhea, and malnutrition in the setting of extensive small bowel resection. Generally, short bowel syndrome that requires prolonged nutritional support may develop when less than 25%, or approximately 120 cm, of functional intestine remains, but the severity of symptoms also depends on the site of resection, the presence of the ileocecal valve and colon, and the functional status and adaptive capacity of the remaining small bowel [53,54]. Major midgut resection may result in rapid intestinal transit and osmotic diarrhea. Distal ileal resection may result in bile acid diarrhea. Removal of the ileocecal valve may result in reflux of bacteria into the small bowel and subsequent bacterial overgrowth. Chronic complications of short bowel syndrome may include malnutrition, cholelithiasis, nephrolithiasis, bacterial overgrowth, and steatohepatitis if parenteral nutrition is required. Short bowel-associated diarrhea in the early postoperative period is frequently impressive, but usually improves with adaptation of the remaining intestine. Early management goals for short bowel syndrome include supportive care with intravenous fluid, electrolyte repletion, and nutritional support with parenteral nutrition. Initial enteral feeding may begin when stool output falls to less than 2.5 L/day [55]. Cholestyramine is often given to patients with distal ileal resection and presumed bile acid-related diarrhea. There is evidence early enteral nutrition has a stimulatory effect on the epithelial cells and the production of trophic hormones and can decrease diarrhea [56].

Complications of bariatric surgery

There is an increasing worldwide epidemic of obesity. The most effective treatment for obesity and its complications is bariatric surgery; these procedures however are associated with a number of nutritional and gastrointestinal complications [57]. Two main types of procedures are most commonly employed; restrictive procedures and restrictive procedures combined with malabsorption procedures. The two main restrictive procedures are vertical gastroplasty and adjustable gastric banding, which is usually placed laparoscopically. The two main malabsorptive procedures are duodenal switch and biliopancreatic diversion.

One of the most common issues found in patients who have undergone bariatric surgery, especially after Roux-en-Y gastric bypass (RYGB) is vitamin deficiency. Almost half of all patients with a RYGB will develop iron deficiency. To be absorbed, the ferric iron in foods must first be reduced to the ferrous state. This reduction occurs in the stomach in the presence of acid. Achlorhydria may develop in RYGB patients, leading to a reduction in iron absorption [58]. Iron supplementation is therefore recommended for all RYGB patients. The absorption of vitamin B_{12} also begins in the stomach, where both pepsin and hydrochloric acid cleave it from foods. This process is also reduced after RYGB, as these patients can also have inadequate secretion of intrinsic factor, a necessary component for vitamin B_{12} absorption [58]. Folic acid deficiency is another common complication of RYGB. This can affect as many as 35% of patients. Folate absorption is facilitated by hydrochloric acid and occurs primarily in the proximal one-third of the small intestine [59]. Furthermore, since vitamin B_{12} acts as a coenzyme in converting methyltetrahydrofolate to tetrahydrofolate, vitamin B_{12} deficiency can lead to folate deficiency. Thiamine (vitamin B_1) is absorbed in the proximal small intestine. Thus, after redirection of the small bowel from a RYGB, patients are at risk of thiamine deficiency [60]. Deficiency of the fat-soluble vitamins (A, C, D, E) may also occur after malabsorptive procedures. Since the duodenum is bypassed, there is delayed mixing of dietary fat with pancreatic enzymes and bile salts. This may lead to malabsorption of fat and fat-soluble vitamins. Treatment of all vitamin deficiencies is through supplementation.

Rapid weight loss, irrespective of the type of bariatric surgery, predisposes patients to the formation of cholesterol gallstones. At 6 months postoperatively, up to one-third of patients develop new gallstones [61]. The administration of ursodeoxycholic acid (UDCA) for 6 months after surgery reduces the incidence of postoperatively formed gallstones to 2% [62]. Due to the difficulty in the optimal performance of ultrasonography in the obese patient, either CT or MRI may need to be utilized in the work-up for gallstones.

Up to 20% of patients who undergo RYGB develop postoperative marginal ulcers. The ulcers usually form on the intestinal side of the gastrojejunostomy anastamosis, occurring a few months after surgery [63]. It is hypothesized that increased acid secretion and local ischemia lead to these marginal ulcers [64]. Patients with marginal ulcers will typically present with dyspepsia or upper gastrointestinal bleeding, but may develop obstructive symptoms due to significant surrounding edema and potentially ischemic fibrosis. The work-up for these symptoms should include an upper endoscopy. NSAID use should be sought and *Helicobactor pylori* should be treated if present to prevent recurrence. If the ulcer is refractory to healing, surgical revision may be needed.

Up to 27% of patients develop stenosis of the gastrojejunal anastomotic site after RYGB. When this occurs, it usually does so within 3 months of surgery. Diagnosis can be made with either barium contrast radiography or upper endoscopy. Stomal stenosis is often amenable to endoscopic balloon dilation [65].

Up to 1% of patients who undergo placement of an inflatable gastric band experience erosion of the band through the gastric wall. On average this complication occurs 19 months postoperatively. Patients most commonly present with refractory port site infection. Other rarer presentations include weight gain, subphrenic abscess, peritonitis, and port-cutaneous fistula. Patients who experience these adverse effects must be treated with surgical band removal. Early band erosion is often the result of intraoperative injury to the stomach wall. The partial stomach wall damage that occurs during surgery may continue to complete penetration under the influence of relative ischemia due to band pressure. A second possible cause for early erosion is microperforation during the primary operation which may result in development of a chronic infectious process which facilitates erosion of the band through the gastric wall [66]. Late erosions are thought to largely be a consequence of chronic ischemia of the stomach wall which could be caused by direct pressure of the band, or may be due to extensive dissection necessary during the primary operation that may impair blood supply rendering the stomach more susceptible to development of pressure necrosis [67].

Gastric reduction with duodenal switch causes moderate intake restriction with substantial calorie malabsorption. The most common complication of this procedure is bowel obstruction, which will often involve the gastric pouch. Approximately two-thirds of the obstructions occur at the level of the proximal anastomosis and the rest in the midbody. There are also rare complications of anastomotic leaks and fistulas [68]. The most common complications of biliopancreatic diversion are nutritional and mineral deficiencies [69,70].

References

1. Egleston CV, Wood AE, Gorey TF, McGovern EM. Gastrointestinal complications after cardiac surgery. *Ann R Coll Surg Engl* 1993; **75**: 52–6.

2. Byhahn C, Strouhal U, Martens S. *et al.* Incidence of gastrointestinal complications in cardiopulmonary bypass patients. *World J Surg* 2001; **25**: 1140–4.

3. Schiessel R, Feil W, Wenzl E. Mechanisms of stress ulceration and implications for treatment. *Gastroenterol Clin North Am* 1990; **90**: 101–20.

4. Pimental M, Roberts DE, Bernstein CN *et al.* Clinically significant gastrointestinal bleeding in critically ill patients in an era of prophylaxis. *Am J Gastroenterol* 2000; **95**: 2801–6.

5. Stremple JF, Mori H, Lev R. *et al.* The stress ulcer syndrome. *Curr Prob Surg* 1973; April: 1–64.

6. Durham RM, Shapiro MJ. Stress gastritis revisited. *Surg Crit Care* 1991; **71**: 791–810.

7. Merki HS, Wilder-Smith CH. Do continuous infusions of omeprazole and ranitidine retain their effect with prolonged dosing? *Gastroenterology* 1994; **106**: 60–4.

8. Levy MJ, Seelig CB, Robinson NJ, Ranney JE. Comparison of omeprazole and ranitidine for stress ulcer prophylaxis. *Dig Dis Sci* 1997; **42**: 1255–9.

9. Yu-feng C, Yi J, Mei M *et al.* Incidence and risk factors of gastrointestinal bleeding in mechanically ventilated patients. *World J Emerg Med* 2010; **1**: 32–6.

10. Quenot J, Thiery N, Barbar S. When should stress ulcer prophylaxis be used in the ICU? *Curr Opin Crit Care* 2009; **15**: 139–43.

11. Martindale RG. Contemporary strategies for the prevention of stress-related mucosal bleeding. *Am J Health Syst Pharm* 2005; **62**: S11–S17.

12. Cook DJ, Reeve BK, Guyatt GH. *et al.* Stress ulcer prophylaxis in critically ill patients. *J Am Med Assoc* 1996; **275**: 308–14.

13. Cook D, Guyatt G, Marshall J *et al.* A comparison of sucralfate and ranitidine for the prevention of upper gastrointestinal bleeding in patients requiring mechanical ventilation. Canadian Critical Care Trials Group. *N Engl J Med* 1998; **338**: 791–7.

14. Lin P, Chang C, Hsu P *et al.* The efficacy and safety of proton pump inhibitors vs histamine-2 receptor antagonists for stress ulcer bleeding prophylaxis among critical care patients: a meta-analysis. *Crit Care Med* 2010; **38**: 1197–205.

15. Schupp KN, Schrand LM, Mutnick AH. A cost-effectiveness analysis of stress ulcer prophylaxis. *Ann Pharmacother* 2003; **37**: 631–5.

16. Cunningham R, Dale B, Undy B, Gaunt N. Proton pump inhibitors as a risk factor for *Clostridium difficile* diarrhea. *J Hosp Infect* 2003; **54**: 243–5.

17. Farrell C, Mercogliano G, Kuntz C. Overuse of stress ulcer prophylaxis in the critical care setting and beyond. *J Crit Care* 2010; **25**: 214–20.

18. Gulmez S, Holm A, Frederiksen H *et al.* Use of proton pump inhibitors and the risk of community-acquired pneumonia. *Arch Intern Med* 2007; **167**: 950–5.

19. Fernández J, Calvo L, Vázquez E *et al.* Risk factors associated with the development of ischemic colitis. *World J Gastroenterol* 2010; **16**: 4564–9.

20. Aranha GU, Pickleman J, Piffare R. *et al.* The reasons for gastrointestinal consultation after cardiac surgery. *Am Surg* 1984; **50**: 301–4.

21. Christerson JT, Schmuziger M, Maurice J *et al.* Postoperative visceral hypotension, the common cause for gastrointestinal complications after cardiac surgery. *Thorac Cardiovasc Surg* 1994; **42**: 152–7.

22. Huddy SPJ, Joyce WP, Pepper JR. Gastrointestinal complications in 4473 patients who underwent cardiopulmonary bypass surgery. *Br J Surg* 1991; **78**: 293–6.

23. Ernst CB, Hagihara PF, Daugherty ME *et al.* Ischemic colitis incidence following abdominal aortic reconstruction: a prospective study. *Surgery* 1976; **80**: 417–21.

24. Hagihara PF, Ernst CB, Griffen WO Jr. Incidence of ischemic colitis following abdominal aortic reconstruction. *Surg Gynecol Obstet* 1979; **149**: 571–3.

25. Longo WE, Lee TC, Barnett MG *et al.* Ischemic colitis complicating abdominal aortic aneurysm surgery in the U.S. veteran. *J Surg Res* 1996; **60**: 351–4.

26. Schiedler MG, Cutler BS, Fiddian-Green RG. Sigmoid intramural pH for prediction of ischemic colitis during aortic surgery. A comparison with risk factors and inferior mesenteric artery

stump pressures. *Arch Surg* 1987; **122**: 881–6.

27. Ernst CB. Prevention of intestinal ischemia following abdominal aortic reconstruction. *Surgery* 1983; **93**: 102–6.

28. Schroeder T, Christoffersen JK, Andersen J. *et al.* Ischemic colitis complicating reconstruction of the abdominal aorta. *Surg Gynecol Obstet* 1985; **160**: 299–303.

29. Boley SJ. Colonic ischemia – 25 years later. *Am J Gastroenterol* 1990; **85**: 931–4.

30. Theodoropoulou A, Koutroubakis IE. Ischemic colitis: clinical practice in diagnosis and treatment. *World J Gastroenterol* 2008; **14**: 7302–8.

31. Elliott JP, Smith RF, Szilagyi DE. Aortoenteric and paraprosthetic-enteric fistulas. *Arch Surg* 1974; **108**: 479–90.

32. Pipinos II, Carr JA, Haithcock BE *et al.* Secondary aortoenteric fistula. *Ann Vasc Surg* 2000; **14**: 688–96.

33. Antoniou G, Koutsias S, Antoniou S *et al.* Outcome after endovascular stent graft repair of aortoenteric fistula: a systematic review. *J Vasc Surg* 2009; **49**: 782–9.

34. Peck JJ, Eidemiler LR. Aortoenteric fistulas. *Arch Surg* 1992; **127**: 1191–4.

35. Kiernan PD, Pairolero PC, Hubert JP. *et al.* Aortic graft-enteric fistula. *Mayo Clin Proc* 1980; **55**: 731–8.

36. Watcha MF, White PF. Postoperative nausea and vomiting. *Anesthesiology* 1992; **77**: 162–84.

37. Gan T, Meyer R, Apfel C *et al.* Society for Ambulatory Anesthesia guidelines for the management of postoperative nausea and vomiting. *Anesth Analg* 2007; **105**: 1615–28.

38. Conway B. Prevention and management of postoperative nausea and vomiting in adults. *AORN J* 2009; **90**: 391–413.

39. Jex RK, van Heerden JA, Wolff BG *et al.* Gastrointestinal anastomoses: factors affecting early complications. *Ann Surg* 1987; **206**: 138–41.

40. Heimburger DC. Diarrhea with enteral feeding: will the real cause please stand up? *Am J Med* 1990; **88**: 89–90.

41. Powell DW. Approach to the patient with diarrhea. In Yamada T, ed. *Gastroenterology*. 3rd edn. Philadelphia, PA: Lippincott, Williams & Wilkins; 1999, pp. 858–909.

42. Hejazi R, Patil H, McCallum R. Dumping syndrome: establishing criteria for diagnosis and identifying new etiologies. *Dig Dis Sci* 2010; **55**: 117–23.

43. Jordan GLJ, Overton RC, DeBakey ME. The postgastrectomy syndrome: studies on pathogenesis. *Ann Surg* 1957; **145**: 471–8.

44. Miholic J, Reilmann L, Meyer HJ *et al.* Extracellular space, blood volume, and the early dumping syndrome after total gastrectomy. *Gastroenterology* 1990; **99**: 923–9.

45. Blackburn AM, Christofides ND, Ghatei MA *et al.* Elevation of plasma neurotensin in the dumping syndrome. *Clin Sci* 1980; **59**: 237–43.

46. Mackie CR, Jenkins SA, Hartley MN. Treatment of severe postvagotomy/ postgastrectomy symptoms with the somatostatin analogue octreotide. *Br J Surg* 1991; **78**: 1338–43.

47. Geer RJ, Richards WO, O'Dorisio TM *et al.* Efficacy of octreotide acetate in treatment of severe postgastrectomy dumping syndrome. *Ann Surg* 1990; **212**: 678–87.

48. Dragstedt LR, Harper PVJ, Tovee EB *et al.* Section of the vagus nerves to the stomach in the treatment of peptic ulcer: complications and end results after four years. *Ann Surg* 1947; **126**: 687–99.

49. Allan JG, Russell RI. Proceedings: double-blind controlled trial of cholestyramine in the treatment of post-vagotomy diarrhoea. *Gut* 1975; **16**: 830.

50. Sawyers JL, Herrington J Jr. Superiority of antiperistaltic jejunal segments in management of severe dumping syndrome. *Ann Surg* 1973; **178**: 311–19.

51. Eamonn M, Quigley, Ahmed A *et al.* Small intestinal bacterial overgrowth. *Infect Dis Clin North Am* 2010; **24**: 943–59.

52. Sauter G, Moussavian A, Meyer G *et al.* Bowel habits and bile acid malabsorption in the months after cholecystectomy. *Am J Gastroenterol* 2002; **97**: 1732–5.

53. Westergaard H. Bile acid malabsorption. *Curr Treat Options Gastroenterol* 2007; **10**: 28–33.

54. Thompson JS. Management of the short bowel syndrome. *Gastroenterol Clin North Am* 1994; **23**: 403–20.

55. Westergaard H. Short bowel syndrome. In Sleisenger MH, Fordtran JS, eds. *Gastrointestinal Disease*. 6th edn. Philadelphia, PA: W. B. Saunders; 1998, pp. 1548–56.

56. Olieman JF. Enteral nutrition in children with short-bowel syndrome: current evidence and recommendations for the clinician. *J Am Diet Assoc* 2010; **110**: 420–6.

57. Buchwald H, Avidor Y, Braunwald E *et al.* Bariatric surgery: a systematic review and meta-analysis. *J Am Med Assoc* 2004; **292**: 1724–37.

58. Smith CD, Herkes SB, Behrns KE *et al.* Gastric acid secretion and vitamin B12 absorption after vertical Roux-en-Y gastric bypass for morbid obesity. *Ann Surg* 1993; **218**: 91–6.

59. Brolin RE, Gorman JH, Gorman RC *et al.* Are vitamin B12 and folate deficiency clinically important after Roux-en-Y gastric bypass? *J Gastrointest Surg* 1998; **2**: 436–42.

60. Halverson JD. Micronutrient deficiencies after gastric bypass for morbid obesity. *Am Surg* 1986; **52**: 594–8.

61. Iglézias Brandão de Oliveira C, Adami Chaim E, Borges da Silva B. Impact of rapid weight reduction on risk of cholelithasis after bariatric surgery. *Obes Surg* 2003; **13**: 625–8.

62. Sugerman HJ, Brewer WH, Shiffman ML *et al.* A multicenter, placebo-controlled, randomized, double-blind, prospective trial of prophylactic ursodiol for the prevention of gallstone formation following gastric-bypass-induced rapid weight loss. *Am J Surg* 1995; **169**: 91–6.

63. Dallal RM, Bailey LA. Ulcer disease after gastric bypass surgery. *Surg Obes Relat Dis* 2006; **2**: 455–9.

64. Sapala JA, Wood MH, Sapala MA *et al.* Marginal ulcer after gastric bypass: a prospective 3-year study of 173 patients. *Obes Surg* 1998; **8**: 505–16.

65. Matthews BD, Sing RF, DeLegge MH *et al.* Initial results with a stapled gastrojejunostomy for the laparoscopic isolated Roux-en-Y gastric bypass. *Am J Surg* 2000; **179**: 476–81.

66. Abu-Abeid S, Keidar A, Gavert N, Blanc A, Szold A. The clinical spectrum of band erosion following laparoscopic adjustable silicone gastric banding for

morbid obesity. *Surg Endosc* 2003; **17**: 861–3.

67. Meir E, Van Baden M. Laparoscopic adjustable silicone gastric banding and band erosion: personal experience and hypotheses. *Obes Surg* 1999; **9**: 191–3.

68. Mitchell M, Carabetta J, Shah R *et al.* Duodenal switch gastric bypass surgery for morbid obesity: imaging of postsurgical anatomy and postoperative gastrointestinal complications. *Am J Roentgenol* 2009; **193**: 1576–80.

69. Luis D, Pacheco D, Izaola O *et al.* Clinical results and nutritional consequences of biliopancreatic diversion: three years of follow-up. *Ann Nutr Metab* 2008; **53**: 234–9.

70. Laurenius A, Taha O, Maleckas A *et al.* Laparoscopic biliopancreatic diversion/ duodenal switch or laparoscopic Roux-en-Y gastric bypass for super-obesity weight loss versus side effects. *Surg Obes Relat Dis* 2010; **6**: 408–14.

Chapter 20

Disorders of red cells

James R. Eckman

Introduction

The primary consideration in medical management of red cell disorders during surgery is to optimize hemoglobin concentration to provide for adequate oxygen delivery to tissues. Blood hemoglobin concentration is a primary direct and indirect determinant of tissue oxygenation. Blood oxygen content increases directly as hemoglobin concentration increases. Tissue oxygen delivery is a complex function of hemoglobin level, cardiac output, hemoglobin oxygen affinity, and tissue oxygen content. As hemoglobin level (more correctly red cell number) increases, blood viscosity increases and cardiac output may decrease so there is an optimal range of hemoglobin concentration that maximizes tissue oxygen delivery. The goal of preoperative and postoperative management is to maintain this optimal level at reasonable cost. Unfortunately, this optimal level is poorly defined in most clinical settings, varies between patients and within individual patients over time, and, even if well defined, cannot be maintained without unacceptable complication rates or costs. Perioperative management involves considering the optimal hemoglobin level for each clinical setting based on an informal cost–benefit analysis that usually is supported by incomplete outcome data.

A number of recent studies have shown that preoperative anemia is independently associated with increased morbidity and mortality in both cardiac and non-cardiac surgery. These studies are retrospective and cannot determine whether the anemia is causal of a worse outcome or a marker for severity of underlying disease. Until prospective controlled studies are completed, it seems prudent to try and identify the causes and correct the anemia before elective surgery. A large retrospective study done in the Veterans Affairs hospitals has shown that elevation in hematocrit above 54% is also associated with increased perioperative mortality and cardiac complications in an older male population.

An initial assessment should be done to determine if the hemoglobin level is too high or too low for the specific patient or surgical procedure. Alterations in hemoglobin level may also suggest underlying clinical conditions that may compromise surgical outcome if not properly diagnosed and treated.

Anemia may require partial correction to prevent cardiac and non-cardiac complications in the perioperative period and may be a manifestation of nutritional problems that may impair healing, hemoglobinopathies that require specific therapy, or autoimmune diseases that may also complicate blood transfusion.

Increased hemoglobin level may also require evaluation and therapy in the preoperative patient. Polycythemia may require correction prior to surgery or could be a sign of acute or chronic volume depletion. Polycythemia may also indicate chronic diseases that are associated with hypoxemia or with increased risk of perioperative thrombosis and bleeding.

Anemia

Anemia is generally defined as a hemoglobin concentration of less than 14 g/dL in males and 12.3 g/dL in females. Corresponding lower limits of normal for hematocrit are 42% in males and 36% in females.

Diagnostic considerations

Evaluation of an anemia caused by decreased production of red cells may reveal nutritional deficiencies that can be treated to maximize hemoglobin level and improve healing. Many microcytic and macrocytic anemias result from specific nutritional deficiencies that cause correctable anemia and may delay healing and predispose to infection. Normocytic anemias may indicate the presence of underlying medical disease or may define patients with marginal marrow reserve. Evaluation of hemolytic anemias must exclude hemoglobinopathies requiring special operative management, immune hemolysis that may complicate blood transfusion and enzyme deficiencies that may influence selection of medications.

Algorithms of use in evaluating anemias are presented in Figures 20.1 through 20.3. Blood loss always must be excluded because it is a common cause of anemia in surgical patients. Studies used to initiate diagnostic testing for most common anemias are presented in Figure 20.1. The reticulocyte count is the initial, and most important, test because it determines if

Medical Management of the Surgical Patient, ed. Michael F. Lubin, Thomas F. Dodson, and Neil H. Winawer. Published by Cambridge University Press. © Cambridge University Press 2013.

the primary cause of the anemia is related to decreased production or increased loss of red cells. Anemias caused by decreased red cell production have a low or normal reticulocyte count (corrected percent < 2% or < 75,000/μL absolute). The mean corpuscular volume (MCV) is the best test to initiate evaluation of anemias caused by decreased red cell production. The diagnostic tests outlined in Figure 20.2 establish the cause of most common anemias with low reticulocyte counts. Tests indicated by the algorithm should be drawn before surgery or transfusion in all but the most urgent surgical emergencies.

When the reticulocyte count is high (corrected percent > 2% or > 75,000/μL absolute), the presence of

hemolytic anemia is confirmed by excluding blood loss and detecting isolated increase in indirect bilirubin, elevated lactic dehydrogenase, decreased haptoglobin, or free hemoglobin in plasma or urine (see Figure 20.1). Once hemolysis is confirmed, preoperative diagnosis of the cause of the hemolytic anemia is particularly important because a number of diseases that cause hemolysis require special management of transfusions during surgery. A careful past medical and family history, a direct antiglobulin (Coombs') test, and examination of the peripheral blood smear in combination with a few confirmatory tests usually results in a diagnosis (see Figure 20.3).

Management considerations

Perioperative management of anemia is not difficult because treatment with transfusion of red cells is readily available. Too often, transfusion of red cells is substituted for thoughtful clinical evaluation and optimal medical therapy. A number of studies have found that perioperative and intraoperative transfusions are associated with a worse outcome in both cardiac and non-cardiac surgery. Prospective studies are needed to determine if this is causal or reflects increased blood loss and severity of comorbid disease, both of which may contribute to morbidity and mortality. Diagnosis and treatment of the cause of the anemia are preferred over transfusion before elective surgery if time permits. If the anemia cannot be corrected or if large blood losses are anticipated, careful planning can allow surgery without transfusion or provide the patient's own blood for transfusion, minimizing the complications. In emergency situations, it is usually best to draw appropriate diagnostic laboratory tests and proceed with transfusion and surgery before the cause of anemia is certain. There are no absolute criteria for management of anemia in the perioperative period, however, a number of useful guidelines have recently been published [1–21].

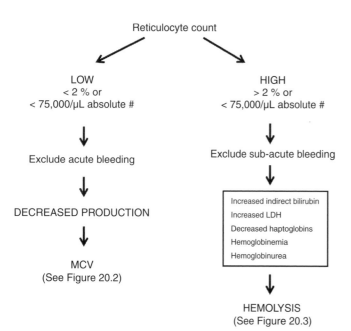

Figure 20.1 Evaluation of anemia. MCV, mean corpuscular volume; LDH, lactate dehydrogenase.

Figure 20.2 Diagnosis of decreased red cell production. MCV, mean corpuscular volume.

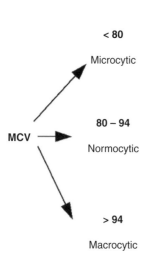

	Diagnosis	Diagnostic tests
< 80 Microcytic	Iron deficiency Anemia of chronic disease Thalassemia Sideroblastic anemia	Serum ferritin Iron, TIBC Red count, Hb ELP, DNA Bone marrow iron stain
80 – 94 Normocytic	Acute blood loss Anemia of chronic disease Renal failure Myelophthisic Leukemia / aplastic Hypothyroidism	Exclude bleeding Iron, TIBC BUN, creatinine Erythropoietin level Bone marrow biopsy Bone marrow with biopsy TSH, T4, T3
> 94 Macrocytic	Vitamin B$_{12}$ deficiency Folic acid deficiency Liver disease Erythroleukemia Hypothyroidism	Serum B12 levels Serum, RBC folate Blood smear, liver profile Bone marrow with biopsy TSH, T4, T3

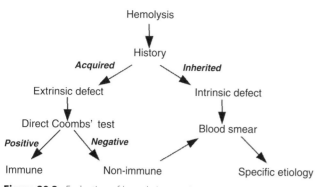

Figure 20.3 Evaluation of hemolytic anemias.

Table 20.1 Approximate complication rates for homologous red cell transfusion.

Immune reaction	
Alloimmunization	1 in 100 to 1 in 150
Acute hemolytic transfusion reaction	1 in 250,000 to 1×10^6
Delayed transfusion reaction	1 in 100,000
Febrile reaction	1 in 1,000
Infection	
HIV	1 in 250,000 to 1 in 2×10^6
Hepatitis B	1 in 30,000 to 1 in 250,000
Hepatitis C (non-A, non-B)	< 1 in 30,000 to 1 in 150,000
Other	
Transfusion-related acute lung injury	1 in 5,000
Bacterial infection	1 in 500,000

Anemia places increased physiologic demands on patients who are undergoing surgery. There is no evidence showing that mild to moderate anemia slows healing, increases infections, or causes bleeding. The approach to preoperative transfusion must be individualized and there is no ideal hemoglobin level required for surgery in all patients. A number of studies suggest that intraoperative transfusion is associated with a poorer outcome, however, cause and effect cannot be assessed in these retrospective studies. Patients without underlying cardiovascular or respiratory problems have considerable physiologic adaptive capacity and can tolerate significant anemia without increasing surgical morbidity or mortality. Patients with underlying medical problems, those with acute anemia, and those experiencing excessive blood losses, however, may be at risk for increased morbidity and mortality and may require more aggressive treatment of anemia.

Factors in addition to hemoglobin level that affect tissue oxygen delivery include cardiac output, vascular volume, blood viscosity, hemoglobin oxygen affinity, and blood oxygen saturation. With chronic anemia many of these factors are modified to provide optimal oxygen delivery to tissues in spite of the anemia. The "magic" hemoglobin level of 10 gm/dL was challenged in a National Institutes of Health Consensus Conference. Indications for perioperative transfusion must be based on careful assessment of coexisting diseases that may cause reduced tolerance for anemia, patient's physiologic adjustments to the anemia, the stress of the surgical procedure, an estimate of potential operative blood loss (based on the nature of the procedure and skill of the surgeon), and the plans for intraoperative procedures to reduce net blood loss (such as hemodilution and intraoperative blood salvage).

Informed consent is required in the perioperative period that documents risks of infection, alloimmunization, volume overload, and immediate and delayed transfusion reactions. Patients' religious and cultural beliefs must be recognized and honored. The risks of direct complications from transfusion are not readily quantifiable and are changing because of evolving blood-banking techniques. Reasonable estimates are presented in Table 20.1. Alternatives to homologous transfusions should be presented to patients who are undergoing elective surgical procedures that will likely require blood administration. Autologous transfusion of blood without or

with administration of erythropoietin is a practical, safe, and underutilized approach to perioperative transfusion. Evidence-based literature indicates that these programs not only provide the safest transfusion for the patient, but they also diminish the need for blood donation both by reducing homologous transfusion and by providing unused units for others. Patients must be informed about autologous donation when the decision for elective surgery is made to allow sufficient time to collect the required blood. In patients with concurrent medical problems, medical consultants should supervise blood collection to prevent complications from donation and optimize blood collection. Because liquid blood can be stored up to 42 days, most needs for surgery can be provided as liquid units, reducing cost. Red cells can be frozen for more than 10 years to meet greater needs, however, this increases costs significantly.

Intraoperative approaches, such as intraoperative autotransfusion or hemodilution, can be advocated by medical consultants but must be implemented by surgeons and anesthesiologists. Intraoperative blood salvage involves aspirating blood lost in the operative site and centrifuging or washing the cells for reinfusion. Numerous devices make this a practical, but somewhat expensive, approach when loss of large amounts of blood is anticipated. Air embolus is a possible complication and this approach is contraindicated if the operative site is contaminated by microorganisms or tumor cells.

Intraoperative hemodilution involves removal of blood after the induction of anesthesia and replacement with colloid or crystalloid solutions to cause acute normovolemic anemia. This allows the blood to be salvaged for reinfusion, decreases surgical loss of red blood cells, and reduces blood viscosity which may result in increased blood flow. Careful monitoring for volume overload during infusion of salvaged units and accurate identification and labeling of units are critical considerations to ensure safe reinfusion.

In patients with chronic anemia, preoperative transfusion must be planned with the understanding that total blood volume may be increased. Transfusions must be started well in advance of elective surgery and given slowly to prevent acute volume overload and to allow physiologic adaptation to the changes in volume status. Transfusion of packed cells causes minimal volume overload, but does increase the total blood volume by an amount equal to the total volume of the unit and this may persist for 24 hours or longer. In general, volume overload can be kept to a minimum by reducing the amount of cells to 250 mL at one time, reducing the rate to 1 mL/kg body wt/hour, and by decreasing right atrial pressure by placing patients in sitting or semiupright position.

Rapid transfusion with diuresis or partial exchange should be reserved for emergent or urgent surgery. Patients with heart failure or renal failure and volume overload, who require rapid transfusion, can be given 20 mg of intravenous furosemide before the transfusion is begun. Additional doses of furosemide can be given by a separate intravenous injection based on urine output and volume of cells infused. Partial exchange transfusion can be used to acutely raise the hemoglobin level in patients with severe anemia and volume overload. One approach is to remove whole blood from one vein as an approximately equal volume of packed red cells is infused through another vein. Severe anemia can be rapidly corrected by infusing a volume of 1,000–1,500 mL of packed red cells as 1,200–1,700 mL of whole blood is removed. The transfused blood should be prewarmed to 37 °C before large volumes are infused rapidly.

In patients with chronic anemia, surgical preparation requires individualized use of transfusion based on the presence of coexisting diseases, chronic hemoglobin levels, and estimates of operative blood losses. If transfusion is required, careful planning may allow use of autologous donation. Preoperative transfusions in patients with chronic anemia should be done well in advance of the surgery to allow physiologic adaptation to the changes in volume and blood viscosity.

Anemias requiring special consideration

Hematologic diseases that require special perioperative management include sickle cell diseases and immune hemolytic anemia. Preoperative screening with a complete blood count, reticulocyte count, and type and cross match will identify most patients with these disorders. The algorithm outlined in Figure 20.3 should be used to establish a definitive diagnosis before surgery in all but the most emergent situations.

Sickle cell diseases

Patients with sickle cell disease are at significantly increased risk for complications during most operative procedures. Individuals with sickle cell anemia (Hb SS) are at greatest risk. Patients who are compound heterozygotes for Hb S and Hb C (Hb SC disease) or Hb S and beta thalassemia (Hb S beta thal) may also be at increased risk; however, the perioperative complication rates are not well defined. Carriers of the sickle gene (Hb AS) are not at increased risk for

complications unless they experience profound hypoxia or undergo prolonged, complicated cardiovascular surgery. Even in these extreme situations, the risks have not been defined by appropriate controlled studies.

The optimal perioperative management of individuals with sickle cell diseases is not clear [22–38]. It is generally agreed that the hemoglobin concentration should be corrected by transfusion of packed red cells to a level of 9–10 g/dL for all but the simplest procedures. A multicenter collaborative trial found that simple transfusion to a hemoglobin level of 10 g/dL was as effective as exchange transfusion to reduce the hemoglobin S level to less than 30%, in reducing complications of surgery and anesthesia, and had lower incidence of transfusion-related complications. Simple transfusion above a hemoglobin level of 10 g/dL should not be done because of the increased viscosity of sickle blood. The level of Hb S can be monitored in the laboratory by using high performance liquid chromatography (HPLC) or by doing standard hemoglobin electrophoresis and estimating the amount of Hb A and Hb S on the membrane using a protein densitometry scanner. This will determine the approximate percentage of erythrocytes with Hb A and Hb S in the patient after transfusion of Hb A-containing erythrocytes. Many advocate transfusion or exchange transfusion to reduce the Hb S level to less than 30% while maintaining the hemoglobin level between 9 and 10 g/dL for cardiovascular bypass surgery, retinal or eye surgery, and major neurosurgery.

There are a number of additional important considerations in planning for transfusion or exchange transfusion in patients with sickle cell disease. The first is the high rate of alloimmunization that accompanies transfusion in these patients. Because up to 20% of patients will develop alloimmunization, some advocate transfusion with red cells that are phenotypically matched for antigens commonly associated with delayed transfusion reactions in this population. Many advocate matching for C, D, E, Kell antigens in all transfused sickle patients. Patients who have developed one alloantibody should receive transfusion with blood matched more extensively for antigen phenotype because of the high probability they will develop multiple alloantibodies and may develop autoantibodies making further transfusion difficult or impossible. This is especially important with exchange transfusions because of the potential increased severity of a delayed transfusion reaction.

Patients can be prepared with multiple transfusions over the weeks prior to elective surgery. The hemoglobin concentration should be measured before each transfusion to avoid hyperviscosity associated with transfusion to levels greater than 10 g/dL. Repeated HPLC or hemoglobin electrophoresis with densitometry scan can be used to document the percentage of Hb S. If there is insufficient time to achieve desired Hb S percentage by simple transfusion, exchange transfusion is best accomplished by red cell pheresis using an automated cell separator. Manual exchange transfusion using published protocols can achieve the same result; however, these are inefficient and labor intensive in adults and large children.

A multicenter transfusion study in sickle cell indicates that complications will still occur even with extensive exchange transfusion. Transfusion or exchange transfusion cannot be substituted for excellent perioperative management to avoid free water dehydration hypoxia, hypothermia, over-sedation, fluid overload, and acidosis. Acute pain episodes, acute chest syndrome, fever or infection, new alloantibodies, and delayed transfusion reactions appear to be among the most common complications. Predisposing factors for these complications are previous history of frequent pain episodes, episodes of acute chest syndrome, and alloimmunization.

Recommendations for the perioperative management of patients with sickle cell diseases are outlined in Table 20.2. Standard practice is to transfuse to a hemoglobin level of 10 g/dL in all patients. Careful preoperative evaluation and optimization of pulmonary, renal, and hepatic function are important, especially in older patients where end-organ damage may have developed. Intravenous hydration must be adequate to avoid free water and intracellular dehydration during the period of restricted oral intake. This is made more important because of the almost universal renal tubular defect that increases obligatory free water loss through the kidneys. Care must also be taken to avoid volume overload in these patients with expanded plasma volumes from chronic anemia. Hypoxia and acidosis should be prevented because of the direct effect of each on the rate of sickling. Decreases in temperature can increase peripheral resistance, reducing local blood flow, and predisposing to pain episodes. Early ambulation and intensive respiratory care are important in preventing acute chest syndrome and other pulmonary complications. Incentive spirometry should be used in all patients. Finally, because postoperative complications appear to be more common, diligent assessment of the cause of fevers and the prompt diagnosis and treatment of infection are important in the postoperative period. Close collaboration between surgeons, anesthesiologists, and hematologists helps improve the operative outcome in these patients with high rates of surgical complications.

Autoimmune hemolytic anemia

The perioperative care of patients with immune hemolysis entails several special considerations. Immune hemolytic anemias are mediated by antibodies directed against red cell membrane components or drugs that interact with the red cell membrane. In general, patients should be treated and the immune hemolytic anemia controlled before surgery is undertaken. Immune hemolytic anemias caused by drugs can be managed by stopping the drug and delaying surgery until the anemia is corrected. Autoimmune hemolytic anemias may pose more difficult problems. The diagnosis of hemolysis is made using the studies outlined in Figure 20.3 and the immune etiology is supported by documenting a positive direct antiglobulin (Coombs) test.

Autoimmune hemolytic anemias may be idiopathic but are also commonly associated with autoimmune diseases, lymphomas, chronic lymphocytic leukemia, HIV disease, other infections, and multiple myeloma. Warm antibody hemolytic anemias are caused by IgG antibodies and usually associated with a positive direct antiglobulin test for IgG, complement, or both. Initial treatment is prednisone 1–1.5 mg/kg/day. Treatment failures are usually treated with splenectomy or immunosuppressive drugs such as cyclophosphamide or azathioprine. Preparation for splenectomy may include the administration of intravenous immunoglobulin, which has been reported to have some activity in controlling immune hemolysis.

Cold reacting autoantibodies are usually IgM antibodies that are associated with positive direct antiglobulin test for complement and high-titer cold agglutinin levels. These antibodies are more commonly caused by infections such as mycoplasma pneumoniae, viruses, or lymphoproliferative disease. Management is difficult if the primary disease can not be treated. Steroids and splenectomy are not effective and immunosuppressive drugs are often required for severe, refractory cases. Avoidance of transfusion and supportive care, including hydration, avoidance of cold, and no infusions of fluids with temperatures of less than 37 °C, are the mainstays of therapy [39–43].

Autoimmune hemolytic anemias are problematic in patients requiring surgery because anemia may be profound and transfusions of red cells can precipitate a number of serious complications. The autoantibody rarely causes accelerated destruction of the transfused cells more than the patient's own erythrocytes but cold antibodies may increase hemolysis causing renal, coagulation, or pulmonary complications. The autoantibody generally causes problems in finding blood for transfusion because autoantibodies can prevent detection of alloantibodies that may precipitate immediate or delayed transfusion reactions and increase hemolysis caused by the autoimmune process.

Table 20.2 Perioperative management of sickle syndromes.

Preoperative transfusion to a hemoglobin level of 10 g/dL using simple transfusion
Preoperative evaluation to exclude pulmonary, renal, hepatic, or CNS complications
Avoidance of hypoxia using careful anesthetic and postoperative respiratory management
Hydration with hypotonic intravenous solutions while not taking oral fluids to avoid cellular dehydration, increased viscosity, hypoperfusion, or acidosis
Careful maintenance of body temperature during and after surgery
Early ambulation and intensive respiratory care
Postoperative vigilance and aggressive evaluation and treatment of fever or infection

Autoantibodies are uncommon, however, and infrequently present preoperative management problems. When present, they require coordinated management by experienced teams of hematologists, clinical pathologists, and anesthesiologists who understand and will coordinate the special management issues. Elective surgery should be delayed if possible until the autoimmune hemolysis is controlled with therapy. If the autoimmune process is resistant to therapy or if the surgery is emergent, the blood bank should be given sufficient time to use special techniques to detect alloantibodies. They also can provide advice when emergent surgery is required. Patients with uncontrolled autoimmune hemolytic anemia require careful monitoring and transfusion of the fewest units possible. Treatment with high-dose steroids is indicated for warm antibodies. Some advocate increasing steroid doses or administering high-dose intravenous immunoglobulin before transfusing patients with poorly controlled autoimmune hemolysis.

Patients with cold antibodies need to be kept warm so the blood temperature exceeds 37 °C throughout the body. All fluids and blood products must be warmed to 37 °C before administration. This may require maintaining the entire operating suite at 37 °C for patients with high-titer cold antibodies. Plasmapheresis is effective for the acute removal of these IgM antibodies and may be considered as emergency treatment before surgery in patients with significant, uncontrolled cold antibody immune hemolysis. Plasmapheresis is technically difficult because fluids, blood, and the patient must be kept warm.

Polycythemia

Elevated hemoglobin or hematocrit levels require preoperative evaluation to exclude conditions that may increase perioperative complications. The upper limits of normal for hemoglobin and hematocrit are 16.5 g/dL and 55% in males and 15.3 g/dL and 52% in females. Polycythemia or erythrocytosis is defined as an elevation above these levels. The elevation may reflect a true polycythemia (erythrocytosis) with increase in red cell mass or a relative increase in hemoglobin and hematocrit levels caused by a reduction in plasma volume. Relative erythrocytosis should be diagnosed and corrected because the low plasma volume is usually associated with a reduced total blood volume. This may predispose to hypotension during induction of anesthesia or performance of surgery. True polycythemia may be caused by polycythemia vera, which must be well controlled before surgery to minimize the high incidence of hemorrhagic and thrombotic complications. Secondary polycythemia results from physiologic processes that may predispose to pulmonary and cardiovascular complications in the perioperative period [44–56].

Diagnostic considerations

The most common cause of elevated hemoglobin is relative polycythemia caused by a reduced plasma volume. This occurs acutely from dehydration or is a chronic state associated with hypertension, adrenergic excess, and increased cardiovascular risk (stress erythrocytosis, Gaisbock's syndrome). If hydration does not return the hemoglobin concentration to normal, a red cell mass should be determined to confirm the presence of true erythrocytosis. Complete blood gas analysis will document chronic hypoxia and detect elevated carbon monoxide in smokers. Exercise-induced hypoxia and sleep apnea should also be considered as a cause of polycythemia because both may increase surgical complications. If there is sufficient time, patients who smoke should stop smoking and be observed to see if the hemoglobin level returns to normal. Determination of carbon monoxide levels may be helpful if the surgery is urgent because the level is usually elevated in smokers with erythrocytosis.

After these more common clinical conditions are excluded, polycythemia vera is now accurately diagnosed directly by determining a mutation in the Janus Kinase 2 (JAK2) gene. JAK2 positivity is diagnostic of polycythemia vera and its absence virtually excludes the diagnosis. Splenomegaly is a cardinal feature of polycythemia vera and may lead to neutropenia and thrombocytopenia in very advanced disease. A very low erythropoietin level supports the diagnosis of polycythemia vera. Determination of erythropoietin level and a search for occult kidney disease or tumors of a number of organs by intravenous pyelography, sonography, or computerized tomography should be considered if a cause of true polycythemia is not defined by the initial evaluation.

Management considerations

Polycythemia vera should be treated to a normal hemoglobin level before surgery because of the high incidence of thrombotic and hemorrhagic perioperative complications in patients with uncontrolled or poorly controlled disease. To assure minimal morbidity and mortality, the general recommendation is that the disease should be well controlled for 4 months before purely elective surgery is undertaken. Before more urgent surgery, the patient should be treated to achieve normal hemoglobin levels. Phlebotomy alone can rapidly control the hemoglobin level in patients with primary elevations. Phlebotomy in combination with hydroxyurea administration should probably be used in patients with elevated hemoglobin levels and platelet counts. The therapeutic goal is a hematocrit level of approximately 45% because of evidence that cerebral blood flow is reduced with higher levels. Phlebotomy can be accomplished rapidly in young individuals by removing 125–200 mL every other day. Patients who have acute orthostatic symptoms may benefit from less frequent phlebotomy or concurrent hydration with an equal volume of normal saline. In older patients or those with underlying cardiovascular disease, slower phlebotomy is prudent, removing 100–150 mL twice a week. Again, concurrent administration of normal saline may prevent acute orthostatic symptoms.

Reduction of the platelet counts to less than 500,000 is advocated, although there are few data that indicate such treatment reduces thrombotic complications. Daily administration of aspirin in a dose of 100 mg daily has been shown to reduce thrombotic complications and improve overall survival.

Patients with polycythemia vera are at higher risk for serious perioperative complications including stroke, myocardial infarction, pulmonary embolus, thrombophlebitis, splenic infarction, and portal or hepatic venous thrombosis. There is also an increased incidence of gastrointestinal and surgical hemorrhage. Alternatives to surgery should be considered. If surgery is necessary, the management plan should be formulated well in advance. Patients require close monitoring for common complications in the perioperative period. For emergency surgery, the hemoglobin level should be returned to normal by removing whole blood and infusion of crystalloid and colloid solutions to maintain blood volume.

Recent publications indicate that patients with relative and secondary polycythemia also may have an increased rate of perioperative complications. It does seem prudent to define the cause of the polycythemia and identify and correct the underlying pathology if possible. Relative polycythemia may indicate acute dehydration that may predispose to hypotension during anesthesia or surgery. Chronic spurious polycythemia is often associated with hypertension and control of blood pressure with antihypertensive agents will often correct the elevated hemoglobin level. Smokers with polycythemia should stop smoking in advance of elective surgery to reduce pulmonary complications. This may also lead to normalization of the hemoglobin concentration.

Secondary polycythemia needs evaluation to detect underlying disease that may require special management in the perioperative period. Hypoxia secondary to pulmonary or cardiac disease is a common cause of secondary polycythemia. Certain types of renal disease which cause ischemia in the juxtaglomerular cells increase erythropoietin resulting in secondary polycythemia. Several uncommon tumors, including renal cell carcinoma, hepatoma, cerebellar hemangioblastoma, uterine fibroids, and ovarian carcinoma may cause polycythemia by increasing erythropoietin. Pheochromocytoma and adrenal cortical carcinoma are rare causes of polycythemia that are important to consider because of the management implications of these tumors during anesthesia and surgery.

If treatment of the underlying condition is impossible or does not correct the polycythemia, phlebotomy to normalize blood viscosity can be considered. Experimental data show that blood flow will be decreased with any true elevation of hemoglobin levels. There is no compelling evidence that phlebotomy is beneficial for either relative or secondary polycythemia with modest elevation of the hemoglobin level. Evidence does suggest that reduction of the hematocrit level may be beneficial if it exceeds 60%, when the elevation is secondary to hypoxia caused by severe pulmonary disease or cyanotic heart disease.

References

1. Allen JB, Allen BA. The minimum acceptable level of hemoglobin. *Int Anesth Clin* 1982; **20**: 1–22.

2. Beattie WS, Karkouti K, Wijeysundera DN, Tait G. Risk associated with preoperative anemia in noncardiac surgery: a single-center cohort study. *Anesthesiology* 2009; **110**: 574–81.

3. Carson JL, Duff A, Poses RM *et al.* Effect of anaemia and cardiovascular disease on surgical mortality and morbidity. *Lancet* 1996; **348**: 1055–60.

4. Consensus Conference. Perioperative red blood cell transfusion. *J Am Med Assoc* 1988; **260**: 2700–3.

5. Council on Scientific Affairs. Autologous blood transfusions. *J Am Med Assoc* 1986; **256**: 2378–80.

6. Etchason J, Petz L, Keeler E. *et al.* The cost-effectiveness of preoperative autologous blood donations. *N Engl J Med* 1995; **332**: 719–24.

7. Glance LG, Dick AW, Mukamel DB *et al.* Association between intraoperative blood transfusion and mortality and morbidity in patients undergoing noncardiac surgery. *Anesthesiology* 2011; **114**: 234–6.

8. Goodnough LT. The role of recombinant growth factors in transfusion medicine. *Br J Anaesth* 1993; **70**: 80–6.

9. Goodnough LT, Rudnick E, Price TH. *et al.* Increased pre-operative collection of autologous blood with recombinant human erythropoietin therapy. *N Engl J Med* 1989; **321**: 1163–8.

10. Goodnough LT, Brecher ME, Kanter MH, AuBuchon JP. Transfusion medicine – blood transfusion. *N Engl J Med* 1999; **340**: 438–47.

11. Herbert PC, Wells G, Blajchman MA *et al.* A multicenter, randomized controlled clinical trial of transfusion requirements in critical care. *N Engl J Med* 1999; **340**: 409–17.

12. Hillyer CD. *Blood Banking and Transfusion Medicine: Basic Principles and Practice.* 2nd edn. Philadelphia, PA: Churchill Livingstone/Elsevier; 2007.

13. Karkouti K, Wijeysundera DN, Beattie WS. Risk associated with preoperative anemia in cardiac surgery: a multicenter cohort study. *Circulation* 2008; **117**: 478–84.

14. Kulier A, Levin J, Moser R *et al.* Impact of preoperative anemia on outcome in patients undergoing coronary artery bypass graft surgery. *Circulation* 2007; **116**: 471–9.

15. Leone BJ, Spahn DR. Anemia, hemodilution, and oxygen delivery. *Anesth Analg* 1992; **75**: 651–3.

16. McFarland JG. Perioperative blood transfusions: indications and options. *Chest* 1999; **115**: 113S–21S.

17. Practice guidelines for perioperative blood transfusion and adjuvant therapies: an updated report by the American Society of Anesthesiologists Task Force on Perioperative Blood Transfusion and Adjuvant Therapies. *Anesthesiology* 2006; **105**: 198–208.

18. Toy PT, Strauss RG, Stehling, LC *et al.* Predeposited autologous blood for elective surgery. A National Multicenter Study. *N Engl J Med* 1987; **316**: 517–20.

19. Wu WC, Schifftner TL, Henderson WG *et al.* Preoperative hematocrit levels and postoperative outcomes in older patients undergoing noncardiac

surgery. *J Am Med Assoc* 2007; **297**: 2481–8.

20. Roback JD, ed. *AABB Technical Manual.* 16th edn. Bethesda, MD: American Association of Blood Banks; 2008.

21. Welch HG, Meehan KR, Goodnough LT. Prudent strategies for elective red blood cell transfusion. *Ann Intern Med* 1992; **116**: 393–402.

22. Adu-Gyamfi Y, Sankarakutty M, Marwa S. Use of a tourniquet in patients with sickle-cell disease. *Can J Anaesth* 1993; **40**: 24–7.

23. Bischoff RJ, Williamson II A, Dalali MJ, Rice JC, Kerstein MD. Assessment of the use of transfusion therapy perioperatively in patients with sickle cell hemoglobinopathies. *Ann Surg* 1988; **207**: 434–8.

24. Burrington JD, Smith MD. Elective and emergency surgery in children with sickle cell disease. *Surg Clin North Am* 1976; **56**: 55–71.

25. Davis SC, Robets-Harewood M. Blood transfusion in sickle cell disease. *Blood Rev* 1997; **11**: 57–71.

26. Esseltine DW, Baster MRN, Bevan JC. Sickle cell states and the anaesthetist. *Can J Anaesth* 1988; **35**: 385–403.

27. Forrester K. Anesthetic implications in sickle cell anemia. *J Assoc Nurs Anesth* 1986; **54**: 314–24.

28. Fullerton MW, Philippart AI, Sarnaik S, Lusher JM. Preoperative exchange transfusion in sickle cell anemia. *J Pediatr Surg* 1981; **16**: 297–300.

29. Gibson JR. Anesthesia for the sickle cell diseases and other hemoglobinopathies. *Semin Anesth* 1987; **6**: 27–35.

30. Janik J, Seeler RA. Perioperative management of children with sickle hemoglobinopathy. *J Pediatr Surg* 1980; **15**: 117–20.

31. Milner PF, Coker NJ. Elective surgery in patients with sickle cell anemia. *Arch Otolaryngol* 1982; **108**: 547–76.

32. Morrison JC, Whybrew WD, Bucovaz ET. Use of partial exchange transfusion preoperatively in patients with sickle cell hemoglobinopathies. *Am J Obstet Gynecol* 1978; **132**: 59–63.

33. Oduro KA, Searle JR. Anaesthesia in sickle-cell states: a plea for simplicity. *Br Med J* 1972; **4**: 596–8.

34. Schlanger M, Cunningham AJ. Intraoperative hypoxemia complicating laparoscopic cholecystectomy in a patient with sickle hemoglobinopathy. *Anesth Analg* 1992; **75**: 838–43.

35. Vichinsky EP, Earles A, Johnson RA *et al.* Alloimmunization in sickle cell anemia and transfusion of racially unmatched blood. *N Engl J Med* 1990; **322**: 1617–21.

36. Vishinsky EP, Haberkern CM, Neumayr L *et al.* A comparison of conservative and aggressive transfusion regimens in the perioperative management of sickle cell disease. *N Engl J Med* 1995; **333**: 206–13.

37. Vichinsky EP. Current issues in blood transfusion in sickle cell disease. *Semin Hematol* 2001; **38**: 14–22.

38. Ware R, Filston HC, Schultz WH, Kinney TR. Elective cholecystectomy in children with sickle hemoglobinopathies. *Ann Surg* 1988; **208**: 17–22.

39. Buetens OW, Ness PM. Red blood cell transfusion in autoimmune hemolytic anemia. *Curr Opin Hematol* 2003; **10**: 429–33.

40. Garratty G, Petz LD. Approaches to selecting blood for transfusion to patients with autoimmune hemolytic anemia. *Transfusion* 2002; **42**: 1390–2.

41. Petz LD. A physician's guide to transfusion in autoimmune haemolytic anaemia *Br J Haematol* 2004; **124**: 712–16.

42. Plapp FV, Beck ML. Transfusion support in the management of immune haemolytic disorders. *Clin Haematol* 1984; **13**: 167–83.

43. Sokol RJ, Hewitt S, Booker DJ, Morris BM. Patients with red cell antibodies: selection of blood for transfusion. *Clin Lab Haematol* 1988; **10**: 257–64.

44. Berk PD, Goldberg JD, Donovan PB *et al.* Therapeutic recommendations in polycythemia vera based on polycythemia vera study group protocols. *Semin Hematol* 1986; **23**: 132–43.

45. DeFilippis AP, Law K, Curtin S, Eckman JR. Blood is thicker than water: the management of hyperviscosity in adults with cyanotic heart disease. *Cardiol Rev* 2007; **15**: 31–4.

46. Fitts WT, Erde A, Peskin GW, Frost JW. Surgical implications of polycythemia vera. *Ann Surg* 1960; **152**: 548–58.

47. Harrison C. Rethinking disease definitions and therapeutic strategies in essential thrombocythemia and polycythemia vera. *Hematology* 2010; **2010**: 129–34.

48. Irving G. Polycythaemia and the anaesthetist. *S Afr Med J* 1991; **80**: 418–19.

49. Fruchtman SM, Wasserman LR. Therapeutic recommendations for polycythemia vera. In Wasserman LR, Berk PD, Berlin NI, eds. *Polycythemia Vera and the Myeloproliferative Syndromes.* Philadelphia, PA: W. B. Saunders; 1995, pp. 337–50.

50. Hoffman R, Wasserman LR. Natural history and management of polycythemia vera. *Adv Intern Med* 1979; **245**: 255–83.

51. Kaplan ME, Mack K, Goldberg JD *et al.* Long-term management of polycythemia vera with hydroxyurea: a progress report. *Semin Hematol* 1986; **23**: 167–71.

52. Lubarsky DA, Gallagher CJ, Berend JL. Secondary polycythemia does not increase the risk of perioperative hemorrhagic or thrombotic complications. *J Clin Anesth* 1991; **3**: 99–103.

53. Tartaglia AP, Goldberg JD, Berk PD, Wasserman LR. Adverse effects of antiaggregating platelet therapy in the treatment of polycythemia vera. *Semin Hematol* 1986; **23**: 172–6.

54. Wallis PJW, Skehan JD, Newland AC *et al.* Effects of erythrapheresis on pulmonary haemodynamics and oxygen transport in patients with secondary polycythaemia and cor pulmonale. *Clin Sci* 1986; **70**: 91–8.

55. Wasserman LR. The treatment of polycythemia vera. *Semin Hematol* 1976; **13**: 57–78.

56. Wasserman LR, Gilbert HS. Surgery in polycythemia vera. *N Engl J Med* 1963; **269**: 1226–30.

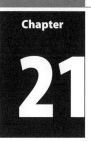

Chapter

21

Perioperative management of hemostasis

Mrinal Dutia, Eve Rodler, and Ted Wun

There is perhaps more money wasted and blood unnecessarily shed in this setting than in any other in medicine.

Sabiston's Textbook of Surgery

Summary

When patients are evaluated for the potential of abnormal bleeding before surgery, the intensity of screening is determined by the hemostatic challenge of the procedure and the likelihood that the patient has an underlying congenital or acquired disorder that would predispose to bleeding. The risk of bleeding associated with the type of surgical procedure ranges from low risk (lymph node biopsies, dental extractions), to moderate risk (laparotomy, thoracotomy, mastectomy), to high risk (neurosurgical, ophthalmic, plastic, cardiopulmonary bypass, prostatic, and surgery to stop bleeding). A screening history should reveal if the patient has experienced any abnormal bleeding or bruising, if there is a history of an acquired medical disorder which could affect hemostasis, if family members have bled abnormally, or if the patient is taking any drugs which could interfere with hemostasis. Physical examination can also provide important information about a patient's surgical bleeding risk. Ecchymoses, petechiae, or purpura may suggest a systemic hemostatic defect. Stigmata of chronic liver disease include hepatomegaly, splenomegaly, jaundice, spider angiomas, palmar erythema, and dilated abdominal veins.

The preoperative hemostatic screening recommendations by Rapaport, based on levels of concern, provide a reasonable basis for selecting laboratories for individual patients [1]. Nearly 30 years old, these recommendations are not obsolete.

Patients at level 1 are those with a reassuring history who are undergoing surgeries with only minimal potential blood loss such as excisional biopsies or dental extractions. No screening is required for these patients as the low predictive value of laboratory screening outweighs the cost of treating minor bleeding episodes in the few individuals who will have mild bleeding disorders undetected by history prior to the operation.

Level 2 indicates patients with a negative bleeding history who have had prior surgical challenges to hemostasis, and are undergoing surgeries such as bowel resection or orthopedic procedures which have a moderate, but not the highest, risk for bleeding. A partial thromboplastin time (PTT) and platelet count are recommended as screening tests to assess the risk of bleeding episode in patients who may have an undiagnosed moderate to severe hemostatic defect.

At level 3 are those patients whose bleeding history suggests a possible defect in hemostasis and who require an operation with a high risk of bleeding. These surgeries include cardiopulmonary bypass in which the pump-oxygenator can damage platelets and coagulation factors, prostatectomies, and all procedures in which even a small amount of bleeding could be catastrophic, e.g., surgeries of the central nervous system. A more extensive evaluation is recommended for these patients. This includes a platelet count and an activated PTT and INR to assess coagulation. The classic template bleeding time has not been shown to be predictive of postprocedural bleeding complications and it should not be performed (and is no longer available in many hospitals).

Level 4 indicates patients whose history is highly suggestive of a bleeding disorder and who should have a thorough evaluation prior to operation, regardless of the type of procedure. The initial laboratory work-up is the same as that for Level 3 patients, but also includes a von Willebrand panel, platelet function test, and specific coagulation factor assays for factors VIII and IX to detect mild hemophilia (in males). A thrombin time can be checked to detect patients with dysfibrinogenemia.

Common causes of unexpected intraoperative and postoperative bleeding and treatment

Most intraoperative and postoperative bleeding is due to a local lesion at the operative site, with minimal or no abnormalities of the hemostatic system. The treatment generally involves surgical intervention to control bleeding vessels. There are specific causes of intra- and postoperative

---

Medical Management of the Surgical Patient, ed. Michael F. Lubin, Thomas F. Dodson, and Neil H. Winawer. Published by Cambridge University Press. © Cambridge University Press 2013.

hemostatic failure related to particular types of surgery where the nature of the surgery itself is a risk factor for bleeding. If unexpected bleeding occurs that is not due to a local lesion or to the specific type of surgery being performed, but rather may be due to an undiscovered preexisting systemic hemostatic defect of the patient, then proper evaluation and management must be undertaken expeditiously.

Cardiopulmonary bypass

The high risk for blood loss during cardiopulmonary bypass surgery is multifactorial: the large size of the surgical wound; exposure of blood to artificial surfaces in the extracorporeal oxygenator; injury to platelets and coagulation factors; activation of fibrinolysis during and after surgery, and medications including anticoagulants and antiplatelet agents. Significant hemorrhage has been reported in 6–25% of patients and bleeding requiring re-exploration occurs in approximately 2–7% [2]. Of those patients who return to the operating room, only half will have an identifiable surgical bleeding source.

Some experts recommend platelet transfusions following cardiac bypass in patients with normal coagulation values and platelet counts below 100,000/uL if unexplained bleeding occurs [3]. However, the value of this strategy is uncertain.

The effect of the vasopressin analog desmopressin (DDAVP) on reducing postoperative blood loss after cardiac surgery has been studied in several randomized studies, with conflicting results. A meta-analysis of 17 randomized, double-blind, placebo-controlled trials showed that DDAVP reduced blood loss by 9%, but had no significant impact on transfusion requirements [4]. Studies have shown that treatment with DDAVP reduced blood loss [5], or transfusion requirements [6] in patients treated with aspirin up to the time of surgery. DDAVP is administered at a dose of 0.3 μg/kg over 30 minutes.

Several prospective trials have found significant decreases in blood loss as well as transfusion requirements with the use of aprotinin, tranexamic acid, and aminocaproic acid [2,7–9]. Several double-blind studies had demonstrated the effectiveness of aprotinin in reducing blood loss in coronary artery bypass operations [10,11]. However, in May 2008 the manufacturer permanently removed aprotinin from the market because of increased adverse events, including mortality.

Aminocaproic acid and tranexamic acid are two synthetic antifibrinolytic agents which can reduce blood loss in cardiac surgery by 30–40%, as demonstrated in clinical trials involving at least 1,000 patients [12]. These agents act by forming a reversible complex with plasminogen, preventing its activation to plasmin. Aminocaproic acid can be given as a bolus intravenous dose of 150 mg/kg before the operation, followed by an infusion of 15 mg/kg/hour during the operation [13] or a bolus intravenous dose of 80 mg/kg, followed by an infusion of 30 mg/kg/hour during the

operation, with an additional 80 mg/kg dose to the pump prime [7]. Tranexamic acid has been administered in a 10-mg/kg bolus followed by continuous infusion of 1–3 mg/kg per hour [14]. Tranexamic acid is no longer available in the USA.

Prophylactic glucocorticoid use has also been studied in this setting and a meta-analysis found that their use resulted in a small but significant decrease in the rate of postoperative bleeding [15,16]. However, these are not generally recommended due to potential side-effects.

If postoperative hemorrhage occurs, ensure that the patient is not hypothermic and that heparin has been fully reversed with protamine sulfate. A full neutralizing dose is 1 mg of protamine sulfate per 100 units of heparin used intravenously. An antifibrinolytic agent can be used along with transfusions of platelets, red blood cells, and cryoprecipitate or fresh frozen plasma as guided by laboratory evaluation.

Fibrin sealants, also referred to as "fibrin glue" or "fibrin tissue adhesives" are used in cardiovascular procedures as well as a broad range of surgeries to control bleeding during and after surgery and reduce blood loss. Those available commercially (e.g., Tisseel, Hemaseel) consist of human fibrinogen and human or bovine thrombin which are applied to the local tissue site. Although pooled plasma has the theoretical risk of viral transmission, only parvovirus B19 has documented transmission from fibrin sealants [17]. Before the introduction of effective viral inactivation techniques, bovine thrombin was used in fibrin sealants to reduce the risk of viral transmission. The use of bovine thrombin carries the risk of coagulopathies due to the development of thrombin and factor V inhibitors. A recent meta-analysis which reviewed the efficacy of fibrin sealants in reducing perioperative blood loss and allogeneic red blood cell transfusion concluded that the use of fibrin sealant resulted in a mean reduction in blood loss of 150 mL per patient, and a reduction in average transfusion requirements by about 0.6 units, though conclusions are weakened due to lack of blinding in most of the studies [18].

Recombinant factor VIIa (rFVIIa) has become increasingly popular to treat perioperative bleeding in various settings, including after cardiac surgery [19]. In a study by Gill et al. the use of rFVIIa in bleeding patients after cardiac surgery resulted in decreased need of blood transfusion; however, use was associated with increased rates of serious complications including death, cerebral infarction, and other thromboembolic events (compared with placebo, patients treated with rFVIIa were at increased risk of these events – 7% vs 12–14%, though this did not meet statistical significance). Hence, use of rFVIIa is often reserved for patients refractory to general measures including other blood product transfusions, and especially used for patients with coagulopathies. The dose remains controversial. A lower dose of 40 μg/kg was found to be effective in one study, although other studies have used doses up to 180 μg/kg in one or two doses safely [20].

Prostatectomy

In prostatectomy, enhanced local fibrinolysis related to high concentrations of urokinase likely contributes to bleeding risk. The use of aminocaproic acid or tranexamic acid resulted in significantly decreased postoperative blood loss compared with placebo [12,21]. These therapies are contraindicated in patients with bleeding from the upper urinary tract because of the risk of clots causing obstruction. Recombinant activated factor VIIa has been utilized in management of bleeding after radical prostatectomy and various studies have shown that it minimizes need for blood transfusions [22,23].

Liver transplantation

Patients undergoing liver transplantation are at high risk for intraoperative blood loss due to coagulopathy and fibrinolysis [24]. Intraoperatively, there is an anhepatic phase during which coagulation factors are not produced and there is excessive fibrinolysis. During the reperfusion phase, t-PA is released from the stored organ and there is proteolytic breakdown of von Willebrand factor. These patients may need replacement with blood products and antifibrinolytic therapy. Recombinant FVIIa has also been approved for liver transplantation [22]. Fibrin sealant has been used successfully in the management of hemorrhage from cut surfaces of parenchymal liver, which is difficult to suture [25].

Major neurosurgery

After head trauma and in patients with brain tumors, disseminated intravascular coagulation (DIC) can occur. A prospective study demonstrated the association of decreased perioperative factor XIII with an increased risk of postoperative hematoma in neurosurgical patients [26]. Neurological surgery may require a platelet count of 100,000/μL [27] although this practice has never been validated in a prospective trial.

Damage control surgery

So-called "damage control surgery" is performed for exsanguinating, major trauma patients. It involves rapid restoration of circulating volume, normothermia, maintenance of oxygen delivery, and correction of transfusion-related coagulopathy so that expeditious re-operation and completion of definitive surgical management can be attained [28–32]. In an effort to save these patients, a three-component damage control surgery was developed originally for patients with massive abdominal trauma with vascular injury. One component of this process is induced hypothermia, which can lead to platelet dysfunction. Hypothermia also impairs the intrinsic and extrinsic coagulation cascades [33]. Laboratory values are not generally helpful in the rapidly exsanguinating patient because the resuscitation proceeds faster than the ability of the laboratory to return information. Platelets and fresh frozen plasma should be transfused after rapid transfusion

of eight or more units of red blood cells in the presence of ongoing bleeding [29]. The use of recombinant factor VIIa has been shown to be effective in coagulopathic trauma patients, and fairly safe for younger, previously healthy patients [30,31]. The optimal dose remains unclear, but a number of studies have utilized a dose of 40 μg/kg which can be repeated to control bleeding.

Massive transfusion

Massive transfusion is defined as replacement of more than 1 blood volume (c. 5,000 mL in a 70 kg adult) within 4 hours. As many as 51% of all deaths in the first 48 hours of hospitalization are related to lack of hemostasis in patients with trauma. Transfusion of fresh frozen plasma is indicated if a patient's history or clinical course suggests coagulopathy and active bleeding is present, or prior to an invasive procedure in the presence of abnormal coagulation factors [27]. If there is excessive operative bleeding, platelet transfusion to greater than or equal to 100,000/μL empirically is indicated [22]. Recombinant factor VIIa has been utilized in severe trauma [22] and appears to be effective despite the presence of a hypothermic and dilutional coagulopathy [34]. Fibrin foams have been used to reduce blood loss by binding to damaged surfaces [35].

An approach to intraoperative or postoperative bleeding

First, it is crucial to determine if bleeding is related to a hemostatic defect or to a local lesion that requires surgical intervention, e.g., "factor XIV (surgical silk) deficiency." Suspect a problem with local control if bleeding is rapid, if it is confined to the operative site, or if there is excessive blood on dressings, in the operative drains or chest tube. In contrast, bleeding is likely due to a systemic hemostatic abnormality if it is generalized, slower, and "oozing" at multiple sites is found.

There are several congenital or acquired hematological abnormalities, which may not have been detected on preoperative personal or family history or labs, which could account for unanticipated perioperative hemorrhage. Mild deficiencies of factor VIII, factor IX, and factor XI can be present without prolongation of aPTT. Factor XIII deficiency requires a specific test for detection. Mild von Willebrand disease or a platelet granule disorder may also be discovered after a surgical procedure. Review of the patient's medication record could reveal an acquired platelet dysfunction from aspirin, antibiotics, or other medications. If a complete blood count was not checked prior to a simple surgical procedure, the patient could have undetected thrombocytopenia.

If possible, review the patient's past medical history, family history, and recent medications for clues to an underlying hemostatic abnormality. Perform a physical examination to see if it is more consistent with a platelet problem (mucosal bleeding) or coagulation problem (soft tissue bleeding), or both. Additional laboratory tests should be sent, including aPTT, PT, thrombin time, fibrinogen, CBC, and peripheral smear. If these laboratory values are all normal, bleeding is unlikely to be due to a systemic bleeding disorder. However, if the clinical suspicion of a hemostatic abnormality is still high, it is reasonable to also test for factor XIII, and von Willebrand disease, although the results of these tests are likely to be delayed unless there is a full-time special coagulation laboratory available. It is important to draw all laboratories through a peripheral venipuncture and not through a catheter, in order to avoid effects of heparin on coagulation testing.

Patients with known disorders of hemostasis
Hemophilia A and B

There are several inherited disorders of blood clotting, but discussion will focus on the four most common: hemophilia A and B; von Willebrand disease; and factor XI deficiency. In general, in the perioperative management of hemophilia A and B, aspirin products, intramuscular and subcutaneous injections should be avoided. It is important to determine if the patient has mild hemophilia (factor VIII or IX level > 5%), moderate (factor level 1–5%) or severe (factor level < 1%) [36]. A baseline factor level and mixing study should be done to determine if a circulating alloantibody or autoantibody (inhibitor) is present.

Therapeutic agents used in patients with hemophilia

If no inhibitors are present, pre- and postoperative recombinant or human factor replacement may be used. For major surgery factor VIII and factor IX levels should be approximately 100% of normal. Continuous infusion with high purity products is recommended to avoid level fluctuations and to decrease overall factor utilization. In patients with hemophilia B, high purity products are preferred to avoid the possible thrombotic side-effects of the less pure factor IX concentrates in hemophilia B. Treatment should begin a few hours before surgery and continue intraoperatively. Postoperative factor levels should be monitored daily. Infusion of factor replacement should continue at least 10–14 days and up to several weeks after major surgery. For moderate risk procedures, such as dental extractions, factor VIII and IX levels should be 50% of normal with perhaps only one additional dose of factor 8–12 hours later.

If factor VIII or IX inhibitors are present, there are several approaches to treatment depending on the level of inhibitor and whether bleeding is minor or major [37,38]. Recombinant factor VIIa (Novoseven; rFVIIa) has been used successfully in the perioperative management of patients with inhibitors [39]. It is hypothesized that factor VIIa activates factor X on the surface of activated platelets without the need for tissue factor [40,41]. Since this is occurring at a localized site of vascular injury, factor VIIa has not been found to cause general activation of coagulation resulting in thrombogenicity, though randomized trials are necessary to test the thrombogenicity of factor VIIa [39,42]. A variety of surgical procedures have been carried out successfully, including amputations, major orthopedic surgeries, and liver biopsies with the use of rFVIIa in hemophiliacs with inhibitors [43,44]. The dosing recommendation is 90–110 µg/kg bolus every 2 hours, followed by the same dose at longer intervals of 3–6 hours thereafter [45]. There are reports of giving rFVIIa as a continuous infusion following surgery, but the target maintenance level has varied and there is no consensus on the optimal regimen for continuous infusion [46]. Porcine factor VIII can sometimes be used in patients with inhibitors to human factor VIII. Hemophilia A patients with inhibitors can be tested to see if their inhibitor cross-reacts with porcine factor VIII, as measured in the Bethesda assay. The recommended starting dose of porcine factor VIII is 100–150 units/kg with measurements of factor VIII levels to guide therapy.

Prothrombin complex concentrates (FEIBA, Autoplex) are products with variable amounts of activated factors, including VIIa, IXa, and Xa. It is postulated that the prothrombin complex concentrate "bypasses" inhibitors by enhancing the tissue factor–factor VIIa pathway of coagulation. The presence of factors in an activated form generates a risk of thrombotic complications [47,48]. The risk is increased in patients receiving high or multiple doses of prothrombin complex concentrates, concurrent antifibrinolytic therapy, or those with significant liver disease. The recommended dose is 75–100 units/kg, which can be repeated after 8–12 hours.

Desmopressin (DDAVP) may be used in patients with mild or moderate hemophilia A, who have shown a capacity to raise the level of factor VIII to a hemostatic level in response to DDAVP. The dose is 30 µg/kg in saline solution given over 30 minutes. DDAVP has no activity in hemophilia B.

Antifibrinolytic agents can be useful as adjunctive therapy, not for initial hemostasis but to prevent clot lysis after hemostasis. These agents are mainly used in cases of mucous membrane bleeding and after dental extractions [49,50]. Aminocaproic acid can be given as an oral tablet or elixir at a dose of 100 mg/kg (maximum 10 g) initially, then 50 mg/kg (maximum 5 g) every 6 hours. Tranexamic acid (if available) can be administered orally at a dose of 25 mg/kg every 6–8 hours, or intravenously at 10 mg/kg every 8 hours.

Local control of bleeding can be improved with fibrin glue as an adjunctive therapy to factor replacement in hemophiliac patients after dental procedures and orthopedic procedures or for other surgical wounds [51].

Factor XI deficiency is the least rare of the non-hemophiliac congenital coagulation factor deficiencies. It occurs most often in Ashkenazi Jews but also in non-Jewish populations [52]. Factor XI deficiency is inherited as an autosomal recessive trait. There is no clear correlation between the genotype and the bleeding tendency; very low factor XI levels are not always associated with a bleeding tendency [53]. The phenotype of the family is important. If a patient with factor XI deficiency is to undergo surgery and has never had surgery, dental extractions, or prior trauma, then the bleeding history of the family provides the only clue whether the patient will bleed. Prior to surgery, perform a specific factor XI assay. Most patients whose levels are below 0.15 IU/mL will experience excessive bleeding after surgery, and some patients with factor XI levels as high as 60–70% of normal will have abnormal bleeding [42].

There is some evidence that desmopressin is effective in patients with partial factor XI deficiency due either to modest increases in factor XI or to larger increases in VIII or von Willebrand factor. Desmopressin may also be used for minor bleeding in mildly affected patients [54]. Antifibrinolytics can be considered for surface or mucosal bleeding. Patients with severe factor XI deficiency often require plasma replacement. The dose of plasma is a loading dose of 15–20 mL/kg body weight, followed by 3–6 mL/kg every 12 hours until hemostasis is achieved. For major surgery, transfusion of fresh frozen plasma should be given for 10–14 days maintaining a trough level of 45% of normal [55]. For minor or moderate risk surgeries fresh frozen plasma can be transfused for 5–7 days with a goal to maintain factor XI levels 30% of normal. Factor XI concentrates from plasma can be used, if available. These products allow efficient replacement therapy but they have thrombogenic potential [56]. Peak levels should not be greater than 0.70 IU/mL, and individual doses should not be greater than 30 IU/kg.

Von Willebrand disease is the most common inherited bleeding disorder with a reported prevalence of 1% of the general population. The treatment of von Willebrand disease depends on the subtype and the response to desmopressin. Factor VIII:C and ristocetin cofactor activity levels are used to monitor the effect of therapy.

Type I von Willebrand disease is the most common type accounting for approximately 90% of patients with von Willebrand disease. Most of these patients will respond to DDAVP with a three- to five-fold increase in plasma vWF [56,57]. It may be given by the intravenous or intranasal route. A single daily infusion is frequently sufficient for minor procedures. The response to DDAVP is variable, but consistent within an individual over time. A trial of desmopressin is recommended prior to a major surgery. If the vWF activity (as measured by the ristocetan cofactor assay) increases to > 100% (u/dL), the patient can be given DDAVP alone. Perioperatively, daily levels of vWF activity should be measured.

For other types of vWD, or if tachyphylaxis develops with DDAVP, a factor VIII concentrate that contains sufficient vWF multimers, such as Humate P or Koate-HP [58], is required. Von Willebrand factor/VIII concentrates are now commonly labeled and prescribed in ristocetan cofactor (RCof) units. The recommended dose is 40–80 RCof units/kg depending on the severity of bleeding. For severe hemorrhage

or major surgery, repeat doses can be given at 8–12-hour intervals until hemostasis is achieved [41]. The target nadir for major surgery is 50% activity. Adjuvant therapies are the same as used for hemophilia A and B.

Thrombocytopenia

The platelet count needed for adequate surgical hemostasis is not well defined. According to the National Institutes of Health Consensus Development Conference, a minimum platelet count of 50,000/mm^3 is recommended for surgery [59]. A reasonable approach is the following: low-risk surgery, either no platelets or transfuse platelets to 50,000; moderate-risk general surgery 50,000 to 100,000/mm^3; and high-risk surgery transfuse to level of 100,000/mm^3 [60]. An exception is immune thrombocytopenia. In this case lower levels of platelets are tolerated, and transfusions generally are not performed unless life-threatening bleeding occurs.

Platelet dysfunction

Patients with platelet dysfunction may be asymptomatic but normally they have a history of excessive mucocutaneous bleeding and bruising, menorrhagia, petechiae, epistaxis, gingival bleeding, or excessive bleeding following surgery or injury. Hereditary causes of platelet dysfunction include Glanzmann's thrombasthenia, Bernard–Soulier disease, Scott syndrome, and storage pool deficiencies and are less common than acquired causes. Transfusion of platelets to the target levels discussed above should provide adequate platelets for primary hemostasis. There are now reports that factor VIIa can be used to stop hemorrhage in this and other intrinsic platelet defect disorders [61].

Medications are the most common reason for an acquired platelet functional defect. The Physicians' Health Study Research Group examined the clinical importance of aspirin on hemostasis in normal individuals by giving aspirin 325 mg every other day or placebo to 22,071 physicians over 5 years. They found a decrease in risk of myocardial infarction for aspirin-treated patients but more patients in the aspirin-treated group had easy bruising, hematemesis, melena, and epistaxis than in the control group (RR1.32, P < 0.00001) and more people in the aspirin group required a blood transfusion over the 5 years (P = 0.02). Thus aspirin does have an impact on normal hemostasis, but it is generally small [62]. For the surgical patient, some, but not all studies have shown that aspirin taken preoperatively increases the amount of blood loss following cardiothoracic surgery [3]. Increased chest tube blood loss in aspirin-treated patients is not associated with worse overall clinical outcomes [63]. Performing epidural and spinal anesthesia in patients who ingested aspirin was found to be safe in a retrospective study [64]. Aspirin should be avoided in patients with known hemostatic defects. It is reasonable to discontinue aspirin ingestion in patients scheduled for non-emergent invasive procedures or surgery

5 days prior to the procedure, as this is enough time for half of the circulating platelets to be replaced by new platelets.

Other non-steroidal anti-inflammatory drugs (NSAIDs) also inhibit platelet cyclooxygenase, thus impairing platelet aggregation and secretion. This effect is reversible and of short duration, so the hemostatic risk with these drugs disappears a few hours after the drug is stopped, with the exception of piroxicam, which has a half-life of greater than 2 days.

Clopidogrel and prasugrel are thienopyridines that are used for secondary prevention of strokes and myocardial infarctions (ticlopidine is another in this class but now not used due to risk of thrombotic microangiopathy). They are prodrugs and when metabolized the active drug irreversibly inhibits platelet P2Y12 ADP receptor. Thienopyridines have an additive effect with aspirin. The effects of oral prasugrel and clopidogrel are seen within hours of the first dose and last for 4–10 days after the drugs have been discontinued [65]. These drugs should be stopped for about 7 days before surgery.

Beta-lactam antibiotics have also been associated with platelet dysfunction. This platelet dysfunction may not subside for several days after the antibiotic is discontinued. It is postulated that these antibiotics inhibit platelet surface receptor functions through a lipophilic association with the plasma membrane [3]. Clinically important bleeding associated with antibiotic-induced platelet dysfunction has mainly occurred in patients with multiple hemostatic defects. Careful observation for important bleeding should be done.

Chronic renal disease

The cause of the bleeding tendency in uremia is multifactorial. Platelet dysfunction has been implicated as a major cause of bleeding risk [3]. However, the relationship between platelet dysfunction and clinical bleeding in patients with renal failure is unclear. Anemia, which correlates with the severity of renal failure, plays a role in the platelet adhesion defect and in the prolonged bleeding time [66]. A prolonged bleeding time (in the era when they were available) in uremic patients was common but did not correlate with the risk for perioperative hemorrhage. The frequency of bleeding in uremic patients after biopsies or surgical procedures is not known but based on reports, it is thought to be uncommon [67]. No prospective randomized study has been done to evaluate the effectiveness of therapeutic regimens for improving hemostasis in the uremic patient. Dialysis can often, but not always, correct the bleeding time and reduce the risk of clinical bleeding in patients with uremia [68,69]. Desmopressin has been reported to shorten the bleeding time in 50–75% of patients with uremia and may be effective in preventing perioperative bleeding in uremic patients [70]. Correction of anemia to a hematocrit > 32% can correct the bleeding time and reduce clinical bleeding in uremic patients [71].

Some uncontrolled studies have found that infusion of cryoprecipitate can correct the bleeding time in uremic patients and decrease bleeding, but other studies have not shown these results. Conjugated estrogens have also been reported to shorten the bleeding time in patients with uremia both in uncontrolled and in double-blind randomized studies [72,73].

Thrombocytosis

Thrombocytosis may be due to a primary myeloproliferative disorder, or to secondary causes such as inflammation, iron deficiency anemia, or the postoperative state. The risk of thrombosis or hemorrhage is low in patients with secondary thrombocytosis or chronic myelogenous leukemia, and there is no correlation between platelet count and thrombotic risk in patients with polycythemia rubra vera (PRV) or essential thrombocytosis (ET). Though counterintuitive, there is actually greater bleeding risk associated with higher platelet counts (> 1 million/mm^3). This is because acquired von Willebrand disease can be seen in patients with very high platelet counts. In PRV and ET, the risk of complications is greater in older patients and in those patients with a history of bleeding or thrombosis [74]. Empirically, in patients with PRV or ET, the platelet count should be lowered to normal or near normal preoperatively with platelet pheresis, hydroxyurea, or anagrelide. Aspirin should be avoided [75].

Polycythemia

Patients with uncontrolled polycythemia vera have a high surgical morbidity and mortality mainly due to thromboembolic events resulting from an increase in blood viscosity. In patients with polycythemia vera, the hematocrit should be reduced to less than 45% by phlebotomy prior to elective surgery. In physiologically inappropriate secondary polycythemia, such as polycystic kidney disease and erythropoietin secreting tumors, the hematocrit should be lowered to 45–50%. In physiologically appropriate polycythemia, usually from diseases causing significant hypoxia such as COPD, patients may need to maintain a higher hematocrit. Therefore, a preoperative hematocrit between 50% and 60% has been suggested [74].

Liver disease

Hemostatic defects of liver disease are complex and include coagulopathy from liver synthetic dysfunction, vitamin K deficiency, thrombocytopenia, and platelet defects. A PT (INR) test is a good measure of the severity of liver dysfunction as it evaluates the vitamin K dependent factors and factor V. Although some have suggested that the measurement of individual procoagulant factors is useful in distinguishing between liver synthetic dysfunction, vitamin K deficiency, and concurrent DIC, in practice this is usually not possible.

If patients with liver disease have a PT prolongation less than 3 seconds, serious surgical bleeding is unlikely unless there are other preexisting hemostatic defects. For patients undergoing high-risk surgery or who have a more prolonged PT, prophylactic fresh frozen plasma is recommended.

If perioperative bleeding occurs, aggressive replacement therapy should be undertaken. Prothrombin complex concentrate is not generally recommended in patients with chronic liver disease because activated factors present in the concentrates are not adequately cleared by the liver and can lead to thrombotic complications [76]. Fibrinogen can be maintained with cryoprecipitate, and vitamin K should be empirically given. The effectiveness of platelet transfusions may be limited by splenic sequestration. Checking the platelet count after transfusion will provide information on the degree of splenic sequestration that is occurring. Recombinant factor VIIa has more recently been found to be useful in this setting but is also associated with thrombotic risk.

Anemia

Although there are data to suggest the preoperative hemoglobin is predictive of surgical mortality, other studies have shown that the degree of perioperative blood loss, rather than the degree of anemia is more predictive of postoperative complications. In a study by Spence et al. [77], 107 patients undergoing elective operations were prospectively studied to evaluate the influence of preoperative hemoglobin level and operative blood loss in patients who refused blood transfusions. They found that mortality was significantly increased with an estimated blood loss of greater than 500 mL, regardless of the preoperative hemoglobin level (P < 0.025). Further, there was no mortality if estimated blood loss was less than 500 mL, regardless of the preoperative hemoglobin level.

The appropriate "transfusion trigger" for preoperative transfusion has not been established in prospective trials. Many physicians have used a threshold hemoglobin of 10 g/dL and a hematocrit of 30% (the "10/30" rule) but practices vary widely [78,79]. In a related area, in a randomized prospective clinical trial [80], 838 patients admitted to the ICU with hemoglobin levels less than 9.0 mg/dL were allocated to a liberal transfusion group (hemoglobin 10–12 g/dL) or to a restrictive group (hemoglobin levels 7–9 g/dL). The study found that the overall in-hospital mortality was significantly lower in the restrictive group, although the 30-day mortality rate was not significantly different. However, in those patients who were less ill (APACHE, 20) or younger (< 55 years of age), the 30-day mortality rates were significantly lower for the patients in the restrictive transfusion group. Interestingly, no difference in mortality between the two groups was seen in cardiac patients.

A similar study was done in patients undergoing elective cardiac bypass surgery, blood transfusions being used either to keep HCT over 30 or 24 [81]. Patients understandably received more transfusions in the arm with higher HCT goal, but there was no difference in the primary endpoint studies, that was a composite endpoint of severe morbidity and mortality: cardiogenic shock, acute respiratory distress syndrome, or acute renal injury requiring dialysis or hemofiltration. A major limitation of the study was lack of use of leukocyte-reduced red blood cells, which has been shown to be superior in terms of risk of infection and surgical morbidity [82]. Regardless, no difference was found in the two study arms, and hence a lower transfusion trigger is considered safe.

The transfusion trigger concept has shifted in the literature from arbitrary levels to that of a level of hemoglobin required to maintain adequate oxygenation of tissues for a particular patient. While minimum hemoglobin levels may be well tolerated in the clinically stable patient, this range might be suboptimal for the critically ill anemic patient. Volume status in anemic patients also appears to influence surgical outcome.

Perioperative erythropoietin

Concern about the risks of allogeneic transfusion is widespread but disproportionate to the risk. Autologous transfusion is misperceived to be safer. In a retrospective analysis, the risk to the donor of a severe reaction requiring hospital admission was 6 : 100,000 when patients made preoperative autologous blood donations (PAD) and 18 : 100,000 if it was the donor's first experience, compared with 0.5 : 100,000 for allogeneic donors. Autologous donors are less likely to receive homologous blood but more likely to be transfused than those who do not donate. The risks of transfusion complications due to clerical error, bacterial contamination, and blood processing are equally great in both groups. Methods of decreasing allogeneic blood transfusion include lowering the "transfusion trigger" when appropriate as discussed above, autologous blood donation techniques, and perioperative erythropoietin therapy [83].

In the USA recombinant human erythropoietin (rHUEpo) has been approved by the FDA for anemic patients scheduled for elective surgery (with the exception of cardiac and vascular surgery). rHUEpo has been used to improve the collection of autologous blood in patients undergoing elective surgery, to correct anemia before surgery, and to hasten the postoperative erythropoietic response [84].

Preoperative autologous blood donation continues to be used as an allogeneic transfusion sparing technique and appears most beneficial for patients at risk for blood transfusion who are undergoing procedures with substantial blood loss [83]. Erythropoietin has been used to augment the number of preoperative autologous units collected. Treatment may also be indicated in patients who reject transfusions because of religious convictions and in bone marrow donors [84]. One treatment schedule is 250 to 300 IU/kg of rHUEpo administered subcutaneously twice weekly over the 3-week period prior to surgery. Intravenous iron supplementation (iron sucrose 200 mg) should be administered at each preoperative autologous donation visit. Alternatively, at least 200 mg of oral elemental iron can be given daily [84].

Patients who do not accept blood products

Surgical experience with Jehovah's Witnesses has demonstrated that people can tolerate very low hemoglobin levels and survive. A review of 16 series published between 1983 and 1990, involving 1,404 operations on Jehovah's Witnesses found that anemia was the primary cause of death in only 8 (0.6%) patients and a contributor to death in an additional 12 patients (0.9%) [85]. Another large review involving 4,722 Jehovah's Witnesses revealed only 23 deaths due to anemia, nearly all of whom had a hemoglobin of less than 5 mg/dL [86]. The general management of these patients includes maximizing preoperative hemoglobin by eliminating any causes of impaired hematopoiesis. Recombinant erythropoietin has human albumin as a stabilizer, so some Jehovah's Witnesses will decline use of this product. Some patients will permit the use of intraoperative cell savers. If abnormal bleeding occurs, permissible hemostatic agents include DDAVP, antifibrinolytic agents, bovine thrombin, and possibly recombinant factor VIIa.

Perioperative DVT prophylaxis

Recent venous thromboembolism greatly increases the risk of postoperative thromboembolism. Recommendations regarding heparin therapy are based on the interval between the thromboembolic event and the operative procedure. Untreated, there is a 50% risk of recurrent thromboembolism in the first month after a deep venous thrombosis (DVT). Warfarin therapy reduces the risk to 5%. Recurrent episodes of thromboembolism have a 6% fatality rate. Similarly, recurrent arterial embolism has a 20% fatality rate and a 40% risk of serious permanent disability. Among patients on anticoagulants the risk of severe postoperative hemorrhage is estimated to be about 3% and, of those, about 3% (0.09% overall) are fatal, making the risk of fatal embolic disease without anticoagulation about 30 times greater than the risk of death from hemorrhage with anticoagulation. However, 50% of major postoperative bleeding events lead to re-operation and 1.5% result in permanent disability.

Total knee and hip replacement surgery is especially thrombogenic, as is neurosurgery. In a meta-analysis, total knee replacement, for example, carried a 64% risk of DVT if no prophylaxis was used, a proximal DVT risk of 15% and a DVT-related fatality rate of 0.2–0.7%. In one study, DVT rates were reduced to 30% by use of low molecular weight heparin (LMWH). It is worth noting that most postoperative DVTs in this setting are asymptomatic. European orthopedists generally begin LMWH therapy 12 hours before surgery at half doses, whereas approved usage in the USA calls for 30 mg LMWH every 12 hours starting 12–24 hours after surgery and continuing for 7–10 days. The bleeding rates are low, 0.9% and 3.5%, respectively. Even so, many American orthopedists are reluctant to use LMWH because of hemorrhagic risk. Prophylactic warfarin therapy in these patients, in contrast, especially if begun just before or immediately after surgery, is less commonly associated with hemorrhage into the replaced knee, but is also less effective in reducing the risk of DVT.

A meta-analysis showed that hip surgery is more commonly associated with symptomatic venous thromboembolic events (VTE) than is knee surgery. Another meta-analysis showed that hip replacement under spinal anesthesia is less

often followed by VTE than when it is performed under general anesthesia. Fondaparinux, a pentasaccharide that binds to and augments that anticoagulant effect of antithrombin can also be used at a fixed dose for postoperative VTE prophylaxis. It is likely that the direct anti-Xa inhibitors and direct thrombin inhibitors, already approved for use in Canada and Europe for VTE prophylaxis, will also be approved in the USA soon. The interested reader is referred to a review [87].

Duration of anticoagulation for surgery-related DVT

Recent data from randomized studies show that indefinite anticoagulation with either moderate intensity vitamin K antagonist (INR 1.5–2.0) or conventional intensity (INR 2.0–3.0) significantly reduces the risk of recurrent VTE in patients with idiopathic DVT (not related to surgery, trauma, or pregnancy). However, the optimal duration of anticoagulation therapy for postoperative VTE without an ongoing risk factor has not been defined in randomized trials. The standard practice is to give secondary prophylaxis with an oral vitamin K antagonist for 3 months.

Asymptomatic coagulopathies

In the course of a preoperative laboratory evaluation or during a hospitalization, it is not unusual to find prolonged aPTT or INR in a patient without a significant bleeding history. In some, a more detailed, focused history may reveal abnormal bleeding. However, for many there will be no such history or a lack of previous hemostatic challenge. The evaluation of these laboratory findings should proceed along the lines of the evaluation of an outpatient with similar findings, with the following points in mind.

1. Minute quantities of heparin in indwelling catheters may prolong coagulation times. Thus, samples for coagulation tests should always be obtained by peripheral venipuncture; even "wasting" the initial blood drawn through a catheter does not ensure lack of contamination.

2. Up to 10% of hospitalized patients will be found to have a slightly prolonged aPTT (up to 40 seconds) without an identifiable cause.

3. A mixing study (1 : 1 dilution) should always be performed in a patient with a new coagulopathy to determine if there is the presence of an inhibitor. Lupus inhibitors (see appropriate section) are common in hospitalized patients and are associated with increased thrombotic risk in certain populations.

4. Mild hemophilia A and B, and especially von Willebrand disease, may not be diagnosed until adulthood in conjunction with a major hemostatic stress (such as postpartum in the case of von Willebrand disease). Thus, if there is a history of bleeding and/or the planned procedure is high-risk for hemorrhage, an appropriate diagnostic evaluation should be performed.

References

1. Rapaport SI. Preoperative hemostatic evaluation–which tests, if any? *Blood* 1983; **61**: 229–31.

2. Katsaros D, Petricevic M, Snow NJ *et al.* Tranexamic acid reduces postbypass blood use: a double-blinded, prospective, randomized study of 210 patients. *Ann Thorac Surg* 1996; **61**: 1131–5.

3. George JN, Shattil SJ. The clinical importance of acquired abnormalities of platelet function. *N Engl J Med* 1991; **324**: 27–39.

4. Cattaneo M, Harris AS, Stromberg U, Mannucci PM. The effect of desmopressin on reducing blood loss in cardiac surgery – a meta-analysis of double-blind, placebo-controlled trials. *Thromb Haemost* 1995; **74**: 1064–70.

5. Sheridan DP, Card RT, Pinilla JC *et al.* Use of desmopressin acetate to reduce blood transfusion requirements during cardiac surgery in patients with acetylsalicylic-acid-induced platelet dysfunction. *Can J Surg* 1994; **37**: 33–6.

6. Dilthey G, Dietrich W, Spannagl M, Richter JA. Influence of desmopressin acetate on homologous blood requirements in cardiac surgical patients pretreated with aspirin. *J Cardiothorac Vasc Anesth* 1993; **7**: 425–30.

7. Menichetti A, Tritapepe L, Ruvolo G. *et al.* Changes in coagulation patterns, blood loss and blood use after cardio-pulmonary bypass: aprotinin vs tranexamic acid vs epsilon aminocaproic acid. *J Cardiovasc Surg (Torino)* 1996; **37**: 401–7.

8. Janssens M, Hartstein G, David JL. Reduction in requirements for allogeneic blood products: pharmacologic methods. *Ann Thorac Surg* 1996; **62**: 1944–50.

9. Rich JB. The efficacy and safety of aprotinin use in cardiac surgery. *Ann Thorac Surg* 1998; **66** (5 Suppl): S6–11.

10. Mannucci PM. Desmopressin: a nontransfusional form of treatment for congenital and acquired bleeding disorders. *Blood* 1988; **72**: 1449–55.

11. Royston D, Bidstrup BP, Taylor KM, Sapsford RN. Effect of aprotinin on need for blood transfusion after repeat open-heart surgery. *Lancet* 1987; **2** (8571): 1289–91.

12. Mannucci PM. Hemostatic drugs. *N Engl J Med* 1998; **339**: 245–53.

13. Vander Salm TJ, Kaur S, Lancey RA *et al.* Reduction of bleeding after heart operations through the prophylactic use of epsilon-aminocaproic acid. *J Thorac Cardiovasc Surg* 1996; **112**: 1098–107.

14. Horrow JC, Van Riper DF, Strong MD *et al.* The dose-response relationship of tranexamic acid. *Anesthesiology* 1995; **82**: 383–92.

15. Whitlock RP, Chan S, Devereaux PJ *et al.* Clinical benefit of steroid use in patients undergoing cardiopulmonary bypass: a meta-analysis of randomized trials. *Eur Heart J* 2008; **29**: 2592.

16. Karkouti K, Cohen MM, McCluskey SA *et al.* A multivariable model for predicting the need for blood transfusion in patients undergoing first-time elective coronary bypass graft surgery. *Transfusion* 2001; **41**: 1193.

17. Reece TB, Maxey TS, Kron IL. A prospectus on tissue adhesives. *Am J Surg* 2001; **182** (2 Suppl): 40S–4S.

18. Carless PA, Anthony DM, Henry DA. Systematic review of the use of fibrin sealant to minimize perioperative allogeneic blood transfusion. *Br J Surg* 2002; **89**: 695–703.

19. Gill R, Herbertson M, Vuylsteke A *et al.* Safety and efficacy of recombinant activated factor VII: a randomized placebo-controlled trial in the setting of bleeding after cardiac surgery. *Circulation* 2009; **120**: 21.

20. van de Garde EM, Bras LJ, Heijmen RH *et al.* Low-dose recombinant factor VIIa in the management of uncontrolled postoperative hemorrhage in cardiac surgery patients. *J Cardiothorac Vasc Anesth* 2006; **20**: 573.

21. Vinnicombe J, Shuttleworth KE. Aminocaproic acid in the control of haemorrhage after prostatectomy. Safety of aminocaproic acid – a controlled trial. *Lancet* 1966; **1**(7431): 232–4.

22. Hedner U. NovoSeven as a universal haemostatic agent. *Blood Coagul Fibrinol* 2000; **11** (Suppl 1): S107–11.

23. Friederich PW, Henny CP, Messelink EJ *et al.* Effect of recombinant activated factor VII on perioperative blood loss in patients undergoing retropubic prostatectomy: a double-blind placebo-controlled randomised trial. *Lancet* 2003; **361**(9353): 201.

24. Porte RJ. Coagulation and fibrinolysis in orthotopic liver transplantation: current views and insights. *Semin Thromb Hemost* 1993; **19**: 191–6.

25. Morikawa T. Tissue sealing. *Am J Surg* 2001; **182** (2 Suppl): 29S–35S.

26. Gerlach R, Tolle F, Raabe A *et al.* Increased risk for postoperative hemorrhage after intracranial surgery in patients with decreased factor XIII activity: implications of a prospective study. *Stroke* 2002; **33**: 1618–23.

27. Lundberg GD. Is there a need for routine preoperative laboratory tests? *J Am Med Assoc* 1985; **253**: 3589.

28. Shapiro MB, Jenkins DH, Schwab CW, Rotondo MF. Damage control: collective review. *J Trauma* 2000; **49**: 969–78.

29. Martin RR, Byrne M. Postoperative care and complications of damage control surgery. *Surg Clin N Am* 1997; **77**: 929–42.

30. Harrison TD, Laskosky J, Jazaeri O *et al.* "Low-dose" recombinant activated factor VII results in less blood and blood product use in traumatic hemorrhage. *J Trauma* 2005; **59**: 150.

31. Bauzá G, Hirsch E, Burke P *et al.* Low-dose recombinant activated factor VII in massively transfused trauma patients with coagulopathy. *Transfusion* 2007; **47**: 749.

32. Johnson JW, Gracias VH, Schwab CW *et al.* Evolution in damage control for exsanguinating penetrating abdominal injury. *J Trauma* 2001; **51**: 261–9.

33. Gubler KD, Gentilello LM, Hassantash SA, Maier RV. The impact of hypothermia on dilutional coagulopathy. *J Trauma* 1994; **36**: 847–51.

34. Martinowitz U, Kenet G, Segal E *et al.* Recombinant activated factor VII for adjunctive hemorrhage control in trauma. *J Trauma* 2001; **51**: 431–8.

35. Holcomb JB, McClain JM, Pusateri AE *et al.* Fibrin sealant foam sprayed directly on liver injuries decreases blood loss in resuscitated rats. *J Trauma* 2000; **49**: 246–50.

36. Lozier JN, Lessler CM. Clinical aspects and therapy of hemophilia. In Hoffman R, Benz EJ, Shattil SJ *et al.*, eds. *Hematology: Basic Principles and Practice*. Philadelphia, PA: Churchill Livingstone; 2000: 1884–5.

37. White GC, Roberts HR. The treatment of factor VIII inhibitors – a general overview. *Vox Sang* 1996; **70** (Suppl 1): 19–23.

38. Roberts HR, Hofmann M. Hemophilia A and hemophilia B. In Beutler E, Lichtman MA, Coller BS *et al.*, eds. *Williams Hematology.* New York, NY: McGraw-Hill; 2001, pp. 1650–5.

39. Lusher JM. Recombinant factor VIIa (NovoSeven) in the treatment of internal bleeding in patients with factor VIII and IX inhibitors. *Haemostasis* 1996; **26** (Suppl 1): 124–30.

40. Monroe DM, Hoffman M, Oliver JA, Roberts HR. A possible mechanism of action of activated factor VII independent of tissue factor. *Blood Coagul Fibrinol* 1998; **9**: S15–20.

41. Kjalke M, Monroe DM, Hoffman M *et al.* Active site-inactivated factors VIIa, Xa, and IXa inhibit individual steps in a cell-based model of tissue factor-initiated coagulation. *Thromb Haemost* 1998; **80**: 578–84.

42. Aledort LM, Green D, Teitel JM. Unexpected bleeding disorders. *Hematology (Am Soc Hematol Educ Program)* 2001; 306–21.

43. Kenet G, Walden R, Eldad A, Martinowitz U. Treatment of traumatic bleeding with recombinant factor VIIa. *Lancet* 1999; **354**(9193): 1879.

44. Ingerslev J. Efficacy and safety of recombinant factor VIIa in the prophylaxis of bleeding in various surgical procedures in hemophilic patients with factor VIII and factor IX inhibitors. *Semin Thromb Hemost* 2000; **26**: 425–32.

45. Hedner U. Recombinant factor VIIa (NovoSeven (R)) as a hemostatic agent. *Semin Hematol* 2001; **38**: 43–7.

46. Schulman S. Continuous infusion of recombinant factor VIIa in hemophilic patients with inhibitors: safety, monitoring, and cost effectiveness. *Semin Thromb Hemost* 2000; **26**: 421–4.

47. Kasper CK. Problems with the potency of factor VIII concentrate. *N Engl J Med* 1981; **305**: 50–1.

48. Chavin SI, Siegel DM, Rocco TA Jr, Olson JP. Acute myocardial infarction during treatment with an activated prothrombin complex concentrate in a patient with factor VIII deficiency and a factor VIII inhibitor. *Am J Med* 1988; **85**: 245–9.

49. Walsh PN, Rizza CR, Matthews JM *et al.* Epsilon-aminocaproic acid therapy for dental extractions in haemophilia and Christmas disease: a double blind controlled trial. *Br J Haematol* 1971; **20**: 463–75.

50. Forbes CD, Barr RD, Reid G *et al.* Tranexamic acid in control of haemorrhage after dental extraction in haemophilia and Christmas disease. *Br Med J* 1972; **2**: 311–13.

51. Martinowitz U, Saltz R. Fibrin sealant. *Curr Opin Hematol* 1996; **3**: 395–402.

52. Asakai R, Chung DW, Davie EW, Seligsohn U. Factor XI deficiency in Ashkenazi Jews in Israel. *N Engl J Med* 1991; **325**: 153–8.

53. Edson JR, White JG, Krivit W. The enigma of severe factor XI deficiency without hemorrhagic symptoms. Distinction from Hageman factor and "Fletcher factor" deficiency; family study; and problems of diagnosis. *Thromb Diath Haemorrh* 1967; **18**: 342–8.

54. Castaman G, Ruggeri M, Rodeghiero F. Clinical usefulness of desmopressin for prevention of surgical bleeding in patients with symptomatic heterozygous factor XI deficiency. *Br J Haematol* 1996; **94**: 168–70.

55. Seligsohn U. Factor XI deficiency. *Thromb Haemost* 1993; **70**: 68–71.

56. Mannucci PM, Bauer KA, Santagostino E *et al.* Activation of the coagulation cascade after infusion of a factor XI concentrate in congenitally deficient patients. *Blood* 1994; **84**: 1314–19.

57. Mannucci PM. Desmopressin (DDAVP) in the treatment of bleeding disorders: the first 20 years. *Blood* 1997; **90**: 2515–21.

58. Mannucci PM, Tenconi PM, Castaman G, Rodeghiero F. Comparison of four virus-inactivated plasma concentrates for treatment of severe von Willebrand disease: a cross-over randomized trial. *Blood* 1992; **79**: 3130–7.

59. Platelet transfusion therapy. National Institutes of Health Consensus Conference. *Transfus Med Rev* 1987; **1**: 195–200.

60. Francis CW, Kaplan KL. Hematologic problems in the surgical patient: bleeding and thrombosis. In Hoffman R, Benz EJ, Shattil SJ *et al.*, eds. *Hematology: Basic Principles and Practice.* Philadelphia, PA: Churchill Livingstone; 2000, pp. 2381–3.

61. Peters M, Heijboer H. Treatment of a patient with Bernard–Soulier syndrome and recurrent nosebleeds with recombinant factor VIIa. *Thromb Haemost* 1998; **80**: 352.

62. Final report on the aspirin component of the ongoing Physicians' Health Study. Steering Committee of the Physicians' Health Study Research Group. *N Engl J Med* 1989; **321**: 129–35.

63. Despotis GJ, Filos KS, Zoys TN *et al.* Factors associated with excessive postoperative blood loss and hemostatic transfusion requirements: a multivariate analysis in cardiac surgical patients. *Anesth Analg* 1996; **82**: 13–21.

64. Horlocker TT, Wedel DJ, Offord KP. Does preoperative antiplatelet therapy increase the risk of hemorrhagic complications associated with regional anesthesia? *Anesth Analg* 1990; **70**: 631–4.

65. McTavish D, Faulds D, Goa KL. Ticlopidine. An updated review of its pharmacology and therapeutic use in platelet-dependent disorders. *Drugs* 1990; **40**: 238–59.

66. Castillo R, Lozano T, Escolar G *et al.* Defective platelet adhesion on vessel subendothelium in uremic patients. *Blood* 1986; **68**: 337–42.

67. Diaz-Buxo JA, Donadio JV Jr. Complications of percutaneous renal biopsy: an analysis of 1,000 consecutive biopsies. *Clin Nephrol* 1975; **4**: 223–7.

68. Castaldi PA, Rozenberg MC, Stewart JH. The bleeding disorder of uraemia. A qualitative platelet defect. *Lancet* 1966; 2(7454): 66–9.

69. Hutton RA, O'Shea MJ. Haemostatic mechanism in uraemia. *J Clin Pathol* 1968; **21**: 406–11.

70. Bolan CD, Alving BM. Pharmacologic agents in the management of bleeding disorders. *Transfusion* 1990; **30**: 541–51.

71. Shattil SJ, Abrams CS, Bennett JS. Acquired qualitative platelet disorders due to diseases, drugs, and foods. In Beutler E, Lichtman MA, Coller BS *et al.*, eds. *Williams Hematology.* New York, NY: McGraw-Hill; 2001, p. 1585.

72. Livio M, Benigni A, Vigano G *et al.* Moderate doses of aspirin and risk of bleeding in renal failure. *Lancet* 1986; **1** (8478): 414–16.

73. Heistinger M, Stockenhuber F, Schneider B *et al.* Effect of conjugated estrogens on platelet function and prostacyclin generation in CRF. *Kidney Int* 1990; **38**: 1181–6.

74. Fellin F, Murphy S. Hematologic problems in the pre-operative patient. *Med Clin North Am* 1987; **71**: 477–87.

75. van Genderen PJ, Mulder PG, Waleboer M *et al.* Prevention and treatment of thrombotic complications in essential thrombocythaemia: efficacy and safety of aspirin. *Br J Haematol* 1997; **97**: 179–84.

76. Marassi A, Manzullo V, di Carlo V, Mannucci PM. Thromboembolism following prothrombin complex concentrates and major surgery in severe liver disease. *Thromb Haemost* 1978; **39**: 787–8.

77. Spence RK, Carson JA, Poses R *et al.* Elective surgery without transfusion: influence of preoperative hemoglobin level and blood loss on mortality. *Am J Surg* 1990; **159**(3): 320–4.

78. Hebert PC, Wells G, Martin C *et al.* A Canadian survey of transfusion practices in critically ill patients. *Crit Care Med* 1998; **26**: 482–7.

79. Hebert PC, Wells G, Martin C *et al.* Variation in red cell transfusion practice in the intensive care unit: a multicentre cohort study. *Crit Care* 1999; **3**: 57–63.

80. Hebert PC, Wells G, Blajchman MA *et al.* A multicenter, randomized, controlled clinical trial of transfusion requirements in critical care. *N Engl J Med* 1999; **340**: 409–17.

81. Karkouti K, Cohen MM, McCluskey SA *et al.* A multivariable model for predicting the need for blood transfusion in patients undergoing first-time elective coronary bypass graft surgery. *Transfusion* 2001; **41**: 1193.

82. van de Watering LM, Hermans J, Houbiers JG *et al.* Beneficial effects of leukocyte depletion of transfused blood on postoperative complications in patients undergoing cardiac surgery: a randomized clinical trial. *Circulation* 1998; **97**: 562.

83. Goodnough LT, Brecher ME, Kanter MH, AuBuchon JP. Transfusion medicine. Second of two parts – blood conservation. *N Engl J Med* 1999; **340**: 525–33.

84. Cazzola M, Mercuriali F, Brugnara C. Use of recombinant human erythropoietin outside the setting of uremia. *Blood* 1997; **89**: 4248–67.

85. Kitchens CS. Are transfusions overrated? Surgical outcome of Jehovah's Witnesses. *Am J Med* 1993; **94**: 117–19.

86. Viele MK, Weiskopf RB. What can we learn about the need for transfusion from patients who refuse blood? The experience with Jehovah's Witnesses. *Transfusion* 1994; **34**: 396–401.

87. Bauer KA. New anticoagulants. *Curr Opin Hematol.* 2008; **15**: 509–15.

Chapter

22

Prophylaxis for deep venous thrombosis and pulmonary embolism in surgery

Taki Galanis and Geno J. Merli

Introduction

Venous thrombosis is a major cause of disability and death in all patient populations. Autopsy studies of hospitalized patients have demonstrated that massive pulmonary embolism (PE) is the cause of death in 5–10% of all hospital deaths and have suggested that two-thirds of all clinically important venous emboli are never recognized during life [1,2]. In a large multi-center study, 30,827 surgical patients were evaluated with respect to venous thromboembolism (VTE) risk and appropriate prophylaxis as recommended by the American College of Chest Physician (ACCP). This study showed that 19,842 surgical patients were considered at risk for VTE but only 11,613 (58.5%) received appropriate ACCP-recommended VTE prophylaxis [3]. More recently, the Surgical Care Improvement Project selected the application of VTE prophylaxis as a nationally reported metric for preventing VTE [4]. The purpose of this chapter is to review the pathophysiology of perioperative deep vein thrombosis (DVT), assess preoperative VTE risk and review the modalities of prophylaxis for preventing postoperative VTE in surgical patients.

Pathophysiology

The pathophysiologic changes of stasis, intimal injury, and hypercoagulability predispose surgical patients to the development of DVT or PE. The supine position on the operating room table, the anatomic position of the extremities for some surgical procedures, and the effect of anesthesia all contribute to stasis during surgery. Venographic contrast studies have shown that the supine position on the operating table decreases venous return [5,6]. In orthopedic, gynecologic, and urologic surgeries, the anatomic position of the body that provides the best surgical access to the operative site impairs adequate venous drainage during the procedure [7]. For example, in total hip replacement and hip fracture repair, the flexion and adduction of the hip that is required for better anatomic access to the surgical field has been shown to impair venous return [7]. Anesthesia causes peripheral venous vasodilation, which results in increased venous capacitance and decreased venous return during the operative procedure [8–10].

Intimal injury may be caused by anatomic positioning and the excessive vasodilation that results from anesthesia. Flexion and adduction of the hip during surgery has been shown to compress the femoral vein. Three intraoperative venographic studies provided clear evidence of distortion of the femoral vein during certain phases of total hip replacement [7,11,12]. The use of a tourniquet on the proximal thigh and flexion of the knee during total knee replacement also compress the underlying venous structures. These positions for prolonged periods may damage the delicate venous endothelium. Anesthesia also contributes to injury by causing excess vasodilation and endothelial damage [13–16]. Comerota and associates demonstrated in dogs that the endothelial lesions occurred as multiple tears around the junction of small side branches with the major receiving veins (jugular and femoral veins) [13]. These tears extended through the endothelium and basement membrane, exposing subendothelial collagen, which is highly thrombogenic. On electron microscopic evaluation, the lesions were infiltrated with leukocytes, platelets, and red blood cells [14]. Limited studies have demonstrated the presence of biologically active substances such as histamine, complement fragment C3a, and leukotrienes, which may contribute to venous vasodilation and endothelial damage [15]. These factors may contribute to thrombus formation at sites distant from the surgical procedure [16]. All these mechanisms produce endothelial cell damage, creating a nidus for clot formation.

The third factor contributing to the development of post-operative DVT is hypercoagulability. Assessing this state has proved to be challenging. The current approach focuses on either coagulation cascade modulators or impairment of the fibrinolytic system. Levels of antithrombin III (AT) have been shown to be decreased for 3–5 days after total hip and knee surgery [17]. This results in impaired modulation of the clotting cascade at the level involving factors Xa and IIa, with an increased propensity toward thrombus formation. The fibrinolytic system also has been evaluated by the measurement of tissue plasminogen activator and plasminogen activator inhibitor-1 levels before and after operation [18]. Several surgical studies have demonstrated a shutdown of the fibrinolytic system as evidenced by alterations in these levels [19]. An increased level of plasminogen activator inhibitor-1 before surgery appears to indicate an increased risk for the development of thrombosis in patients undergoing orthopedic procedures [20]. Another marker of an altered fibrinolytic system is the presence of alpha 2-antiplasmin, the primary function of which is to inactivate plasmin. Increased levels of alpha 2-antiplasmin complexes are indicative of active fibrinolysis, which is an indirect measure of active thrombus formation [20]. This radioimmunoassay requires further study as a predictor of postoperative DVT. Coupled with stasis and intimal injury, however, it seems to suggest an increased risk for DVT or PE. As Virchow postulated in 1856, the three factors (stasis, intimal injury, hypercoagulability) as described above increase the risk for the development of DVT and PE. Our responsibility as consultants is to ameliorate these risk factors wherever possible.

VTE risk factor assessment prior to surgery

The American College of Chest Physicians advocates a unified approach to VTE risk assessment by assigning risk according to the type of surgery, mobility, and individual risk factors [1,21] (Tables 22.1 and 22.2). The patient can be classified as being at low, moderate, or high risk for the development of VTE. Low-risk patients are those who are mobile and are having minor surgery. Medical patients who are fully ambulatory are also considered to be at low risk. Based on studies utilizing objective, diagnostic screening for asymptomatic DVT in patients not receiving prophylaxis, the approximate DVT risk is less than 10% in patients assigned to the low risk category. Moderate-risk patients are those undergoing general, open gynecologic, or urologic surgery. The approximate incidence of DVT without thromboprophylaxis in this group is 10–40%. The high-risk group includes patients having hip or knee replacement, fractured hip surgery, major trauma, and acute spinal cord injury. The DVT risk without thromboprophylaxis in this category is between 40% and 80%.

Another approach to risk assessment is the Caprini Risk Assessment Model [17,22] (Figure 22.1). This method consists of a list of exposing risk factors (genetic and clinical characteristics), each with an assigned relative risk score. The scores are summed to produce a cumulative score which is used to classify the patient into 1 through 4 risk levels and determines the type and duration of VTE prophylaxis. This risk assessment tool was validated by Bahl *et al.* [18,23].

Table 22.1 Risk factors for venous thromboembolism.

1. Surgery
2. Trauma (major trauma or lower extremity injury)
3. Immobility; lower extremity paresis
4. Cancer (active or occult)
5. Cancer therapy (hormonal, chemotherapy, angiogenesis inhibitors or radiotherapy)
6. Venous compression (tumor, hematoma, arterial abnormality)
7. Previous deep vein thrombosis or pulmonary embolism
8. Increasing age
9. Pregnancy and the postpartum period
10. Estrogen containing oral contraceptives or hormone replacement therapy
11. Selective estrogen receptor modulators
12. Erythropoiesis-stimulating agents
13. Acute medical illness
14. Inflammatory bowel disease
15. Nephrotic syndrome
16. Myeloproliferative disorders
17. Paroxysmal nocturnal hemoglobinuria
18. Obesity
19. Entral venous catheter
20. Inherited or acquired thrombophilia

Modified from Geerts WH, Bergqvist D, Pineo GF *et al.* Prevention of venous thromboembolism. *Chest* 2008; **133**: S381–453.

Table 22.2 Classification of the risk of postoperative venous thrombosis and pulmonary embolism.

Level of risk	Approximate risk with no prophylaxis	Prophylaxis options
High risk Total hip or knee arthroplasty Hip fracture Major trauma Spinal cord injury	40–80%	LMWH, fondaparinux, warfarin
High VTE risk plus high bleeding risk		Intermittent pneumatic compression
Moderate risk Most general, open gynecologic or urologic surgery patients, medical patients, bed rest or sick	10–40%	LMWH, Fondaparinux, UFH (BID/TID)
Moderate VTE risk plus high bleeding risk		Intermittent pneumatic compression
Low risk Minor surgery in mobile patients, Medical patients who are fully mobile	<10%	No specific thromboprophylaxis. Early and aggressive ambulation

LMWH, low molecular weight heparin; UFH, unfractionated heparin.
Modified from Geerts WH, Bergqvist D, Pineo GF *et al.* Prevention of venous thromboembolism. *Chest* 2008; **133**: S381–453.

Deep Vein Thrombosis (DVT)
Prophylaxis Orders
(For use in Elective General Surgery Patients)

Thrombosis Risk Factor Assessment
(Choose all that apply)

BIRTHDATE

NAME

CPI No.

SEX M F   VISIT No. _____

Each Risk Factor Represents 1 Point

☐ Age 41-60 years
☐ Swollen legs (current)
☐ Varicose veins
☐ Obesity (BMI >25)
☐ Minor surgery planned
☐ Sepsis (<1 month)
☐ Serious Lung disease including pneumonia (<1 month)
☐ Oral contraceptives or hormone replacement therapy
☐ Pregnancy or postpartum (<1 month)
☐ History of unexplained stillborn infant, recurrent spontaneous abortion (≥ 3), premature birth with toxemia or growth-restricted infant
☐ Other risk factors_____

☐ Acute myocardial infarction
☐ Congestive heart failure (<1 month)
☐ Medical patient currently at bed rest
☐ History of inflammatory bowel disease
☐ History of prior major surgery (<1 month)
☐ Abnormal pulmonary function (COPD)

Subtotal:

Each Risk Factor Represents 2 Points

☐ Age 61-74 years
☐ Arthroscopic surgery
☐ Malignancy (present or previous)
☐ Laparoscopic surgery (>45 minutes)
☐ Patient confined to bed (>72 hours)
☐ Immobilizing plaster cast (<1 month)

☐ Central venous access
☐ Major surgery (>45 minutes)

Subtotal:

Each Risk Factor Represents 3 Points

☐ Age 75 years or older   ☐ Family History of thrombosis*
☐ History of DVT/PE   ☐ Positive Prothrombin 20210A
☐ Positive Factor V Leiden ☐ Positive Lupus anticoagulant
☐ Elevated serum homocysteine
☐ Heparin-induced thrombocytopenia (HIT)
    (Do not use heparin or any low molecular weight heparin)
☐ Elevated anticardiolipin antibodies
☐ Other congenital or acquired thrombophilia
If yes: Type_____
* most frequently missed risk factor

Subtotal:

Each Risk Factor Represents 5 Points

☐ Stroke (<1 month)   ☐ Multiple trauma (<1 month)
☐ Elective major lower extremity arthroplasty
☐ Hip, pelvis or leg fracture (<1 month)
☐ Acute spinal cord injury (paralysis) (<1 month)

Subtotal:

TOTAL RISK FACTOR SCORE:

FACTORS ASSOCIATED WITH INCREASED BLEEDING
Patient may not be a candidate for anticoagulant therapy & SCDs should be considered.
Active Bleed, Ingestion of Oral Anticoagulants, Administration of glycoprotein IIb/IIIa inhibitors, History of heparin induced thrombocytopenia

CLINICAL CONSIDERATIONS FOR THE USE OF SEQUENTIAL COMPRESSION DEVICES (SCD)
Patient may not be a candidate for SCDs & alternative prophylactic measures should be considered.
Patients with Severe Peripheral Arterial Disease, CHF, Acute Superficial DVT

Total Risk Factor Score	Risk Level	Incidence of DVT	Prophylaxis Regimen
0-1	Low Risk	2%	☐ Early ambulation
2	Moderate Risk	10-20%	Choose the following medication **OR** compression devices: ☐ Sequential Compression Device (SCD) ☐ Heparin 5000 units SQ BID
3-4	Higher Risk	20-40%	Choose **ONE** of the following medications + / - compression devices: ☐ Sequential Compression Device (SCD) ☐ Heparin 5000 units SQ TID ☐ Enoxaparin/Lovenox: ☐ 40mg SQ daily (WT < 150kg, CrCl > 30mL/min) ☐ 30mg SQ daily (WT < 150kg, CrCl = 10-29mL/min) ☐ 30mg SQ BID (WT > 150kg, CrCl > 30mL/min) (Please refer to Dosing Guidelines on the back of this form)
5 or more	Highest Risk	40-80%	Choose **ONE** of the following medications **PLUS** compression devices: ☐ Sequential Compression Device (SCD) ☐ Heparin 5000 units SQ TID (Preferred with Epidurals) ☐ Enoxaparin/Lovenox (Preferred): ☐ 40mg SQ daily (WT < 150kg, CrCl > 30mL/min) ☐ 30mg SQ daily (WT < 150kg, CrCl = 10-29mL/min) ☐ 30mg SQ BID (WT > 150kg, CrCl > 30mL/min) (Please refer to Dosing Guidelines on the back of this form)

☐ Ambulatory Surgery - No orders for venous thromboembolic prophylaxis required
☐ VTE Prophylaxis Contraindicated, Reason: _____

Joseph A. Caprini, MD, MS, FACS, RVT
VTE Risk Factor Assessment Tool

Physician Signature	Dr. #	Date	Time

Processed By: Date/Time:

White-Medical Record
Yellow-MIS   Pink-Pharmacy

M University of Michigan Health System

DVT Prophylaxis Regimen

Figure 22.1 Caprini Risk Index.

Prophylaxis modalities

A number of modalities are used for the prophylaxis of DVT and PE in patients undergoing surgery. Each approach is reviewed with respect to dosage, administration, and length of therapy (Table 22.3).

Unfractionated heparin

Unfractionated heparin (UFH) is administered at an initial dose of 5,000 U given subcutaneously 2 hours before surgery. After surgery, 5,000 U is given subcutaneously every 8–12 hours until patients are discharged from the hospital. In double-blind trials, the incidence of major hemorrhagic events using this regimen was 1.8% compared with 0.8% in the control group [24]. This difference was not statistically significant. The incidence of minor bleeding such as injection site and wound hematomas, however, was significant with heparin prophylaxis (6.3% compared with 4.1% in the control group).

Table 22.3 Pharmacologic modalities of venous thrombosis prophylaxis.

Agent	Dose and schedule
1. Unfractionated heparin	5,000 U, SC 2 hours prior to surgery then Q8 or 12 hours postoperative. Continue until discharge
2. Low molecular weight heparin a. Dalteparin Orthopedic Surgery TKA, THA, FH General Surgery b. Enoxaparin Orthopedic Surgery TKA, THA, FH General Surgery c. Fondaparinux Orthopedic Surgery TKA, THA, FH	
3. Warfarin	5 mg, p.o. the evening of surgery then adjust for INR 2–3
4. Aspirin	325 mg, BID starting day of surgery and continue 6 weeks or 81 mg, once daily if gastrointestinal symptoms develop. Continue for 6 weeks

Dalteparin: 5,000 units subcutaneously every 24 hours (initiated evening of surgery).
Fondaparinux: 2.5 mg, subcutaneously beginning 6 hours following surgery then once daily.
Enoxaparin: orthopedic surgery 30 mg subcutaneously every 12 hours (initiated evening of surgery) and all other surgeries 40 mg subcutaneously every 24 hours (initiated evening of surgery).
TKA, total knee arthroplasty; THA, total hip arthroplasty; FH, hip fracture.

Low molecular weight heparin

Low molecular weight heparin (LMWH; dalteparin, enoxaparin, tinzaparin) preparations have become the primary agents for the prevention of postoperative DVT/PE in orthopedic surgery and cancer surgery. Low molecular weight heparin have been observed to have a more significant inhibitory effect on factor Xa than on factor IIa, as well as a lower bleeding risk than standard heparin [25]. Each of these LMWH preparations has a different molecular weight, anti-Xa to anti-IIa activity, rate of plasma clearance, and recommended dosage regimen [26]. When considering the safety and efficacy of LMWH preparations for the prevention of postoperative DVT, the clinician must keep in mind that these agents are distinct compounds with unique properties and different dosage regimens.

Low molecular weight heparin preparations are fragments of commercial-grade standard heparin prepared by either chemical or enzymatic depolymerization. The resulting LMWH contains the pentasaccharide required for specific binding to AT [27]. This binding inhibits Xa and IIa without forming the complex that occurs when standard heparin binds with these factors. Unfractionated heparin molecules with fewer than 18 saccharides (molecular weight less than 5,400 daltons) are unable to simultaneously bind thrombin and AT but retain their ability to catalyze the inhibition of factor Xa by AT [27]. Low molecular weight heparin formulations are not bound to plasma proteins (histidine-rich glycoprotein, platelet factor 4, vitronectin, fibronectin, and von Willebrand factor), endothelial cells, or macrophages as is standard heparin [25,26]. This lower affinity contributes to a longer plasma half-life, more complete plasma recovery at all concentrations, and clearance that is independent of dose and plasma concentration. In comparing the potential for hemorrhagic complications with standard heparin and LMWH, three factors must be considered. Standard UFH inhibits both collagen-induced and von Willebrand factor-dependent platelet aggregation and increases vascular permeability [25]. These three qualities result in a higher bleeding potential with standard UFH than with LMWH, which does not have these effects.

In contrast to UFH, the LMWHs are administered 6–12 hours following the surgical procedure. The dose of dalteparin for general surgical and orthopedic surgery is 5,000 units, subcutaneous once daily. Enoxaparin is administered at 40 mg, subcutaneous, once daily for general surgery whereas the orthopedic dose used in the USA is 30 mg, subcutaneous every 12 hours. In Europe the dose for orthopedic surgery is 40 mg subcutaneous given 12 hours prior to surgery followed by 40 mg subcutaneous once daily. Dose reductions are necessary in patients with a creatinine clearance less than 30 and these medications are contraindicated in patients who require dialysis or have a creatinine clearance less than 15.

Fondaparinux is a synthetically prepared molecule of the active pentasaccharide sequence of unfractionated heparin [27]. Like unfractionated heparin and LMWHs, this drug binds to AT which inhibits factor Xa. Fondaparinux occupies only a part of the heparin-binding site on antithrombin and the conformational change induced by this binding differs from UFH [27]. Because this medication is a catalyst, each molecule serves several times in activating AT. Peak plasma levels are obtained around 2 hours after subcutaneous injection, and significant levels are reached within 25 minutes [27]. This indicates a rapid onset of antithrombotic activity. The elimination half-life is dose-independent and ranges from 17–21 hours. Fondaparinux is renally excreted and should be avoided in patients with a creatinine clearance of less than 30 cc/min. It is administered 2.5 mg, subcutaneously beginning 6 hours after surgery and subsequently once daily.

Warfarin

Warfarin has been studied and approved for use in patients undergoing orthopedic surgery [21,28]. It can be administered by two methods. The first approach is to begin warfarin on the evening prior to the day of surgery while the second method involves the initiation of the drug on the day of the procedure. This latter schedule is the most commonly used in the USA. The usual starting dose of warfarin is 5 mg and the dose is adjusted for a goal INR between 2 to 3. The American Academy of Orthopedic Surgeons (AAOS) recommends an INR of less than 1.5 [28]. A loading dose of warfarin in excess of 5 mg is generally not recommended and lower starting doses may be considered in patients who are elderly or who have certain comorbidities including impaired nutrition, liver disease or congestive heart failure [21]. The duration of prophylaxis is maintained for up to 35 days at an INR goal of 2 to 3 with some studies using an INR of 1.8 to 2.5. The rare complication of warfarin-induced skin necrosis has never been reported in studies using this agent as prophylaxis for DVT and PE.

In some institutions, a debate exists regarding the most appropriate VTE prophylaxis in orthopedic patients that adequately balances the risk of bleeding with efficacy. A meta-analysis by Mismetti *et al.* concluded that LMWH is more effective in reducing the risk of venographically detected proximal DVT compared with vitamin K antagonists [29]. There was, however, no difference in the rate of PE between these two classes of medications with a similar to slightly greater risk of bleeding associated with LMWH. The ACCP guidelines have also acknowledged a greater efficacy of LMWH and, by indirect comparisons, fondaparinux in preventing both asymptomatic and symptomatic VTE in orthopedic patients at a cost of a slight increase in surgical site bleeding [21]. The postulated reason for this finding is a quicker onset of action with LMWH and fondaparinux compared with warfarin.

Mechanical prophylaxis modalities

Various forms of mechanical prophylaxis exist and include intermittent pneumatic compression, graduated compression stockings, and venous foot pumps. The main advantage of these products is the lack of a potential for bleeding with their use. Studies have shown them to be effective in reducing the rate of DVT, but not PE or death, in various surgical populations and they may provide additive efficacy when combined with anticoagulants. However, they have generally been found to be less effective than the pharmacologic prophylactic modalities and have not been as vigorously studied as the anticoagulants. A lack of compliance with these devices has been observed and should be taken into account, along with their respective costs, prior to their utilization [21].

External pneumatic compression sleeves are mechanical methods of improving venous return from the lower extremities [30]. They reduce stasis in the gastrocnemius-soleus pump. They are placed on the patient on the morning of surgery and are worn throughout the surgical procedure and continuously in the postoperative period until the patient is ambulatory or an anticoagulant is started. The most common complaints pertain to local discomfort caused by increased warmth, sweating, or disturbance of sleep. If a patient has been on bed rest or immobilized for more than 72 hours without any form of prophylaxis, it is our practice to perform lower extremity non-invasive testing to ensure that the patient does not have a DVT prior to the application of the sleeves.

Mechanical foot compression operates by compressing the sole of the foot, which activates a physiologic pump mechanism and improves venous return in the lower extremity [31]. The arteriovenous impulse system (foot pump, A-V Impulse System) was developed to accomplish this function. Like the external pneumatic compression sleeves, this device is worn during and after the surgery until the patient is ambulatory or the device is replaced by a pharmacologic agent. The A-V Impulse System has not been shown to be as effective as the external pneumatic compression sleeves [32,33].

A recent study randomized 410 patients to low molecular weight heparin versus a new external pneumatic compression device plus aspirin 81 mg daily [34]. The new device is called the synchronized flow technology compression device which is portable and operated by either battery or electrical power. This allows patient ambulation while wearing the device. The clinical outcomes of the study were symptomatic DVT/PE and major bleeding. The compression group had a 5% (10/197) incidence of DVT/PE while the LMWH cohort also had a 5% (10/192) thromboembolic event rate. The rate of major bleeding was 0% in the compression group and 6% with LMWH. In this protocol the compression sleeves were worn for a mean of 11 days with a mean of 24 hours per day.

Calf-length gradient elastic stockings are worn during surgery and are maintained until the patient is discharged. There are no known complications from their use. These mechanical methods of prophylaxis are effective for low-risk procedures. As with all other mechanical modes of prophylaxis, these products must be worn continuously to be effective. Practically speaking the use of mechanical devices poses a significant challenge with patient compliance. We see this as another option for patients who have a very high bleeding risk.

Aspirin

There is a lack of consensus on the role of aspirin for the prevention of VTE in the orthopedic population. The American Academy of Orthopedic Surgeons (AAOS) endorses the use of aspirin for certain patients who undergo non-traumatic hip or knee arthroplasty whereas the American College of Chest Physicians (ACCP) recommends against the use of aspirin for any patient undergoing a joint replacement procedure [21,33]. Warfarin, low molecular weight heparin, and the synthetic pentasaccharide have been shown to more effectively reduce this risk, and thus are recommended by the ACCP. The AAOS, however, recommends the use of aspirin in patients with a standard risk of both PE and major bleeding or in those with an elevated risk of major bleeding with a standard risk of PE since there is evidence to suggest a decrease in the rate of symptomatic events with the use of aspirin. There are no recommendations for aspirin use in the other surgical groups.

New oral anticoagulants

The new oral anticoagulants may prove to be one of the most significant innovations in clinical practice in the past 60 years (Table 22.4). Apixaban and rivaroxaban are specific inhibitors of Factor Xa while dabigatran inhibits Factor IIa. The predictable pharamacological profile of these new agents will allow physicians to use these drugs without the need for routine coagulation monitoring which is the mainstay of warfarin therapy. In addition, these new medications have not been shown to have any major food interactions and limited drug–drug interactions due to their limited metabolism through the CYP450 system. This unique pharmacokinetic profile may usher in for clinicians a new era of managing thromboembolic disorders. In this section, the pharmacology of these new oral anticoagulants is reviewed along with the major clinical trial results for VTE prevention.

Apixaban

Apixaban is a selective, reversible, direct inhibitor of Factor Xa. Its time to maximum plasma concentration is 30 minutes to 2 hours (Table 22.4). The half-life of the drug is 8–15 hours [35]. Apixaban is metabolized by CYP3A4 in the CYP450 system and the route of elimination is 30% renal and 70% fecal [35]. Apixaban showed moderate selectivity for clot-bound over free factor Xa and also inhibits thrombin generation [35]. In addition, apixaban is a substrate for the transport protein p-glycoprotein (p-GP) which functions as an efflux pump to prevent the absorption or increase the secretion of certain drugs known as p-GP substrates [36,37]. Apixaban has not been reported to have any food interactions. In healthy volunteers, the aPTT and modified PT were dose-dependently prolonged and correlated with the determined plasma concentrations of the drug [38]. Apixaban has a minimal impact on the prothrombin time (INR) and aPTT at therapeutic concentrations, but Factor Xa inhibition appears sensitive to detect its presence.

Rivaroxaban

Rivaroxaban is a selective, reversible direct inhibitor of Factor Xa. The time to maximum plasma concentration is 30 minutes to 3 hours (Table 22.4). Rivaroxaban's half-life has been reported to be 3–9 hours [39,40]. Three aspects of the pharmacologic profile of rivaroxaban are its concentration-dependent inhibition of Factor Xa with high potency and selectivity, its inhibition of thrombin generated from prothrombin and a dose-dependent inhibition of tissue factor [41]. This agent is metabolized by CYP3A4 in the CYP450 system and the route of elimination is 70% renal and 30% fecal [42]. Rivaroxaban does interact with the CYP450 system with specific interactions with CYP3A4 and CYP2J2 [43]. In addition, this agent is a substrate for transport p-GP and subject to interaction with drugs that interact with this protein. Studies reported the lack of any clinically relevant interaction of rivaroxaban with salicylic acid or naproxen [43]. Rivaroxaban's bioavailability was increased by about 2.5-fold upon co-administration of CYP3A4/p-GP inhibitors such as ketoconazole or ritonavir and decreased by about 50% after administration of the CYP3A4 inducer rifampicin [39]. Concomitant food intake only marginally increased rivaroxaban's bioavailability in healthy subjects [44]. Changes in gastric pH by antacids or ranitidine did not significantly affect absorption. There have not been any relevant effects of extreme body weight, age or gender on the pharmacological profile of this drug that has facilitated fixed-dose prescribing recommendations. Rivaroxaban prolongs the prothrombin time (INR) with the sensitivity dependent on the reagent being used. Factor Xa inhibition may be a more appropriate surrogate marker for evaluating the plasma concentration of rivaroxaban.

Table 22.4 Comparison of new oral antithrombotic agents.

Characteristic	Dabigatran	Rivaroxaban	Apixaban
1. Target	IIa	Xa	Xa
2. Bioavailability	7%	60–80%	80%
3. Half-life	12–17 hours	7–11 hours	12 hours
4. Clearance	80% renal	60% renal 33% biliary	25% renal 75% biliary
5. Metabolism	Conjugation to active glucuronides	CYP3A4 CYP2J2	CYP3A4
6. p-GP interaction	Yes	Yes	Minimal

p-GP = transport glycoproteins which prevent the absorption or increase secretion of certain drugs known as p-GP substrates. Dabigatran and rivaroxaban are p-GP substrates. Amiodarone, verapamil, and clarithromycin inhibit p-GP therefore increase the anticoagulant effect of dabigatran and rivaroxaban.

Recently, evidence has suggested that prothrombin complex concentrate (PCC) will cause a decrease in bleeding time and PT after administration of rivaroxaban [45]. These are promising, but due to lack of large studies and varying composition and availability of PCCs, more research will have to be performed to identify a reliable antidote for rivaroxaban.

Dabigatran

Dabigatran etexilate is the prodrug of dabigatran that selectively and reversibly inhibits both free and clot-bound thrombin by binding to the active site of the thrombin molecule (Table 22.4). The time to maximum plasma concentration is 1.25–1.5 hours with maximum effect in 2 hours [46]. Its half-life is about 12 hours. In human studies, over 90–95% of systemically available dabigatran was eliminated unchanged via renal excretion with the remaining 5–10% excreted in bile [47]. A unique aspect of this drug is that it is neither metabolized by nor induced or inhibited by the cytochrome P450 drug metabolizing enzymes. Because this drug exhibits low plasma protein binding (35%), it is a dialyzable agent with few displacement interactions to affect its pharmacodynamics [44]. In cases of overdose or severe bleeding, where more rapid reversal of the anticoagulant effects is required, hemodialysis could be effective in accelerating plasma clearance of dabigatran, especially in patients with renal impairment [48].

Food prolongs the time to peak plasma dabigatran levels by approximately 2 hours without significantly influencing overall bioavailability in healthy volunteers [47,49]. There have been no reported food interactions with dabigatran. Dabigatran is a substrate for transporter p-glycoprotein that could lead to changes in bioavailability of the drug. Drug interaction studies of dabigatran etexilate in combination with atorvastatin (CYP3A4 and p-GP substrate), diclofenac (CYP2C9 substrate), and digoxin (p-GP substrate) did not result in any significant pharmacokinetic changes of dabigatran or co-administered drugs [46,47,50–52]. Amiodarone, a p-GP inhibitor, increased the bioavailability of dabigatran by about 50% to 60% which may require an appropriate reduction in dosing [44]. In contrast, dabigatran's bioavailability was about 20–30% lower when pantoprazole was co-administered indicating its decreased oral bioavailability at elevated gastric pH [47,49]. Both the thrombin clotting time (TT) and ecarin clotting time (ECT) are highly sensitive tests for quantitating the anticoagulant effects of dabigatran [53]. The prothrombin time (INR) is prolonged by dabigatran, but it is not sensitive enough to detect clinically relevant changes in drug concentration and the aPTT is prolonged but not in a dose-dependent manner. Thus, the aPTT may serve as a qualitative test because it is less sensitive at supra-therapeutic concentrations of dabigatran. Reports on dabigatran using activated prothrombin complex (aPCC) concentrate and recombinant Factor VII (VIIa) have shown mixed results on the impact of aPTT and bleeding times; therefore, the role of these factors has yet to be determined [45].

Venous thromboembolism prophylaxis for surgery

General surgery

The incidence of DVT in general surgery has been documented to be 15–30% while the rates of fatal PE ranged between 0.2% and 0.9% [21]. These studies evaluated a wide age group of patients undergoing a variety of procedures and studies without VTE prophylaxis are no longer performed. A meta-analysis of 46 randomized clinical trials in general surgery compared thromboprophylaxis using unfractionated heparin (5,000 U Q8hours or Q12hours) with no thromboprophylaxis or with placebo [54]. The rate of DVT was significantly reduced from 22% to 9% (odds ratio 0.3; NNT 7) as were the rates of symptomatic PE from 2.0% to 1.3% (OR 0.5; NNT 143), fatal PE 0.8% to 0.3% (OR 0.4; NNT 182), and all cause mortality from 4.2% to 3.2% (OR 0.8; NNT 97). The above meta-analysis concluded that, based on indirect comparisons, unfractionated heparin 5,000 U Q8hours was more efficacious than 5,000 U Q12hours and there was no increase in the incidence of bleeding. There are no head-to-head studies comparing unfractionated heparin 5,000 U Q8hours versus Q12hours.

Table 22.5 Venous thrombosis prophylaxis: general surgery.

I. **Low risk general surgery (minor procedures with no thromboembolic risk factors) [Grade 1A]**
  A. Early and frequent ambulation
II. **Moderate-risk general surgery (major procedures for benign disease) [Grade 1A]**
  A. Heparin 5,000 units, subcutaneous every 12 hours until discharge
  B. Enoxaparin 40 mg, subcutaneous, beginning 12 hours post procedure followed by 40 mg, subcutaneous, Qdaily, until discharge
  C. Dalteparin 2,500 IU, subcutaneous, 1–2 hours prior to surgery, 2,500 IU, subcutaneous 12 hours postoperative, followed by 5,000 IU, subcutaneous, every 24 hours, until discharge
III. **High-risk general surgery (major procedures for cancer) [Grade 1A]**
  A. Heparin 5,000 units every 8 hours until discharge
  B. Enoxaparin 40 mg, subcutaneous, beginning 12 hours post procedure followed by 40 mg, subcutaneous, Qdaily, until discharge
  C. Dalteparin 2,500 IU, subcutaneous, 1–2 hours prior to surgery, 2,500 IU, subcutaneous 12 hours postoperative, followed by 5,000 IU, subcutaneous, every 24 hours, until discharge
IV. **High-risk general surgery with multiple thromboembolic risk factors [Grade 1C]**
  A. Heparin or LMWH combined with intermittent pneumatic compression sleeves until discharge [Grade 1C]
V. **High bleeding risk general surgery [Grade 1A]**
  A. Intermittent compression until bleeding risk lower then initiate pharmacologic prophylaxis as above

In evaluating LMWHs in general surgery, a meta-analysis demonstrated a reduction in asymptomatic DVT and symptomatic VTE by greater than 70% compared with patients not receiving prophylaxis [55]. When UFH and LMWHs were compared, there was no difference in the rates of symptomatic VTE. A large randomized trial in major abdominal surgery compared fondaparinux (2.5 mg started 6 hours postoperatively and then once daily) with dalteparin (5,000 U given preoperatively then once daily) [56]. There was no significant differences between the groups in the rates of VTE (4.6% vs 6.1%), major bleeding (3.4% vs 2.4%), or death (1.6% vs 1.4%).

The mechanical methods of prophylaxis are recommended for patients with a high perioperative bleeding risk and are replaced with a pharmacologic agent once the bleeding risk subsides. As stated above, the combined use of mechanical and pharmacologic prophylaxis may be considered for patients considered to have a high VTE risk. Table 22.5 outlines the recommendations for VTE prophylaxis in the general surgery population.

Urologic surgery

A review of the prophylaxis studies in urologic surgery has shown that the average patient was a male in the 50- to 70-year-old age group. The incidence of DVT has varied in these studies, with a reported rate between 31% and 51% in open prostatectomies to 7–10% in transurethral resections of the prostate [21]. The subject population of these studies had a mixture of benign and malignant diseases. This factor could have potentially introduced bias into the outcome of these studies. A clinical trial by Soderdahl et al. in major urologic surgery randomized 90 patients to receive thigh length or calf length intermittent pneumatic compression (IPC) stockings [56]. Venous compression ultrasound was the trial endpoint. One patient in the thigh length group developed a PE while only one patient in the calf length group developed a proximal thrombotic event. Thus, both mechanical methods were effective. The optimal prophylactic modality for VTE in urologic surgery, however, is not known because of the lack of well-controlled trials. Table 22.6 outlines the current recommendations for VTE prophylaxis in urologic surgery.

Neurosurgery

Craniotomies and spinal surgeries have been the predominant neurosurgical procedures evaluated for prophylaxis. In several randomized clinical trials, which included a variety of neurosurgical procedures, the rate of DVT detected by fibrinogen uptake testing among the control subjects was 22% with 5% of thrombotic events located proximally [21]. The two largest studies performed in neurosurgical patients compared graduated compression stockings (GCS) alone versus GCS with LMWH initiated post procedure with venography as the endpoint of the trial. There was a significant reduction in DVT in the GCS plus LMWH compared with GCS alone [57,58]. Goldhaber et al. randomized 150 brain tumor patients

Table 22.6 Prophylaxis for urologic surgery.

I. **Urologic surgery (transurethral or other low risk urologic procedures) [Grade 1A]**
   A. Early and frequent ambulation

II. **Major urologic surgery (major open procedures)**
   A. Heparin 5,000 units, subcutaneous every 8 or 12 hours until discharge [Grade 1B]
   B. Intermittent pneumatic compression sleeves initiated just prior to surgery and maintained while patient is not ambulating [Grade 1B]
   C. Enoxaparin 40 mg, subcutaneous, beginning 12 hours post procedure followed by 40 mg, subcutaneous, Qdaily, until discharge [Grade 1C]
   D. Dalteparin 2,500 IU, subcutaneous, 1–2 hours prior to surgery, 2,500 IU, subcutaneous 12 hours postoperative, followed by 5,000 IU, subcutaneous, every 24 hours, until discharge [Grade 1C]
   E. Intermittent pneumatic compression sleeves initiated just prior to surgery and maintained while patient is not ambulating plus heparin or LMWH
      1. Heparin 5,000 units, SC, beginning 8 to 12 hours postoperative then every 8 or 12 hours until discharge [Grade 1C]
      2. Enoxaparin 40 mg, subcutaneous, beginning 12 hours post procedure followed by 40 mg, subcutaneous, Qdaily, until discharge [Grade 1C]
      3. Dalteparin 2,500 IU, subcutaneous 12 hours postoperative, followed by 5,000 IU, subcutaneous, every 24 hours, until discharge [Grade 1C]

III. **High bleeding risk urologic surgery [Grade 1A]**
   A. Intermittent pneumatic compression until bleeding risk lower then initiate pharmacologic prophylaxis as above

IV. **Laparoscopic urologic procedures**
   A. Patients without thromboembolic risk factors: Early and frequent ambulation [Grade 1B]
   B. Patients with additional thromboembolic risk factors:
      1. Heparin 5,000 units, subcutaneous every 12 hours until discharge [Grade 1C]
      2. Enoxaparin 40 mg, subcutaneous, beginning 12 hours post procedure followed by 40 mg, subcutaneous, Qdaily, until discharge [Grade 1C]
      3. Dalteparin 2,500 IU, subcutaneous, 1–2 hours prior to surgery, 2,500 IU, subcutaneous 12 hours postoperative, followed by 5,000 IU, subcutaneous, every 24 hours, until discharge [Grade 1C]
      4. Intermittent pneumatic compression sleeves initiated just prior to surgery and maintained while patient is not ambulating [Grade 1C]
      5. Gradient elastic stockings placed prior to the procedure and maintained as outpatient

undergoing craniotomy to receive IPC plus either UFH (5,000 U BID) or enoxaparin (40 mg daily) [59]. The UFH group had a 7% incidence of DVT while the enoxaparin cohort had 12% DVT. Proximal DVT was found in 3% of patients in both groups. There was no difference in major bleeding between the groups. Although the reported incidence of major

Table 22.7 Prophylaxis for neurosurgery.

I. **High-risk neurosurgery (major procedures)**
   A. Intermittent pneumatic compression sleeves initiated just prior to surgery and maintained while patient is not ambulating [Grade 1A]
   B. Heparin 5,000 units, SC, beginning 8 to 12 hours postoperative then every 8 or 12 hours until discharge [Grade 2B]
   C. Enoxaparin 40 mg, subcutaneous, beginning 12 hours post procedure followed by 40 mg, subcutaneous, Qdaily, until discharge [Grade 2A]
   D. Dalteparin 2,500 IU, subcutaneous 12 hours postoperative, followed by 5,000 IU, subcutaneous, every 24 hours, until discharge [Grade 2A]

II. **High-risk neurosurgery (major procedure with additional thromboembolic risk factors)**
   A. Intermittent pneumatic compression sleeves initiated just prior to surgery and maintained while patient is not ambulating plus heparin or LMWH
      1. Heparin 5,000 units, SC, beginning 8 to 12 hours postoperative then every 8 or 12 hours until discharge [Grade 2B]
      2. Enoxaparin 40 mg, subcutaneous, beginning 12 hours post procedure followed by 40 mg, subcutaneous, Qdaily, until discharge [Grade 2B]
      3. Dalteparin 2,500 IU, subcutaneous 12 hours postoperative, followed by 5,000 IU, subcutaneous, every 24 hours, until discharge [Grade 2B]

Table 22.8 LMWH, low molecular weight heparin. Prophylaxis for gynecologic surgery.

I. **Low-risk gynecologic surgery (minor procedures without thromboembolic risk factors) [Grade 1A]**
   A. Early and frequent ambulation
II. **Moderate-risk gynecologic surgery (major procedures for benign disease without additional thromboembolic risk factors)**
   A. Heparin 5,000 units, subcutaneous every 12 hours until discharge [Grade 1A]
   B. Enoxaparin 40 mg, subcutaneous, beginning 12 hours post procedure followed by 40 mg, subcutaneous, Qdaily, until discharge [Grade 1A]
   C. Dalteparin 2,500 IU, subcutaneous, 1–2 hours prior to surgery, 2,500 IU, subcutaneous 12 hours postoperative, followed by 5,000 IU, subcutaneous, every 24 hours, until discharge [Grade 1A]
   D. Intermittent pneumatic compression sleeves initiated just prior to surgery and maintained while patient is not ambulating [Grade 1B]
III. **High-risk gynecologic surgery (major procedures for malignancy and for patients with additional thromboembolic risk factors)**
   A. Heparin 5,000 units every 8 hours until discharge [Grade 1A]
   B. Enoxaparin 40 mg, subcutaneous, beginning 12 hours post procedure followed by 40 mg, subcutaneous, Qdaily, until discharge [Grade 1A]
   C. Dalteparin 2,500 IU, subcutaneous, 1–2 hours prior to surgery, 2,500 IU, subcutaneous 12 hours postoperative, followed by 5,000 IU, subcutaneous, every 24 hours, until discharge [Grade 1A]
   D. Intermittent pneumatic compression sleeves initiated just prior to surgery and maintained while patient is not ambulating [Grade 1A]
   E. Alternative considerations would be heparin or LMWH with intermittent pneumatic compression sleeves or gradient elastic stockings or fondaparinux 2.5 mg, Qday [Grade 1C]
IV. **High bleeding risk gynecologic surgery [Grade 1A]**
   A. Intermittent pneumatic compression until bleeding risk lower then initiate pharmacologic prophylaxis as above
V. **Laparoscopic procedures**
   A. Patients without thromboembolic risk factors: Early and frequent ambulation [Grade 1B]
   B. Patients with additional thromboembolic risk factors:
      1. Heparin 5,000 units, subcutaneous every 12 hours until discharge [Grade 1C]
      2. Enoxaparin 40 mg, subcutaneous, beginning 12 hours post procedure followed by 40 mg, subcutaneous, Qdaily, until discharge [Grade 1C]
      3. Dalteparin 2,500 IU, subcutaneous, 1–2 hours prior to surgery, 2,500 IU, subcutaneous 12 hours postoperative, followed by 5,000 IU, subcutaneous, every 24 hours, until discharge [Grade 1C]
      4. Intermittent pneumatic compression sleeves initiated just prior to surgery and maintained while patient is not ambulating [Grade 1C]
      5. Gradient elastic stockings placed prior to the procedure and maintained as outpatient

bleeding was not increased, clinicians hesitate to use pharmacologic prevention. The pooled rates of intracranial hemorrhage in randomized trials of neurosurgery patients were 2.1% for postoperative LMWH and 1.1% for mechanical or no thromboprophylaxis [58,59]. Most of these bleeds occurred within the first 2 days after surgery. However, a meta-analysis for intracranial hemorrhage did not demonstrate significant differences for comparisons of LMWH versus UFH, or between LMWH and no heparin [61]. Table 22.7 outlines the recommendations for DVT prophylaxis in neurosurgery patients.

Gynecologic surgery

The incidence of DVT, PE, and fatal PE in major gynecologic surgery is similar to those following general surgical procedures. A Cochrane Database review by Oates-Whitehead *et al.* identified 11 studies and six of them were randomized controlled trials [61]. The trials included a total of 7,431 patients. Compared with compression alone, the use of combined modalities reduced significantly the incidence of both symptomatic PE (from about 3% to 1%; odds ratio (OR) 0.39, 95% confidence interval (CI) 0.25 to 0.63) and DVT (from about 4% to 1%; OR 0.43, 95% CI 0.24 to 0.76). Compared with pharmacological prophylaxis alone, the use of combined modalities significantly reduced the incidence of DVT (from 4.21% to 0.65%; OR 0.16, 95% CI 0.07–0.34) but the included studies were underpowered with regard to PE. The comparison of compression plus pharmacological prophylaxis versus compression plus aspirin showed a non-significant reduction in PE and DVT in favor of the former group. Four randomized clinical trials compared UFH given three times daily versus LMWH in gynecologic cancer surgery. Both agents were effective and safe in preventing postoperative VTE [63–66].

The current recommended options for DVT prophylaxis (Table 22.8) are UFH, LMWHs and intermittent pneumatic compression. The issue of extended VTE prevention in the outpatient setting was studied by Bergqvist *et al.* [66]. In this double-blind multicenter trial, 322 patients undergoing abdominal or pelvic surgery were randomized to receive enoxaparin (40 mg once daily) versus placebo for 25–31 days after the initial procedure. Venography at the completion of the trial was the endpoint of the study. The enoxaparin group had a 5% incidence of DVT while the placebo cohort had a 12% incidence (OR 0.36, P = 0.02). The rate of proximal DVT was low in both groups with calf vein thrombosis being the predominant finding.

Orthopedic surgery

Prophylaxis for VTE in orthopedic surgery patients has been strongly advocated by the American College of Chest Physicians' (ACCP) Consensus Conference on Antithrombotic Therapy 2008 and the American Academy of Orthopedic Surgeons (AAOS) [21,28]. Joint replacement procedures and hip fracture repair comprise the predominant procedures performed in patients with degenerative joint disease or rheumatoid arthritis. The incidence of fatal pulmonary embolism in patients undergoing joint replacements who have not received prophylaxis has been reported to be 5% [21]. This high incidence of fatal pulmonary embolism is not an acceptable outcome in patients undergoing these procedures. In order to understand the approach to prophylaxis, joint replacement procedures and fractured hip repair will be reviewed.

Without prophylaxis, the overall incidence of DVT following total hip replacement (THR) procedures has ranged from 42% to 57% and this complication has been reported to occur in 41% to 85% of patients undergoing total knee replacement (TKR). The rate of proximal DVT has ranged from 18% to 36% in THR and 5% to 22% in TKR. Fatal pulmonary embolism has occurred in 0.1% to 2.0% in the THR patient group whereas the incidence of this complication has ranged from 0.1% to 1.7% in patients undergoing TKR. Without VTE prophylaxis, the incidence of total DVT in hip fracture (FH) patients has ranged from 46% to 60% with 23–30% of these thrombotic events located proximally [21]. In a study by Eriksson *et al.*, 1,711 hip fracture patients were randomized to receive enoxaparin 40 mg once daily beginning 12–24 hours postoperatively or fondaparinux 2.5 mg once daily starting 4–8 hours after surgery [67]. The rates of VTE by postoperative day 11 were 19.1% in the enoxaparin group and 8.3% in the fondaparinux cohort (P < 0.001). Proximal DVT occurred in 4.3% of those taking enoxaparin versus 0.9% in the fondaparinux group (P < 0.001).

Table 22.9 Deep vein thrombosis/pulmonary embolism prophylaxis for orthopedic surgery.

Total hip replacement prophylaxis

I. Low molecular weight heparin (dalteparin, enoxaparin, fondaparinux) [Grade 1A]
   1. Dalteparin: 2,500 IU, SC, 4–8 hours postoperative then 5,000 IU, SC, Qdaily
   2. Enoxaparin: 30 mg, SC, 12 hours postoperative then 30 mg, SC, Q12hours (creatinine clearance < 30 cc/mL, 30 mg, SC, Qdaily)
   3. Fondaparinux: 2.5 mg, SC, 6 hours postoperative, then 2.5 mg, Qdaily
II. Warfarin (INR 2–3) [Grade 1A]
III. ASA, dextran, LDUFH, IPC, or VFP should not be used as the only method of VTE prophylaxis [Grade 1A]

Fractured hip

I. Low molecular weight heparin (LMWH)
   1. Fondaparinux 2.5 mg, SC, 6 hours postoperative, then 2.5 mg, Qdaily [Grade 1A]
   2. Dalteparin 2,500 IU, SC, 4–8 hours postoperative then 5,000 IU, SC, Qdaily (Grade 1C+)
   3. Enoxaparin 30 mg, SC, 12 hours postoperative then 30 mg, SC, Q12hours creatinine clearance < 30 cc/mL, 30 mg, SC, Qdaily [Grade 1C+]
II. Warfarin (INR 2–3) [Grade 2B]
III. Unfractionated heparin (UFH) 5,000 U, SC, Q8hours [Grade 1B]
IV. Delayed surgery prophylaxis: UFH or LMWH should be applied between the time of hospital admission and surgery [Grade 1C+]
V. External pneumatic compression if anticoagulation is contraindicated [Grade 1C+]
VI. ASA should not be used as the only method of VTE prophylaxis [Grade 1A]

Total knee replacement

I. Low molecular weight heparin (LMWH) [Grade 1A]
   1. Enoxaparin: 30 mg, SC, 12 hours postoperative then 30 mg, SC, Q12hours Creatinine clearance < 30 cc/mL, 30 mg, SC, Qdaily
   2. Fondaparinux: 2.5 mg, SC, 6 hours postoperative, then 2.5 mg, Qdaily
II. Warfarin (INR 2–3) [Grade 1A]
III. External pneumatic compression [Grade 1B]
IV. ASA [Grade 1A], UFH [Grade 1A], VFP [Grade 1B] should not be used as the only method of VTE prophylaxis.

ASA, aspirin; LDUFH, low dose unfractionated heparin; IPC, intermittent pneumatic compression stockings; VFP, venous foot pump; VTE, venous thromboembolism.

There was no difference in major bleeding between the two groups. The fatal PE rate has ranged from 0.3% to 7.5% [21]. Low molecular weight heparin, fondaparinux, and warfarin are currently the pharmacologic agents of choice for DVT prophylaxis according to the ACCP for the aforementioned procedures and should be administered as described above. External pneumatic compression sleeves can be used in combination with an anticoagulant in those patients considered to have a high risk of developing a VTE [21].

On the basis of the results of a phase II study in patients undergoing knee arthroplasty, the phase III Apixaban for the Prevention of Thrombosis-Related Events (ADVANCE) program compared a 2.5-mg twice-daily dose of apixaban (started in the morning of the day after surgery) with enoxaparin in patients undergoing knee arthroplasty. In Tables 22.10 and 22.11 the three ADVANCE trials are outlined. For both trials, the primary efficacy outcome (total event rate) was a composite of asymptomatic and symptomatic deep-vein thrombosis, non-fatal pulmonary embolism, and death from any cause during treatment. In ADVANCE 1, which involved 3,195 patients, a 10–14 day course of apixaban was compared with a similar duration of enoxaparin (30 mg twice daily). Apixaban had efficacy similar to enoxaparin with total event rates of 9.0% and 8.8%, respectively [68]. Major bleeding rates were 0.7% with apixaban and 1.4% with enoxaparin ($P = 0.05$). Despite similar efficacy, apixaban did not meet the prespecified non-inferiority goal because the event rates were lower than expected. The ADVANCE 2 trial, which included 3,057 patients, compared the same apixaban regimen with an equal duration of treatment with enoxaparin at a dose of 40 mg once daily [70]. In this trial, apixaban significantly reduced total event rates compared with enoxaparin (15.1% and 24.4%, respectively; $P < 0.0001$) and was associated with a trend for less major bleeding (0.6% and 0.9% respectively; $P = 0.3$). ADVANCE 3 treated 5,407 total hip arthroplasty patients for 32–38 days with apixaban (2.5 mg twice daily) versus enoxaparin (40 mg once daily). Apixaban (1.4%) was superior to enoxaparin (3.9%) for the primary outcome. Major bleeding rates were the same in apixaban (0.8%) and enoxaparin (0.7%) [70].

The phase II Oral Direct Factor Xa Inhibitor (ODIXa) VTE prevention studies established the dose for rivaroxaban that was used in the phase III RECORD trial program [71–74].

Table 22.10 Apixaban: total knee arthroplasty (TKA) study designs.

Key points	ADVANCE 1 (n 3,195)	ADVANCE 2 (n 3,057)	ADVANCE 3 (n 5,407)
1. Surgery	TKA	TKA	THA
2. Apixaban	2.5 mg BID	2.5 mg BID	2.5 mg BID
3. First dose apixaban	12–24 hours postop.	12–24 hours postop.	12–24 hours postop.
4. Comparator	Enoxaparin 30 mg BID started 12–24 hours postop	Enoxaparin 40 mg Qday started 12 hours preop	Enoxaparin 40 mg Qday started 12 hours preop.
5. Duration of prophylaxis	10–14 days	10–14 days	32–38 days
6. DVT endpoint	Venogram	Venogram	Venogram
7. Primary outcome	Total VTE* + all-cause mortality	Total VTE* + all-cause mortality	Total VTE* + all-cause mortality
8. Analysis	Apixaban inferior to enoxaparin	Apixaban not inferior to enoxaparin	Apixaban not inferior and superior to enoxaparin

* Total VTE = symptomatic and asymptomatic DVT plus non-fatal PE.

Table 22.11. Apixaban study results.

Study	Primary outcome		Major bleeding	
	Apixaban	Enoxaparin	Apixaban	Enoxaparin
ADVANCE 1	9%	8.8%	0.7%	1.4%
ADVANCE 2	15%	24%	0.6%	0.9%
ADVANCE 3	1.4%	3.9%	0.8%	0.7%

ADVANCE 1 and 2 = TKA
ADVANCE 3 = THA
Primary outcome: Symptomatic and asymptomatic DVT, non-fatal PE, and all-cause death.
Major bleeding: Acute clinically overt bleeding accompanied by one or more of the following: a decrease in blood hemoglobin concentration of 2 g/dL or more during 24 hours; transfusion of two or more units of packed red blood cells; critical site bleeding (including intracranial, intraspinal, intraocular, pericardial, or retroperitoneal bleeding); bleeding into the operated joint needing reoperation or intervention; intramuscular bleeding with compartment syndrome; or fatal bleeding.

Table 22.12 Rivaroxaban: total knee and hip arthroplasty study designs.

Key Points	RECORD1 (n 4,541)	RECORD2 (n 2,509)	RECORD3 (n 2,531)	RECORD4 (n 3,148)
1. Surgery	THA	THA	TKA	TKA
2. Rivaroxaban	10 mg Qday	10 mg Qday	10 mg Qday	10 mg Qday
3. First dose of rivaroxaban	6–8 hours postop.	6–8 hours postop	6–8 hours postop.	6–8 hours postop.
4. Comparator	Enoxaparin 40 mg Qday started 12 hours preop.	Enoxaparin 40 mg Qday started 12 hours preop.	Enoxaparin 40 mg Qday started 12 hours preop.	Enoxaparin 30 mg BID started 12–24 hours postop.
5. Duration of prophylaxis[*]	34 days	34 days R[**] 12 days E[***]	12 days	11 days
6. DVT endpoint	Venogram	Venogram	Venogram	Venogram
7. Primary outcome	Total VTE[****] + all-cause mortality	Total VTE+ all-cause mortality	Total VTE+ all-cause mortality	Total VTE + all-cause mortality
8. Analysis	Rivaroxaban superior	Rivaroxaban superior	Rivaroxaban superior	Rivaroxaban superior

[*] Mean duration of treatment.
[**] Rivaroxaban.
[***] Enoxaparin.
[****] Total VTE = asymptomatic and symptomatic DVT plus non-fatal PE.

Table 22.13 Rivaroxaban RECORD study results.

Study	Primary outcome		Major bleeding	
	Rivaroxaban	Enoxaparin	Rivaroxaban	Enoxaparin
RECORD 1: THA	1.1%	3.7%	0.3%	0.1%
RECORD 2: THA	2%	9.3%	< 0.1%	< 0.1%
RECORD 3: TKA	9.6%	18.9%	0.6%	0.5%
RECORD 4: TKA	6.9%	10.1%	0.7%	0.3%

Primary endpoint of study: DVT, non-fatal pulmonary embolism, death.
Major bleeding: Bleeding that was fatal, occurred in a critical organ (retroperitoneal, intracranial, intraocular, and intraspinal), or required reoperation or extrasurgical site bleeding that was clinically overt and was associated with a fall in the hemoglobin level of at least 2 g/dL or that required transfusion of two or more units of whole blood or packed cells.

This program evaluated the efficacy and safety of rivaroxaban compared with enoxaparin in over 12,000 patients undergoing hip or knee arthroplasty. Tables 22.12 and 22.13 outline the design of the above trials as well as the primary outcomes. The dose of rivaroxaban in all four RECORD trials was 10 mg once daily, started 6 to 8 hours after wound closure. The European-approved dose of enoxaparin (40 mg once daily with the first dose given in the evening before surgery) was used as the comparator in the first three RECORD trials, whereas the North American-approved dose of enoxaparin (30 mg twice daily starting 12–24 hours after surgery) was the comparator in the RECORD 4 trial [75–78]. The primary efficacy outcome (total event rate) in all of the trials was the composite of deep vein thrombosis (either symptomatic or detected by bilateral venography if the patient was asymptomatic), non-fatal pulmonary embolism, or death from any cause.

In the RECORD 1 trial, which included 4,541 patients undergoing hip arthroplasty, a 31–39-day course of rivaroxaban significantly reduced the total event rate compared with an equal duration of treatment with enoxaparin (1.1% and 3.7%, respectively; P < 0.001) [75] [Tables 22.12 and 22.13]. In the RECORD 2 trial involving 2,509 patients undergoing total hip arthroplasty, a 31–39-day course of rivaroxaban significantly reduced the total event rate compared with a 10–14-day course of enoxaparin followed by 21–25 days of placebo (2.0% and 9.3%, respectively; P < 0.0001) [76]. The RECORD 3 trial included 2,531 patients undergoing knee arthroplasty. A 10–14-day course of treatment with rivaroxaban

Table 22.14 Dabigatran: total knee and hip arthroplasty study designs.

Key points	RE-MOBILIZE (n 2,615)	RE-MODEL (n 2,101)	RE-NOVATE (n 3,494)	RE-NOVATE II (n 2,055)
1. Surgery	TKA	TKA	THA	THA
2. Dabigatran	150 mg or 220 mg once daily	150 mg or 220 mg once daily	150 mg or 220 mg once daily	220 mg once daily
3. First dose dabigatran	6–12 hours postop. (1/2 dose on day 1)	1–4 hours postop. (1/2 dose on day 1)	1–4 hours postop. (1/2 dose on day 1)	(1/2 dose on day 1)
4. Comparator	Enoxaparin 30 mg BID started 12–24 hours postop.	Enoxaparin 40 mg Qday started 12 hours preop.	Enoxaparin 40 mg Qday started 12 hours preop.	Enoxaparin 40 mg Qday started 12 hours preop.
5. Duration of prophylaxis	12–15 days	6–10 days	28–35 days	28–35 days
6. DVT endpoint	Venogram	Venogram	Venogram	Venogram
7. Primary outcome	Total VTE + all-cause mortality	Total VTE + all-cause mortality	Total VTE + all-cause mortality	Total VTE + all-cause mortality
8. Analysis	Dabigatran inferior to enoxaparin	Dabigatran non-inferior to enoxaparin	Dabigatran non-inferior to enoxaparin	Dabigatran non-inferior to enoxaparin

Total VTE events = symptomatic or venographically detected deep vein thrombosis and/or symptomatic pulmonary embolism.

Table 22.15 Dabigatran study results.

Study	Primary outcome			Major bleeding		
	Dabi-220 mg	Dabi-150 mg	Enoxaparin	Dabi-220 mg	Dabi-150 mg	Enoxaparin
RE-NOVATE	6.0%	8.6%	6.7%	2%	1.3%	1.6%
RE-MODEL	36.4%	40.5%	37.7%	1.5%	1.3%	1.3%
RE-MOBILIZE	31.1%	33.7%	25.3%	0.6%	0.6%	1.4%
RE-MOBILIZE II	7.7%		8.8%	1.4%		0.9%

Primary outcome = asymptomatic and symptomatic deep vein thrombosis, non-fatal pulmonary embolism, all-cause death.
Major bleeding: Fatal bleeding, clinically overt bleeding in excess of expected and associated with a fall of 2 g/dL, or leading to transfusion of > 2 units packed red cells or whole blood; symptomatic retroperitoneal, intracranial, intraocular, or intraspinal bleeding; bleeding requiring treatment cessation and/or operation.

significantly reduced the total event rate compared with an equal duration of treatment with enoxaparin (9.6% and 18.9%, respectively, P < 0.001) [69]. Finally, in the RECORD 4 trial involving 3,148 patients undergoing knee arthroplasty, a 10–14-day course of treatment with rivaroxaban significantly reduced the total event rate compared with an equal duration of enoxaparin at the higher 30 mg BID dose (6.9% and 10.1%, respectively; P < 0.012) [77]. In both the RECORD 2 and 3 trials, rivaroxaban significantly reduced the incidence of symptomatic VTE compared with enoxaparin [76,77]. Rivaroxaban did not increase major bleeding in any of the trials, but a pooled analysis performed by the FDA of the four RECORD trials revealed a small but significant increase in major plus clinically relevant non-major bleeding with rivaroxaban. On the basis of these results, rivaroxaban 10 mg once daily

has been recently approved for VTE prophylaxis in patients undergoing hip or knee replacement procedures in the USA.

Based on results from phase II studies, two doses of dabigatran were investigated in the phase III trials for thromboprophylaxis after hip or knee arthroplasty: 220 mg or 150 mg (both given once daily) which was initiated at half the usual dose on the first day [Tables 22.14 and 22.15] [79–82]. The European-approved dose of enoxaparin (40 mg once daily with the first dose given in the evening before surgery) was used as the comparator in the RE-MODEL study after total knee replacement and RE-NOVATE and RE-NOVATE II studies after total hip replacement [81,82]. The North American-approved dose of enoxaparin (30 mg twice daily starting 12 to 24 hours after surgery) was the comparator in the RE-MOBILIZE study after total knee replacement [79].

In all three trials, the primary efficacy endpoint (total event rate) was a composite of venographically detected or symptomatic DVT, non-fatal PE, and all-cause mortality. Table 22.16 outlines the design of the above trials as well as the primary outcomes.

In the RE-MODEL trial involving 2,076 patients undergoing knee arthroplasty, 6–10 days of either dose of dabigatran etexilate had efficacy similar to that of enoxaparin (dabigatran 220 mg, 36.4%; dabigatran 150 mg, 40.5%; enoxaparin 37.7%). The incidence of major bleeding did not differ significantly among the three groups (1.5%, 1.3%, and 1.3%, respectively) [79]. In the RE-NOVATE trial involving 3,494 patients undergoing hip arthroplasty, treatment with either dose of dabigatran etexilate for 28–35 days had efficacy similar to that of enoxaparin (dabigatran 220 mg, 6.0%; dabigatran 150 mg,

8.6%; enoxaparin, 6.7%) [81]. The incidence of major bleeding did not differ significantly among the three groups (2.0%, 1.3%, and 1.6%, respectively) [81]. In the RE-MOBILIZE study of 2,615 patients undergoing knee arthroplasty, treatment with either dose of dabigatran etexilate for 12–15 days was statistically inferior to a similar duration of treatment with enoxaparin (dabigatran 220 mg, 31%; dabigatran 150 mg, 34%; enoxaparin, 25%). The incidence of major bleeding did not differ significantly among the three groups (0.6%, 0.6%, and 1.4%, respectively) [79]. The RE-NOVATE II study evaluated 2,055 patients undergoing total hip arthroplasty treated with dabigatran (220 mg once daily) versus enoxaparin (40 mg once daily) for 28–35 days [82]. Dabigatran (7.7%) was not inferior to enoxaparin (8.8%) for the primary outcome [82]. The incidence of major bleeding did not differ significantly among the two groups (1.4% dabigatran, 0.9% enoxaparin) [82].

Dabigatran etexilate is approved in Europe and Canada for VTE prevention after elective hip or knee arthroplasty. Per the European label, the 220-mg dose of dabigatran etexilate is recommended for the majority of patients, whereas the 150-mg dose is reserved for patients also taking amiodarone and for those at higher risk for bleeding, such as patients older than 75 years or with a creatinine clearance < 50 mL/min.

Extended prophylaxis for DVT and PE

Despite our most effective DVT and PE prophylaxis regimens, the incidence of DVT has not been reduced to zero. The duration of risk for the development of DVT after release from hospital following surgery has become an important issue (Table 22.16). The topic of extended VTE prevention in the outpatient setting was studied by Bergqvist et al. [82]. In this double-blind, multicenter trial of 322 patients undergoing abdominal or pelvic surgery, patients were randomized to receive enoxaparin (40 mg once daily) versus placebo for 25–31 days after the initial procedure. Venography at the completion of the trial was the endpoint of the study. The enoxaparin group had a 5% incidence of DVT while the placebo cohort had 12% (OR 0.36, P = 0.02). The rate of proximal DVT was low in both groups with calf vein thrombosis being the predominant finding. In another open-label study conducted in 233 major abdominal surgery patients, LMWH (dalteparin 5,000 IU Q24hours) was administered once daily for 1 or 4 weeks [83]. All patients completed bilateral lower extremity venography at day 28 +/− 2 days. DVT was detected in 16% of patients who had 7 days of prophylaxis versus 6% in those receiving LMWH for 4 weeks (P = 0.09). The proximal DVT incidence was 9% in the former and 0% in the latter group.

More recently, two studies evaluated total hip replacement patients for 21 days following discharge [84,85]. Both studies were randomized, double-blind, placebo-controlled trials using enoxaparin (40 mg daily). All study patients underwent bilateral lower extremity venography at the completion of 21 days of prophylaxis. Planes and colleagues reported a 19.3% incidence of DVT in the placebo group and a 7.1% incidence in the

Table 22.16 Extended venous thromboembolism prophylaxis for general, gynecologic and orthopedic surgery.

General surgery
In selected high-risk general surgery patients, including those who have undergone major cancer surgery, extended prophylaxis for 28–30 days should be provided (2A)
Low molecular weight heparin
1. Enoxaparin 40 mg, SC, Qdaily
2. Dalteparin 5,000 IU, SC, Qdaily

Gynecologic surgery
In selected high-risk gynecologic surgery patients, including those who have undergone cancer surgery, are > 60 years of age, or have had previous VTE, extended prophylaxis for 28–30 days are recommended (2C)
1. Enoxaparin 40 mg, SC, Qdaily
2. Dalteparin 5,000 IU, SC, Qdaily

Orthopedic surgery
Total hip replacement or hip fracture surgery patients should receive extended VTE prophylaxis for up to 35 days following surgery (1A)

Total hip replacement
Low molecular weight heparin (1A)
1. Enoxaparin 40 mg, SC, Qdaily
2. Dalteparin 5,000 IU, SC, Qdaily
3. Fondaparinux: 2.5 mg, SC, Qdaily (1C+)

Warfarin: INR 2–3 range (1A)

Hip fracture surgery
I. Low molecular weight heparin (1C+)
   1. Enoxaparin 40 mg, SC, Qdaily
   2. Dalteparin 5,000 IU, SC, Qdaily
   3. Fondaparinux: 2.5 mg, SC, Qdaily (1A)
II. Warfarin INR 2–3 (1C+)

Total knee arthroplasty
I. Low molecular weight heparin (1C+)
   1. Enoxaparin 40 mg, SC, Qdaily
   2. Dalteparin 5,000 IU, SC, Qdaily
   3. Fondaparinux: 2.5 mg, SC, Qdaily (1C+)
II. Warfarin INR 2–3 (1C+)

enoxaparin patients [85]. Bergqvist and coworkers showed a 39% incidence of DVT in the placebo-treated patients and an 18% incidence in those receiving enoxaparin [86]. Three meta-analyses of patients undergoing THR and TKA found that post-hospital discharge VTE prophylaxis was both effective and safe [86–88]. Major bleeding did not occur in any groups receiving extended prophylaxis with LMWH. Those who underwent THR derived greater protection from symptomatic VTE using extended prophylaxis (pooled OR, 0.33; 95% CI, 0.19–0.56; NNT 62) than patients who underwent TKA (pooled OR, 0.74; 95% CI, 0.26–2.15; NNT, 250). A recent double-blinded clinical trial treated 656 hip fracture surgery patients with fondaparinux or placebo for an additional 3 weeks following discharge [91]. Venography documented DVT occurred in 1.4% of the extended prophylaxis group and 35% in the placebo cohort. The major bleeding rates were the same in both groups. The recent *Chest* guidelines have defined the risk period following discharge to be 21–42 days [21]. It is recommended that prophylaxis with LMWH or warfarin be provided for this time period in patients undergoing major orthopedic procedures (Table 22.9). As for the non-orthopedic surgery population, those who have undergone surgery for a malignancy are considered high risk for VTE and should be considered for extended VTE prophylaxis for 21–30 days following the procedure. Considering the above, we recommend LMWH (enoxaparin 40 mg Q24hours or dalteparin 5,000 U Q24hour) for 30 days following the procedure for patients undergoing abdominal or pelvic surgery for cancer. In orthopedic surgery, patients should receive extended prophylaxis with warfarin (INR 2 to 3), LMWH (enoxaparin 40 mg, dalteparin 5,000 IU) or fondaparinux 2.5 mg every 24 hours for up to 35 days.

Conclusion and clinical considerations

As the population ages and innovations in healthcare improve survival, the frequency of patients undergoing surgical procedures will increase in this country. Preoperative venous thromboembolism risk assessment in the above population will require the application of appropriate DVT/PE prophylaxis. The new oral anticoagulants introduced in this chapter have the potential to play a significant role in the orthopedic joint replacement population. The studies presented above in joint replacement surgery demonstrated the efficacy and safety of these new oral agents (direct Xa inhibitors apixaban and rivaroxaban; direct IIa inhibitor dabigatran) in preventing venous thromboembolism.

References

1. Carter C, Gent M. The epidemiology of venous thrombosis. In Colman R, Hirsh J, Marder V, Salzman E, eds. *Hemostasis and Thrombosis*. Philadelphia, PA: JB Lippincott; 1982, pp. 805–19.

2. Dismuke S, Wagner E. Pulmonary embolism as a cause of death: the changing mortality in hospitalized patients. *J Am Med Assoc* 1986; **255**: 2039–42.

3. Cohen A, Tapson V, Bergmann J *et al.* Venous thromboembolism risk and prophylaxis in the acute hospital care setting (ENDORSE Study): a multi-national cross sectional study. *Lancet* 2008; **371**: 387–94.

4. Surgical Care Improvement Project. Joint Commission website: www.jointcommission.org.

5. Nicolaides A, Kakkar V, Renney J. Soleal sinuses and stasis. *Br J Surg* 1970; **57**: 307.

6. Nicolaides A, Kakkar V, Field E *et al.* Venous stasis and deep vein thrombosis. *Br J Surg* 1972; **59**: 713–16.

7. Stamatakis J, Kakkar V, Sagar S *et al.* Femoral vein thrombosis and total hip replacement. *Br Med J* 1977; **112**: 223–5.

8. Clark C, Cotton L. Blood flow in deep veins of the legs: recording technique and evaluation of method to increase flow during operation. *Br J Surg* 1968; **55**: 211–14.

9. Lindstrom B, Ahlman H, Honsson O *et al.* Blood flow in the calves during surgery. *Acta Chir Scand* 1977; **143**: 335–9.

10. Linstrom B, Ahlman H, Jonsson O *et al.* Influence of anesthesia on blood flow to the calves during surgery. *Acta Anaesthesiol Scand* 1984; **28**: 201–3.

11. Johnson R, Carmichael J, Almond H *et al.* Deep vein thrombosis following Charneley arthroplasty. *Clin Orthop* 1978; **132**: 24–30.

12. Planes A, Vochelle N, Fagola M. Total hip replacement and deep vein thrombosis: a venographic and necropsy study. *J Bone Joint Surg* 1990; **72B**: 9–13.

13. Comerota A, Stewart G, Alburger P *et al.* Operative venodilation: a previously unsuspected factor in the cause of postoperative deep vein thrombosis. *Surgery* 1989; **106**: 301–9.

14. Schaub P, Lynch P, Stewart G. The response of canine veins to three types of abdominal surgery: a scanning and transmission electron microscope study. *Surgery* 1978; **83**: 411–22.

15. Stewart G, Schaub R, Niewiarowske S. Products of tissue injury: their induction of venous endothelial damage and blood cell adhesion in the dog. *Arch Pathol Lab Med* 1980; **104**: 409–13.

16. Stewart G, Alburger P, Stone E *et al.* Total hip replacement induces injury to remote veins in a canine model. *J Bone Joint Surg* 1983; **65A**: 97–102.

17. Gitel S, Salvanti E, Wessler S *et al.* The effect of total hip replacement and general surgery on antithrombin III in relation to venous thrombosis. *J Bone Joint Surg* 1979; **61A**: 653–6.

18. Eriksson B, Eriksson E, Wessler S *et al.* Thrombosis after hip replacement: relationship to the fibrinolytic system. *Acta Orthop Scand* 1989; **60**: 159–63.

19. Kluft C, Verheijen J, Jie A *et al.* The postoperative fibrinolytic shutdown: a rapidly reverting acute phase pattern for the fast acting inhibitor of tissue type plasminogen activator after trauma. *Scand J Clin Lab Invest* 1985; **45**: 605–10.

20. D'Angelo A, Kluft C, Verheijen J *et al.* Fibrinolytic shut down after surgery: impairment of the balance between tissue plasminogen activator and its specific inhibitors. *Eur J Clin Invest* 1985; **15**: 308–12.

21. Geerts WH, Bergqvist D, Pineo GF et al. Prevention of venous thromboembolism. *Chest* 2008; **133**: S381–453.

22. Caprini J. Risk assessment as a guide for the prevention of the many faces of venous thromboembolism. *Am J Surg* 2010; **199**: S3–10.

23. Bahl V, Hu HM, Henke PK et al. A valid study of a retrospective venous thromboembolism risk scoring method. *Ann Surg* 2010; **2**: 344–50.

24. Clagett G, Reisch J. Prevention of venous thromboembolism in general surgical patients: results of meta-analysis. *Ann Surg* 1988; **208**: 227–40.

25. Hirsh J, Levine M. Low molecular weight heparin. *Blood* 1992; **79**: 1–17.

26. Weitz J. Low molecular weight heparins. *N Engl J Med* 1997; **337**: 688–98.

27. Samama M. Synthetic direct and indirect factor Xa inhibitors. *Thrombosis Res* 2002; **106**: 267–73.

28. Johanson N, Lachiewicz PF, Lieberman JR et al. Prevention of symptomatic pulmonary embolism in patients undergoing total hip or knee arthroscopy. *J Am Acad Ortho Surg* 2009; **17**: 183–96.

29. Mismetti P, Laporte S, Zufferey P et al. Prevention of venous thromboembolism in orthopedic surgery with vitamin K antagonists: a meta analysis. *J Thromb Haemost* 2004; **2**: 1058–70.

30. Caprini J, Scurr J, Hasty J. Role of compression modalities in a prophylactic program for deep vein thrombosis. *Semin Thromb Hemost* 1988; **14**: 77–87.

31. Gardner A, Fox R. The venous pump of the human foot: a preliminary report. *Bristol Med Chir J* 1983; **98**: 109–14.

32. Fordyce M, Ling R. A venous foot pump reduces thrombosis after total hip replacement. *J Bone Joint Surg* 1992; **74B**: 45–9.

33. Wilson N, Das S, Kakkar V et al. Thrombo-embolic prophylaxis in total knee replacement: evaluation of the A-V impulse system. *J Bone Joint Surg* 1992; **74B**: 50–2.

34. Colwell C, Froimson M, Mont M et al. Thrombosis prevention after total hip arthroplasty: a prospective, randomized trial comparing a mobile compression device with low molecular weight heparin. *J Bone Joint Surg Am* 2010; **92**: 527–35.

35. Raghavan N, Frost CE, Yu Z et al. Apixaban metabolism and pharmacokinetics after oral administration to humans. *Drug Metab Dispos* 2009; **37**: 74–81.

36. Jiang X, Crain EJ, Luettgen JM et al. Apixaban, an oral direct factor Xa inhibitor, inhibitis human clot-bound factor Xa activity in vitro. *Thromb Haemost* 2009; **101**: 780–2.

37. Luettgen JM, Wang Z, Seiffer DA et al. Inhibition of measured thrombin generation in human plasma by apixaban: a predictive mathematical model based on experimentally determined rate constants. *J Thromb Haemost* 2007; **5** (Suppl. 2): p-T-633.

38. Frost C, Yu Z, Moore K et al. Apixaban, an oral direct factor Xa inhibitor: multiple-dose safety, pharmacokinetics and pharmacodynamics in healthy subjects. *J Thromb Haemost* 2007; **5**: P-M-664.

39. Kubitza D, Becka M, Wensing G et al. Safety, pharmacodynamics, and pharmacokinetics of BAY 59–7939: an oral, direct Factor Xa inhibitor after multiple dosing in healthy male subjects. *Eur J Clin Pharmacol* 2005; **61**: 873–80.

40. Kubitza D, Becka M, Voith B et al. Safety, pharmacodynamics, and pharmacokinetics of single doses of BAY 59–7939, an oral, direct Factor Xa inhibitor. *Clin Pharmacol Ther* 2005; **78**: 412–21.

41. Perzborn E, Strassburger J, Wilmen A et al. In vitro and in vivo studies of the novel antithrombotic agent BAY 59–7939, an oral, direct Factor Xa inhibitor. *J Thromb Haemost* 2005; **3**: 514–21.

42. Weinz C, Schwartz T, Kubitza D et al. Metabolism and excretion of rivaroxaban, an oral, direct Factor Xa inhibitor, in rats, dogs, and humans. *Drug Metab Dispos* 2009; **37**: 1056–64.

43. Ufer M. Comparative efficacy and safety of the novel oral anticoagulants dabigatran, rivaroxaban and apixaban in preclinical and clinical development. *Thromb Haemost* 2010; **103**: 572–85.

44. Kubitza D, Becka M, Zuehlsdorf M et al. Effects of food, an antacid, and the H2 antagonist ranitidine on the absorption of BAY 59–7939 (rivaroxaban), an oral direct Factor Xa inhibitor, in healthy subjects, *J Clin Pharmacol* 2006; **46**: 549–58.

45. Stangier J, Rathgen K, Stahle H et al. Pharmacokinetics and pharmacodynamics of the direct oral thrombin inhibitor dabigatran in healthy elderly subjects. *Clin Pharmacokinet* 2008; **47**: 47–59.

46. Stangier J, Rathgen K, Stahle H et al. The pharmacokinetics, pharmacodynamics and tolerability of dabigatran etexilate, a new oral direct thrombin inhibitor, in healthy male subjects. *Br J Clin Pharmacol* 2007; **64**: 292–303.

47. European Medicines Agency (EMEA). European public assessment report: Pradaxa. www/emea.europa.eu/humandocs/PFFs/EPAR/pradaxa/H-829-PI-en.pdf.

48. Stangier J, Eriksson BI, Dahl OE et al. Pharmacokinetic profile of the oral direct thrombin inhibitor dabigatran etexilate in healthy volunteers and patients undergoing total hip replacement. *J Clin Pharmacol* 2005; **45**: 555–63.

49. Stangier J, Rathgen K, Stahle H et al. Coadministration of dabigatran etexilate and atorvastatin: assessment of potential impact on pharmacokinetics and pharmacodynamics. *Am J Cardiovasc Drugs* 2009; **9**: 59–68.

50. Stangier J, Stahle H, Rathgen K et al. Coadministration of the oral direct thrombin inhibitor dabigatran etexilate and diclofenac has little impact on the pharmacokinetics of either drug (abstract). XXIst Congress of the International Society of Thrombosis and Haemostasis 2007; P-T-677. Available at: http://isth2007. abstractsondemand.com/. Accessed 7/21/2011.

51. Stangier J, Stahle H, Rathgen K et al. No interaction of the oral direct thrombin inhibitor dabigatran etexilate and digoxin (abstract) XXIst Congress of the International Society of Thrombosis and Haemostasis 2007; P-W-672. Available at http://isth2007. abstractsondemand.com/.

52. Van Ryn J, Stangier J, Naertter S et al. Dabigatran etexilate: a novel, reversible, oral direct thrombin inhibitor: interpretation of coagulation assays and reversal of anticoagulant activity.

Thromb Haemost 2010; **103**(6): 1116–27.

53. Collins R, Scrimogeour A, Yusuf S *et al.* Reduction in fatal pulmonary embolism and venous thrombosis by perioperative administration of subcutaneous heparin: overview of results of randomized trials in general, orthopedic, and urologic surgery. *N Engl J Med* 1988; **318**: 1162–73.

54. Mismetti P, Laporte S, Darmon JY *et al.* Meta-analysis of low molecular weight heparin in the prevention of venous thromboembolism in general surgery. *Br J Surg* 2001; **88**: 913–30.

55. Agnelli G, Bergqvist D, Cohen AT *et al.* Randomized clinical trial of postoperative fondaparinux versus perioperative dalteparin for prevention of venous thromboembolism in high risk abdominal surgery. *Br J Surg* 2005; **92**: 1212–20.

56. Soderdahl DW, Henderson SR, Hansberry KL. A comparison of intermittent pneumatic compression of the calf and whole leg in preventing deep venous thrombosis in urologic surgery. *J Urol* 1997; **157**: 1774–6.

57. Nurmohamed MT, van Riel AM, Henkens CM *et al.* Low molecular weight heparin and compression stockings in the prevention of venous thromboembolism in neurosurgery. *Thromb Haemost* 1996; **75**: 233–8.

58. Agnelli G, Piovella F, Buoncristiani P *et al.* Enoxaparin plus compression stockings compared with compression stockings alone in the prevention of venous thromboembolism after elective neurosurgery. *N Engl J Med* 1998; **339**: 80–5.

59. Goldhaber SZ, Dunn K, Gerhard-Herman M *et al.* Low rate of venous thromboembolism after craniotomy for brain tumor using multimodality prophylaxis. *Chest* 2002; **122**: 1933–7.

60. Collen JF. Prevention of venous thromboembolism in neurosurgery: a metaanalysis. *Chest* 2008; **134**(2): 237–49.

61. Oates-Whitehead RM, D'Angelo A, Mol B. Anticoagulant and aspirin prophylaxis for preventing thromboembolism after major gynecological surgery. *Cochrane Database Syst Rev* 2003; **4**: CD003679.

62. ENOXACAN Study Group. Efficacy and safety of enoxaparin versus unfractionated heparin for prevention of deep vein thrombosis in elective cancer surgery: a double blind randomized multicenter trial with venographic assessment *Br J Surg* 1997; **84**: 1099–103.

63. Baykal C, Al A, Demirtas E *et al.* Comparison of enoxaparin and standard heparin in gynecologic oncologic surgery: a randomized prospective double blind clinical study. *Eur J Gynaec Oncol* 2001; **22**: 127–30.

64. Fricker JP, Vergnes Y, Schach R *et al.* Low dose heparin versus low molecular weight heparin (Fragmin) in the prophylaxis of thromboembolic complications of abdominal oncological surgery. *Eur J Clin Invest* 1988; **18**: 561–7.

65. Heilmann L, von Templehoff GF, Kirkpatrick C *et al.* Comparison of unfractionated versus low molecular weight heparin for deep vein thrombosis prophylaxis during breast and pelvic cancer surgery: efficacy, safety, and follow up. *Clin Appl Thromb Hemost* 1998; **4**: 268–73.

66. Bergqvist D, Agnelli G, Cohen AT *et al.* Duration of prophylaxis against venous thromboembolism with enoxaparin after surgery for cancer. *N Engl J Med* 2002; **346**: 975–80.

67. Eriksson BI, Lassen MR, the PENTassacharide in HIpFRActure Surgery Plus (PENTHIFRA Plus) Investigators. Duration of prophylaxis against venous thromboembolism with fondaparinux after hip fracture surgery: a multi-center, randomized, placebo-controlled, double-blind study. *Arch Intern Med* 2003; **163**: 1337–42.

68. Lassen MR, Raskob GE, Gallus A *et al.* Apixaban or enoxaparin for thromboprophylaxis after knee replacement. *N Eng J Med* 2009; **361**: 594–604.

69. Lassen MR, Raskob GE, Gallus A *et al.* Apixaban versus enoxaparin for thromboprophylaxis after knee replacement (ADVANCE-2): a randomised double-blind trial. *Lancet* 2010; **375**: 807–15.

70. Lassen MR, Gallus A, Raskob GE *et al.* Apixaban versus enoxaparin for thromboprophylaxis after hip replacement. *N Engl J Med* 2010; **363**: 2487–98.

71. Turpie AG, Fisher WD, Bauer KA *et al.* BAY 59-7939: an oral, direct factor Xa inhibitor for the prevention of venous thromboembolism in patients after total knee replacement: a phase II dose-ranging study. *J Thromb Haemost* 2005; **3**: 2479–86.

72. Eriksson BI, Borris LC, Dahl OE *et al.* A once-daily, oral, direct factor Xa inhibitor, rivaroxaban (BAY 59-7939), for thromboprophylaxis after total hip replacement. *Circulation* 2006; **114**: 2374–81.

73. Eriksson BI, Borris L, Dahl OE *et al.* Oral, direct factor Xa inhibition with BAY 59-7939 for the prevention of venous thromboembolism after total hip replacement. *J Thromb Haemost* 2006; **4**: 121–8.

74. Eriksson BI, Borris LC, Friedman RJ *et al.* Rivaroxaban versus enoxaparin for thromboprophylaxis after hip arthroplasty. *N Engl J Med* 2008; **358**: 2765–75.

75. Lassen MR, Ageno W, Borris LC *et al.* Rivaroxaban versus enoxaparin for thromboprophylaxis after total knee arthroplasty. *N Engl J Med* 2008; **358**: 2776–86.

76. Kakkar AK, Brenner B, Dahl OE *et al.* Extended duration rivaroxaban versus short-term enoxaparin for the prevention of venous thromboembolism after total hip arthroplasty: a double-blind, randomised controlled trial. *Lancet* 2008; **372**: 31–9.

77. Turpie AG, Lassen MR, Davidson BL *et al.* Rivaroxaban versus enoxaparin for thromboprophylaxis after total knee arthroplasty (RECORD4): a randomised trial. *Lancet* 2009; **373**: 1673–80.

78. Ginsberg JS, Davidson BL, Comp PC *et al.* Oral thrombin inhibitor dabigatran etexilate vs North American enoxaparin regimen for prevention of venous thromboembolism after knee arthroplasty surgery. *J Arthroplasty* 2009; **24**: 1–9.

79. Eriksson BI, Dahl OE, Rosencher N *et al.* Oral dabigatran etexilate vs. subcutaneous enoxaparin for the prevention of venous thromboembolism after total knee replacement: the RE-MODEL randomized trial. *J Thromb Haemost* 2007; **5**: 2178–85.

80. Eriksson BI, Dahl OE, Rosencher N *et al.* Dabigatran etexilate versus enoxaparin for prevention of venous thromboembolism after total hip

replacement: a randomised, double-blind, non-inferiority trial. *Lancet* 2007; **370**: 949–56.

81. Eriksson BI, Dahl OE, Huo MH *et al.* Oral dabigatran versus enoxaparin for thromboprophylaxis after primary total hip arthroplasty (RE-NOVATE II). *Thromb Haemost* 2011; **105**(4): 721–9.

82. Bergqvist D, Agnelli G, Cohen AT *et al.* Duration of prophylaxis against venous thromboembolism with enoxaparin after surgery for cancer. *N Engl J Med* 2002; **346**: 975–80.

83. Rasmussen MS, Jorgensen LM, Wille-Jorgensen P *et al.* Prolonged prophylaxis with dalteparin to prevent late thromboembolic complications in patients undergoing major abdominal surgery: a multicenter randomized open label study. *J Thromb Haemost* 2006; **4**: 2384–90.

84. Planes A, Vochelle N, Darmon J *et al.* Risk of deep venous thrombosis after hospital discharge in patients having undergone total hip replacement: double-blind randomized comparison of enoxaparin versus placebo. *Lancet* 1996; **348**: 224–8.

85. Bergqvist D, Benoni G, Bjorgell O *et al.* Low molecular weight heparin (enoxaparin) as prophylaxis against venous thromboembolism after total hip replacement. *N Engl J Med* 1996; **335**: 696–700.

86. Eikelboom JW, Quinlan DJ, Douketis JD. Extended-duration prophylaxis against venous thromboembolism after total hip or knee replacement: a meta-analysis of the randomized trials. *Lancet* 2001; **358**: 9–15.

87. Douketis JD, Eikelboom JW, Quinlan DJ *et al.* Short duration prophylaxis against venous thromboembolism after total hip or knee replacement: a meta-analysis of prospective studies investigating symptomatic outcomes. *Arch Intern Med* 2002; **162**: 1465–71.

88. Cohen AT, Bailey CS, Alikhan R *et al.* Extended thromboprophylaxis with low molecular weight heparin reduces symptomatic venous thromboembolism following lower limb arthroplasty: a meta-analysis. *Thromb Haemost* 2001; **85**: 940–1.

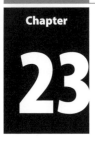

Blood transfusion: preoperative considerations and complications

Julie Katz Karp, Christopher D. Hillyer, and Beth H. Shaz

Introduction

In the USA, blood transfusion is the most common procedure performed in hospitals [1]. Component therapy is the preferred method of blood administration, as it allows blood transfusion to be individualized to the patient's specific needs. Blood components include red cells, platelets, plasma, and cryoprecipitate. Although transfusion is often essential to effective patient care, it is not without risk. Blood transfusion is associated with multiple adverse outcomes, including both non-infectious and infectious complications. Thus, benefits and risks of transfusion must be considered for each patient.

Preoperative blood product ordering
Maximum surgical blood order

A maximum surgical blood order schedule (MSBOS) is used to predict surgical blood needs and to reserve blood products for transfusion for surgery. A MSBOS is created by reviewing institutional blood utilization for each type of surgical procedure and usually set at the number of products required for 80–90% of the procedures. The MSBOS will dictate if either a type and screen (T/S) or a type and cross (T/C) is indicated, as well as the number and type of blood products to be reserved for a particular surgical procedure.

A MSBOS is important because it serves to limit pretransfusion testing and avoid blood wastage. After the creation of an institutional MSBOS, blood utilization is commonly monitored with a crossmatch-to-transfusion (C : T) ratio for each surgical procedure and/or each surgeon. The C : T ratio helps to refine the MSBOS and identify opportunities for blood utilization improvement. A C : T ratio of less than 2 is generally considered optimal. If the patient is anemic or has a clinically significant antibody more red cell products may be crossmatched for the surgical procedure than dictated by the MSBOS [3].

Pretransfusion testing

In order to have blood products ready to be transfused to the patient in the operating room a number of steps must occur. First, an appropriately labeled patient specimen must

be received in the transfusion service. Second, the patient's specimen must be tested for ABO group and D type and for the presence of unexpected antibodies. Lastly red cell products need to be crossmatched with the patient's sample and other components may need to be prepared as ordered.

Recipient identification and labeling of samples

A properly labeled pretransfusion blood specimen from the intended transfusion recipient is crucial to safe blood transfusion. The majority of hemolytic transfusion reactions are due to patient misidentification or labeling errors in pretransfusion blood specimens.

Phlebotomists drawing pretransfusion blood specimens must definitively confirm the identity of the patient. This may involve examining a patient wristband and asking the patient to verbally confirm his/her identity. Other systems of patient identification and blood specimen collection may include bar-code identification systems, radio frequency tags, or pre-prepared labels.

Once the patient's identity is confirmed, the phlebotomist must indelibly label each specimen at the patient's bedside with two independent patient identifiers and the date of collection. Additionally, the identity of the phlebotomist must be documented on the specimen itself, on the requisition, or electronically.

Upon receipt by the blood bank, the labeled pretransfusion blood specimen and the information on the pretransfusion testing request must be confirmed to be identical. If any discrepancies are identified or there is any question as to the identity of the patient, a new specimen must be obtained. Strict labeling policies protect the patient from blood typing errors and ABO incompatible transfusions [2].

Type and screen/type and crossmatch

A type and screen (T/S) involves typing the patient's red cells for ABO and D type (also known as the Rh type), as well as screening the patient's plasma for clinically significant red cell antibodies. A type and crossmatch (T/C) is equivalent to a

Medical Management of the Surgical Patient, ed. Michael F. Lubin, Thomas F. Dodson, and Neil H. Winawer. Published by Cambridge University Press. © Cambridge University Press 2013.

T/S, but also includes the process of selecting, crossmatching, and reserving appropriate red cell products for the patient.

Typing the patient for ABO and D type is done both by testing the patient's red cells with commercial antisera (called a forward type) and testing the patient's plasma for the presence of anti-A and anti-B (called a reverse type). If the forward and reverse types agree, an ABO and D type can be determined.

The patient's plasma is screened for the presence of unexpected antibodies prior to red cell transfusion. Screening the patient for clinically significant red cell antibodies requires the patient's plasma and commercially prepared red cells from 2–3 different people with known red cell antigens. The patient's plasma is added to each of these 2–3 commercially prepared red cells and assessed for agglutination. If no agglutination is observed, the screen is considered negative. If agglutination is observed, the screen is considered positive and further investigation is initiated to determine the identity of the patient's red cell antibody.

Once the identity of the patient's red cell antibody has been established, the transfusion service will determine if the antibody is clinically significant. Although not all antibodies identified are clinically significant, those that are may cause red cell hemolysis or shortened survival of transfused red cells. If the antibody is clinically significant, the transfusion service will select and reserve red cell products for the patient that do not carry the reciprocal antigen. Additionally, the blood bank will automatically increase the number of products crossmatched for the surgical procedure.

Determining the identity of a patient's red cell antibody and crossmatching the appropriate red cell products can take several hours and, rarely, days, depending upon the antibody or antibodies identified. To prevent delays, patients should have a T/S or T/C blood specimen sent to the blood bank well in advance of any scheduled surgical procedure. Because the majority of clinically significant antibodies are formed in response to previous pregnancy or transfusion, this is particularly true in the case of patients with a history of previous surgery, pregnancy, or transfusion. Institutional policies will dictate how far in advance a specimen can be drawn, however in patients with a negative antibody screen and no history of transfusion or pregnancy in the preceding 3 months, blood bank specimens may be drawn up to 1 month before surgery. If the patient has been transfused or pregnant in the preceding 3 months, a pre-transfusion specimen is valid only for 3 days [2,3].

Blood products

Whole blood is typically divided into red cell product, platelet product, and plasma product. Plasma products can then be divided into cryoprecipitate and cryoprecipitate reduced plasma. In addition, products can be collected through automated apheresis instruments. In the USA, the majority of platelet products are collected through apheresis and a growing number of red cell products are collected through apheresis.

Plasma collected through apheresis is usually used for manufacturing plasma derivatives, such as intravenous immunoglobulin and human derived factor concentrates (Table 23.1). Granulocytes, which are beyond the scope of this chapter, are usually collected through apheresis and used in patients with severe infection and profound neutropenia.

Whole blood

Whole blood refers to a blood product in which the red cells, platelets, and plasma have not been divided into separate components. While whole blood provides both oxygen-carrying capacity (red cells) and coagulation factors (plasma), few viable platelets are present in whole blood after more than 24 hours of refrigerated storage. By contrast, stable clotting factors are well preserved in stored whole blood. Whole blood must be ABO identical to that of the recipient [2].

Whole blood has largely been replaced by individual blood components, as most patients only require one component (red cells, platelets, or plasma). Although controversial, whole blood is still used in complex pediatric cases primarily to decrease donor exposure and in military combat due to lack of available platelet products [3].

Red cell products

Red cell products are most commonly made from whole blood by removing 200–250 mL plasma. Red cell products can also be made using apheresis technology, by which two products are collected from a single donor in one collection. Regardless of the method of collection, red cell products are stored at 1–6 °C in one of several anticoagulant preservative solutions.

Each of these anticoagulant-preservative solutions contain variable amounts and types of anticoagulants and preservatives, including citrate, dextrose, adenine, and mannitol. The type of preservative solution used determines the hematocrit and shelf life of the product. Red cells stored in CPD (sodium citrate, citric acid, dextrose, monobasic sodium phosphate) have a hematocrit of 65–80% and a shelf life of 21 days. Red cells stored in CPDA-1 (sodium citrate, citric acid, dextrose, monobasic sodium phosphate, adenine) also have a hematocrit of 65–80% and a shelf life of 35 days. Red cells stored in additive solution (AS-1: dextrose, adenine, mannitol, sodium chloride; AS-3: dextrose, adenine, monobasic sodium phosphate, sodium chloride, sodium citrate, citric acid; AS-5 dextrose, adenine, manitol, sodium chloride) have a lower hematocrit of 55–65% and the longest shelf life of 42 days. In the USA, the majority of red cell products are stored in additive solutions.

Red cells are indicated for treatment of anemia (decreased red cell mass) in patients who require increased oxygen-carrying capacity. Although much research has been devoted to determining optimal red cell transfusion triggers, red cell transfusion requirements should be based on the clinical status of the patient and related medical conditions. A number of randomized clinical trials in ICU patients have demonstrated

Table 23.1 Blood product characteristics.

Product	Volume	Composition	Storage conditions	Storage length	Comments
Red cells	300–350 mL	200 mL red cells, 50–100 mL plasma, 50–100 mL anticoagulant and additive solution	1–6 °C	• CPD: 21 days • CPDA-1: 35 days • AS: 42 days	• Leukoreduced: $< 5 \times 10^6$ leukocytes • Red cells must be ABO compatible with patient plasma
Platelets	50 mL per unit; 200–400 mL per apheresis unit	Platelets suspended in sufficient plasma or platelet additive solution	20–24 °C with constant gentle agitation	• 5 days • Pooled in an open system: 4 hours	• Whole blood-derived platelets: $> 5.5 \times 10^{10}$ platelets per unit • Whole blood-derived platelets into pools of 4–6 units • Apheresis platelets: $> 3 \times 10^{11}$ platelets • Pool or apheresis, leukoreduced: $< 5 \times 10^6$ leukocytes • ABO compatibility is not required
Plasma	200–250 mL	One mL of FFP contains one unit of coagulation factor activity	−18 °C; 1–6 °C after thawing	• Frozen shelf life: 1 year • FFP/FP24 after thaw: 24 hours • Thawed plasma: 5 days	• FFP: Plasma frozen within 8 hours of phlebotomy • FP24: Plasma frozen within 24 hours of phlebotomy • Thawed plasma: FFP/FP24 stored for up to 4 days beyond outdate • Plasma must be ABO compatible with patient red cells
Cryoprecipitate	10–15 mL per unit	80–120 units factor VIII, > 150 mg fibrinogen, factor XIII, von Willebrand factor	−18 °C; room temperature after thawing	• Frozen shelf life: 1 year • Thawed/pooled in an open system: 4 hours • Thawed/pooled in a closed system: 6 hours	• ABO compatibility is not required

Table 23.2 Red cell products and compatibility with plasma.

Patient type	Red cell product type			
	O	A	B	AB
O	yes	no	no	no
A	yes	yes	no	no
B	yes	no	yes	no
AB	yes	yes	yes	yes

that a hemoglobin threshold of 7 g/dL results in an equivalent patient outcome as threshold of 10 g/dL. Thus, a hemoglobin of 7 g/dL is typically used as a threshold in a non-bleeding patient without active cardiac disease. Red cell transfusion is also indicated in sickle cell patients requiring simple transfusion or red cell exchange, as well as in patients with parasitized red cells secondary to babesiosis or malaria. In an average adult, one red cell product will increase the hemoglobin by about 1 g/dL and the hematocrit by about 3%. In children 10–15 mL/kg of RBCs raises the hemoglobin about 2–3g/dL [4]. Red cell products must be compatible with the recipient's plasma (Table 23.2) [2].

Product modification

Red cells and other blood products can be modified to decrease the adverse effects of transfusion, including the transmission of disease, and facilitate the availability of rare products. Blood product modifications include leuko-reduced, irradiated, frozen volume reduced, and washed products.

Over 85% of red cell and platelet products transfused in the USA are leuko-reduced, a process by which 99.9% of the white blood cells (WBCs) are removed. Leuko-reduction of blood components reduces the incidence of febrile non-hemolytic transfusion reactions (FNTRs) and decreases the risk of transfusion transmitted cytomegalovirus (CMV) and other infections transmitted by WBCs. Leuko-reduction also decreases the incidence of HLA alloimmunization and may decrease the incidence of transfusion related immunomodulation (TRIM), which is a transient depression of the immune system following transfusion [5,6].

Irradiation of cellular blood products (typically defined as red cell, platelet, and granulocyte products) prevents transfusion-associated graft-versus-host-disease (TA-GVHD). Transfusion-associated graft-versus-host-disease occurs when donor lymphocytes engraft in the recipient, resulting in tissue damage with nearly uniform fatality. It is seen in immunocompromised recipients who cannot mount an immunological response against donor lymphocytes or in recipients who do not recognize donor lymphocytes as foreign. Irradiation of red cells shortens their storage period to 28 days from irradiation, or their original outdate, whichever comes first [7].

Red cells are frozen to increase length of storage, which can be up to 10 years or more. Thus, red cell products with rare phenotypes can be frozen for a decade or more for use by patients with red cell antibodies to high frequency antigens or rare combinations of antigens. Frozen red cells must be thawed and thoroughly washed to remove the cryoprotectant (usually glycerol). Since washed cellular blood products are devoid of plasma and supernatant, they are indicated for patients who have a history of severe allergic, anaphylactoid, or anaphylactic reactions. Washed components can also be used for patients at risk for transfusion related hyperkalemia. Washed red cells expire 24 hours after washing [8]. Volume reduction of products also removes plasma/supernatant and can be used for volume-sensitive patients, and to decrease risk of hyperkalemia.

Alternatives to allogeneic red cell transfusion

Alternatives to allogeneic red cell transfusion are usually considered in patients at risk for a substantial blood loss during the procedure (usually defined as more than one liter). Each of these alternatives has a potential benefit and cost.

Preoperative autologous donation

Patients may donate their own blood in the weeks prior to a scheduled surgery, a process referred to as preoperative autologous donation (PAD). The advantages of PAD include: reduced risk of infectious disease transmission, reduced risk of alloimmunization to donor antigens, and availability of compatible products, if the patient requires rare red cell products. Disadvantages include: increased cost relative to allogeneic products, adverse reactions associated with autologous blood donation, and iatrogenic preoperative anemia secondary to the autologous donation. Preoperative autologous donation products are more expensive because special handling ensures they are only transfused to the intended recipient and they are frequently wasted. The wastage rate for autologous products is about 60%, suggesting that most preoperative autologous donations are unnecessary.

Patients donating a preoperative autologous product should have a hematocrit of at least 33% (hemoglobin 11 g/dL). Contraindications to PAD include: infection or risk of bacteremia, active seizure disorder, uncontrolled hypertension, recent myocardial infarction, aortic stenosis, cerebrovascular accident, and severe cardiopulmonary disease. The PAD product should be collected more than 72 hours prior to the scheduled surgery. Preoperative autologous donations products are stored at 1–6 °C for 35 to 42 days, depending on the preservative solution.

It is important to remember that there is risk associated with the transfusion of autologous blood. Clerical errors may result in the patient receiving the wrong product. Furthermore, bacterial contamination and transfusion associated circulatory overload remain a concern with autologous transfusion [3].

Directed blood donation

Directed donors are individuals who donate blood products for use by a specific patient, typically a family member or friend. Although directed donors are typically motivated by compassion for the patient, it is important to note that products from directed donations are not safer than those from volunteer donations. In particular, it is thought that in their enthusiasm to help the patient, the directed donor may intentionally or unintentionally omit facts that might defer them from donating. This omission may compromise the safety of the resulting directed donation. By contrast, directed donations from relatives may be medically indicated when a patient requires HLA-matched products or red cells with a rare phenotype. To prevent TA-GVHD, all directed donations from blood relatives should be irradiated [3].

Intraoperative blood recovery

Intraoperative blood recovery may utilize several techniques to salvage and reinfuse blood lost during a surgical procedure. The simplest approach to intraoperative blood recovery is direct reinfusion of recovered blood without washing. In this method, recovered blood is collected, anticoagulant is added, and blood is reinfused within 4 hours of the end of collection.

Alternatively, devices are available that can wash the recovered blood with saline prior to reinfusion. These devices are able to collect and process large volumes quickly, making intraoperative blood salvage practical in surgical procedures with rapid blood loss. Blood recovered by these methods must be reinfused within 4 hours of the end of collection, or, if stored at 1–6 °C, within 24 hours of the start of collection.

Intraoperative blood recovery has several limitations that may compromise the safety of the collected product. Contraindications for intraoperative blood recovery include blood recovery from contaminated surgical sites, blood recovery from surgical procedures for neoplastic processes (possible risk of tumor cells in the recovered blood), and blood collected in surgical sites treated with medications. These increased risks must be balanced by the patient's need for blood and their willingness to receive allogeneic transfusions [4].

Acute normovolemic hemodilution

Acute normovolemic hemodilution (ANH) involves the intraoperative removal of whole blood into standard collection bags with concomitant crystalloid or colloid volume replacement to the patient. Hemodilution reduces red cell loss, as a bleeding patient with an iatrogenically lowered hematocrit loses fewer red cells.

The patient's cardiovascular status is monitored closely during the intraoperative hemodilution process. The removed whole blood products are stored in the operating room and are reinfused in reverse order of collection. This allows for the products with the highest hematocrit to be transfused last, presumably when surgical bleeding has been controlled. In addition, ANH products have coagulation factors and functioning platelets, if stored at room temperature. The iatrogenic anemia introduced by ANH can affect oxygen transport, but this is usually offset by the decrease in blood viscosity and compensatory cardiac output. If stored at room temperature, the collected products must be used within 8 hours of the start of collection. If stored at 1–6 °C, the collected product must be used within 24 hours of the start of collection [4].

Postoperative blood collection

Both canister systems and red cell processors can be used to collect postoperative blood drainage from serosal cavities. Because blood salvaged from serosal cavities typically has little residual fibrinogen or platelets, the addition of anticoagulants to collected blood is typically not necessary.

Collected blood will contain free hemoglobin, as well as contaminants like tissue exudate, bone, bone marrow, and other biological and surgical materials. Adverse effects of collected postoperative blood transfusion can include respiratory distress, hypotension with anaphylaxis, and fever. Blood collected postoperatively must be used within 6 hours of the start of collection [4].

Platelet products

Platelet products can be manufactured from whole blood or apheresis collections. Platelets derived from whole blood are called *platelets* by the FDA, but are also commonly referred to as *whole blood derived platelets*, *random donor platelets*, or *platelet concentrates*. Each platelet unit derived from whole blood contains approximately 5.5×10^{10} platelets, and usually five of these units are pooled together to make a therapeutic dose. Platelets collected by apheresis are called *platelets, pheresis* by the FDA, but are also commonly referred to as *single donor platelets*, *apheresis platelets*, and *plateletpheresis*. The required minimum content for a platelet product collected by apheresis is 3.0×10^{11} platelets. Many apheresis-derived platelet collections contain 2 or 3 times the required minimum and are subsequently split to make multiple platelet products from a single donation.

Platelet transfusions are used for prophylaxis to prevent bleeding or as treatment for bleeding in thrombocytopenic patients. Platelet transfusion is also indicated in patients with qualitative defects in platelet function, either inherited or acquired secondary to disease or anti-platelet medications. The threshold to transfuse platelets is determined by the patient's platelet count in addition to the underlying disease and the presence of bleeding.

In adults, a typical platelet dose is a single apheresis product or 4–6 whole blood-derived platelet units pooled. Most ordering physicians will transfuse a single platelet dose in non-bleeding thrombocytopenic patients at platelet counts below 10,000/μL, with higher thresholds in patients with fever, sepsis, or coagulopathy. Platelet transfusion is also indicated during surgery or before invasive procedures at platelet counts below 50,000/μL. In children, transfusion of 10 mL/kg of platelets generally results in an increase in platelet count of 50,000–100,000/μL. If platelet products are pooled in an open system, the product must be transfused within 4 hours of pooling. Although platelet products from all ABO groups are acceptable for all recipients, whenever possible, platelet products should be compatible with the recipient's red cells. The particular risk is for group O platelets being transfused into group A, B, or AB patients and resulting in hemolysis. Many blood banks are now titering their group O platelet products in order to prevent these reactions. High-titer products (usually defined as anti-A titer greater than 1 : 100) are then transfused to group O patients only.

Response to platelet transfusion can be assessed by improvement of bleeding and through measuring the post-transfusion increment typically collected 15–60 minutes after transfusion. A typical dose of platelets, as described above, can be expected to increase the patient's platelet count by 30,000–60,000/μL. A significant number of clinical conditions can be expected to decrease the expected post-transfusion increment. These conditions can include fever, sepsis, disseminated intravascular coagulation, and bleeding as well as HLA and/or platelet antibodies. A more formal evaluation of the platelet increment can be performed using the corrected count increment (CCI). The CCI accounts for both the patient's size (via body surface area) and the number of platelets in the transfused product.

$$CCI = \frac{\text{Body surface area}(\text{m}^2) \times \text{Platelet count increment} \times 10^{11}}{\text{Number of platelets transfused}}$$

Each unit of platelets contains a minimum of 5.5×10^{10} platelets and a unit of apheresis platelets contains at least 3.0×10^{11} platelets. A 1 hour CCI > 7.5 is considered acceptable. A CCI < 7.5 is suggestive of platelet refractoriness and the patient should be evaluated for an underlying cause. Evaluation of platelet refractoriness usually includes HLA and platelet antibody screens. If the patient has HLA or platelet-specific antibodies, HLA-matched, antigen negative, or cross-matched platelets can be transfused [4].

Platelet products can be modified to decrease the risk of adverse events from transfusion, in addition to leuko-reduction, irradiation, and washing/volume reduction as described above.

First, platelet products are screened for the presence of bacteria to decrease the risk of septic transfusion reactions. Bacteria screening has decreased septic reactions by over 50%. Second, the risk of TRALI (transfusion related acute lung injury) can be mitigated by testing platelet donors for human leukocyte antigen (HLA) antibodies or using smaller amounts of plasma. Lastly, platelet products can be stored in platelet additive solutions, decreasing the risk of allergic transfusion reactions or hemolytic transfusion reactions due to ABO incompatibility between the donor and recipient. Current FDA-approved platelet additive solution is 35% plasma and 65% platelet additive solution (acetate, phosphate, citrate, and sodium chloride). Alternative platelet additive solutions will likely be FDA approved in the future.

Plasma products

Plasma products can be manufactured from whole blood donations after centrifugation and red cell removal or by apheresis. Plasma products referred to as *fresh frozen plasma* (FFP) are frozen at −18 °C or colder within 8 hours of collection. Alternatively, if plasma is frozen at −18 °C or colder within 24 hours of collection, it is referred to as *plasma frozen within 24 hours after phlebotomy* (FP24). Once frozen, both FFP and FP24 have a frozen shelf life of 1 year. Prior to transfusion, FFP and FP24 must be thawed in a 30–37 °C water bath for 20–30 minutes. Thawed FFP or FP24 should be transfused immediately or stored at 1–6 °C for up to 24 hours. The storage of FFP or FP24 can be extended up to four additional days at 1–6 °C to prevent wastage, and is referred to as *thawed plasma* and is required to be labeled as such. An additional plasma product, referred to as *plasma, cryoprecipitate-reduced*, is the plasma that remains after removal of cryoprecipitate. Plasma, cryoprecipitate reduced (also known as cryoprecipitate reduced plasma) is indicated only for use in the treatment of thrombocytopenic thrombotic purpura (TTP), since it is lacking fibrinogen, von Willebrand factor and other coagulation factors.

Fresh frozen plasma contains approximately 1 IU/mL of each clotting factor. By comparison, FP24 has approximately 20% less factor VIII, which in non-hemophilia A patients is clinically insignificant. Thawed plasma has further decreased levels of factors VII, V, and VII, but these differences are not usually clinically significant. Thus, for most clinical purposes, FFP, FP24, and thawed plasma are considered equivalent and interchangeable.

Plasma transfusions are usually used to either prevent bleeding or treat hemorrhage in patients with congenital or acquired coagulopathies, as measured by the prothrombin time (PT), international normalized ratio (INR), and activated partial thromboplastin time (aPTT). There is no defined laboratory value that serves as a trigger for plasma transfusion. Minor prolongations in coagulation tests are uncommonly associated with bleeding. As such, plasma transfusion is indicated only when the PT and aPTT suggest factor levels less than 30% or the INR is 1.6 or higher. Plasma is indicated for acute reversal of warfarin in patients with life-threatening bleeding. Plasma is also indicated as replacement fluid for plasma exchange in patients with thrombotic thrombocytopenic purpura (TTP) and other diseases.

The typical dose of plasma is 10–20 mL/kg for adults and children. As each single plasma unit product is 200–300 mL, an average adult dose is 2–4 plasma products. Coagulation factors are expected to increase by 20% immediately after infusion [4]. Plasma products must be compatible with the recipient's red cells (Table 23.3) [2].

Table 23.3 Plasma products and red cell compatibility.

Patient type	Plasma product type			
	O	A	B	AB
O	yes	yes	yes	yes
A	no	yes	no	yes
B	no	no	yes	yes
AB	no	no	no	yes

Alternatives to plasma transfusion

Desmopressin

Desmopressin (DDAVP) is primarily used for treatment of von Willebrand disease, but also has been reported to be effective in treating bleeding associated with uremia and congenital platelet function abnormalities. DDAVP can be administered via nasal spray or intravenous dosing, and test doses should be given to confirm patient responsiveness. Tachyphylaxis is well documented with DDAVP treatment. Patients unresponsive to DDAVP can be treated with exogenous von Willebrand factor concentrates [3].

Prothrombin complex concentrates

Prothrombin complex concentrates (PCCs) offer an alternative to plasma transfusion for rapidly replacing clotting factors and correcting the INR. Prothrombin complex concentrates (PCCs) contain a combination of vitamin K-dependent clotting factors (factors II, VII, IX, and X), with factor content varying by the type of PCC. PCCs currently available in the USA include a non-activated factor IX complex, Profilnine, and an activated PCC with factor VIII inhibitor bypassing activity, FEIBA. Both are approved for use primarily in hemophilia patients with factor inhibitors, but off-label use is not uncommon.

The use of PCCs is not without risk. Thrombosis and DIC have been reported, as have allergic reactions. Additionally, viral inactivation processes applied to PCCs are less effective at the removal of parvovirus B19 and Hepatitis A. As such, infusion of PCCs carries a risk of infection with these viruses [4].

Recombinant factor VIIa

Recombinant factor VIIa (rFVIIa, NovoSeven) is approved to treat patients with inhibitors to factor VIII or factor IX and in patients with congenital factor VII deficiency. However, like PCCs, it is not infrequently used off-label to treat patients with a variety of bleeding complications. rFVIIa directly activates factor X, causing a thrombin burst and clot formation. Appropriate dosing is controversial, and rFVIIa should be used in consultation with a physician experienced in its use. Adverse effects of rFVIIa include venous and arterial thromboembolism [3].

Cryoprecipitate

Cryoprecipitate is also known as *cryoprecipitated antihemophilic factor* (AHF). Cryoprecipitate is made by thawing fresh frozen plasma at 1–6 °C. During this thawing process, a precipitate forms (the cryoprecipitate) which is subsequently removed and refrozen. Cryoprecipitate contains fibrinogen, fibronectin, factor VIII, von Willebrand factor, and factor XIII. Cryoprecipitate and the supernatant (cryoprecipitate poor plasma) are both refrozen and stored up to 1 year from collection.

Historically, cryoprecipitate was used as factor VIII replacement in hemophilia A patients and as von Willebrand factor replacement in patients with von Willebrand disease. Currently, there are purified and virally inactivated products for both of these indications (and recombinant products for factor VIII), thus cryoprecipitate is no longer indicated for the treatment of these conditions. Cryoprecipitate is used primarily for fibrinogen replacement. Cryoprecipitate is also occasionally used as factor XIII replacement and in the manufacture of fibrin sealants and glue. In the USA, human purified and virally inactivated fibrinogen concentrate and fibrin sealants are available.

Cryoprecipitate is used for fibrinogen replacement in acquired hypofibrinogenemia with disseminated intravascular coagulopathy, liver failure, the anhepatic phase of liver transplantation, and massive transfusion with dilutional coagulopathy. Cryoprecipitate should be given when fibrinogen levels fall below 100 mg/dL. Cryoprecipitate is also used for fibrinogen replacement in patients with dysfibrinogenemia, where fibrinogen is present but functionally defective. Cryoprecipitate was previously used for congenital hypofibrinogenemia. However, in January 2009, the FDA approved a human-derived, lyophilized, fibrinogen concentrate for this indication.

Per AABB Standards for Blood Banks and Transfusion Services, each unit of cryoprecipitate must contain a minimum of 150 mg fibrinogen and 80 IU of factor VIII. Each single 10–15 mL unit of cryoprecipitate will increase the fibrinogen concentration by approximately 50 mg/dL per 10 kg of body weight. For adult patients, a typical dose is 10 units of cryoprecipitate, which are pooled into a single bag for transfusion. For children, the typical dose is 1–2 units per 10 kg. Each unit of cryoprecipitate takes 10–15 minutes to thaw in a 30–37 °C water bath, although several units can be thawed at one time. Pooling may take an additional 10–15 minutes. Alternatively, some institutions now have pre-pooled cryoprecipitate. These pre-pooled units are usually composed of five single units of cryoprecipitate pooled prior to freezing, and thus, do not require pooling post thaw. Once thawed, a single or pre-pooled unit of cryoprecipitate expires in 6 hours; pooled units using an open system expire in 4 hours. Cryoprecipitate from all ABO groups are acceptable for all recipients since cryoprecipitate contains 10–15 mL of plasma [4].

Transfusion in emergency situations
Massive transfusion

Massive transfusion is defined as transfusion of 10 or more red cell products within 24 hours. Other definitions of massive transfusion include replacement of 50% of total blood volume within 3 hours or blood loss exceeding 150 mL per minute.

Historically, volume resuscitation during severe hemorrhage involved significant crystalloid or colloid infusion and many red cell products. This initial resuscitation was then followed by component therapy, given as needed and guided by laboratory values. Laboratory directed component therapy has now been replaced by massive transfusion protocols (MTPs), which employ specified numbers of blood products issued at predetermined ratios early in the resuscitation period. The ratios of blood products used reflect that of whole blood. In addition, crystalloid infusion is minimized due to studies demonstrating an association between volume of crystalloid resuscitation and adverse outcomes. Early reports in the military theater, as well as more recent studies in civilian healthcare, have demonstrated improved mortality with these protocols.

A multidisciplinary symposium held at the US Army Institute of Surgical Research in 2005 led to the recommendation of a 1 : 1 : 1 ratio of red cells, plasma, and platelets during massive transfusion. A 2007 retrospective study demonstrated improved survival with more plasma transfused per each RBC product in damage-control resuscitation [9]. Studies are currently underway to further refine blood product ratios in MTPs.

Aside from the quantities of blood products to be administered, MTPs also define communication pathways between the laboratory, transfusion service, and clinical team, the timing of blood product availability, laboratory testing algorithms, and other patient care needs. MTPs are designed to ensure optimal transfusion therapy to prevent and treat the coagulopathy that can occur in the minutes to hours after injury.

Massive transfusion is frequently complicated by a multifactorial coagulopathy. The patient's underlying condition results in the consumption of platelets and coagulation factors. Transfusion of red cell products often causes a dilutional coagulopathy, as red cell products contain minimal amounts of clotting factors. Furthermore, transfusion of stored, refrigerated red cell products can cause hypothermia, impaired metabolism of citrate and lactate, release of potassium (which subsequently returns to the red cells), and reduced ability of the transfused RBCs to release oxygen due to decreased 2,3-DPG levels. All of these changes may adversely affect the recipient during massive transfusion [4].

Emergency release of blood products

The emergent release of blood products is required when the urgency of the clinical situation and the need for transfusion precludes completion of pretransfusion testing, including T/C. This is most commonly encountered when resuscitating trauma patients or other patients who acutely require transfusion. In these instances, uncross-matched group O red cells and group AB plasma should be issued. D-negative red cells should be used for female patients with childbearing potential in order to prevent formation of anti-D.

Each organization should have a policy for emergency issue of blood products. A physician signature is required for the emergent release of blood products and to indicate the nature of the emergency. A pretransfusion patient sample should also be obtained as soon as possible after patient arrival. Uncross-matched blood products will continue to be issued until cross-matched type-specific products can be identified. This will allow for emergent patient treatment while preserving the limited type O red cell and AB plasma product supply [3].

Non-infectious adverse effects of blood transfusion

The adverse effects of blood transfusion can be classified as acute (within 6 hours) or delayed (days to years) and infectious versus non-infectious [10].

Acute transfusion reactions

Acute hemolytic transfusion reaction

Acute hemolytic transfusion reactions (AHTRs) occur when preformed recipient red cell antibodies bind to transfused red cell antigens resulting in antigen-antibody complex formation. This complex formation activates the complement cascade and causes intravascular hemolysis. Most commonly, AHTRs are severe reactions due to ABO incompatibility. This occurs when transfused red cell antigens are incompatible with the recipient's plasma (e.g., group A red cells into group O recipient) or, less commonly, when transfused plasma contains antibodies against the recipient's red cell antigens (e.g., group O plasma into group A recipient). Acute hemolytic transfusion reactions can also be associated with antigen-antibody complex formation outside of the ABO system, patients with ongoing hemolytic disease, and non-immune causes.

The incidence of ABO incompatible red cell transfusion is approximately 1 in 50,000 transfusions. Approximately 50% of ABO incompatible red cell transfusions have no adverse effect, while 5% are fatal. ABO incompatible red cell transfusions

most commonly occur with mis-transfusion, when the patient receives the wrong blood. Mis-transfusion is usually caused by human error, including improper identification of the intended recipient during pretransfusion sample collection, improper ABO typing of the blood component or the intended recipient, or improper identification of the recipient and/or the blood product at the time of transfusion.

The signs and symptoms of AHTRs are fever, chills/rigors, anxiety, chest and abdominal pain, flank and back pain, nausea, vomiting, dyspnea, hemoglobinuria, diffuse bleeding, and oliguria/anuria. If an AHTR is suspected, the transfusion should be stopped immediately and reported to the blood bank for investigation. Diagnosis is based on laboratory evidence of hemolysis and evidence of incompatible blood transfusion [4].

Acute hemolytic transfusion reactions can be prevented by ensuring proper pretransfusion sample, transfusion recipient, and blood product identification. Each institution must develop and implement policies and procedures to identify patients, specimen tubes, and blood products. These policies and procedures are varied, but may include barcode based identification systems, non-barcode based identification systems, and radiofrequency identification systems, as briefly described above [2].

Febrile non-hemolytic transfusion reaction

Febrile non-hemolytic transfusion reactions (FNTRs) are defined as a temperature increase of ≥ 1 °C associated with transfusion and/or chills/rigor. By definition, the temperature increase cannot be attributed to other etiologies.

Febrile non-hemolytic transfusion reactions occur in approximately 1% of platelet transfusions and 0.2% of red cell transfusions. In platelet products, FNTRs are caused by leukocyte-derived cytokines which accumulate in the product during storage. In red cell products, these reactions are caused by donor leukocytes interacting with patient white cell antibodies. Of note, the incidence of FNTRs has significantly decreased with the widespread use of leuko-reduction.

If a FNTR is suspected, the transfusion should be stopped and reported to the blood bank for investigation. Supportive care should be given to the patient. Some providers provide prophylactic antipyretics for all transfusions in all patients, while others only order antipyretics in patients with prior FNTRs. Still others are opposed to the use of prophylactic antipyretics, because data do not support its use in prevention of reactions [2,4].

Allergic transfusion reaction

Allergic transfusion reactions occur when pre-formed recipient antibodies bind to transfused allergens. Allergic transfusion reactions occur in approximately 0.5% of red cell transfusions and 1% of platelet and plasma transfusions. Anaphylactic reactions occur in approximately 1 in 20,000 transfusions.

The majority of allergic transfusion reactions are mild. Mild reactions consist of urticaria with or without generalized pruritus or flushing. More severe symptoms include hoarseness, stridor, wheezing, dyspnea, hypotension, gastrointestinal symptoms and shock. Mild reactions can be treated with antihistamines, while more severe reactions can be treated with epinephrine, H1-receptor antagonists, and steroids.

Anaphylactic reactions may be secondary to anti-IgA, usually found in patients with IgA deficiency. Patients who have severe allergic reactions should be tested for IgA deficiency and the presence of anti-IgA. If anti-IgA is identified, the patient should receive plasma products from IgA deficient donors or washed red cell and platelets products.

Allergic transfusion reactions can be mitigated with premedication with antihistamines, but only in patients with a history of allergic reactions. Oral premedication with antihistamines should be given 30–60 minutes before transfusion, while intravenous premedication should be given 10 minutes before transfusion [2,4].

Transfusion-associated circulatory overload

Transfusion-associated circulatory overload (TACO) results from circulatory overload following the transfusion of blood products, and is most common in very young or very old patients with cardiac dysfunction or positive fluid balance. The incidence of TACO is unknown, but it is increasingly recognized clinically. Studies have reported the incidence to be as high as 1 in 700 to 1 in 5,000 blood products transfused. One study reported a mortality rate of 1.3% [2].

Symptoms include dyspnea, orthopnea, cough, chest tightness, cyanosis, hypertension, and headache. Symptoms usually present at the end of transfusion but may occur up to 6 hours post-transfusion. Diagnosis is based on the presence of cardiogenic pulmonary edema. Management includes discontinuing transfusion, diuretic therapy, oxygen supplementation, and sitting the patient upright. Transfusion-associated circulatory overload can be prevented by avoiding rapid transfusion, unless clinically indicated. Transfusions should be administered slowly, usually 1 mL/kg per hour, particularly in patients at risk for TACO [4].

Transfusion-related acute lung injury

Transfusion-related acute lung injury (TRALI) is noncardiogenic pulmonary edema associated with the transfusion of blood products. Transfusion-related acute lung injury is caused by neutrophil and pulmonary endothelial activation, usually caused by transfused donor white cell antibodies, including human leukocyte antigen (HLA) antibodies and human neutrophil antigen (HNA) antibodies. These donor antibodies react with the recipient's white cells in the pulmonary vasculature causing leuko-agglutination, activation of the complement cascade, cytokine release, and pulmonary edema. Approximately 5% of TRALI is caused by the opposite mechanisms, which are recipient white cell antibodies against transfused donor white cells. Non-immune mechanisms are also thought to mediate TRALI, including bioactive lipids and CD40 ligand.

Although TRALI is believed to be underdiagnosed and underreported, TRALI is the most common cause of transfusion-associated mortality in the USA. It is usually associated with transfusion of blood products containing large volumes of plasma. Signs and symptoms appear within 2–6 hours of transfusion and include respiratory distress with dyspnea, tachypnea, hypoxia, fever, tachycardia, and hypotension. Bilateral pulmonary infiltrates on chest X-ray may be seen with no evidence of left atrial hypertension. In cases of suspected TRALI, the transfusion should be discontinued. Medical management is primary supportive, commonly with supplemental oxygen and endotracheal intubation, if needed. Diuresis is not indicated, and the role of steroids is unclear. The majority of patients improve within 2 days, although TRALI has a 5–10% mortality rate [4].

In the USA, multiple strategies have been implemented to reduce the risk of TRALI. First, donors implicated in prior TRALI reactions are deferred from further blood donation. Second, multiparous female donors can be tested for HLA and HNA antibodies, as these are most commonly identified in this population. Female donors with high-titer antibodies are typically deferred from platelet and plasma donation. Third, plasma supplied to hospitals for transfusion can be all male; and female plasma is diverted for fractionation. These strategies have significantly reduced the risk of TRALI without significantly reducing blood product availability [2].

Hypotensive transfusion reactions

Hypotensive transfusion reactions have been reported, usually associated with red cell or platelet transfusions. These reactions appear to be related to the generation of bradykinin, resulting in vasodilation and hypotension. Hypotensive reactions have most commonly been reported in association with the use of negatively charged bedside leuko-reduction filters in patients being treated with ACE inhibitors.

Hypotensive transfusion reactions typically resolve with cessation of transfusion. Furthermore, the use of pre-storage leuko-reduction, in lieu of bedside leuko-reduction, also limits the incidence of these reactions.

Delayed transfusion reactions
Delayed hemolytic transfusion reaction

Delayed hemolytic transfusion reactions (DHTRs) occur when red cell transfusion precipitates an alloantibody response, resulting in hemolysis and decreased red cell survival. If an alloantibody response is noted in the absence of red cell destruction, it is termed a delayed serologic transfusion reaction (DSTR). Delayed serologic transfusion reactions occur four times more often than DHTRs. If alloantibodies are formed within days of transfusion, it is presumed to be an anamnestic alloantibody response in an individual who had previously formed antibodies. If alloantibodies are formed within weeks of transfusion, it is presumed to be a primary alloantibody response.

Delayed hemolytic transfusion reactions are characterized by an unexpected decrease in hemoglobin or less than expected increase in hemoglobin post-transfusion. Other signs and symptoms include fever, chills, jaundice, malaise, back pain, and rarely renal failure. The incidence of delayed hemolytic and serologic transfusion reactions is about 1 in 1,500 red cell transfusions. To prevent future reactions, the patient should receive red cells lacking the reciprocal antigen for future transfusions.

Post-transfusion purpura

Post-transfusion purpura (PTP) is an immune thrombocytopenia caused by antiplatelet alloantibodies, most often anti-HPA-1a. All types of blood products have been implicated in PTP, with transfusion triggering an antibody response to platelet antigen. The incidence of PTP is approximately 1 in 330,000 transfusions. Diagnosis is based on the clinical presentation and the identification of platelet-specific alloantibodies.

Post-transfusion purpura is characterized by acute, profound thrombocytopenia ($< 10,000/\mu L$), unexplained purpuric rash, bruising, or mucosal bleeding 1–3 weeks post-transfusion. Thirty percent of affected patients have major hemorrhage and 10% of patients have fatal hemorrhage. The primary treatment for PTP is intravenous immunoglobulin.

Transfusion-associated graft-versus-host-disease

Transfusion-associated graft-versus-host-disease (TA-GVHD) results from the engraftment of transfused viable donor lymphocytes in a recipient. The donor lymphocytes subsequently mount an immune response against the recipient, resulting in pancytopenia, erythemia, liver dysfunction, and gastrointestinal symptoms. Unlike GVHD associated with hematopoietic stem cell transplantation, TA-GVHD has nearly a 100% fatality rate due to the profound pancytopenia.

Patients at increased risk for TA-GVHD include those with congenital immunodeficiencies, Hodgkin's disease, acute leukemia, or other hematologic malignancies, as well as patients undergoing hematopoietic stem cell transplantation. Patients also at increased risk are those receiving HLA-matched blood products or blood products from close relatives, granulocyte transfusions, intrauterine transfusions, or neonatal red cell exchange. Patients at increased risk for TA-GVHD should receive irradiated cellular blood products. Irradiation results in the inability of leukocytes to replicate, and hence prevents TA-GVHD [4].

Infectious complications of transfusion

Ensuring blood component safety is critical to any medical system. Blood safety relies upon several measures, including the appropriate selection of donors, careful donor screening by questionnaire, the use of good manufacturing practices, and blood product testing for infectious disease markers. Although all of these measures are important, the latter will be discussed here.

Table 23.4 Residual risk of transfusion.

Test	Residual risk of transfusion/unit transfused
HIV	1 : 1,467,000
HCV	1 : 1,149,000
HBV	1 : 282,000–1 : 357,000
HTLV	1 : 2,993,000
Syphilis	Last reported case in the USA in 1966
Chagas' disease	Seven reported cases in the USA
WNV NAT	Six reported cases in the USA 2004–11
Sepsis (bacterial)	1 : 25,350 whole blood-derived platelets & 1 : 74,807 apheresis platelets

Blood donor screening tests were introduced and improved incrementally over the last several decades. Currently in the USA, blood donations are screened for infection with Hepatitis B virus, Hepatitis C virus, HIV-1 and -2, Human T-cell lymphotrophic viruses (HTLV) types I and II, West Nile virus (WNV), syphilis, and *Trypanosoma cruzi*. In addition, platelet components are screened for bacterial contamination (Table 23.4).

Hepatitis B virus

Hepatitis B virus (HBV) is a double-stranded DNA virus and is transmitted via parenteral, sexual, and vertical (pregnant mother to infant) routes. Seroprevalence in the USA is about 5.6%. In the USA, blood components are screened for HBV by testing for Hepatitis B surface antigen (HBsAg), anti-HBc, and HBV nucleic acid amplification testing (NAT). The estimated risk of HBV transmission per product transfused is approximately 1 in 282,000–357,000 products [2,11,12].

Hepatitis C virus

Hepatitis C virus (HCV) is single-stranded RNA virus and is transmitted primarily via parenteral routes, through intravenous drug use, infected transfusions, and clotting factor use prior to effective screening tests and viral inactivation methods. Sexual and vertical transmission of HCV is uncommon. In the USA, blood components are screened for HCV by testing for anti-HCV and HCV NAT. The estimated risk of HCV transmission per product transfused is approximately 1 in 1,149,000 products [2,13].

Human immunodeficiency virus

Human immunodeficiency virus (HIV) is single-stranded RNA virus and is transmitted via parenteral, sexual, and vertical routes. HIV-1 is found worldwide, with subtype B being most common in North America and Europe. HIV-2 is found mainly in West Africa. In the USA, blood components are screened for HIV-1 and HIV-2 by testing for anti-HIV-1/2 and

HIV-1 nucleic acid amplification testing (NAT), which have 9 and 21 days window periods, respectively. The estimated risk of HIV transmission per product transfused is approximately 1 in 1,467,000 products [2,11].

Human T-cell lymphotrophic virus

Human T-cell lymphotrophic virus (HTLV) is a member of the *Retroviridae* family, like HIV. HTLV is primarily transmitted via parenteral routes, although transmission is thought to occur from mother to infant through breastfeeding. Infected individuals are commonly asymptomatic. HTLV-I infection is associated with increased risk of T-cell leukemia/lymphoma, HTLV-associated myelopathy/tropical spastic paraparesis, and immunologic disease. HTLV-II infection is associated with non-specific immunosuppression. In the USA, blood components are screened for HTLV-I and -II by testing for anti-HTLV-I/II. This test has a window period of 80 days. The estimated risk of HTLV transmission per product transfused is approximately 1 in 2,993,000 products. Leukocyte reduction is thought to provide additional protection against HTLV transmission [2,14].

West Nile virus

West Nile virus (WNV) is a single-stranded RNA virus that is predominantly found in birds and transmitted to humans via bites from infected mosquitoes. Eighty percent of WNV cases are asymptomatic. Common symptoms include fever and rash, with encephalitis and meningitis occurring in 0.7% of those infected. In the USA, blood components are screened for WNV by testing for WNV NAT. To improve testing sensitivity, WNV NAT on pooled samples continues until increased regional disease activity is detected. At that time, testing is converted to WNV NAT on individual donors. Donor screening has substantially reduced the number of transfusion transmitted cases of WNV, with six cases reported between 2004 and 2011 [2,15,16].

Syphilis

Syphilis is caused by the spirochete *Treponema pallidum* and is typically sexually transmitted. In addition to being a rare infection in the US population, only one transfusion-transmitted syphilis infection has been reported in the last 50 years. In the USA, blood components are screened for syphilis by nontreponemal or treponemal tests [2,17].

Trypanosoma cruzi

Chagas' disease is caused by the flagellate protozoan parasite *Trypanosoma cruzi*. Chagas' disease is endemic to Central and South America and is transmitted through bites of infected Reduviid bugs, as well as vertically. Beyond the acute symptomatic infection, chronic infection typically persists for life with asymptomatic, low-level, intermittent parasitemia. These chronically infected, asymptomatic donors are of concern, and, as such, blood components in the USA are screened for *T. cruzi* by testing for anti-*T. cruzi*. Seven cases of transfusion-transmitted Chagas' disease were reported in the USA prior to initiation of screening in 2006 [2,18].

Bacterial contamination

Bacterial contamination of blood products is a significant concern given the morbidity and mortality associated with sepsis. The most common sources of bacterial contamination are donor skin and donors with asymptomatic bacteremia. Platelet products are of particular concern because of their room temperature storage conditions. Bacterial detection methods include culture of the product and point of issue testing. The residual risk of bacterial contamination of whole blood-derived platelets is 1 in 25,350 products. The residual risk of bacterial contamination of apheresis platelets is 1 in 74,807 products [2,18–21].

Pathogen reduction and inactivation

Despite major advances in blood donor screening and infectious disease testing, a risk of transfusion-transmitted infection remains. Transfusion-transmitted infections may still occur during the "window period," when infection is present but testing is negative. Transfusion-transmitted infections may also occur due to infectious agents which have not yet been identified or for which testing is not routinely available.

In light of these concerns, pathogen reduction and inactivation methods further reduce the risk of transfusion-transmitted infections by reducing the pathogenicity of a variety of organisms, including viruses, bacteria, protozoa, and fungi. Pathogen reduction and inactivation methods include heat, solvent/detergent treatment chemical, UVC, and photochemical treatments where photosensitive compounds are added to the product and exposed to light of a specific wavelength. Although pathogen reduction and inactivation is widely used in Europe for plasma and platelet products, these technologies are not currently available in the USA [2,3].

References

1. Agency for Healthcare Research and Quality, Overview of Hospitals. 2003. www.ahrq.gov/data/hcup/factbk7/factbk7b.htm.

2. Roback JD, Combs MR, Grossman BJ *et al. AABB Technical Manual.* 16th edn. Bethesda, MD: AABB; 2008.

3. Karen E, King MD, Gottschall J *et al. Blood Transfusion Therapy: A Physician's Handbook.* 9th edn. Bethesda, MD: AABB; 2008.

4. Hillyer CD, Shaz BH, Zimring JC, Abshire TC, eds. *Transfusion Medicine and Hemostasis: Clinical and*

Laboratory Aspects. Philadelphia, PA: Elsevier; 2009.

5. Blajchman MA. The clinical benefits of the leukoreduction of blood products. *J Trauma* 2006; **60**: s83–90.

6. Nichols WG, Price TH, Gooley T, Corey L, Boeckh M. Transfusion-transmitted cytomegalovirus infection after receipt of leukoreduced blood products. *Blood* 2003; **1010**: 4195–220.

7. Schroeder ML. Transfusion-associated graft-versus-host disease. *Br J Haematol* 2002; **117**: 275–87.

8. Popovsky MA. Frozen and washed red blood cells: new approaches and applications. *Transfus Apher Sci* 2001; **25**: 193–4.

9. Borgman MA, Spinella PC, Perkins JG *et al.* The ratio of blood products transfused affects morality in patients receiving massive transfusions at a combat support hospital. *J Trauma* 2007; **62**: 805–13.

10. The National Healthcare Safety Network (NHSN) Manual: Biovigilance Component. Centers for Disease Control and Prevention, June 2011. www.cdc.gov/nhsn/PDFs/Biovigilance/ BV-Protocol-1–3–1-June-2011.pdf.

11. Zou S, Stramer SL, Notari EP *et al.* Current incidence and residual risk of hepatitis B infection among blood donors in the United States. *Transfusion* 2009; **49**: 1609–20.

12. Commanor L, Holland P. Hepatitis B virus blood screening: unfinished agendas. *Vox Sanguinis* 2006; **91**: 1–123.

13. Zou S, Dorsey KA, Notari EP *et al.* Prevalence, incidence, and residual risk of human immunodeficiency virus and hepatitis C virus infections among United States blood donors since the introduction of nucleic acid testing. *Transfusion* 2010; **50**: 1495–504.

14. Dodd RY, Notari EP, Stramer SL. Current prevalence and incidence of infectious disease markers and estimated window-period risk in the American Red Cross blood donor population. *Transfusion* 2002; **42**: 975–9.

15. US Food and Drug Administration. Guidance for Industry: Use of Nucleic Acid Tests to Reduce the Risks of Transmission of West Nile Virus from Donors of Whole Blood and Blood Components intended for Transfusion. November 2009.

16. Centers for Disease Control and Prevention. West Nile Virus Transmission via Organ Transplantation and Blood Transfusion – Louisiana, 2008. *Morbid Mortal Weekly Rep* 2009; **58** (45): 1263–7.

17. Perkins HA, Busch MP. Transfusion-associated infections: 50 years of relentless challenges and remarkable progress. *Transfusion* 2010; **50**: 2080–99.

18. Young C, Losikoff P, Chawla A, Glasser L, Forman E. Transfusion-acquired *Trypanosoma cruzi* infection. *Transfusion* 2007; **47**: 540–4.

19. AABB Association Bulletin #10–02 – Interim Standard 5.1.5.1.1. www.aabb. org/resources/publications/bulletins/ Pages/ab10–02.aspx.

20. Benjamin RJ, Kline L, Dy BA *et al.* Bacterial contamination of whole-blood-derived platelets: the introduction of sample diversion and prestorage pooling with culture testing in the American Red Cross. *Transfusion* 2008; **48**(11): 2348–55.

21. Eder AF, Kennedy JM, Dy B *et al.* Bacterial screening of apheresis platelets and the residual risk of septic transfusion reactions: the American Red Cross experience (2004–6). *Transfusion* 2007; **47**: 1134–42.

Chapter

24

Preventive antibiotics in surgery

Stuart H. Cohen and Jennifer Brown

Introduction

In 1867, British surgeon Joseph Lister published his landmark series *On the Antiseptic Principle of the Practice of Surgery* in which he presented his novel technique of applying carbolic acid on surgical wounds to destroy "septic germs" [1]. This "aseptic" technique markedly decreased the incidence of gangrene and death and helped solidify the belief that "minute organisms" were the cause of suppuration. Rapid progress in aseptic technique followed and, coupled with the discovery of antibiotics such as penicillin in the mid-1900s, revolutionized the field of surgery from a practice that had been plagued by frequent infection and death into the discipline it is today. Yet, despite more than a century of great improvements in the prevention of surgical site infections (SSIs) and antimicrobial prophylaxis, surgery-related infections remain a problem.

Over 30 million operative procedures are performed in US hospitals each year, with an overall postsurgical infection rate of 2–5% [2,3]. Among healthcare-associated infections, surgical site infections (SSIs) are the second most common, accounting for 17–20% of all nosocomial infections [2,4]. The US Centers for Disease Control and Prevention (CDC) reports that about 500,000 SSIs occur yearly, but this number is likely an underestimation of the true burden. This underestimation probably can be attributed to the rapid proliferation of outpatient/ambulatory surgeries and shorter postoperative inpatient days, which, in turn, have made the detection of SSIs more difficult. In fact, outpatient operations accounted for 63% of all surgeries performed in US community hospitals in 2002, compared with just 16% in 1980 [5]. In 2006, an estimated 53.3 million surgical and non-surgical procedures were performed in ambulatory surgery centers, yet there is no standardized method for SSI surveillance in these venues [2,6]. Globally, the lack of surveillance systems for SSIs in developing countries makes it difficult to gauge the worldwide burden of SSIs. However, in their meta-analysis of 220 studies of healthcare-associated infections in developing countries, Allegranzi and colleagues estimate that SSIs are the leading cause of nosocomial infections with an incidence up to three times higher than that recorded in developed countries [7].

Surgical site infections are a substantial cause of postoperative morbidity and mortality. In comparison to patients who do not experience SSIs, those who do, have a 60% greater risk of being admitted to the ICU, a 3% higher mortality rate, and a 2–11 times higher risk of death. In fact, 75% of deaths among patients with SSIs are directly attributable to the SSI [2,8]. Surgical site infections also have profound effects on patients' quality of life and mental health. Using the Medical Outcome Study Short Form Health Survey, several studies have found that SSIs negatively impact quality of life and mental health scores [9,10].

Surgical site infections negatively affect healthcare costs and resource utilization. Each SSI can extend a patient's hospital stay by 7–10 additional postoperative days, amounting to over 3 million excess hospital days annually in the USA [2,8,11]. The attributable costs of each SSI depend on the type of operative procedure and infecting pathogens, but are reported to range from $3,000–29,000 [2]. Broex and colleagues, in their review of 16 studies of SSIs from 2004 to 2009, determined that the healthcare costs and length of hospital stay incurred by a patient with a SSI are at least twice those incurred by a patient without a SSI [12]. In total, the inpatient costs of SSIs in the USA are believed to account for up to $10 billion annually in healthcare expenditures, but this does not take into consideration the additional costs for services rendered post-discharge. In 2003, Perencevich and colleagues published their study of the health and economic effects of SSIs recognized over a 2-month post-discharge period; they found that patients with SSIs required significantly more outpatient and emergency room visits, radiology services, readmissions, and home-health services than did patients without SSIs. The average total cost during the 8 weeks after discharge was nearly three times greater for patients who had SSIs than those who did not [10]. Thus, the prevention of post-surgical infections would be expected to improve, not only quality of life and mortality, but also healthcare economics.

While the benefits of administering antibiotics to help prevent surgical infections are apparent, the disadvantages of antimicrobial use, especially overuse, must be appreciated. It is

Medical Management of the Surgical Patient, ed. Michael F. Lubin, Thomas F. Dodson, and Neil H. Winawer. Published by Cambridge University Press. © Cambridge University Press 2013.

overly simplistic to believe we can prevent all SSIs from occurring. Humans are not sterile beings; surgery is not performed in a vacuum; and each patient has a unique set of immune defenses and risks for infection. The goal of antimicrobial prophylaxis is not to sterilize a patient but rather to decrease the bacterial burden at the surgical site. Prophylaxis augments the host's natural immune defense mechanisms by increasing the inoculum size of bacteria needed to cause an infection. However, it is important to consider the negative impact of the overuse of antibiotics, including the development of multidrug-resistant organisms, adverse reactions from antibiotics, and the development of *Clostridium difficile* infection. Therefore, the use of antimicrobial agents to prevent infection must be weighed against the untoward effects of antibiotic use and overuse.

Fortunately, studies performed over the past 60 years have helped formulate guidelines for appropriate antimicrobial prophylaxis. This section provides general principles for the use of antibiotic prophylaxis, other considerations to decrease the rate of postsurgical infections, and evidence-based antimicrobial prophylaxis for specific operations.

Antimicrobial prophylaxis for surgery: general principles

Antimicrobial prophylaxis is defined as the administration of antibiotics at the time of surgery to patients who do not have evidence of established infection in order to prevent infection. Patients who have a preexisting infection such as pneumonia, a ruptured appendix, or an infected heart valve, where the use of antibiotics is considered therapeutic, are excluded from this discussion. General principles to consider in antibiotic prophylaxis include (a) assessing a patient's underlying risk of SSI, (b) weighing the risks and benefits of prophylaxis, (c) understanding the microbiology of the surgical site and resultant infections, and (d) choosing the dose and timing of the antimicrobic administration.

Assessing patient risk

In the prevention of surgical infections, it is first important to understand the limitations of antimicrobial prophylaxis and the inherent infection risk. Historically, a patient's risk of developing a postoperative infection correlated with the type of surgical procedure being performed and the bacterial load already present within the surgical field. For that reason, surgical wounds are divided into four different categories (Table 24.1), according to the potential for infection [13]. The potential ranges from low for clean procedures, where reservoirs of endogenous patient flora are not encountered, to very high for dirty procedures where there may be, for example, clinical infection or a perforated viscus.

While this classification crudely ranks infection risk, it does not take into account individual patient or procedural risk factors for infection which should be evaluated when deciding how aggressive to be in trying to prevent a SSI. Epidemiologic studies have identified a number of patient-centered risk factors associated with SSIs, including extremes of age, diabetes, use of corticosteroids, prior site irradiation, hypoxemia, nicotine use, low preoperative serum albumin level, positive allergen skin test, prolonged preoperative hospitalization, severe malnutrition or obesity, and the presence of a remote infection at the time of surgery [2]. In order to assess the independent importance of each of these factors, the Study on the Efficacy of Nosocomial Infection Control (SENIC) was conducted in 1985. In the study, Haley *et al.* established, by use of multivariate analysis, that operations involving the abdomen, procedures lasting longer than two hours, and the presence of three or more discharge diagnoses (as a surrogate for identifying patients with complicated illnesses) were independent risk factors for infection. When these factors were incorporated into the traditional wound classification system, a paradigm that stratified patients further into low, medium, and high risk of infection was developed. As a result, the ability to identify risk of infection for individual patients improved by two-fold when compared with the traditional classification of wound contamination [14].

Subsequently, the grading of SSI risk was further refined through construction of the National Nosocomial Infection Surveillance (NNIS) risk index, which incorporates three criteria of increased risk: (1) patients with American Society of Anesthesia (ASA) scores of ≥ 3; (2) procedures involving contaminated or dirty-infected wounds; and (3) operations lasting longer than the 75th percentile for that specific procedure [15]. Each risk factor increases the rates of infection significantly. The ASA score, which is compiled at the time of operation, is regarded as a more accurate measure of a patient's underlying health status than is the number of diagnoses at discharge. The customized time representative of the 75th percentile of the average time required for each type of operation accounts for procedures that traditionally take a longer or shorter time to complete. Of note, the laparoscopic approach for colonic surgery and cholecystectomy is associated with fewer SSIs (regardless of underlying risk for SSI) as it is for appendectomy and gastric surgery (with no risk factors for SSI). Thus, for these laparoscopic procedures, one point of risk is subtracted in the NNIS risk index.

Cost (risk)–benefit assessment

As detailed above, all surgical procedures do not carry the same risk of infection. Therefore, the potential benefit of preventing infection in individual circumstances must be balanced against the risk and cost of surgical prophylaxis. The administration of antibiotics routinely in all surgical settings is not cost effective. Antimicrobial utilization can account for high percentages of hospital pharmacy budgets, with prophylactic antibiotics constituting about one-third of all antimicrobials administered [16,17]. Much of this use is deemed inappropriate, particularly in the setting of unwarranted surgical prophylaxis.

Table 24.1 Classification of surgical wounds and risk of subsequent infection.

Wound classification	Definition	Infection rate (%)	
		Without preoperative antibiotics	With preoperative antibiotics
Clean wound	A non-traumatic wound in which no inflammation was encountered, no break in surgical technique occurred, and the respiratory, gastrointestinal, and genitourinary tracts were not entered	5.1	0.8
Clean-contaminated wound	A non-traumatic wound in which a break in surgical technique occurred or the respiratory, gastrointestinal, or genitourinary tracts were entered without significant spillage	10.1	1.3
Contaminated wound	A fresh, traumatic wound from a relatively clean source or an operative wound with a major break in technique such as gross spillage from the gastrointestinal tract or entrance into infected urinary or biliary tract. This includes incisions encountering acute non-purulent inflammation	21.9	10.2
Dirty wound	Traumatic wounds from a dirty source or with delayed treatment, fecal contamination, foreign bodies, a devitalized viscus, or pus from any source that is encountered	40	10

In addition to the tremendous financial cost, other forms of "collateral damage" resulting from antimicrobial prophylaxis are much more difficult to quantify. With each dose of antibiotic there is an ecological cost in the development of antimicrobial resistance. The use, and particularly misuse, of antibiotics significantly contributes to the development of multidrug-resistant organisms [18]. It is difficult to weigh the future risk of antimicrobial resistance against the immediate benefit of preventing a SSI, thus attempts to assign an overall value to the ecologic cost of antimicrobial resistance are challenging. However, the past two decades have seen an epidemic rise in the incidence of antibiotic-resistant organisms, such as methicillin-resistant *Staphylococcus aureus* (MRSA) and multidrug-resistant gram negative bacilli throughout the world [19,20]. In conjunction with this rise, the striking decline in the development of new antibiotics has ignited alarms, prompting many organizations, including the CDC and the Institute of Medicine, to declare this a substantial public health threat [20].

Beyond the mounting public health crisis, infections due to drug-resistant organisms are associated with significantly worse clinical outcomes and increased healthcare costs. For example, in 2003, Engemann and colleagues published their study of 479 patients with SSIs due to MRSA; they found that patients with SSIs due to MRSA had a greater mortality rate and a 1.19-fold increase in hospital charges compared with patients who had methicillin-susceptible *S. aureus* SSIs [21]. Similarly, negative outcomes have been reported for infections due to drug-resistant gram-negative bacilli, such as extended-spectrum beta-lactamase-producing organisms, as well as *Acinetobacter* and *Enterobacter* species [22].

Antibiotic usage also can change the normal bacterial flora in the gastrointestinal tract, which, in turn, can promote the development of *C. difficile* infection (CDI). *Clostridium difficile* infection can be associated with the use of any antimicrobial agent, including, of course, those used for antibiotic prophylaxis. Indeed, the rate of CDI in surgical patients whose only antibiotic exposure was that for surgical prophylaxis has been reported to be as high as 14.9 cases per 1,000 [23]. The complications of CDI, including toxic megacolon and bowel perforation, can be devastating if not fatal. In a retrospective study of cardiac surgery patients, CDI was associated with a two-fold increase in duration of mechanical ventilation and ICU stay and a significant increase in length of hospital stay [24]. In recent years, there has been a striking increase in mortality due to CDI, from 5.7 deaths per million in 1999 to 23.7 deaths per million in 2004 [25]. Therefore, it is evermore essential to weigh the benefits and risks of antibiotic prophylaxis and to administer antibiotics only when appropriate.

Bearing the aforementioned issues in mind, one must answer the cost–benefit question by assessing the specifics for each surgical procedure and reviewing the results of rigorous clinical trials. In general, since clean surgeries carry a low risk of infection (approximately 5%), the risks of antimicrobial prophylaxis in these cases usually outweigh the benefits of their use. Indeed, Knight *et al.* retrospectively reviewed clean general surgery operations from a private hospital, comparing cases that received antibiotic prophylaxis with cases that did not [26]. Although there may be some patient-selection bias, infection rates did not differ significantly whether the patients received prophylactic antibiotics or not. Thus, except in a few defined circumstances discussed below (see section "Clean surgical procedures"), prophylaxis is not indicated in most clean surgeries. Neither are prophylactic antibiotics indicated for surgeries classified as contaminated or dirty since patients undergoing these operations usually are already receiving

Table 24.2 Likely pathogens for specific surgeries.

Operation	Likely pathogens
Clean surgeries	
Orthopedic	S. aureus; coagulase-negative staphylococci; gram-negative bacilli
Total joint replacement	
Closed fractures/use of nails, bone plates	
Functional repair without implant	
Neurosurgical	S. aureus; coagulase-negative staphylococci
Cardiothoracic	S. aureus; coagulase-negative staphylococci
Vascular	S. aureus; coagulase-negative staphylococci
Clean-contaminated surgeries	
Head and neck	S. aureus; streptococci; oropharyngeal anaerobes (e.g., peptostreptococci)
Incisions through the oropharyngeal mucosa	
Gastrointestinal	Gram-negative bacilli; enterococci; group B streptococci; anaerobes
Biliary	Gram-negative bacilli; anaerobes
Colorectal	Gram-negative bacilli; anaerobes
Genitourinary	Gram-negative bacilli
May not have pathogens if urine is sterile	
Gynecologic and obstetric	Gram-negative bacilli; enterococci; group B streptococci; anaerobes
Trauma	S. aureus; coagulase-negative staphylococci; gram-negative bacilli

therapeutic antibiotics. Prophylactic antibiotics are indicated, though, for most clean-contaminated surgeries.

Microbiology of prophylaxis

Integral in the choosing of antimicrobial agents must be an understanding of the microorganisms that commonly cause SSIs. For clean surgical procedures, wound infections are, by definition, caused by airborne microorganisms or those residing on the skin since other reservoirs of bacteria, such as the gastrointestinal tract, are not entered. For other procedures, endogenous polymicrobial flora are potential pathogens, depending on the location. For example, when oropharyngeal mucous membranes are surgically manipulated, staphylococci, streptococci, and oropharyngeal anaerobes (e.g., peptostreptococci) usually are isolated. For procedures involving the gastrointestinal tract, gram-negative organisms (e.g., *Escherichia coli*), gram-positive organisms (e.g., enterococci), and anaerobes (e.g., *Bacteroides fragilis*) typically are implicated. Infections associated with procedures performed in the perineum or groin may be due to fecal flora. Table 24.2 lists the likely pathogens associated with individual procedures. Seeding of the surgical site from a distant focus is not common, but this route of infection may be important when prosthetic material, which can be a site for attachment for microorganisms, is inserted. Additionally, fungi causing infections may originate either from exogenous or endogenous sources.

Hidron and colleagues have published data regarding the pathogens implicated in SSIs: from January 2006 to October 2007 a total of 5,291 cases of SSIs were reported by participating US hospitals to the National Healthcare Safety Network [27]. Overall, *S. aureus* (30%) and coagulase-negative staphylococci (13.7%) were still the most prevalent pathogens causing SSIs for most types of surgery. Gram-negative rods and enterococci remained the most prevalent after abdominal surgery. Enterococci were associated with about one-third of cases after transplant surgery. Twenty percent of SSIs were polymicrobial, and *Candida* species made up about 2% of isolates. With respect to antimicrobial resistance, 49% of *S. aureus* isolates were resistant to oxacillin. For enterococci, 56% of *Enterococcus faecium* isolates were resistant to vancomycin and 71% were resistant to ampicillin while 4.7% of *Enterococcus faecalis* isolates were resistant to vancomycin and 4.1% were resistant to ampicillin. Nearly 16% of *Pseudomonas aeruginosa* isolates were resistant to fluoroquinolones, 5.7% were resistant to cefepime and 11.8% were resistant to imipenem or meropenem. Of *Acinetobacter baumanii* isolates, 30.6% were resistant to imipenem or meropenem. Nearly 23% of *E. coli* isolates were resistant to fluoroquinolones. These data confirmed the increasing emergence of resistant organisms, thus heightening concerns that antibiotics currently used for prophylaxis will become increasingly ineffective.

While the patient's endogenous flora deserves much attention for their role in causing SSIs, the behavior of operating-room personnel also merits discussion. Those who have direct contact with the operating field must observe strict sterile precautions. Some outbreaks of SSIs due to *Serratia marcescens* in cardiovascular surgery patients, and *Candida albicans* osteomyelitis in spinal surgery patients, have been linked to the use of artificial nails [28,29]. Consequently, many hospitals now prohibit healthcare workers from wearing them. Anesthesia personnel also may play a role in causing postsurgical infections. Although they are not directly involved in the surgical field, they perform a variety of procedures that may be implicated. For example, outbreaks of bloodstream infections and SSIs have been linked to anesthesiologists' re-use of propofol vials and to other breaks in aseptic technique [30].

Choosing an antibiotic

This section will focus on the key principles of selecting an appropriate antibiotic regimen for surgical prophylaxis; specific antibiotic choices will be reviewed later. In addition to the general issues to be considered in selecting antibiotics (drug allergies, drug interactions, or other contraindications), certain considerations are especially applicable to prophylaxis for surgical procedures. Foremost is the spectrum of activity of the drug. The chosen antibiotic need not be active against the entire gamut of organisms that may be encountered, but it must provide effective coverage against the most common SSI pathogens for each specific operation. Ideally, the antibiotic chosen for prophylaxis should not be the same as that which would be used should an infection occur. For this reason, broad-spectrum antibiotics typically are not recommended for prophylaxis because that use may compromise their effectiveness as therapeutic agents.

The pharmacokinetics and pharmacodynamics of the various antibiotics must also be taken into account. Specifically, the agent must achieve and maintain therapeutic tissue concentrations above the minimum inhibitory concentration (MIC) of the probable pathogens from the time of incision to the time of closure [13]. Re-dosing of antibiotics during the operation may be necessary if the procedure is long and exceeds the time in which therapeutic drug levels can be maintained; this will be discussed further below. Re-dosing may also be indicated if multiple transfusions are required or if the antibiotic is cleared rapidly. For instance, the use of cardiopulmonary bypass in cardiothoracic surgery can alter the volume of distribution and clearance of vancomycin, resulting in markedly decreased serum concentrations of the drug [31]. Finally, the cost of the antibiotic (including drug monitoring, administration, re-dosing, and adverse effects) must also be considered when selecting the antibiotic.

Given all of these factors, narrow-spectrum cephalosporins have traditionally been the recommended choice for prophylaxis for most surgical procedures because they have an acceptable safety profile, good tissue penetration, sufficient spectrum of action, and reasonable cost. Specifically, cefazolin is generally the preferred antibiotic for most clean procedures [13]. For procedures that require additional coverage against anaerobic organisms (e.g., operations on the distal intestinal tract, major head and neck operations, and biliary or gynecologic procedures) the addition of metronidazole or the use of a cephalosporin with anaerobic activity is recommended.

Increasingly, consideration must be given also to local resistance patterns and nosocomial wound pathogens. Historically, vancomycin was not routinely recommended for prophylaxis for any procedure; it was reserved for circumstances such as outbreaks of SSIs due to methicillin-resistant *Staphylococcus aureus* (MRSA) or methicillin-resistant coagulase-negative staphylococci. Over the past two decades, though, escalating rates of multidrug-resistance in gram-positive pathogens have triggered a re-examination of the use of glycopeptides (vancomycin or teicoplanin) for prophylaxis [32,33]. In 2004, Bolon and colleagues published their meta-analysis of seven randomized trials of SSIs in cardiac surgery patients [34]. They determined that glycopeptides were no more effective than beta-lactams in preventing SSIs and concluded that beta-lactams should remain the preferred prophylaxis for most cardiac operations. However, the majority of these studies were conducted at institutions with low rates of MRSA and prior to the emergence of community-acquired MRSA. More recent guidelines uphold that vancomycin should not be administered routinely for surgical prophylaxis, although indications for its use have expanded to include, in addition to proven outbreaks of SSIs due to MRSA: (1) "high endemic rates of MRSA," (2) certain patients who are at high risk for SSIs due to MRSA (including cardiothoracic surgical patients and elderly patients with diabetes), and (3) high-risk surgical procedures in which an implant is placed [2,35]. The definition of "high endemic rates of SSIs due to MRSA" has not been established, but if a hospital's prevalence of MRSA exceeds 20%, or if the patient has known MRSA colonization, the use of vancomycin may be indicated. Another consideration for the use of vancomycin in groups 2 and 3 is the role of coagulase-negative staphylococci as a cause of infection in these populations since the large majority of coagulase-negative staphylococci are resistant to methicillin. Nevertheless, it is critical to remember that glycopeptides are not active against gram-negative pathogens, which account for up to 20–30% of SSIs; hence, some authorities recommend adding vancomycin to standard antimicrobial prophylaxis rather than using it as a sole prophylactic agent [2,36].

Timing and re-dosing of prophylaxis

The appropriate timing of antimicrobial administration is one of the most important determinants of successful perioperative antibiotic use. Burke first observed this phenomenon in a guinea pig model, in which administration of antibiotics before or soon after inoculation with *S. aureus* helped to reduce the extent of subcutaneous *S. aureus* infection [37]. A delay in administration of an hour resulted in a more severe infection, and the longer the delay, the greater the severity of infection. Classen and colleagues made similar observations in a clinical setting: the administration of antibiotics after the start of a procedure or too long beforehand resulted in more postsurgical infections [38].

In the USA, the Surgical Care Improvement Project (SCIP) recommends that prophylactic antimicrobials be administered within 1 hour before incision for cephalosporins and within 2 hours for vancomycin or a fluoroquinolone [2,36]. These requirements are one component of the quality measure set of the Centers for Medicare and Medicaid Services' prospective payment system. Some authorities favor an even shorter interval between antibiotic administration and incision. In 2009, the results of The Trial to Reduce Antimicrobial Prophylaxis Errors were published. In this multicenter study of cardiac, hysterectomy, and knee/hip arthroplasty operations, the authors found that the risk of developing a SSI was lowest for patients who received cephalosporins within 30 minutes before incision (and within 1 hour for vancomycin or a fluoroquinolone) [39]. Thus, the optimal timing of antimicrobial administration continues to evolve.

As mentioned above, re-dosing of antibiotics may be necessary if the procedure is of long duration. To ensure that tissue concentrations of the antibiotic remain above the MIC for expected pathogens, additional intraoperative doses should be given at intervals of one or two times the half-life of the drug [40]. For example, in patients with normal renal function, cefazolin should be re-dosed at 3–4 hour intervals. If the operation requires the use of a tourniquet placed proximal to the site of administration, the entire dose of antibiotic should be administered prior to tourniquet inflation. Higher doses of antibiotics may be required for obese patients. Forse and colleagues found that a 1 g dose of cefazolin produced lower tissue and serum concentrations in morbidly obese patients than in non-obese patients [41] and Edmiston and colleagues, in their study of obese patients given 2 g of cefazolin, found that therapeutic tissue levels of the antibiotic were achieved in less than 50% of persons with a BMI between 40 and 49 and in only about 10% of those with a BMI over 59 [42]. Consequently, it may be necessary to use a continuous infusion of cefazolin in morbidly obese patients.

Duration of prophylaxis

The duration of antimicrobial prophylaxis is one of the most difficult areas for physician adherence to published guidelines. The general misconception is, if antibiotics were useful in preventing infection at the time of incision, their continued administration would be of further benefit. However, evidence suggesting that postoperative doses of antibiotics are unnecessary continues to grow. Burke's seminal paper clearly showed that antibiotics administered more than 3 hours after inoculation of S. aureus did not prevent infection [37]. Clinical studies, summarized by Dipiro, have shown that, for most surgical procedures, the use of single-dose antibiotic prophylaxis is as effective in the prevention of SSIs as multiple doses given for as long as 24–48 hours after the procedure [43]. (This observation does not apply to procedures in which the re-dosing of an antibiotic may be necessary because of lengthy operation time or the need for transfusion.)

Most guidelines recommend that antibiotics given for surgical prophylaxis should be discontinued within 24 hours after the operation, and ideally, should be terminated by the end of the operation. However, continuation of antibiotic administration for 48 hours is allowable in cardiothoracic surgery patients, since SSIs in these cases can be especially devastating, and the optimal duration of antibiotic prophylaxis is still under debate [2,44]. The SCIP performance measures also target these indices of appropriate duration of prophylaxis.

In cardiothoracic operations, patients often require monitoring with more invasive devices (e.g., central venous and arterial catheters) and have drains left in place postoperatively. Some surgeons believe that a longer period of antimicrobial prophylaxis is warranted in these patients because the foreign materials may promote hematogenous seeding of newly repaired/replaced heart valves and also may elevate the risk of SSIs such as mediastinitis. Studies aimed at defining the optimal duration of antibiotic administration in this population have produced conflicting results. Hall and colleagues reported that infection rates were two times higher in patients who received only short courses of prophylactic antibiotics than in patients whose antibiotics were continued until lines and drains were removed [45]. Subsequently, an observational cohort study of 2,641 patients undergoing coronary artery bypass graft operations found that continuing antibiotic prophylaxis beyond 48 hours not only was ineffective in reducing SSIs, but was associated with a 1.6 times higher probability of patients acquiring an antibiotic-resistant pathogen [46]. In 2006, after an extensive review of major trials, The Society of Thoracic Surgeons released guidelines which state that the duration of antibiotic prophylaxis should not be based on the presence of indwelling catheters of any type [44]. They also concluded that 24-hour prophylaxis may be as effective as 48-hour prophylaxis, but additional studies of this issue are still needed.

Additional prophylactic measures: preoperative skin antisepsis and decolonization of *S. aureus* carriers

The prevention of SSIs requires a multifaceted approach. In addition to antimicrobial prophylaxis, infection rates are influenced by many other variables: patient-centered factors, surgeons' skill, and the operating room environment; these variables are beyond the scope of this chapter, but two measures, preoperative skin antisepsis and S. aureus decolonization will be reviewed.

Bacterial flora on the skin is a major source of SSI pathogens. The benefit of preoperative cleansing of the skin at the surgical site is widely accepted and numerous organizations, including the CDC and the London-based National Institute for Health and Clinical Excellence (NICE), recommend using an antiseptic agent for preoperative skin preparation [13,47].

Many investigators have sought to determine which antiseptic agent is the most efficacious [48,49]. Recently, Darouiche and colleagues randomly assigned 849 adults undergoing clean-contaminated surgeries in six hospitals to preoperative skin preparation with either chlorhexidine-alcohol scrub or povidone-iodine scrub and paint. They found that the overall rate of SSIs was significantly lower in the chlorhexidine-alcohol group than in the povidone-iodine group (9.5% vs 16.1%) [48]. As a result, chlorhexidine-containing antiseptics are preferred for preoperative skin preparation.

Intuitively, it would seem that extending preoperative cleansing to include showering or bathing of the entire body with antiseptic agents would further decrease SSIs. Whereas this practice does reduce the bacterial burden of the skin flora, it has not been shown to decrease SSIs. In fact, Webster and Osborne, in their review of seven trials that compared chlorhexidine gluconate with other wash products (e.g., bar soap or placebo) for preoperative bathing, found no clear evidence that the use of chlorhexidine gluconate over other wash products was superior in reducing SSIs [50]. Nevertheless, the CDC recommends that patients shower or bathe with an antiseptic agent on at least the night before an operation [13]. In contrast, the NICE recommends using soap (not defined as antiseptic) [47].

The aforementioned skin antiseptics are effective against a host of gram-positive and gram-negative organisms, including *S. aureus*. However, because *S. aureus* is a particularly virulent organism, and over half of SSIs attributed to *S. aureus* may arise from endogenous flora, strategies directed toward the preoperative eradication of nasal and extranasal reservoirs of this organism have intensified [3]. One approach is the intranasal application of the topical antibiotic mupirocin. Results of a meta-analysis of nine trials showed that the treatment of *S. aureus* carriers with intranasal mupirocin significantly reduced the development of *S. aureus* infections [51]. However, Perl and colleagues, in their trial comparing surgical patients who received intranasal mupirocin with those who received placebo, found that, while prophylactic intranasal mupirocin reduced the rate of *S. aureus* nosocomial infections, it did not reduce the rate of *S. aureus* SSIs [52]. In contrast, other studies have noted that intranasal mupirocin use did decrease the rate of SSIs following non-general surgeries such as cardiothoracic, orthopedic, and neurosurgery operations [53,54].

Subsequently, Bode and coworkers published the results of their multicenter trial in which nasal carriers of *S. aureus* were rapidly identified, then treated with either intranasal mupirocin ointment and chlorhexidine soap or placebo ointment and placebo soap [55]. The authors found a significantly lower incidence of *S. aureus* infections in the mupirocin-chlorhexidine group. In subset analysis of the surgical patients in this study, it was found that deep SSIs occurred less frequently in the mupirocin-chlorhexidine group (0.9% vs 4.4% in the placebo group). Although this study demonstrates that SSIs can be reduced by a comprehensive program that includes the rapid detection of *S. aureus* followed by intranasal mupirocin and chlorhexidine gluconate baths, the relative contributions of each of these measures has been questioned. One expert's analysis suggests that, in contrast to chlorhexidine skin preparation (where the number of patients who would need be to treated to prevent one SSI is estimated to be 17), a total of 250 patients would need to be screened and 23 carriers would need to be treated with intranasal mupirocin in order to prevent one *S. aureus* infection [3]. Thus, routine administration of intranasal mupirocin to all surgery patients is not practical. This reality, in combination with the fact that strains of *S. aureus* have already developed resistance to mupirocin, has led to the recommendation that preoperative intranasal mupirocin therapy should be reserved for *S. aureus* carriers who undergo procedures associated with a high risk for deleterious sequelae (e.g., cardiothoracic operations, procedures where an implant is placed, and operations involving immunosuppressed patients) should a *S. aureus* infection occur [3,56].

Antimicrobial prophylaxis for specific surgical procedures

This section will first review recommendations for patient groups who may require additional measures to prevent infections when undergoing operations. Then, recommendations for specific surgeries will be discussed.

Prophylaxis for infective endocarditis

In 2007, the American Heart Association released new guidelines for the prevention of infective endocarditis (IE) [57]. This document contains major revisions from the previous guidelines; both the types of cardiac conditions and the types of procedures for which IE prophylaxis is indicated were narrowed. In general, IE prophylaxis now is recommended only for patients who have underlying cardiac conditions associated with the highest risk of adverse outcomes from IE who are undergoing: (1) dental procedures that involve manipulation of gingival tissue or the periapical region of the teeth, or (2) procedures that involve perforation of the oral mucosa. Infective endocarditis is no longer recommended for patients undergoing genitourinary or gastrointestinal tract procedures (Table 24.3).

The primary reason for these revisions is that IE is much more likely to result from the frequent exposure to random bacteremias associated with daily activities, such as teeth brushing, than from bacteremia caused by a dental, genitourinary, or gastrointestinal procedure. Also, prophylaxis may prevent only a few, if any, cases of IE in these settings and the overall risk of antibiotic-associated adverse events exceeds the benefit from prophylactic antibiotics [57].

The cardiac conditions for which IE prophylaxis is considered reasonable include: (1) prosthetic cardiac valves or cardiac valves repaired with prosthetic material, (2) previous IE, (3) cardiac transplant recipients with valvulopathy, (4) certain congenital heart diseases (CHD) such as unrepaired

Table 24.3 Prophylaxis for endocarditis.

Procedure	Regimen for adults	Comments
Dental procedures that involve manipulation of gingival tissue or periapical region or perforation of oral mucosa	Amoxicillin 2 g orally 30–60 minutes before the procedure For penicillin or ampicillin allergy; cephalexin 2 g OR clindamycin 600 mg OR azithromycin 500 mg OR clarithromycin 500 mg 30–60 minutes before the procedure*	For patients unable to take oral medication; ampicillin 2 g IM/IV OR cefazolin 1 g IM/IV OR ceftriaxone 1g IM/IV 30–60 minutes before the procedure For penicillin or ampicillin allergy and unable to take oral medications; cefazolin 1 g IM/IV OR ceftriaxone 1 g IM/IV OR clindamycin 600 mg IM/IV 30–60 minutes before the procedure[a]
Incision or biopsy of respiratory mucosa/tonsillectomy/adenoidectomy	Prophylaxis can be considered; use same regimens as for dental procedures	
Bronchosopy/gastrointestinal/genitourinary procedures	Prophylaxis no longer recommended	

IM, intramuscular; IV, intravenous.
[a] Cephalosporins should not be used if patient has a history of anaphylaxis, angioedema, or urticaria with penicillins or ampicillin.

cyanotic CHD, congenital heart defects completely repaired with prosthetic material/device for the first 6 months post-procedure, repaired CHD with residual defects at or adjacent to the site of a prosthetic patch/device. Most notably, IE prophylaxis is no longer recommended for patients with mitral valve prolapse.

Distant site infections

Infections remote from the operative site (e.g., infections of the urinary tract, skin, or respiratory tract) may increase the risk of SSIs. Valentine and colleagues retrospectively studied the impact of remote infections on SSIs in clean surgeries. They concluded that antibiotic treatment of a remote infection initiated more than 24 hours before surgery decreased the rate of SSIs to that in patients without remote infections [58]. Consequently, whenever possible, remote infections should be treated prior to an elective operation. It is not necessary to perform routine preoperative screening (e.g., urine or blood cultures) for remote infections in patients who do not have signs or symptoms of infection.

Clean surgical procedures

Most clean operations do not require the use of prophylactic antibiotics. Clean operations for which antimicrobial prophylaxis has been shown to be beneficial include: (1) procedures in which an implant is placed, (2) procedures in which a SSI would result in a grave consequence for the patient, and (3) procedures involving the placement of intravascular prosthetic material (Table 24.4). Elek and Conen clarified the role of prosthetic material in the pathogenesis of wound infection. They showed that the inoculum of bacteria needed to cause an infection was reduced 10,000-fold in the presence of foreign material [59]. Examples of operations in which a SSI would pose a catastrophic risk to the patient include all types of cardiac surgeries, including cardiac pacemaker placement.

Orthopedic surgery

The placement of a foreign body during most orthopedic operations predisposes to SSIs. Moreover, because of the severe consequences of infection after joint replacement, prophylaxis is recommended [40]. Most postoperative infections of prosthetic joints result from the seeding of microorganisms during the operation. While the majority of infections will manifest clinically within the first month after the procedure, many infections will take years to become apparent. Infections occurring over 2 years after the operation are usually attributed to hematogenous seeding of the joint, rather than direct inoculation of bacteria at the time of surgery. *Staphylococcus aureus* and coagulase-negative staphylococci account for up to 90% of the orthopedic SSIs that occur within the first 2 years. Cefazolin is the antibiotic usually recommended for prophylaxis due to its efficacy against gram-positive pathogens, reasonable cost, and favorable safety profile. However, in centers where the prevalence of methicillin resistance in *S. aureus* or coagulase-negative staphylococci is high, the addition of vancomycin for prophylaxis is warranted. Intranasal mupirocin may be considered for patients who are nasal carriers of *S. aureus*, however there is controversy regarding its impact on the rates of orthopedic SSIs [53,60].

The sole use of an antibiotic cement does not seem to alter the rate of SSIs or the rate of revisions required for previously replaced joints. However, the use of an antibiotic cement, in addition to systemic antimicrobial prophylaxis, seems to be better than the use of systemic antibiotics alone. Espenhaug's study of nearly 11,000 primary total hip arthroplasty patients showed that the rates of infection or revision were lower in patients who received a combined regimen (antibiotic cement plus systemic antibiotics) as compared with systemic antibiotics alone. These positive results were seen in early infection, and the difference was even greater over an 8-year follow-up period [61]. Guidelines for the use of antimicrobial cements do

Table 24.4 Prophylaxis for clean surgical procedures.

Orthopedic surgery	Recommended regimen	Comments
Arthroplasty of joints including joint replacements	Cefazolin 1–2 g or cefuroxime 1.5 g preoperatively; re-dose every 3–5 hours for patients with normal renal function	Use vancomycin if beta-lactam allergy Consider addition of vancomycin in hospitals with rates of MRSA > 20% and in MRSA carriers When using a tourniquet, a higher cefazolin dose should be considered (2 g); the entire dose should be administered prior to tourniquet inflation
Open reduction of fracture	Cefazolin 1–2 g or cefuroxime 1.5 g preoperatively; re-dose every 3–5 hours for patients with normal renal function	Complex (open) fractures are not considered clean procedures; they require treatment as contaminated procedures with a full course of antimicrobials
Lower limb amputation	Cefoxitin 2 g preoperatively; re-dose every 2–4 hours for patients with normal renal function	Other combinations of 3rd generation cephalosporin and metronidazole would also be acceptable

Laminectomy, spinal fusion without prosthesis placement do not require prophylaxis in non-compromised patients

Neurosurgery	Recommended regimen	Comments
Craniotomy or shunt placement	Cefazolin 1–2 g preoperatively; re-dose every 3–5 hours for patients with normal renal function	Use vancomycin if beta-lactam allergy Consider addition of vancomycin in hospitals with rates of MRSA > 20% and in MRSA carriers If surgery crosses the sinuses or nasopharynx; clindamycin 900 mg IV

Cardiothoracic surgery	Recommended regimen	Comments
Median sternotomy, coronary artery bypass surgery, or repair of a valve	Cefazolin 1–2 g or cefuroxime 1.5 g preoperatively; re-dose every 3–5 hours for patients with normal renal function or if massive hemorrhage occurs	Use vancomycin if beta-lactam allergy Consider addition of vancomycin in hospitals with rates of MRSA > 20% and in MRSA carriers
Pacemaker insertion	Cefazolin 1–2 g or cefuroxime 1.5 g preoperatively	With beta-lactam allergy, due to low incidence of infection, may be reasonable to give no prophylaxis
Thoracic surgery, including lobectomy and pneumonectomy	Cefazolin 1–2 g or cefuroxime 1.5 g preoperatively; re-dose every 3–5 hours for patients with normal renal function	Use vancomycin if beta-lactam allergy Consider addition of vancomycin in hospitals with rates of MRSA > 20% and in MRSA carriers Can also consider clindamycin for beta-lactam allergy

Vascular surgery	Recommended regimen	Comments
Aortic and femoral vascular procedures, including bypass and reconstruction	Cefazolin 1–2 g or cefuroxime 1.5 g preoperatively; re-dose every 3–5 hours for patients with normal renal function	Use vancomycin if beta-lactam allergy Consider addition of vancomycin in hospitals with rates of MRSA > 20% and in MRSA carriers Vein stripping and carotid endarterectomy do not require prophylaxis unless baseline infection rates are high

not exist, however the US Food and Drug Administration has approved several antibiotic cement preparations for use in the second stage of a two-stage revision of previously infected joint prostheses.

Neurosurgery

The infection rate associated with clean neurosurgical operations is very low. Antimicrobial prophylaxis is not necessary for all neurosurgical procedures. Meta-analyses by Barker found that, when antibiotic prophylaxis in specific neurosurgical operations is analyzed, a significant benefit is seen with antibiotic prophylaxis for craniotomies and spinal surgery

[62,63]. With respect to craniotomies, it is clear that antimicrobial prophylaxis reduces postoperative wound infections, but its effect on post-craniotomy meningitis is unclear [64]. However, one meta-analysis of six studies of post-craniotomy meningitis found that the administration of prophylactic antibiotics does significantly reduce the rates of postoperative meningitis [65].

The use of antimicrobial prophylaxis has also been shown to decrease SSIs after ventricular shunt placements. Ratial and colleagues, in their review of 17 trials of intracranial ventricular shunt placements, established that antimicrobial prophylaxis decreases the rate of shunt infections diagnosed within the first postoperative day [66]. A similar benefit was not seen with shunt revisions. This study did not evaluate for SSIs beyond the initial 24-hour postoperative period, nor did it evaluate all-cause mortality. Nevertheless, many authorities now include ventricular shunt placement as an indication for antibiotic prophylaxis.

Cardiothoracic surgery

Although regarded as clean operations, the risks of infection associated with open-heart operations, such as mediastinitis or pericarditis, are life-threatening and justify the use of prophylactic antibiotics. Early studies of antibiotic prophylaxis in cardiac surgery did not show a benefit with antibiotic prophylaxis [67]. However, a later study by Fong and colleagues, which applied more stringent experimental methods, showed a significant benefit with a short course of antibiotics over placebo [68]. Cefazolin remains the recommended antibiotic, but the addition of vancomycin may be indicated in specific clinical situations [35]. (See section "Choosing an antibiotic" for further discussion.) Antimicrobial prophylaxis should be discontinued within 48 hours of the operation and should not be continued even if indwelling catheters or drains remain in place after this period [44]. Intranasal mupirocin should be considered for *S. aureus* carriers.

Vascular surgery

Surgical site infection rates in vascular operations differ greatly and are dependent on the surgical site. Operations that involve an incision in the groin area have a higher infection rate than that for operations that occur in the carotid or upper extremities. Thus, prophylaxis is recommended for all aortic or femoral reconstructions. The benefit of prophylactic antibiotics in aortic or femoral vascular procedures was shown by Hasselgren and colleagues. In their study of patients undergoing lower extremity vascular reconstructive surgery, the use of cefuroxime for 24 hours decreased the wound infection rate from 16.7% to 3.8% [69]. Extension of antibiotics to 72 hours showed no difference when compared with 24 hours.

Though uncommon, prosthetic graft (e.g., aortic endograft) infections carry a high mortality rate. Thus, any vascular operation that involves the placement of a prosthetic graft requires antibiotic prophylaxis. Antimicrobial prophylaxis is also recommended for peripheral endografts such as hemodialysis grafts [70]. Bennion and colleagues showed that the use of antibiotic prophylaxis reduced the rate of infection in patients undergoing placement of hemodialysis grafts [71].

Lower extremity amputations for ischemia should also receive prophylaxis. Sonne-Holm and coworkers studied 152 patients undergoing lower extremity amputation for ischemia. They found that postoperative wound infection rates decreased from 38.7% in the placebo arm to 16.9% in the antibiotic group [72]. Prophylaxis for lower extremity amputations should include coverage for anaerobic flora.

Head and neck surgery

Clean head and neck operations, such as thyroidectomy, parotidectomy, or submandibular gland resection for benign disease, have very low postoperative infection rates (< 2%) and do not require antimicrobial prophylaxis [73]. On the other hand, prophylactic antibiotics may be useful in clean oncologic neck dissections where the incidence of infection is higher [74].

Clean-contaminated surgical procedures

Clean-contaminated surgeries are those that involve nontraumatic wounds during which: (1) a break in surgical technique occurs, or (2) the respiratory, gastrointestinal, or genitourinary tracts are entered without significant spillage. Antimicrobial prophylaxis is recommended for most clean-contaminated surgeries (Table 24.5).

Head and neck surgery

In clean-contaminated head and neck operations, surgical wounds become contaminated because the oropharyngeal mucosa is entered. In these operations, the rate of infection can be as high as 87%, thus the use of antimicrobial prophylaxis is required [74,75]. Factors associated with an increased risk for head and neck SSIs include bilateral neck dissection, advanced cancer, total laryngectomy, and prior tracheostomy [76,77]. It may be that more extensive procedures carry an increased risk of infection because of the inability to achieve a watertight closure, the closing of mucosal suture lines under tension, and/or the need for complex reconstruction. A prior tracheostomy increases the burden of bacteria in the upper airway, which may lead to increased rates of infection.

The antibiotics chosen for prophylaxis should address the pathogens most commonly associated with head and neck SSIs, including *S. aureus*, streptococcal species, and anaerobes. Rubin and colleagues reviewed the cases of head and neck SSIs at their institution: Almost all infections were polymicrobial and, in 74% of polymicrobial infections, anaerobic organisms were found [78]. Lower rates of SSIs occur when the combination of metronidazole (which has anaerobic coverage) and cefazolin is used for prophylaxis, as compared with cefazolin alone (11.9% vs 23.9%) [79]. Hence antimicrobial prophylaxis for clean-contaminated head and neck surgeries should include adequate anaerobic coverage.

The role of gram-negative organisms in the development of head and neck SSIs is controversial. Studies comparing the use of clindamycin (which has no gram-negative coverage) to the regimen of clindamycin plus an agent with gram-negative activity for prophylaxis, show equal efficacy in reducing SSIs, suggesting that a broader agent with gram-negative coverage is not necessary [80,81].

The use of topical antibiotics (e.g., topical clindamycin or piperacillin-tazobactam) either alone, or in combination with

Table 24.5 Prophylaxis for clean-contaminated surgical procedures.

Head and neck surgery	Recommended regimen	Comments
Major procedures involving contamination with oropharyngeal secretions	Cefazolin 1–2 g preoperatively; re-dose every 3–5 hours AND metronidazole 0.5 g preoperatively; re-dose every 8 hours	Consider addition of vancomycin in hospitals with rates of MRSA > 20% and in MRSA carriers Alt: Clindamycin 600 mg preoperatively; re-dose every 6–8 hours
Gastroduodenal surgery	**Recommended regimen**	**Comments**
Procedures involving the esophagus or stomach, with risk factors for decreased acid production	Cefazolin 1–2 g preoperatively; re-dose every 3–5 hours	Risk factors for decreased acid production: elderly, tumor, use of antacids, disease states with decreased acid production (i.e., pernicious anemia or atrophic gastritis)
General/colorectal surgery	**Recommended regimen**	**Comments**
Biliary tract surgery in high-risk patients	Cefazolin 1–2 g preoperatively; re-dose every 3–5 hours	1st generation cephalosporins as effective as 2nd generation cephalosporins. With beta-lactam allergy, can use gentamicin 80 mg IV preoperatively; re-dose every 8 hours. Acute cholecystitis or ascending cholangitis need full-course treatment
Colorectal surgery	Oral: Neomycin and erythromycin base 1 g of each at 1, 2, 11 pm the day prior to surgery	Alt: Neomycin and metronidazole 2 g of each at 7, 11 pm the day prior to surgery
	IV: Cefazolin 1–2 g preoperatively; re-dose every 3–5 hours AND metronidazole 0.5 g preoperatively; re-dose every 8 hours	Alt: Ceftizoxime or gentamicin plus metronidazole; or cefoxitin; or ampicillin-sulbactam; or ertapenem If beta-lactam allergy: Clindamycin plus gentamicin or ciprofloxacin or aztreonam; metronidazole plus gentamicin or ciprofloxacin
Genitourinary surgery	**Recommended regimen**	**Comments**
Open operations with opening of genitourinary tract	Oral: Trimethoprim-sulfamethoxazole 1 DS; or ciprofloxacin 500 mg IV: 1st or 2nd generation cephalosporin	Alt: Aminoglycoside plus metronidazole; or amoxicillin-clavulanate Must know local patterns of resistance
Open operations with opening of gastrointestinal tract	Same as colorectal surgery	
Cystoscopy in high-risk patients or with manipulation/transurethral resection of prostate	Oral: Trimethoprim-sulfamethoxazole 1 DS; or ciprofloxacin 500 mg	Alt: Aminoglycoside plus ampicillin; or amoxicillin-clavulanate; or 1st or 2nd generation cephalosporin
Transrectal prostate biopsy	Oral: Ciprofloxacin 500 mg	Alt: 2nd or 3rd generation cephalosporin; or aminoglycoside plus metronidazole
Gynecologic/obstetric surgery	**Recommended regimen**	**Comments**
Hysterectomy	Cefazolin 1–2 g preoperatively; re-dose every 3–5 hours	Alt: Cefoxitin or cefuroxime or ampicillin-sulbactam If beta-lactam allergy: Clindamycin plus gentamicin, aztreonam, or ciprofloxacin Treat bacterial vaginosis if present
Cesarean section	Cefazolin 1–2 g	Administration prior to incision may be superior to administration after cord clamping

IV, intravenous.

systemic antibiotics has not been shown to reduce infection rates and this practice is discouraged [74,82].

Extending the duration of prophylactic antibiotics beyond 24 hours or until drains have been removed is not beneficial [74,77].

Gastro-duodenal surgery

The risk of developing a SSI following a gastro-duodenal operation is inversely related to the presence of gastric acid and the degree of motility within the stomach prior to surgery.

Patients with normal gastric acid output and normal gastric motility harbor few bacteria in the stomach and proximal intestine. This scarcity of bacteria, which is attributed to the bacteriostatic action of stomach acid, as well as the mechanical cleansing action of normal motility, results in a decreased risk for SSIs [83]. Conversely, patients with obstructing ulcers, tumors, or decreased acidity of the stomach (e.g., upper gastrointestinal bleeding, elderly patients, use of antacid medications) may have an overgrowth of endogenous bacteria and, therefore, an increased risk of infection. Antimicrobial prophylaxis has been shown to be beneficial for these high-risk individuals [84,85]. Prophylaxis with an agent that has activity against oral flora and coliforms, such as a first- or second-generation cephalosporin is efficacious.

Biliary surgery

Clean-contaminated operations involving the biliary system are limited to elective cholecystectomies and prophylaxis is not always required. In their study of patients who did not receive antibiotic prophylaxis prior to undergoing biliary surgery, Keighley and colleagues defined a set of clinical features that were associated with an increased risk for SSIs: (1) age > 70 years old, (2) history or presence of jaundice, (3) previous biliary tract surgery, (4) chills or fevers within one week of surgery, (5) common duct disease, (6) those with operations performed within 1 month of an attack of acute cholecystitis, and/or (7) diabetes mellitus [86]. Patients who have one or more of these characteristics should receive antibiotic prophylaxis with cefazolin (or a second-generation cephalosporin). Otherwise, antimicrobial prophylaxis is typically not recommended.

The use of laparoscopic surgery has dramatically decreased the rates of infection associated with elective cholecystectomies to < 0.5% [87]. Randomized controlled trials comparing antibiotic prophylaxis to placebo or to no prophylaxis in patients undergoing uncomplicated, elective laparoscopic cholecystectomy have not shown a benefit for prophylactic antibiotics [88]. Thus, antimicrobial prophylaxis is generally not recommended for patients undergoing elective laparoscopic cholecystectomy.

Colorectal surgery

Of the clean-contaminated surgeries, colorectal operations encounter the largest amount of bacteria and thus present a formidable task in the prevention of SSIs. Among patients who undergo colorectal operations, the rate of SSIs can be as high as 30% [89,90]. Prophylaxis for colorectal surgery may involve several components: (1) oral antibiotics for bowel preparation, (2) parenteral antibiotics, and (3) mechanical bowel preparation [13,40].

Mechanical preparation of the bowel (by use of enemas or cathartics) has traditionally been employed to reduce colonic bacterial counts prior to surgery. Increasingly, however, the utility of mechanical preparation is being questioned. Guenaga and colleagues conducted a meta-analysis of 14 trials that examined mechanical bowel preparation versus no preparation in elective colorectal operations. The authors did not find a significant difference in the rates of peritonitis, wound infection, or mortality [91]. Thus, many experts have now abandoned the use of mechanical preparation altogether [89].

Conversely, studies have demonstrated that both oral antibiotics (used to reduce the bacterial burden within the bowel lumen) and parenteral antibiotics (to achieve adequate tissue concentrations) are effective in lowering the rates of SSIs in colorectal surgery [92,93]. With respect to whether oral antibiotics or parenteral antibiotics are more efficacious, there has been debate. However, a meta-analysis of 13 studies comparing a combination of oral plus parenteral antimicrobial prophylaxis to parenteral prophylaxis in colorectal surgery, found that the combined use of oral plus parenteral prophylaxis resulted in a 49% risk reduction for SSIs [94].

The parenteral antibiotics chosen for prophylaxis for colorectal operations should have activity against both the facultative anaerobes (e.g., *E. coli*) and anaerobes (e.g., *Bacteroides* spp.) that reside within the bowel. A variety of antibiotic regimens are equally efficacious in reducing colorectal SSIs. Recommended regimens include: (1) a second-generation cephalosporin that has anaerobic activity, such as cefoxitin, or (2) ampicillin-sulbactam, or (3) one antibiotic that has facultative anaerobic activity (e.g., cefazolin, cefotaxime, ceftriaxone, gentamicin) plus one antibiotic that has anaerobic activity (e.g., metronidazole or clindamycin) [40,89]. Recently, Itani and colleagues found that colorectal surgery patients who received ertapenem (a broad-spectrum carbapenem) for prophylaxis had lower rates of SSIs as compared with those who received cefotetan (17.1% vs 26.2%) [95]. However, some authorities have cautioned that the use of ertepenem for prophylaxis may lead to higher rates of *C. difficile* colitis and an increase in the emergence of antibiotic-resistant organisms [89].

For oral prophylaxis, neomycin plus erythromycin or neomycin plus metronidazole is recommended. These should be initiated no more than 18–24 hours before the operation [40].

Urologic surgery

Postoperative infections in urologic surgery include surgical wound infections, urinary tract infections, pyelonephritis, prostatitis, bacteremia, and sepsis. This diversity of infections, along with a lack of uniform clinical trials, has made antibiotic prophylaxis for urologic surgery a challenge. The American Urological Association (AUA) and the European Association of Urology (EAU) have each released guidelines for antibiotic prophylaxis for urologic procedures; for the most part, these are based on limited data [96,97].

Both organizations recommend antimicrobial prophylaxis for open or laparoscopic surgeries that penetrate the urinary tract or the gastrointestinal tract. If the urinary tract is entered, the prophylactic antibiotics should cover the common genitourinary organisms (e.g., *E. coli*, *Proteus* spp., *Klebsiella* spp.,

Enterococcus spp.) and if the gastrointestinal tract is entered (e.g., urinary diversion operations), the prophylactic antibiotics should have activity against both urinary organisms and gastrointestinal organisms.

The frequency of infectious complications following cystoscopy or ureteroscopy is low. In patients with sterile urine prior to these procedures, antibiotic prophylaxis is not necessary unless a manipulation is performed or if the patient has risk factors for infection (e.g., advanced age, anatomic anomalies of the urinary tract, chronic corticosteroid use, immunodeficiency, externalized catheters, or proximal/impacted stone).

Transrectal prostate biopsy and transurethral resection of the prostate are indications for antibiotic prophylaxis. Oral trimethoprim-sulfamethoxazole or a fluoroquinolone is usually sufficient for transrectal prostate biopsy. A meta-analysis of 32 studies of antimicrobial prophylaxis for transurethral prostate resection, which included over 4,000 patients, found that antibiotic prophylaxis decreased both bacteriuria (relative risk reduction of 65%) and clinical septicemia (relative risk reduction of 77%) [98]. No standards have been established for the topical preparation (e.g., povidine-iodine enema, sodium biphosphate enema, bisacodyl suppository) of the rectum prior to transurethral resection of the prostate.

Patients who have preexisting infections (e.g., clinically significant bacteriuria or colonized stone at the time of the procedure) should complete a therapeutic course of antibiotics prior to an elective procedure. However, if the infection cannot be eradicated prior to the operation, a therapeutic course of antibiotics may need to be completed after the operation. Otherwise, prophylaxis should not extend beyond 24 hours after a procedure.

For the urinary tract, cephalosporins, fluoroquinolones, trimethoprim-sulfamethoxazole, and aminoglycosides are efficacious. However, given the rising rates of organisms with antibiotic resistance, it is crucial to consider local patterns of resistance prior to choosing an antibiotic for prophylaxis.

Gynecologic surgery

The overall infection rate for gynecologic operations is about 5% [99]. Operations that are performed through a vaginal approach have a higher risk of infection than those performed through a trans-abdominal approach. Procedures involving the vagina can expose wounds to both aerobic and anaerobic bacteria, and procedures that penetrate the endocervix may distribute these organisms to the endometrium and fallopian tubes.

Antimicrobial prophylaxis is recommended for both transvaginal and trans-abdominal hysterectomy [99]. For abdominal or vaginal hysterectomy, cefazolin is as efficacious as cefoxitin (which have improved activity against anaerobic bacteria). Metronidazole is recommended as an alternative for patients undergoing hysterectomy, but it may be less effective as a single agent for prophylaxis [40,99]. In patients who have a beta-lactam allergy, reasonable alternatives include: clindamycin combined with gentamicin, aztreonam, or ciprofloxacin. The

presence of bacterial vaginosis can increase the risk of post-hysterectomy cuff cellulitis, therefore patients with bacterial vaginosis should be treated prior to hysterectomy.

Procedures that do not require antimicrobial prophylaxis include intrauterine device insertion, routine hysteroscopy, hysterosalpingography, endometrial biopsy, and laparoscopic surgery [99]. Litta and colleagues, in their study of women who underwent laparoscopic surgery for benign gynecologic conditions, found no difference in the rate of SSIs in those who received cefazolin prophylaxis as compared with no antibiotic prophylaxis [100]. In fact, there were no SSIs diagnosed in either group, hence the risk of infection following laparoscopic surgery is very low. Patients with a history of pelvic inflammatory disease or who are found to have fallopian tube damage during trans-cervical procedures have a greater risk for post-procedure pelvic inflammatory disease; women with these findings should receive doxycycline for 5 days after the procedure [99].

Obstetric surgery

Cesarean sections have a 5–20-fold greater risk of infectious complications than do vaginal deliveries. Smaill and Gyte, in their review of 86 studies of prophylactic antibiotics versus no antibiotics in women undergoing cesarean section, determined that prophylactic antibiotics reduced the rates of both endometritis and wound infection [101]. Therefore, prophylactic antibiotics are recommended for women undergoing elective or non-elective cesarean sections [102,103]. The benefits of antimicrobial prophylaxis are greatest for high-risk patients, such as those undergoing cesarean section for emergent delivery or after rupture of membranes [40]. A narrow-spectrum first-generation cephalosporin, such as cefazolin, provides adequate prophylaxis.

Traditionally, the administration of antimicrobial prophylaxis in cesarean section has been delayed until the umbilical cord is clamped because of concerns about drug delivery to the neonate or the potential masking of signs of neonatal sepsis. However, this strategy does not provide the mother with optimal tissue concentrations of antibiotics at the time of incision. Sullivan and colleagues, in their study of 357 women undergoing cesarean section, found that the administration of cefazolin prior to skin incision resulted in a decrease in both endomyometritis and post-cesarean infectious morbidity, but no increase in neonatal sepsis or sepsis work-ups [104]. These data suggest that administering antibiotic prophylaxis prior to the skin incision, as with other surgical procedures, may be a better strategy.

Trauma surgery

Ten to fifteen percent of trauma victims with penetrating abdominal injuries develop infections. In those patients who develop severe abdominal infections, the attributable mortality rate is about 30% [105]. In addition to perioperative antibiotics, other variables (e.g., surgical technique, the number of red cell transfusions, and the penetrating abdominal trauma index score) are important factors in post-trauma infections [106].

For chest trauma, antimicrobial prophylaxis should be considered for esophageal injuries, especially when repair is delayed for more than 12 hours. One day of cefazolin is recommended for patients with little or no contamination. A longer course may be given if there is extensive mediastinal spillage. Similarly, due to the risk of sternal wound infection, patients with cardiac trauma may receive prophylaxis with cefazolin for 24 hours.

For abdominal trauma, the spectrum of activity of the antibiotic(s) chosen for prophylaxis should have activity against both skin and bowel flora. The regimens recommended for use in colorectal operations are also appropriate in the setting of abdominal trauma.

The use of antibiotics in traumatic injuries has been traditionally considered therapeutic rather than prophylactic because the wounds are often grossly contaminated. However, prolonged courses of antibiotics are usually not necessary. Kirton and colleagues, in their study comparing 1 day or 5 days of perioperative antibiotics in patients with penetrating hollow viscus injuries, found that there was no difference in the rates of SSIs or non-surgical-site infections [106]. Thus, in most instances, < 24 hours of antibiotic therapy is appropriate.

Conclusions

Antimicrobial prophylaxis is an important component of a comprehensive approach to SSI prevention. The benefits of antimicrobial prophylaxis must be balanced with its risks, including adverse effects and the emergence of antimicrobial resistance. Whenever possible, the evaluation of antimicrobial prophylaxis should be based on evidence-based data from clinical studies.

References

1. Lister J. On the antiseptic principle in the practice of surgery. *Br Med J* 1867; **2**: 246–8.

2. Anderson DJ, Kaye KS, Classen D *et al.* Strategies to prevent surgical site infections in acute care hospitals. *Infect Control Hosp Epidemiol* 2008; **29** (Suppl 1): S51–61.

3. Wenzel RP. Minimizing surgical-site infections. *N Engl J Med* 2010; **362**: 75–7.

4. Klevens RM, Edwards JR, Richards CL Jr *et al.* Estimating health care-associated infections and deaths in U.S. hospitals, 2002. *Public Health Rep* 2007; **122**: 160–6.

5. Agency for Healthcare Research and Quality. Ambulatory Surgery in U.S. Hospitals, 2003 Executive Summary. 2003. www.ahrq.gov/data/hcup/factbk9a.htm.

6. Cullen KA, Hall MJ, Golosinskiy A. Ambulatory surgery in the United States, 2006. *Natl Health Stat Report* 2009; **11**: 1–25.

7. Allegranzi B, Bagheri Nejad S, Combescure C *et al.* Burden of endemic health-care-associated infection in developing countries: systematic review and meta-analysis. *Lancet* 2011; **377**(9761): 228–41.

8. Kirkland KB, Briggs JP, Trivette SL *et al.* The impact of surgical-site infections in the 1990s: attributable mortality, excess length of hospitalization, and extra costs. *Infect Control Hosp Epidemiol* 1999; **20**: 725–30.

9. Whitehouse JD, Friedman ND, Kirkland KB *et al.* The impact of surgical-site infections following orthopedic surgery at a community hospital and a university hospital: adverse quality of life, excess length of stay, and extra cost. *Infect Cont Hosp Epidemiol* 2002; **23**: 183–9.

10. Perencevich EN, Sands KE, Cosgrove SE *et al.* Health and economic impact of surgical site infections diagnosed after hospital discharge. *Emerg Infect Dis* 2003; **9**: 196–203.

11. Martone WJ, Nichols RL. Recognition, prevention, surveillance, and management of surgical site infections: introduction to the problem and symposium overview. *Clin Infect Dis* 2001; **33** (Suppl 2): S67–8.

12. Broex EC, van Asselt AD, Bruggeman CA *et al.* Surgical site infections: how high are the costs? *J Hosp Infect* 2009; **72**: 193–201.

13. Mangram AJ, Horan TC, Pearson ML *et al.* Guideline for prevention of surgical site infection, 1999. Hospital Infection Control Practices Advisory Committee. *Infect Control Hosp Epidemiol* 1999; **20**: 250–78.

14. Haley RW, Culver DH, Morgan WM *et al.* Identifying patients at high risk of surgical wound infection. *A J Epidemiol* 1985; **121**: 206–15.

15. Culver DH, Horan TC, Gaynes RP and the National Nosocomial Infections Surveillance Systems (NNIS): surgical wound infection rates by wound class, operation and risk index in U.S. Hospitals. *Am J Med* 1991; **91** (Suppl 3B): 152S–7S.

16. John JF Jr, Fishman NO. Programmatic role of the infectious diseases physician in controlling antimicrobial costs in the hospital. *Clin Infect Dis* 1997; **24**: 471–85.

17. Sasse A, Mertens R, Sion JP *et al.* Surgical prophylaxis in Belgian hospitals: estimate of costs and potential savings. *J Antimicrob Chemother* 1998; **41**: 267–72.

18. Goldstein EJ. Beyond the target pathogen: ecological effects of the hospital formulary. *Curr Opin Infect Dis* 2011; **24** (Suppl 1): S21–31.

19. McDonald LC. Trends in antimicrobial resistance in health care-associated pathogens and effect on treatment. *Clin Infect Dis* 2006; **42** (Suppl 2): S65–71.

20. Spellberg B, Guidos R, Gilbert D *et al.* The epidemic of antibiotic-resistant infections: a call to action for the medical community from the Infectious Diseases Society of America. *Clin Infect Dis* 2008; **46**: 155–64.

21. Engemann JJ, Carmeli Y, Cosgrove SE *et al.* Adverse clinical and economic outcomes attributable to methicillin resistance among patients with *Staphylococcus aureus* surgical site infection. *Clin Infect Dis* 2003; **36**: 592–8.

22. Cosgrove SE. The relationship between antimicrobial resistance and patient outcomes: mortality, length of hospital stay, and health care costs. *Clin Infect Dis* 2006; **42** (Suppl 2): S82–9.

23. Carignan A, Allard C, Pépin J *et al.* Risk of *Clostridium difficile* infection after perioperative antibacterial prophylaxis before and during an outbreak of infection due to a hypervirulent strain. *Clin Infect Dis* 2008; **46**: 1838–43.

24. Crabtree T, Aitchison D, Meyers BF *et al. Clostridium difficile* in cardiac surgery: risk factors and impact on postoperative outcome. *Ann Thorac Surg* 2007; **83**: 1396–402.

25. Redelings MD, Sorvillo F, Mascola L. Increase in *Clostridium difficile*-related mortality rates, United States, 1999–2004. *Emerg Infect Dis* 2007; **13**: 1417–19.

26. Knight R, Charbonneau P, Ratzer E *et al.* Prophylactic antibiotics are not indicated in clean general surgery cases. *Am J Surg* 2001; **182**: 682–6.

27. Hidron AI, Edwards JR, Patel J *et al.*; National Healthcare Safety Network Team; Participating National Healthcare Safety Network Facilities. NHSN annual update: antimicrobial-resistant pathogens associated with healthcare-associated infections: annual summary of data reported to the National Healthcare Safety Network at the Centers for Disease Control and Prevention, 2006–2007. *Infect Control Hosp Epidemiol* 2008; **29**: 996–1011.

28. Passaro DJ, Waring L, Armstron R *et al.* Postoperative *Serratia marcescens* wound infections traced to an out-of-hospital source. *J Infect Dis* 1997; **175**: 992–5.

29. Parry MF, Grant B, Yukna M *et al.* Candida osteomyelitis and diskitis after spinal surgery: an outbreak that implicates artificial nail use. *Clin Infect Dis* 2001; **32**: 352–7.

30. Bennett SN, McNeil MM, Bland LA *et al.* Postoperative infections traced to contamination of an intravenous anesthetic, propofol. *N Engl J Med* 1995; **333**: 147–54.

31. Ortega GM, Martí-Bonmatí E, Guevara SJ *et al.* Alteration of vancomycin pharmacokinetics during cardiopulmonary bypass in patients undergoing cardiac surgery. *Am J Health Syst Pharm* 2003; **60**: 260–5.

32. Finkelstein R, Rabino G, Mashiah T *et al.* Vancomycin versus cefazolin prophylaxis for cardiac surgery in the setting of a high prevalence of methicillin-resistant staphylococcal infections. *J Thorac Cardiovasc Surg* 2002; **123**: 326–32.

33. Garey KW, Lai D, Dao-Tran TK *et al.* Interrupted time series analysis of vancomycin compared to cefuroxime for surgical prophylaxis in patients undergoing cardiac surgery. *Antimicrob Agents Chemother* 2008; **52**: 446–51.

34. Bolon MK, Morlote M, Weber SG *et al.* Glycopeptides are no more effective than beta-lactam agents for prevention of surgical site infection after cardiac surgery: a meta-analysis. *Clin Infect Dis* 2004; **38**: 1357–63.

35. Engelman R, Shahian D, Shemin R *et al.*; Workforce on Evidence-Based Medicine, Society of Thoracic Surgeons. The Society of Thoracic Surgeons practice guideline series: Antibiotic prophylaxis in cardiac surgery, Part II: Antibiotic choice. *Ann Thorac Surg* 2007; **83**: 1569–76.

36. Bratzler DW, Hunt DR. The surgical infection prevention and surgical care improvement projects: national initiatives to improve outcomes for patients having surgery. *Clin Infect Dis* 2006; **43**: 322–30.

37. Burke JF. The effective period of preventive antibiotic action in experimental incisions and dermal lesions. *Surgery* 1961; **50**: 161–8.

38. Classen DC, Evans RS, Pestotnik SL *et al.* The timing of prophylactic administration of antibiotics and the risk of surgical-wound infection. *N Engl J Med* 1992; **326**: 281–6.

39. Steinberg JP, Braun BI, Hellinger WC *et al.*; Trial to Reduce Antimicrobial Prophylaxis Errors (TRAPE) Study Group. Timing of antimicrobial prophylaxis and the risk of surgical site infections: results from the Trial to Reduce Antimicrobial Prophylaxis Errors. *Ann Surg* 2009; **250**: 10–16.

40. Bratzler DW, Houck PM; Surgical Infection Prevention Guidelines Writers Workgroup. Antimicrobial prophylaxis for surgery: an advisory statement from the National Surgical Infection Prevention Project. *Clin Infect Dis* 2004; **38**: 1706–15.

41. Forse RA, Karam B, MacLean LD *et al.* Antibiotic prophylaxis for surgery in morbidly obese patients. *Surgery* 1989; **106**: 750–6.

42. Edmiston CE, Krepel C, Kelly H *et al.* Perioperative antibiotic prophylaxis in the gastric bypass patient: do we achieve therapeutic levels? *Surgery* 2004; **136**: 738–47.

43. Dipiro JT, Cheung RP, Bowden TA *et al.* Single dose systemic antibiotic prophylaxis of surgical wound infections. *Am J Surg* 1986; **152**: 552–9.

44. Edwards FH, Engelman RM, Houck P *et al.*; Society of Thoracic Surgeons. The Society of Thoracic Surgeons practice guideline series: Antibiotic prophylaxis in cardiac surgery, Part I: Duration. *Ann Thorac Surg* 2006; **81**: 397–404.

45. Hall JC, Christiansen KJ, Goodman M *et al.* Duration of antimicrobial prophylaxis in vascular surgery. *Am J Surg* 1998; **175**: 87–90.

46. Harbarth S, Samore MH, Lichtenberg D *et al.* Prolonged antibiotic prophylaxis after cardiovascular surgery and its effect on surgical site infections and antimicrobial resistance. *Circulation* 2000; **101**: 2916–21.

47. National Institute for Health and Clinical Excellence. Surgical site infection: Prevention and treatment of surgical site infection. 2008. www.nice.org.uk/nicemedia/live/11743/42379/42379.

48. Darouiche RO, Wall MJ Jr, Itani KM *et al.* Chlorhexidine-alcohol versus povidone-iodine for surgical-site antisepsis. *N Engl J Med* 2010; **362**: 18–26.

49. Saltzman MD, Nuber GW, Gryzlo SM *et al.* Efficacy of surgical preparation solutions in shoulder surgery. *J Bone Joint Surg Am* 2009; **91**: 1949–53.

50. Webster J, Osborne S. Preoperative bathing or showering with skin antiseptics to prevent surgical site infection. *Cochrane Database Syst Rev* 2007; **2**: CD004985.

51. van Rijen MM, Bonten M, Wenzel RP *et al.* Intranasal mupirocin for reduction of *Staphylococcus aureus* infections in surgical patients with nasal carriage: a systematic review. *J Antimicrob Chemother* 2008; **61**: 254–61.

52. Perl TM, Cullen JJ, Wenzel RP *et al.* Mupirocin And The Risk Of *Staphylococcus aureus* Study Team. Intranasal mupirocin to prevent postoperative *Staphylococcus aureus* infections. *N Engl J Med* 2002; **346**: 1871–7.

53. Wilcox MH, Hall J, Pike H *et al.* Use of perioperative mupirocin to prevent methicillin-resistant *Staphylococcus*

aureus (MRSA) orthopaedic surgical site infections. *J Hosp Infect* 2003; **54**: 196–201.

54. Kallen AJ, Wilson CT, Larson RJ. Perioperative intranasal mupirocin for the prevention of surgical-site infections: systematic review of the literature and meta-analysis. *Infect Control Hosp Epidemiol* 2005; **26**: 916–22.

55. Bode LG, Kluytmans JA, Wertheim HF *et al*. Preventing surgical-site infections in nasal carriers of *Staphylococcus aureus*. *N Engl J Med* 2010; **362**: 9–17.

56. Yokoe DS, Mermel LA, Anderson DJ *et al*. A compendium of strategies to prevent healthcare-associated infections in acute care hospitals. *Infect Control Hosp Epidemiol* 2008; **29** (Suppl 1): S12–21.

57. Wilson W, Taubert KA, Gewitz M *et al*.; American Heart Association. Prevention of infective endocarditis: guidelines from the American Heart Association: a guideline from the American Heart Association Rheumatic Fever, Endocarditis and Kawasaki Disease Committee, Council on Cardiovascular Disease in the Young, and the Council on Clinical Cardiology, Council on Cardiovascular Surgery and Anesthesia, and the Quality of Care and Outcomes Research Interdisciplinary Working Group. *Circulation* 2007; **116**: 1736–54. Erratum in: *Circulation* 2007; **116**: e367.

58. Valentine RJ, Weigelt JA, Dryer D *et al*. Effect of remote infections on clean wound infection rates. *Am J Infect Control* 1986; **14**: 64–7.

59. Elek SD, Conen PE. The virulence of *Staphylococcus pyogenes* for man. A study of the problems of wound infection. *Br J Exp Pathol* 1957; **38**: 573–86.

60. Kalmeijer MD, Coertjens H, van Nieuwland-Bollen PM *et al*. Surgical site infections in orthopedic surgery: the effect of mupirocin nasal ointment in a double-blind, randomized, placebo-controlled study. *Clin Infect Dis* 2002; **35**: 353–8.

61. Espenhaug B, Engesaeter LB, Vollset SE *et al*. Antibiotic prophylactics in total hip arthroplasty. *J Bone Joint Surg* 1997; **79**: 590–5.

62. Barker FG 2nd. Efficacy of prophylactic antibiotics for craniotomy: a meta-analysis. *Neurosurgery* 1994; **35**(3): 484–90.

63. Barker FG 2nd. Efficacy of prophylactic antibiotic therapy in spinal surgery: a meta-analysis. *Neurosurgery* 2002; **51**: 391–400.

64. Korinek AM, Baugnon T, Golmard JL *et al*. Risk factors for adult nosocomial meningitis after craniotomy: role of antibiotic prophylaxis. *Neurosurgery* 2006; **59**: 126–33.

65. Barker FG 2nd. Efficacy of prophylactic antibiotics against meningitis after craniotomy: a meta-analysis. *Neurosurgery* 2007; **60**: 887–94.

66. Ratilal B, Costa J, Sampaio C. Antibiotic prophylaxis for surgical introduction of intracranial ventricular shunts. *Cochrane Database Syst Rev* 2006; **3**: CD005365.

67. Fekety FR, Cluff LE, Sabiston DC *et al*. A study of antibiotic prophylaxis in cardiac surgery. *J Thorac Cardiovasc Surg* 1969; **57**: 757–63.

68. Fong IW, Baker CB, McKee DC. The value of prophylactic antibiotics in aortacoronary bypass operations. *J Thorac Cardiovasc Surg* 1979; **78**: 908–13.

69. Hasselgren P, Ivarsson L, Risberg B *et al*. Effects of prophylactic antibiotics in vascular surgery. *Ann Surg* 1984; **200**: 86–92.

70. Venkatesan AM, Kundu S, Sacks D *et al*.; Society of Interventional Radiology Standards of Practice Committee. Practice guidelines for adult antibiotic prophylaxis during vascular and interventional radiology procedures. *J Vasc Interv Radiol* 2010; **21**: 1611–30.

71. Bennion RS, Hiatt JR, Williams RA *et al*. A randomized, prospective study of perioperative antimicrobial prophylaxis for vascular access surgery. *J Cardiovasc Surg* 1985; **26**: 270–4.

72. Sonne-Holm S, Boeckstyns M, Menck H *et al*. Prophylactic antibiotics in amputation of the lower extremity for ischemia. *J Bone Joint Surg* 1985; **67**A: 800–3.

73. Johnson JT, Wagner RL. Infection following uncontaminated head and neck surgery. *Arch Otolaryngol Head Neck Surg* 1987; **113**: 368–9.

74. Simo R, French G. The use of prophylactic antibiotics in head and neck oncological surgery. *Curr Opin Otolaryngol Head Neck Surg* 2006; **14**: 55–61.

75. Becker GD, Parell GJ. Cefazolin prophylaxis in head and neck cancer surgery. *Ann Otol Rhinol Laryngol* 1979; **88**: 183–6.

76. Coskun H, Erisen L, Basut O. Factors affecting wound infection rates in head and neck surgery. *Otolaryngol Head Neck Surg* 2000; **123**: 328–33.

77. Tabet JC, Johnson JT. Wound infection in head and neck surgery: prophylaxis, etiology, and management. *J Otolaryngol* 1990; **19**: 197–200.

78. Rubin J, Johnson JT, Wagner RL *et al*. Bacteriologic analysis of wound infection following major head and neck surgery. *Arch Otolaryngol Head Neck Surg* 1988; **114**: 969–72.

79. Robbins KT, Byers RM, Cole R *et al*. Wound prophylaxis with metronidazole in head and neck surgical oncology. *Laryngoscope* 1998; **98**: 803–6.

80. Piccart M, Dor P, Klastersky J. Antimicrobial prophylaxis of infections in head and neck cancer surgery. *Scand J Infect Dis Suppl* 1983; **39**: 92–6.

81. Johnson JT, Yu V, Myers EN *et al*. An assessment of the need for gram-negative coverage in antibiotic prophylaxis for oncological head and neck surgery. *J Infect Dis* 1987; **155**: 331–3.

82. Simons JP, Johnson JT, Yu VL *et al*. The role of topical antibiotic prophylaxis in patients undergoing contaminated head and neck surgery with flap reconstruction. *Laryngoscope* 2001; **111**: 329–35.

83. LoCicero J, Nichols RJ. Sepsis after gastroduodenal operations: relationship to gastric acid, motility, and endogenous microflora. *South Med J* 1980; **73**: 878–80.

84. Lewis RT, Allan CM, Goodall RG *et al*. Discriminate use of antibiotic prophylaxis in gastroduodenal surgery. *Am J Surg* 1979; **138**: 640–3.

85. Nichols RL, Webb WR, Jones JW *et al*. Efficacy of antibiotic prophylaxis in high risk gastroduodenal operations. *Am J Surg* 1982; **143**: 94–8.

86. Keighley MRB, Flinn R, Alexander-Williams J. Multivariate analysis of clinical and operative findings associated with biliary sepsis. *Br J Surg* 1976; **63**: 528–31.

87. McGuckin M, Shea JA, Schwartz JS. Infection and antimicrobial use in

laparoscopic cholecystectomy. *Infect Control Hosp Epidemiol* 1999; **20**: 624–6.

88. Sanabria A, Dominguez LC, Valdivieso E *et al.* Antibiotic prophylaxis for patients undergoing elective laparoscopic cholecystectomy. *Cochrane Database Syst Rev* 2010; **12**: CD005265.

89. Fry DE. Preventive systemic antibiotics in colorectal surgery. *Surg Infect (Larchmt)* 2008; **9**: 547–52.

90. Fry DE. Surgical site infections and the surgical care improvement project (SCIP): evolution of national quality measures. *Surg Infect (Larchmt)* 2008; **9**: 579–84.

91. Guenaga KK, Matos D, Wille-Jørgensen P. Mechanical bowel preparation for elective colorectal surgery. *Cochrane Database Syst Rev* 2009; **1**: CD001544.

92. Clarke JS, Condon RE, Barlett JG *et al.* Preoperative oral antibiotics reduce septic complications of colon operations: results of prospective, randomized, double-blind clinical study. *Ann Surg* 1977; **186**: 251–9.

93. Song F, Glenny AM. Antimicrobial prophylaxis in colorectal surgery: a systematic review of randomized controlled trials. *Health Technol Assessm* 1998; **2**: 1–110.

94. Lewis RT. Oral versus systemic antibiotic prophylaxis in elective colon surgery: a randomized study and meta-analysis send a message from the 1990s. *Can J Surg* 2002; **45**: 173–80.

95. Itani KM, Wilson SE, Awad SS *et al.* Ertapenem versus cefotetan prophylaxis in elective colorectal surgery. *N Engl J Med* 2006; **355**: 2640–51.

96. American Urological Association. *Best Practice Statement on Urologic Surgery Antimicrobial Prophylaxis.* 2008. www.auanet.org/content/media/antimicroprop08.

97. European Association of Urology. *Guidelines on Urological Infections.* 2010. www.uroweb.org/gls/pdf/Urological%20Infections%202010.

98. Berry A, Barratt A. Prophylactic antibiotic use in transurethral prostatic resection: a meta-analysis. *J Urol* 2002; **167**: 571–7.

99. ACOG Committee on Practice Bulletins-Gynecology. ACOG Practice Bulletin No. 104. Antibiotic prophylaxis for gynecologic procedures. *Obstet Gynecol* 2009; **113**: 1180–9.

100. Litta P, Sacco G, Tsiroglou D *et al.* Is antibiotic prophylaxis necessary in elective laparoscopic surgery for benign gynecologic conditions? *Gynecol Obstet Invest* 2010; **69**: 136–9.

101. Smaill FM, Gyte GM. Antibiotic prophylaxis versus no prophylaxis for preventing infection after cesarean section. *Cochrane Database Syst Rev* 2010; **1**: CD007482.

102. American College of Obstetricians and Gynecologists. ACOG Practice Bulletin No. 47. Prophylactic antibiotics in labor and delivery. *Obstet Gynecol* 2003; **102**: 875–82.

103. van Schalkwyk J, Van Eyk N; Society of Obstetricians and Gynaecologists of Canada Infectious Diseases Committee. Antibiotic prophylaxis in obstetric procedures. *J Obstet Gynaecol Can* 2010; **32**: 878–92.

104. Sullivan SA, Smith T, Chang E *et al.* Administration of cefazolin prior to skin incision is superior to cefazolin at cord clamping in preventing postcesarean infectious morbidity: a randomized, controlled trial. *Am J Obstet Gynecol* 2007; **196**: 455.e1–5.

105. Fabian TC. Infection in penetrating abdominal trauma: risk factors and preventive antibiotics. *Am Surg* 2002; **68**: 29–35.

106. Kirton OC, O'Neill PA, Kestner M *et al.* Perioperative antibiotic use in high-risk penetrating hollow viscus injury: a prospective randomized, double-blind, placebo-control trial of 24 hours versus 5 days. *J Trauma* 2000; **49**: 822–32.

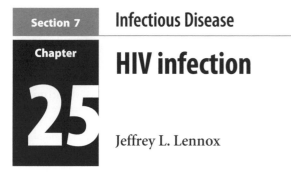

Chapter

25

HIV infection

Jeffrey L. Lennox

The epidemic of human immunodeficiency virus (HIV) infection that began in the late twentieth century has become one of the dominant health issues worldwide for the early twenty-first century. Advances in the prevention of HIV infection have reduced the global incidence of infection and advances in treatment have dramatically extended the lifespan of infected patients. In the developed world a 20-year-old who begins antiretroviral therapy is estimated to have a life expectancy of an additional 43.1 years while a treated patient in the developing world has an additional life expectancy of 26.7 years [1,2]. In 2009 of the estimated 33.3 million people worldwide living with HIV approximately 5 million were on antiretroviral therapy [3]. Since an additional 1.8 million people become infected with HIV each year, the effect of increased longevity will produce increasing opportunities for internists and surgeons to collaborate in the management of HIV-infected patients.

The clinical course of HIV infection has been well described and should be familiar to most physicians. HIV infection is associated with abnormalities in the number and function of CD4-positive T-lymphocytes. Because the CD4-positive T-lymphocytes are essential to the regulation of the human immune system, progressive immune dysfunction is a natural consequence of HIV infection in most patients. This progressive immune dysregulation is associated with decreased cell-mediated immune function, alterations in the humoral immune response, chronic inflammation and depressed mucosal immunity. The late stages of HIV infection are associated with pathologic processes in many organ systems and eventual death due to opportunistic infections or tumors. This natural history of the disease has been dramatically altered by the widespread use in the developed world of highly active antiretroviral therapy (HAART). HAART is an acronym that refers to combinations of antiretroviral agents that have been shown in clinical trials to result in undetectable plasma HIV RNA levels in the majority of patients. These combinations may include two nucleoside analogs plus either a protease inhibitor, an integrase inhibitor or a non-nucleoside reverse transcriptase inhibitor. Guidelines

for the use of these agents in HIV-infected adults and children have been developed, are frequently updated, and are available through the Internet [4].

The use of HAART is associated with significant increases in the levels of CD4-positive T-lymphocytes, decreases in levels of inflammatory markers, decreases in lymphocyte activation and apoptosis, improvement in antibody-mediated immune responses and reductions in infections and tumors. In HAART-treated patients CD4-positive T-lymphocytes will increase by approximately 50–150 cells/mm^3 over the first year of therapy, then by about 50 cells/mm^3 until a steady state is reached after 3–4 years [5]. Patients who in an earlier era would have died of AIDS-related complications may present for surgical care with conditions which are related to the normal aging process, or to other underlying risk factors such as smoking. There is also evidence that survival on HAART is associated with an increased risk for diabetes, certain malignancies, cardiovascular disease, osteoporosis, and cirrhosis in those with concomitant chronic viral hepatitis [6–8]. It is therefore likely that surgeons and internists will be called upon to care for an increasing number of patients undergoing typical surgical interventions that have been used in their HIV-uninfected brethren.

Perioperative evaluation and care

Surgical risk

The risk of surgical procedures in HIV-infected patients is influenced by many of the same factors that determine risk for uninfected patients. Age, operative procedure, other underlying diseases, and the experience of the surgical team are but a few of these factors. In addition, the immunodeficiency caused by HIV may pose an increased risk for infected patients. Most of the data regarding operative risk in patients with HIV infection was collected in the pre-HAART era. Considering the profound effect of HAART on immune function in HIV-infected patients, it is likely that any assessment of surgical risk that relies on these data is an overestimate. In general, studies from the pre-HAART era indicated that HIV-infected patients are at a somewhat increased risk for postoperative morbidity and mortality [9–11]. However, the absolute degree and clinical significance of this risk is controversial. The majority of the studies were retrospective, case-control reports that included small numbers of patients. In addition, staging of the degree of immunosuppression was not routinely reported in all series.

Perioperative mortality

An estimation of the maximal likely risk of perioperative mortality attributable to AIDS may be made by determining the mortality associated with urgent abdominal surgery. In four studies reported between 1994 and 1999, 205 patients underwent urgent abdominal surgery [12–15]. The majority of these patients had an AIDS-defining illness prior to the operation. The most common reasons for abdominal operation were appendicitis (93 patients) and cholecystitis/cholangitis (66 patients). In these 159 patients, the operative mortality was 3%. The remaining 46 patients had undergone surgery for intestinal bleeding (10 patients), intestinal obstruction (12 patients), perforation (8 patients), trauma (6 patients), and other causes (10 patients). In many of these patients the underlying reason for the operation was either an obstructive tumor or an infectious complication of HIV infection. Of these 46 patients, 17 (37%) died in the 30-day postoperative period.

Based on these studies, most of the increased risk associated with urgent surgery in the pre-HAART era was likely to occur in patients who had an active opportunistic infection or a tumor causing obstruction or bleeding. In addition to active infections and tumors, hypoalbuminemia and leukopenia were also associated in some series with an increased operative mortality [12,13]. Surprisingly, there have been few comparative studies of outcomes of surgery in the modern era. The best study is by Horberg, who performed a matched case-control study in a large insured population in California [16]. They selected cases of HIV-infected patients who had undergone surgery between 1997 and 2002, and matched them 1:1 to control patients by age, sex, hospital, and type of operative procedure. Of the 332 matched pairs approximately 80% had abdominal procedures, 11% orthopedic procedures, 6% cardiothoracic procedures and 5% other procedures. The mean CD4 count of the 332 patients with HIV infection was 418 cells/mm^3, and approximately 68% were on antiretroviral therapy. Thirty-day hospital mortality was 0.0% in the HIV negative population and 0.6% in the HIV positive population, a non-statistically significant difference. Similar findings were reported in a case-control study from France and Italy of HIV-positive patients and matched controls who underwent coronary artery bypass grafting [17]. In this population 96% were on antiretroviral therapy, with a mean CD4 count of 502 cells/mm^3, and 30-day mortality was 0.0% in both groups. Based on these two studies it appears that patients who are on treatment with antiretroviral therapy have operative mortality similar to that of HIV-uninfected patients.

Wound infections

Given the dysregulation of immune function associated with HIV infection, it has been suggested that HIV-infected patients may have an increased risk for postoperative wound infections. The literature on this subject suffers again from its retrospective nature, poor controls, and limited sample sizes. The results of analyses reported in the literature are conflicting, with some papers indicating a marked increased risk of wound infection and others indicating no increased risk.

Buehrer et al. reported on 169 invasive procedures performed in patients with hemophilia or other clotting disorders between 1979 and 1988 [18]. The wound infection rate in the HIV-infected patients was 1.4%, which was not statistically significantly different from that reported in the HIV-uninfected patients. In the Horberg study summarized above, the wound infection rate was 3.9% among the HIV-infected patients and 4.8% among the uninfected patients [16]. Similarly, there were no differences in wound infection rates or mediastinitis in the comparative study among patients undergoing CABG [17]. These studies may be viewed as a best-case scenario since they do not involve the implantation of large prosthetic or foreign devices. Reports of orthopedic treatment of traumatic fractures in the pre-HAART era indicated that HIV-infected patients were at a high risk of infection [19–21]. A recent study of orthopedic implants questions the relevance of these early studies. Bahebeck performed a study of wound infections among 74 HIV-infected patients and 572 HIV-uninfected patients receiving an orthopedic implant between 2004 and 2007 [22]. For patients who had less than 500 T cells/mm^3 they began antiretroviral therapy and gave 10 days of twice-daily cefuroxime pre- and postoperatively. Patients who had greater than 500 T cells/mm^3 or who were HIV-uninfected received one dose of cefuroxime preoperatively. The wound infection rate was 4.5% in the lowest T cell group, 6.6% in the higher T cell group and 6.4% in the HIV-negative group. Based on the recent literature, patients with HIV infection who are on antiretroviral therapy appear to have little increased risk for surgical wound infections.

If there is an increased risk, it may be mostly found in those with an AIDS-defining condition. Patients with AIDS have been shown to have an increased carriage rate of Staphylococcus aureus compared with HIV-uninfected controls [23]. This may account for some of the possible increased risk. A recent study indicates that preoperative reduction in staphylococcus colonization rates may reduce postoperative wound infection rates and bacteremia [24]. A randomized placebo-controlled trial of monthly intranasal mupirocin among HIV-positive, non-surgical outpatients demonstrated a reduced rate of nasal S. aureus colonization, but did not decrease infection rates [25]. Given the contradictory data regarding wound infection rates, and the paucity of data regarding the efficacy of colonization eradication preoperatively in this patient population, no formal recommendations can be made regarding this strategy.

Other complications

Other operative complications besides mortality and wound infection have also been the subject of concern. Albaran *et al.* studied all operative complications in 43 patients who underwent abdominal surgery [26]. In the 11 patients who had greater than 200 CD4 positive lymphocytes/mm^3 there were only two postoperative complications. In the 32 patients who had less than 200 T cells/mm^3, there were a total of 31 major complications in 19 patients. The most common complication was pneumonia, which sometimes resulted in respiratory failure. Other complications included pancreatitis, intravenous line infections, and pseudomembranous colitis. These findings are somewhat contradicted by a meta-analysis published by Rose *et al.* [27]. In their analysis of 22 studies that compared outcomes in HIV-infected and uninfected patients, no difference in postoperative complications was found in 15 of the 22 studies. In the large comparative study of Horberg there was a trend towards an increased complication rate in those who had a HIV RNA level of greater than 30,000 copies/mL (OR 2.96, CI 0.91–9.65, P = 0.07) [16]. An analysis of the United States National Trauma Data Bank found that HIV-infected patients hospitalized for trauma had an average length of stay that was 2 days longer than uninfected patients, and increased rates of bacteremia and pneumonia [28]. Similarly, in a study examining the rate of fracture non-union there was no difference in fracture union between the 829 HIV uninfected patients and the 729 HIV-infected patients [29]. However, restricting the analysis to those who had World Health Organization stage IV HIV disease (severe immunodeficiency) there did appear to be an increased rate of non-union compared with HIV-infected patients.

Taken together, the available data indicate that the presence of HIV infection itself is not a contraindication to surgical intervention. It is likely, however, that patients in advanced stages of untreated HIV infection are at increased risk for postoperative complications. The internist and the surgeon must therefore evaluate the degree of immunosuppression, concurrent disease processes and the inherent risk of the surgical procedure in order to adequately inform the patient of the anticipated likelihood of major complications. For patients who have advanced immunosuppression, in whom elective surgery is being considered, it seems prudent to recommend that HAART be instituted in anticipation of the immunologic benefits that have been noted in the majority of treated patients. It must be recognized, however, that this recommendation is not based on a randomized study, nor is it likely that any such study will ever be done. For patients requiring immediate surgery, additional attention should be given to *Pneumocystis* pneumonia prophylaxis, airway management, and antibiotic utilization.

General assessment

A thorough medical history should be performed prior to elective surgery in any HIV-infected patient. It is essential that the degree of the patient's current immune function be determined. The most reliable determinant of this function is the total CD4-positive T-lymphocyte count. For patients who are on HAART, an existing CD4 count and viral load may be used if the results have been obtained within the last 4–6 months prior to operation. In patients who are on a stable antiretroviral regimen, which has fully suppressed the viral load to less than 50 copies of HIV RNA/mL, it is unlikely that the CD4 lymphocyte count will vary significantly over this period of time. In patients who are not on therapy, a CD4 cell count should be performed within 4 weeks prior to surgery in order to determine if the patient is at an increased risk for postoperative complications and to assess for the need for prophylactic therapy to prevent opportunistic infections. In addition, patients should be questioned closely to determine whether they have received immunization against pneumococcal and influenza associated disease, and for the need for prophylactic therapy to prevent *Pneumocystis* pneumonia as recommended by the Public Health Service [30].

Given the widespread use of antivirals and antibiotic therapy, a thorough medication history should be documented for each patient. Certain medications have important drug interactions and the interactions must be anticipated prior to the operative intervention. Table 25.1 lists the antiretroviral medications and potential drug interactions that should be anticipated in the operative setting. In general, the antiretroviral drugs that are of the greatest concern are those that primarily act as inhibitors of the cytochrome P450 enzyme system. These drugs include the class of antiretroviral protease inhibitors, and also certain members of the azole family of antifungal agents. Medications which fall into these two categories may be anticipated to prolong the effects of any other medications which are metabolized by CYP450 3A enzymes. Since many other drug interactions too numerous to enumerate in this table are possible, a search of a drug interaction resource should be undertaken prior to prescribing any medication to a patient on antiretroviral therapy.

In general, the strongest inhibitors of this system include one HIV protease inhibitor that is combined with a second protease inhibitor, ritonavir, specifically to inhibit the metabolism of the first drug. These so-called "boosted protease inhibitors" may prolong the effects of the analgesics meperidine and fentanyl, and may have variable effects on Codone derivatives. Certain anxiolytics such as midazolam, diazepam, alprazolam and others may also be affected. If anxiolytics must be used in the operative setting, an alternative is lorazepam, which is not metabolized by the CYP450 system.

In addition to the interactions noted above, certain patients will require anticoagulation in the postoperative setting. Warfarin, which is metabolized by the cytochrome isoenzymes, will have its activity increased by the protease inhibitors. Careful monitoring of the international normalized ratio (INR) or the prothrombin time (PT) should be undertaken in patients who are receiving coumadin in the postoperative setting.

In contrast to the inhibition of liver cytochromes as outlined above, some medications are primarily inducers of

Table 25.1 Selected interactions between antiretrovirals and medications potentially used in the operative setting.[a]

Drug A	Drug B					
	Analgesics		**Barbiturates**	**Benzodiazepines**		**Other**
	Codones Propofol	Meperidine Fentanyl	Phenobarbital Pentobarbital Thiopental	Alprazolam Midazolam Triazolam	Diazepam Flurazepam	Ketamine
Atazanavir/r	B Decreased	B Increased	C	C	B Increased	
Darunavir/r	B Decreased	B Increased	C	C	B Increased	
Fosamprenavir/r	B Decreased	B Increased	C	C	B Increased	
Indinavir/r	B Decreased	B Increased Avoid M	C	C	B Increased	
Lopinavir/r	B Decreased	B Increased Avoid M	C	C	B Increased	B Increased
Saquinavir/r	B Decreased	B Increased	C	C	B Increased	
Tipranavir/r	B Decreased	B Increased	C	C	B Increased	
Nelfinavir		B Increased	C	C	B Increased	
Efavirenz		B Decreased	A Decreased	C	B Increased	B Decreased
Etravirine		B Decreased	C	B Decreased		
Nevirapine	P Decreased	B Decreased	A Decreased	B Decreased	B Decreased	
Maraviroc	B Decreased		A Decreased			

[a] Based on pharmacokinetics, and the package inserts for each drug. Interactions with other medications exist, see reference [1] for more details.
Drug/r = Drug A used in conjunction with ritonavir; C, Contraindicated; M, Meperidine; P, Propofol.

the cytochrome system. These medications include the non-nucleoside reverse transcriptase inhibitors efavirenz and nevirapine, and both rifampin and rifabutin. These medications would be expected to decrease the activities of many of the same medications listed in Table 25.1. In addition to these important drug interactions, many of the medications used in the setting of HIV infection have toxicities that may become apparent during the perioperative and postoperative setting. Table 25.2 gives a listing of some of the commonly used medications and their associated toxicities. For simplicity's sake the common side-effects of nausea, headache and malaise are not included in this table.

Immune reconstitution inflammatory syndrome (IRIS)

The immune improvements experienced as a result of HAART may also give rise to certain conditions that can necessitate surgical intervention. It is important to recognize these conditions in order to help guide the proper surgical approach. In those individuals who begin HAART at a time when their T-helper cell count is < 200 cells/mm^3 there may occur a syndrome of immune response to occult infections. This syndrome, sometimes referred to as the immune reconstitution inflammatory syndrome (IRIS), is most likely to occur in the first 16 weeks following HAART initiation [31]. In most

treated patients the plasma HIV RNA level will fall by 90% and the CD4-positive T-cell counts in peripheral blood will rise following the initiation of HAART. The most frequently described manifestations of IRIS are painful inflammatory lymphadenitis due to mycobacterial infection, retinitis due to cytomegalovirus (CMV), meningitis due to cryptococcus, worsening tuberculosis and hepatitis due to chronic hepatitis C or B [32,33]. After 16 weeks, late manifestations include thyroiditis and sarcoidosis [34,35]. Optimal management of these conditions has not been elucidated, but in general the severity of the disorder dictates the approach. In patients with mild symptoms, simple observation or anti-inflammatory medication may suffice. In patients with severe inflammatory manifestations, corticosteroids may be beneficial to reduce the inflammation [36]. Surgery may be indicated to drain large abscesses, to place lumbar–peritoneal shunts to relieve intracranial hypertension, or to do a biopsy to aid in diagnosis. In general it is recommended that there be no interruption of antiretroviral therapy in patients with IRIS [4].

Hematopoietic disorders

Patients with advanced HIV infection frequently have leukopenia, anemia, and thrombocytopenia. These hematological abnormalities may increase the likelihood of postoperative

Table 25.2 Adverse effects of medications commonly used to treat HIV infection or its complications.[a]

Acidosis, hepatic steatosis	All nucleoside reverse transcriptase inhibitors
Bleeding	Protease inhibitors (in hemophiliacs)
Bone marrow suppression	Cidofovir, dapsone, flucytosine, ganciclovir, interferon, lamivudine (rare), linezolid, primaquine, pyrimethamine, ribavirin, rifabutin, sulfadiazine, TMP-SMX, valganciclovir, zidovudine
Bronchospasm	Pentamidine
Cardiovascular	Atazanavir (PR interval prolongation)
Dermatologic – rash	Abacavir, atovaquone, dapsone, delavirdine, darunavir, etravirine, fosamprenavir, efavirenz, nevirapine, pyrimethamine, ribavirin, rifabutin, rifampin, rilpivirine, sulfadiazine, TMP-SMX
Dermatologic – other	Fluconazole (hair loss at high dose), emtricitabine (hyperpigmentation), foscarnet (genital ulcers), indinavir (hair loss, ingrown toenails), zidovudine (hyperpigmentation)
Diabetes/glucose intolerance	Didanosine, growth hormone, pentamidine, protease inhibitors
Diarrhea	Atovaquone, clindamycin, protease inhibitors, tenofovir
Hepatotoxicity	All antiretrovirals, all azole antifungals, azithromycin, clarithromycin, isoniazid, pyrazinamide, rifabutin, rifampin, TMP-SMX
Hyperlipidemia	Delavirdine, efavirenz, nevirapine, protease inhibitors, stavudine
Hypersensitivity – fever, rash, multiorgan failure	Abacavir, etravirine
Lipodystrophy	Protease inhibitors, stavudine, zidovudine
Myopathy	All nucleoside analog antiretrovirals
Nephrotoxicity	Acyclovir (high-dose), adefovir, aminoglycosides, amphotericin B, cidofovir, foscarnet, ganciclovir, indinavir (nephrolithiasis), pentamidine, tenofovir, TMP-SMX, valganciclovir
Neurotoxicity – central	Acyclovir (high-dose), azithromycin, clarithromycin, efavirenz, interferon, quinolones
Neurotoxicity – peripheral	Didanosine, growth hormone (carpal tunnel syndrome), isoniazid, metronidazole, ritonavir (paresthesias), stavudine
Ocular toxicity	Cidofovir (hypotony), didanosine, ethambutol (color blindness), interferon (retinal lesions), rifabutin (uveitis), voriconazole
Ototoxicity	Azithromycin, clarithromycin
Pancreatitis	Didanosine, lamivudine (rare), pentamidine, ritonavir, stavudine, TMP-SMX, zalcitabine

[a] This table does not include common upper gastrointestinal, electrolyte or psychiatric disorders.
TMP-SMX, trimethoprim-sulfamethoxazole.

complications. Such conditions may also be worsened by certain antivirals and prophylactic antibiotics (see Table 25.2). The antibiotic dapsone can also cause methemoglobinemia, which at high levels may result in cyanosis. In general, any medication that is being used to prevent or to suppress an opportunistic infection may be safely withheld for a brief period of time (i.e., 2–3 days) if necessary. Longer periods of interruption should prompt the selection of alternative regimens that have fewer hematological side-effects.

In addition to the above abnormalities, some HIV-infected patients may have an increased propensity for thrombosis. Conditions associated with thrombosis include acquired deficiencies of Protein S and Protein C, anticardiolipin antibodies, and nephrotic syndrome [37]. The efficacy of screening for these conditions prior to surgery has not been studied. Thrombotic complications have primarily been described in patients who are not being treated with antiretroviral therapy. Patients with untreated HIV infection should therefore be considered at increased risk for thrombosis, and appropriate preventive measures instituted.

Respiratory disorders

It is important to assess for upper airway disease prior to the intubation of an HIV-infected patient. The physician should examine for oral candidiasis and treat it appropriately if possible prior to the procedure. In addition, patients with advanced immunosuppression are at an increased risk for aphthous ulceration. This painful condition impairs the ability of the patient to tolerate food and oral medications. Aphthous ulceration may be treated with either systemic corticosteroids or with thalidomide [38].

Patients with HIV infection are also at an increased risk for pulmonary complications in the postoperative setting [26,28]. All patients who have a CD4-positive T-lymphocyte count < 200 cells/mm^3, or a CD4-positive T-lymphocyte percentage of < 14%, or who have a history of oral candidiasis should receive prophylaxis to prevent Pneumocystis pneumonia [30]. For patients who have not received prophylaxis, a high degree of suspicion must be maintained for pneumocystosis if pulmonary complications are noted in the postoperative setting.

Since pneumonia is the most commonly reported post-operative complication, physicians should be familiar with the spectrum of HIV-associated pathogens. Common bacterial etiologies of pneumonia in HIV-infected patients include *Streptococcus pneumoniae*, *Hemophilus influenzae*, *Legionella pneumophila*, and *Pseudomonas aeruginosa*. Common opportunistic infections include *Mycobacterium tuberculosis*, *Mycobacterium kansasii*, Cytomegalovirus, *Aspergillus* species, *Cryptococcus neoformans*, *Coccidioides immitis*, and *Histoplasma capsulatum*. Patients who have suffered recurrent episodes of opportunistic pulmonary infections may develop chronic obstructive pulmonary disease. It should also be noted that patients with HIV infection have an increased risk for primary pulmonary hypertension, and although rare, this disorder should be considered in any patient with unexplained dyspnea [39].

Cardiovascular disorders

The spectrum of cardiac disease associated with HIV infection is broad. HIV-1 infection itself and many opportunistic infections have been reported to cause either cardiac dysfunction or pericardial effusion. These include tuberculosis, toxoplasmosis, cytomegalovirus, cryptococcosis, and others.

In addition to these infectious complications, nucleoside reverse transcriptase inhibitors may be associated with cardiac dysfunction. This cardiomyopathy is felt to be due to mitochondrial dysfunction [26]. Tissues that have an increased need for mitochondrial activity, particularly muscle and liver, are more likely to be adversely affected by long-term nucleoside analog use [40]. Such patients may present with isolated signs of cardiac failure, or may present with signs or symptoms of more extensive mitochondrial dysfunction (see Hepatobiliary disorders).

Untreated HIV infection is known to be associated with elevated triglyceride levels. Certain antiretrovirals can cause additional elevations in LDL cholesterol and triglycerides (Table 25.2). Protease inhibitors may also be associated with reduced arterial endovascular function, glucose intolerance and diabetes. Given the presence of these factors, it is likely that HIV-infected patients who are receiving antiretroviral therapy may be at an increased risk for cardiovascular disease [6,8,41]. Given the lipid abnormalities observed with certain HAART regimens, a cardiac risk assessment should be performed prior to elective surgery. In general, such assessment

should follow the guidelines for operative risk as outlined in Chapter 9.

Hepatobiliary disorders

Patients with HIV infection utilize a variety of medications which are potentially hepatotoxic, as outlined in Table 25.2. Nevirapine, in particular, may cause severe hepatitis, especially in women with CD4 and T-cell counts > 250 cells/mm^3 and men with CD4 counts > 400 cells/mm^3. This affliction is usually observed in the first few months of therapy. Careful follow-up and weekly or every other week monitoring of liver transaminases for the first 16 weeks should be routine. There is also an increased prevalence of hepatitis B and hepatitis C virus infection in patients with HIV infection. In patients who are seropositive for hepatitis B surface antigen or for hepatitis C virus antibodies, a history and physical assessment to determine the likelihood of liver disease should be performed.

Physicians should also be aware of the signs and symptoms of hepatic steatosis due to nucleoside-induced mitochondrial dysfunction [42]. This disorder is less common since modern therapy does not usually include the nucleosides most closely associated with mitochondrial dysfunction, stavudine, didanosine and zidovudine. Symptoms of this disorder include fatigue, malaise, weakness, and abdominal pain. In the late stages of mitochondrial dysfunction patients present with lactic acidosis, hepatic steatosis, myopathy, and at times with pancreatitis. Patients who have symptoms or signs of mitochondrial dysfunction should have a resting serum lactate level determined and an ultrasound or CAT scan of the liver. Appropriate management should be instituted prior to surgery if at all possible. Such management should include the withholding of antiretroviral therapy if the lactate level is greater than 2–5 times the upper limit of normal, the patient is symptomatic, and no other cause of lactic acidemia is present [43]. Recovery of full mitochondrial function may take several weeks, and as such may delay elective surgery.

Late-stage, HIV-infected patients are also at an increased risk for biliary tract disease. This typically presents in patients who have < 100 CD4-positive T-lymphocytes/mm^3. Common complaints include right upper quadrant pain (88%), nausea (83%), diarrhea (59%), and weight loss (41%) [44]. Biliary tract disease may be due to cholelithiasis (33%), opportunistic infection (34%), or be idiopathic (acalculous) (33%). The opportunistic infections most commonly associated with biliary tract disease include CMV, *Cryptosporidium* and Microsporidiosis. In patients with an opportunistic infection the alkaline phosphatase level tends to be elevated to a greater degree than that observed in patients with acalculous cholecystitis [45]. Patients with acalculous cholecystitis are more likely to have a normal right upper quadrant ultrasound and a normal HIDA scan than patients who have an opportunistic infection. In contrast, patients with opportunistic infections are more likely to have a thickened gallbladder wall or sludge noted by ultrasound [45]. Patients with an opportunistic infection of the biliary tree may present with worsening of this condition in the setting of the immune reconstitution syndrome. Operative intervention in late stage patients with an opportunistic infection of the biliary system is prone to complications. However, laparoscopic cholecystectomy is a safe procedure in HIV-infected patients and should be considered for any patient in whom there are operative indications [46].

Gastrointestinal disorders

Candidiasis, aphthous ulceration, and CMV are common causes of esophageal disease in HIV-infected patients who are immunosuppressed. In a patient who complains of odyno-phagia or dysphagia, a course of oral azole antifungal therapy should be given, whether or not oral candidiasis is present. If there is no improvement after 48–72 hours, an esophagoscopy should then be performed.

Kaposi's sarcoma and many opportunistic infections may be associated with diarrhea. These infections include bacterial pathogens (Shigella, Salmonella, Campylobacter, *Clostridium difficile*), viruses (CMV, HSV), parasites (Giardia, Microspor-idiosis, Isospora), and mycobacteria (tuberculosis, disseminated *Mycobacterium avium–intracellulare* complex (DMAC)). Protease inhibitors are also noted for their propensity to cause diarrhea. Patients who complain of diarrhea should have an evaluation for infectious causes prior to elective surgery. In residents of the developed world in whom symptoms of proctitis are absent, it is reasonable to perform stool cultures and a stool smear for Giardia. A stool smear for Microspor-idiosis and other intestinal parasites should be done for those in whom these initial results are negative. A stool test for *C. difficile* toxin should be performed if the patient is febrile or has a peripheral blood leukocytosis. Patients with symptoms of proctitis should initially be tested for HSV, gonorrhea and Chlamydia by collecting rectal swab specimens. If these are negative, then further testing as outlined above, and a proctoscopy or flexible sigmoidoscopy, may be performed.

Patients with DMAC or CMV frequently complain of abdominal pain. For DMAC a blood mycobacterial culture should be performed. For CMV a computer-assisted tomography scan of the abdomen may reveal thickening of the colonic wall. A colonoscopy with biopsy is the typical diagnostic procedure. However, for patients who refuse this procedure and who have active ophthalmic CMV, a presumptive diagnosis may be made if there is a symptomatic response to therapy. Whether a blood CMV PCR is useful for diagnosing CMV colitis has not been determined since many HIV-infected patients who have low T-cell counts may have a positive result [47].

Renal disorders

African-American patients with HIV infection are at an increased risk for renal dysfunction due to HIV-associated nephropathy (HIVAN) [48]. This condition is rare in Caucasians and other racial groups. HIVAN is characterized by focal and segmental glomerulosclerosis, glomerular collapse, and progressive azotemia. In the early stages, HIVAN may be detected by increased protein excretion in the urine. In the later stages nephrotic range proteinuria and renal dysfunction become evident. Ultrasound examination of the kidneys will frequently reveal enlarged kidneys with increased echogenicity. There is no known effective treatment, although reports from patient cohorts have indicated likely benefit of HAART in delaying the onset and progression [49,50]. Patients who have asymptomatic proteinuria may be at an increased risk for medication induced renal toxicity. A screening urinalysis should be performed in HIV-infected, African-American patients in order to assess for this potential complication. Table 25.2 includes a listing of commonly used medications that are potentially nephrotoxic.

Miscellaneous disorders

Since HIV infection can affect every organ system of the body, the internist should perform a thorough assessment for miscellaneous conditions. These include adrenal insufficiency, pancreatic disease, central nervous system disease, peripheral nervous system disease and musculoskeletal disease. All of these general conditions are noted to be more prevalent in HIV-infected patients either due to the disease process or due to medications.

Occupational transmission of HIV

HIV can be transmitted from infected patients to healthcare workers. However, the risk of acquiring infection in the surgical setting is small. For example, in the first 19 years of the HIV epidemic, during the time when antiretroviral therapy was only marginally effective, only 56 US healthcare personnel were documented to have occupationally acquired HIV infection [38]. In addition, another 138 healthcare workers had a possible work-related infection. However, the majority of the healthcare workers infected as a result of an occupational exposure were not physicians or operating room personnel.

The risk of developing HIV infection in the healthcare setting includes several elements. Among these are the prevalence of HIV infection in the patient population, the size of the blood inoculum, the depth of penetration and the duration of contact with the inoculum. Another important factor is the stage of illness of the patient. Patients with advanced stages of HIV infection typically have higher plasma viral loads than patients with earlier stages. High-risk needle sticks are caused by hollow bore needles that have been in the vein of an HIV-infected patient, and which cause a deep penetrating injury to the healthcare worker. Factors that reduce the infectious inoculum include injury from a solid needle or instruments, the use of antiretroviral therapy in the source patient and the wearing of gloves. Laboratory studies have suggested that double gloving has the potential to additionally reduce HIV transmission.

The Centers for Disease Control and Prevention estimates that the average rate of transmission of HIV after a percutaneous exposure is approximately 0.32%, and for mucous membrane exposures 0.09% [52]. These estimates are derived from data collected during an era when HAART therapy was not available for either patients or healthcare workers. The risk should be much lower if the source patient and the healthcare worker are appropriately treated. Concern about the potential transmission of HIV should therefore not be a significant consideration of whether to perform an operative procedure. However, since even one high-risk exposure can result in infection, appropriate measures to reduce the risk to operating room personnel should be utilized. These universal precautions, which should be used for all patients, involve the use of fluid-resistant gowns, gloves, masks and eyewear that reduce contact with infectious fluids.

The risk of infection for healthcare workers can be reduced further by the appropriate administration of postexposure prophylaxis. Based on available data, postexposure prophylaxis reduces the risk of transmission by approximately 80%. In general, the efficacy of postexposure prophylaxis is dependent upon rapid evaluation and appropriate medical treatment. The Public Health Service recommendations indicate that all healthcare workers who sustain percutaneous injuries from HIV-infected patients should be considered for postexposure prophylaxis [52]. For small-volume percutaneous injuries, such as solid needle and a superficial injury, two to three drugs are recommended depending on the stage of illness of the patient. For patients with > 500 CD4 T-cells, or for those known to have a low viral load, a regimen of two nucleoside analogs is considered acceptable. For advanced stage patients, or for more severe injuries, an expanded three-drug regimen is recommended. The guidelines recommend that three-drug regimens include two nucleoside analog inhibitors and either a protease inhibitor or efavirenz. However, it is also recommended that the regimen be tailored to the virus harbored by the individual source patient. There are documented cases where postexposure prophylaxis was administered, but failed due to resistant virus present in the source patient's blood. Healthcare workers should receive postexposure medications to which the source patient's virus is likely to be sensitive. A useful resource for those involved in the management of occupational exposures is the National HIV/AIDS Clinicians' Consultation Center hotline. This hotline is available 24 hours a day and may be reached at 001–888–448–4911, and the website for this organization is http://www.nccc.ucsf.edu.

The optimal duration of prophylaxis is unknown. Based on the available data, the Public Health Service recommends that healthcare workers who receive prophylaxis be treated for 4 weeks. Cohort studies have indicated that approximately 50% of healthcare workers will experience drug-associated adverse events. The majority of these are gastrointestinal upset, although more severe toxicities have also been reported. In general, nevirapine should be avoided for prophylaxis due to the potential for hepatitis and Stevens–Johnson syndrome. Unusual or severe toxicity should be reported to the Food and Drug Administration at 001–800–332–1088. Occupationally acquired HIV infection or failure of postexposure prophylaxis should be reported to the CDC at 001–800–893–0485.

References

1. The Antiretroviral Therapy Cohort Collaboration. Life expectancy of individuals on combination antiretroviral therapy in high-income countries: a collaborative analysis of 14 cohort studies. *Lancet* 2008; **372**: 293–9.

2. Mills EJ, Bakanda C, Birungi J *et al.* Life expectancy of persons receiving combination antiretroviral therapy in low-income countries: a cohort analysis from Uganda. *Ann Intern Med* 2011; **155**: 209–16.

3. UNAIDS report on the global AIDS epidemic 2010. www.unaids.org/documents/20101123_GlobalReport_em.pdf.

4. Panel on Antiretroviral Guidelines for Adults and Adolescents. Guidelines for the use of antiretroviral agents in HIV-1-infected adults and adolescents. Department of Health and Human Services. January 10, 2011; 1–166. www.aidsinfo.nih.gov/ContentFiles/AdultandAdolescentGL.pdf.

5. Kaufmann GR, Perrin L, Pantaleo G *et al.* CD4 T-lymphocyte recovery in individuals with advanced HIV-1 infection receiving potent antiretroviral therapy for 4 years: the Swiss HIV Cohort Study. *Arch Intern Med* 2003; **163**: 2187–95.

6. Beherns G, Schmidt H, Meyer D *et al.* Vascular complications associated with use of HIV protease inhibitors. *Lancet* 1998; **351**: 1958.

7. Allison GT, Bostrom MP, Glesby MJ. Osteonecrosis in HIV disease: epidemiology, etiologies, and clinical management. *AIDS* 2003; **17**(1): 1–9.

8. The Data Collection on Adverse Events of anti-HIV drugs Study Group. Combination antiretroviral therapy and the risk of myocardial infarction. *N Engl J Med* 2003; **349**: 1993–2003.

9. Ferguson CM. Surgical complications of human immuno-deficiency virus infection. *Am Surg* 1988; **54**: 4–9.

10. Wexner SD, Smithy WB, Trillo C *et al.* Emergency colectomy for cytomegalovirus ileocolitis in patients with the acquired immune deficiency syndrome. *Dis Colon Rectum* 1988; **31**: 755–61.

11. Robinson G, Wilson SE, Williams RA. Surgery in patients with acquired immunodeficiency syndrome. *Arch Surg* 1987; **122**: 170–5.

12. Whitney TM, Brunel W, Russell TR *et al.* Emergent abdominal surgery in AIDS: experience in San Francisco. *Am J Surg* 1994; **168**: 239–43.

13. Bizer LS, Pettorino R, Ashikari A. Emergency abdominal operations in the patient with acquired immunodeficiency syndrome. *J Am Coll Surg* 1995; **180**: 205–9.

14. Flum DR, Steinberg SD, Sarkis AY *et al.* Appendicitis in patients with acquired immunodeficiency syndrome. *J Am Coll Surg* 1997; **184**: 481–6.

15. Ricci M, Puente AO, Rothenberg RE *et al.* Open and laparoscopic cholecystectomy in acquired immunodeficiency syndrome: indications and results in fifty-three patients. *Surgery* 1999; **125**: 172–7.

16. Horberg MA, Hurley LB, Klein DB *et al.* Surgical outcomes in human immunodeficiency virus-infected patients in the era of highly active antiretroviral therapy. *Arch Surg* 2006; **141**: 1238–45.

17. Filsoufi F, Salzberg SP, von Harbou KTJ, Neibart E, Adams DH. Excellent outcomes of cardiac surgery in patients infected with HIV in the current era. *Clin Infect Diseas* 2006; **43**: 532–6.

18. Buehrer JL, Weber DJ, Meyer AA *et al.* Wound infection rates after invasive procedures in HIV-1 seropositive versus HIV-1 seronegative hemophiliacs. *Ann Surg* 1990; **211**: 492–8.

19. Paiement GD, Hymes RA, LaDouceur MS *et al.* Postoperative infections in asymptomatic HIV-seropositive orthopedic trauma patients. *J Trauma* 1994; **37**: 545–51.

20. Hoekman P, Van de Perre P, Nelissen J *et al.* Increased frequency of infection after open reduction of fractures in patients who are seropositive for human immunodeficiency virus. *J Bone Joint Surg [Am]* 1991; **73**: 675–9.

21. Jellis JE. Orthopaedic surgery and HIV disease in Africa. *Int Orthop* 1996; **20**: 253–6.

22. Bahebeck J, Eone DH, Nonga BN, Kingue TN, Sosso M. Implant orthopaedic surgery in HIV asymptomatic carriers: management and early outcome. *Injury* 2009; **40**: 1147–50.

23. Ganesh R, Castle D, McGibbon D *et al.* Staphylococcal carriage and HIV infection. *Lancet* 1989; **2**: 558.

24. Kalmeijer MD, Coertjens H, van Nieuwland-Bollen PM *et al.* Surgical site infections in orthopedic surgery: the effect of mupirocin nasal ointment in a double-blind, randomized, placebo-controlled study. *Clin Infect Dis* 2002; **35**: 353–8.

25. Gordon RJ, Chez N, Jia H, Zeller B *et al.* The NOSE study (nasal ointment for *Staphylococcus aureus* eradication): a randomized controlled trial of monthly mupirocin in HIV-infected individuals. *J Acquir Immune Defic Syndr* 2010; **55**: 466–72.

26. Albaran RG, Webber J, Steffes CP. CD4 cell counts as a prognostic factor of major abdominal surgery in patients infected with the human immunodeficiency virus. *Arch Surg* 1998; **133**: 626–31.

27. Rose DN, Collins M, Kleban R. Complications of surgery in HIV-infected patients. *AIDS* 1998; **12**: 2243–51.

28. Morrison CA, Wyatt MM, Carrick MM. Effects of human immunodeficiency virus status on trauma outcomes: a review of the National Trauma Database. *Surg Infect* 2010; **11**: 41–7.

29. Kamat AS, Govender M. The effects of HIV/AIDS on fracture union. *J Bone Joint Surg [BR]* 2010; **92**-B: S228.

30. Centers for Disease Control and Prevention. Guidelines for prevention and treatment of opportunistic infections in HIV-infected adults and adolescents. *Morb Mortal Wkly Rep* 2009; **58**: 1–207.

31. Müller M, Wandel S, Colebunders R *et al.* Immune reconstitution inflammatory syndrome in patients starting antiretroviral therapy for HIV infection: a systematic review and meta-analysis. *Lancet Infect Dis* 2010; **10**: 251–61.

32. Ofotokun I, Smithson SE, Lu C, Easley KA, Lennox JL. Liver enzymes elevation and immune reconstitution among treatment-naïve HIV-infected patients instituting antiretroviral therapy. *Am J Med Sci.* 2007; **334**: 334–41.

33. Anderson AM, Mosunjac MB, Palmore MP, Osborn MK, Muir AJ. Development of fatal acute liver failure in HIV-HBV coinfected patients. *World J Gastroenterol* 2010; **16**: 4107–11.

34. Crum N, Ganesan A, Johns S, Wallace MR. Graves disease: an increasingly recognized immune reconstitution syndrome. *AIDS* 2006; **20**: 466–9.

35. Naccache JM, Antoine M, Wislez M *et al.* Sarcoid-like pulmonary disorder in human immunodeficiency virus-infected patients receiving antiretroviral therapy. *Am J Respir Crit Care Med* 1999; **159**: 2009–13.

36. Meintjes G, Wilkinson RJ, Morroni C *et al.* Randomized placebo-controlled trial of prednisone for paradoxical tuberculosis-associated immune reconstitution inflammatory syndrome. *AIDS* 2010; **24**: 2381–90.

37. Saif MW, Bona R, Greenberg B. AIDS and thrombosis: retrospective study of 131 HIV-infected patients. *AIDS Patient Care Stds* 2001; **15**: 311–20.

38. Patton LL, van der Horst C. Oral infections and other manifestations of HIV disease. *Infect Dis Clin North Am* 1999; **13**: 879–900.

39. Mehta NJ, Khan IA, Mehta RN, Sepkowitz DA. HIV-related pulmonary hypertension: analytic review of 131 cases. *Chest* 2000; **118**: 1133–41.

40. Lewis W, Dalakas MC. Mitochondrial toxicity of antiviral drugs. *Nature Med* 1995; **1**: 417–22.

41. Friis-Møller N, Weber R, Reiss P *et al.* Cardiovascular disease risk factors in HIV patients- association with antiretroviral therapy. Results from the DAD study. *AIDS* 2003; **17**: 1179–93.

42. Fortgang IS, Belitsos PC, Chaisson RE *et al.* Hepatomegaly and steatosis in HIV-infected patients receiving nucleoside analog antiretroviral therapy. *Am J Gastroenterol* 1995; **90**: 1433–6.

43. Carr A. Lactic acidemia in Human Immunodeficiency Virus. *Clin Infect Dis* 2003; **36** (Suppl 2): S96–100.

44. Nash JA, Cohen SA. Gallbladder and biliary tract disease in AIDS. *Gastroenterol Clin North Am* 1997; **26**: 323–35.

45. French AL, Beaudet LM, Benator DA *et al.* Cholecystectomy in patients with AIDS: clinicopathologic correlations in 107 cases. *Clin Infect Dis* 1995; **21**: 852–8.

46. Ricci M, Puente AO, Rothenberg RE *et al.* Open and laparoscopic cholecystectomy in acquired immunodeficiency syndrome: indications and results in fifty-three patients. *Surgery* 1999; **125**: 172–7.

47. Deayton JR, Sabin CA, Johnson MA *et al.* Importance of cytomegalovirus viraemia in risk of disease progression and death in HIV-infected patients

receiving highly active antiretroviral therapy. *Lancet* 2004; **363**: 2116–21.

48. Gupta SK, Eustace JA, Winston JA *et al.* Guidelines for the management of chronic kidney disease in HIV-infected patients: recommendations of the HIV Medicine Association of the Infectious Diseases Society of America. *Clin Infect Dis* 2005; **40**: 1559–85.

49. Smith MC, Austen JL, Carey JT. Prednisone improves renal function and proteinuria in human immunodeficiency virus-associated nephropathy. *Am J Med* 1996; **101**: 41–8.

50. Szczech LA. Renal diseases associated with human immunodeficiency virus infection: epidemiology, clinical course, and management. *Clin Infect Dis* 2001; **33**: 115–19.

51. Cardo DM, Culver DH, Ciesielski CA *et al.* A case-control study of HIV seroconversion in health care workers after percutaneous exposure. *N Engl J Med* 1997; **337**: 1485–90.

52. Centers for Disease Control and Prevention. Updated U.S. Public Health Service guidelines for the management of occupational exposures to HBV, HCV, and HIV and recommendations for postexposure prophylaxis. *Morb Mortal Wkly Rep* 2005; **54**: 1–17.

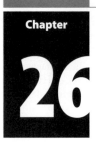

Chapter 26

Fever and infection in the postoperative setting

James P. Steinberg and Shanta M. Zimmer

Fever is common in the postoperative period, and its causes are diverse (Table 26.1). Fever may result from a benign process such as the release of pyrogens from traumatized tissue and have little bearing on the clinical outcome. Alternatively, fever may be an early sign of a potentially life-threatening infection. The clinician's challenge is to identify those important fevers early, while avoiding the excessive use of diagnostic resources and therapeutic interventions such as unnecessary antibiotics.

Evaluation of a febrile surgical patient begins with a careful history and review of the medical record. The presence of symptoms or signs of infection before the operative procedure or underlying medical problems that increase the likelihood of postoperative complications are valuable clues. The type of surgical procedure performed, operative findings, and the temporal relationship between the operation and the onset of fever are also important. Although prolonged endotracheal intubation, indwelling bladder catheters, and intravascular catheters may be important components of patient care, they violate normal host defenses and increase the likelihood of postoperative infection. When a patient has a significant infection, symptoms and signs in addition to fever usually are present. Thus, a careful physical examination is essential. Laboratory and radiographic studies should be directed by the relevant clinical data and not obtained by an undirected "shotgun" approach.

The incidence of postoperative fever varies widely depending on the surgical procedure performed and the definition of fever used. There is no consensus regarding what constitutes fever in the postoperative setting. Investigators have used temperatures ranging from 37.5 °C to 38.5 °C to define fever with 38 °C as the most common cut-off point. In addition, some investigators require that the temperature be elevated on consecutive measurements to meet their definition of fever, whereas others require that the temperature be elevated for 2 consecutive days. Thus, it is not surprising that the reported incidence of postoperative fever ranges from 13.7% after general surgery to nearly 100% following cardiac surgery [1,2]. Even among studies that involve only abdominal

operations, there still is a considerable variation in the reported incidence of fever (Table 26.2) [3–6].

Temporal aspects of postoperative fever

The time of onset of postoperative fever is a helpful clue that can suggest a particular cause. Fever that develops within 24 hours after surgery usually is not caused by infection (Figure 26.1). The time-honored dogma that atelectasis causes most early postoperative fever [7,8] may be incorrect [2,9]. Garibaldi and colleagues found that unexplained (and presumed non-infectious) early postoperative fever did not occur more frequently after thoracic and upper abdominal surgeries, procedures that predispose to atelectasis and pneumonia [9]. In addition, Roberts and associates did not find a strong correlation between early fever (48 hours or less) following abdominal surgery and radiographic evidence of atelectasis [10]. Cytokine release during surgery appears to be the major cause of early postoperative fevers. A shift in the core temperature curve has been observed in all postoperative patients (Figure 26.2) [11], with the highest temperature occurring 11.5 ± 5.8 hours after surgery. Tissue trauma during surgery causes a release of proinflammatory cytokines, the levels of which correlate with increases in core temperature [11]. Duration and perhaps extent of surgical intervention appear to impact the degree of temperature elevation. Other non-infectious causes of early postoperative fever include drug hypersensitivity reactions (including anesthetic agents) and transfusion reactions, which may cause hemolysis. Malignant hyperthermia usually manifests with high fever (39 °C to 44 °C) beginning within 30 minutes of the administration of an anesthetic agent. Rarely, the fever associated with malignant hyperthermia is delayed and develops several hours after operation.

On occasion, infection does occur within 1 to 2 days after surgery. *Streptococcus pyogenes* and *Clostridium perfringens* infections, although rare, are the classic causes of early postoperative wound infections and can produce high fever within 24 hours of surgery. With streptococcal infections, erythema around the

Medical Management of the Surgical Patient, ed. Michael F. Lubin, Thomas F. Dodson, and Neil H. Winawer. Published by Cambridge University Press. © Cambridge University Press 2013.

Table 26.1 Causes of postoperative fever.

Non-infectious	Infectious
Adrenal insufficiency	Abscess
Alcohol withdrawal	Bloodstream infections
Atelectasis	Cholecystitis
Blood (hematoma/ CSF)	*Clostridium difficile* colitis
Dehydration	Endocarditis
Drug fever (including anesthetics)	Infusion-related infections Intravascular device infections
Factitious	Parotitis
Malignant hyperthermia	Peritonitis
Myocardial infarction	Pneumonia
Neoplasms	Prostatitis
Pancreatitis	Surgical site infections
Pheochromocytoma	
Pericarditis/Dressler's syndrome	
Pulmonary embolism	Transfusion-related infection (cytomegalovirus, hepatitis)
Thrombophlebitis	
Thyrotoxicosis	Urinary tract infection
Tissue trauma	
Transfusion reaction	

Postoperative fever can be divided into two broad categories – infectious and non-infectious. The reported proportion of febrile episodes attributed to bacterial infection also varies widely. In general, high fevers are more likely caused by infection, but considerable overlap exists.

Table 26.2 Incidence of fever and infection causing fever following abdominal surgery.

Procedure [reference]	Definition of fever	N	% with fever	% of those febrile with infection
Major abdominal [3]	≥ 38.5 °C (rectally) on two consecutive measurements during first 6 postoperative days	464	15	27[a]
Cholecystectomy [4]	≥ 38.4 °C or ≥38.0 °C (orally) on consecutive measurements 4 hours apart	176	16	7[b,c]
Abdominal [5]	≥ 38.1 °C during first 7 postoperative days	434	38	16[a]
Intra-abdominal, duration > 1 hour [6]	≥ 38.0 °C (rectally) on two measurements > 1 hour apart	608	43	36
	Group A – 38°–38.4 °C		A–15	A–19
	Group B – ≥ 38.5 °C		B–27	B–45

[a] Required culture confirmation.
[b] Eight other patients had infection but were afebrile.
[c] Uses CDC definition of infection.

surgical site develops early and spreads rapidly. Clostridial wound infections typically occur after biliary tract or intestinal surgery. Severe pain is present and tense edema develops at the surgical site. A bronze or violaceous hue may develop followed by hemorrhagic bullae and the formation of tissue gas.

Toxic shock syndrome also produces high fever early in the postoperative period. Hypotension, diffuse erythematous rash, confusion, and other signs of toxemia often are present. In contrast to other wound infections, signs of local inflammation are absent, even though the surgical site harbors the toxigenic *Staphylococcus aureus*.

If significant aspiration of oropharyngeal or gastric contents occurred during induction of anesthesia, a postoperative pneumonia may manifest within 1 or 2 days of surgery. If the surgery is prompted by infection (such as peritonitis following a ruptured viscus), fever can antedate or occur shortly after the procedure. On occasion, an unrelated infection is incubating at the time of surgery and produces early fever. Accurate

diagnosis can be difficult, especially when patients are intubated or sedated after operation and are unable to relate their histories.

Fever that develops 72 hours or more after operation suggests the presence of infection. Rates of infection vary considerably with the type of operation performed, ranging from 2% after herniorrhaphy to 20.8% after gastric surgery [12]. Although the causes of postoperative infection are numerous (Table 26.1), surgical site infections, bloodstream infections, pneumonia, and urinary tract infections (UTIs) account for 80–90% of all cases. Surgical site infections are most common overall but the distribution of infections depends on the type of operation performed. Surgical site infections typically manifest themselves 5 to 10 days after operation, although deep organ space abscesses may appear later. Infections involving implanted devices may become evident weeks to months following implantation. Bacterial pneumonias are often precipitated by perioperative aspiration or early postoperative atelectasis and, consequently, tend to occur within the first week after surgery. Urinary tract

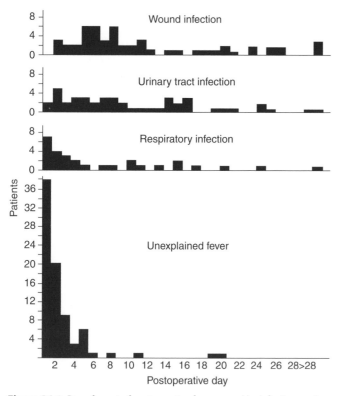

Figure 26.1 Day of onset of postoperative fever caused by infections and unexplained fever [9].

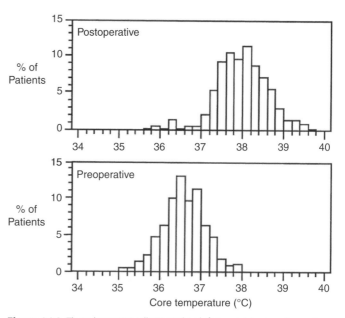

Figure 26.2 These histograms illustrate the shift in maximum postoperative core temperatures in the first 24 hours following surgery patients compared with preoperative core temperatures (N = 271) [11].

infections can appear at any time; the major risk factors for UTI development are instrumentation of the urinary tract and indwelling urinary catheters. The probability of bacterial colonization in the bladder increases with duration of catheterization. Bloodstream infections may result from any of these infections but are most commonly caused by intravascular devices. The risk of bloodstream infection increases with the duration of intravascular access.

Fever may accompany postoperative myocardial infarction, which occurs most commonly within 72 hours. Clinical clues may be difficult to assess in the intubated and sedated patient but include tachycardia, arrhythmia, congestive heart failure, and diaphoresis. Postpericardiotomy syndrome, including Dressler's syndrome, is another non-infectious cause of postoperative fever; careful auscultation for a pericardial friction rub aids in this diagnosis.

Thrombophlebitis, pulmonary embolism, and pulmonary infarction are important causes of postoperative fever that can occur early or late in the postoperative period, depending on the clinical situation. Diagnosis can be difficult and a high index of suspicion is necessary. Hematomas can produce occult fevers or mimic an intra-abdominal abscess. The possibility of a hematoma should be considered when the hematocrit continues to decline after the operation in the absence of other explanations such as gastrointestinal blood loss. Resorption of blood can produce hyperbilirubinemia and an elevated lactate dehydrogenase level. Hematomas also can become secondarily infected, further complicating the clinical picture.

Medications are an important cause of postoperative fever. Drug fever caused by antibacterial agents classically develops 7–10 days after starting the medication [13]. Misconceptions abound regarding drug fever; rash, eosinophilia, and other signs of drug allergy are frequently absent. In addition, drug fever can produce a variety of fever patterns including a hectic fever curve.

Late fever, developing more than 2 weeks after surgery, usually occurs in patients with underlying medical problems or complicated hospital courses. Prolonged intravenous access, bladder catheterization, or endotracheal intubation presents ongoing risks for infection. Transient bacteremias can lead to metastatic foci of infection that declare themselves in the late postoperative period. Drug fevers can occur several weeks or longer after a new medication is introduced. Transfusion-related infections, particularly cytomegalovirus infection, can produce fever weeks to months after the receipt of blood products. Screening of blood products for human immunodeficiency virus, hepatitis B and C has reduced transfusion-associated infection to extremely low levels. *Clostridium difficile* diarrhea occurs days to several weeks after antibiotics are administered. Single-dose surgical antibiotic prophylaxis is less likely to induce this infection than longer courses of antibiotics.

Surgical site infections

The term *surgical site infection* is preferred to *surgical wound infection* because it allows for a more precise categorization of infections. According to the CDC definitions, surgical site infections are divided into incisional or organ/space infections [14]. Superficial incisional infections involve the skin and subcutaneous tissues whereas deep incisional infections involved the fascia and muscle. Organ/space surgical site infections involve any anatomic part other than the incised body wall layers opened or manipulated during the procedure. The term surgical "wound" in standard parlance extends from the skin to the deep soft tissues and not to the organ space. Thus, the term *deep wound infection*, referring to infections at or deep to the fascial layers, is ambiguous. The distinction between incisional and organ/space infections has relevance because certain procedures (e.g., cesarean section) are more likely to lead to organ/space infection, whereas other procedures (e.g., herniorrhaphy, appendectomy) are complicated more often by incisional infections.

The standard classification of surgical wounds has four categories – clean, clean–contaminated, contaminated, and infected – based on the degree of bacterial contamination at the time of the procedure. Although it is helpful, this system has limited capability to stratify the risk of surgical site infections [15]. Host factors that contribute to the development of postoperative infections include diabetes, advanced age, obesity, tobacco use, malnutrition, other immunosuppression, and infection or colonization at other body sites [16]. Prolonged duration of the operation independently predicts risk of infection. For some operations including cholecystectomy and colon resection, the laparoscopic approach is associated with lower infection rates compared with open surgery [17]. Prolonged hospital stay prior to surgery or prolonged stay in intensive care following surgery also increases the likelihood of surgical site infection [18].

Superficial surgical site infections are heralded by pain at the surgical site disproportionate to usual postoperative pain. Edema, tenderness, erythema, and purulent drainage are frequently evident on inspection of the wound. The wound should be examined closely for areas of fluctuance. Occasionally, crepitus is present and suggests the involvement of anaerobic organisms. Deep incisional infections may not show the typical local signs and diagnosis may be delayed. Fever and leukocytosis are usually present but are not invariable.

Effective drainage, which usually includes suture removal, is the cornerstone of therapy for incisional infections. Purulent drainage should be sent to the microbiology laboratory for Gram stain and culture. If cellulitis and systemic signs of infection are absent, drainage is usually curative. Antibiotic selection should be based on Gram stain results, if these are available. Staphylococci and streptococci are the major causes of superficial incisional infections. Approximately half of *S. aureus* isolates causing surgical site infections in the USA are methicillin-resistant *S. aureus* (MRSA) [12]. The need to consider vancomycin as part of empiric therapy depends on the prevalence of methicillin-resistant *S. aureus* at the particular institution, the severity of the infection, the duration of hospitalization, and previous antibiotic administration.

Organ/space infections involving the peritoneal cavity or the pelvis are frequently polymicrobial, and empiric antibiotics should have activity against gram-negative and anaerobic pathogens. Peritonitis typically occurs following procedures that enter contaminated areas such as the bowel or the biliary tract. Procedures that include anastomoses of the gastrointestinal tract pose an increased risk of peritonitis. Anastomotic leaks usually occur between the third and fifth postoperative days, when edema of the suture line begins to resolve. The diagnosis of peritonitis in the postoperative period is usually straightforward. Signs of peritoneal irritation are often heralded by fever, tachycardia, and abdominal pain.

Intra-abdominal or pelvic abscesses occurring after gastrointestinal or gynecologic surgery can have a subtle presentation. Abdominal pain and other localizing signs may or may not be present. Persistent or recurrent fever and leukocytosis may be early clues. Computed tomography is invaluable, both for diagnosis and percutaneous drainage of abscesses. Computed tomographic scans are typically obtained about one week after the initial surgery if abscess is suspected. During this interval, some of the expected inflammatory changes in the operative area should resolve, whereas any infection that is present may evolve into a discrete abscess.

Infection after median sternotomy may be superficial, involve the sternum, or result in mediastinitis. After the procedure, the sternum is contiguous with the deeper mediastinal structures and the pericardium. Thus, differentiating superficial from deep infection may be difficult. When mediastinitis is present, patients are often critically ill with accompanying bacteremia. On occasion, fever and systemic signs of infection develop before other clinical signs of wound infection such as purulent drainage. *Staphylococcus aureus* and coagulase-negative staphylococci are common causes of sternal wound infections. Therapy involves prolonged administration of intravenous antibiotics and aggressive surgical debridement. Prolonged surgery, reoperation, underlying diseases such as diabetes mellitus, cigarette smoking, obesity, and use of internal mammary arteries are risk factors for the development of sternal wound infections. Postoperative stays in the ICU of more than 72 hours have also been associated with an increased risk of sternal wound infection [18].

Bloodstream infections

Bloodstream infections in the postoperative setting can result from localized processes such as surgical site infections, pneumonias, or UTIs. The rate of secondary bloodstream infection varies considerably depending on the operative procedure performed. Rates of bacteremia accompanying incisional and organ/space infections are the highest (13.2% and 39.7%, respectively) after cardiac surgery [12]. Postoperative pneumonia is more likely to lead to secondary bacteremia in patients who are mechanically ventilated than in those who are not.

Primary bloodstream infections, usually a consequence of intravascular access devices [19], are more common than secondary bloodstream infections and account for 7% of nosocomial infections in surgical patients [12]. Although any device can serve as the source for a bacteremia or fungemia, most device-related bloodstream infections in the postoperative setting are caused by central venous catheters. Careful attention to optimal central line insertion practices and prompt removal of devices can decrease the risk of line-related bloodstream infection. Femoral venous catheters are also associated with a higher rate of infection and a higher rate of non-infectious complications, primarily thrombosis, compared with subclavian catheters [20]. The catheter insertion site may show erythema or purulence, although these findings are often absent with catheter-associated bacteremia.

Peripheral catheters can be the source of phlebitis and bloodstream infection [21]. Phlebitis manifests with pain, erythema, tenderness, and an indurated thrombosed vein. Phlebitis is a reaction to the catheter material or the infusate and does not imply that infection is present. However, phlebitis predisposes to the development of catheter-related infection and should prompt catheter removal. The inflammation associated with phlebitis can produce fever. The absence of phlebitis does not exclude a catheter-related bloodstream infection. An erythematous or indurated catheter site should be assessed for signs of suppurative phlebitis which include fluctuance over the course of the vein and purulence that can be expressed from the insertion site by milking the vein. Suppurative phlebitis is the cause of a sustained bacteremia; patients frequently appear septic with high spiking fevers. Excision of the involved vein is often necessary.

In the assessment of febrile postoperative patients, any intravascular catheter should be considered a potential source of infection, especially if no other site of infection is apparent. Two sets of blood cultures should be obtained, at least one by peripheral venipuncture. A negative line-drawn blood culture is evidence against an intravascular catheter-related infection. However, blood cultures obtained through the device have a higher contamination rate, emphasizing the importance of clinical interpretation of a positive line culture [22].

If intravascular catheter-related bacteremia is suspected, empiric antibiotic therapy is warranted. Coagulase-negative staphylococci and *S. aureus* are the most common pathogens but many types of bacteria and fungi have been associated with catheter-related infections. Prolonged antibiotic therapy, hyperalimentation, acute renal failure, underlying medical problems such as diabetes mellitus, central venous access, and previous surgery are risk factors for catheter-related fungemia [23]. If patients with central venous catheter-related bacteremia remain febrile despite the administration of appropriate antibiotics and if follow-up blood cultures show a sustained bacteremia, an infected thrombus or endocarditis should be suspected. Unlike septic phlebitis of peripheral veins, there are few clues on the physical examination to suggest septic thrombosis of a central vein.

Pneumonia

Pneumonia and other pulmonary sources of postoperative fever are discussed in Chapter 15.

Urinary tract infections

According to CDC data, UTIs account for 27% of postoperative infections [12]. Although they are the second most common infection in surgical patients, UTIs cause less morbidity and mortality than do pneumonias, bloodstream infections, or surgical site infections. Urinary tract infections occur almost exclusively in patients with bladder catheterization or previous urinary tract manipulation. The risk of bacteriuria increases with duration of catheterization. The microbiology of nosocomial UTIs is much broader than that of community-acquired UTIs, with *Escherichia coli* accounting for only about 30%. The intensive use of broad-spectrum antibiotics, including third-generation cephalosporins, in the postoperative setting has contributed to the increase in the number of UTIs caused by enterococci, resistant gram-negative bacilli, and yeast. Removal of the bladder catheter as soon as feasible is the best means of minimizing the risk of UTI. Current best practices call for removal of a bladder catheter within 2 days after an operation or documentation of a compelling reason for continued catheter use.

Seventy to 80% of patients with catheter-associated bacteriuria are asymptomatic. The presence of the bladder catheter obscures the symptoms of lower tract infection. Pyuria is common even when symptoms are absent. Signs of upper tract infection, including fever and flank pain, are rare; secondary bacteremia occurs in about 1% of patients with bacteriuria. Because bacteriuria is common and the course usually benign, other sources of infection should be considered in febrile postoperative patients who have positive results on urine cultures. After the removal of short-term urinary catheters, symptomatic lower UTIs developed in seven of 42 patients (17%) with catheter-associated bacteriuria [24]. However, at this time there are insufficient data to recommend routine screening for postcatheterization bacteriuria.

Candida species are commonly isolated from the urine in post-surgical patients with indwelling catheters but determining the clinical significance of funguria in the febrile postoperative patient is problematic. Funguria rarely leads to systemic infection and often clears after removal of the indwelling catheter. However, candida can seed the urinary tract through hematogenous dissemination. Thus, in the patient at risk for disseminated fungal infection, the presence of funguria may be a clue to bloodstream infection and disseminated candidiasis. In asymptomatic patients with funguria, there is no benefit of antifungal therapy. A randomized controlled trial did not find a sustained clearance of candiduria in patients receiving fluconazole compared with placebo [25]. In general, antifungal therapy should be reserved for those patients with documented infection (pyuria and funguria on more than one urine specimen) who are symptomatic or have unexplained fever. The high prevalence of funguria underscores the importance of minimizing risk factors such as inappropriate antibiotic use and indwelling urinary catheters.

Other infections

Ten to 20% of infections in the surgical patient are from sources other than the surgical site, lung, urinary tract or device-associated bloodstream infection. The diagnosis may be cryptic, especially in critically ill patients in ICUs. Physical examination, although difficult to perform, is nonetheless essential. Careful inspection of the skin, including the sacrum, for evidence of decubitus ulcers, phlebitis, or rashes is important. Maxillary sinusitis, often staphylococcal, occurs in patients with nasotracheal intubation or nasogastric tubes. Sinus tenderness may be present, even in obtunded patients. A boggy, tender, and enlarged parotid gland suggests parotitis, an uncommon complication seen in sick patients with volume depletion. A careful funduscopic examination should be performed to search for evidence of fungal endophthalmitis, especially in patients with risk factors for candidemia. Acute cholecystitis can occur following surgery remote to the gall bladder. Right upper quadrant pain is usually present but recognition can be delayed in the sedated and paralyzed patients. Calculi may be absent on imaging studies. Without prompt diagnosis and surgical intervention, perforation, peritonitis, and sepsis can develop. Diarrhea is sometimes absent or mild with *C. difficile* colitis; this diagnosis should be considered in any postoperative patient with fever and abdominal tenderness.

Antibiotic usage in the perioperative and postoperative setting

Perioperative antimicrobial prophylaxis reduces the postoperative infection rates following most operative procedures [26]. (See Chapter 24 for a more detailed discussion of surgical prophylaxis.) One pre-incisional dose administered within 60 minutes of incision (120 minutes for antibiotics requiring prolonged infusion including vancomycin) is usually sufficient with intraoperative re-dosing for prolonged operations based on the half-life of the drug [27]. While there are no compelling data that any postoperative doses prevent infection, current guidelines allow up to 24 hours of antibiotics for most procedures [26]. Prolonging antibiotic therapy in the absence of established infection should be avoided because of the increased likelihood of colonization and infection with antibiotic-resistant bacteria, increased risk of *C. difficile* diarrhea and increased cost. There is temptation to continue the administration of perioperative antibiotics because of early postoperative fever. This temptation should be balanced by the realization that fever on the first postoperative day is rarely due to infection and by knowledge of the hazards of prolonged antibiotic coverage. In choosing an antibiotic regimen for a postoperative infection, the clinician must be cognizant not only of the likely pathogens but also of the previous antibiotics administered to the patients and resistance trends in the hospital.

References

1. Galicier C, Richet H. A prospective study of postoperative fever in a general surgery department. *Infect Control* 1985; **6**: 487–90.

2. Livelli FD Jr, Johnson RA, McEnany MT *et al.* Unexplained in-hospital fever following cardiac surgery. *Circulation* 1978; **57**: 968–75.

3. Freischlag J, Busuttil RW. The value of postoperative fever evaluation. *Surgery* 1983; **94**: 358–63.

4. Giangobbe MJ, Rappaport WD, Stein B. The significance of fever following cholecystectomy. *J Fam Pract* 1992; **34**: 437–40.

5. Mellors JW, Kelly JJ, Gusberg RJ, Horwitz SM, Horwitz RI. A simple index to estimate the likelihood of bacterial infection in patients developing fever after abdominal surgery. *Am Surg* 1988; **54**: 558–64.

6. Jorgensen FS, Sorensen CG, Kjaergaard J. Postoperative fever after major abdominal surgery. *Ann Chir Gynaecol* 1988; **77**: 47–50.

7. Hiyama DT, Zinner MJ. Surgical complications. In Schwartz SI, ed. *Principles of Surgery.* 6th edn. New York, NY: McGraw-Hill; 1994, p. 455.

8. Fry DE. Postoperative fever. In Mackowiak PA, ed. *Fever: Basic Mechanisms and Management.* New York, NY: Raven Press; 1991, p. 243.

9. Garibaldi RA, Brodine S, Matsumiya S, Coleman M. Evidence for the non-infectious etiology of early postoperative fever. *Infect Control* 1985; **6**: 273–7.

10. Roberts J, Barnes W, Pennock M, Browne G. Diagnostic accuracy of fever as a measure of postoperative pulmonary complications. *Heart Lung* 1988; **17**: 166–70.

11. Frank SM, Kluger MJ, Kunkel SL. Elevated thermostatic setpoint in post-operative patients. *Anesthesiology* 2000; **93**: 1426–31.

12. Hidron AI, Edwards JR, Patel J *et al.* Antimicrobial resistant pathogens associated with healthcare-associated infections: annual summary of data reported to the National Healthcare Safety Network at the Centers for Disease Control and Prevention, 2006–2007. *Infect Control Hosp Epidemiol* 2008; **29**: 996–1011.

13. Mackowiak PA. Drug fever. In Mackowiak PA, ed. *Fever: Basic Mechanisms and Management.* New York, NY: Raven Press; 1991, p. 255.

14. Horan T.C, Gaynes RP, Martone WJ, Jarvis WR, Emori TG. CDC definitions of nosocomial surgical site infections, 1992: a modification of CDC definitions of surgical wound infections. *Infect Control Hosp Epidemiol* 1992; **13**: 606–8.

15. Culver DH, Horan TC, Gaynes RP *et al.* Surgical wound infection rates by wound class, operative procedure, and patient risk index. National Nosocomial Infections Surveillance System. *Am J Med* 1991; **91**: 152S–7S.

16. The Society for Hospital Epidemiology of America; The Association for Practitioners in Infection Control; The Centers for Disease Control; The Surgical Infection Society. Consensus paper on the surveillance of surgical wound infections. *Infect Control Hosp Epidemiol* 1992; **13**: 599–605.

17. Gaynes RP, Culver DH, Horan TC *et al.* Surgical site infection rates in the United States, 1992–1998: The National Nosocomial Infections Surveillance

System basic SSI risk index. *Clin Infect Dis* 2001; **33** (Suppl 2): S69.

18. Kohli M, Yuan L, Escobar M *et al.* A risk index for sternal surgical wound infection after cardiovascular surgery. *Infect Control Hosp Epidemiol* 2003; **24**: 17–25.

19. Maki DG. Infections due to infusion therapy. In Bennett JV, Brachman PS, eds. *Hospital Infections.* 3rd edn. Boston, MA: Little, Brown; 1992, p. 849.

20. Merrer J, DeJonghe B, Golliot F *et al.* Complications of femoral and subclavian venous catheterization in critically ill patients. *J Am Med Assoc* 2001; **286**: 700–7.

21. Mermel LA, McCormick RD, Springman SR, Maki DG. The pathogenesis and epidemiology of catheter-related infection with pulmonary artery Swan–Ganz catheters: a prospective study utilizing molecular subtyping. *Am J Med* 1991; **91** (Suppl 3B): 197S–205S.

22. Mermel LA, Allon M, Bouza E *et al.* Clinical practice guidelines for the diagnosis and management of intravascular catheter-related infections: 2009 update by the Infectious Diseases Society of America. *Clin Infect Dis* 2009; **49**: 1–45.

23. Blumberg HM, Jarvis WR, Soucie JM *et al.*; NEMIS Study Group. Risk factors for candidal bloodstream infections in surgical intensive care unit patients: the NEMIS Prospective Multicenter Study. *Clin Infect Dis* 2001; **33**: 177–86.

24. Harding GKM, Nicolle LE, Ronald AR *et al.* How long should catheter-acquired urinary tract infections in women be treated? *Ann Intern Med* 1991; **114**: 713–19.

25. Sobel JD, Kauffman CA, McKinsey D *et al.* Candiduria: a randomized, double-blind study of treatment with fluconazole and placebo. *Clin Infect Dis* 2000; **30**: 19–24.

26. Bratzler DW, Houck PM. for the Surgical Infection Prevention Guidelines Writers Group. Antimicrobial prophylaxis for surgery: an advisory statement from the National Surgical Infection Prevention Project. *Clin Infect Dis* 2004; **38**: 1706–15.

27. Steinberg JP, Braun BI, Hellinger WC *et al.* Timing of antimicrobial prophylaxis and the risk of surgical site infections: results from the Trial to Reduce Antimicrobial Prophylaxis Errors (TRAPE). *Ann Surg* 2009; **250**: 10–16.

27

Surgery in the patient with renal disease

Andrew I. Chin, Jane Y. Yeun, and Burl R. Don

Introduction

Kidney disease encompasses a wide spectrum of disorders, ranging from those with normal glomerular filtration rates (GFR) but with urinary abnormalities (nephrotic syndrome or nephritic syndrome), to those with GFR impairments. Patients with a long-standing history (months to years) of renal disease are deemed to have chronic kidney disease (CKD). A staging system has been developed by the National Kidney Foundation to categorize CKD by GFR levels: Stage 1 (GFR $\geq$ 90 mL/min, but with persistent urinary abnormalities such as proteinuria); Stage 2, mild CKD (GFR 60–89 mL/min); Stage 3, moderate CKD (GFR 30–59 mL/min); Stage 4, severe CKD (GFR 15–29 mL/min); and finally Stage 5, kidney failure or end-stage renal disease (ESRD) (GFR < 15 mL/min *or* on some form of renal replacement therapy). There is clinical rationale in dividing CKD into these stages; patients with more advanced stages, especially those at stage 3 or higher, have higher rates of death, cardiovascular events, and hospitalizations [1]. In contrast to established kidney disease, acute kidney injury (AKI), previously termed "acute renal failure," reflects renal dysfunction that arises in the span of hours to days. AKI can develop in those with previously normal kidney function or can be superimposed upon existing CKD. More advanced CKD stages 3 through 5 and AKI are most commonly associated with perioperative complications, and these patients will be the focus of this chapter.

Patients with CKD and ESRD are becoming increasingly common in the USA and around the world. Newly diagnosed ESRD develops in about 350 patients per 1 million Americans each year [2]. This affects the non-Caucasian population at a disproportionately higher rate [2]. Diabetes mellitus and hypertension remain the major causes of CKD and ESRD in the USA. Almost 398,000 individuals are now on dialysis, most of them on hemodialysis, with a prevalence of around 1,700 patients per million population [2]. Additionally, another 172,000 have a functional renal allograft. Just like for ESRD, CKD prevalence is also on the rise, with a recent cross-sectional survey of the US adult population demonstrating greater than 8% prevalence of CKD stage 3 or higher [3]. In

the older population > 69 years of age, the prevalence of stage 3 or higher is close to 38% [3]. Therefore, almost all clinicians and specialists will encounter ESRD and CKD patients in their practice. Despite the increase in these populations, most of the literature specific to their perioperative care is anecdotal and based on rather limited evidence-based data.

While patients with CKD, ESRD, and AKI are subject to many similar potential perioperative complications, there are significant clinical care issues that are specific for each group. For instance, in patients with CKD, avoiding additional renal insult is of primary importance in the perioperative period because episodes of AKI, especially those requiring dialysis, are associated with increased mortality and progression of CKD [4,5]. Therefore, prevention of contrast-induced nephropathy, avoidance of hypotension and renal hypo-perfusion, and not using renal toxic medications are vital. In patients with ESRD, there are other challenges to contend with such as volume and electrolyte disturbances as well as fluctuations of hemodynamics due to the dialysis modalities. Patients with functioning renal allografts pose other unique problems. In this chapter, we will focus on some of these care issues with an emphasis on avoiding AKI in the perioperative period.

Perioperative morbidity and mortality

The perioperative mortality is 4% for ESRD patients undergoing general surgery and 10–18% for cardiac surgery [6–9]. It is now fairly well established that patients with CKD also have a higher mortality for surgical procedures, with recent studies showing a step-wise increase in risk for each advancing stage of CKD [10,11]. Postoperative mortality is usually due to a cardiovascular or infectious complication. Just as importantly, perioperative morbidity in ESRD patients is extremely high at > 54% for general surgery and > 46% for cardiac surgery [6]. Patients with kidney disease may face morbidity related to electrolyte disturbances, infections, blood pressure instability, bleeding, cardiac arrhythmias, and dialysis access problems. The hope is that reducing perioperative morbidity will be a step in the right direction in reducing postoperative mortality.

Medical Management of the Surgical Patient, ed. Michael F. Lubin, Thomas F. Dodson, and Neil H. Winawer. Published by Cambridge University Press. © Cambridge University Press 2013.

Cardiac preoperative evaluation

One of the major reasons for a thorough preoperative evaluation is risk stratification for an acute cardiac event. Pre-test probability for cardiovascular disease is high in the CKD and ESRD population [1,2,12–15]. However, cardiac disease in these groups differs in many ways from the typical atherosclerotic coronary artery disease that clinicians encounter in those without kidney disease. For example, cardiac-related causes account for around 50% of all deaths in the United States ESRD patient population [2]. About half of those are categorized as sudden cardiac death, a rate that is not only significantly greater than that seen in other populations with known coronary artery disease, but also greater than what is expected given the underlying traditional risk factors in these ESRD patients. Misclassification of sudden cardiac death notwithstanding, the rate of this is fairly consistent in large, prospective trials in ESRD patients [12–14]. Even in patients with CKD, there is growing evidence that sudden cardiac death occurs at a higher rate in those with impaired GFR, and CKD appears to be an independent risk factor [15–20]. Some of this cardiovascular mortality risk is decreased after renal transplantation, but even those with a functional allograft have a higher prevalence of heart disease [21,22].

Other sections of this textbook have detailed the preoperative cardiac evaluation of the general population undergoing surgery. We would like to point out several important differences in the presentation and underlying pathology of cardiac disease between patients with kidney disease and the general population. One of the difficulties in preoperative evaluation of CKD and ESRD patients is the lack of correlation of clinical symptoms with typical atherosclerotic coronary artery disease. Patients with renal disease can have significant acute cardiac ischemia without symptoms [17,18], possibly due to uremic and/or diabetic neuropathy. Notably, ESRD patients with acute coronary syndrome may present with atypical symptoms such as heart failure or syncope [18]. The converse is also observed in advanced kidney disease – patients with typical angina but with no significant coronary artery disease on evaluation. Observational studies have suggested that 25–50% of ESRD patients with angina [19–22] do not have major epicardial arterial lesions, possibly reflecting symptoms due to small vessel disease as a result of severe left ventricular hypertrophy (LVH) or diabetes mellitus.

Concentric LVH is also highly prevalent in CKD and ESRD patients, found in 70–90% of subjects in some studies [22–25]. Thus, the use of electrocardiography (ECG) in preoperative evaluation for acute ischemic changes may be masked by the strain patterns seen with LVH. Lastly, traditional cardiac risk factors such as hypertension, smoking, and hyperlipidemia poorly predict the presence of coronary artery disease in patients with kidney disease, and studies that intervene have not shown significant benefits [14,26,27]. Indeed, non-traditional risk factors such as hyperuricemia, hyperphosphatemia, hyperparathyroidism, elevated C reactive protein, and other inflammatory agents may be actively affecting cardiac risk [28]. Specifically, hyperphosphatemia has been implicated as a major risk factor for the accelerated vascular calcification seen in both CKD and ESRD patients and is a strong predictor of cardiovascular mortality in this population.

Despite the major differences in cardiac symptomatology and pathology between those with kidney disease and the general population, the decision to obtaining additional cardiac testing usually hinges on patient symptoms and risk factors. Table 27.1 outlines reported criteria for ordering additional cardiac screening tests; it is probably the minority of ESRD patients who do not have at least one of these risk factors. West et al. only screened high-risk patients, defined as individuals having diabetes mellitus, prior myocardial infarction, age ≥ 50 years, cerebral and/or peripheral vascular disease, congestive heart failure, class I or II angina, or on dialysis > 5 years [29]. Dobutamine stress echocardiography was ordered prior to kidney transplantation. Unfortunately, the authors do not report on the cardiovascular outcome of the 91 out of 133 dialysis patients who did not undergo non-invasive studies to assess for coronary artery disease. Le et al. also looked at kidney transplant candidates and recommended screening if the patients were at high risk for a cardiac event based on any of the following characteristics: age ≥ 50 years, history of angina, insulin-dependent diabetes mellitus, congestive heart failure, or an abnormal electrocardiogram (other than left ventricular hypertrophy) [30]. After 4 years of follow-up, patients in the low-risk group (e.g., none of the above characteristics) had a 1% cardiac mortality, compared with

Table 27.1 Criteria for obtaining additional cardiac screening tests in kidney patients. Reference numbers are given in brackets.

West [29]	Le [30]	UC Davis
Age ≥ 50 years	Age ≥ 50 years	Age ≥ 65 years
Diabetes mellitus	Diabetes mellitus I	Diabetes mellitus and peripheral vascular disease
Class I or II angina	Angina	
Myocardial infarction	Congestive heart failure	Functional class III or IV angina
Peripheral vascular disease	Abnormal ECG (other than left ventricular hypertrophy)	Congestive heart failure from systolic dysfunction
Cerebral vascular disease		
Congestive heart failure		
Dialysis > 5 years		

17% in the high-risk group. At our center, in collaboration with cardiology and transplant surgery, we recently established new guidelines to screen for patients at high risk of cardiovascular complications in preparation for vascular access surgery: age > 65 years, history of angina, history of congestive heart failure due to systolic dysfunction, class III or IV symptoms of angina (symptoms of chest discomfort or dyspnea with daily activity or at rest, respectively), and a combination of diabetes and peripheral vascular disease.

Additional preoperative cardiac studies are often obtained in kidney disease patients. Although several studies have addressed the issue of cardiac evaluation in patients with kidney disease [31–34], all have significant confounding variables. Many studies were small and retrospective in nature. Many included only ESRD and not CKD patients, dealt only with diabetic patients, or included only patients undergoing evaluation for renal transplantation. The "gold standard" employed in the studies also differed significantly, ranging from subsequent clinical cardiac events to angiographic coronary artery lesions with varying degrees of stenosis. Most importantly, the outcome measures for these studies are long-term all cause and/or cardiac mortality, which may differ from immediate postoperative mortality.

There is no ideal choice for cardiac testing in the CKD and ESRD population. Coronary angiography, usually considered the "gold standard" of all tests, has been used to screen patients with CKD. However, the high prevalence of demand ischemia from LVH and microvascular disease should make one question the appropriateness of angiography as the comparative standard. The bulk of studies using coronary angiography were performed for pre-kidney transplant evaluation in patients who were either asymptomatic or with stable symptoms. In one such study, 151 diabetic patients being evaluated for renal transplantation underwent coronary angiography, revealing 31 patients (20.5%) with at least one > 75% stenotic vessel [35]. Twenty-six of these patients were randomized to medical versus revascularization, and the group in the medical management (medical management was not well standardized) had a worse long-term outcome.

In contrast to this result, major studies in patients without advanced kidney disease suggest that not all patients with significant coronary artery disease benefit from preoperative revascularization. For example, in a study of older men in the Veterans Affairs system who were randomized to medical management versus revascularization prior to major elective vascular surgery, no difference in the primary outcome of long-term mortality was noted between the treatment strategies, 22% in the medical treatment arm and 23% in the revascularization arm at 2.7 years follow-up [36]. There was a similar rate of perioperative non-fatal myocardial infarctions at 12% and 14%, respectively. While this study did not include any patients on dialysis, the cohort did have extensive coronary artery disease, with 15% of patients having had coronary artery bypass surgery in the past and 33% with 3-vessel lesions on angiography at the time of randomization. A subsequent

prospective randomized study, arguably with an even higher risk cohort (43% with left ventricular ejection < 35%; 75% with 3-vessel disease) came to a similar conclusion [37]. As with most such studies, renal status of the participants was not clearly delineated even though CKD with a creatinine of > 1.6 mg/dL was considered a cardiac risk factor in the latter study. As always, applicability of these findings to CKD and ESRD patients must be done with caution.

The results of the above studies suggest no significant benefit of preoperative revascularization in patients with coronary disease and stable symptoms. This basic sentiment is reflected in the American College of Cardiology/American Heart Association guidelines for perioperative cardiovascular evaluation [38]. This implies that identifiable epicardial artery lesions may not be the culprit in the perioperative period. Indeed, histologic autopsy and functional cardiac study correlations of perioperative myocardial infarction locations to preoperative determination of culprit lesions are poor [39,40], suggesting a different mechanism of injury in the perioperative period. Proposed pathologic underpinnings to explain this finding revolve around perioperative stress responses, which include cytokine release, catecholamine surge, hemodynamic stress, vasospasm and hypercoagulable state. These factors may be quite pertinent in CKD and ESRD patients, especially since non-traditional cardiac risk factors appear to be powerful in this population. However, many ESRD patients have very poor exercise tolerance and often function at relatively low metabolic equivalents, thus never provoking symptoms even if they do have significant cardiac disease. This brings us to the discussion of non-invasive functional studies, which may provide better insight into cardiac susceptibility to stressors.

A host of non-invasive tests is available with few fully vetted out in the ESRD or CKD population. Institutional preference and experience dictates what is appropriate. We will briefly cover the commonly utilized studies. In our opinion, there is little role of exercise ECG as a preoperative screening tool in the ESRD population. The preponderance of preexisting ECG abnormalities due to bundle branch blocks, left ventricular hypertrophy (LVH), chronic T wave changes makes interpretation difficult [41]. One study that examined exercise ECG in ESRD patients undergoing pretransplant evaluation found that the resting portion, not the exercise part, was more predictive of coronary artery disease, but with overall moderate sensitivity and poor specificity [42]. Additionally, many patients with advanced kidney disease cannot exercise to a level required for this test. Exercise stress testing with thallium administration [32,43–49], the dipyridamole thallium stress test [22,30,31,33,34,43,45,50,51], dobutamine stress echocardiography [42,52–56], combined dipyridamole and stress echocardiography [31], and single-photon emission computed tomography (SPECT) [57,58] are additional cardiac screening tests. Exercise stress with thallium has the same pitfall as exercise ECG, in that many dialysis patients are unable to exercise sufficiently to achieve target heart rate and blood pressure. Studies reporting the sensitivity,

Table 27.2 Sensitivity and specificity of cardiac screening tests in patients with kidney disease. Reference numbers are given in brackets.

Cardiac screening	Comparative standard	Sensitivity (%)	Specificity (%)	NPV (%)
Exercise thallium	Coronary angiogram [49]	50	67	
	Cardiovascular events [234]	88	70	86
Persantine thallium	Coronary angiogram [33,49,50,235]	37–92	37–89	61–98
	Cardiovascular events [235,236]	67–100	81–88	91–100
Dobutamine stress echocardiography	Coronary angiogram [29,42,53–55,223]	44–95	60–94	57–97
	Cardiovascular events [52–54,56]	31–82	74–95	80–94
Persantine and exercise stress echocardiography	Coronary angiogram [31]	83	84	93
	Cardiovascular events [31]	86	94	96
SPECT	Coronary angiogram [53]	64	53	66
	Cardiovascular events [53]	63	58	90

SPECT, single-photon emission computed tomography; NPV, negative predictive value.

specificity, and negative predictive values or containing sufficient detail to allow their calculation are summarized in Table 27.2. Notably, sensitivity and specificity vary tremendously given the heterogeneity of the populations, the sample sizes, and the method or duration of follow-up.

None of the screening modalities offers absolute confidence in predicting the absence of significant coronary artery disease (defined as stenosis of > 50–75%). Additionally, 25–50% of renal failure patients with an abnormal functional study do not have significant coronary artery disease on subsequent angiography [32–34,45]. As noted previously, the mechanism of acute perioperative myocardial infarction may be quite different from that of plaque rupture in culprit lesions found on coronary angiography, thus the poor sensitivity of many non-invasive studies for coronary angiographic lesions. A negative non-invasive, functional screening test offers a modicum of reassurance (negative predictive values ranging in 80–100% range) that the patient will not have an adverse cardiovascular event in the near future.

There are clear long-term benefits of beta-blockers and aspirin use in non-renal disease patients with established coronary artery disease. In addition, perioperative use of beta-blockers in the general population has also been studied. In the CKD and ESRD populations, conclusive evidence of benefit from these classes of medications is lacking. We will spend a bit more time going over the use of perioperative beta-blockers in the later section on hypertension control in the perioperative period.

We should also mention the use of perioperative aspirin in the kidney patient. There are no good data on the efficacy of aspirin in primary prevention of cardiac events in this population. Results of a large meta-analysis suggest a possible advantage to aspirin use in patients on hemodialysis [59]. However, the bleeding risks, especially in the ESRD patients, may be problematic in the surgical patient. Therefore, we cannot recommend its routine use in the perioperative period.

In summary, renal disease is now considered an independent cardiac risk factor in the preoperative scenario. Given the high pretest probability of cardiovascular disease in CKD and ESRD patients, they frequently receive additional cardiac studies. Asymptomatic kidney patients at lower risk (Table 27.1) probably need no further cardiac evaluation prior to surgery. Patients at high risk but without symptoms can be further stratified using a non-invasive functional test. Keep in mind that the correlation with angiographic coronary disease is poor as evidenced by the overall low sensitivity and specificity of available screening modalities. Limited data exist as to whether angiographic disease should be treated or not in stable patients with renal disease, though growing evidence suggests treatment may not change short-term outcomes in the non-kidney disease population. A subgroup of patients at very high risk of an adverse cardiac event (symptoms of unstable angina) should be considered for coronary angiography without non-invasive testing, recalling that a good percentage of ESRD patients can be symptomatic without significant coronary artery disease.

Perioperative considerations
Management of volume status

Perioperatively, it is important to ensure that the patient is euvolemic. Excessive volume overload may lead to poorly controlled hypertension and hypoxia either during surgery or afterwards. Conversely, significant volume depletion will make the patient more susceptible to hypotension and the possibility of end organ injury such as AKI. Typically, volume assessment in the preoperative period is based on basic physical examination and review of systems data. If dependent edema in the lower extremities or the sacral area is present, it may be accompanied by hypertension, pulmonary congestion, and distended jugular veins. If pulmonary edema is present, congestive heart failure must be ruled out since congestive heart failure will require therapy in addition to diuretics.

In CKD or AKI patients not requiring dialysis, volume overload is managed with salt and fluid restriction (2 g sodium diet, 1 L fluid per day) and diuretics, administered either orally or intravenously. Loop diuretics are the most potent and are the diuretic of choice. Since diuretics must be filtered by the glomeruli and/or secreted by the tubular cells into the tubular lumen to be effective, the dose of diuretic given must be appropriate for the degree of kidney failure. The worse the kidney function, the higher the dose of diuretics needed for the desired effect [48]. When GFR is less than 25 mL/min, furosemide dose in excess of 120 mg and bumetanide dose in excess of 3 mg *may* be required. Occasionally, metolazone (5–10 mg orally) or chlorothiazide (250–500 mg intravenously) is given 30 minutes before the loop diuretic to augment the diuretic response. Although loop diuretics, particularly in high doses, are associated with ototoxicity, toxicity is generally in the setting of concomitant administration of other ototoxic drugs or bolus injection of the loop diuretic [48,60]. The high peak serum level after intravenous bolus is thought to be the most important factor. Doses in excess of 80 mg should be infused over 30 minutes in a small amount of fluid. When high doses of loop diuretics are necessary to maintain diuresis, a continuous infusion may be preferable because it decreases the total daily dose required to achieve the same diuretic response. After a bolus of 40–80 mg to help achieve steady state blood levels, furosemide is administered continuously at a rate of 10–20 mg/hour. If the desired diuresis is not achieved after 2 hours, a repeat bolus should be given and the infusion rate increased by 10–20 mg/hour. If excessive diuresis ensues, the infusion rate can be decreased.

Routine use of salt-poor albumin either infused prior to the diuretic dose or at the same time as diuretic infusion is generally not warranted. The rationale behind this approach is based on the theory that patients with very low serum albumin (nephrotic syndrome and liver cirrhosis patients) may benefit from receiving a colloid such as albumin or fresh frozen plasma (FFP) to keep the diuretic in the vascular space and/or to increase intravascular oncotic pressure to promote water movement from the interstitial space back into the vascular space, both allowing for better diuretic response [61]. Recall that almost all diuretics need to remain in the vascular space to be filtered by the glomeruli into the kidney urinary space for the drug to reach its target. However, in clinical studies of both nephrotic syndrome and liver cirrhosis patients, the concomitant use of albumin with loop diuretics has had mixed results, and was not found to routinely increase diuresis [62–65]. Therefore, we cannot recommend the use of albumin with loop diuretics on a routine basis. However, severely hypoalbuminemic patients may require higher diuretic doses to achieve an adequate diuresis.

Based on clinical experience, patients with ESRD should undergo dialysis within 24 hours of surgery to optimize volume status. Concomitant dietary sodium (2 g) and fluid (1 L) restrictions are very important adjuncts to dialysis. Patients on peritoneal dialysis should have their peritoneal dialysate drained shortly before going to the operating room. Prolonged dwelling time of dialysate in the peritoneum will dissipate the glucose gradient and result in absorption of the peritoneal fluid, contributing to volume overload. In addition, the presence of a large amount of fluid in the abdomen may compromise lung function during surgery.

Conversely, excessive fluid removal with diuretics or dialysis before surgery may lead to perioperative hypotension, increasing susceptibility to end-organ dysfunction including development of AKI in those not already on dialysis. Anesthetics administered during surgery may cause vasodilation, which will aggravate hypotension if the patient is already volume depleted. This may be even more apparent in patients receiving angiotensin converting enzyme (ACE) inhibitors as part of their anti-hypertensive regimen (see section below on hypertension). Fluid sequestration after surgery will further deplete the intravascular volume and also exacerbate hypotension. Special attention to volume status should be paid to those with CKD and requiring presurgical radiocontrast studies. The section on medical imaging in kidney disease will address methods of minimizing renal risk for such procedures.

In ESRD patients who are volume replete, maintenance intravenous fluids should be no more than 0.5 L a day to replace insensible fluid losses. Of course, if the patient has large amounts of fluid loss through nasogastric suctioning, high fevers, abdominal drainage, significant urine output, diarrhea, or other additional sources of fluid loss, these also should be replaced. Otherwise, the reflexive used 75–125 mL/hour of maintenance fluid may lead to pulmonary edema and hypertension in patients on dialysis or with oliguric AKI. The type of crystalloid fluid used is also important. If the patient has hypotonic losses, then replacement fluid should be with a hypotonic solution such as 0.45% sodium chloride. If only the minimal maintenance fluid (0.5 L a day) is required, 0.9% NaCl solution may be more appropriate to prevent development of hyponatremia.

There remains ongoing debate over use of crystalloid fluids versus colloid fluids for hospitalized patients, especially in those in the intensive care setting. However, recent large observational studies in heterogeneous ICU patients and large meta-analyses have suggested no benefit of colloid over crystalloid fluid with perhaps even an increase in AKI associated with some colloid formulations [66–70]. It should be noted that these studies included the most critically ill of medical and surgical patients and by nature of these studies, there was no standardization of fluids. Given the overall findings, we recommend crystalloid fluids for basic preoperative and postoperative care.

Control of hypertension

In general, hypertension in patients with kidney disease may be managed in the same manner as for patients without kidney disease. However, there are a number of points that bear special emphasis. First, CKD and ESRD patients have a high prevalence of cardiovascular disease, but the influences of traditional risk factors such as hypertension and hypercholesterolemia are tempered. Second, the benefits of what are commonly thought of as cardio-protective medications such as beta-blockers, ACE inhibitors and HMG-CoA reductase inhibitors (statins) are not universally seen in this population. Third, ESRD patients on hemodialysis have a very large fluctuation of blood pressures due to the effects of their dialysis treatments which oftentimes causes hypotension during the treatment due to intravascular volume depletion (ultrafiltration during dialysis) and vasodilation. A significant minority of dialysis patients actually have an increase in blood pressure during dialysis. These patients may be at greater risk for long-term cardiovascular morbidity and mortality.

Given the high incidence of cardiovascular disease in patients with renal disease, patients on beta-blockers preoperatively should be kept on them intraoperatively and postoperatively. This recommendation is based on studies that suggest lower mortality in patients on beta-blockers in non-cardiac surgical patients [71–73]. However, additional analysis has demonstrated mixed results [74,75], with some randomized trials suggesting a lower perioperative rate of myocardial infarction but a higher rate of mortality and stroke [76]. No good studies have focused on patients with advanced CKD or ESRD. We recommend CKD or ESRD patients who have been on beta-blockers in the past to continue on them through the perioperative period. If patients cannot take their usual oral beta-blockers, metoprolol and esmolol are available as intravenous preparations. Esmolol is usually given as a continuous intravenous infusion because of its very short half-life.

Many kidney patients are on medications that block the effects of the renin-angiotensin II system, including ACE (angiotensin converting enzyme) inhibitors and ARBs (angiotensin receptor blockers). These classes of medications have not only renal protective effects in many patients with CKD, but may also improve their cardiac outcomes. While the long-term benefits are fairly well established, some studies have found that perioperative ACE inhibitors and ARBs may be associated with a higher rate of AKI after cardiothoracic surgery [77]. Additionally, there is evidence that preoperative use of these medications may also lead to postoperative hypotension and hemodynamic instability at the time of anesthesia induction [78–80]. Holding or reducing the dose of ACE inhibitor or ARB has been advised by some authors [81]. However, there are no good studies looking at this effect in the CKD or ESRD population, and even some authors who have led the cited studies suggest that the evidence is too weak to provide firm recommendations. Nonetheless, it would be quite reasonable to hold ACE inhibitors and ARBs on the day of their procedure.

Other commonly used medications for hypertension control also require some comment. In patients on clonidine preoperatively, severe rebound hypertension may occur if clonidine is stopped abruptly. Rebound hypertension is especially a concern at a dose of ≥ 0.6 mg/day. Such patients should have a clonidine patch substituted for the oral medication at least 1 day before the surgery, to allow the patch to achieve therapeutic blood levels of clonidine prior to surgery.

Frequently used intravenous medications for treating hypertension postoperatively include beta-blockers (metoprolol, esmolol, and labetalol), enalaprilat, hydralazine, and nitroprusside [82]. Beta-blockers are first-line agents in patients with tachycardia or ischemia postoperatively, or a history of coronary artery disease and angina. Patients with a history of systolic dysfunction can be treated with enalaprilat for blood pressure control if intravenous medications are needed, unless there is intervening AKI or poorly controlled hyperkalemia. Hydralazine and an oral long-acting nitrate are often substituted for an ACE inhibitor or ARB if these classes of drugs cannot be used. We advise being cautious about using hydralazine without concomitant use of beta-blockers because it may cause significant reflex tachycardia and aggravate cardiac ischemia. Lastly, nitroprusside should be reserved for severe hypertension that cannot be controlled by other means, because of the increased risk of thiocyanate and cyanide toxicity in patients with impaired kidney function [83]. In general, nitroprusside should not be administered continuously for more than 48 hours in patients with renal failure. If longer administration is required, close monitoring of thiocyanate level is mandatory. If and when nitroprusside is initiated, simultaneous initiation or dose escalation of oral or other intravenous antihypertensive medications is mandatory to allow titration off of nitroprusside as soon as possible.

Postoperative hypertension may be difficult to control in patients with renal disease [82]. Pain, anxiety, and volume overload may be significant contributing factors. Adequate pain control and judicious use of anti-anxiety medications and loop diuretics may help to control blood pressure in the immediate postoperative period. For ESRD patients, dialysis is indicated for control of hypertension if there is also significant volume overload.

The ideal blood pressure in the advanced CKD and ESRD population is an area of ongoing investigation. Most outcome-based studies have suggested that hypertension control benefits these patients, and goal blood pressures of 130–140 mmHg systolic, 80–90 mmHg diastolic, may be very reasonable ranges for the perioperative period. Excessively low blood pressures may be counterproductive. Keeping in mind that patient diet and adherence to medications in the perioperative period may be quite different from their usual patterns, clinicians may need to watch out for hypotension and adjust accordingly and not simply restart all of the usual blood pressure-lowering medications. The ESRD patient on dialysis is particularly challenging in that volume shifts with ultrafiltration on hemodialysis treatments will make blood pressure vary significantly. Low blood pressures in ESRD patients also place hemodialysis arteriovenous shunts at greater risk for thrombosis [84].

Electrolyte, mineral, and acid–base status
Sodium and water disorders

Patients with kidney disease generally do not have problems handling water until creatinine clearance (C_{Cr}) is below 10–15 mL/min, by which time they are generally on dialysis. However, patients with severe renal failure ($C_{Cr} < 25$ mL/min) have little renal reserve and may not be able to excrete an acute water load rapidly [82], leading to hyponatremia. Factors commonly seen in the postoperative setting such as pain, stress, and nausea may lower serum sodium further by increasing the release of antidiuretic hormone. Because of an intact thirst mechanism in ambulatory patients, hypernatremia is usually not a problem in patients with renal failure. In a postoperative patient in the ICU, hypernatremia may ensue, especially in the setting of significant free water losses from diarrhea, continuous nasogastric suctioning, diuresis with loop diuretics, insensible fluid losses (fever, open wound), osmotic diuresis from hyperglycemia or other osmotic agents (mannitol, contrast). Factors such as intubation and altered mental status may further contribute to the problem by blunting thirst. In such cases of worsening hypernatremia where the patient cannot correct the water deficit by him or herself, free water, intravenously as 5% dextrose or via the gastrointestinal tract feeding tube as flushes every 4–6 hours, should be provided to prevent further worsening of the hypernatremia and to correct the water deficit.

Postoperative patients with impaired kidney function should receive sufficient intravenous fluids for (a) insensible fluid losses, approximately 0.5 L of 0.45% NaCl solution, and (b) replacement of fluids lost from other sources, such as urine, wound drainage, fistula drainage, and gastrointestinal tract [85]. Close monitoring of serum chemistries and volume status will allow adjustment of the rate of intravenous infusion as well as type of fluid administered. Dialysis patients without urine output should receive no more than 1 L of fluid a day, unless there are significant fluid losses from other sources. If more than 0.5 L of intravenous fluid is necessary in a dialysis patient, it should be administered as an isotonic solution such as 0.9% NaCl unless there are significant hypotonic fluid losses. The anuric patient is unable to excrete the excess free water present in 0.45% NaCl beyond the 0.5 L or so of insensible fluid loss and will develop hyponatremia. When the patient resumes oral intake, intravenous fluids should be discontinued and the patient placed on a 1 L/day fluid restriction to avoid volume overload or water balance disorders. The daily fluid restriction encompasses both the patient's oral intake as well as any intravenous fluids accompanying administration of heparin, antibiotics, parenteral nutrition, or other medication. Increasing the concentration of these intravenous medications may at times be needed to limit daily fluid administration.

Patients with renal failure and volume overload and/or congestive heart failure being treated with loop diuretics should have serum electrolytes monitored closely, because loop diuretics tend to generate a hypotonic urine [82]. If hypernatremia ensues, the patient should receive an infusion of at least 0.5 mL of 5% dextrose in water for each milliliter of urine to prevent worsening hypernatremia. Additional free water must be administered to correct the hypernatremia. Often, there is concern that administration of 5% dextrose in water will worsen the congestive heart failure, but theoretically only 83 mL of one liter of water

remains in the intravascular space. The remainder distributes to the interstitial and intracellular fluid compartments.

Potassium disorders

Disturbances of potassium balance are not uncommon in patients with advanced CKD or ESRD. While hypokalemia may be seen in some CKD patients who require high doses of diuretics, perioperatively, hyperkalemia is more common than hypokalemia in patients with kidney disease. In addition, hyperkalemia is associated with increased mortality in hospitalized CKD patients, though they also seem to be able to tolerate a higher level [86,87].

Barring any medications that inhibit renal potassium excretion or a Type IV renal tubular acidosis, hyperkalemia generally does not occur until GFR or C_{Cr} is below 20 mL/min [86]. Nonetheless, renal reserve is decreased and the diseased kidneys may not be able to excrete an acute potassium load. In addition, patients with CKD and ESRD may have a defect in non-renal potassium homeostasis (impaired response to insulin, catecholamines, and/or aldosterone), such that potassium shifts less readily from the intravascular into the intracellular compartment [88]. These two impaired limbs of potassium homeostasis may act in concert to cause life-threatening hyperkalemia in the postoperative period.

Sources of potassium in perioperative patients include (a) administration in intravenous fluid, total parenteral nutrition, or enteral nutrition, (b) increased catabolism, (c) red blood cell transfusion, (d) reabsorption of hematoma, (e) tissue breakdown, and (f) red blood cell salvage and re-infusion intraoperatively (Table 27.3). If hypokalemia is not present, routine supplementation of intravenous fluids and total parenteral nutrition with potassium should be avoided. Therefore, the routine use of lactated Ringer's or Plasmalyte® intravenous fluids (whose potassium contents are 4 mmol/L and 5 mmol/L,

Table 27.3 Causes of perioperative hyperkalemia.

Mechanism	Cause
Increased potassium load	Increased catabolism Blood transfusion Reabsorption of hematoma Tissue breakdown Red blood cell salvage Potassium administration
Impaired transcellular potassium shift	Fasting state (insulinopenia) beta-blockers
Decreased potassium excretion	Volume depletion Constipation Medications Trimethoprim-sulfamethoxazole Potassium sparing diuretics Angiotensin converting enzyme inhibitors Angiotensin receptor blockers

respectively) should be avoided. With advanced CKD and ESRD, enteral nutrition preparations containing the least amount of potassium are preferred. Dialysis patients should receive the freshest blood available to minimize the amount of potassium infused. If possible, blood should be transfused during dialysis to allow simultaneous removal of the excess volume and potassium. However, blood transfusion during heparin-free dialysis can increase the risk of dialyzer thrombosis because of the high viscosity of packed red blood cells.

Potassium elimination may be reduced perioperatively through volume depletion in patients with CKD. Volume depletion limits renal potassium excretion because distal sodium delivery is required to allow exchange of potassium for sodium [82]. Constipation is another important cause of hyperkalemia in patients with severe CKD and ESRD [82,89]. Unlike subjects with normal kidney function who eliminate 10% of their daily potassium load through the gastrointestinal tract, patients with advancing renal failure secrete 30–40% of their daily potassium load in the colon. Constipation limits potassium secretion into the gastrointestinal tract. Medications that limit renal potassium secretion, such as trimethoprim/sulfamethoxazole, potassium sparing diuretics, ACE inhibitors, angiotensin receptor blockers, and calcineurin inhibitors will worsen hyperkalemia. Medications that antagonize aldosterone action also will exacerbate hyperkalemia through inhibition of colonic secretion of potassium.

A basal level of insulin is vital to the cellular uptake of potassium (Table 27.3) [88,90]. When patients with CKD and ESRD fast, insulin release is suppressed, leading to hyperkalemia [91]. Administering a glucose-containing solution to fasting patients will prevent this occurrence.

Previously, metabolic acidosis was thought to cause hyperkalemia through shift of potassium from the intracellular to the extracellular compartment. It is now clear that organic metabolic acidosis (lactic acidosis, ketoacidosis alone, and acidosis from renal failure) does not cause such a potassium shift [86,92]. The major cause of hyperkalemia seen in the initial phases of diabetic ketoacidosis is more likely due to potassium shift from intracellular compartment to the circulation due to solvent drag induced by hyperglycemia. The hyperglycemic/hyperosmolar environment causes water to shift from the intracellular to the extracellular compartment and potassium is passively pulled with the water from intracellular to extracellular space (solvent drag).

Treatment of hyperkalemia in the postoperative period is identical to that in other situations [82,93]. The first step is to minimize the acute risks of cardiac arrhythmia. Intravenous calcium gluconate is administered acutely to stabilize the myocardial cell membrane should there be electrocardiographic changes. Insulin and 50% dextrose are administered intravenously to shift the potassium intracellularly. Inhaled beta-agonists will shift potassium intracellularly as well but should be used with caution in patients with an extensive cardiac history since tachycardia may occur with its use. Intravenous bicarbonate may not lower the potassium level and should be used only as an adjunct to other treatments for hyperkalemia [88,92,93].

Once the immediate dangers of cardiac arrhythmias are mitigated with the above measures, ridding the body of the excess potassium is required. The use of loop diuretics in conjunction with a rate of fluid infusion to match urine output can also be used in non-oliguric patients to initiate a diuresis and urinary potassium loss. Cation exchange resins such as sodium polystyrene sulfonate (SPS), known more familiarly as Kayexalate®, to remove potassium can be given either orally or as a retention enema if oral therapy is not possible. When given orally, sorbitol must accompany the polystyrene. There has been recent concern about the risk of bowel necrosis and perforation with SPS. In particular, the risk may be higher with formulations that contain larger amounts of sorbitol and when SPS is given with sorbitol as an enema [94,95]. However, the incidence rate is most likely quite low as estimated by some authors [96]. It is our opinion that SPS can still be safely given with certain precautions. We would advise not using it in the immediate postoperative state where bowel function has yet to return or in situations where bowel surgery has just occurred. Additionally, sorbitol should not exceed 30%. If the SPS is given as a retention enema, we would advise mixing with water instead of sorbitol, though the amount of potassium removal may be much less with the water formulation. In cases of severe hyperkalemia (> 7 meq/L) or a contraindication to the use of SPS, dialysis should be instituted.

As noted earlier, hypokalemia is less common in patients with advanced CKD or ESRD, and usually results from aggressive diuresis or diarrhea in the perioperative period. Frequent use of inhaled beta-agonists for reactive airway disease may also cause hypokalemia mainly due to intracellular shift of potassium. Therefore, in this scenario, potassium may revert back to near normal levels after the acute effect of the beta-agonist has worn off. Given the high incidence of cardiovascular disease in patients with renal disease, moderate hypokalemia, even in dialysis patients, may be treated with cautious potassium repletion. The impaired transcellular shift of potassium makes it imperative that only small doses of potassium be given at a time, not to exceed 40 meq orally or 10 meq intravenously, with sufficient elapsed time between doses and preferably a follow-up blood test. Rapid administration of potassium will result in iatrogenic hyperkalemia. Nonetheless, if the patient is able to eat and the potassium is ≥ 3.5 meq/L, we would not replenish with potassium unless ongoing cardiac arrhythmias attributable to the potassium level are of concern.

Magnesium disorders

Patients with severe CKD and ESRD are unable to adequately excrete magnesium. Therefore, medications such as milk of magnesia, magnesium citrate, and magnesium-containing antacids should not be used. Constipation may be treated with sorbitol, lactulose, and polyethylene glycol solutions (Colyte®, Miralax®), or with enemas that do not contain phosphorus.

Aluminum-containing antacids may be used in the short term instead of magnesium-containing antacids, but will result in aluminum toxicity with prolonged use (more than 3–6 months). If stronger anti-acid treatment is needed, proton pump inhibitors and H_2-blockers may be used, keeping in mind that cimetidine and ranitidine are cleared by the kidney and may cause altered mental status. Additionally, cimetidine, but not ranitidine, impairs renal tubular secretion of creatinine which accounts for 5–20% of daily excreted creatinine. Therefore, a patient with CKD may have a mild elevation of serum creatinine after a few doses of cimetidine, without an actual decrease in GFR.

Low serum magnesium is rarely encountered in the advanced CKD or ESRD patient. Recently, proton pump inhibitors have been associated with severe hypomagnesemia [97,98] with the mechanism thought due to impaired gastrointestinal tract magnesium absorption or loss [99]. However, most cases are associated with chronic use of proton pump inhibitors for years. The literature describes this mainly in patients with fairly normal renal function, though cases involving advanced CKD are noted as well [99].

Phosphorus disorders

Impaired phosphorus excretion occurs at a GFR < 40 mL/min, but hyperphosphatemia is not seen clinically until a GFR < 25 mL/min. The main concern of acute hyperphosphatemia is symptomatic hypocalcemia, sufficient to cause cardiac arrhythmias [100]. Chronic hyperphosphatemia causes secondary hyperparathyroidism, increased bone turnover, and metastatic calcification in tissues, including accelerated vascular calcification [101]. Calcium phosphate may deposit in the skin causing pruritus, in the eye giving conjunctivitis, in the heart leading to conduction system disease, in the joint causing a crystalline arthropathy, and in blood vessels leading to cardio- and cerebrovascular ischemia and peripheral vascular disease.

As soon as patients with severe renal function impairment begin eating, phosphate binders should be restarted. The binders must be given with meals to precipitate with the phosphorus in food and prevent its absorption [102].

Many different types of binders are available including: calcium carbonate, calcium acetate, aluminum hydroxide, sevelamer (chloride and carbonate), and lanthanum carbonate. The only ones presently available in liquid form are aluminum hydroxide and calcium acetate. Because calcium carbonate is not very effective at phosphate binding [103] compared with calcium acetate or aluminum hydroxide, more of the calcium is available for absorption and may give rise to hypercalcemia. This is obviously undesirable if the phosphorus levels are elevated since this may exacerbate metastatic calcification in various tissues noted above, most notably in blood vessels. Aluminum hydroxide is the most effective phosphate binder, but long-term use (> 3–6 months) may result in aluminum toxicity [104]. Aluminum toxicity can occur acutely if a citrate-

containing medication (sodium, potassium, or calcium citrate) is given concomitantly with the aluminum [105]. Citrate chelates calcium in the gastrointestinal tract, thereby opening up tight junctions in the mucosa and allowing rapid absorption of aluminum. Sevelamer is a non-calcium and non-aluminum containing resin that selectively binds phosphate, avoiding the problems of excessive calcium and aluminum administration. Unlike aluminum hydroxide solutions or calcium tablets or solutions, sevelamer cannot be administered via a nasogastric tube and would be of no use as a phosphate binder in postoperative patients receiving nasogastric feeding. Like all resins, sevelamer quickly becomes a gelatinous mass when exposed to water. Lanthanum is a rare earth element and is a capable phosphorus binder. Like sevelamer, it does not contain calcium which may have some advantages in certain patients. In general, if phosphate is < 6 mg/dL and the product < 60, any of the above binders may be used. If either is high, then aluminum hydroxide or sevelamer is the initial choice, keeping in mind that sevelamer is not as effective as aluminum at phosphate binding. Once the phosphate and the calcium/phosphate product are lower, another binder should be substituted for aluminum hydroxide.

Dietary phosphorus intake must be restricted to less than 700 mg a day. Common sources of phosphorus include cola drinks, milk products, and protein sources including beans and legumes. In addition, some enemas and oral medications used for constipation or bowel prep such as Fleet® enema or Phospho-soda® contain large amounts of phosphorus and must be avoided in patients with renal failure. Recently, the US FDA has placed a warning on the use of phosphorous-containing enemas and bowel preps due to cases of AKI induced by the large absorbed phosphorus load. Elderly patients and those with CKD are noted to be at high risk. We recommend using other means for either bowel prep or the treatment of constipation in all patients with CKD or ESRD. In severe cases of hyperphosphatemia, continuous dialysis or extended daily dialysis (see below) will effectively correct the phosphate within two to three days [106,107].

Rarely, hypophosphatemia occurs. Refeeding hypophosphatemia is the likely cause if the patient is nutritionally depleted and begins feeding [108]. Another common cause is the use of continuous or extended hemodialysis treatments since these modalities may remove large amounts of phosphorus [106]. Our protocols allow the addition of phosphorus into the dialysate to limit removal. If that is not available, providing phosphorus infusion during the treatment may be an option. Lastly, sucralfate, used in the ICU as gastrointestinal bleeding prophylaxis, is an excellent phosphate binder and can cause hypophosphatemia [109].

Calcium disorders

New-onset hypercalcemia is unusual in the perioperative patient with AKI or CKD, since patients with renal failure tend to have lower serum calcium. Hypercalcemia noted preoperatively is likely due to: (a) continued use of calcium-containing phosphate binders despite poor oral intake, allowing the calcium to be absorbed, (b) excessive calcitriol administration which responds quickly to withholding the calcitriol, and (c) severe secondary or tertiary hyperparathyroidism, as in the ESRD patient awaiting parathyroidectomy. De novo hypercalcemia rarely may be seen in the setting of prolonged immobilization [110]. Treatment consists of removing calcium-containing drugs, vitamin D analogs, and dialysis against a low calcium dialysate in severe cases. The hypercalcemia from prolonged immobilization may respond to bisphosphonate therapy [111], such as pamidronate or alendronate, although long-term benefits remain unknown. Renal dose adjustment for alendronate is 5 mg orally daily or 35 mg once a week, though the long-term risks and benefits of bisphosphonate therapy in CKD and ESRD patients are unclear. We would not advocate starting these medications without a very compelling indication other than just a higher blood calcium level.

Hypocalcemia most commonly occurs as a result of hyperphosphatemia, and should not be treated with intravenous calcium because of the risk of precipitating metastatic calcification, unless life-threatening arrhythmias are present. Instead, efforts should be directed at correcting the hyperphosphatemia. Use of regional citrate anticoagulation (see below) may also lead to symptomatic and/or life-threatening hypocalcemia and should be corrected by raising the calcium infusion rate. Finally, patients who undergo parathyroidectomy to treat severe secondary or tertiary hyperparathyroidism can develop severe hypocalcemia from the "hungry bone syndrome" [112]. They require large amounts of elemental calcium and calcitriol. Initially, the calcium may need to be administered as an intravenous infusion repeated over days, until the patient stabilizes on oral doses of calcium administered apart from meals and oral calcitriol. Hemodialysis against a higher dialysate calcium concentration will correct severe hypocalcemia quickly, though the amount of calcium needed to replenish the mineral bone is usually not correctable by hemodialysis treatments alone.

Acid–base status

Patients with renal failure usually have a mild metabolic acidosis because of the accumulation of non-volatile acids resulting from the metabolism of food (about 1 mmol/kg/day). In most cases, the acidosis can be corrected easily by oral base supplementation (e.g., sodium bicarbonate) or by dialysis. If stable patients with renal failure develop progressive acidosis, other causes should be vigorously investigated. These include lactic acidosis, ketoacidosis, intoxications (e.g., ethylene glycol), and severe diarrhea.

A fall in arterial pH to less than 7.10 can precipitate potentially fatal ventricular arrhythmias and reduce both cardiac contractility and inotropic response to catecholamines [113–115]. Neurologic symptoms ranging from lethargy to

coma have been described in patients with metabolic acidosis, which appear to be related to a decrease in cerebrospinal fluid pH [116]. The initial goal in the management of severe metabolic acidosis (blood pH less than 7.2) is to treat the underlying cause. The next important step in managing profound metabolic acidosis in a ventilated patient is vigorous use of the ventilator to augment carbon dioxide excretion by the lungs. Rapid assessment of inadequate ventilation and subsequent ventilator adjustments to lower the pCO_2 is a very powerful treatment in ameliorating the severity of the metabolic acidosis and is frequently underutilized in the ICU for the management of metabolic acidosis. For example, a patient with a pCO_2 of 38 mmHg (which is in the normal range for most blood gas labs) and serum bicarbonate level of 10 mmol/L will have an arterial blood pH of 7.04. Such a patient would be suffering from a combined metabolic acidosis and a respiratory acidosis; the pCO_2 inappropriately normal for the degree of metabolic acidosis. Simply increasing the minute ventilation to lower the pCO_2 to 25 mmHg will increase the pH to 7.23 and quickly attenuates the severity of the profound metabolic acidosis.

Metabolic acidosis in the perioperative patient with either acute or chronic renal failure can be effectively treated with acute hemodialysis or hemofiltration with bicarbonate-containing replacement fluids, which is the treatment of choice. If the patient has a profound metabolic acidosis with serum bicarbonate < 10 mmol/L (and arterial pH < 7.10) and dialysis treatment has not been initiated, administering intravenous sodium bicarbonate may help raise the pH to a safer level (> 7.20) at which abnormalities in cardiovascular function become less likely. Another indication for sodium bicarbonate therapy is in patients with metabolic acidosis due to massive gastrointestinal bicarbonate loss from severe diarrhea. Bicarbonate can be given as a "push" of 50 mmol of bicarbonate in each 50 mL ampule. However, rapid intravenous administration of bicarbonate can lead to fluid overload, worsening tissue oxygenation, hypokalemia, and worsening cerebrospinal fluid acidosis (because the blood–brain barrier is more permeable to CO_2 than to bicarbonate) [115,116]. To minimize these complications, intravenous bicarbonate therapy either should be stopped or infused at a much slower rate once the blood pH has reached 7.20. Other complications of treatment with sodium bicarbonate include hypernatremia (if hypertonic bicarbonate solutions are used), hyponatremia (if hypotonic solutions are used), and metabolic alkalosis (if excessive bicarbonate is given). In addition, there is ongoing controversy concerning the use of sodium bicarbonate therapy in patients with lactic acidosis. Based on a number of experimental and clinical studies, bicarbonate therapy in the setting of lactic acidosis only transiently increases serum bicarbonate levels but worsens intracellular acidosis [117]. However, if the lactic acidosis is profound (pH < 7.10), bicarbonate should be administered judiciously to attenuate the severity of the acidosis and its untoward effects on cardiovascular function [118,119]. It is important to note the dialysis does not correct lactic acidosis except to provide additional bicarbonate that would help raise serum pH, much like what a bicarbonate infusion would accomplish. The main advantage of doing this on dialysis is that the bicarbonate can be diffused during the treatment without the sodium and volume loads commonly of concern in such critically ill patients. Although equations exist to allow calculations of the bicarbonate deficit [119], serial measurements of the blood pH and serum bicarbonate are mandatory to monitor the rate and extent of correction of the metabolic acidosis.

Another option for the treatment of metabolic acidosis is the use of tromethamine or tris-hydroxymethyl amino-methane (THAM). THAM is an inert amino alcohol that buffers both acids and CO_2 by binding a proton and forming $THAM-NH_3^+$ [120]. The main theoretical advantages of THAM over bicarbonate include: (1) no sodium load, THAM may actually bind sodium; and (2) there is no generation of CO_2. The drug has been used to treat severe acidosis but its clinical efficacy compared with the use of sodium bicarbonate is unproven. In addition, serious side-effects including hyper-kalemia, hypoglycemia, and respiratory depression have been attributed to THAM. Most notably, there is a relative contra-indication to its use in patients with advanced CKD and ESRD as over 70% of the drug is excreted by the kidneys.

The choice of intravenous fluids may also play a role in acid–base balance. As noted in the above section on sodium and potassium disorders, we generally recommend normal saline as the choice for maintenance intravenous fluids, if needed. In patients with kidney disease, the higher chloride load of saline may exacerbate a metabolic acidosis. In a ran-domized study of patients at the time of renal transplant, patients on lactated Ringer's and Plasmalyte® (which contain base equivalents of lactate and acetate) had higher serum bicarbonate levels than those patients randomized to saline [121]. However, all groups had similar arterial pH levels, and the fluid volumes used were modest. Since CKD and ESRD patients are at risk for hyperkalemia, these potassium-containing fluids may create additional electrolyte issues. An alternative, if control of metabolic acidosis is required, would be the addition of bicarbonate into a potassium-free solution. As noted above, if urgent correction of a severe hyperchlore-mic metabolic acidosis is needed, bicarbonate push may quickly stabilize the scenario. If slower administration of bicar-bonate is desired, adding 3 ampules of 50 mmol of bicarbonate into a 5% dextrose and water solution will provide an approxi-mate 150 mmol/L saline solution with bicarbonate which can be infused at an hourly rate.

Metabolic alkalosis in patients with renal failure is usually caused by acid losses from vomiting, nasogastric suction, or diuretic use (in those with CKD). The administration of exces-sive alkali (e.g., sodium bicarbonate, citrate-anticoagulated blood transfusion) also causes metabolic alkalosis because excretion of bicarbonate is markedly reduced in patients with renal failure. Treatment must be directed at the underlying cause. If patients are volume depleted or hypokalemic, then careful volume expansion with isotonic saline or supplemen-tation with potassium chloride is indicated, and such maneu-vers will allow appropriate renal excretion of accumulated bicarbonate in those with CKD not on dialysis. There are limited studies on the use of acetazolamide, a carbonic anhy-drase inhibitor, in the setting of metabolic alkalosis and CKD. Hemodialysis or hydrochloric acid administration can be used to treat symptomatic or severe alkalosis [122].

Management of nutrition in the perioperative patient

Malnutrition is a common problem in patients with either acute or chronic renal failure. Approximately one-third of chronic dialysis patients are malnourished, due to a combin-ation of factors including poor nutritional intake, protein losses during dialysis, and increased catabolism [123]. Decreased serum albumin levels are strong predictors of mor-tality and hospitalization in chronic dialysis patients. The risk of mortality increases as serum albumin decreases below 4.0 g/dL, doubles in patients with a serum albumin between 3.5 and 4.0 g/dL, and is 15-fold higher when albumin falls below the 3.0 g/dL range [124]. Recently, it has been recognized that a substantial number of ESRD patients appear to have serologic evidence of an augmented inflammatory state with activation of the systemic inflammatory response. Moreover, it appears that inflammation may be as or more important than protein intake in causing hypoalbuminemia [125].

Patients with ESRD undergoing surgical procedures need to receive adequate protein and calorie intake. One problem with dietary intake recommendations for malnourished dialy-sis patients is choosing the appropriate weight to compute protein and caloric needs, since the actual body weight reflects the effects of malnutrition. Protein and caloric intake estimates should be based on average body weight for healthy subjects of the same sex, height, age, and body frame [126]. The Kidney and Dialysis Outcomes Quality Initiative (K-DOQI™) [127] recommends that stable hemodialysis patients should ingest 1.2 g of protein per kilogram of average body weight per day (g/kg/day), and peritoneal dialysis patients 1.5 g/kg/day because of increased protein losses in the dialysate. At least 50% of the protein should be of high biologic value. Caloric intake should be 35 kcal/kg/day in dialysis patients less than 60 years of age and 30–35 kcal/kg/day in those over 60 years [127], because this level of caloric intake is necessary to main-tain neutral nitrogen balance and prevent protein breakdown in dialysis patients. At least half of the calorie intake should be from carbohydrates. Patients with advanced CKD but not on dialysis do require adequate nutritional support, though the recommendations are less defined. We would advocate at least 0.8–1.0 g of protein per kilogram per day, with attention paid to keeping potassium and phosphorus contents on the lower side. Many hospital renal diets may not fulfill all of these requirements and individualized adjustments are sometimes needed.

Table 27.4 Adjustment factors for determining energy requirements.

Clinical condition	Adjustment factor
Mechanical ventilation	
Without sepsis	1.10–1.20
With sepsis	1.25–1.35
Peritonitis	1.15
Infection	
Mild	1.00–1.10
Moderate	1.10–1.20
Sepsis	1.20–1.30
Soft-tissue trauma	1.10
Bone fractures	1.15
Burns (% of body surface area)	
0–20%	1.15
20–40%	1.50
40–100%	1.70

Source: From Rocco MV, Blumenkrantz MJ. Nutrition. In Daugirdas JT, Blake PG, Ing TS, eds. *Handbook of Dialysis*. Philadelphia: Little Brown & Co; 2001, pp. 420–45.

For the surgical patient with acute renal failure or ESRD, both the caloric and protein requirements are much greater because of increased catabolism, protein losses, and higher energy demands. Rocco and Blumenkrantz [126] have adapted adjustment factors from the literature for determining energy requirements (non-protein calories) in patients with renal failure (Table 27.4). The amino acid or protein requirements for these patients should be in the range of 1.2–2.0 g/kg/day. For patients with acute renal failure, augmenting protein intake beyond these levels does not improve nitrogen balance or survival [128] and serves only to increase nitrogenous waste products and hence the uremic environment. Perioperative patients with either acute or chronic renal failure who are unable to ingest sufficient calories and protein may require nasogastric or parenteral nutritional support. When initiating nutritional support, special attention should be given to the potassium, sodium, phosphorus, and free water content of the solution to avoid precipitating electrolyte disturbances (see prior sections).

Management of anemia in the perioperative patient

Anemia in renal disease is due mainly to insufficient production of erythropoietin by the diseased kidney. Other factors may contribute to the anemia including folate and vitamin B_{12} deficiency, chronic gastrointestinal bleeding, shortened red blood cell survival, and uremic inhibition of red cell synthesis [129]. The development of recombinant erythropoietin (EPO) was one of the greatest advances in the care of this population since the advent of chronic dialysis [130]. In the past few years, clinical trials using EPO to achieve hemoglobin values > 12 g/dL in both ESRD and CKD patients have found a higher rate of adverse events including all-cause mortality and stroke [131–133]. None of these studies addressed specifically the

use of EPO in the perioperative scenario. Guidelines and practice patterns have changed after the results of these studies were announced, and goal hemoglobin levels have been modified to < 12 g/dL. At this time, we would advise patients with ESRD admitted for surgical procedures to be maintained on their outpatient EPO regimen, generally administered 1–2 times a week subcutaneously if their hemoglobin level is < 12 g/dL and to hold the EPO if hemoglobin is higher. Patients with CKD may only be receiving their EPO every 1–2 weeks, and depending on the length of hospital stay may not need to have EPO given in the perioperative period, at least for anemia management (see section on bleeding diathesis for additional EPO effects). While some may advocate a temporary increase in EPO administration prior to surgery to raise hemoglobin above the usual target goals in anticipation of blood loss, we do not favor this approach in most patients. In the exception that the patient has a religious belief against receiving blood products, the risks of temporarily raising the blood count versus those related to perioperative bleeding need to be weighed on a case by case basis.

The rate of rise in hematocrit is dose dependent but should not exceed 1–3% per week, since higher rates of rise may result in severe hypertension and seizures. If the perioperative patient with renal disease is profoundly anemic (hematocrit < 25%), treatment with EPO may not raise the hematocrit fast enough to prevent perioperative complications from the anemia, especially in patients with underlying cardiac disease or where significant surgical blood loss is anticipated. Blood transfusions are usually required for these patients to raise the hematocrit quickly to a safer level (> 27%). Patients who are or may become candidates for renal transplantation should receive irradiated packed blood cells and infusion via a white cell filter in order to minimize exposure to nucleated cells and thus immune sensitization, though evidence of effectiveness of this approach in lacking.

Perioperative patients with either acute or chronic renal failure may be resistant to EPO if infection or surgery-induced inflammation is present. Higher doses of EPO may overcome such resistance. The stimulation of erythropoiesis usually depletes iron stores and periodic parenteral iron administration may be required. Percent iron saturation and ferritin levels should be obtained to evaluate iron stores since relative or absolute iron deficiency is another major cause of EPO resistance. Criteria and treatment protocols for management of iron deficiency are discussed in the DOQI guidelines [134]. Erythropoietin has been used in patients with AKI, although there is a paucity of studies evaluating its use in this setting with no data suggesting improved outcomes. In general, we do not recommend the use of EPO in the setting of anemia with AKI.

Bleeding diathesis

Patients with either acute or chronic renal failure can manifest derangement in hemostasis with impairment in clot formation in response to vascular injury [135]. Many factors contribute to impairment in clot formation, which largely revolve around defects in platelet function. Platelet aggregation is abnormal in patients with renal failure and may be due to reduced intra-platelet adenosine diphosphate (ADP) and serotonin levels, and defective thromboxane A_2 production. An adhesion receptor, the glycoprotein IIb-IIIa complex is a key component in controlling the formation of platelet thrombi. For patients with either acute or chronic renal failure, activation of this receptor complex is impaired leading to prolonged bleeding time [136–138]. In addition, abnormalities in von Willebrand factor and increased production of nitric oxide have been implicated and contribute to the bleeding diathesis of uremia [139]. Finally, anemia, especially when the hemoglobin < 10 g/dL, appears to impair platelet aggregation leading to prolonged bleeding time [135].

The perioperative evaluation of any potential coagulopathy in the patient with either acute or chronic renal failure should entail measurement of the platelet count, prothrombin time (INR) and partial thromboplastin time. These values should be within the normal range even for patients with renal failure unless there is an additional pathologic process such as liver disease or disseminated intravascular clotting. An important point is that patients with renal failure have a qualitative disorder and platelet counts are normal in this population unless another disease process is present. This bleeding diathesis can be assessed by measuring skin bleeding time [140]. The risk for hemorrhage is increased when the bleeding time exceeds 10 minutes. Practically, bleeding times are not commonly performed perioperatively, because of the general assumption that there is a bleeding diathesis and that active bleeding should be treated promptly and not delayed by tests. Moreover, bleeding times do not necessarily correlate with clinical bleed events.

Preoperatively, the bleeding diathesis can be mitigated to some extent by performing hemodialysis prior to surgery. Patients who are markedly uremic with very high blood urea nitrogen levels (>100 mg/dL) may benefit from more than one dialysis treatment prior to a major surgical procedure, if time permits, to minimize whatever component the uremic milieu may be contributing to the bleeding diathesis. Postoperatively, if bleeding is still an active issue, intensive dialysis support should be continued to help improve platelet function [141].

Severely anemic patients with renal failure should receive blood transfusions prior to surgery to achieve hemoglobin of > 10 g/dL, though risks for immune sensitization should be considered in those who are viable renal transplant candidates. The increase in hematocrit forces the platelets to flow along the periphery of the blood vessel, making the platelets readily available should the blood vessel become disrupted. This hematocrit should be maintained during the perioperative period in order to minimize bleeding.

Erythropoietin is often used in the CKD and ESRD patient to treat anemia as discussed in the prior section. Erythropoietin may also decrease bleeding risks in the CKD population by means other than its effect on red blood cell production.

Erythropoietin may improve platelet–platelet and platelet–endothelium interactions, improve platelet signaling, and increase the relative number of reticulated platelets that are more active [142]. Therefore, continuation of EPO, as long as hemoglobin does not exceed 12 g/dL, may not only maintain the red cell mass, but may also aid in controlling postoperative bleeding.

For the perioperative patient with renal failure who is either actively bleeding or at high risk for bleeding during a major surgical procedure, the administration of either cryoprecipitate or 1-desamino-8-D-arginine vasopressin (DDAVP) can be effective in improving the qualitative platelet defect of uremia [135,138,143]. Cryoprecipitate is a pooled plasma fraction enriched with factor VIII and von Willebrand factor and has been demonstrated to improve bleeding times. The effect is apparent 1 hour after infusion of 10 units with a peak effect between 4 and 12 hours. DDAVP induces the release of endogenous von Willebrand factor. When given intravenously in a dose of 0.3 μg/kg, the bleeding time begins to decrease within 1 hour and remains effective for 6–8 hours. A similar effect can be achieved with subcutaneous administration, but the onset of action is delayed by 2 hours. Repeated administration of DDAVP, more often than every 48 hours, results in decreased efficacy due to depletion of endogenous stores of von Willebrand factor.

Conjugated estrogens also improve bleeding times in patients with renal failure. Although the onset of action is much slower with estrogens compared with DDAVP or cryoprecipitate, the duration of action is much longer (7–10 days). The use of conjugated estrogens may be helpful in improving the bleeding diathesis in renal failure patients undergoing elective procedures with a high risk for bleeding, since the drug can be started 1 week prior to the planned surgery. It may also be beneficial in improving the bleed diathesis in renal failure patients with prolonged postoperative bleeding and is given as conjugated estrogen 0.6 mg/kg intravenously daily for 5 days [138,144]. The use of anticoagulation during hemodialysis for the perioperative patient with either acute or chronic renal failure may contribute to the bleeding diathesis. For a full discussion, see the section below.

Medical imaging

Medical imaging is frequently performed during the perioperative period, including magnetic resonance imaging or angiography (MRI, MRA). Gadolinium is commonly administered intravenously as a contrast agent during MR imaging. Over the past 10 years, a devastating systemic fibrosing disorder has been identified in patients with advanced chronic renal insufficiency that has been attributed to use of gadolinium in this population. This disorder, known as nephrogenic systemic fibrosis (NSF) develops insidiously (months to years) after exposure to gadolinium in patients with advanced CKD [145]. The clearance of gadolinium is decreased in the setting of reduced GFR. The half-life is 1.5 hours in normal subjects,

10 hours for CKD stage III–IV and 34 hours for ESRD [146]. Free gadolinium is poorly soluble and forms toxic precipitates. The pathogenesis of NSF is not well understood but may be due to gadolinium-induced stimulation of the bone marrow to produce CD34+ fibrocytes. These fibrocytes accumulate in affected tissues (skin predominantly) and produce collagen [147]. The clinical result of this is development of subcutaneous fibrotic indurated plaques and nodules that begin in the feet, legs, and hands and can expand to arms, buttocks, and torso. Movement of the joints becomes limited by the fibrosis and patients complain of pain and burning in the affected areas [148]. The diagnosis of NSF is based on histopathologic examination of a skin biopsy. Unfortunately, NSF is a progressive disorder with no proven therapy.

The main issue for the surgical patient with either CKD or AKI is prevention of NSF. The current recommendation is that gadolinium should not be administered to patients with a GFR less than 30 mL/hour (CKD stages IV and V) and alternate medical imaging be considered [149]. The recommendations for CKD stage III (30–60 mL/hour) are vague since the risk for NSF for this group is not well defined. In our practice, we tend to avoid use of gadolinium in stage III CKD [149].

If gadolinium must be given in a patient with reduced renal function, there are some general considerations. First, the patient must be informed of the risks. Second, there is an observation that of the gadolinium preparations, gadodiamide may be more toxic, and other gadolinium preparations such as gadoteridol should be used [150]. Third, the dose of gadolinium should be given in the lowest amount possible to perform the study. Finally, hemodialysis does remove gadolinium, and if a patient with a GFR less than 15 mL/min is given gadolinium, performing hemodialysis immediately after the MR scan should be strongly considered [151]. There is no evidence, however, that hemodialysis will prevent NSF in patients with reduced kidney function. The low risk of performing dialysis in a patient with a GFR less than 15 mL/min and potential benefit of preventing NSF in this high-risk group supports this recommendation.

The administration of iodinated contrast agents can worsen renal function, especially in patients with CKD. This topic is discussed in detail in "Risk of acute kidney injury with medical imaging" below.

Perioperative acute kidney injury

Prevention of kidney injury is the perioperative goal in the management of patients with functioning kidneys. Acute kidney injury that develops after anesthesia and surgery is associated with increased mortality. Mortality rates for acute postoperative AKI requiring dialysis has ranged from 47% to 81% in a number of clinical series [152]. A retrospective cohort of 10,518 patients suggests that development of AKI after surgery worsens long-term survival [153]. Risk factors for increased mortality for patients with AKI include male gender, presence of oliguria, mechanical ventilation, acute myocardial infarction, acute stroke or seizure, and chronic immunosuppression [154]. Despite advances in intensive care and dialysis technology, the outcome in perioperative patients with AKI has not improved. In addition to facing increased mortality, patients who survive after developing AKI post-surgery have three possible outcomes: (1) return to baseline renal function, (2) development of chronic kidney disease in previously normal kidneys, and (3) accelerated progression of underlying chronic kidney disease [155].

The two major causes of AKI developing in the perioperative period are prerenal disease and acute tubular necrosis (ATN). Decreased kidney function due to prerenal disease occurs when renal ischemia is part of a generalized decrease in tissue perfusion and when there is selective renal ischemia that is generally reversible with fluid administration and restoration of renal blood flow. Acute tubular necrosis can occur with prolonged and/or severe ischemia. This can result in histologic changes, including necrosis and have a more prolonged clinical course that is generally not responsive to fluid therapy and may require renal replacement therapy.

Both prerenal disease and ATN can occur in a variety of perioperative settings. Prerenal disease may result from true volume depletion, hypotension, edematous states, and selective renal ischemia, while ATN is principally due to all the same causes of severe prerenal disease, particularly hypotension, and nephrotoxins. In evaluating a patient with AKI, the clinician needs to determine if the etiology is prerenal, ATN, or a combination of both given that therapy for each etiology will be different. A careful history and physical examination can frequently categorize a patient's volume status and identify events or risk factors that would suggest the etiology for the AKI. The first diagnostic tool in evaluating a patient with AKI is the performance of a urinalysis. The urinalysis is normal or near-normal in prerenal disease; hyaline casts may be seen, but these are not an abnormal finding. In comparison, the classic urinalysis in ATN reveals muddy brown granular and epithelial cell casts and free epithelial cells.

The perioperative patient with a clinical history consistent with fluid loss, a physical examination consistent with hypovolemia (hypotension and tachycardia) and/or oliguria should be administered intravenous fluid therapy, unless contraindicated. This fluid challenge attempts to identify prerenal failure that can progress to ATN if not treated promptly. The fractional excretion of sodium (FENa) and/or urea can be helpful as supportive (not diagnostic) data in evaluating a patient with oliguria and AKI. The FENa is typically less than 1% in prerenal disease (indicative of the sodium retention) and above 2% in ATN. The fractional excretion of urea may be a more sensitive and specific test compared with the FENa to differentiate prerenal versus ATN in oliguric patients, especially if diuretics have been administered to the patient [156]. In prerenal states, the fractional excretion of urea is generally less than 35%. Unfortunately, the FENa can have a prerenal pattern in many forms of ATN such as contrast-induced or myoglobinuric-induced ATN and can be misleading in these clinical conditions. Moreover, the use of the FENa should only be used in oliguric forms of AKI and its utility in non-oliguric AKI is suspect. It is our opinion, that there has been too heavy reliance on the FENa as the primary diagnostic test in evaluating patients with AKI. The etiology of AKI should be made by a history, physical exam, and urinalysis performed by a trained healthcare professional familiar with identifying components of the urinary sediment [157].

Because there has not been a uniform consensus on the definition of AKI, there has been an attempt in recent years to develop a standard definition and staging system for AKI. The impetus for a staging system for AKI was motivated, in part, by the acceptance and popularity of the CKD staging system and in part, by the need for a consensus definition of AKI for clinical research purposes.

One of the earlier classification systems developed by the Acute Dialysis Quality Initiative used the acronym RIFLE for risk, injury, failure, loss of function and ESRD [158]. This classification system was later modified by the Acute Kidney Injury Network (AKIN). According to the AKIN criteria, AKI is defined as an abrupt (within 48 hours) absolute increase in serum concentration of creatinine ≥ 0.3 mg/dL from baseline, a percentage increase in serum concentration 50%, or oliguria of less than 0.5 mL/kg/hour for more than 6 hours [159]. These diagnostic criteria should only be applied after volume status has been optimized and urinary tract obstruction has been ruled out as a cause for AKI. The AKIN classification for AKI comprises three stages (Table 27.5) [160].

At present, the greatest utility for the AKIN staging systems is for clinical research in which standard definitions of AKI will facilitate epidemiologic analysis and provide uniform inclusion criteria and end-points for clinical trials. At present, the utility of this staging system for medical and surgical services caring for patients with AKI is not clear. In addition to the development of a staging system for AKI, there is currently an active area of research measuring a number of biomarkers, such as neutrophil gelatinase associated lipocalin (NGAL), that may identify patients at risk for AKI before there are changes in serum creatinine levels and urine output [161].

A number of risk factors have been identified as contributing to perioperative AKI, most often due to acute tubular necrosis (Table 27.6). These can be broadly divided into two categories: decreased renal perfusion (ischemia) and exposure to nephrotoxins. Postoperative patients are at increased risk for ATN because preoperative fluid depletion, anesthesia, and intraoperative fluid losses can lead to volume depletion and reduction in renal blood flow and glomerular filtration rate. Most patients can tolerate these procedures, but the likelihood of tubular injury is increased if the patient has preexisting CKD. In addition, the presence of hypotension and hemolysis exacerbates tubular injury.

Surgical risk factors

Three surgical procedures are associated with the highest risk for developing acute tubular necrosis: abdominal aortic aneurysm repair, surgery to correct obstructive jaundice and

Table 27.5 Classification and staging system for acute kidney injury (AKI).

Stage	Serum creatinine criteria	Urine output criteria
1	Increase in serum creatinine of more than or equal to 0.3 mg/dL or increase to more than or equal to 150–200% (1.5- to 2-fold) from baseline	Less than 0.5 mL/kg per hour for more than 6 hours
2	Increase in serum creatinine to more than 200–300% (> 2- to 3-fold) from baseline	Less than 0.5 mL/kg/ hour for more than 12 hours
3	Increase in serum creatinine to more than 300% (> 3-fold) from baseline or a serum creatinine of more than or equal to 4.0 mg/dL with an acute increase of at least 0.5 mg/dL	Less than 0.5 mL/kg/ hour for 24 hours or anuria for 12 hours

Adapted from [159,160].

Table 27.6 Causes of perioperative acute kidney injury.

Decreased renal perfusion
    Intravascular volume depletion
    Congestive heart failure
    Sepsis
    Cardiopulmonary bypass
    Anesthetic effects on renal blood flow
    Aortic cross-clamping
    Use of non-steroidal anti-inflammatory drugs or cyclooxygenase inhibitors
    Use of angiotensin converting enzyme inhibitors/angiotensin receptor blockers

Nephrotoxin exposure
    Aminoglycosides
    Radiocontrast agents
    Anesthetic agents
    Myoglobin/rhabdomyolysis

cardiac surgery with cardiopulmonary bypass [162]. In abdominal aortic aneurysm repair, the kidneys may receive no blood flow for prolonged periods if the aorta is clamped above the renal arteries during surgery [163]. Surgery to correct obstructive jaundice is associated with greater decreases in glomerular filtration rate than other types of abdominal surgery, perhaps due to higher rates of sepsis and increased gut absorption of endotoxin [164]. Finally, in the setting of cardiac surgery, underlying heart disease with impaired left ventricular function plus hypotension contributes to the increased risk for AKI from acute tubular necrosis. Furthermore, prolonged cardiopulmonary bypass and hemolysis during bypass may contribute further to acute tubular necrosis.

Table 27.7 Cleveland Clinic clinical scoring system for acute kidney injury (AKI) after cardiac surgery.

Risk factor	Points
Female gender	1
Congestive heart failure	1
Left ventricular ejection fraction < 35%	1
Preoperative use of IABP	2
COPD	1
Insulin-requiring diabetes	1
Previous cardiac surgery	1
Emergency surgery	2
Valve surgery only (reference to CABG)	1
CABG + valve (reference to CABG)	2
Other cardiac surgeries	2
Preoperative creatinine 1.2 to < 2.1 mg/dL (reference to 1.2)	2
Preoperative creatinine ≥ 2.1 (reference to 1.2)	5
Minimum score, 0; maximum score, 17	

IABP, intra-aortic balloon pump; COPD, chronic obstructive pulmonary disease; CABG, coronary artery bypass grafting.
Adapted from reference [166].

Common themes that appear as risk factors for perioperative AKI include older age, preexisting CKD, diabetes mellitus, intravascular volume depletion, presence of congestive heart failure, emergency surgery, high-risk surgery (intraperitoneal, intrathoracic, or suprainguinal vascular procedures) and history of cardio- and cerebrovascular ischemia [165]. A clinical scoring system has been developed to predict postoperative AKI after cardiac surgery that required dialysis based on over 15,000 patients who underwent open-heart surgery at the Cleveland Clinic. The risk factors and point system are listed in Table 27.7, which is used to develop an acute renal score ranging from 0 to a maximum value of 17. Based on the scores, four risk categories were analyzed (scores 0–2, 3–5, 6–8 and 9–13). The frequency of developing AKI requiring dialysis was 0.4%, 1.8%, 9.5%, and 21.3%, respectively for the four risk groups [166]. Recent data suggest that on-pump coronary artery bypass graft surgery is more deleterious to renal function compared with off-pump surgery, especially in diabetic patients with CKD [167].

Sepsis with and without hypotension is an important cause of acute tubular necrosis in the perioperative patient. Multiple organ dysfunction and probable endotoxemia frequently accompany the sepsis syndrome in this population [68]. The mechanism by which sepsis causes acute tubular necrosis is not well understood, but may involve systemic hypotension with tubular ischemia, direct renal vasoconstriction, the release of a number of cytokines such as tumor necrosis factor, and activation of neutrophils which leads to direct renal injury.

Use of drugs that affect renal hemodynamics

Many anesthetic agents have been associated with decreases in renal blood flow, glomerular filtration rate, and urine output. It is not clear if these decreases in renal function reflect direct effects of the anesthetic or indirect effects of sympathetic and neurohumoral activation and anesthetic-induced hypotension. Although the role of anesthetics in causing AKI is not well understood, surgical anesthesia combined with hypotension appear to increase the risk for acute tubular necrosis.

A number of pharmacologic agents such as non-steroidal anti-inflammatory drugs (NSAIDs), cyclooxygenase-2 (COX-2) inhibitors, ACE inhibitors, and angiotensin receptor blockers (ARBs) can impair renal perfusion. NSAIDs and COX-2 inhibitors block the production of important vasodilatory prostaglandins such as prostaglandin E_2. In the setting of impaired renal perfusion as seen in the perioperative patient, the kidney augments the production of these locally produced autacoids to enhance renal blood flow and maintain glomerular filtration rate. NSAIDs and COX-2 inhibitors prevent this adaptive vasodilatory response leading to relative renal vasoconstriction and decrease in renal blood flow and glomerular filtration rate [169,170]. These drugs should not be used in the perioperative patient, especially in the setting of major surgery where decreased renal perfusion or elevated serum creatinine concentration is present.

ACE inhibitors and ARBs are commonly used antihypertensive agents, especially in patients with left ventricular dysfunction, diabetes mellitus, and CKD. Although there are no national or international guidelines that delineate a standard of care for the use of these agents in the perioperative period, there have been a number of reports of significant hypotension developing in the first 30 minutes of anesthesia in patients taking either ACE inhibitors or ARBs. These hypotensive episodes frequently require the use of systemic vasopressor drugs to maintain blood pressure. Preoperative use of ACE inhibitors has been associated with a doubling of the mortality risk in patients undergoing coronary artery bypass graft surgery [171]. In addition, there is increased risk of developing postoperative AKI in patients taking ACE inhibitors or ARBs preoperatively [171]. We generally recommend holding ACE inhibitors and ARBs preoperatively and in the immediate postoperative period.

In addition, the worsening of renal function perioperatively associated with inhibitors of the renin-angiotensin system may be exacerbated by volume depletion. During intravascular volume depletion and/or impaired renal perfusion, the renin–angiotensin system is stimulated and angiotensin II production increased. By selectively increasing efferent arteriolar vasoconstriction, angiotensin II maintains intraglomerular capillary pressure and glomerular filtration rate despite reduced renal blood flow. ACE inhibitors or ARBs block, respectively, the production and action of angiotensin II [172,173].

Nephrotoxins

The perioperative patient is frequently exposed to a number of nephrotoxins that can cause acute tubular necrosis. Aminoglycoside antibiotics are used perioperatively, especially in the setting of trauma and abdominal surgery. Volume depletion, hypotension, sepsis, and preexisting renal disease appear to act synergistically with aminoglycosides to cause acute tubular necrosis [174–176]. Additional risk factors for aminoglycoside nephrotoxicity include dose and plasma levels, concomitant use of penicillins or cephalosporins, and duration of therapy. Acute renal failure generally develops after at least 5–7 days of treatment. However, in the setting of hypotension or volume depletion, the combined insults may lead to earlier development of acute tubular necrosis. Close monitoring of peak and trough plasma levels and adjustment of the dose are key components of aminoglycoside therapy. Recently, there has been evidence that once-daily dosing of aminoglycosides may be less nephrotoxic than the traditional divided dose regimens. However, in the setting of preexisting CKD, the divided dose regimens with appropriate dose reduction or interval lengthening should be used to avoid toxic peak and trough levels. Most patients with aminoglycoside-induced acute tubular necrosis are non-oliguric and generally do not require dialysis support unless they have prior renal failure and marginal renal reserve or are oliguric because of multiple nephrotoxic insults.

Radiocontrast agent is another nephrotoxin that can cause AKI and will be discussed below.

Rhabdomyolysis and myoglobinuria

Surgery services frequently manage patients who have sustained major trauma and accompanying severe muscle injury (rhabdomyolysis). The resulting myoglobinuria causes acute tubular necrosis, because the heme moiety separates from the globin in acidic urine (pH 5–5.5) and releases free iron. In addition, the filtered myoglobin may precipitate in the renal tubules causing intrarenal obstruction. Finally, volume depletion with third space sequestration of fluid leads to impaired renal blood flow and renal ischemia [177–179].

Early and vigorous intravenous fluid therapy to correct hypovolemia and renal ischemia is important in attenuating renal injury [180]. Since myoglobin is more nephrotoxic in acid urine, most groups advocate the addition of sodium bicarbonate to the intravenous fluids to alkalinize the urine [177,178,181], which also may ameliorate the hyperkalemia. Mannitol is used in combination with fluid/alkaline therapy to prevent renal injury in rhabdomyolysis [181]. Potential benefits of mannitol include: (a) increase in urine flow and prevention of obstructing cast formation, (b) reduction in renal tubular epithelial swelling and injury, and (c) scavenging of oxygen free radicals [182].

Although there are no controlled trials to show a direct benefit of forced alkaline-mannitol diuresis in preventing AKI in rhabdomyolysis, there are many case reports suggesting such therapy was instrumental in averting renal injury. We recommend the infusion of both mannitol and sodium bicarbonate solutions if the patient remains oliguric after adequate volume resuscitation with isotonic crystalloid solutions, usually normal saline. The mannitol-bicarbonate solution, made by adding 25 g mannitol (12.5 g/50 mL) and 100 meq $NaHCO_3$ (50 meq/50 mL) to 800 mL of 5% dextrose in water, is infused at 250 mL/hour. If urine flow rate increases after 4 hours, the infusion rate should be adjusted to equal urine output and to achieve a urine pH > 6.5 until azotemia improves and all evidence of myoglobinuria disappear. If urine flow does not increase after 4 hours, the patient has established oliguric AKI. The mannitol-bicarbonate solution should be discontinued and the patient treated conservatively until dialysis is required [179]. This approach corrects oliguria, hastens the clearing of azotemia, and avoids the need for dialysis in roughly half of the patients with myoglobinuric AKI. Patients who responded have less muscle damage and better preservation of renal function than those that did not respond [183]. Whether this reflects earlier intervention, a less severe degree of muscle injury, or just vigorous volume expansion is not known.

Once AKI is established, dialysis may be required. Daily hemodialysis or some form of continuous renal replacement therapy (CRRT) is often required for the first several days, because these patients tend to be quite catabolic and develop metabolic acidosis, hyperkalemia, hyperphosphatemia, and concomitant hypocalcemia. Full recovery of renal function is the rule, provided other coexisting organ-system dysfunction resolves.

Risk of acute kidney injury with medical imaging (contrast-induced nephropathy)

Medical imaging in the perioperative patients with and without chronic kidney disease may result in worsening renal function because of the use of iodinated radiocontrast agents. The mechanism is not well understood but is probably due to intense renal vasoconstriction and/or direct tubular toxicity. The renal vasoconstriction may result from contrast-induced release of endothelin and adenosine, although there is controversy as to the role of endothelin in AKI.

Risk factors for developing AKI following iodinated radiocontrast agents include: (a) underlying CKD (plasma creatinine >1.5 mg/dL), (b) diabetic nephropathy with renal insufficiency, (c) hypovolemia or impaired renal perfusion, (d) volume of contrast administered, and (e) presence of multiple myeloma [184,185]. Since perioperative patients may be intravascularly volume depleted, especially in the setting of trauma, they are at increased risk for contrast-induced AKI. The risk increases further if the patient has concomitant preexisting CKD and/or diabetic nephropathy.

Worsening of renal function from radiocontrast agents usually begins soon after the infusion of the contrast (< 24 hours), peaks in 2–3 days, and resolves over the next 3–5 days. Complete recovery with renal function returning to baseline levels is the norm. Patients are usually non-oliguric and the majority does not require dialysis. However, if the patient has advanced renal failure (creatinine > 4 mg/dL) at baseline, there may be insufficient renal reserve to avoid dialysis.

The use of iodinated contrast agents is not contraindicated in dialysis patients since they are committed already to long-term renal replacement therapy. However, contrast may reduce further any residual renal function of the native kidneys. It is important for the non-nephrologist to appreciate that residual renal function does help in the overall solute clearance and volume removal and may be critical in peritoneal dialysis patients. In addition, the belief that dialysis should be performed immediately following contrast administration is unfounded [186]. By the time dialysis begins (at least 30 minutes after contrast administration), the contrast has circulated already through the kidneys innumerable times. The effectiveness of hemodialysis in removing contrast media depends on many factors, including the protein binding, hydrophilicity, and electrical charge of the contrast medium, and several sessions are required to remove the contrast completely.

Prevention and treatment of contrast-induced acute renal failure

As discussed above, the use of iodinated radiocontrast agents mainly impacts patients with CKD and/or diabetic nephropathy, exacerbated in the perioperative patient by the potential for intravascular volume depletion. When one or more risk factors are present in a perioperative patient, use of an alternative medical imaging test such as ultrasound or magnetic resonance imaging should be considered.

If medical imaging requiring iodinated radiocontrast is deemed essential in the evaluation of a high-risk perioperative patient, some measures can be undertaken to help prevent or attenuate the severity of the AKI. First, use of non-ionic low osmolal or iso-osmolal iodinated contrast agents may be associated with less risk for contrast-induced nephropathy in high-risk patients compared with ionic hyper-osmolal agents [187,188]. Second, a number of studies have demonstrated that adequate hydration with either 0.45% or 0.9% saline prior to administering a radiocontrast agent attenuates or prevents AKI in high-risk patients [184,185,189]. Saline may be preferable to half-normal saline based on a recent study [190]. Most studies infused saline starting 12 hours before the contrast administration and continuing for 12 hours afterwards, at a rate of 75–125 mL/hour. Despite potential theoretical benefits, recent studies have failed to show any benefit in the use of mannitol or furosemide to prevent contrast-induced AKI [189]. In fact, furosemide was associated with a worse outcome compared with saline alone. Using lower volumes of contrast may be beneficial. In addition, the newer non-ionic iso-osmolar agents may be associated with less nephrotoxicity [187].

Two popular agents for the prevention of contrast-induced AKI in high-risk patients are the use of oral N-acetylcysteine

and intravenous sodium bicarbonate given prior to radiocontrast study. Acetylcysteine is a thiol compound with antioxidant and vasodilatory properties, thus the theoretical benefit of this agent may be due to reducing vasoconstriction and free radical generation in the setting of radiocontrast administration. Initial studies suggested acetylcysteine was beneficial in preventing contrast-induced nephropathy in high-risk patients, but other studies and meta-analyses have been less supportive of the salutatory effect of this agent [190–193]. Different dosing regimens have been studied, but acetylcysteine given 1,200 mg orally the day before and 1,200 mg orally on the day of the contrast study has yielded the best results [194]. Administration of isotonic sodium bicarbonate solution intravenously may be superior to normal saline based on a number of studies and meta-analyses [195,196]. Isotonic bicarbonate solution is prepared by adding three 50 mL ampules of sodium bicarbonate (150 mmol) to a liter of D5-water and giving this solution at 3 mL/kg, one hour prior to the contrast study, and then 1 mL/kg/hour for 6 hours after the study.

Although some studies suggest that acetylcysteine and $NaHCO_3$ prophylaxis reduce the incidence of acute deterioration of renal function in high-risk patients [197,198], other studies did not [199–201]. Since acetylcysteine and sodium bicarbonate have little or no toxicity, it seems reasonable to continue using them for prophylaxis against contrast nephropathy despite ambivalent studies. Adequate hydration is probably the most important prophylactic maneuver.

A number of other measures have been tried to prevent contrast-induced acute renal failure with no clear-cut benefits, including dopamine, fenoldopam, atrial natriuretic peptide, and endothelin antagonists. In addition, it has been proposed that acute hemodialysis after the contrast study may help prevent AKI through removing the radio-contrast agent. Despite this potential theoretical benefit, no definitive study has shown any value for prophylactic hemodialysis after a radio-contrast study.

In summary, it appears that the most beneficial measures to help prevent contrast-induced AKI in high-risk patients are: (a) intravenous hydration with saline, (b) use of a non-ionic low or iso-osmolal iodinated contrast agent, (c) use of acetylcysteine and/or $NaHCO_3$, and (d) reduced amount of contrast.

General measures for prevention of perioperative AKI

As noted in the previous section, volume expansion with saline is effective in lowering the risk or attenuating the severity of ATN related to the exposure to radiocontrast agents and myoglobin. There is, unfortunately, a paucity of data on the role of volume expansion in preventing or attenuating AKI in the setting of ischemia, hypotension, and sepsis. Despite adequate data, most agree that optimizing volume status in high-risk patients is preferred. The problem is that use of saline hydration for patients with CKD and/or congestive heart failure to prevent AKI could lead to volume overload, pulmonary edema and decompensated congestive heart failure. Thus, volume expansion in high-risk patients with CHF and/or CKD needs to be done with judicious amounts of fluids and monitored closely. In addition, excessive volume expansion leading to peripheral edema may impair post-surgical wound healing.

There is no role for the use of diuretics in the prevention of AKI. In one study, the use of furosemide actually worsened renal function post-cardiac surgery [202]. When infused at low doses (0.5 to 3 μg/kg/min), dopamine dilates renal arteries and arterioles including the afferent and efferent arterioles, which results in an increase in renal blood flow and may increase GFR. This effect has led to its use in preventing AKI in postoperative patients. Despite its popularity in surgical and some medical ICUs, the use of low-dose dopamine has not been shown to be effective in preventing AKI in patients at increased risk for ATN [203,204]. Moreover, there may be risks to the use of dopamine including tachycardia, arrhythmias, myocardial ischemia, and intestinal ischemia. There has been interest whether the specific dopamine receptor-1 agonist, fenoldopam may have a salutatory effect in preventing or ameliorating AKI. A meta-analysis of 16 randomized trials [205] has suggested there may be a significant benefit in the use of fenoldopam in preventing AKI and the need for renal replacement therapy. There are major limitations to this meta-analysis, and a large randomized controlled study is needed to confirm this observation.

Other therapies have been studied to prevent or attenuate AKI including atrial natriuretic peptides, intensive insulin therapy, and statins. Atrial natriuretic peptides vasodilate the afferent arteriole and block sodium reabsorption and thus theoretically may be beneficial in preventing or treating AKI. A meta-analysis of 23 randomized control trials suggest there may be a benefit in patients with renal dysfunction associated with cardiovascular surgery requiring dialysis therapy [206]. Given the limitations of this meta-analysis, the use of natriuretic peptides is generally not recommended to prevent AKI until there is validation by a large randomized control trial. Intensive glucose control with insulin has been associated with better outcomes in critically ill patients, including improved renal outcomes. Despite this association, a number of randomized trials have not shown a significant renal benefit of intensive insulin therapy, specifically regarding need for renal replacement therapy [207,208]. Finally, there has been a suggestion that statins may reduce the risk of AKI after elective surgery [209]. This observation is based on retrospective data and will need further validation prior to routine use of this class of drugs for AKI prevention [210].

There is some controversy whether patients having coronary artery bypass surgery may have less AKI when the surgery is performed without the use of the heart lung pump (off pump) [211]. A meta-analysis of 37 randomized and 22 observational studies noted that off pump bypass surgery had a non-significant decrease in AKI in the randomized trials and a significant reduction in the observational studies [212]. The decision to perform off-pump cardiac surgery is dependent on a number of factors including the complexity of the surgery, expertise of the surgeon and additional studies supporting beneficial effect of this modality of cardiothoracic surgery.

Dialytic management of the surgery patient with kidney disease

For patients with CKD V (ESRD)

Patients with CKD V on chronic hemodialysis usually will receive dialysis the day prior to elective surgery to minimize the risks for volume overload and hypertension, hyperkalemia, and metabolic acidosis. The dialysis treatment preceding surgery also will optimize control of the uremic environment, which in turn mitigates platelet dysfunction (as noted above), impaired immune function, malnutrition, and possibly impaired wound healing. The goals of dialysis therapy for these patients are to achieve euvolemia or "dry weight," normalize serum potassium level, and increase serum bicarbonate levels to attenuate metabolic or respiratory acidosis. As discussed above, maintaining euvolemia will improve blood pressure control and reduce congestive heart failure.

Patients who are chronically under dialyzed (blood urea nitrogen > 100 mg/dL) and hypervolemic may benefit from daily dialysis for a few days preceding elective surgery. Reducing nitrogenous waste products may improve immune function, malnutrition, and wound healing. Whether intensive dialysis actually improves these parameters has not been proven rigorously, but most nephrologists agree that the degree of azotemia should be minimized prior to surgery. Under-dialyzed patients are at increased risk of developing pericarditis, which obviously should be avoided perioperatively.

Approximately 10% of the CKD V population in the USA is on peritoneal dialysis. Patients can continue on peritoneal dialysis perioperatively to manage volume overload and electrolyte and acid–base abnormalities. Before surgery, all of the peritoneal dialysis fluid is drained from the abdominal cavity, to allow ease of surgery for abdominal procedures and to prevent respiratory compromise intraoperatively from increased abdominal pressure. For simple abdominal procedures, the peritoneal dialysis catheter can be left in place and the patient should receive hemodialysis via a temporary venous catheter until the abdominal incision has healed sufficiently to permit resumption of peritoneal dialysis. For abdominal procedures in which the catheter may be contaminated, such as perforated bowel cases, it is probably prudent to remove the peritoneal dialysis catheter and switch the patient to hemodialysis temporarily. Other situations when a peritoneal dialysis patient will require surgical removal of the catheter are recurrent bacterial peritonitis, a peritoneal catheter tunnel infection, and fungal peritonitis. When the patient has completely healed from the abdominal surgery and/or peritonitis and there is no issue of continued intra-abdominal infection, a new peritoneal dialysis catheter can be placed and peritoneal dialysis resumed.

Table 27.8 Indications for acute dialysis.

Symptoms and signs associated with uremia in patients with GFR < 20–25 mL/min per 1.73 m [2]

Nausea, vomiting, anorexia
  Other gastrointestinal symptoms (gastritis with hemorrhage, colitis with or without hemorrhage)
  Altered mental status (lethargy, somnolence, malaise, stupor, coma, or delirium)
  Signs of uremic encephalopathy (asterixis, multifocal clonus, or seizures)
  Pericarditis
  Bleeding diathesis from uremic platelet dysfunction

Refractory or progressive fluid overload
Uncontrolled hyperkalemia
Severe metabolic acidosis, especially in an oliguric patient

Acute and progressive worsening of renal function with
  Blood urea nitrogen levels > 70–100 mg/dL
  Measured creatinine clearance < 15–20 mL/min

For patients with AKI

Acute renal failure can develop during the preoperative, intra-operative, or the postoperative period in high-risk patients, especially in the setting of trauma and major vascular procedures during which renal blood flow is compromised. The AKI is usually due to the development of acute tubular necrosis (see above). Important questions are: (a) what are the indications for dialysis therapy in patients with AKI, and (b) which renal replacement modality should be used to treat such patients?

The indications for dialysis and other forms of renal replacement therapy (RRT) (see below) in a perioperative patient with AKI are the same as for any patient with AKI. The most common indication is the presence of the signs and symptoms of uremia (Table 27.8), such as pericarditis and an otherwise unexplained worsening of mental status. Hyperkalemia, severe acidosis, and volume overload that cannot be managed with drugs are common indications for acute dialysis. Patients with perioperative AKI are generally quite catabolic and are receiving large volumes of fluid in the form of total parenteral nutrition and various medications. Thus, RRT, and more specifically ultrafiltration is crucial in preventing or attenuating volume overload and congestive heart failure. The goal of therapy is to maintain adequate oxygenation while keeping the inspired oxygen concentration below 50% to minimize pulmonary oxygen toxicity.

Many nephrologists will initiate RRT in patients with AKI when the blood urea nitrogen level reaches 70–100 mg/dL or when the creatinine clearance is below 15 mL/min, even if the patient has no overt clinical indications for dialysis. This practice is common and has been the practice at our center, especially in catabolic and oliguric patients with a rapid rise in blood urea nitrogen (>20 mg/dL/day) and serum creatinine (>2 mg/dL/day). There have been a number of recent studies that suggest that earlier RRT was associated with improved

survival. The Program to Improve Care in Acute Renal Disease (PICARD), assessing a large multicenter database, noted that mortality in AKI was lower when the blood urea nitrogen (BUN) at start of dialysis was less than 76 mg/dL. This and other studies have been the basis for the general recommendation to initiate dialysis/renal replacement therapy when the BUN reaches 80–100 mg/dL. There has been some concern that early dialysis may be detrimental to renal function because of hypotension [213] or use of bio-incompatible dialysis membranes (see below) [214].

The optimal timing for initiation of renal replacement therapy requires an adequately powered prospective trial. This is currently not available and thus the recommendations noted above are opinion-based on current literature. There is general consensus among nephrologists that the synthetic and more biocompatible hemodialysis membranes should be used in treating patients with AKI, and not the older bio-incompatible cuprophane membranes. The cuprophane membranes are associated with complement activation and upregulation of adhesion molecules [214], and clinically with a delay in recovery from AKI and worse survival when compared with bio-compatible membranes [215,216]. Current practice is to use biocompatible dialysis membranes also when treating perioperative patients with ESRD.

Renal replacement therapy modalities

There are three general therapeutic modalities that can be used for treatment of renal failure (either acute or chronic) in the perioperative patient: peritoneal dialysis, intermittent hemodialysis, and CRRT. Most patients with AKI in the perioperative period are catabolic, resulting in high urea, potassium, and phosphate levels. They are also frequently volume overloaded because of the administration of total parenteral nutrition, antibiotics, blood products, and pressor agents. The discussion that follows focuses on dialytic management of catabolic patients with AKI, but the discussion applies equally to ESRD patients who are catabolic in the perioperative period.

Although peritoneal dialysis is rarely used in the USA to treat AKI, there are some theoretical advantages to its use in such patients. Since solute and volume removal is much slower with peritoneal dialysis, it may be more desirable in hemodynamically unstable patients. Moreover, systemic anticoagulation is not required. However, there are also major disadvantages. Acute peritoneal dialysis is contraindicated after major abdominal surgery because of the need for abdominal wound healing, the presence of drains, and the increased risk for infection. There may be pleuro-peritoneal communications after thoracic surgery, leading to large pleural effusions with peritoneal dialysis. Moreover, instillation of fluid in the peritoneal cavity may increase intra-abdominal pressure and compromise respiratory effort, a major issue in the perioperative patient with AKI who frequently has concomitant respiratory failure and adult respiratory distress syndrome. Finally, the slow nature of peritoneal dialysis renders it inefficient in treating the catabolic and hyperkalemic perioperative patient with AKI and pulmonary edema. For these reasons, it is not our practice to use peritoneal dialysis in the treatment of AKI.

The major modalities used to treat AKI are either intermittent hemodialysis or some form of CRRT. CRRT includes a variety of modalities that provide continuous support for patients with severe AKI including continuous hemofiltration, continuous hemodialysis, and continuous hemodialfiltration. The modalities can be delivered by either venovenous or arteriovenous circuits. The most popular method is using a pump-driven venovenous circuit employing double-lumen catheters placed in the large bore vein (internal jugular, femoral, subclavian). Hemofiltration is associated with better clearance of large molecular weight molecules (convective clearance) compared with hemodialysis (diffusive clearance). Despite these differences, there is no apparent clinical advantage to hemofiltration compared with hemodialysis.

One major question nephrologists have had over the past 20 years is what is the optimal modality of renal replacement therapy in a patient with severe AKI; continuous versus intermittent. Review of the various studies addressing this question is beyond the scope of this chapter. Most studies suggest that patient survival and recovery of renal function is similar with both CRRT and intermittent hemodialysis. No survival benefit can be attributed to either modality. The decision should be based on local expertise and tailoring therapy to the specific needs/goals of a given patient.

Another question that has been raised in the management of patients with AKI requiring renal replacement therapy is what is the optimal dose or intensity of renal replacement therapy that should be used for these patients. The VA/NIH Acute Renal Failure Trial Network study did not find a difference in mortality between intensive therapy (hemodialysis, SLED, six times per week, CRRT at effluent rate of 35 mL/kg/hour) versus less intensive therapy (hemodialysis, SLED at three times per week, or CRRT at 20 mL/kg/hour). These results have been supported by subsequent studies and two meta-analyses. Our general recommendation is to individualize renal replacement therapy based on the specific metabolic and volume needs of the patient using either intermittent hemodialysis provided on a minimum of at least three times per week schedule achieving adequate urea clearance per session (Kt/V > 1.2), or CRRT.

Anticoagulation during hemodialysis

Heparin is used routinely during hemodialysis to prevent clotting of blood through the dialysis circuit. Postoperatively, hemodialysis can be performed without heparin to help minimize bleeding, using periodic saline flushes during the procedure to help prevent clotting of the circuit. It is our practice to avoid heparin use in the perioperative patient with either acute or chronic kidney disease. In perioperative patients with active bleeding requiring daily dialysis or CRRT yet who have frequent clotting of the dialysis circuit,

an alternative to systemic heparin is regional citrate anti-coagulation. This procedure involves administering citrate into the blood in the extracorporeal circuit and using a calcium-free dialysate. By chelating all available calcium, coagulation is prevented in the extracorporeal circuit. When the blood is returned to the patient, the process is reversed by infusing calcium to prevent hypocalcemia and systemic anticoagulation. Approximately one-third of the citrate is dialyzed off, and the remaining two-thirds is metabolized quickly by the patient to form bicarbonate. Although regional citrate anticoagulation is very effective in preventing clotting of the extracorporeal circuit, the major disadvantages are symptomatic and possibly life-threatening hypocalcemia and metabolic alkalosis. Serum calcium levels must be monitored very closely and the calcium infusion must be adjusted to maintain normal calcium levels [217]. Since perioperative patients with acute or chronic renal failure and multi-organ failure tend to have higher risks for bleeding, the use of periodic saline flushes or regional citrate anticoagulation may be preferable to heparin.

Care of the dialysis access

Peritoneal dialysis catheters must receive daily care to the exit site, consisting of washing the area with soap and water, thoroughly drying it, and then applying a new dressing over the exit site. Such exit site care is best provided by someone with expertise. Each time the peritoneal dialysis catheter is manipulated to start or complete an exchange everyone in the room should wear a mask. In addition, thorough hand washing should precede handling of the peritoneal dialysis catheter.

A common complication in hemodialysis patients post-operatively is thrombosis of the vascular access, either due to hypotension or applying a tourniquet or blood pressure cuff above the arteriovenous fistula or graft. Preventing hypotension and conspicuous labeling of the access arm may help to avoid access thrombosis and delay in subsequent dialysis. If the vascular access for dialysis is a tunneled catheter, then the catheter should be labeled clearly that it is for dialysis use only. Frequent accessing of the dialysis catheter increases the risk of catheter-related infection and catheter thrombosis, because non-dialysis personnel are unfamiliar with use of the catheter. We currently use citrate locks in our dialysis catheters to avoid systemic anticoagulation that has been associated with heparin locks.

Surgery in the patient with a stable kidney transplant

A full discussion of perioperative care in the kidney transplant recipient in the immediate post-transplant period is beyond the scope of this chapter, as is a full discussion of perioperative care in the patient with a stable kidney transplant. Nephrology or transplant nephrology consultation must be obtained. However, a few points deserve emphasis.

Immunosuppressive regimens differ among transplant centers and among patients. These medications generally should be continued in the perioperative period, according to the outpatient schedule. Usually, prednisone (unless the patient is on a steroid-sparing protocol) is taken early in the morning, along with the morning dose of a calcineurin inhibitor (either cyclosporine or tacrolimus) or mTOR inhibitor (sirolimus), and an antimetabolite (usually azathioprine or mycophenolate mofetil). The evening dose of the calcineurin inhibitor and antimetabolite must be given 12 hours later. If the patient cannot take medications orally, the steroid must be given intravenously at an equivalent dose (e.g., convert prednisone orally to solumedrol intravenously). Cyclosporine and tacrolimus may be administered intravenously as an infusion, but the dose is one-third of the oral dose because of increased bioavailability. Stress dose steroids should be considered in most patients who are not on a steroid-sparing protocol to prevent adrenal insufficiency, since chronic suppression of the adrenal glands renders them less capable of mounting a stress response.

Clinicians also need to be wary of drug interactions in patients with transplants. Because many of the medications are metabolized via the cytochrome P450 system, medications which are removed from or added to the usual regimen of these patients during hospitalization could alter the levels of calcineurin inhibitors. For example, verapamil and diltiazem inhibit the cytochrome system. If a patient is usually on one of these medications and it is stopped in the perioperative period, the levels of the calcineurin inhibitors may drop. Conversely, if cytochrome inhibiting medications are started in the hospital, tacrolimus and cyclosporine levels rise. Therefore, following 12-hour trough levels may be necessary when such medications are stopped or added to a patient's usual regimen.

If the patient is maintained on sirolimus, a discussion with the transplant specialist should be considered, as sirolimus is associated with a greater risk of lymphoceles and wound dehiscence [218]. The type of surgery, preexisting risks and immunosuppressive needs must all be examined, and consideration of transition from sirolimus to either cyclosporine or tacrolimus in the perioperative period requires close interaction between surgeon and transplant specialist. Finally, an indwelling urinary catheter should be avoided if at all possible or removed as soon as possible, due to the increased risk of and susceptibility to urinary tract infection and pyelonephritis.

Drugs

The kidneys eliminate many drugs either primarily or secondarily. Secondary clearance occurs in drugs that require hepatic metabolism to render the drug water soluble; the kidney then clears this metabolite. Some of these metabolites may be physiologically active. Therefore, many drugs or their metabolites accumulate in renal failure and can cause significant side-effects. Furthermore, the volume of distribution of some drugs may be affected by renal disease because of alteration in protein binding, increasing the free drug level and its clinical efficacy. We will discuss briefly some of the frequently encountered problems in the perioperative period.

General principles of drug therapy in kidney disease

Drug toxicity is an important cause of morbidity in patients with kidney disease, and there are several responsible mechanisms. First, drugs that are cleared by the kidney will accumulate in kidney failure. The dose and/or frequency of administration of such medications must be adjusted. While some medications, such as some of the penicillins and cephalosporins, require dose adjustment only when kidney function is severely impaired ($C_{Cr} < 25$ mL/min), others require dose adjustment even at higher levels of kidney function. Second, medications that are cleared by the liver may be metabolized into conjugated moieties that then require renal clearance. If these metabolites have activity or serious side-effects, such effects will be prolonged because of the delay in clearance. Examples of such medications are procainamide and morphine (see below). Procainamide is metabolized in the liver to N-acetylprocainamide, which accumulates in renal failure and can induce torsade de pointe [219,220]. A third mechanism is decreased absorption via the gastrointestinal tract because of concomitant use of phosphate binders, which may also bind medications [221,222]. Coumadin, immunosuppressive medications used in kidney transplant, and ferrous sulfate are some examples that exhibit this interaction.

The volume of distribution of some drugs is altered in kidney failure because of altered protein binding. Classic examples include digoxin [223] and phenytoin [224]. Both drugs are protein-bound to significant degrees in health, and free levels of both drugs are increased in patients with renal failure. Therefore, the loading dose of such medications must be reduced, since the volume of distribution effectively has decreased. In addition, maintenance levels should also be lower than the target for the general population to avoid toxicity, especially when the drug has a narrow therapeutic index. Checking drug levels, when available, will aid in the correct dosing of these protein-bound drugs.

Appropriate dosing of medications in kidney failure requires an estimated creatinine clearance. Serum creatinine is a poor indicator of kidney function, especially in elderly patients and chronically ill patients who have significant loss of lean muscle mass. A reasonable estimate of creatinine clearance (C_{Cr}) that does not require a 24-hour urine collection is the Cockcroft–Gault equation that is based on age, body weight in kilograms (BW – preferably ideal body weight as opposed to actual body weight), and serum creatinine (S_{Cr}):

$$C_{Cr} = \frac{(140 - age)(BW)}{S_{Cr}}$$

or the MDRD equation using serum creatinine, age, ethnicity, and gender [225]. A recent study in geriatric patients receiving medical care at a tertiary care institution shows that medications are frequently not well adjusted in elderly patients with even mild degrees of renal impairment [226].

In addition to non-renal side-effects, certain classes of drugs can cause acute deterioration of kidney function in patients with preexisting CKD. In postoperative patients already experiencing renal perfusion problems, aminoglycosides, radiographic contrast, NSAIDs, ACE inhibitors, and ARBs can further reduce perfusion to the kidneys and cause either pre-renal azotemia or acute tubular necrosis if ischemia is prolonged. Certain antibiotics (penicillins and sulfamethoxazole) and NSAIDs also can induce acute interstitial nephritis. Lastly, overly aggressive use of diuretics can lead to volume depletion, hypotension, and AKI. ESRD patients with residual renal function, as evidenced by > 500 mL of urine output a day, may suffer loss of this remaining renal function if given NSAIDs or aminoglycosides. Maintaining residual renal function may be especially important to patients on peritoneal dialysis. On the other hand, in ESRD patients without substantial residual renal function, traditionally renal toxic medications may be used if indicated, though the drugs frequently require dose adjustments. For example, if aminoglycosides are administered, the dosing may need to be timed after hemodialysis, since much of the drug is removed by the treatment. Drug levels are useful to follow if prolonged use is needed. Some of the medications commonly used in the perioperative situation are listed in Table 27.9.

Anesthesia

In general, regional anesthesia is preferred in patients with renal failure because of the increased risk of general anesthesia and the difficulty in selecting the right combination of general anesthetics. These are particularly useful for insertion of arteriovenous grafts and fistulae for dialysis access. Spinal and epidural anesthesia, however, are less desirable because of the potential for severe hypotension in patients with autonomic neuropathy, and the risk for spinal hematoma from platelet dysfunction.

Many of the agents used in inducing general anesthesia have altered protein binding in renal failure (thiopental, methohexital, diazepam, etomidate, midazolam) (Table 27.9) [227,228]. Therefore, the dose of such drugs should be reduced when renal failure is present.

Many muscle relaxants are partially or completely renally cleared, leading to a prolonged half-life in patients with renal failure [227,228]. Some have active metabolites, further prolonging the drug action (vecuronium and pancuronium). In addition, succinylcholine as a depolarizing agent may result in significant hyperkalemia especially with repeated dosing and is contraindicated in advanced renal failure. Atracurium and cistracurium do not rely on renal elimination, and the metabolite of atracurium has limited activity [227]. Therefore, these are the drugs of choice for muscle relaxants in patients with renal failure.

Some volatile anesthetic agents (enflurane and sevoflurane) are contraindicated in renal failure because of the production of fluoride and the potential for developing fluoride-induced acute renal failure [228], although there is some controversy [229,230]. Isoflurane, desflurane, and halothane are better tolerated and preferred in renal failure [228,231]. Propofol appears to be safe in patients with renal failure. Hepatic clearance is unaffected in renal failure, and its metabolite lacks activity. However, ESRD patients may require higher induction doses of propofol [113]. The negative correlation of propofol dose with preoperative hemoglobin concentration suggested that the increased requirement may be a consequence of anemia-induced hyperdynamic circulation. The rare condition of propofol related infusion syndrome (PRIS) which can lead to rhabdomyolysis and lactic acidosis has not been shown to be related to CKD or ESRD, though clearly renal failure can be a manifestation of the syndrome [232]. Fentanyl and sufentanil are commonly used as adjuncts though some elimination may be impaired in renal failure [228]. Remifentanil is preferred because it is rapidly inactivated by nonspecific esterases in blood and does not depend on either renal or hepatic elimination [228]. However, we have extensive experience with the use of fentanyl in ESRD and feel that a limited dose in conjunction with a sedating agent is quite safe (see the next section on analgesia). Finally, the half-life of drugs that are used to reverse anesthesia, anticholinergic agents and anticholinesterases, are prolonged in patients with renal disease [227,228]. After reversal, patients may develop excessive muscarinic effects to include bradyarrhythmias, increased respiratory secretions, and bronchospasm, because the half-life of the anticholinesterases is more prolonged than that of the anticholinergic agents.

Pain management/analgesia

Pain control is obviously an important issue in the postoperative patient. However, many pain medications are contraindicated in the patient with renal disease. Non-steroidal anti-inflammatory drugs should not be administered in the patient with advanced CKD because of the risk of AKI. Ketorolac, in particular, appears to be a common offending agent in the perioperative period, because it is the only NSAID that can be given parenterally. While we would advise against using NSAIDs in ESRD patients who still have residual renal function (see above discussion with aminoglycosides), they may be used in ESRD patients if there is no gastrointestinal contraindication.

Although narcotics are the mainstay of pain management in the postoperative period, all narcotic drugs may have a prolonged half-life to one degree or another when renal failure is present. However, two drugs are well known for their adverse central nervous system effects in patients with renal failure. Morphine is metabolized in the liver to morphine-6-glucuronide, a metabolite with 40 times the activity of morphine, which then requires renal elimination [228]. Meperidine

Table 27.9 Commonly used medications in the perioperative period that may need special attention in the chronic kidney disease (CKD) or end-stage renal disease (ESRD) patient.

Drug class	Drug	Route of elimination	Toxic metabolite	Altered protein binding	Dose adjustment
Anesthetics	Enflurane	Respiratory	Fluoride		Avoid
	Sevoflurane	Respiratory	Fluoride		Avoid
	Etomidate	Hepatic		Yes	Reduced dose
Muscle relaxants	Gallamine	Renal			Avoid
	Demethyl tubocurarine	Renal			Avoid
	Pancuronium	Partial renal	3-Hydroxy-pancuronium		Avoid
	Pipecuronium	Partial renal			Avoid
	d-Tubocurarine	Partial renal			Avoid
	Vecuronium	Partial renal	Desacetyl-vecuronium		Avoid
	Doxacurium	Partial renal			Avoid
	Succinylcholine	Hepatic			Avoid
Barbiturates	Thiopental	Hepatic		Yes	Reduce dose
	Methohexital	Hepatic		Yes	Reduce dose
	Phenobarbital	Partial renal			Reduce dose
Anticholinergic	Atropine	Partial renal			Reduce dose
	Glycopyrrolate	Partial renal			Reduce dose
Cholinergic	Neostigmine	Partial renal			Reduce dose
	Pyridostigmine	Partial renal			Reduce dose
	Edrophonium	Partial renal			Reduce dose
Antibiotics	Vancomycin	Renal			Reduce dose/interval
	Aminoglycosides	Renal			Reduce dose/interval
	Cephalosporins	Renal			Variable
	Penicillins	Renal			Variable
	Imipenem	Renal			Reduce dose/interval
	Fluconazole	Renal			Reduce dose/interval
	Acyclovir	Renal			Reduce dose/interval
	Ganciclovir	Renal			Reduce dose/interval
Cardiovascular	Digoxin	Renal		Yes	Reduce dose/interval
	Procainamide	Renal/Hepatic	N-acetylprocainamide		Avoid
	Quinidine	Partial renal			Reduced dose
	Nitroprusside	Hepatic	Thiocyanate		Avoid after 24–48 hours
	ACE inhibitor	Variable renal			
	ARB	Variable renal			
	Atenolol	Renal			Avoid
Diuretics	Hydrochlorothiazide	Renal			Avoid (ineffective)
	Furosemide	Renal			Increase dose
Psychoactive	Diazepam	Hepatic	Oxazepam	Yes	Reduce dose/interval
	Midazolam	Hepatic	1-Hydroxy-midazolam		Reduce dose/interval
Analgesics	Morphine	Hepatic	Morphine-6-glucuronide		Avoid
	Meperidine	Hepatic	Normeperidine		Avoid
	Other narcotics	Hepatic			Reduce dose/caution
Anti-seizure	Phenytoin	Hepatic		Yes	Reduce dose
H$_2$ blockers	Cimetidine	Renal			Reduce dose
	Ranitidine	Renal			Reduce dose
	Famotidine	Renal			Reduce dose

Table 27.9 (*cont.*)

Drug class	Drug	Route of elimination	Toxic metabolite	Altered protein binding	Dose adjustment
Hypoglycemics	Glyburide	Renal			Avoid
	Insulin	Renal			Reduce dose
Others	Allopurinol	Partial renal			Reduce dose

is also hepatically metabolized to normeperidine, which has neuroexcitatory effects and requires renal excretion [228]. Both morphine and meperidine are relatively contraindicated in patients with ESRD and advanced CKD. If they have to be used, patients must be monitored carefully and the drug discontinued at the first sign of undesirable neurologic effects. In our experience, it is often not until the patient is ready to be weaned off of the ventilator that the over-sedation with morphine becomes apparent, delaying spontaneous breathing trials by days until the active metabolites are finally eliminated. Other narcotics also must be administered with caution because disposition may vary from individual to individual.

For minor procedures that require only sedation and analgesia, there are good data suggesting that CKD and ESRD patients can be safely managed with a rapid-onset, short-acting benzodiazepine and a short-acting narcotic that are both primarily cleared by the liver. We have extensive experience with midazolam and fentanyl given intravenously for outpatient vascular access procedures performed by the interventional nephrologist in our ESRD population. A recently published retrospective study of over 12,000 patients who received these same two medications for their interventional hemodialysis access procedures also concludes that they are both safe and efficacious in renal failure patients [233].

References

1. Go AS, Chertow GM, Fan D *et al.* Chronic kidney disease and the risks of death, cardiovascular events, and hospitalization. *N Engl J Med* 2004; **351**: 1296–305.

2. US Renal Data System, USRDS 2010 Annual Data Report. *Atlas of Chronic Kidney Disease and End-Stage Renal Disease in the United States*; 2011.

3. Coresh J, Selvin E, Stevens LA *et al.* Prevalence of chronic kidney disease in the United States. *J Am Med Assoc* 2007; **298**: 2038–47.

4. Hsu CY, Chertow GM, McCulloch CE *et al.* Nonrecovery of kidney function and death after acute on chronic renal failure. *Clin J Am Soc Nephrol* 2009; **4**: 891–8.

5. Lo LJ, Go AS, Chertow GM *et al.* Dialysis-requiring acute renal failure increases the risk of progressive chronic kidney disease. *Kidney Int* 2009; **76**: 893–9.

6. Kellerman PS. Perioperative care of the renal patient. *Arch Intern Med* 1994; **154**: 1674–88.

7. Bechtel JF, Detter C, Fischlein T *et al.* Cardiac surgery in patients on dialysis: decreased 30-day mortality, unchanged overall survival. *Ann Thorac Surg* 2008; **85**: 147–53.

8. Rahmanian PB, Adams DH, Castillo JG *et al.* Early and late outcome of cardiac surgery in dialysis-dependent patients: single-center experience with 245 consecutive patients. *J Thorac Cardiovasc Surg* 2008; **135**: 915–22.

9. Thourani VH, Sarin EL, Kilgo PD *et al.* Short- and long-term outcomes in patients undergoing valve surgery with end-stage renal failure receiving chronic hemodialysis. *J Thorac Cardiovasc Surg* 2012; **144**: 117–23.

10. Diez C, Mohr P, Kuss O *et al.* Impact of preoperative renal dysfunction on in-hospital mortality after solitary valve and combined valve and coronary procedures. *Ann Thorac Surg* 2009; **87**: 731–6.

11. Howell NJ, Keogh BE, Bonser RS *et al.* Mild renal dysfunction predicts in-hospital mortality and post-discharge survival following cardiac surgery. *Eur J Cardiothorac Surg* 2008; **34**: 390–5; discussion 395.

12. Eknoyan G, Beck GJ, Cheung AK *et al.* Effect of dialysis dose and membrane flux in maintenance hemodialysis. *N Engl J Med* 2002; **347**(25): 2010–19.

13. Wang AY, Lam CW, Chan IH *et al.* Sudden cardiac death in end-stage renal disease patients: a 5-year prospective analysis. *Hypertension* 2010; **56**: 210–16.

14. Wanner C, Krane V, Marz W *et al.* Atorvastatin in patients with type 2 diabetes mellitus undergoing hemodialysis. *N Engl J Med* 2005; **353**: 238–48.

15. Goldenberg I, Moss AJ, McNitt S *et al.* Relations among renal function, risk of sudden cardiac death, and benefit of the implanted cardiac defibrillator in patients with ischemic left ventricular dysfunction. *Am J Cardiol* 2006; **98**: 485–90.

16. Pun PH, Smarz TR, Honeycutt EF *et al.* Chronic kidney disease is associated with increased risk of sudden cardiac death among patients with coronary artery disease. *Kidney Int* 2009; **76**: 652–8.

17. Herzog CA, Littrell K, Arko C *et al.* Clinical characteristics of dialysis patients with acute myocardial infarction in the United States: a collaborative project of the United States Renal Data System and the National Registry of Myocardial Infarction. *Circulation* 2007; **116**: 1465–72.

18. Sosnov J, Lessard D, Goldberg RJ *et al.* Differential symptoms of acute myocardial infarction in patients with kidney disease: a community-wide perspective. *Am J Kidney Dis* 2006; **47**: 378–84.

19. Rostand SG, Brunzell JD, Cannon RO 3rd *et al.* Cardiovascular complications in renal failure. *J Am Soc Nephrol* 1991; **2**: 1053–62.

20. Rostand SG, Kirk KA, Rutsky EA. Dialysis-associated ischemic heart disease: insights from coronary

angiography. *Kidney Int* 1984; **25**: 653–9.

21. Rostand SG, Kirk KA, Rutsky EA. The epidemiology of coronary artery disease in patients on maintenance hemodialysis: implications for management. *Contrib Nephrol* 1986; **52**: 34–41.

22. Schmidt A, Stefenelli T, Schuster E *et al.* Informational contribution of noninvasive screening tests for coronary artery disease in patients on chronic renal replacement therapy. *Am J Kidney Dis* 2001; **37**: 56–63.

23. Foley RN, Parfrey PS, Harnett JD *et al.* Clinical and echocardiographic disease in patients starting end-stage renal disease therapy. *Kidney Int* 1995; **47**: 186–92.

24. Foley RN, Parfrey PS, Sarnak MJ. Epidemiology of cardiovascular disease in chronic renal disease. *J Am Soc Nephrol* 1998; **9** (12 Suppl): S16–23.

25. Nally JV Jr. Cardiac disease in chronic uremia: investigation. *Adv Ren Replace Ther* 1997; **4**: 225–33.

26. Agarwal R. Blood pressure and mortality among hemodialysis patients. *Hypertension* 2010; **55**: 762–8.

27. Isbel NM, Haluska B, Johnson DW *et al.* Increased targeting of cardiovascular risk factors in patients with chronic kidney disease does not improve atheroma burden or cardiovascular function. *Am Heart J* 2006; **151**: 745–53.

28. Karthikeyan V, Ananthasubramaniam K. Coronary risk assessment and management options in chronic kidney disease patients prior to kidney transplantation. *Curr Cardiol Rev* 2009; **5**: 177–86.

29. West JC, Napoliello DA, Costello JM *et al.* Preoperative dobutamine stress echocardiography versus cardiac arteriography for risk assessment prior to renal transplantation. *Transpl Int* 2000; **13** (Suppl 1): S27–30.

30. Le A, Wilson R, Douek K *et al.* Prospective risk stratification in renal transplant candidates for cardiac death. *Am J Kidney Dis* 1994; **24**: 65–71.

31. Dahan M, Viron BM, Poiseau E *et al.* Combined dipyridamole-exercise stress echocardiography for detection of myocardial ischemia in hemodialysis patients: an alternative to stress nuclear imaging. *Am J Kidney Dis* 2002; **40**: 737–44.

32. Holley JL, Fenton RA, Arthur RS. Thallium stress testing does not predict cardiovascular risk in diabetic patients with end-stage renal disease undergoing cadaveric renal transplantation. *Am J Med* 1991; **90**: 563–70.

33. Marwick TH, Steinmuller DR, Underwood DA *et al.* Ineffectiveness of dipyridamole SPECT thallium imaging as a screening technique for coronary artery disease in patients with end-stage renal failure. *Transplantation* 1990; **49**: 100–3.

34. Mistry BM, Bastani B, Solomon H *et al.* Prognostic value of dipyridamole thallium-201 screening to minimize perioperative cardiac complications in diabetics undergoing kidney or kidney-pancreas transplantation. *Clin Transplant* 1998; **12**: 130–5.

35. Manske CL, Thomas W, Wang Y *et al.* Screening diabetic transplant candidates for coronary artery disease: identification of a low risk subgroup. *Kidney Int* 1993; **44**: 617–21.

36. McFalls EO, Ward HB, Moritz TE *et al.* Coronary-artery revascularization before elective major vascular surgery. *N Engl J Med* 2004; **351**: 2795–804.

37. Poldermans D, Schouten O, Vidakovic R *et al.* A clinical randomized trial to evaluate the safety of a noninvasive approach in high-risk patients undergoing major vascular surgery: the DECREASE-V Pilot Study. *J Am Coll Cardiol* 2007; **49**: 1763–9.

38. Fleisher LA, Beckman JA, Brown KA *et al.* ACC/AHA 2007 Guidelines on perioperative cardiovascular evaluation and care for noncardiac surgery: executive summary: a report of the American College of Cardiology/ American Heart Association Task Force on Practice Guidelines (Writing Committee to Revise the 2002 Guidelines on Perioperative Cardiovascular Evaluation for Noncardiac Surgery) developed in collaboration with the American Society of Echocardiography, American Society of Nuclear Cardiology, Heart Rhythm Society, Society of Cardiovascular Anesthesiologists, Society for Cardiovascular Angiography and Interventions, Society for Vascular Medicine and Biology, and Society for Vascular Surgery. *J Am Coll Cardiol* 2007; **50**: 1707–32.

39. Cohen MC, Aretz TH. Histological analysis of coronary artery lesions in fatal postoperative myocardial infarction. *Cardiovasc Pathol* 1999; **8**: 133–9.

40. Poldermans D, Boersma E, Bax JJ *et al.* Correlation of location of acute myocardial infarct after noncardiac vascular surgery with preoperative dobutamine echocardiographic findings. *Am J Cardiol* 2001; **88**: 1413–14, A6.

41. Abe S, Yoshizawa M, Nakanishi N *et al.* Electrocardiographic abnormalities in patients receiving hemodialysis. *Am Heart J* 1996; **131**: 1137–44.

42. Sharma R, Pellerin D, Gaze DC *et al.* Dobutamine stress echocardiography and the resting but not exercise electrocardiograph predict severe coronary artery disease in renal transplant candidates. *Nephrol Dial Transplant* 2005; **20**: 2207–14.

43. Brown KA, Rimmer J, Haisch C. Noninvasive cardiac risk stratification of diabetic and nondiabetic uremic renal allograft candidates using dipyridamole-thallium-201 imaging and radionuclide ventriculography. *Am J Cardiol* 1989; **64**: 1017–21.

44. Cottier C, Pfisterer M, Muller-Brand J *et al.* Cardiac evaluation of candidates for kidney transplantation: value of exercise radionuclide angiocardiography. *Eur Heart J* 1990; **11**: 832–8.

45. Iqbal A, Gibbons RJ, McGoon MD *et al.* Noninvasive assessment of cardiac risk in insulin-dependent diabetic patients being evaluated for pancreatic transplantation using thallium-201 myocardial perfusion scintigraphy. *Clin Transplant* 1991; **5**: 13–19.

46. Morrow CE, Schwartz JS, Sutherland DE *et al.* Predictive value of thallium stress testing for coronary and cardiovascular events in uremic diabetic patients before renal transplantation. *Am J Surg* 1983; **146**: 331–5.

47. Philipson JD, Carpenter BJ, Itzkoff J *et al.* Evaluation of cardiovascular risk for renal transplantation in diabetic patients. *Am J Med* 1986; **81**: 630–4.

48. Suki WN. Use of diuretics in chronic renal failure. *Kidney Int Suppl* 1997; **59**: S33–5.

49. Vandenberg BF, Rossen JD, Grover-McKay M et al. Evaluation of diabetic patients for renal and pancreas transplantation: noninvasive screening for coronary artery disease using radionuclide methods. *Transplantation* 1996; **62**: 1230–5.

50. Boudreau RJ, Strony JT, duCret RP et al. Perfusion thallium imaging of type I diabetes patients with end stage renal disease: comparison of oral and intravenous dipyridamole administration. *Radiology* 1990; **175**: 103–5.

51. Trochu JN, Cantarovich D, Renaudeau J et al. Assessment of coronary artery disease by thallium scan in type-1 diabetic uremic patients awaiting combined pancreas and renal transplantation. *Angiology* 1991; **42**: 302–7.

52. Bates JR, Sawada SG, Segar DS et al. Evaluation using dobutamine stress echocardiography in patients with insulin-dependent diabetes mellitus before kidney and/or pancreas transplantation. *Am J Cardiol* 1996; **77**: 175–9.

53. De Lima JJ, Sabbaga E, Vieira ML et al. Coronary angiography is the best predictor of events in renal transplant candidates compared with noninvasive testing. *Hypertension* 2003; **42**: 263–8.

54. Herzog CA, Marwick TH, Pheley AM et al. Dobutamine stress echocardiography for the detection of significant coronary artery disease in renal transplant candidates. *Am J Kidney Dis* 1999; **33**: 1080–90.

55. Reis G, Marcovitz PA, Leichtman AB et al. Usefulness of dobutamine stress echocardiography in detecting coronary artery disease in end-stage renal disease. *Am J Cardiol* 1995; **75**: 707–10.

56. Tita C, Karthikeyan V, Stroe A et al. Stress echocardiography for risk stratification in patients with end-stage renal disease undergoing renal transplantation. *J Am Soc Echocardiogr* 2008; **21**: 321–6.

57. Hase H, Tsunoda T, Tanaka Y et al. Risk factors for de novo acute cardiac events in patients initiating hemodialysis with no previous cardiac symptom. *Kidney Int* 2006; **70**: 1142–8.

58. Siedlecki A, Foushee M, Curtis JJ et al. The impact of left ventricular systolic dysfunction on survival after renal transplantation. *Transplantation* 2007; **84**: 1610–17.

59. Antithrombotic Trialists' Collaboration. Collaborative meta-analysis of randomised trials of antiplatelet therapy for prevention of death, myocardial infarction, and stroke in high risk patients. *Br Med J* 2002; **324** (7329): 71–86.

60. Greenberg A. Diuretic complications. *Am J Med Sci* 2000; **319**: 10–24.

61. Inoue M, Okajima K, Itoh K et al. Mechanism of furosemide resistance in analbuminemic rats and hypoalbuminemic patients. *Kidney Int* 1987; **32**: 198–203.

62. Akcicek F, Yalniz T, Basci A et al. Diuretic effect of frusemide in patients with nephrotic syndrome: is it potentiated by intravenous albumin? *Br Med J* 1995; **310**(6973): 162–3.

63. Chalasani N, Gorski JC, Horlander JC Sr et al. Effects of albumin/furosemide mixtures on responses to furosemide in hypoalbuminemic patients. *J Am Soc Nephrol* 2001; **12**: 1010–16.

64. Fliser D, Zurbruggen I, Mutschler E et al. Coadministration of albumin and furosemide in patients with the nephrotic syndrome. *Kidney Int* 1999; **55**: 629–34.

65. Gentilini P, Casini-Raggi V, Di Fiore G et al. Albumin improves the response to diuretics in patients with cirrhosis and ascites: results of a randomized, controlled trial. *J Hepatol* 1999; **30**: 639–45.

66. Brunkhorst FM, Engel C, Bloos F et al. Intensive insulin therapy and pentastarch resuscitation in severe sepsis. *N Engl J Med* 2008; **358**: 125–39.

67. Bunn F, Trivedi D, Ashraf S. Colloid solutions for fluid resuscitation. *Cochrane Database Syst Rev* 2008; **1**: CD001319.

68. Perel P, Roberts I. Colloids versus crystalloids for fluid resuscitation in critically ill patients. *Cochrane Database Syst Rev* 2007; **4**: CD000567.

69. Schortgen F, Girou E, Deye N et al. The risk associated with hyperoncotic colloids in patients with shock. *Intensive Care Med* 2008; **34**: 2157–68.

70. Westphal M, James MF, Kozek-Langenecker S et al. Hydroxyethyl starches: different products – different effects. *Anesthesiology* 2009; **111**: 187–202.

71. Auerbach AD, Goldman L. Beta-blockers and reduction of cardiac events in noncardiac surgery: scientific review. *J Am Med Assoc* 2002; **287**: 1435–44.

72. Mangano DT, Layug EL, Wallace A et al. Effect of atenolol on mortality and cardiovascular morbidity after noncardiac surgery. Multicenter Study of Perioperative Ischemia Research Group. *N Engl J Med* 1996; **335**: 1713–20.

73. Poldermans D, Boersma E, Bax JJ et al. The effect of bisoprolol on perioperative mortality and myocardial infarction in high-risk patients undergoing vascular surgery. Dutch Echocardiographic Cardiac Risk Evaluation Applying Stress Echocardiography Study Group. *N Engl J Med* 1999; **341**: 1789–94.

74. Devereaux PJ, Beattie WS, Choi PT et al. How strong is the evidence for the use of perioperative beta blockers in non-cardiac surgery? Systematic review and meta-analysis of randomised controlled trials. *Br Med J* 2005; **331**: 313–21.

75. Juul AB, Wetterslev J, Gluud C et al. Effect of perioperative beta blockade in patients with diabetes undergoing major non-cardiac surgery: randomised placebo controlled, blinded multicentre trial. *Br Med J* 2006; **332**: 1482.

76. Devereaux PJ, Yang H, Yusuf S et al. Effects of extended-release metoprolol succinate in patients undergoing non-cardiac surgery (POISE trial): a randomised controlled trial. *Lancet* 2008; **371**(9627): 1839–47.

77. Arora P, Rajagopalam S, Ranjan R et al. Preoperative use of angiotensin-converting enzyme inhibitors/angiotensin receptor blockers is associated with increased risk for acute kidney injury after cardiovascular surgery. *Clin J Am Soc Nephrol* 2008; **3**: 1266–73.

78. Comfere T, Sprung J, Kumar MM et al. Angiotensin system inhibitors in a general surgical population. *Anesth Analg* 2005; **100**: 636–44.

79. Coriat P, Richer C, Douraki T et al. Influence of chronic angiotensin-converting enzyme inhibition on anesthetic induction. *Anesthesiology* 1994; **81**: 299–307.

80. Raja SG, Fida N. Should angiotensin converting enzyme inhibitors/angiotensin II receptor antagonists be

omitted before cardiac surgery to avoid postoperative vasodilation? *Interact Cardiovasc Thorac Surg* 2008; 7: 470–5.

81. Marik PE, Varon J. Perioperative hypertension: a review of current and emerging therapeutic agents. *J Clin Anesth* 2009; 21: 220–9.

82. Yee J, Parasuraman R, Narins RG. Selective review of key perioperative renal-electrolyte disturbances in chronic renal failure patients. *Chest* 1999; 115 (5 Suppl): 149S–57S.

83. Rindone JP, Sloane EP. Cyanide toxicity from sodium nitroprusside: risks and management. *Ann Pharmacother* 1992; 26: 515–19.

84. Chang TI, Paik J, Greene T *et al.* Intradialytic hypotension and vascular access thrombosis. *J Am Soc Nephrol* 2011; 22: 1526–33.

85. Burke JF Jr, Francos GC. Surgery in the patient with acute or chronic renal failure. *Med Clin North Am* 1987; 71: 489–97.

86. Bia MJ, DeFronzo RA. Extrarenal potassium homeostasis. *Am J Physiol* 1981; 240: F257–68.

87. Einhorn LM, Zhan M, Hsu VD *et al.* The frequency of hyperkalemia and its significance in chronic kidney disease. *Arch Intern Med* 2009; 169: 1156–62.

88. Salem MM, Rosa RM, Batlle DC. Extrarenal potassium tolerance in chronic renal failure: implications for the treatment of acute hyperkalemia. *Am J Kidney Dis* 1991; 18: 421–40.

89. Martin RS, Panese S, Virginillo M *et al.* Increased secretion of potassium in the rectum of humans with chronic renal failure. *Am J Kidney Dis* 1986; 8: 105–10.

90. Ferrannini E, Taddei S, Santoro D *et al.* Independent stimulation of glucose metabolism and Na⁺-K⁺ exchange by insulin in the human forearm. *Am J Physiol* 1988; 255: E953–8.

91. Allon M, Takeshian A, Shanklin N. Effect of insulin-plus-glucose infusion with or without epinephrine on fasting hyperkalemia. *Kidney Int* 1993; 43: 212–17.

92. Allon M, Shanklin N. Effect of bicarbonate administration on plasma potassium in dialysis patients: interactions with insulin and albuterol. *Am J Kidney Dis* 1996; 28: 508–14.

93. Blumberg A, Weidmann P, Shaw S *et al.* Effect of various therapeutic approaches on plasma potassium and major regulating factors in terminal renal failure. *Am J Med* 1988; 85: 507–12.

94. Pirenne J, Lledo-Garcia E, Benedetti E *et al.* Colon perforation after renal transplantation: a single-institution review. *Clin Transplant* 1997; 11: 88–93.

95. Sterns RH, Rojas M, Bernstein P *et al.* Ion-exchange resins for the treatment of hyperkalemia: are they safe and effective? *J Am Soc Nephrol* 2010; 21: 733–5.

96. Watson M, Abbott KC, Yuan CM. Damned if you do, damned if you don't: potassium binding resins in hyperkalemia. *Clin J Am Soc Nephrol* 2010; 5: 1723–6.

97. Cundy T, Dissanayake A. Severe hypomagnesaemia in long-term users of proton-pump inhibitors. *Clin Endocrinol (Oxf)* 2008; 69: 338–41.

98. Kuipers MT, Thang HD, Arntzenius AB. Hypomagnesaemia due to use of proton pump inhibitors – a review. *Neth J Med* 2009; 67: 169–72.

99. Hoorn EJ, van der Hoek J, de Man RA *et al.* A case series of proton pump inhibitor-induced hypomagnesemia. *Am J Kidney Dis* 2010; 56: 112–16.

100. Van Der Klooster JM, Van Der Wiel HE, Van Saase JL *et al.* Asystole during combination chemotherapy for non-Hodgkin's lymphoma: the acute tumor lysis syndrome. *Neth J Med* 2000; 56: 147–52.

101. Levin NW, Hoenich NA. Consequences of hyperphosphatemia and elevated levels of the calcium-phosphorus product in dialysis patients. *Curr Opin Nephrol Hypertens* 2001; 10: 563–8.

102. Schiller LR, Santa Ana CA, Sheikh MS *et al.* Effect of the time of administration of calcium acetate on phosphorus binding. *N Engl J Med* 1989; 320: 1110–13.

103. Sheikh MS, Maguire JA, Emmett M *et al.* Reduction of dietary phosphorus absorption by phosphorus binders. A theoretical, in vitro, and in vivo study. *J Clin Invest* 1989; 83: 66–73.

104. Cannata-Andia JB, Fernandez-Martin JL. The clinical impact of aluminium overload in renal failure. *Nephrol Dial Transplant* 2002; 17 (Suppl 2): 9–12.

105. Molitoris BA, Froment DH, Mackenzie TA *et al.* Citrate: a major factor in the toxicity of orally administered aluminum compounds. *Kidney Int* 1989; 36: 949–53.

106. Kumar VA, Yeun JY, Vu JT *et al.* Extended daily dialysis (EDD) rapidly reduces serum phosphate levels in intensive care unit (ICU) patients with acute renal failure (ARF). *Am Soc Artif Internal Organs* 2001; 47: 150.

107. Tan HK, Bellomo R, M'Pis DA *et al.* Phosphatemic control during acute renal failure: intermittent hemodialysis versus continuous hemodiafiltration. *Int J Artif Organs* 2001; 24: 186–91.

108. Crook MA, Hally V, Panteli JV. The importance of the refeeding syndrome. *Nutrition* 2001; 17: 632–7.

109. Hemstreet BA. Use of sucralfate in renal failure. *Ann Pharmacother* 2001; 35: 360–4.

110. Mechanick JI, Brett EM. Endocrine and metabolic issues in the management of the chronically critically ill patient. *Crit Care Clin* 2002; 18: 619–41, viii.

111. Gallacher SJ, Ralston SH, Dryburgh FJ *et al.* Immobilization-related hypercalcaemia – a possible novel mechanism and response to pamidronate. *Postgrad Med J* 1990; 66: 918–22.

112. Cruz DN, Perazella MA. Biochemical aberrations in a dialysis patient following parathyroidectomy. *Am J Kidney Dis* 1997; 29: 759–62.

113. Goyal P, Puri GD, Pandey CK *et al.* Evaluation of induction doses of propofol: comparison between endstage renal disease and normal renal function patients. *Anaesth Intensive Care* 2002; 30: 584–7.

114. Mitchell JH, Wildenthal K, Johnson RL Jr. The effects of acid-base disturbances on cardiovascular and pulmonary function. *Kidney Int* 1972; 1: 375–89.

115. Orchard CH, Kentish JC. Effects of changes of pH on the contractile function of cardiac muscle. *Am J Physiol* 1990; 258: C967–81.

116. Posner JB, Plum F. Spinal-fluid pH and neurologic symptoms in systemic acidosis. *N Engl J Med* 1967; 277: 605–13.

117. Adrogue HJ, Madias NE. Management of life-threatening acid-base disorders.

First of two parts. *N Engl J Med* 1998; **338**: 26–34.

118. Narins RG, Cohen JJ. Bicarbonate therapy for organic acidosis: the case for its continued use. *Ann Intern Med* 1987; **106**: 615–18.

119. Rose BD, Post TW. Metabolic acidosis. In *Clinical Physiology of Acid–Base and Electrolyte Disorders*. New York: McGraw Hill, 2001, pp. 578–646.

120. Holmdahl MH, Wiklund L, Wetterberg T *et al.* The place of THAM in the management of acidemia in clinical practice. *Acta Anaesthesiol Scand* 2000; **44**: 524–7.

121. Hadimioglu N, Saadawy I, Saglam T *et al.* The effect of different crystalloid solutions on acid-base balance and early kidney function after kidney transplantation. *Anesth Analg* 2008; **107**: 264–9.

122. Swartz RD, Rubin JE, Brown RS *et al.* Correction of postoperative metabolic alkalosis and renal failure by hemodialysis. *Ann Intern Med* 1977; **86**: 52–5.

123. Hakim RM, Levin N. Malnutrition in hemodialysis patients. *Am J Kidney Dis* 1993; **21**: 125–37.

124. Lowrie EG, Lew NL. Death risk in hemodialysis patients: the predictive value of commonly measured variables and an evaluation of death rate differences between facilities. *Am J Kidney Dis* 1990; **15**: 458–82.

125. Don BR, Kaysen GA. Assessment of inflammation and nutrition in patients with end-stage renal disease. *J Nephrol* 2000; **13**: 249–59.

126. Rocco MV, Blumenkrantz MJ. Nutrition. In Daugirdas JT, Blake PG, Ing TS, eds. *Handbook of Dialysis*. Philadelphia: Little Brown & Co.; 2001, pp. 420–45.

127. National Kidney Foundation Dialysis Outcomes Quality Initiative. Clinical practice guidelines for nutrition in chronic renal failure. *Am J Kidney Dis* 2000; **35** (6 Suppl 2): S1–140.

128. Feinstein EI, Kopple JD, Silberman H *et al.* Total parenteral nutrition with high or low nitrogen intakes in patients with acute renal failure. *Kidney Int Suppl* 1983; **16**: S319–23.

129. Eschbach JW, Adamson JW. Anemia of end-stage renal disease (ESRD). *Kidney Int* 1985; **28**: 1–5.

130. Eschbach JW, Egrie JC, Downing MR *et al.* Correction of the anemia of end-stage renal disease with recombinant human erythropoietin. Results of a combined phase I and II clinical trial. *N Engl J Med* 1987; **316**: 73–8.

131. Besarab A, Bolton WK, Browne JK *et al.* The effects of normal as compared with low hematocrit values in patients with cardiac disease who are receiving hemodialysis and epoetin. *N Engl J Med* 1998; **339**: 584–90.

132. Pfeffer MA, Burdmann EA, Chen CY *et al.* A trial of darbepoetin alfa in type 2 diabetes and chronic kidney disease. *N Engl J Med* 2009; **361**: 2019–32.

133. Singh AK, Szczech L, Tang KL *et al.* Correction of anemia with epoetin alfa in chronic kidney disease. *N Engl J Med* 2006; **355**: 2085–98.

134. National Kidney Foundation Dialysis Outcomes Quality Initiative: Clinical practice guidelines for anemia of chronic kidney disease: update 2000. *Am J Kidney Dis* 2001; **37** (1 Suppl 1): S182–238.

135. Eberst ME, Berkowitz LR. Hemostasis in renal disease: pathophysiology and management. *Am J Med* 1994; **96**: 168–79.

136. Escolar G, Cases A, Bastida E *et al.* Uremic platelets have a functional defect affecting the interaction of von Willebrand factor with glycoprotein IIb-IIIa. *Blood* 1990; **76**: 1336–40.

137. Koch M, Gradaus F, Schoebel FC *et al.* Relevance of conventional cardiovascular risk factors for the prediction of coronary artery disease in diabetic patients on renal replacement therapy. *Nephrol Dial Transplant* 1997; **12**: 1187–91.

138. Rabelink TJ, Zwaginga JJ, Koomans HA *et al.* Thrombosis and hemostasis in renal disease. *Kidney Int* 1994; **46**: 287–96.

139. Noris M, Remuzzi G. Uremic bleeding: closing the circle after 30 years of controversies? *Blood* 1999; **94**: 2569–74.

140. Steiner RW, Coggins C, Carvalho AC. Bleeding time in uremia: a useful test to assess clinical bleeding. *Am J Hematol* 1979; **7**: 107–17.

141. Lindsay RM, Friesen M, Aronstam A *et al.* Improvement of platelet function by increased frequency of hemodialysis. *Clin Nephrol* 1978; **10**: 67–70.

142. Hedges SJ, Dehoney SB, Hooper JS *et al.* Evidence-based treatment recommendations for uremic bleeding. *Nat Clin Pract Nephrol* 2007; **3**: 138–53.

143. Mannucci PM. Hemostatic drugs. *N Engl J Med* 1998; **339**: 245–53.

144. Vigano G, Gaspari F, Locatelli M *et al.* Dose-effect and pharmacokinetics of estrogens given to correct bleeding time in uremia. *Kidney Int* 1988; **34**: 853–8.

145. Moschella SL, Kay J, Mackool BT *et al.* Case records of the Massachusetts General Hospital. Weekly clinicopathological exercises. Case 35–2004. A 68-year-old man with end-stage renal disease and thickening of the skin. *N Engl J Med* 2004; **351**: 2219–27.

146. Joffe P, Thomsen HS, Meusel M. Pharmacokinetics of gadodiamide injection in patients with severe renal insufficiency and patients undergoing hemodialysis or continuous ambulatory peritoneal dialysis. *Acad Radiol* 1998; **5**: 491–502.

147. Mendoza FA, Artlett CM, Sandorfi N *et al.* Description of 12 cases of nephrogenic fibrosing dermopathy and review of the literature. *Semin Arthritis Rheum* 2006; **35**: 238–49.

148. Cowper SE, Su LD, Bhawan J *et al.* Nephrogenic fibrosing dermopathy. *Am J Dermatopathol* 2001; **23**: 383–93.

149. Perazella MA. How should nephrologists approach gadolinium-based contrast imaging in patients with kidney disease? *Clin J Am Soc Nephrol* 2008; **3**: 649–51.

150. Grobner T. Gadolinium – a specific trigger for the development of nephrogenic fibrosing dermopathy and nephrogenic systemic fibrosis? *Nephrol Dial Transplant* 2006; **21**: 1104–8.

151. Saitoh T, Hayasaka K, Tanaka Y *et al.* Dialyzability of gadodiamide in hemodialysis patients. *Radiat Med* 2006; **24**: 445–51.

152. Miller CF. Renal failure. In Breslow MJ, Miller CF, Rogers MC, eds. *Perioperative management*. St. Louis: C.V. Mosby Co.; 1990, pp. 327–42.

153. Bihorac A, Yavas S, Subbiah S *et al.* Long-term risk of mortality and acute kidney injury during hospitalization after major surgery. *Ann Surg* 2009; **249**: 851–8.

154. Chertow GM, Lazarus JM, Paganini EP *et al.* Predictors of mortality and the provision of dialysis in patients with

acute tubular necrosis. The Auriculin Anaritide Acute Renal Failure Study Group. *J Am Soc Nephrol* 1998; **9**: 692–8.

155. Borthwick E, Ferguson A. Perioperative acute kidney injury: risk factors, recognition, management, and outcomes. *Br Med J* 2010; **341**: c3365.

156. Carvounis CP, Nisar S, Guro-Razuman S. Significance of the fractional excretion of urea in the differential diagnosis of acute renal failure. *Kidney Int* 2002; **62**: 2223–9.

157. Tsai JJ, Yeun JY, Kumar VA *et al.* Comparison and interpretation of urinalysis performed by a nephrologist versus a hospital-based clinical laboratory. *Am J Kidney Dis* 2005; **46**: 820–9.

158. Bellomo R, Ronco C, Kellum JA *et al.* Acute renal failure – definition, outcome measures, animal models, fluid therapy and information technology needs: the Second International Consensus Conference of the Acute Dialysis Quality Initiative (ADQI) Group. *Crit Care* 2004; **8**: R204–12.

159. Mehta RL, Kellum JA, Shah SV *et al.* Acute Kidney Injury Network: report of an initiative to improve outcomes in acute kidney injury. *Crit Care* 2007; **11**: R31.

160. Bagshaw SM, George C, Bellomo R. A comparison of the RIFLE and AKIN criteria for acute kidney injury in critically ill patients. *Nephrol Dial Transplant* 2008; **23**: 1569–74.

161. Devarajan P. NGAL in acute kidney injury: from serendipity to utility. *Am J Kidney Dis* 2008; **52**: 395–9.

162. Rose BD. Postischemic and postoperative acute tubular necrosis. In Rose BD, ed. *Up To Date*, Vol. 10.**3**. Wellesley, MA: Up to Date; 2002, pp. 320–42.

163. Myers BD, Miller DC, Mehigan JT *et al.* Nature of the renal injury following total renal ischemia in man. *J Clin Invest* 1984; **73**: 329–41.

164. Dawson JL. Post-operative renal function in obstructive jaundice: effect of a mannitol diuresis. *Br Med J* 1965; **1**: 82–6.

165. Abelha FJ, Botelho M, Fernandes V *et al.* Determinants of postoperative acute kidney injury. *Crit Care* 2009; **13**: R79.

166. Thakar CV, Arrigain S, Worley S *et al.* A clinical score to predict acute renal failure after cardiac surgery. *J Am Soc Nephrol* 2005; **16**: 162–8.

167. Sajja LR, Mannam G, Chakravarthi RM *et al.* Coronary artery bypass grafting with or without cardiopulmonary bypass in patients with preoperative non-dialysis dependent renal insufficiency: a randomized study. *J Thorac Cardiovasc Surg* 2007; **133**: 378–88.

168. Wardle EN. Acute renal failure and multiorgan failure. *Nephron* 1994; **66**: 380–5.

169. Patrono C, Dunn MJ. The clinical significance of inhibition of renal prostaglandin synthesis. *Kidney Int* 1987; **32**: 1–12.

170. Perazella MA, Eras J. Are selective COX-2 inhibitors nephrotoxic? *Am J Kidney Dis* 2000; **35**: 937–40.

171. Auron M, Harte B, Kumar A *et al.* Renin-angiotensin system antagonists in the perioperative setting: clinical consequences and recommendations for practice. *Postgrad Med J* 2011; **87**: 472–81.

172. Bakris GL, Weir MR. Angiotensin-converting enzyme inhibitor-associated elevations in serum creatinine: is this a cause for concern? *Arch Intern Med* 2000; **160**: 685–93.

173. Oster JR, Materson BJ. Renal and electrolyte complications of congestive heart failure and effects of therapy with angiotensin-converting enzyme inhibitors. *Arch Intern Med* 1992; **152**: 704–10.

174. Humes HD. Aminoglycoside nephrotoxicity. *Kidney Int* 1988; **33**: 900–11.

175. Meyer RD. Risk factors and comparisons of clinical nephrotoxicity of aminoglycosides. *Am J Med* 1986; **80**: 119–25.

176. Moore RD, Smith CR, Lipsky JJ *et al.* Risk factors for nephrotoxicity in patients treated with aminoglycosides. *Ann Intern Med* 1984; **100**: 352–7.

177. Zager RA. Studies of mechanisms and protective maneuvers in myoglobinuric acute renal injury. *Lab Invest* 1989; **60**: 619–29.

178. Zager RA. Rhabdomyolysis and myohemoglobinuric acute renal failure. *Kidney Int* 1996; **49**: 314–26.

179. Don B, Rodriguez RA, Humphreys MH. *Diseases of the Kidney and Urinary Tract*. Philadelphia, PA: Lippincott, Williams & Wilkins; 2001, pp. 1299–1326.

180. Bywaters EG, Beall D. Crush injuries with impairment of renal function. 1941. *J Am Soc Nephrol* 1998; **9**: 322–32.

181. Better OS, Stein JH. Early management of shock and prophylaxis of acute renal failure in traumatic rhabdomyolysis. *N Engl J Med* 1990; **322**(12): 825–9.

182. Zager RA. Combined mannitol and deferoxamine therapy for myohemoglobinuric renal injury and oxidant tubular stress. Mechanistic and therapeutic implications. *J Clin Invest* 1992; **90**(3): 711–19.

183. Eneas JF, Schoenfeld PY, Humphreys MH. The effect of infusion of mannitol-sodium bicarbonate on the clinical course of myoglobinuria. *Arch Intern Med* 1979; **139**(7): 801–5.

184. Barrett BJ. Contrast nephrotoxicity. *J Am Soc Nephrol* 1994; **5**(2): 125–37.

185. Solomon R. Contrast-medium-induced acute renal failure. *Kidney Int* 1998; **53**(1): 230–42.

186. Morcos SK, Thomsen HS, Webb JA. Dialysis and contrast media. *Eur Radiol* 2002; **12**(12): 3026–30.

187. Aspelin P, Aubry P, Fransson SG *et al.* Nephrotoxic effects in high-risk patients undergoing angiography. *N Engl J Med* 2003; **348**(6): 491–9.

188. Rudnick MR, Goldfarb S, Wexler L *et al.* Nephrotoxicity of ionic and nonionic contrast media in 1196 patients: a randomized trial. The Iohexol Cooperative Study. *Kidney Int* 1995; **47**(1): 254–61.

189. Solomon R, Werner C, Mann D *et al.* Effects of saline, mannitol, and furosemide to prevent acute decreases in renal function induced by radiocontrast agents. *N Engl J Med* 1994; **331**(21): 1416–20.

190. Weisbord SD, Palevsky PM. Prevention of contrast-induced nephropathy with volume expansion. *Clin J Am Soc Nephrol* 2008; **3**(1): 273–80.

191. Zagler A, Azadpour M, Mercado C *et al.* N-acetylcysteine and contrast-induced nephropathy: a meta-analysis of 13 randomized trials. *Am Heart J* 2006; **151**(1): 140–5.

192. Pannu N, Manns B, Lee H et al. Systematic review of the impact of N-acetylcysteine on contrast nephropathy. *Kidney Int* 2004; **65**(4): 1366–74.

193. Nallamothu BK, Shojania KG, Saint S et al. Is acetylcysteine effective in preventing contrast-related nephropathy? A meta-analysis. *Am J Med* 2004; **117**(12): 938–47.

194. Marenzi G, Assanelli E, Marana I et al. N-acetylcysteine and contrast-induced nephropathy in primary angioplasty. *N Engl J Med* 2006; **354**(26): 2773–82.

195. Zoungas S, Ninomiya T, Huxley R et al. Systematic review: sodium bicarbonate treatment regimens for the prevention of contrast-induced nephropathy. *Ann Intern Med* 2009; **151**(9): 631–8.

196. Merten GJ, Burgess WP, Gray LV et al. Prevention of contrast-induced nephropathy with sodium bicarbonate: a randomized controlled trial. *J Am Med Assoc* 2004; **291**(19): 2328–34.

197. Diaz-Sandoval LJ, Kosowsky BD, Losordo DW. Acetylcysteine to prevent angiography-related renal tissue injury (the APART trial). *Am J Cardiol* 2002; **89**(3): 356–8.

198. Tepel M, van der Giet M, Schwarzfeld C et al. Prevention of radiographic-contrast-agent-induced reductions in renal function by acetylcysteine. *N Engl J Med* 2000; **343**(3): 180–4.

199. Boccalandro F, Amhad M, Smalling RW et al. Oral acetylcysteine does not protect renal function from moderate to high doses of intravenous radiographic contrast. *Catheter Cardiovasc Interv* 2003; **58**(3): 336–41.

200. Briguori C, Manganelli F, Scarpato P et al. Acetylcysteine and contrast agent-associated nephrotoxicity. *J Am Coll Cardiol* 2002; **40**(2): 298–303.

201. Durham JD, Caputo C, Dokko J et al. A randomized controlled trial of N-acetylcysteine to prevent contrast nephropathy in cardiac angiography. *Kidney Int* 2002; **62**(6): 2202–7.

202. Lassnigg A, Donner E, Grubhofer G et al. Lack of renoprotective effects of dopamine and furosemide during cardiac surgery. *J Am Soc Nephrol* 2000; **11**(1): 97–104.

203. Friedrich JO, Adhikari N, Herridge MS et al. Meta-analysis: low-dose dopamine increases urine output but does not prevent renal dysfunction or death. *Ann Intern Med* 2005; **142**(7): 510–24.

204. Szerlip HM. Renal-dose dopamine: fact and fiction. *Ann Intern Med* 1991; **115**(2): 153–4.

205. Landoni G, Biondi-Zoccai GG, Tumlin JA et al. Beneficial impact of fenoldopam in critically ill patients with or at risk for acute renal failure: a meta-analysis of randomized clinical trials. *Am J Kidney Dis* 2007; **49**(1): 56–68.

206. Nigwekar SU, Hix JK. The role of natriuretic peptide administration in cardiovascular surgery-associated renal dysfunction: a systematic review and meta-analysis of randomized controlled trials. *J Cardiothorac Vasc Anesth* 2009; **23**(2): 151–60.

207. Finfer S, Chittock DR, Su SY et al. Intensive versus conventional glucose control in critically ill patients. *N Engl J Med* 2009; **360**(13): 1283–97.

208. Thomas G, Rojas MC, Epstein SK et al. Insulin therapy and acute kidney injury in critically ill patients: a systematic review. *Nephrol Dial Transplant* 2007; **22**(10): 2849–55.

209. Molnar AO, Coca SG, Devereaux PJ et al. Statin use associates with a lower incidence of acute kidney injury after major elective surgery. *J Am Soc Nephrol* 2011; **22**(5): 939–46.

210. Waikar SS, Brunelli SM. Peri-surgical statins lessen acute kidney injury. *J Am Soc Nephrol* 2011; **22**(5): 797–9.

211. Stallwood MI, Grayson AD, Mills K et al. Acute renal failure in coronary artery bypass surgery: independent effect of cardiopulmonary bypass. *Ann Thorac Surg* 2004; **77**(3): 968–72.

212. Wijeysundera DN, Beattie WS, Djaiani G et al. Off-pump coronary artery surgery for reducing mortality and morbidity: meta-analysis of randomized and observational studies. *J Am Coll Cardiol* 2005; **46**(5): 872–82.

213. Myers BD, Moran SM. Hemodynamically mediated acute renal failure. *N Engl J Med* 1986; **314**(2): 97–105.

214. Schulman G, Fogo A, Gung A et al. Complement activation retards resolution of acute ischemic renal failure in the rat. *Kidney Int* 1991; **40**(6): 1069–74.

215. Hakim RM, Wingard RL, Parker RA. Effect of the dialysis membrane in the treatment of patients with acute renal failure. *N Engl J Med* 1994; **331**(20): 1338–42.

216. Schiffl H, Lang SM, Konig A et al. Biocompatible membranes in acute renal failure: prospective case-controlled study. *Lancet* 1994; **344**(8922): 570–2.

217. Hertel J, Keep DM, Caruana RJ. Anticoagulation. In Daugirdas JT, Blake PG, Ing TS, eds. *Handbook of Dialysis*. Philadelphia, PA: Lippincott, Williams & Wilkins; 2001, pp. 182–98.

218. Troppmann C, Pierce JL, Gandhi MM et al. Higher surgical wound complication rates with sirolimus immunosuppression after kidney transplantation: a matched-pair pilot study. *Transplantation* 2003; **76**(2): 426–9.

219. Connolly SJ, Kates RE. Clinical pharmacokinetics of N-acetylprocainamide. *Clin Pharmacokinet* 1982; **7**(3): 206–20.

220. Vlasses PH, Ferguson RK, Rocci ML Jr et al. Lethal accumulation of procainamide metabolite in severe renal insufficiency. *Am J Nephrol* 1986; **6**(2): 112–16.

221. Maton PN, Burton ME. Antacids revisited: a review of their clinical pharmacology and recommended therapeutic use. *Drugs* 1999; **57**(6): 855–70.

222. Pruchnicki MC, Coyle JD, Hoshaw-Woodard S et al. Effect of phosphate binders on supplemental iron absorption in healthy subjects. *J Clin Pharmacol* 2002; **42**(10): 1171–6.

223. Cheng JW, Charland SL, Shaw LM et al. Is the volume of distribution of digoxin reduced in patients with renal dysfunction? Determining digoxin pharmacokinetics by fluorescence polarization immunoassay. *Pharmacotherapy* 1997; **17**(3): 584–90.

224. Borga O, Hoppel C, Odar-Cederlof I et al. Plasma levels and renal excretion of phenytoin and its metabolites in patients with renal failure. *Clin Pharmacol Ther* 1979; **26**(3): 306–14.

225. Levey AS, Bosch JP, Lewis JB et al. A more accurate method to estimate glomerular filtration rate from serum creatinine: a new prediction equation. Modification of diet in Renal Disease Study Group. *Ann Intern Med* 1999; **130**(6): 461–70.

226. Hu KT, Matayoshi A, Stevenson FT. Calculation of the estimated creatinine clearance in avoiding drug dosing

errors in the older patient. *Am J Med Sci* 2001; **322**(3): 133–6.

227. Cranshaw J, Holland D. Anaesthesia for patients with renal impairment. *Br J Hosp Med* 1996; **55**(4): 171–5.

228. Sladen RN. Anesthetic considerations for the patient with renal failure. *Anesthesiol Clin North America* 2000; **18**(4): 863–82.

229. Conzen PF, Nuscheler M, Melotte A *et al.* Renal function and serum fluoride concentrations in patients with stable renal insufficiency after anesthesia with sevoflurane or enflurane. *Anesth Analg* 1995; **81**(3): 569–75.

230. Nishimori A, Tanaka K, Ueno K *et al.* Effects of sevoflurane anaesthesia on renal function. *J Int Med Res* 1997; **25** (2): 87–91.

231. Litz RJ, Hubler M, Lorenz W *et al.* Renal responses to desflurane and isoflurane in patients with renal insufficiency. *Anesthesiology* 2002; **97** (5): 1133–6.

232. Roberts RJ, Barletta JF, Fong JJ *et al.* Incidence of propofol-related infusion syndrome in critically ill adults: a prospective, multicenter study. *Crit Care* 2009; **13**(5): R169.

233. Beathard GA, Urbanes A, Litchfield T *et al.* The risk of sedation/analgesia in hemodialysis patients undergoing interventional procedures. *Semin Dial* 2011; **24**(1): 97–103.

234. Brown JH, Vites NP, Testa HJ *et al.* Value of thallium myocardial imaging in the prediction of future cardiovascular events in patients with end-stage renal failure. *Nephrol Dial Transplant* 1993; **8**(5): 433–7.

235. Dahan M, Viron BM, Faraggi M *et al.* Diagnostic accuracy and prognostic value of combined dipyridamole-exercise thallium imaging in hemodialysis patients. *Kidney Int* 1998; **54**(1): 255–62.

236. Camp AD, Garvin PJ, Hoff J *et al.* Prognostic value of intravenous dipyridamole thallium imaging in patients with diabetes mellitus considered for renal transplantation. *Am J Cardiol* 1990; **65**(22): 1459–63.

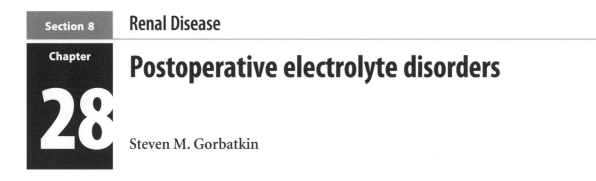

Chapter

28

Postoperative electrolyte disorders

Steven M. Gorbatkin

A variety of electrolyte disorders are common postoperatively due to a combination of the specific surgical procedure, fluid losses, IV fluid infusion, fluid shifts including third spacing, and medication or blood product administration. Since patients must remain fasting until bowel function has returned, many first-line oral remedies for electrolyte disorders cannot be used in the immediate postoperative period. Acid–base status is also frequently altered and has specific interactions with cation and anion concentrations.

Units

Millimoles (mmol), milliequivalents (mEq), and milligrams (mg) are used as units for electrolytes. For potassium (K^+), since the ionic charge is 1, 1 mmol = 1 mEq. Calcium (Ca^{2+}) and magnesium (Mg^{2+}) both have ionic charges of 2, and so there are 2 mEq per mmol. Phosphorus exists as two separate anions with different charges ($H_2PO_4^-$ and HPO_4^{2-}), so mmol rather than mEq is the unit used. Units of mg/dL are used for serum and plasma concentrations of magnesium, phosphorus, and calcium, with mg referring to elemental mass. Medication masses expressed in mg or grams often refer to molecular or compound mass rather than elemental mass. For example, 8.1 mEq (= 4.05 mmol) of elemental Mg^{2+} corresponds to 1 gram of magnesium sulfate ($MgSO_4 7H_2O$) and 98.4 mg of elemental Mg^{2+}.

Sodium disorders

Abnormalities of plasma sodium are disorders of water balance [1–6]. Hyponatremia occurs when there is excess free water compared with total body sodium, and hypernatremia occurs in patients who have a deficit of water compared with sodium. A key point in consideration of mechanisms and dangers of sodium disorders is that hypotonic IV fluids should not be routinely used in the perioperative period. Rather, they should be used to correct hypernatremic states or to balance known large free water losses.

Hyponatremia ($Na^+ < 135$ mmol/L)

Plasma sodium concentration $[Na^+]$ is a main component of plasma osmolality (P_{osm}), defined by the equation:

$$P_{osm} = 2 \times [Na^+] + glucose/18 + BUN/2.8 \qquad (28.1)$$

Normal plasma osmolality ranges from 280 to 295 mosm/kg. Plasma osmolality is carefully regulated by osmoreceptors in the anterior hypothalamus and osmolality above 280–290 causes increased thirst and increased output of anti-diuretic hormone (ADH) from the posterior lobe of the pituitary. Anti-diuretic hormone acts in the kidney on the collecting tubules, causing resorption of water and a decrease in plasma sodium. Volume depletion, decreased blood pressure, pain, or emotional stress can also cause ADH release.

The nature of a solute contributing to osmolality determines whether increasing its plasma concentration will alter plasma sodium. Solutes that are permeable across cell membranes including urea, methanol, ethanol, and ethylene glycol do not cause water movement across cell membranes. Solutes such as glucose, mannitol, maltose, and glycine are not permeable across cell membranes, contribute to "effective osmolality," and if increased in the plasma will cause water movement to decrease plasma sodium concentration. The terms "effective osmolality" and "tonicity" are often used interchangeably.

Hyponatremia can coexist with normal or elevated osmolality when, for example, there is hyperglycemia. The osmotically active glucose pulls water out of the cell, and the decrease in plasma sodium is approximately 1.6 mEq/L for every 100 mg/dL increase in plasma glucose.

Mannitol infusion or absorption of glycine during transurethral prostate resection (TURP) or hysterectomies can also increase effective osmolality, causing movement of water from the intracellular to the extracellular space and "translocational" hyponatremia. Irrigant solutions may be either hypotonic or isotonic and the resultant hyponatremia may be hypo-, iso-, or hyperosmolar, depending on the solution used, the degree of absorption, the ability of the solution

Medical Management of the Surgical Patient, ed. Michael F. Lubin, Thomas F. Dodson, and Neil H. Winawer. Published by Cambridge University Press. © Cambridge University Press 2013.

components to diffuse across the cell membrane, and the degree of osmotic diuresis induced.

Development of hyponatremic symptoms following use of irrigant solution for TURP is referred to as "post-TURP syndrome" or simply "TURP syndrome." Normal saline irrigation has been used to prevent this complication [7].

Pseudohyponatremia, rarely seen, is associated with severe elevation in lipids or proteins and the use of a flame photometer, which measures the sodium concentration in the entire plasma volume rather than just the concentration in the liquid portion. The current use of ion-specific electrodes eliminates this problem.

Hyponatremia is usually associated with hypo-osmolality, and the combination of hyponatremia and hypo-osmolality is further characterized based on the volume status of the patient – hypovolemic, normovolemic, or hypervolemic. History and clinical examination with orthostatic blood pressure, orthostatic pulse measurement, assessment of jugular venous distension, and evaluation of edema are used to assess volume status.

Hypovolemic hyponatremia is associated with total body deficits of both Na^+ and water, with the Na^+ deficit exceeding the water deficit. A spot urine sodium of > 20 mmol/L suggests renal losses, with a common cause being thiazide diuretics. Loop diuretics tend to cause hypovolemic hypernatremia rather than hyponatremia. Osmotic diuresis can cause hyponatremia when combined with free water intake. Other sources of renal loss leading to hypovolemic hyponatremia include salt-losing nephropathy (which can be associated with obstructive uropathy), mineralicorticoid deficiency, and cerebral salt wasting described most commonly in subarachnoid hemorrhage. Distinguishing salt wasting nephropathy from the syndrome of inappropriate antidiuretic hormone secretion (SIADH) can be difficult. Volume depletion, which is not characteristic of SIADH, is a key component of cerebral salt wasting.

A spot urine $Na^+ < 20$ mmol/L in hypovolemic hyponatremia suggests non-renal losses. Diarrhea, pancreatitis, trauma, burns, and bowel obstruction are examples. Contributing factors include direct gastrointestinal losses, direct skin losses, blood loss, and third spacing of fluids. Vomiting is associated with non-renal loss, but it can also be seen with a urine $Na^+ > 20$ mmol/L and hypovolemia when the associated metabolic alkalosis requires simultaneous cation (such as Na^+) excretion.

Patients with euvolemic hyponatremia have no evidence of increased total body sodium and are not edematous. Glucocorticoid deficiency, hypothyroidism, stress, medications (including desmopressin, haloperidol, carbamazepine, opiate derivatives, and SSRIs), and SIADH are causes of euvolemic hyponatremia, with SIADH a diagnosis of exclusion.

Hypervolemic hyponatremia is seen with decreased effective circulating volume and low urine sodium (< 20 mmol/L) in congestive heart failure, cirrhosis, and nephrotic syndrome. Urine sodium > 20 mmol/L and hypervolemic hyponatremia

can be seen in acute or chronic renal failure where fewer nephrons are available to excrete sodium and the kidneys have difficulty excreting free water (even with complete vasopressin suppression).

Development of hyponatremia can also be analyzed by considering causes of impaired renal free water excretion plus sources of excessive water intake. Excess free water intake may be iatrogenic or through self-induced increased oral intake. Hyponatremia may occur in the postoperative state due to the administration of excessive amounts of hypotonic intravenous fluids or absorption of irrigant solutions along with increased secretion of ADH related to postoperative pain, anesthesia, analgesic use, and third spacing of fluid.

A 1980s prospective study on postoperative hyponatremia demonstrated that it occurred in 4.4% of operations [8]. It was particularly common following cardiovascular and gastrointestinal or biliary surgeries, where it occurred 23.1% and 18.9% of the time respectively; 21% of patients were volume overloaded, 42% were euvolemic, and 94% were receiving hypotonic fluids at the time of development of hyponatremia.

Postoperative hyponatremia may also arise with the administration of isotonic fluid. In these cases elevated plasma ADH levels may lead to excretion of hypertonic urine [9].

The symptoms of hyponatremia, primarily of central nervous system dysfunction and related to cerebral edema, include headache, lethargy, nausea, vomiting, and ataxia. More severe symptoms include seizures, respiratory depression or arrest, brain-stem herniation, coma, and death. Patients are generally asymptomatic if plasma sodium is greater than 125 mEq/L, but symptoms at higher sodium concentrations can occur if hyponatremia has developed rapidly.

Young menstruating women are at increased risk of permanent brain injury or death related to hyponatremia [10,11].

Management of hyponatremia

The initial step in management of hyponatremia is to assess for an emergency related to hyponatremia, and if one exists to treat with hypertonic saline. Acute hyponatremia has been defined as a fall of more than 12 mEq/L/24 hour of less than 48 hour duration. Emergency treatment is warranted for "all symptomatic patients with acute hyponatremia, for hyponatremia associated with underlying neurologic or neurosurgical conditions, and for all hyponatremic patients with seizures or coma regardless of the duration of the electrolyte disturbance" [6]. Examples of neurologic or neurosurgical disease include intracranial hemorrhage, brain tumors, and central nervous system infections.

For seizures or coma, a 4–6 mEq/L increase in plasma sodium is estimated to be enough to rescue the most severely affected patients. An example regimen is a 2 mL/kg bolus of 3% saline up to a maximum of 100 mL over 10 minutes, repeated up to two additional times at 10-minute intervals if no clinical improvement [12]. This high rate of initial correction is only used in the early stages of emergency treatment.

One author has emphasized "confusion was created when a proposed limit of 12 mEq/L per day was expressed as an hourly rate. In fact, there is no evidence that a rapid hourly rate of correction is harmful as long as the total increase in plasma sodium concentration over a 24 hour period is not excessive" [13].

Osmotic demyelination (central pontine myelinolysis) may occur with correction of plasma sodium that is too rapid and is associated with deteriorating mental status one to several days later. It can cause quadriparesis, pseudobulbar palsy, coma, and even death [14]. Patients who have developed hyponatremia on a chronic basis are at higher risk of developing complications relating to the rapid correction of plasma sodium than patients who have developed acute hyponatremia. Also, liver transplant patients have been identified as a high-risk group.

Desired rates of plasma sodium changes of 8–12 mEq/L/24 hour have been proposed, with 8 mmol/L/24 hour a more conservative target to prevent complications [4]. The target rate of increase on subsequent days is less, with one review proposing upper limits of correction of 10 mmol/L, 18 mmol/L, and 20 mmol/L for 24, 48, and 72 hours respectively, and lower therapeutic targets of 6–8 mmol/L in the first 24 hours, 12–14 mmol/L in 48 hours, and 14–16 mmol/L in 72 hours [6]. If the initial rate of correction is too rapid, for example the plasma sodium has already increased or is projected to increase by more than 10 mmol/L in the first 24 hours, it may be necessary to administer free water as 5% dextrose or give IV or SQ desmopressin to yield a net 24-hour change of plasma sodium in the desired range [15].

The initial goal plasma sodium if asymptomatic is approximately 125 mmol/L, but for patients with acute neurologic or neurosurgical conditions, a consensus has developed for treating hyponatremia when the plasma sodium is less than 131 mmol/L regardless of the duration of the hyponatremia [16].

An example sliding scale protocol developed for neurologic and neurosurgical patients is started for plasma Na $\leq$ 133 mmol/L or a fall of plasma Na^+ by > 6 mmol/L over 24–48 hours [17]. The protocol includes administration of NaCl tablets 3 g every 6 hours orally or per nasogastric tube combined with IV 3% NaCl initially at 20 mL/hour. Depending on the plasma Na, the 3% NaCl is increased every 6 hours by 10 to 20 mL/hour to a maximum of 80 mL/hour. The rate is kept constant for Na 136 to 140 mmol/L and held for 6 hours for plasma sodium > 140 mmol/L.

For non-emergency correction, the treatment depends on the source of hyponatremia. For patients who are hypovolemic, normal saline should be administered initially to restore volume with plasma sodium monitored frequently. In the case of hypervolemic patients with hyponatremia, loop diuretics along with free water restriction to less than 1 L per day are standard treatments. Recent approval of vasopressin antagonists such as tolvaptin provides another option for treatment of hypervolemic hyponatremia, particularly in patients with heart failure.

For patients who are euvolemic with SIADH, free water restriction is the mainstay of therapy but 3% saline may be needed initially for severe hyponatremia [18,19]. Loop diuretics may be used to increase the excretion of dilute urine but caution must be used to avoid volume depletion. Demeclocycline, a tetracycline derivative, has been used in a dose of 600–1200 mg/day to decrease renal sensitivity to ADH, producing a nephrogenic diabetes insipidus, but due to its side-effect profile, including the possibility of renal toxicity, it should not be used first line. Vasopressin antagonists may also have a role in SIADH treatment in the future.

A commonly used calculation is the change in plasma sodium produced by administering one liter of an infusate [4]. It may be estimated as:

Change in plasma sodium after one litre of infusate

$$= ((\text{infusate } Na^+ + \text{infusate } K^+) - \text{plasma } Na^+) \\ /(\text{Total Body Water} + 1) \qquad (28.2)$$

The above equation should only be used as an initial estimate, since losses of free water through urine, stool, and insensible routes will also contribute to rises in plasma sodium. Frequent measurement of plasma sodium, as often as every 1–2 hour, is indicated during the initial management phase of severe hyponatremia.

Urine osmolality cannot be used to accurately predict the effect of the urine water content on plasma sodium. The electrolyte free water clearance (C_{water}), which quantitates the amount of free water produced in the urine, is used to predict the contribution of urination to changes in plasma sodium and is given by:

$$C_{water} = \text{Urine Volume} \times (1 - (\text{Urine } Na^+ + \text{Urine } K^+) \\ /\text{Plasma } Na^+) \qquad (28.3)$$

If the (Urine Na^+ + Urine K^+) is less than the plasma Na^+, the plasma Na^+ concentration increases. If (Urine Na^+ + Urine K^+) is greater than the plasma Na^+, plasma Na^+ concentration decreases.

Hypernatremia (Na^+ > 145 mmol/L)

Hypernatremia most often occurs as a postoperative complication in patients who are unable to drink adequately to meet their free water needs. Patients who are on ventilators or elderly patients who have delirium or dementia are commonly affected. In one study of patients with hospital-acquired hypernatremia, 86% of patients lacked access to free water [20].

Hypernatremia can be classified according to volume status as hypovolemic, euvolemic, or hypervolemic.

Hypovolemic hypernatremia is the result of losses of both sodium and water, with the loss of water exceeding sodium loss. It can occur with excess renal excretion such as with loop diuretic administration, osmotic diuresis from hyperglycemia, post obstructive diuresis, or with intrinsic renal disease. It is associated with a spot urine Na^+ greater than 20 mmol/L. Sources of extrarenal losses, for which the spot urine sodium is less than 20 mmol/L, include burns, fistulae, and osmotic diarrhea.

Euvolemic hypernatremia occurs when patients lose free water but there is minimal total body Na$^+$ loss. Hypodypsia, insensible dermal and pulmonary losses, and diabetes insipidus are typical causes.

Diabetes insipidus (DI) can be central (neurogenic) or nephrogenic. Central DI may be seen in a variety of forms of neurogenic trauma, infiltration, infection, and bleeding. It was found in 18% of patients immediately following transsphenoidal surgery [21]. Nephrogenic DI occurs when the collecting tubules are resistant to the effects of ADH. In addition to renal disease and medications, nephrogenic DI may be caused by hypercalcemia or hypokalemia. In DI, the patient may be able to keep up with free water losses and avoid hypernatremia provided there is an intact sensorium and access to water.

Hypervolemic hypernatremia is less common and is associated with sodium administration without an accompanying proportional increase in total body water. Excess oral NaCl or NaHCO$_3$, intravenous 3% saline, intra-amniotic instillation for therapeutic abortions, or dialysis against a high Na concentration are possible causes.

Symptoms of hypernatremia, including weakness, seizures, and coma, result from cellular dehydration and depend on the acuity of the change in plasma sodium concentration. Brain shrinkage caused by hypernatremia can cause vascular rupture including cerebral bleeding and subarachnoid hemorrhage.

Management of hypernatremia

The management of hypernatremia involves first correcting any severe volume deficit with normal saline or blood products, followed by correction of the free water deficit using hypotonic fluid administration with a goal plasma Na of 145 mmol/L. Intravenous repletion can be performed with hypotonic saline or 5% dextrose in water. Pure water cannot be administered intravenously because the local hypotonicity can produce severe hemolysis.

It has been suggested that the rate of lowering of plasma sodium should not exceed 0.5 mEq/L/hour with a target fall in plasma sodium of 10 mmol/L/24 hours; a more rapid initial rate of correction of 1–2 mmol/L/hour can be used in those patients in whom the hypernatremia has developed over a period of hours. The primary risks of correcting hypernatremia too quickly are cerebral edema and cerebral hemorrhage.

Equation 28.2 in the section on management of hyponatremia can also be used to estimate the effect of infusion of various hypotonic solutions on the plasma sodium [3]. With hypotonic solutions, the equation will yield a negative value for the change in plasma sodium, consistent with the goal of treatment. Insensible free water losses (10–15 mL/kg/day for women and 15–20 mL/kg/day for men) as well as free water excretion in urine and stool must be accounted for and replenished, and frequent measurement of plasma sodium is

indicated. Equation 28.3 is useful to estimate free water loss in the urine, and high output of dilute urine is a frequent cause of a much lower rate of sodium change than expected using Equation 28.2.

Free water administered orally or through feeding tubes can contribute to correction of hypernatremia, but uncertainties in absorption make initial correction with hypotonic IV fluids more reliable. Another approach to estimating the total amount of free water that must be administered in addition to replenishment of ongoing losses is to calculate the water deficit using:

$$\text{Water deficit} = (0.6 \text{ for males}, 0.5 \text{ for females}) \times [\text{body mass}][([\text{Na}^+]/140) - 1] \quad (28.4)$$

Addressing the underlying cause of the hypernatremia is the other key factor in management, and may involve stopping gastrointestinal fluid losses, eliminating glucosuria, withholding lactulose to prevent osmotic diarrhea, or adding free water to the daily feeding regimen which for alert patients includes providing access to free water.

In central, or "neurogenic" diabetes insipidus, desmopressin (dDAVP) may be administered. It comes in nasal and oral forms with a nasal dose ranging from 5 to 20 μg once or twice a day, or an oral dose of 0.1–0.8 mg/day divided in two or three doses daily. Nephrogenic diabetes insipidus may be treated with thiazide diuretics and a low protein, low sodium diet.

Potassium disorders

Hyperkalemia (K$^+$ > 5 mmol/L)

Hyperkalemia results from increased potassium intake, decreased excretion, or transcellular shift [22–25]. Although hyperkalemia is defined as K$^+$ > 5 mmol/L, mild hyperkalemia in the low to mid 5 mmol/L is often well tolerated unless there has been an acute rise in potassium. Plasma K$^+$ ≥ 6 mmol/L or any level of hyperkalemia accompanied by electrocardiogram (ECG) changes requires prompt intervention. K$^+$ ≥ 7.0 mmol/L, marked ECG changes at any K$^+$ level, or severe muscle weakness from hyperkalemia require emergent and immediate treatment.

Hyperkalemia may be caused by excessive intravenous infusion or oral supplementation of potassium, particularly in a patient with impaired renal function. One may see transcellular shift causing hyperkalemia in the patient with hyperglycemia and insulin deficiency. In such patients, although plasma potassium levels are high, total body potassium is usually low as a result of increased renal excretion of potassium and correction may lead to hypokalemia.

Hyperkalemia also may result from tissue breakdown in rhabdomyolysis, tissue necrosis, or tumor lysis syndrome during treatment of hematologic malignancies. Reperfusion of ischemic areas as well as rewarming from hypothermic states can result in significant hyperkalemia.

Drugs classes such as potassium-sparing diuretics, ACE inhibitors, NSAIDS, and angiotension receptor blockers are generally well recognized as causes of hyperkalemia. Succinylcholine causes hyperkalemia through transcellular shifts. Trimethoprim, pentamidine, beta-blockers, heparin, penicillin G, digoxin, and the immunosuppressive medications tacrolimus and cyclosporin also contribute to hyperkalemia.

Symptoms of severe hyperkalemia include paresthesias and fasciculations in the arms and legs, and ascending paralysis. Respiratory, trunk, and head muscles are usually spared, but rarely respiratory failure can occur.

The major danger of severe hyperkalemia is a cardiac arrhythmia. The changes seen in the ECG from hyperkalemia include the initial appearance of narrow and peaked T waves, followed by PR prolongation, flattening of the P waves, and QRS widening. Eventually, a sine wave ECG pattern can be seen, with possible impending ventricular fibrillation or asystole. Hypocalcemia increases susceptibility to hyperkalemic ECG changes.

Management of hyperkalemia

The first steps in managing hyperkalemia include checking an ECG, discontinuing any IVs or medications which can contribute to hyperkalemia, and rechecking the potassium to make sure hemolysis or extending tourniquet time are not giving a false reading. A complete blood count should be reviewed for leukocytosis and thrombocytosis, since these abnormalities can cause pseudohyperkalemia. The initial management of life-threatening hyperkalemia, which includes $K^+ \geq 7.0$ or any K^+ level with significant ECG changes such as QRS prolongation, is the administration of IV calcium, which acts to stabilize the myocardium. Calcium may be administered in the form of calcium gluconate, 10 mL of 10% solution (90 mg elemental calcium per 10 mL) over 2–3 minutes. Calcium gluconate can be given through a peripheral line. Calcium chloride, which has a higher concentration of elemental calcium (272 mg per 10 mL in 10% solution), requires a central venous line. Calcium gluconate is preferred over calcium chloride, because extravasation of calcium chloride can cause severe tissue necrosis.

Administration of intravenous calcium to patients taking digoxin requires extreme caution. The risk of calcium administration can be reduced by infusing calcium over 30 minutes rather than as a rapid bolus. Digoxin immune FAB may be indicated, especially in the setting of digitalis toxicity which itself can cause hyperkalemia.

The next step in treatment is to shift potassium from the extracellular to the intracellular space using insulin, given as 10 units of IV regular insulin. If the blood glucose is less than 250 mg/dL, 25–50 g of glucose, usually as an IV bolus of 50% dextrose, accompanies the insulin. Albuterol nebulizers also cause shift of potassium to the intracellular space when given at doses of 10–20 mg, which is significantly higher than the dose used for respiratory treatments. Albuterol should not be used in patients with unacceptably high risk for cardiac events from the tachycardia associated with albuterol treatment.

Sodium bicarbonate, although it has a role in treatment of chronic conditions that cause metabolic acidosis and hyperkalemia such as type IV renal tubular acidosis, is not a reliable treatment for hyperkalemia in the acute setting. It has minimal effect for patients with advanced kidney disease, and in cases of high anion gap acidosis, mechanisms other than exchange transfer of K^+ and H^+ dominate as causes of hyperkalemia, making sodium bicarbonate minimally effective.

Loop diuretics and thiazide or thiazide-like diuretics will often assist in causing renal potassium excretion, however they may not have a significant effect on potassium in cases of reduced renal function or volume depletion and should not be relied upon to treat hyperkalemia in the acute setting. They should be prescribed as needed for volume overload with other treatments used first for hyperkalemia.

Sodium polystyrene sulfonate (Kayexalate™) is a cation exchange resin that causes removal of potassium through exchange of Na^+ for K^+ in the gastrointestinal tract. It should be avoided postoperatively due to an increased risk of colonic necrosis when there is limited bowel motility. It is typically given orally in doses of 15–60 g, mixed with sorbitol to aid passage through the gastrointestinal tract, as often as every 4–6 hours. It can also be administered by gravity as a retention enema, 30–60 g in 250 mL of water, retained for 30–60 minutes. Sorbitol increases risk of colonic necrosis in the enema form. If it is only available premixed with sorbitol, then 50 mL of solution with sorbitol should be mixed with at least 200 mL of tap water. Enema administration should be followed by 250–1000 mL of a non-sodium irrigant solution to reduce the risk of colonic toxicity.

Dialysis may be necessary to treat hyperkalemia refractory to more conservative measures. In some patients surgical intervention may be necessary to remove ongoing sources of potassium shift such as large hematomas or tissue necrosis from conditions including gangrene and ischemic bowel.

Plasma potassium should be monitored frequently until ongoing sources of hyperkalemia have been eliminated and the plasma potassium is 5.8 mmol/L or less.

Hypokalemia ($K^+ < 3.5$ mmol/L)

Losses of potassium are categorized as renal or extrarenal [22–25]. Extrarenal losses may be from the GI tract, especially from diarrhea, or from skin losses, especially severe burns. Vomiting and gastric tube drainage deplete some potassium through the loss of gastrointestinal fluids containing potassium, however a majority of the potassium is lost through the kidneys because of the metabolic alkalosis induced by decreased gastric acid.

Renal wasting of potassium commonly occurs as a result of loop and thiazide diuretics, or in states of mineralocorticoid or cortisol excess such as primary hyperaldosteronism or

Cushing's syndrome. Another condition leading to hypokalemia in the hospitalized patient is treatment with amphotericin B, which leads to enhanced secretion of K^+ from the distal tubule and causes a type I renal tubular acidosis.

Severe magnesium deficiency can also precipitate hypokalemia and reduce the response to IV repletion, thus magnesium levels should be checked early during evaluation of hypokalemia.

Patients can experience weakness and constipation with potassium levels between 2.5 and 3.0 mmol/L. With K^+ < 2.5 mmol/L, there is an increased risk of muscle necrosis and rhabdomyolysis. At K^+ < 2.0 mmol/L, ascending paralysis and respiratory failure can occur.

Management of hypokalemia

The management of hypokalemia involves the oral supplementation or intravenous infusion of potassium, along with addressing the underlying problem that caused the potassium deficiency.

Potassium chloride is the treatment of choice for intravenous repletion, however potassium phosphate can be used for simultaneous potassium and phosphorus repletion. The recommended rate of IV correction through a peripheral line is 10 mEq/hour, with no more than 60 mmol of KCl placed in a 1-liter bag of IV fluid (to prevent excessive administration). Higher infusion rates require a central venous line, and infusion rates of 20–40 mmol/hour are reserved for life-threatening hypokalemia requiring emergent treatment. Hourly plasma potassium checks are appropriate in cases of severe depletion. As discussed in the previous section, severe hypomagnesemia must be corrected to expedite correction of hypokalemia.

Oral potassium supplementation is preferred if there are no immediate health threats. Potassium chloride is indicated for hypokalemia associated with diuretic use or volume depletion. Liquid KCl may be difficult to tolerate due to strong taste. The microencapsulated formulation is associated with fewest complications. A typical initial dose in a patient with normal renal function is 40–100 mmol/day in 2–3 divided doses.

Extreme care must be exercised in considering potassium replacement during hypothermic states because of the hyperkalemia associated with rewarming.

Calcium disorders

Forty percent of total calcium in the plasma is bound to protein, mostly albumin, and the measured concentration will decrease with hypoalbuminemia. The corrected calcium is equal to the measured plasma calcium plus 0.8 mg/dL for every 1 mg/dL decrease in albumin (below the normal albumin of 4 mg/dL). Normal corrected calcium is 8.6–10.2 mg/dL. Ionized calcium is the biologically active form, and normal ionized calcium is approximately 4.0–5.0 mg/dL (1.0–1.25 mmol/L).

Hypercalcemia (corrected Ca^{2+} > 10.2 mg/dL)

Malignancy is the most common cause of hypercalcemia, followed by hyperparathyroidism [26–30]. In the perioperative setting, volume depletion, immobility, and the commonly used thiazide diuretics will exacerbate hypercalcemia. Hypercalcemia itself stimulates urinary losses of sodium and water, volume contraction, decreased urinary loss of calcium, and further aggravation of hypercalcemia. The effect of immobility on calcium is most prominent for patients with underlying disorders associated with increased bone turnover such as Paget disease.

Symptoms of hypercalcemia include fatigue, somnolence, muscle weakness, depression, constipation, nausea, vomiting, polyuria and if severe, stupor and coma. Electrocardiography may show a shortened QT interval, and hypercalcemia increases digitalis toxicity.

Management of hypercalcemia

The first crucial step is aggressive volume repletion as allowed by any reduction in cardiac or renal function. Although loop diuretics such as furosemide should not be used first line for calcium reduction, if patients suffer from volume overload as a result of IV fluid administration, then a loop diuretic can be used both to reduce volume and to increase urinary calcium excretion. Volume repletion is often adequate for initial treatment of patients with corrected plasma calcium less than 12 mg/dL.

For patients with corrected calcium greater than 14 mg/dL or with symptomatic hypercalcemia, in addition to aggressive volume repletion, it is appropriate to initiate bisphosphonate treatment early with an onset of action of approximately 72 hour. A common contraindication to bisphosphonates is reduced renal function with GFR < approximately 35 mL/min/1.73 m^2. Calcitonin is an option for a more immediate effect, however it becomes minimally effective after a few doses. Glucocorticoids are useful for vitamin D intoxication, granulomatous diseases such as sarcoid, and some malignancies and the effect is seen 1–2 days after starting therapy. Dialysis is required in extreme cases of hypercalcemia.

Hypocalcemia (corrected Ca^{2+} < 8.6 mg/dL)

Surgery can contribute to hypocalcemia if it results in vitamin D deficiency or secondary hypoparathyroidism. Hypocalcemia is associated with acute pancreatitis, although the mechanism is not well understood. Gastrectomy or intestinal bypass can reduce absorption of vitamin D.

Hypocalcemia from hypoparathyroidism is associated with intentional or accidental removal of the parathyroid glands or by interruption of the blood supply. Acute postoperative hypocalcemia should be anticipated in patients undergoing elective parathyroidectomy since it has the potential to be life threatening without close monitoring and treatment [26–30].

Citrate binding of free calcium can cause hypocalcemia, and citrate is used to anticoagulate blood given for transfusion [31]. Significant hypocalcemia should not develop from routine transfusions, but as the volume of transfused blood increases, particularly at a level of massive transfusions defined as the replacement of more than 50% of the blood volume in 12–24 hours, the risk of hypocalcemia also increases. The likelihood of hypocalcemia is further increased for patients with preexisting liver disease or acute hepatic dysfunction since the citrate is metabolized in the liver.

The symptoms of hypocalcemia depend both on rate of change of calcium and calcium level. Symptoms of hypocalcemia include fatigue, muscular weakness, irritability, confusion, hallucinations, paranoia, and depression. If acute or severe, there may be paresthesias of lips or extremities, muscle cramps, tetany, laryngeal stridor, or seizures.

Management of hypocalcemia

Symptomatic hypocalcemia should be treated with IV calcium; 10% calcium gluconate (90 mg elemental calcium per 10 mL) or calcium chloride (272 mg elemental calcium per 10 mL). As mentioned earlier in the section on hyperkalemia treatment, calcium gluconate is preferred because calcium chloride causes tissue necrosis if there is accidental extravasation. Calcium chloride requires a central venous line. An example regimen for active seizures or tetany is an IV bolus of 10 mL of 10% calcium gluconate (90 mg Ca^{2+}) over approximately 4 min followed by 30–60 mL of 10% calcium gluconate mixed in 500–1000 mL of 5% dextrose infused over 6–12 hours [32].

Oral treatment should be initiated when the patient is able to eat with calcium carbonate, calcium gluconate, or calcium lactate. Loop diuretics should be avoided if possible because of their hypercalciuric action. If the oral calcium is insufficient, then vitamin D is often required, especially post-parathyroidectomy.

Hypocalcemia responds poorly to IV calcium administration if there is associated magnesium deficiency. Interestingly, therapeutic use of magnesium sulfate causing supernormal plasma magnesium levels may cause severe hypocalcemia because of suppression of parathyroid hormone (PTH) secretion.

Magnesium disorders

Specific cutoffs for hypomagnesemia and hypermagnesemia are difficult to establish because of poor correlation between total body stores and extracellular concentration, but plasma magnesium levels of 1.7–2.3 mg/dL (0.70–0.95 mmol/L, 1.4–1.9 mEq/L) are considered normal [22,27,29,30,33].

Hypermagnesemia

Hypermagnesemia commonly results from iatrogenic administration including treatment for preeclampsia or eclampsia, or inadvertent administration of excessive doses of magnesium-containing laxatives, supplements, Epsom salts, antacids, or enemas. Clinical manifestations are unusual with plasma magnesium levels < 4.5–5 mg/dL. Nausea, vomiting, cutaneous flushing hyporeflexia, and hypotension may be seen, with hypotension becoming more severe and accompanied by loss of tendon reflexes and muscle weakness for levels > 7–10 mg/dL. Respiratory muscle paralysis is seen with magnesium > 12–15 mg/dL. Complete heart block is seen for Mg^{2+} > 10–15 mg/dL, with cardiac arrest for levels > 15 mg/dL.

Management of hypermagnesemia

Dialysis can be performed for extreme hypermagnesemia. Intravenous calcium (100–200 mg of elemental calcium given over 5–10 min) can be used for temporary stabilization until dialysis can be performed. Additional details on calcium administration can be found in sections on hyperkalemia and hypocalcemia treatment.

Hypomagnesemia

Hypomagnesemia can be caused by decreased intake, increased gastrointestinal losses, or increased renal losses. It is also associated with acute pancreatitis, hungry bone syndrome after parathyroidectomy, diabetic ketoacidosis, and medications such as osmotic diuretics, loop diuretics, and long-term thiazide use.

Decreased oral intake of magnesium is common in alcoholics, and patients who rely on intravenous nutritional support can suffer from inadequate magnesium supplementation in total parenteral nutrition (TPN) or IV fluids. Causes of impaired absorption in the gastrointestinal tract include diarrhea, inflammatory bowel disease, laxative abuse, and surgical resection such as ileostomies.

Neuromuscular abnormalities include hyperreflexia, carpopedal spasm, seizures, and tetany. There is an increase risk of digitalis cardiac toxicity, and ECG manifestations include torsades de pointes, premature ventricular contractions, ventricular tachycardias, and ventricular fibrillation.

Management of hypomagnesemia

Symptomatic or severe hypomagnesemia is treated with intravenous magnesium. Mg^{2+} less than 1.2 mg/dL (1.0 mEq/L = 0.5 mmol/L) should be considered severe. For active seizures or cardiac arrhythmias, an initial dose of 8–16 mEq of Mg^{2+} (1–2 g of $MgSO_4 7H_2O$) given over 2–10 minutes is appropriate. For non-emergent repletion, 64 mEq of Mg^{2+} over 24 hours followed by 32 mEq Mg^{2+} over the subsequent 24 hours is a reasonable regimen. Up to 6 days of 32 mEq may be required. The dose should be reduced by 25–50% with close monitoring of plasma magnesium for GFR < 20–30 mL/min/1.73 m^2.

Oral repletion can be given as magnesium oxide (242 mg = 20 mEq Mg^{2+} per 400 mg tablet) with a typical dose of 400 mg 2–3 times daily. Diarrhea is a common side-effect. Mg chloride, Mg gluconate, Mg lactate, and Mg L-aspartate are other formulations used.

Phosphorus disorders

Hyperphosphatemia (phosphorus > 4.5 mg/dL)

Hyperphosphatemia can result from increased intestinal absorption, intracellular to extracellular shifts, or from decreased renal excretion [26–30,33]. Treatment with excessive phosphorus laxatives or the use of phosphate-containing enemas, particularly in patients with reduced renal function, is a perioperative cause of hyperphosphatemia. Rhabdomyolysis, hemolysis, hyperthermia, tumor lysis, and severe catabolic stress can cause cellular shifts. Acute hyperphosphatemia may cause pruritus but otherwise is generally asymptomatic unless accompanied by a rapid change in plasma calcium.

Management of hyperphosphatemia

For normal renal function or mild to moderate decreases in renal function, the kidneys can often readily excrete phosphorus and the key intervention is to reduce phosphorus load. Ensuring adequate volume repletion is useful for patients with normal renal function. In patients with reduced renal function, dietary restriction is combined with administration of oral phosphate binders such as calcium acetate, sevelamer, or lanthanum carbonate, which must be taken with meals to be effective. Dialysis removes phosphorus, although hemodialysis performed 3 times per week removes an amount of phosphorus less than typical weekly intake, and dialysis is predominantly performed for indications other than hyperphosphatemia.

Hypophosphatemia (phosphorus < 2.5 mg/dL)

Hypophosphatemia can occur with decreased intestinal absorption, increased gastrointestinal losses, excess renal wasting, or extracellular to intracellular shifts. Phosphorus levels less than 2.5 mg/dL are considered moderate and levels less than 1.0 mg/dL are considered severe. Respiratory alkalosis can cause a cellular shift and decrease plasma phosphorus to severe levels. A sudden influx of phosphorus into cells may be induced by feeding a malnourished patient (refeeding syndrome). Moderate to severe hypophosphatemia can cause muscle weakness and contribute to difficulty weaning from a vent. It is also a risk factor for rhabdomyolysis. Hemolysis, impaired white blood cell and platelet function, and rarely neurologic disorders can also occur.

Management of hypophosphatemia

For patients who can tolerate oral nutrition, milk is a preferred treatment since it includes both phosphorus and vitamin D, which assists with phosphorus absorption. Sodium or potassium phosphate salts are other options. Intravenous phosphorus can be given as sodium phosphate (4.0 mEq/mL of sodium per 3 mmol/mL of phosphorus), or for patients who also need potassium, as potassium phosphate (4.4 mEq/mL of potassium per 3 mmol/mL of phosphorus). An appropriate rate for initial IV repletion in a patient with severe hypophosphatemia (< 1 mg/dL) without renal insufficiency is 15–30 mmol infused over 6 hours. Doses up to 15 mmol infused over 6 hours can be used for patients with decreased renal function or who are on dialysis.

Acid-base disorders

Definitions

Blood pH is maintained between 7.35 and 7.45, with pH below 7.35 referred to as acidemia and pH greater than 7.45 referred to as alkalemia. The metabolic and respiratory abnormalities that contribute include metabolic acidosis, metabolic alkalosis, respiratory acidosis, and respiratory alkalosis [34–38].

Respiratory and metabolic components are related by the modified Henderson–Hasselbalch equation, which can be used to check for internal consistency between measured quantities. pCO_2 is the arterial CO_2 in mmHg and $[HCO_3^-]$ is the plasma concentration of bicarbonate in mmol/L (= mEq/L).

$$pH = -\log[H^+] = -\log[24 \times 10^{-9}(pCO_2)/[HCO_3^-]] \quad (28.5)$$

For normal values of $pCO_2 = 40$ mmHg and $[HCO_3^-] = 24$ mmol/L, Equation 28.5 yields pH $= -\log[40 \times 10^{-9}] = 7.40$. If values of pH and pCO_2 from an arterial blood gas (ABG) and the $[HCO_3^-]$ from a plasma chemistry are not internally consistent, then improper collection or different collection times with a change in clinical status are likely explanations.

Metabolic acidosis

Calculation of the plasma anion gap ($[Na^+] - [Cl^-] - [HCO_3^-]$) assists in establishing a differential diagnosis for metabolic acidosis [39]. The average anion gap measured in healthy individuals has ranged from 6–15 mEq/L, with lower values seen with the recent use of ion selective electrodes. Elevation of the anion gap is generally due to the production of organic acids or decreased excretion of anions and net acid with renal failure. The most common anions are lactate (lactic acidosis) and beta-hydroxybutyrate plus acetoacetate (ketoacidosis). There is a significant reduction in the chance of identifying the identity of the anion causing an elevated anion gap acidosis for anion gaps less than approximately 24 mEq/L.

A non-anion gap metabolic acidosis is also referred to as a hyperchloremic metabolic acidosis because of the increase in $[Cl^-]$ accompanying the decrease in $[HCO_3^-]$. Bowel fluids, pancreatic secretions, and biliary secretions are high in HCO_3^-, so diarrhea, GI drainage or fistulae, and urinary diversion to bowel are associated with postoperative hyperchloremic metabolic acidosis.

Renal loss of $[HCO_3^-]$ is another cause of hyperchloremic metabolic acidosis that leads to a renal tubular acidosis (RTA). In some cases, such as when GI losses are not severe, it may be difficult to distinguish GI losses from renal losses as the cause of the acidosis. The urine anion gap (UAG) is given by: UAG = $[Na^+] + [K^+] - [Cl^-]$ and is useful in this setting [40].

A negative UAG reflects an ability of the kidney to produce NH_4^+ and is consistent with a non-renal cause such as GI loss. A positive UAG reflects an inability of the kidney to produce adequate NH_4^+ and suggests a renal cause such as an RTA.

Another potential cause of postsurgical hyperchloremic metabolic acidosis is the infusion of large volumes of normal saline. Dilution and renal wasting of $[HCO_3^-]$ are thought to be contributing mechanisms. Recent British consensus guidelines [41] include the recommendation "because of the risk of inducing hyperchloraemic acidosis in routine practice, when crystalloid resuscitation or replacement is indicated, balanced salt solutions, e.g., Ringer's lactate/acetate or Hartmann's solution should replace 0.9% saline, except in cases of hypochloraemia, e.g., from vomiting or gastric drainage." This recommendation, however, has been challenged and the evidence for harm from normal saline called "circumstantial and inconsequential" [42].

Hyperchloremic metabolic acidosis can also result from administration of parenteral nutrition with a high $[Cl^-]$/acetate ratio. Increasing the amount of acetate and reducing the $[Cl^-]$ will result in less acid build-up.

With severe acidemia associated with lactic acidosis or ketoacidosis, the key to treatment is elimination of the source of the organic anions, but clinicians are often faced with a decision regarding administration of base. Decreased cardiac function is often cited as a reason to treat, but clear evidence of benefit is lacking. Base such as bicarbonate is administered with or without dialysis depending on clinical conditions.

Without clear guidelines, a previous survey of critical care specialists and nephrologists sheds light on current practice [43]. Eighty-six percent of nephrologists and 67% of critical care specialists would administer base to patients with severe lactic acidosis, while 60% of nephrologists and 28% of critical care specialists would administer base for severe ketoacidosis. Of those who would give base, a cumulative (summing those who would require pH < 7.1, < 7.0, or < 6.9) 63% of critical care specialists and 40% of nephrologists would require pH < 7.1, including 35% of critical care specialists and only 6% of nephrologists who would require pH < 7.0. A majority of practitioners would target a pH of 7.2 as the goal once the decision to administer base is made.

Metabolic alkalosis

Gastric drainage, usually through a nasogastric tube, or vomiting cause depletion of H^+ and simultaneous loss of Na^+ and Cl^- that result in metabolic alkalosis. The accuracy of the term "contraction alkalosis" has been questioned with a recommendation to replace it with "Cl depletion metabolic alkalosis" to emphasize the role of Cl^- loss [44].

Metabolic alkalosis associated with loss of chloride (chloride responsive) can be distinguished from metabolic alkaloses not associated with chloride loss (chloride resistant) by measuring the urine chloride. A spot urine chloride < 10–20 mmol/L is associated with chloride responsive metabolic alkalosis such as vomiting or nasogastric suction and the alkalosis will improve with normal saline treatment. A spot urine chloride > 20–30 mmol/L is associated with sources of metabolic alkaloses which will not respond to administration of normal saline such as hyperaldosteronism or the use of high doses of glucocorticoids.

Metabolic alkalosis can also be seen in surgical patients after rapid correction of hypercapnia (but before renal correction, which requires Cl^-), from loop or thiazide diuretic use, from excess acetate in parenteral nutrition, or due to the infusion of large amounts of blood products [31] as a result of production of HCO_3^- from the citrate anticoagulant.

Treatment of metabolic alkalosis generally involves addressing the underlying cause and infusion of normal saline if chloride responsive. For life-threatening metabolic alkalosis, for example pH > 7.6 with seizures and ventricular arrhythmias, intubation with controlled hypoventilation is an option to raise the arterial CO_2 concentration and lower the blood pH rapidly. This approach has been proposed over sole use of acidic solutions such as HCl because of the potential for a more rapid response with fewer complications [34]. HCl, 0.10–0.15 mol/L infused through a central venous line, can be used as an adjuvant for treatment of severe metabolic alkalosis. Dialysis is another option.

Respiratory acidosis

Respiratory acidosis is associated with an increase in arterial pCO_2 to greater than 45 mmHg. A variety of acute causes can be seen in surgical patients including decreased central drive secondary to anesthesia, narcotics, other sedatives, or cerebral pathology, and suboptimal ventilation from lung injury, pulmonary edema, or airway obstruction. Electrolyte abnormalities discussed earlier in this chapter can be involved, including acute hyponatremia causing cerebral edema and decreased respiratory drive, and severe hypokalemia, causing muscle dysfunction and respiratory failure. Numerous chronic causes of respiratory acidosis can also be encountered, including chronic obstructive pulmonary disease, chronic upper airway flow limitations, or depressed central drive.

A priority in management of respiratory acidosis is maintenance of adequate oxygenation in addition to reversing underlying etiologies when possible. Additional management steps require a careful balance including avoidance of pulmonary trauma from large tidal volumes (if intubated), considering and minimizing the negative effect of elevated $PaCO_2$ on brain pathology, especially when there is increased intracranial pressure, and avoidance of severe posthypercapnic alkalosis which can result from overly rapid correction.

Respiratory alkalosis

Respiratory alkalosis is associated with a decrease in arterial pCO_2 to less than 35 mmHg and is a result of increased ventilation. Examples of causes include stimulated respiratory drive secondary to hypoxemia, iatrogenic hyperventilation, hepatic failure, or septicemia; increased central drive from pain, anxiety, or brain pathology; pregnancy; and a variety of pulmonary abnormalities including pulmonary embolism.

Correction of the cause of respiratory alkalosis and management includes a priority of maintaining adequate oxygenation plus avoidance of too rapid a correction, which can lead to reperfusion injury in the brain and lung.

References

1. Berl T, Schrier RW. Disorders of water homeostasis. In Schrier RW, ed. *Renal and Electrolyte Disorders*. 7th edn. Philadelphia, PA: Lippincott Williams & Wilkins; 2010.

2. Parikh C, Berl T. Disorders of water metabolism. In Feehally J, Floege J, Johnson RJ, eds. *Comprehensive Clinical Nephrology*. 3rd edn. Philadelphia, PA: Mosby; 2007.

3. Adrogue HJ, Madias NE. Hypernatremia. *N Engl J Med* 2000; **342**: 1493–9.

4. Adrogue HJ, Madias NE. Hyponatremia. *N Engl J Med* 2000; **342**: 1581–9.

5. Dennen P, Linas S. Hypernatremia. In Greenberg A, ed. *Primer on Kidney Diseases*. 5th edn. Philadelphia, PA: Elsevier; 2009.

6. Sterns RH, Nigwekar SU, Hix JK. The treatment of hyponatremia. *Semin Nephrol* 2009; **29**: 282–99.

7. Issa MM, Young MR, Bullock AR, Bouet R, Petros JA., Dilutional hyponatremia of TURP syndrome: a historical event in the 21st century. *Urology* 2004. **64**: 298–301.

8. Chung HM, Kluge R, Schrier RW, Anderson RJ. Postoperative hyponatremia. A prospective study. *Arch Intern Med* 1986; **146**: 333–6.

9. Steele A, Gowrishankar M, Abrahamson S *et al.* Postoperative hyponatremia despite near-isotonic saline infusion: a phenomenon of desalination. *Ann Intern Med* 1997; **126**: 20–5.

10. Arieff AI. Hyponatremia, convulsions, respiratory arrest, and permanent brain damage after elective surgery in healthy women. *N Engl J Med* 1986; **314**: 1529–35.

11. Ayus JC, Wheeler JM, Arieff AI. Postoperative hyponatremic encephalopathy in menstruant women. *Ann Intern Med* 1992; **117**: 891–7.

12. Moritz ML, Ayus JC. 100 cc 3% sodium chloride bolus: a novel treatment for hyponatremic encephalopathy. *Metab Brain Dis* 2010; **25**: 91–6.

13. Sterns RH, Emmett M. Fluid, electrolyte, and acid-base disturbances. *NephSap* 2011; **10**: 147.

14. Laureno R, Karp BI. Myelinolysis after correction of hyponatremia. *Ann Intern Med* 1997; **126**: 57–62.

15. Sterns RH, Hix JK. Overcorrection of hyponatremia is a medical emergency. *Kidney Int* 2009; **76**: 587–9.

16. Rahman M, Friedman WA. Hyponatremia in neurosurgical patients: clinical guidelines development. *Neurosurgery* 2009; **65**: 925–35; discussion 935–6.

17. Woo CH, Rao VA, Sheridan W, Flint AC. Performance characteristics of a sliding-scale hypertonic saline infusion protocol for the treatment of acute neurologic hyponatremia. *Neurocrit Care* 2009; **11**: 228–34.

18. Fenske W, Allolio B. The syndrome of inappropriate secretion of antidiuretic hormone: diagnostic and therapeutic advances. *Horm Metab Res* 2010; **42**: 691–702.

19. Ellison DH, Berl T. Clinical practice. The syndrome of inappropriate antidiuresis. *N Engl J Med* 2007; **356**: 2064–72.

20. Palevsky PM, Bhagrath R, Greenberg A. Hypernatremia in hospitalized patients. *Ann Intern Med* 1996; **124**: 197–203.

21. Nemergut EC, Zuo Z, Jane JA Jr, Laws ER Jr. Predictors of diabetes insipidus after transsphenoidal surgery: a review of 881 patients. *J Neurosurg* 2005; **103**: 448–54.

22. Gorbatkin SM, Schlanger L, Bailey JL. Potassium and magnesium disorders. In McKean SM, Dressler JRD, Brotman D, Ginsberg J, eds. *Principles and Practice of Hospital Medicine*. New York, NY: McGraw-Hill; 2011.

23. Weiner ID, Linas SL, Wingo CS. Disorders of potassium metabolism. In Feehally J, Floege J, Johnson RJ, eds.

Comprehensive Clinical Nephrology. 3rd edn. Philadelphia, PA: Mosby; 2007.

24. Kamel KS, Oh MS, Lin S-H, Halperin ML. Treatment of hypokalemia and hyperkalemia. In Wilcox CS, ed. *Therapy in Nephrology and Hypertension*. 3rd edn. Philadelphia, PA: Elsevier; 2008.

25. Palmer BF, Dubose TD. Disorders of potassium metabolism. In Schrier RW, ed. *Renal and Eletrolyte Disorders*. 7th edn. Philadelphia, PA: Lippincott; 2010.

26. Popovtzer MM. Disorders of calcium, phosphorus, vitamin D, and parathyroid hormone activity. In Schrier RW, ed. *Renal and Eletrolyte Disorders*. 7th edn. Philadelphia, PA: Lippincott; 2010.

27. Pollak MR, Yu ASL, Taylor EN. Disorders of calcium, magnesium, and phosphate balance. In Brenner BM, Levine SA, eds. *Brenner and Rector's The Kidney*. 8th edn. Philadelphia, PA: Elsevier; 2008.

28. Saifullah A, Moe SM. Disorders of calcium and phosphorus. In Greenberg A, ed. *Primer on Kidney Diseases*. 5th edn. Philadelphia, PA: Elsevier; 2009.

29. Nouri P, Llach F. Hypercalcemia, hypocalcemia, and other divalent cation disorders. In Wilcox CS, ed. *Therapy in Nephrology & Hypertension*. 3rd edn. Philadelphia, PA: Elsevier; 2008.

30. Drueke TB, Lacour B. Disorders of calcium, phosphate, and magnesium metabolism. In Feehally J, Floege J, Johnson RJ, eds. *Comprehensive Clinical Nephrology*. 3rd edn. Philadelphia, PA: Elsevier; 2007.

31. Sihler KC, Napolitano LM. Complications of massive transfusion. *Chest* 2010; **137**: 209–20.

32. Pak CYC. Calcium disorders: hypercalcemia and hypocalcemia. In Kokko JP, Tannen RL, eds. *Fluids and Electrolytes*. 2nd edn. Philadelphia, PA: W.B. Saunders; 1990, p. 596.

33. Yu ASL. Disorders of magnesium and phosphorus. In Goldman L, Ausiello D, eds. *Cecil Medicine*. 23rd edn. Philadelphia, PA: Elsevier, 2008.

34. Ratnam S, Kaehny W, Shapiro JI. Pathogenesis and management of metabolic acidosis and alkalosis. In Schrier RW, ed. *Renal and Electrolyte Disorders*. 7th edn. Philadelphia, PA: Lippincott; 2010.

35. Kaehny WD. Pathophysiology and management of respiratory and mixed acid-base disorders. In Schrier RW, ed. *Renal and Electrolyte Disorders*. 7th edn. Philadelphia, PA: Lippincott; 2010.

36. Androgue HJ, Madias NE. Respiratory acidosis, respiratory alkalosis, and mixed disorders. In Feehally J, Floege J, Johnson RJ, eds. *Comprehensive Clinical Nephrology*. Philadelphia, PA: Elsevier; 2007.

37. Kaplan LJ, Kellum JA. Fluids, pH, ions and electrolytes. *Curr Opin Crit Care* 2010; **16**: 323–31.

38. Tanrikut C, McDougal WS. Acid-base and electrolyte disorders after urinary diversion. *World J Urol* 2004; **22**: 168–71.

39. Kraut JA, Madias NE. Serum anion gap: its uses and limitations in clinical medicine. *Clin J Am Soc Nephrol* 2007; **2**: 162–74.

40. Batlle DC, Hizon M, Cohen E, Gutterman C, Gupta R. The use of the urinary anion gap in the diagnosis of hyperchloremic metabolic acidosis. *N Engl J Med* 1988; **318**: 594–9.

41. Powell-Tuck J, Gosling P, Lobo D *et al.* Summary of the British Consensus Guidelines on Intravenous Fluid Therapy for Adult Surgical Patients (GIFTASUP) – for comment. *J Intensive Care Soc* 2009; **10**: 13–15.

42. Soni, N. British Consensus Guidelines on Intravenous Fluid Therapy for Adult Surgical Patients (GIFTASUP): Cassandra's view. *Anaesthesia* 2009; **64**: 235–8.

43. Kraut JA, Kurtz I. Use of base in the treatment of acute severe organic acidosis by nephrologists and critical care physicians: results of an online survey. *Clin Exp Nephrol* 2006; **10**: 111–17.

44. Galla JH, Luke RG. We come to bury contraction alkalosis, not to praise it. *NephSap* 2011; **10**: 91–5.

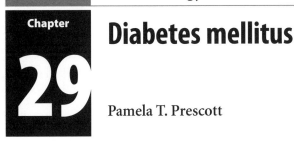

Diabetes mellitus

Pamela T. Prescott

Surgery has major effects on carbohydrate metabolism and thus presents special risks for patients with diabetes. Surgical mortality rates for patients with diabetes have declined but the successful perioperative care of these patients requires close cooperation between surgeons, anesthesiologists, and primary physicians to prevent complications. There are 25.8 million children and adults in the USA with diabetes – 8.3% of the population [1]. Diabetes is listed as a diagnosis on 23% of hospital discharges [2]. At least half of these patients will require surgery at some point in their lives. In addition to surgical conditions typical of the general population, patients with diabetes have an increased incidence of occlusive vascular disease; cholelithiasis; ophthalmic disease (i.e., cataract extraction, vitrectomy); renal disease; and infection. Three of four patients with diabetes are older than 40 years and are approaching a time of life when surgical indications increase. The presence of diabetes typically is known prior to surgery, although a new diagnosis of diabetes is made in the perioperative period in as many as 12% of cases [3].

Hyperglycemia in the hospital is common and may result from stress, infection, effect of procedures, or is iatrogenic [4]. Previously, glucose levels between 100 and 200 mg/dL were not treated in the perioperative period. This practice was challenged by studies suggesting that more aggressive treatment of elevated glucose levels with insulin reduces infectious complications, decreases mortality, and decreases length of hospital stay [5–7]. Many hospitals developed programs, and started treating both medical and surgical patients with intensive insulin therapy to maintain blood glucose at or below 110 mg/dL, particularly in ICU settings. But, following studies performed in other ICUs, particularly medical ones, failed to reproduce the beneficial effects of intensive insulin therapy. In fact, intensive insulin therapy increased the risk of death [8–11]. One study demonstrated a 2.6% absolute increase in 90-day mortality in patients randomized to tight glucose control [10]. This may have been related to the increased risk for hypoglycemia in the intensive insulin group [12].

There is insufficient evidence at this time to support strict glycemic control in the intra- and postoperative period among surgical patients [13]. The current recommendations are the following [4,14]:

1. In critically ill patients, insulin therapy should be started for persistent hyperglycemia > 180 mg/dL.
2. Once insulin therapy is started, a goal is a glucose level in the range of 140–180 mg/dL.
3. In non-critically ill patients on insulin, goal pre-meal blood glucose targets are generally < 140 mg/dL with random blood glucose < 180 mg/dL.

Pathophysiology

The endocrine pancreas, which consists of the islets of Langerhans, accounts for less than 3% of the total pancreatic mass in adults. The islets are unevenly distributed through the pancreas and contain four cell types: A (α) cells, which secrete glucagons; B (β) cells, which secrete insulin; D (δ) cells, which secrete somatostatin; and F cells, which secrete pancreatic polypeptide. Insulin, the major secretory product, is synthesized as a precursor molecule, preproinsulin, in the endoplasmic reticulum and is cleaved by microsomal enzymes to proinsulin. Proinsulin is then converted by proteolysis to insulin and an amino acid residue, c-peptide. After secretion into the portal venous system, insulin passes through the liver and the portion that is not extracted enters the peripheral circulation. There it binds to specific cell-surface receptors, initiating multiple phosphorylations of receptor and intra-cellular proteins and the internalization of the insulin–receptor complex.

The normal basal production of insulin is about 1 U/hour, with an additional 3 to 5 U produced after meals. The usual fasting serum insulin concentration is 10 μU/mL; peak postprandial values rarely exceed 100 μU/mL. Endogenous insulin, which has a half-life of less than 5 minutes in plasma, is metabolized by hepatic and renal insulinases [15]. Its major function is to promote the storage of ingested nutrients in many tissues, especially the liver, muscle, and fat. The major biologic effects are outlined in Table 29.1. Deficiency or reduced effectiveness of insulin has profound consequences on metabolism.

Medical Management of the Surgical Patient, ed. Michael F. Lubin, Thomas F. Dodson, and Neil H. Winawer. Published by Cambridge University Press. © Cambridge University Press 2013.

Table 29.1 Major biologic effects of insulin.

Organ or system	Effect
Liver	Promotes glycogen synthesis and storage, inhibits glycogenolysis Promotes triglyceride, very low-density lipoprotein, and cholesterol synthesis Inhibits ketogenesis Promotes glycolysis, inhibits gluconeogenesis
Fat	Promotes triglyceride storage, inhibits lipolysis
Muscle	Promotes protein synthesis Promotes glycogen synthesis and storage
Vascular	Promotes lipoprotein lipase activity

Diabetes mellitus is a metabolic condition characterized by elevated glucose levels resulting from defects in insulin secretion, insulin action, or both. Diabetes mellitus is classified as type 1 diabetes (caused by an absolute deficiency of insulin secretion), and type 2 diabetes (caused by a combination of insulin resistance to insulin action and inadequate insulin secretory response). Occasionally, hyperglycemia can occur in individuals who have other conditions and who have a predisposition for diabetes mellitus. These conditions include sepsis, pancreatitis, corticosteroid use, Cushing's syndrome, pregnancy (gestational diabetes), thyrotoxicosis, acromegaly, glucagonoma, pheochromocytoma, cirrhosis, and obesity [16,17]. Diabetes mellitus is diagnosed when [4]:

1. HbA1c > 6.5%, or
2. The fasting glucose level is > 126 mg/dL, or
3. Random glucose is > 200 mg/dL with classic symptoms (polyuria, polydipsia, unexplained weight loss), or
4. 2-hour glucose tolerance test glucose of > 200 mg/dL (glucose load 75 g).

Patients with type 1 diabetes (10–20% of all patients with diabetes in the USA) typically have circulating antibodies to islet cells and insulin that precedes the clinical manifestations of the disease and persists for a few years after the onset of illness. Patients with type 1 diabetes secrete little insulin, are prone to ketosis, and require insulin for treatment. Patients with type 2 diabetes commonly are obese (85%), are not prone to ketosis, and demonstrate insulin resistance that precedes impaired insulin secretion.

Effects of diabetes on surgery

Surgical mortality rates for patients with diabetes have declined substantially over the years with improved perioperative care. Uncomplicated diabetes is no longer associated with an increased mortality rate after cholecystectomy or peripheral vascular surgery and is associated with only a slightly increased risk after coronary artery bypass grafting. Nonetheless,

multiple anatomic and functional complications of the disease do introduce specific problems during surgery.

Infection and poor wound healing are the most common postoperative complications in patients with diabetes. Diabetic patients who undergo major surgery are at increased risk for postoperative infections compared with non-diabetic patients. Several factors may contribute to the increased incidence of infection in diabetic patients, including impairment of the immune response, especially the response of neutrophils. Neutrophils isolated from diabetic patients demonstrate impaired activity in chemotaxis, oxidative burst, and phagocytosis [18]. Perioperative stress also can worsen hyperglycemia. Counter-regulatory hormone, tumor necrosis factors, and cytokines can impair the function of insulin and cause hyperglycemia [19,20]. Stress-induced hyperglycemia can worsen ischemic events following myocardial infarction and cerebral stroke.

The mechanisms causing the increased incidence may include impairment of cardiac contractility, increase in the frequency of arrhythmias, impairment of the endothelium-dependent vasorelaxation and increased thrombosis. Controlling or normalizing the glucose levels before, during, and after surgery significantly decreases mortality, decreases myocardial infarction and reinfarction rates, decreases incidence of congestive heart failure (CHF), and cerebral vascular events [16–20]. Controlling blood glucose levels also shortens hospital stay.

The chronic complications of diabetes may also complicate surgery. The presence of neuropathy, particularly autonomic neuropathy, places patients at increased risk for perioperative cardiac arrest. Resting tachycardia or little compensatory change in the pulse (with deep inspiration or exercise) are warning signs and should encourage close postoperative cardiac and respiratory monitoring. The presence of gastroparesis increases the risk of aspiration, and appropriate perioperative therapy with metoclopramide and H_2 blockers is indicated. Ileus and urinary retention are additional complications of autonomic neuropathy. Renal disease can complicate fluid and electrolyte management. Of critical importance is macrovascular disease affecting coronary, cerebral, and peripheral vessels. Cardiac morbidity and death are also predicted by preexisting CHF and valvular disease. Non-cardiac vascular complications are best predicted by the presence of retinopathy, neuropathy, nephropathy, CHF, and peripheral vascular disease.

Effects of surgery (stress) on diabetes

Patients who do not have diabetes sometimes develop hyperglycemia due to the stress of surgery. Marked elevations are reached in intraoperative and postoperative levels of the counter-regulatory hormones (glucagons, catecholamines, cortisol, and growth hormone). Experimental data indicate that the effects of these hormones are synergistic. In diabetes, the effects of stress are magnified by limited insulin availability or effectiveness. Furthermore, insulin release is significantly depressed during surgery. The hormonal milieu fosters hyperglycemia, and the markedly increased ratio of glucagon to insulin can result in ketoacidosis.

Care of surgical patients with diabetes

A careful history, physical examination, and selected laboratory tests (e.g., blood count, urinalysis, fasting blood glucose level, electrolyte levels, creatinine level, hemoglobin A_{1c}, electrocardiogram, home glucose monitoring records) provide information regarding specific risk factors and assist in the care of surgical patients with diabetes. When possible, optimal control of diabetes should be achieved before surgery, although early admission to the hospital for this purpose often is not possible because of diagnosis-related group regulations.

Surgery should be performed early in the day to limit the time that patients are without food and are not receiving their usual treatment regimens. The goal of diabetes management in the perioperative period is to prevent marked hyperglycemia, ketosis, postoperative infections, and impaired wound healing, while also preventing unrecognized and potentially fatal hypoglycemia. This requires an intensive, coordinated effort between the internist or endocrinologist, surgeon, anesthesiologist, and nursing staff. Frequent and precise monitoring of the perioperative glucose level is the most important factor in achieving optimal control.

Patients with type 1 diabetes

Patients with type 1 diabetes always require insulin before, during, and after surgery. Insulin cannot be withheld, even if the patient is not eating and is NPO. Insulin can be administered subcutaneously (by injection or via an insulin pump), intramuscularly, or intravenously. Several approaches exist for preoperative insulin management. If the patient is using an insulin pump, the insulin pump can be left to infuse at the patient's usual basal rate preoperatively. If the patient takes intermediate acting insulin in the morning, one-third to one-half the usual dose could be given. If the patient takes short-acting insulin before each meal and intermediate acting insulin at night, the intermediate acting insulin should be given the night before the surgical procedure, and half the usual short-acting insulin dose should be given on the morning of the procedure. An infusion including 5% dextrose should be started while the patient is NPO to prevent catabolism. The blood glucose should be monitored every 1–2 hours and supplemental insulin should be given to maintain normal glycemia.

Treatment with a regular insulin intravenous infusion can be started at any time. Guidelines for adjusting the insulin infusion include the following.

1. Increased insulin needs to be expected with the stress of surgery, sepsis, surgical procedures, glucose-containing intravenous solutions, and hypothermia.

2. Until patients can resume their usual diets, intravenous insulin therapy remains the optimal mode of therapy.

3. Insulin half-life is about 5–10 minutes and the biological half-life is 20–30 minutes. Total discontinuation of the insulin drip is promptly associated with catabolism leading to hyperglycemia and subsequent ketosis.

4. Thus, a dose or subcutaneous regular insulin should be given 30 minutes before the insulin infusion is stopped.

Patients with type 2 diabetes

For minor surgery, most patients with diet-controlled type 2 diabetes do not require insulin treatment. Patients who are taking the shorter-acting sulfonylureas (glipizide, tolbutamide, tolazimide), glinides (repaglinide, nateglinide), alpha-glucocidase inhibitors (acarbose), and biguanides (metformin) should hold the doses the day of surgery. Patients who are taking the longer-acting agents (glimepiride, glyburide) should hold the doses the day before and the day of surgery. Blood glucose levels should be checked every 6 hours. When perioperative insulin is required, it should be giving using a sliding scale with intravenous dextrose running at 100 mL/hour.

Patients with type 2 diabetes who normally use insulin can be treated in the perioperative period by the traditional method using sliding-scale regular insulin (see section on insulin therapy below). Patients with type 2 diabetes who are undergoing major surgery are best treated with continuous intravenous insulin infusion if adequate glucose monitoring is available.

Postoperative care

In the postoperative period, all patients with diabetes must be closely monitored to prevent both hyperglycemia and hypoglycemia. As soon as possible, patients should resume their usual diets and regimens of insulin or oral hypoglycemic agents. Because of the increased risk of postoperative infection, wound care must be assiduous and devices such as Foley and vascular catheters should be removed as soon as possible. In patients at high risk for coronary events, postoperative electrocardiographic monitoring can be helpful to monitor for new changes. With careful glucose monitoring and insulin infusions as needed, patients with diabetes can safely undergo major surgical procedures.

Insulin therapy

The following are definitions and guidelines for starting and adjusting subcutaneous and intravenous insulin [22–26].

1. Definitions

| **Basal insulin** | intermediate or long-acting insulin required for continuous 24-hour coverage, e.g., Lantus® (glargine), NPH and Levemir (detemir). No relationship to food intake. |

Nutrition insulin scheduled short-acting insulin given to cover for meals, tube feedings, or parenteral nutrition, e.g., regular (Novolin®), Novolog® (aspart), and Humalog® (lispro).

Correction insulin short-acting insulin that is given in addition to scheduled prandial insulin (or given at other times of the day) as a response to pre-existing high blood glucose levels.

Total Daily Dose of Insulin (TDDI) is calculated by adding all prescribed insulin types (basal, prandial, and correction insulin).

2. Bedside blood glucose monitoring.

- If the patient is eating or receiving bolus tube feedings: QAC (before meals) and QHS (at bedtime).
- If patient is NPO: every 6 hours.
- If patient receives continuous tube feedings or parenteral nutrition (PN): every 6 hours.
- For unstable patients, when their condition is fluctuating: four to five times a day (before meals, at bedtime, and at 3:00 in the morning).
- When correction insulin is given at bedtime additional mandatory blood glucose (BG) check at 3:00 in the morning.

3. Approach to ordering a subcutaneous insulin regimen:

A. Calculate the estimated Total Daily Dose of Insulin (TDDI) patient may require.

It can be done in one of three different ways:

i. You may use a patient's total home dose (if on insulin).
ii. If you don't know where to start, calculate a weight-based TDDI:

Weight-based estimation: TDDI (in units) = the patient's weight (in kg) × N (see Table 29.2).

iii. Calculate TDDI based on recent insulin infusion requirement: use an average insulin infusion rate during a relatively steady-state period in the last 6 hours, and multiply this hourly rate by 24 (hours). Patient with type 2 diabetes will require 80% and with type 1 approximately 60–70% of what you have calculated:

Type 2: TDDI = unit/hour × 24 × 0.8.
Type 1: TDDI = unit/hour × 24 × 0.7.

B. Calculate the basal insulin requirement. Most patients with diabetes require basal insulin. In general, insulin-dependent patients or patients with persistent hyperglycemia on short-acting insulin must have basal insulin. Some patients with mild hyperglycemia/type 2 diabetes may not require basal insulin.

In patients who are eating, about half the TDDI is basal and the other half is for nutrition. A good estimate is 50% of the total daily insulin need is basal insulin when using Lantus® and 66% (two-thirds) when using twice daily NPH insulin as the basal insulin. When using Lantus® the 50/50 rule has the advantage of being easy to remember and to calculate (Table 29.3). However, in some settings, a ratio of 40/60 (or lower) is preferred.

Lantus®: basal insulin = TDDI × 0.5; give once daily.
NPH: basal insulin = TDDI × 0.66; divide between two injections/day.

Table 29.2 Calculation of "N" for estimation of Total Daily Dose of Insulin.

Patients who are:	N =
Malnourished, elderly, chronic kidney disease (on dialysis), severe liver disease, or insulin naïve	0.3
Without clear features of insulin sensitivity or resistance (most patients)	0.4
Overweight	0.5
Obese, receiving high doses of corticosteroids or known to be insulin resistant	0.6–0.8

Table 29.3 Lantus® insulin adjustment schedule.

Fasting blood glucose (mg/dL)	Current Lantus® dose (units)/adjustment dose (units)			
	< 30 units	30–60 units	61–90 units	90 + units
< 60	Decrease 3 units	Decrease 5 units	Decrease 6 units	Decrease 8 units
60–79	Decrease 1 units	Decrease 2 units	Decrease 3 units	Decrease 4 units
80–110	no change	no change	no change	no change
111–160	+ 1 unit	+ 2 units	+ 3 units	+ 4 units
161–210	+ 2 units	+ 4 units	+ 6 units	+ 8 units
211–260	+ 3 units	+ 6 units	+ 9 units	+ 12 units
261–310	+ 4 units	+ 8 units	+ 12 units	+ 16 units
> 310	+ 5 units	+ 10 units	+ 15 units	+ 20 units

C. Calculate the nutrition insulin requirement.
For patients who are not eating/receiving nutrition, they should not receive nutrition insulin. Basal insulin represents 100% of the total daily insulin needs in NPO patients not receiving nutrition.

Estimation of nutrition insulin dosage can be done in three different ways:

i. Give 50% of TDDI in equally divided doses with each meal. Remember to reduce the insulin dose proportionate to nutritional intake. When patient takes 50% of PO diet, nutrition insulin dose has to be cut by half.

> For example: TDDI (calculated above) = 60 units.
> Basal = 50% TDDI = 30 units Lantus® insulin nightly.
> Bolus = 50% TDDI = 30 units Novolog® total daily, divided amongst meals; = 10 units Novolog® before each meal three times daily.

ii. For each meal, use carbohydrate counting to more accurately determine the amount of nutrition insulin to be given. This approach is preferred in the patient who is transitioning from NPO status or intermittently taking a PO diet.

> For example: TDDI (calculated above) = 60 units.

> Basal insulin = 50% TDDI = 30 units Lantus® insulin nightly.
> Nutrition insulin dose (bolus): use carbohydrate to insulin ratio (CIR).
> CIR can be estimated by 500/TDDI, where CIR is g carb/unit insulin.
> CIR = 500/60 = ~8 g carb/unit Novolog® for a 64 g carb meal.
> Novolog® dose would be: 64 g carb/8 g carb/unit = 8 units Novolog®.

iii. Patients on continuous tube feedings or parenteral nutrition may initially be placed on IV insulin infusion or insulin sliding scale, usually during initiation phase (24–48 hours), to more accurately determine the amount of TDDI the patient requires.

Correction insulin (formerly sliding scale insulin (SSI))

1. Further downward adjustment of elevated blood glucose is achieved through the use of correction doses of short-acting insulin, which may be given at the same time, and in addition to scheduled nutrition insulin. It functions as a third layer of insulin supplementing the basal and nutrition insulin doses. To do this, "correction" doses of the *same* insulin type can be added to adjust for pre-meal hyperglycemia. If the pre-meal BG were higher (or lower) than target, additional insulin would be added to (or subtracted; see correction factor, above).

Correction factor insulin: administer the same type of short-acting insulin in addition to scheduled nutrition insulin (Table 29.4). Rapid-acting analogs (RAA) insulin is preferred.

Bedtime correction insulin (if bedtime correction dose insulin is used, 3:00 am fingerstick blood glucose *must* be monitored): RAA, regular, or NPH insulin can be used as bedtime correction dose insulin depending on the clinical situation (Table 29.5).

2. Prolonged use of insulin sliding scale as the sole form of insulin therapy is strongly discouraged in hospitalized patients. However, in certain patients who are NPO, or in those in whom it is difficult to predict insulin dosing requirements, also patients who are initiated on continuous tube feeding or parenteral nutrition, using SSI for 24–48 hours may be necessary. Consider increasing thresholds for scale initiation in those at high risk of hypoglycemia, such as the malnourished patient with deteriorating renal function, adrenal insufficiency, gastroparesis, hypoglycemia unawareness, or a prior history of "brittle" diabetes. Regular insulin is conventionally used for sliding scale every 6 hours. If RAA insulin is used (not preferred in this setting), dosing should be every 4 hours or QAC.

Table 29.4 Correction doses of insulin.

Total Daily Dose of Insulin (TDDI) (units)	Blood glucose (mg/dL)/subcutaneous insulin dose (units)							
	120–150	151–180	181–210	211–240	241–270	271–300	301–330	331+
≤ 40	-----	1	1	2	2	3	3	4
41–80	1	2	3	4	5	6	7	8
81–120	1	3	4	6	7	9	10	12
121–160	2	4	6	8	10	12	14	16
161+	3	6	9	12	15	18	21	24

RAA insulin not to be given more frequently than every 4 hours and Regular insulin more than every 6 hours.

Table 29.5 Bedtime correction insulin.

Total Daily Dose of Insulin (TDDI) (units)	Blood glucose (mg/dL)/subcutaneous insulin dose (units)					
	181–210	211–240	241–270	271–300	301–330	331+
≤ 40	1	1	2	2	3	3
41–80	2	3	4	5	6	7
81–120	3	4	6	7	9	10
121–160	4	6	8	10	12	14
161+	6	9	12	15	18	21

Table 29.6 Regimen for type 2 diabetes only.

Insulin sensitivity	Blood glucose (mg/dL)/subcutaneous insulin dose (units)							
	< 100	100–150	151–180	181–210	211–250	251–300	301–350	351+
High	0	0	1	1	2	3	4	5
Normal (most patients)	0	0	2	3	4–5	6	8	10
Resistant	0	1	3	4	6–8	10	15	20

Regular insulin is preferred for patients who are NPO, on continuous tube feeding, or TPN (Table 29.6). RAA insulin can be used in patients who are eating, usually as a dose-finding strategy and for a short period of time.

3. Assess and adjust insulin dose daily. Increase TDDI by 20–30% for consistently poor control and decrease by 20–50% for any hypoglycemia. If correction insulin scale is not matching your patient's needs, consider calculating the expected decrease in blood glucose level for one unit of insulin (correction factor (CF)) by using 1,700/TDDI given = correction factor. The correction factor is used to determine the correction dose of insulin for a given blood sugar:

Correction dose insulin = Desired drop (or increase) in blood glucose/CF.

4. Management of hypoglycemia (blood glucose less than 70 mg/dL). Hypoglycemia is commonly over-treated. Intravenous dextrose should only be used if mental status is altered or patient is NPO. Standard treatment is the following.

Patient who is taking food by mouth:

- Give 15 g of fast-acting carbohydrate (150 mL of fruit juice/non-diet soda, 240 mL of non-fat milk, or 3–4 glucose tablets).
- For blood glucose 50–60 mg/dL, give 6 glucose tablets or 240 mL of juice or 25 mL of D50 as IV push.
- For blood glucose less than 50 mg/dL, give 50 mL of D50 as IV push.
- Check BG glucose every 15 minutes and repeat above if BG < 100 mg/dL.
- Start dextrose-containing IV fluid if significant risk of recurrent hypoglycemia.

Patients who are NPO:

- If no IV access give 1 mg of glucagon subcutaneously once and start IV.
- Patient with IV access, give 25 mL of D50 as slow IV push.
- Check BG glucose every 15 minutes and repeat above if BG < 100 mg/dL.
- Start dextrose-containing IV fluid if significant risk of recurrent hypoglycemia.

References

1. 2011 National Diabetes Fact Sheet. American Diabetes Association. www.diabetes.org/diabetes-basics/diabetes-statistics.
2. Newton CA, Young S. Financial implications of glycemic control: results of an inpatient diabetes management program. *Endocr Pract* 2006; **12** (Suppl 3): 43–8.
3. Levetan CS, Passaro M, Jablonski K, Kass M, Ratner RE. Unrecognized diabetes among hospitalized patients. *Diabetes Care* 1998; **21**: 246–9.
4. American Diabetes Association. ADA Clinical Practice Guidelines, 2013. *Diabetes Care* 2013; **36**: 511–66.
5. van den Berghe G, Wouters P, Weekers F *et al.* Intensive insulin therapy in the critically ill patient. *N Engl J Med* 2001; **345**: 1359–67.

6. Garber AJ, Moghissi ES, Bransome ED Jr et al.; American College of Endocrinology Task Force on Inpatient Diabetes Metabolic Control. American College of Endocrinology position statement on inpatient diabetes and metabolic control. *Endocr Pract* 2004; **10**: 77–82.

7. Clement S, Braithwaite SS, Magee MF et al.; American Diabetes Association Diabetes in Hospitals Writing Committee. Management of diabetes and hyperglycemia in hospitals. *Diabetes Care* 2004; **27**: 553–91.

8. van den Berghe G, Wilmer A, Hermans G et al. Intensive insulin therapy in the medical ICU. *N Engl J Med* 2006; **354**: 449–61.

9. Arabi YM, Dabbagh OC, Tamim HM et al. Intensive versus conventional insulin therapy: a randomized controlled trial in medical and surgical critically ill patients. *Crit Care Med* 2008; **36**: 3190–7.

10. Finfer S, Chittock DR, Su SY et al. NICE-SUGAR Study Investigators. Intensive versus conventional glucose control in critically ill patients. *N Engl J Med* 2009; **360**: 1283–97.

11. Lena D, Kalfon P, Preiser JC, Ichai C. Glycemic control in the intensive care unit and during the postoperative period. *Anesthesiology* 2011; **114**: 438–44.

12. Marik PE. Glycemic control in critically ill patients: what to do post NICE-SUGAR? *World J Gastrointest Surg* 2009; **1**: 3–5.

13. Kao LS, Meeks D, Moyer VA, Lally KP. Peri-operative glycaemic control regimens for preventing surgical site infections in adults. *Cochrane Database Syst Rev*. 2009; **3**: CD006806.

14. Qaseem A, Humphrey LL, Chou R, Snow V, Shekelle P; Clinical Guidelines Committee of the American College of Physicians. Use of intensive insulin therapy for the management of glycemic control in hospitalized patients: a clinical practice guideline from the American College of Physicians. *Ann Intern Med* 2011; **154**: 260–7.

15. Grodsky GM, Curry D, Landahl H, Bennett L. Further studies on the dynamic aspects of insulin release in vitro with evidence for a two-compartmental storage system. *Acta Diabetol Lat* 1969; **6** (Suppl 1): 554–78.

16. Preiser JC, Devos P, Van den Berghe G. Tight control of glycaemia in critically ill patients. *Curr Opin Clin Nutr Metab Care* 2002; **5**: 533–7.

17. Golden, SH, Peat-Vigilance C, Kao WH, Brancati FL. Perioperative glycemic control and the risk of infectious complications in a cohort of adults with diabetes. *Diabetes Care* 1999; **22**: 1408–14.

18. Rassias AJ, Givan AL, Marrin CA et al. Insulin increases neutrophil count and phagocytic capacity after cardiac surgery. *Anesth Analg* 2002; **94**: 1113–19.

19. Mizock BA. Alterations in carbohydrate metabolism during stress: a review of the literature. *Am J Med* 1995; **98**: 75–84.

20. McCowen KC, Malhotra A, Bistrian BR. Stress-induced hyperglycemia. *Crit Care Clin* 2001; **17**: 107–24.

21. Capes SE, Hunt D, Malmberg K, Gerstein HC. Stress hyperglycaemia and increased risk of death after myocardial infarction in patients with and without diabetes: a systematic overview. *Lancet* 2000; **355**: 773–8.

22. Bode BW, Braithwaite SS, Steed RD, Davidson PC. Intravenous insulin infusion therapy: indications, methods, and transition to subcutaneous insulin therapy. *Endocr Pract* 2004; **10** (Suppl 2): 71–80.

23. Brown G, Dodek P. Intravenous insulin nomogram improves blood glucose control in the critically ill. *Crit Care Med* 2001; **29**: 1714–19.

24. Beyer J, Krause U, Dobronz A et al. Assessment of insulin needs in insulin-dependent diabetics and healthy volunteers under fasting conditions. *Horm Metab Res* 1990; **24** (Suppl): 71–7.

25. Mokan M, Gerich JE. A simple insulin infusion algorithm for establishing and maintaining overnight near-normoglycemia in type I and type II diabetes. *J Clin Endocrinol Metab* 1992; **74**: 943–5.

26. Chen HJ, Steinke DT, Karounos DG, Lane MT, Matson AW. Intensive insulin protocol implementation and outcomes in the medical and surgical wards at a Veterans Affairs Medical Center. *Ann Pharmacother* 2010; **44**: 249–56.

Chapter

30

Disorders of the thyroid

Pamela T. Prescott

Because thyroid hormones exert regulatory effects on multiple organ systems, thyroid function should be aggressively evaluated and abnormal function treated in patients who require surgery. Thyroid hormones also significantly affect the metabolism of many drugs, and dose adjustments may be required when function is abnormal. Medical consultants performing preoperative evaluations should include clinical assessments of thyroid function and perform confirmatory tests when indicated.

The adult thyroid gland weighs 15–20 g, typically consists of two lobes connected by an isthmus, and is located just below the cricoid cartilage. A remnant of the thyroglossal duct, the pyramidal lobe may be noted arising superiorly from the isthmus or medial side of a lobe. Enlargement of the pyramidal lobe indicates a diffuse thyroidal abnormality. The thyroid gland consists of follicles, which are spheres lined by a single layer of cuboidal cells and are filled with a colloid that is composed primarily of thyroglobulin. A rich capillary network surrounds the follicles, explaining why a bruit is sometimes heard over hyperactive, enlarged thyroid glands. Scattered throughout the thyroid are calcitonin-secreting perifollicular cells. Hyperplasic or malignant transformation of these cells does not result in abnormalities of thyroid function [1–3].

Inorganic iodide is actively transported from the blood into the follicular cells, immediately oxidized by perioxidase, and is rapidly incorporated into the tyrosine residues of thyroglobulin. These monoiodotyrosine and diiodotyrosine residues couple to form the iodothyronines thyroxine (T_4) and triiodothyronine (T_3), which are stored in the follicles. In response to thyroid-stimulating hormone (TSH), follicular cells extend pseudopods into the colloid and take it up by endocytosis. Subsequent hydrolysis of thyroglobulin in cellular lysosomes yields T_4 and, to a lesser extent, T_3, which are then secreted into the blood [4,5].

Thyroid function is closely regulated by the hypothalamic–pituitary–thyroidal axis. Hypothalamic thyrotropin-releasing hormone (TRH) stimulates the synthesis and release of TSH. Secretion of TSH is modulated by negative feedback from T_3 produced in the pituitary by monodeiodination of T_4. The thyroid gland also exhibits autoregulation in response to iodine availability [6,7]. Only 0.03% of T_4 and 0.3% of T_3 circulates as free hormones. The remainder is bound to thyroid-binding globulin (TBG), T_4 binding prealbumin, and albumin. Virtually all circulating T_4 is secreted from the thyroid gland, whereas 85% of T_3 is derived from peripheral deiodination of T_4. Deiodination at the 5′ and 5 positions on T_4 yields T_3 and the biologically inactive reverse T_3 (rT_3), respectively.

A wide variety of tests are available to evaluate thyroid function and effect in individuals with known or suspected thyroid disease. Tests may be classified as those that:

1. Measure the concentration and binding of thyroid products.
2. Directly test thyroid function or anatomy.
3. Assess the hypothalamic pituitary access [5,8].

Measuring thyroid products

The first thyroid test of choice is the highly sensitive TSH assay with a lower detection limit of < 0.01 µU/mL. The TSH measurement can be combined with a single measurement of a free T_4 to improve the detection of thyroid abnormalities. If total T_4 is measured, a T_3 uptake assay is done at the same time to measure the effect of or changes in thyroid-binding proteins. A free thyroid index (FTI) is then calculated [8,9]. The FTI is an estimation of free T_4. If the TSH is low, but the free T_4 is normal, then a free T_3 assay should be obtained. Thyroid antibody assays (antithyroid peroxidase antibodies, antithyroglobulin antibodies, and thyroid-stimulating antibodies) can be done to help determine the cause of a thyroid abnormality. If the TSH, free T_4, and free T_3 are normal, and thyroid antibodies are negative, thyroid disease can be excluded. Measurement of rT_3 is usually not necessary but can help differentiate severe non-thyroidal illness from hypothyroidism because levels are normal to elevated in the former and decreased in the latter [9].

Thyroglobulin is detectable in the serum and is usually elevated in hyperthyroidism and subacute thyroiditis, while being decreased in hypothyroidism and excessive use of

Medical Management of the Surgical Patient, ed. Michael F. Lubin, Thomas F. Dodson, and Neil H. Winawer. Published by Cambridge University Press. © Cambridge University Press 2013.

thyroxine. It is used after thyroid cancer surgery and Iodine 131 ablation to detect residual or recurrent disease [10].

Interpretation of thyroid tests, when a patient is overtly hypothyroid or hyperthyroid, is usually straightforward. The TSH and free T_4 are usually all that is needed to make the diagnosis. There are several conditions, when thyroid antibodies or free T_3 are needed to more clearly identify the condition. Table 30.1 describes six patterns of thyroid function tests and the associated thyroid diseases [11.]

In addition, there are other conditions not mentioned above that can have varying effects on thyroid function tests: these are pregnancy, psychiatric decompensation, chronic renal failure, and non-thyroid illness.

Pregnancy can have significant, but reversible changes in thyroid function tests. Both normal pregnancy, and pregnancy complicated by conditions such as hyperemesis gravidarium can be associated with thyroid function study changes that are strongly suggestive of hyperthyroidism in the absence of thyroid disease. The earliest and most marked change is an elevation in the serum concentrations of T_4 and T_3. The free T_4 and free T_3 are generally in the normal range although they may be slightly elevated in the first trimester and slightly reduced in the third trimester. Placental human chorionic gonadotropin (hCG) shares a common alpha subunit with TSH, but having a unique beta subunit. During gestation hCG acts as a TSH agonist so that elevated levels contribute to a transient increase in thyroid hormone seen in about 0.3% of pregnancies [12]. A TSH level provides the most sensitive index to reliably detect thyroid function abnormalities [13,14].

In the first trimester TSH levels are low when hCG levels are the highest and then gradually return to normal after the second trimester. Persistently suppressed TSH into the second trimester can be seen with molar pregnancies and with hyperemesis gravidarum. Serum thyroglobulin levels gradually elevate throughout the pregnancy and are generally proportional to thyroid mass. Anti-thyroid antibody levels fall through the last trimester of pregnancy, but they can rise during the postpartum period [15,16].

Acute psychiatric decompensation (schizophrenia, major depression, bipolar disorder) causes transient elevation in serum-free T_4 with a suppressed or normal TSH. Individuals with a rapidly cycling bipolar disorder may have a slightly low total T_4 and a high TSH [17,18].

Chronic renal failure can affect thyroid tests. Both plasma T_3 and T_4 are reduced. The low T_3 is due to impaired extrathyroidal T_4 to T_3 conversion, and the reduction in T_4 is due to circulating inhibitors that impair binding of T_4 to TBG. Despite decreased T_4 and T_3, TSH levels are normal. The hypothalamo-pituitary axis remains normal. When renal failure patients become hypothyroid the TSH is elevated and when hyperthyroid, the TSH is suppressed. Thyroid hormone is minimally lost during hemodialysis and peritoneal dialysis and does not require replacement.

Elderly individuals have decreased T_3 levels and lower mean TSH concentrations. Autoimmune thyroid disease is

Table 30.1 Six patterns of thyroid function tests and the associated thyroid diseases [12].

Low TSH, raised free T_3 or T_4	Primary hyperthyroidism (Graves' multinodular goiter, toxic nodule) Subacute, painful thyroiditis (postviral or de Quervain's) Subacute, painless thyroiditis (postpartum) Drug-induced (amiodarone, lithium) Therapeutic (thyroxine ingestion) Factitious Ectopic (struma ovarii, molar pregnancy, choriocarcinoma, gestational hyperthyroidism) Excess iodine ingestion (Jod–Basedow effect)
Low TSH, normal free T_3 or T_4	Therapeutic (thyroxine ingestion, high-dose glucocorticoids, dopamine and dobutamine infusions) Subclinical hyperthyroidism Non-thyroidal illness (euthyroid sick syndrome)
Low or normal TSH, low free T_3 or T_4	Non-thyroidal illness (euthyroid sick syndrome) Pituitary disease (secondary hypothyroidism) Treated hyperthyroidism[a]
Raised TSH, low free T_3 or T_4	Primary hypothyroidism (autoimmune, postsurgical, postablative) Excess iodine ingestion (Wolff–Chaikoff effect) Drug induced (amiodarone, lithium) Reidel's thyroiditis Pendred syndrome
Raised TSH, normal free T_3 or T_4	Subclinical hypothyroidism Antimouse immunoglobulin[b] Malabsorption of thyroxine Amiodarone Pendred syndrome TSH resistance
Normal or raised TSH, raised free T_3 or T_4	Ingestion of high-dose thyroxine just before tests Antibodies to T_4 or T_3 Familial dysalbuminemic hyperthyroxinemia Amiodarone Acute psychiatric disorders Methamphetamines (acute response) TSH-secreting pituitary tumors Thyroid hormone resistance Recovery from non-thyroidal illness

TSH, thyroid-stimulating hormone.
[a] As hyperthyroidism is treated, TSH levels may remain suppressed despite low levels of free T_3 or T_4. The pituitary response may be delayed and the TSH remains suppressed even if the hyperthyroid treatment causes low levels of free T_3 or T_4. During this 2- to 3-month period, the treatment is adjusted according to the free T_3 or T_4 levels.
[b] When TSH does not return to normal after treatment, but T_4 is normal, there may be an anti-mouse immunoglobulin interfering with the TSH assay. Need to repeat with a different assay.

particularly prevalent because the frequency of thyroid antibodies increases with age [19,20].

Non-thyroidal illness (euthyroid sick syndrome) causes change in hormone production so interpretation of thyroid function studies can be difficult [21,22]. In any critical illness there can be a drop in both serum T_3 and T_4 as well as an increase in rT_3. The values of TSH at the onset of the illness are usually normal, but with progression and increasing severity the TSH can become suppressed [23]. With recovery the TSH and free T_4 rise and return to normal [24,25].

Evaluating thyroid anatomy and function

Although the radioactive iodine uptake test is typically increased in hyperthyroidism and decreased in hypothyroidism it is not commonly used for differentiation. A low radioactive iodine uptake test result accompanying hyperthyroidism suggests subacute thyroiditis, exogenous thyroid administration, resolving hyperthyroidism, struma ovarii, iodine-induced thyrotoxicosis, or functional thyroid cancer metastases after thyroidectomy. Radionuclide scanning with iodine or technetium isotopes provides information regarding the functional status of nodules and thyroid size but is not helpful with respect to metabolic status [26]. Thyroid ultrasound does not give functional information but does define nodules to help determine whether they are cystic, mixed, or solid, or have grown. Fine-needle aspiration of thyroid nodules has decreased the need. Ultrasound radionuclide scanning is typically the first test performed in the evaluation of a thyroid nodule [27].

Assessing the hypothalamic–pituitary thyroidal axis

The measurement of TSH by radioimmunoassay is of great utility in evaluating thyroid function. The new "supersensitive" assays distinguish hyperthyroidism as well as hypothyroidism from normal thyroid activity. A normal or low TSH accompanying hypothyroidism is evidence for hypothalamic or pituitary disease.

Indications for surgery

The most common reasons for recommending surgery are marked thyroid enlargement, rapidly growing goiter, substernal extension of a goiter, compressive symptoms, an abnormal finding on a fine needle aspiration, failure of medical therapy for the treatment of hyperthyroidism, and patient preference. Patients presenting with well-controlled hypo- and hyperthyroidism do not usually have increased risk of complications during and after surgery. However, patients with uncontrolled hyper- and hypothyroidism are at considerable risk [28–30].

Preparation for surgery

The history and physical examination of patients scheduled for thyroidectomy should include identification of abnormalities of thyroid function. Besides symptoms and signs of hypo- and hyperthyroidism, evidence for other medical conditions should be sought, including cardio-respiratory disease and associated endocrine disorders. For example, patients who require thyroidectomy for medullary cancer may have an associated pheochromocytoma [31].

Routine laboratory tests include thyroid function tests, hemoglobin, white cell and platelet count, urea and electrolytes, and serum calcium. If liver abnormalities or clotting disorders are suspected, prothrombin time (PT) and international normalized ratio (INR) should be included in the initial laboratory evaluation. Patients may have a fine needle aspiration as a diagnostic test prior to surgery. A chest X-ray may be needed to show evidence of tracheal compression or deviation, and extension of the thyroid tissue into the mediastinum. An ECG should generally be performed, particularly in those with a history of hypertension, cardiac disease, diabetes mellitus or hyperthyroidism [31,32].

Complications of surgery

Postoperative complications of surgery in patients with thyroid disease may include difficulty with extubation, hemorrhage, laryngeal or pharyngeal edema, nerve damage (recurrent laryngeal, superior laryngeal, or phrenic nerve), tracheal collapse, pneumothorax, hypocalcemia, vomiting, wound infection, pain, and thyroid storm in hyperthyroid patients. During extubation, care should be taken to decrease coughing because of the risk of bleeding. Injury to the recurrent and superior laryngeal nerves can be temporary or permanent. Temporary recurrent laryngeal nerve damage occurs in 3–4% and can cause minor voice hoarseness. Patients usually require only observation. Permanent unilateral vocal cord paralysis occurs in < 1% and can lead to hoarseness, aspiration, breathlessness, and stridor. It is usually treated with silicone injections, or vocal cord fixation. Bilateral vocal cord paralysis is extremely rare, and usually requires tracheotomy. Tracheal collapse is rare, but usually occurs upon resection from prolonged compression of a large goiter. Typical features include stridor and respiratory compromise. Patients may require reintubation and a tracheotomy. Pneumothorax usually results if lower neck dissection is required [33–35].

Hypocalcium from parathyroid stunning or unintentional parathyroidectomy can cause temporary or permanent hypocalcemia. Patients may develop perioral numbness, carpopedal spasms, and anxiety. Symptoms usually appear within 1–7 days after surgery. If patients are screened early, within the first 12–24 hours after surgery, they then can be treated with oral calcium and vitamin D before hypocalcemic symptoms occur [36]. Severe hypocalcemia is treated with intravenous calcium gluconate 10% (2 g over 2 hours) until calcium is consistently greater than 7.5 mg/dL. Intravenous calcium can irritate the veins, and cause skin necrosis if the intravenous solution extravasates. Mild hypocalcemia is treated with oral calcium carbonate (starting at 1 g 2–3 times a day). In patients with severe and/or prolonged hypocalcemia 1–2 g calcium is given

3 times daily along with calcitriol (0.25–1 μg 2–3 times daily) [37]. Permanent hypocalcemia requires chronic treatment with calcium and vitamin D (see Chapter 28).

Patients undergoing thyroidectomy have a high rate of nausea and vomiting following thyroidectomy (as high as 71% in some studies). Nausea or vomiting with retching is uncomfortable and in severe cases can lead to postoperative bleeding with development of a hematoma or hemorrhage. This can lead to airway obstruction and the need for surgical revision [38].

Hyperthyroidism

Hyperthyroidism results from Graves' disease (the most common cause), toxic adenoma, toxic multinodular goiter, subacute thyroiditis, the hyperthyroid phase of Hashimoto's thyroiditis (reflecting overlap with Graves' disease), thyrotoxicosis factitia from exogenous hormone, and iodine-induced thyrotoxicosis. Rare causes include ovarian struma, hydatidiform mole, metastatic follicular carcinoma, and a TSH-producing adenoma. Measurement in serum of free T_4 or of the free T_4 index (total T_4 with T_3 resin uptake) plus a sensitive TSH should confirm the diagnosis. Serum T_3 is increased in hyperthyroidism but may be normal after iodine ingestion or

Table 30.2 Symptoms and signs of hyperthyroidism.

Eye	Upper lid retraction
Cardiovascular	Decreased peripheral vascular resistance Tachycardia Atrial fibrillation Congestive heart failure Cardiomyopathy Thromboembolic events
Respiratory	Respiratory muscle weakness
Gastrointestinal	Hyperdefecation Elevated alanine amniotransferase (ALT) Elevated alkaline phosphatase Hepatomegaly Depletion of hepatic glycogen stores
Nervous system	Nervousness Emotional lability Hyperkinesia Fatigue
Muscle	Muscle weakness
Skeletal	Bone loss
Metabolic	Hypercalcemia Hyperglycemia Relative or true adrenal insufficiency
Hematopoietic	Neutropenia Thrombocytopenia
Reproductive	Menstrual irregularity Infertility Increased incidence of miscarriages

when severe non-thyroidal illness is present. A flat TSH response to TRH is confirmatory when the TSH level is equivocal or sensitive measurements are not available. An increased serum thyroid-stimulating immunoglobulin level is seen with Graves' disease. In younger patients, the clinical presentation of hyperthyroidism is typically dramatic with obvious signs of increased sympathetic activity. The diagnosis is often more subtle in elderly patients who may be markedly apathetic with weight loss, weakness, poor appetite, and congestive heart failure without tachyarrhythmias or goiter [39].

Multiple organs are influenced by hyperthyroidism. The most common alterations with hyperthyroidism include those listed in Table 30.2 [40.]

Surgery in patients with hyperthyroidism

The preoperative diagnosis and treatment of hyperthyroidism is of great importance to prevent tachyarrhythmias and life-threatening thyroid storm [41]. If surgery is not emergent patients should be rendered euthyroid. Beta-adrenergic blockade provides prompt symptomatic relief but does not significantly affect thyroid hormone levels. Some beta-blockers (e.g., propranolol, atenolol) block the peripheral conversion of T_4 to T_3 but the therapeutic importance of this is questionable and beta-blockers without this action are equally effective. The risks and benefits of beta-blockade must be weighed in patients with congestive heart failure or bronchospasm. Both propylthiouracil (300–600 mg in three divided doses daily) and methimazole (30–40 mg in two divided doses daily), are effective inhibitors of thyroid hormone synthesis. Propylthiouracil (PTU) blocks peripheral conversion of T_4 to T_3 and is favored by some endocrinologists for this reason, but then again, this effect may be of little clinical consequence. The decreased frequency of dosing required with methimazole may improve compliance. Propylthiouracil is preferred during pregnancy and nursing because it crosses the placenta one-fourth the amount of methimazole and enters breast milk one-tenth the amount. With adequate doses of antithyroid drugs, patients may be nearly euthyroid within 3 weeks. The clearance of beta-blockers is increased in hyperthyroidism. Thus dose reductions are needed as the euthyroid state is approached [42].

Emergent surgery in hyperthyroid patients requires a different approach. Rapid preparation for surgery may be needed, and the goals are rapid lowering of thyroid hormone levels, decrease in thyroid hormone release, and control of peripheral effects of the thyroid hormone. The therapeutic steps for surgical preparation are given in Table 30.3 [43,44.]

The antithyroid drugs that only block organification and thyroid hormone synthesis are ineffective because of their slow onset of action. Beta-adrenergic blockade alone has been used successfully. If propranolol is selected, it should be given at the dose of 40–80 mg orally every 6 hours and continued after surgery because fever, tachycardia, and thyroid storm can occur with inadequate dosing or too rapid discontinuation. Propranolol, 1–5 mg can be given slowly by the intravenous

Table 30.3 Therapeutic steps for surgical preparation.

		Special considerations
Step 1. Start beta-adrenergic blockade	Propranolol 40–80 mg PO TID–QID.	Decrease T_4-to-T_3 conversion
Step 2. Stop hormone synthesis and release (choose one)	PTU 200 mg PO every 4 hours	Inhibition of new thyroid hormone synthesis and decreases T_4-to-T_3 conversion
	Methimazole 20 mg p.o. every 4 hours	Inhibition of new thyroid hormone synthesis only
Step 3. Stabilize the B/P and maintain vasomotor stability (choose one)	Hydrocortisone 100 mg PO or IV every 8 hours	Decreases T_4-to-T_3 conversion
	Dexamethasone 2 mg PO or IV Q 6 hours	Decreases T_4-to-T_3 conversion
Step 4. Block release of thyroid hormone iodine (choose one)	Potassium iodide SSKI 5 drops PO Q 6 hours	Should be administered at least 1 hour after PTU or methimazole
	Lugol's solution 4–8 drops PO Q 6–8 hours	Should be administered at least 1 hour after PTU or methimazole

route if time does not permit oral administration, and this should be continued every 6 hours as needed through the perioperative period [42,44].

There are rare and serious side-effects associated with PTU and methimazole, including agranulocytosis, hepatotoxicity, and vasculitis. Agranulocytosis occurs in 0.1–0.5% of patients [45,46]. PTU-related severe liver damage is approximately 0.1–0.2% in adults [47–50].

There is now a Food and Drug Administration black box warning about the hepatic effects of PTU. Side-effects of methimazole are dose-related, whereas those of PTU are less clearly related to dose. Methimazole is better than PTU in controlling more severe hyperthyroidism because it has less toxicity, especially when prescribed in lower doses. Propylthiouracil should be used as a second-line agent, except in thyroid storm and in pregnancy [47]. Propylthiouracil should never be used in children. Data for children suggest that the risk of drug-induced liver failure may be greater for children than for adults [51].

Iodide should be used in conjunction with beta-blockade in emergency preparation for surgery. Iodide acutely blocks the release of thyroid hormone from the gland as well as inhibiting organification. A decline of T_4 levels to normal may be reached in a week using 10 drops of an oral saturated solution of potassium iodide or 1 g of intravenous sodium iodide daily.

Occasionally, other agents are needed to quickly prepare patients for surgery when conventional agents like PTU and methimazole cannot be used or have failed. Iopanoic acid, which is an oral iodinated cholecystographic agent that inhibits 5′-deiodinase and causes a reduction in the peripheral conversion of T_4 to T_3, has been used in a small number of patients. There are reports of its use to successfully prepare patients with amiodarone-induced thyrotoxicosis for surgery when they were unresponsive to PTU, methimazole or steroids. Mean dose was 1 g/day for 13 days [44]. Very rarely, lithium is used for intractable hyperthyroidism, including

amiodarone induced hyperthyroidism that is resistant to usual therapies. Usual clinical response is seen with 900–1500 mg/day [52–54].

Although they are not immediately effective, therapy with antithyroid drugs should be initiated in patients who are undergoing emergent surgery. The rectal route has been shown to provide adequate serum levels when oral administration is precluded [55]. If patients develop signs of thyroid storm (e.g., hyperthermia, vomiting, hypertension, tachycardia, altered mental state, impending vascular collapse), prompt treatment with beta-blockers, iodide, antithyroid drugs, and glucocorticoids (hydrocortisone, 75–100 mg intravenously every 8 hours) is required. Glucocorticoids cover potential inadequate adrenal reserve as well as inhibit 5′-monodeiodinase, thereby lowering T_3 levels. Salicylates should not be used because they displace thyroid hormone from binding proteins resulting in increased free levels. The diagnosis of thyroid storm is a clinical one. Thyroid hormone levels are not higher than those in hyperthyroidism without storm. Presumably concomitant stress increases catecholamine levels, with a profound effect on the already increased beta-adrenergic receptor activity characteristic of the hyperthyroid state.

Hypothyroidism

The clinical presentation of hypothyroidism ranges from mild symptoms of fatigue to myxedema coma. A higher index of suspicion of the disease is required in the elderly because many mild symptoms and signs of hypothyroidism may be attributed to the aging process. The diagnosis of hypothyroidism is made by measuring free T_4 and TSH. An increase in TSH precedes the decline in circulating thyroid hormone levels; a low TSH suggests a hypothalamic–pituitary cause. The most common cause of hypothyroidism, Hashimoto's thyroiditis, is associated with high levels of antimicrosomal and antithyroglobulin antibodies.

The results of thyroid hormone deficiency are varied and affect surgery. Cardiovascular manifestations include bradycardia, decreased cardiac output, atrioventricular conduction defects, and pericardial effusions. Respiratory effects include decreased alveolar ventilation (due to blunted responsiveness to anoxia and hypercarbia) and pleural effusions. Delayed gastric emptying and intestinal mobility can lead to abdominal distension and ileus. Women may have menorrhagia or amenorrhea. Decreased metabolism of administered drugs may lead to toxicity and trigger respiratory failure [56].

Surgery in patients with hypothyroidism

When possible, surgery should be postponed until hypothyroidism can be corrected. Studies have shown a small increase in intraoperative hypotension and postoperative congestive heart failure, ileus, and confusion when patients were moderately hypothyroid. These studies support the need for close monitoring of respiratory status, attention to fluid balance, and cautious use of narcotics and sedatives. If surgical patients demonstrate signs of myxedema coma (e.g., stupor, hypothermia, hypoventilation, hypoglycemia, hyponatremia, hypotension), emergency treatment is required [57,58]. Levothyroxine is given intravenously at a dosage of 400 µg. Glucocorticoids (hydrocortisone, 75–100 mg intravenously every 8 hours) are administered because relative adrenal insufficiency may be present (e.g., hypopituitarism, coincident autoimmune Addison's disease).

In young patients without evidence of cardiac disease, full replacement with levothyroxine 100–125 µg intravenously or orally per day, may be initiated and continued through the perioperative period. A 50% reduction in dose is appropriate when long-term parenteral administration is needed. When coronary artery disease is present, a starting dose of 25 µg/day is more appropriate. If angina or arrhythmias occur, the dose should be reduced. For patients undergoing coronary revascularization surgery, thyroid replacement is best not initiated. These patients do well with surgery and the replacement of thyroid hormone often increases angina and induces arrhythmias. If thyroid function tests are inconclusive or not available, and hypothyroidism is clinically suspected, it is prudent to treat patients with replacement doses of levothyroxine and re-evaluate when they are stable [57,58].

Patients who are euthyroid while receiving replacement therapy can be maintained on parenteral therapy through the perioperative period. Alternatively, interruption of thyroid replacement for as long as 1 week is not detrimental [59].

Effect of surgery on thyroid function

Non-thyroidal surgery is associated with several changes in circulating thyroid hormone levels. Most profoundly an abrupt decline in T_3 levels occurs within 24 hours as a result of inhibition of 5′-monodeiodinase. Reverse T_3 levels rise for the same reason. The effect on T_4 levels is less predictable but a decline is usually noted when the procedure is prolonged and associated with greater stress and extended fasting. Free T_4 and TSH levels are typically normal. These patients are considered to be euthyroid (the "euthyroid sick" syndrome) and should not be treated with thyroid hormone.

Discharge planning after thyroid surgery

Patients are ready for discharge after thyroidectomy when the patient has no breathing difficulties, the wound drain has been removed, there is no evidence of a hematoma, and the calcium level is normal [60]. Routine calcium and vitamin D supplementation has been shown to reduce the risk of hypocalcemia [61,62].

References

1. Larsen PR, Davies T, Hay ID. Thyroid gland. In Wilson JD, Foster DW, Kronenberg HM et al., eds. Williams Textbook of Endocrinology. 9th edn. Philadelphia, PA: W. B. Saunders; 1998, pp. 389–515.
2. Summers JE. Surgical anatomy of the thyroid gland. Am J Surg 1950; 80(1): 35–43.
3. van de Graaf SA, Ris-Stalpers C, Pauws E et al. Structure update: up to date with human thyroglobulin. J Endocrinol 2001; 170: 307–21.
4. Rokita SE, Adler JM, McTamney PM, Watson JA Jr. Efficient use and recycling of the micronutrient iodide in mammals. Biochimie 2010; 92: 1227–35.
5. Pilo A, Iervasi G, Vitek F et al. Thyroidal and peripheral production of 3,5,3′-triiodothyronine in humans by multicompartmental analysis. Am J Physiol 1990; 258: E715–26.
6. Ridgway EC, Weintraub BD, Maloof F. Metabolic clearance and production rates of human thyrotropin. J Clin Invest 1974; 53: 895–903.
7. Eisenberg MC, Santini F, Marsili A, Pinchera A, DiStefano JJ 3rd. TSH regulation dynamics in central and extreme primary hypothyroidism. Thyroid 2010; 20: 1215–28.
8. Dufour DR. Laboratory tests of thyroid function: uses and limitations. Endocrinol Metab Clin North Am. 2007; 36: 579–94.
9. Surks MI, Chopra IJ, Mariash CN, Nicoloff JT, Solomon DH. American Thyroid Association guidelines for use of laboratory tests in thyroid disorders. J Am Med Assoc 1990; 263: 1529–32.
10. Malandrino P, Latina A, Marescalco S et al. Risk-adapted management of differentiated thyroid cancer assessed by a sensitive measurement of basal serum thyroglobulin. J Clin Endocrinol Metab 2011; 96: 1703–9.
11. Dayan CM. Interpretation of thyroid function tests. Lancet 2001; 357: 619–24.
12. Lazarus JH. Thyroid function in pregnancy. Br Med Bull. 2011; 97: 137–48.
13. Glinoer D, Spencer CA. Serum TSH determinations in pregnancy: how, when and why? Nat Rev Endocrinol 2010; 6: 526–9.

14. Brent GA. Maternal thyroid function: interpretation of thyroid function tests in pregnancy. *Clin Obstet Gynecol* 1997; **40**: 3–15.

15. Weetman AP. Immunity, thyroid function and pregnancy: molecular mechanisms. *Nature Rev Endocrinol* 2010; **6**: 311–18.

16. Galofre JC, Davies TF. Autoimmune thyroid disease in pregnancy: a review. *J Womens Health (Larchmt)* 2009; **18**: 1847–56.

17. Cassidy F, Ahearn EP, Carroll BJ. Thyroid function in mixed and pure manic episodes. *Bipolar Disord* 2002; **4**: 393–7.

18. Gold PW, Goodwin FK, Wehr T, Rebar R. Pituitary thyrotropin response to thyrotropin-releasing hormone in affective illness: relationship to spinal fluid amine metabolites. *Am J Psychiatry* 1977; **134**: 1028–31.

19. Lim VS. Thyroid function in patients with chronic renal failure. *Am J Kidney Dis* 2001; **38**: S80–4.

20. Zoccali C, Mallamaci F, Tripepi G, Cutrupi S, Pizzini P. Low triiodothyronine and survival in end-stage renal disease. *Kidney Int* 2006; **70**: 523–8.

21. Langton JE, Brent GA. Nonthyroidal illness syndrome: evaluation of thyroid function in sick patients. *Endocrinol Metab Clin North Am* 2002; **31**: 159–72.

22. Bello G, Ceaichisciuc I, Silva S, Antonelli M. The role of thyroid dysfunction in the critically ill: a review of the literature. *Minerva Anesthesiol* 2010; **76**: 919–28.

23. Warner MH, Beckett GJ. Mechanisms behind the non-thyroidal illness syndrome: an update. *J Endocrinol* 2010; **205**: 1–13.

24. Stockigt J. Assessment of thyroid function: towards an integrated laboratory – clinical approach. *Clin Biochem Rev* 2003; **24**: 109–22.

25. De Groot LJ. Dangerous dogmas in medicine: the nonthyroidal illness syndrome. *J Clin Endocrinol Metab* 1999; **84**: 151–64.

26. Vazquez BJ, Richards ML. Imaging of the thyroid and parathyroid glands. *Surg Clin North Am* 2011; **91**: 15–32.

27. Luster M, Verburg FA, Scheidhauer K. Diagnostic imaging work up in multi-nodular goiter. *Minerva Endocrinol* 2010; **35**: 153–9.

28. Mittendorf EA, McHenry CR. Thyroidectomy for selected patients with thyrotoxicosis. *Arch Otolaryngol Head Neck Surg* 2001; **127**: 61–5.

29. Alsanea O, Clark OH. Treatment of Graves' disease: the advantages of surgery. *Endocrinol Metab Clin North Am* 2000; **29**: 321–37.

30. Okamoto T, Iihara M, Obara T. Management of hyperthyroidism due to Graves' and nodular diseases. *World J Surg* 2000; **24**: 957–61.

31. Farling PA. Thyroid disease. *Br J Anaesth* 2000; **85**: 15–28.

32. Graham GW, Unger B, Coursin DB. Perioperative management of selected endocrine disorders. *Int Anesthesiol Clin* 2000; **38**: 31–67.

33. Grodski S, Stalberg P, Robinson BG, Delbridge LW. Surgery versus radioiodine therapy as definitive management for Graves' disease: the role of patient preference. *Thyroid* 2007; **17**: 157–60.

34. Liu J, Bargren A, Schaefer S, Chen H, Sippel RS. Total thyroidectomy: a safe and effective treatment for Graves' disease. *J Surg Res* 2011; **168**: 1–4

35. McHenry CR. Patient volumes and complications in thyroid surgery. *Br J Surg* 2002; **89**: 821.

36. Roh JL, Park JY, Park CI. Prevention of postoperative hypocalcemia with routine oral calcium and vitamin D supplements in patients with differentiated papillary thyroid carcinoma undergoing total thyroidectomy plus central neck dissection. *Cancer* 2009; **115**: 251–8.

37. Khan MI, Waguespack SG, Hu MI. Medical management of postsurgical hypoparathyroidism. *Endocr Pract* 2010; **6**: 1–19.

38. Sonner JM, Hynson JM, Clark O, Katz JA. Nausea and vomiting following thyroid and parathyroid surgery. *J Clin Anesth* 1997; **9**: 398–402.

39. Effraimidis G, Strieder TG, Tijssen JG, Wiersinga WM. Natural history of the transition from euthyroidism to overt autoimmune hypo- or hyperthyroidism: a prospective study. *Eur J Endocrinol* 2011; **164**: 107–13.

40. Pulli RS, Coniglio JU. Surgical management of the substernal thyroid gland. *Laryngoscope* 1998; **108**: 358–61.

41. Shindo M. Surgery for hyperthyroidism [review]. *ORL J Otorhinolaryngol Relat Spec* 2008; **70**: 298–304.

42. Nayak B, Burman K. Thyrotoxicosis and thyroid storm. *Endocrinol Metab Clin North Am* 2006; **35**: 663–86.

43. Langley RW, Burch HB. Perioperative management of the thyrotoxic patient. *Endocrinol Metab Clin North Am* 2003; **32**: 519–34.

44. Bogazzi F, Miccoli P, Berti P *et al.* Preparation with iopanoic acid rapidly controls thyroxicosis in patients with amiodarone-induced thyrotoxicosis before thyroidectomy. *Surgery* 2002; **132**: 1114–17.

45. Cooper DS. Antithyroid drugs. *N Engl J Med* 2005; **352**: 905–17.

46. Cooper DS. The side effects of antithyroid drugs. *Endocrinologist* 1999; **9**: 457–76.

47. Bartalena L, Bogazzi F, Martino E. Adverse effects of thyroid hormone preparations and antithyroid drugs. *Drug Saf* 1996; **15**: 53–63.

48. Carrion AF, Czul F, Arosemena LR *et al.* Propylthiouracil-induced acute liver failure: role of liver transplantation. *Int J Endocrinol.* 2010; 2010: 910636. doi: 10.1155/2010/910636.

49. Kim HJ, Kim BH, Han YS *et al.* The incidence and clinical characteristics of symptomatic propylthiouracil-induced hepatic injury in patients with hyperthyroidism: a single-center retrospective study. *Am J Gastroenterol* 2001; **96**: 165–9.

50. Primeggia J, Lewis JH. Gone (from the Physicians' desk reference) but not forgotten: propylthiouracil-associated hepatic failure: a call for liver test monitoring. *J Natl Med Assoc* 2010; **102**: 531–4.

51. Cooper DS, Rivkees SA. Putting propylthiouracil in perspective. *J Clin Endocrinol Metab* 2009; **94**: 1881–2.

52. Osman F, Franklyn JA, Sheppard MC, Gammage MD. Successful treatment of amiodarone-induced thyrotoxicosis. *Circulation* 2002; **105**: 1275–7.

53. Dickstein G, Shechner C, Adawi F *et al.* Lithium treatment in amiodarone-induced thyrotoxicosis. *Am J Med* 1997; **102**: 454–8.

54. Kauschansky A, Genel M. Preoperative treatment of intractable

hyperthyroidism with acute lithium administration. *Eur J Pediatr Surg* 1996; **6**: 301–2.

55. Zweig SB, Schlosser JR, Thomas SA, Levy CJ, Fleckman AM. Rectal administration of propylthiouracil in suppository form in patients with thyrotoxicosis and critical illness: case report and review of literature. *Endocr Pract* 2006; **12**: 43–7.

56. Devdhar M, Ousman YH, Burman KD. Hypothyroidism. *Endocrinol Metab Clin North Am* 2007; **36**: 595–615.

57. Schiff RL, Welsh GA. Perioperative evaluation and management of the patient with endocrine dysfunction. *Med Clin North Am* 2003; **87**: 175–92.

58. Kohl BA, Schwartz S. Surgery in the patient with endocrine dysfunction. *Med Clin North Am* 2009; **93**: 1031–47.

59. Spell NO 3rd. Stopping and restarting medications in the perioperative period. *Med Clin North Am* 2001; **85**: 1117–28.

60. Aslam R, Steward D. Surgical management of thyroid disease.

Otolaryngol Clin North Am 2010; **43**: 273–83.

61. Roh JL, Park CI. Routine oral calcium and vitamin D supplements for prevention of hypocalcemia after total thyroidectomy. *Am J Surg* 2006; **192**: 675–78.

62. Sanabria A, Dominguez LC, Vega V, Osorio C, Duarte D. Routine postoperative administration of vitamin D and calcium after total thyroidectomy: a meta-analysis. *Int J Surg* 2011; **9**: 46–51.

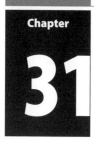

Disorders of the adrenal cortex

Pamela T. Prescott

During surgery there is a coordinated response to stress that includes the nervous, endocrine, and immune systems. Inappropriately low response or inappropriately excessive response to stress may lead to disease and possible premature death [1,2]. The hypothalamic–pituitary–adrenal (HPA) axis and the sympathetic nervous system react to stress by releasing hypothalamic CRH and vasopressin (AVP). These hormones synergistically stimulate systemic ACTH secretion, which, in turn, stimulates the adrenal cortexes to secrete glucocorticoids. Central activation of the sympathetic neurons leads to activation of both the systemic sympathetic nervous system and the adrenal medullae [2,3]. The immune system through inflammatory mediators, especially cytokines, stimulates the release of corticotropin-releasing factor from hypothalamic neurons. This central activation of the HPA axis and the direct stimulation of the adrenal glands by the sympathetic system may be a regulatory mechanism for preventing an excessive immune reaction [4,5].

Adrenocorticotropic hormone (ACTH) is released in quick, pulsatile bursts followed by a slower, more sustained rise in cortisol and metabolites [6,7]. Free cortisol is the active hormone and acts directly on tissues [6]. Normal ACTH release and production of cortisol follows a circadian rhythm and is connected to light. It is the highest on awakening in the morning (peaking about 8 hours after the onset of sleep), declines over the day, and is lowest in the middle of the night [7]. The cortisol secretory pattern is usually resistant to acute change. Prolonged bed rest, continuous feeding, or 5 days of fasting, do not alter the rhythm [8]. Occasionally, abrupt time changes of the sleep–awake cycle, as during shift work rotations and jet lag, may have some effect on the 24-hour cortisol patterns [9–11]. Critical illness, chronic inflammatory conditions, chronic insomnia, coronary artery disease, and severe stress often alter the daily rhythm [12–14]. These conditions exert their effect by cytokines, interleukins, and tumor necrosis factors. Circulating interleukin-6 is a potent activator of the HPA axis. By stimulating pituitary ACTH and therefore cortisol, response to inflammation can enhance resistance to inflammatory

disease, while a decreased or defective response can increase susceptibility [4,5,13].

Glucocorticoids have multiple actions and affect every system of the body. In broadest terms, glucocorticoids affect the metabolism of glucose, protein and lipids, and the function of the immune, renal, and circulatory systems [15]. Glucocorticoids increase blood glucose levels by increasing hepatic glucose production, decreasing insulin action, and increasing glucagon secretion. Glucocorticoids increase the availability and release of amino acids, and lipids that are used as substrate for glucose production [16]. During fasting, these processes protect against hypoglycemia. With endogenous or exogenous glucocorticoid excess, hyperglycemia can occur; with glucocorticoid deficiency, hypoglycemia can occur.

Glucocorticoids can cause redistribution of immune cells. They increase intravascular polymorphonuclear cell release from the bone marrow, but cause temporary sequestration of lymphocytes and monocytes into the spleen, lymph nodes, and bone marrow [16]. Glucocorticoids increase glomerular filtration by a direct effect, and in conjunction with mineralocorticoid activity, affect electrolyte and water balance [2,17]. When in excess, glucocorticoids with mineralocorticoid activity (i.e., cortisol), can cause sodium retention, hypokalemia, and hypertension. Glucocorticoids in conjunction with catecholamines maintain vascular tone, vascular permeability, and the vascular distribution of water [2]. Deficiency can result in refractory shock in the stressed state, and excess can cause hypertension. Excess glucocorticoids inhibit connective tissue and bone formation, decrease gastrointestinal absorption of calcium, and increase calciuria. Both excess and deficiency of glucocorticoids have major effects on the central nervous system [7].

Cortisol is the most important glucocorticoid. Cortisol synthesis proceeds through several steps, the final being the hydroxylation in mitochondria of 11-deoxycortisol to cortisol. Adrenal androgen synthesis in adults is stimulated by ACTH. The physiological effects of adrenal androgens in adult men are inconsequential. In women, however (in whom the adrenal androgen supply is roughly 50%), excess adrenal production

Medical Management of the Surgical Patient, ed. Michael F. Lubin, Thomas F. Dodson, and Neil H. Winawer. Published by Cambridge University Press. © Cambridge University Press 2013.

results in acne, hirsutism, and virilization. Most of the circulating cortisol is bound to corticosteroid-binding globulin, with < 10% in the free, biologically active form [2]. Corticosteroid-binding globulin is the predominant binding protein, with albumin binding a lesser amount. During acute illness, particularly sepsis, corticosteroid-binding globulin levels fall by as much as 50%, resulting in a significant increase in the percentage of free cortisol [18–21].

Glucocorticoid levels increase immediately with surgery, severe injury, burns, pain, fever, hypothermia, emotional distress, and hemorrhage with subsequent hypotension or hypovolemia [3–7]. Surgery is a potent activator of the HPA axis. ACTH rises with the incision and during surgery. The highest rise in ACTH is with extubation and the immediate postoperative period [18,19]. During surgical procedures such as laparotomy, glucocorticoid levels rise immediately, peaking in the immediate postoperative period and decline to baseline over 24–48 hours [18,19]. After surgery and with severe illness there is no circadian variation. Glucocorticoid levels tend to be higher than baseline. The normal cortisol response to stress is usually considered to be a level > 18 to 20 μg/dL. In patients with traumatic injuries, cortisol levels can peak between 30–45 μg/dL [18]. In patients with severe illness and in those shortly before death, the cortisol levels can be as high as 30–260 μg/dL [18]. The level of the cortisol response is related to the severity of the illness. There is no precisely known level that distinguishes an adequate from an inadequate adrenal response. Previously, many believed that a random cortisol level in a stressed patient should achieve a threshold of at least 25 μg/dL [19].

The production of aldosterone by the adrenal cortex is controlled primarily by the renin-angiotensin system and secondarily by ACTH. Acute increases in serum potassium, depletion of body sodium, and renin production by the kidneys are also potent stimulators of aldosterone production. Excess production is manifested by hypertension, hypokalemia, suppression of the renin system, and normal to low cortisol secretion.

Adrenal insufficiency

Given that the stress response associated with surgery requires adequate adrenal reserves, it is critical that adrenal insufficiency be diagnosed and treated preoperatively. Medical consultants should always inquire about a history of glucocorticoid use in patients undergoing surgery. Although the inhaled steroids used to treat obstructive pulmonary disease are usually not associated with adrenal suppression, high doses of these drugs can result in suppression sufficient enough to require perioperative systemic glucocorticoids.

In the USA, 80% of primary adrenocortical insufficiency (Addison's disease) is a result of autoimmune adrenalitis. This is often associated with other autoimmune disorders, including Hashimoto's thyroiditis, Graves' disease, type 1 diabetes mellitus, premature ovarian failure, hypoparathyroidism,

and rarely, testicular failure. Associated non-endocrine conditions include mucocutaneous candidiasis, vitiligo, alopecia, pernicious anemia, and chronic active hepatitis. Worldwide, tuberculosis remains the most common cause of Addison's disease; it is the second most common cause in the USA. Rare causes include hemorrhage (a risk of anticoagulant therapy), fungal infections, tumor metastases, surgical adrenalectomy, radiation, amyloidosis, sarcoidosis, hemochromatosis, congenital enzyme defects, and medications (e.g., metyrapone, ketoconazole, aminoglutethimide, etopamide, mitotane) [22–27].

The most common cause of secondary adrenal insufficiency is ACTH deficiency resulting from exogenous glucocorticoid therapy. The administration of replacement doses of glucocorticoids (i.e., 5 mg of prednisone or 20 mg of hydrocortisone daily) for more than 2 weeks is sufficient to suppress the hypothalamic–pituitary–adrenal axis. Subnormal cortisol responses to stimuli can persist for as long as 1 year after the discontinuation of glucocorticoid therapy. Pituitary recovery precedes adrenal recovery by months. Endogenous secondary adrenal insufficiency is most commonly caused by pituitary or hypothalamic tumors [22].

Critical illness adrenal insufficiency varies widely (0–77%), depending on the population of patients studied and the diagnostic criteria. However, the overall prevalence of adrenal insufficiency in critically ill medical patients approximates 10–20%, with a rate as high as 60% in patients with septic shock. The mechanisms leading to dysfunction of the HPA axis during critical illness are complex and poorly understood and likely include decreased production of corticotropin-releasing hormone, ACTH, cortisol and the dysfunction of their receptors. A subset of patients may have structural damage to the adrenal gland from either hemorrhage or infarction, and this may result in long-term adrenal dysfunction [21]. Decreased production of cortisol or ACTH is particularly common in patients with severe sepsis and septic shock [24].

Patients with primary adrenal insufficiency are weak and fatigued. Appetite is decreased despite increased taste and smell sensation. Nausea, vomiting, and weight loss are common. Hyperpigmentation, hyponatremia, and fasting hypoglycemia (especially in children) can occur. Because of the associated mineralocorticoid deficiency, volume depletion with orthostatic hypotension, hyperkalemia, and acidosis occur. Acute adrenal crisis is characterized by fever, volume depletion with refractory hypotension, nausea, weakness, depressed mentation, and hypoglycemia. Patients with secondary adrenocortical insufficiency have most of the same symptoms but are not hyperpigmented because the production of ACTH and beta-lipotropin is reduced. Because aldosterone production typically remains intact they do not have volume depletion, hyperkalemia, or acidosis. Hyponatremia from impaired excretion of water does occur, and there is the potential for hypotension with a stress-induced crisis [22,23].

Primary adrenal insufficiency is best diagnosed with the ACTH stimulation test. A normal serum cortisol response is at least 20 µg/dL 30–60 minutes after a 250 µg dose of intravenous or intramuscular synthetic ACTH (cosyntropin) [22]. To rule out the diagnosis of Addison's disease in patients who have been receiving glucocorticoids, several daily doses of synthetic ACTH or an 8-hour infusion of ACTH may be needed to achieve a normal cortisol response because of superimposed secondary adrenal insufficiency [12]. In secondary adrenal insufficiency the serum cortisol response to ACTH is frequently blunted but can be normal [7].

Hypothalamic–pituitary–adrenal (HPA) axis function can be evaluated by the overnight metyrapone test. After bedtime administration of 30 mg/kg of oral metyrapone (an agent that blocks the conversion of 11-deoxycortisol), cortisol levels are measured at 8:00 am the following morning. A cortisol level of less than 5 µg/dL indicates that the level of blockade was adequate and a marked increase (80-fold) in 11-deoxycortisol confirms that the adrenal response was normal [7].

Alternatively the HPA axis can be tested with insulin-induced hypoglycemia. After the intravenous injection of 0.1 U/kg of regular insulin, a serum glucose nadir occurs in 20–30 minutes. The serum cortisol should increase to more than 20 µg/dL, 30–60 minutes after the glucose nadir. Because of the potential morbidity of hypoglycemia this test requires the presence of a physician and should not be performed in the elderly or in patients with significant cardiovascular or cerebrovascular disease. Measurement of plasma ACTH and serum cortisol after CRH administration has been disappointing in distinguishing between hypothalamic and pituitary disease. Predictably, the ACTH response to CRH is exaggerated in primary adrenal insufficiency [7,22,23,25].

Critical illness-related corticosteroid insufficiency is diagnosed by a change in cortisol levels of < 9 µg/dL (after 250 µg dose of intravenous or intramuscular synthetic ACTH, cosyntropin), or a random total cortisol of < 10 µg/dL [21].

Patients receiving long-term glucocorticoid therapy can develop secondary adrenal insufficiency. Any long-term use of topical, inhaled, or oral glucocorticoids, can increase the risk for HPA suppression. Chronic oral glucocorticoid use, however, is more likely to cause HPA axis suppression and a blunted response to stress [22,23]. If glucocorticoids are abruptly discontinued, then adrenal insufficiency can occur and the patient may develop hypotension, hypoglycemia, dehydration, altered mental status, or death. Chronic glucocorticoid use can also increase infection rate, osteoporosis, and poor wound healing [23].

Preoperative assessment of HPA axis function is not needed if the patient's glucocorticoid dose will be continued before and after surgery. Hypothalamic–pituitary–adrenal axis testing will be needed if the patient's steroids have been discontinued just prior to surgery, or if there are no plans to continue them after surgery. As with any patient with adrenal insufficiency, the clinical diagnosis must be entertained if, off the glucocorticoid, the 8:00 am cortisol level is less than 5 mg/dL. If a random cortisol or Cortrosyn (250 ug 1–24

ACTH) stimulated cortisol is greater than 25 mg/dL, adrenal insufficiency is unlikely [24].

Treatment for secondary adrenal insufficiency is influenced by the underlying disease being treated, the long-term dose being used prior to surgery and the type of procedure that will be done [25].

If the patient's glucocorticoid preoperative dose is equivalent to or higher than the dose needed for stress found in Table 31.2, then the preoperative dose of glucocorticoid should be continued. If the preoperative dose is lower then

Table 31.1 Management of adrenal insufficiency.

	Hydrocortisone dose adjustment
Strenous activities	Do not increase for emotional stress, common cold, or exercise
Fever > 100.5°	Double the dose
Fever > 102°	Triple the dose
Vomiting, diarrhea	Double or triple the dose depending on severity
Minor surgery	Intravenous 25–75 mg
Major surgery	100–150 mg 1 hour prior to procedure, then hydrocortisone 100 mg intravenously q 8 hour
Acute adrenal crisis	100–200 mg intravenously
Recovery from stress	Once the patient is stable, taper the hydrocortisone dose over 3–4 days to maintenance levels (30 mg/day in at least two divided doses) or to the patient's preoperative dose of glucocorticoid
Intravenous fluid needs	Prevent volume depletion and hypoglycemia with the use of intravenous saline and glucose

If the adrenal status is not known, or critical illness-related corticosteroid insufficiency is suspected in a patient with severe stress, a random serum cortisol should be drawn, and hydrocortisone 100 mg every 8 hours started. If the serum cortisol level subsequently is found to be < 10 µg/dL, the hydrocortisone is continued and tapered as the condition warrants.

Table 31.2 Interpretation of Cushing's screening tests [42–44].

Test	Cushing's syndrome is likely if results are:
24 hour UFC	Above the upper limit of normal More than 4 times the normal value is considered diagnostic of Cushing syndrome Up to 3-fold elevation can be associated with pseudoCushing's
1 mg overnight DST 8:00 am cortisol level	< 1.8 µg/dL
Midnight salivary cortisol	Greater than twice the upper limit of the reference range

the stress dose, then the glucocorticoid dose will need to be increased to meet the stress demand.

Treatment of adrenal insufficiency

Adrenal insufficiency is treated with steroid replacement. The mean total cortisol production in an unstressed individual is 10 mg/m^2 [7,24,28–30]. For primary adrenal insufficiency maintenance doses are 20–30 mg/day of hydrocortisone in 2–3 divided doses or 5–7.5 mg/day of prednisone in a single or divided dose [24]. Patients who are also receiving drugs such as rifampin, barbiturates, pioglitazone and phenytoin which induce hepatic metabolism of glucocorticoids, may require modest increases in the glucocorticoid dosage. Drugs that impair metabolism are itraconazole, ritonavir, fluoxetine, diltiazem, and cimetidine [31]. The necessity for mineralocorticoid replacement with Florinef (9α-fluorocortisol) at a dosage of 0.05–0.2 mg/day is determined by assessment of the blood pressure and serum potassium level [35].

During stress, patients may need adjustment in their hydrocortisone dose. For increased physical activity patients may have to add 5–10 mg of hydrocortisone to their usual dose. For severe stress such as fever or gastroenteritis they may need to double their usual dose. For extreme stress, procedures, or adrenal crisis 100–200 mg of intravenous hydrocortisone should be given [32–35].

Surgery is a major form of stress and traditionally patients are given the maximal stress dose (ten times the maintenance dose or 300 mg of hydrocortisone per day) starting in the perioperative period. Hydrocortisone 100 mg is given intravenously with induction of anesthesia, and 100 mg every 8 hours for at least 24 hours. The patient's status is determined and, if stable, the hydrocortisone is tapered over 4–5 days, (i.e., 50 mg every 8 hours for 1 day, 25 mg every 8 hours for 1 day, 25 mg BID for 1 day, then down to maintenance 10–20 mg in the morning and 5–10 mg in the afternoon). There is some evidence that smaller doses of hydrocortisone can be given, thus avoiding some of the adverse effects of high-dose steroids [36–38]. The dosing of the hydrocortisone depends on the stress produced by the surgery. For low-stress procedures (like an inguinal hernia repair) 25 mg on the day of the procedure for moderate stress (open cholecystectomy or colon resection), 50–75 mg on the day of surgery, and for 1–2 days after; and for major surgery (cardiothoracic surgery or esophagectomy) 100–150 mg on day of surgery and for 1–2 days after [36,37]. Daily doses of hydrocortisone exceeding 50 mg supply adequate mineralocorticoid replacement, but comparable doses of methylprednisolone and dexamethasone do not have the same degree of mineralocorticoid activity [24]. Blood pressure, electrolyte, and glucose measurements, as well as fluid status, must be carefully monitored. If patients develop any signs suggestive of acute adrenal crisis, intravenous hydrocortisone at a dosage of 300 mg/day (100 mg every 8 hours) plus glucose and saline infusions must be given emergently [39]. Once the acute stress has passed, patients can be weaned over several days to maintenance doses. Table 31.1 outlines the management of adrenal insufficiency.

Cushing's syndrome

The most common cause of Cushing's syndrome (the term for any state characterized by increased glucocorticoid effect) is exogenous glucocorticoid administration, which results in pituitary adrenal suppression. Cushing's disease, adrenal hyperplasia resulting from excess pituitary production of ACTH, is the cause of 70% of all cases of endogenous Cushing's syndrome. A pituitary adenoma is identified in most cases. Autonomous adrenal hyperfunction resulting from an adrenal adenoma or carcinoma, and ectopic production of ACTH by tumors (especially small cell carcinomas of the lung), each account for about 15% of all cases of endogenous Cushing's syndrome. Common signs and symptoms include obesity, facial plethora, hirsutism, menstrual irregularities, hypertension, proximal muscle weakness, back pain, and skin stria. Psychologic symptoms (e.g., euphoria, mania, psychosis) are probably under-reported. Patients with ectopic ACTH production have fewer chronic signs of glucocorticoid excess but demonstrate more mineralocorticoid effect with hypertension and hypokalemia associated with weight loss [40]. Adrenal carcinomas often are accompanied by signs of marked androgenicity as well as glucocorticoid effect, but often patients are diagnosed incidentally [41].

The initial testing for Cushing's syndrome includes one of the following [42]:

Urinary free cortisol (UFC) (at least two separate collections).

Late night salivary cortisol (at least two separate measurements).

1 mg overnight dexamethasone suppression test (DST).

Longer low-dose DST (0.5 mg every 6 hours for 48 hours = total 2 mg/48 hours).

If any of the tests are in the normal range, Cushing's syndrome is unlikely. The diagnosis of Cushing's syndrome is likely if two screening tests are abnormal [43–46]. If any of the tests are positive then localization studies are needed. Interpretation of the initial testing is listed in Table 31.2. If test results are equivocal then one of the tests needs to be repeated or dexamethasone suppression with CRH should be performed [43].

There are many substances that can interfere with the evaluation of Cushing's syndrome testing; they are listed in Table 31.3 [42].

Therapy for Cushing's syndrome involves surgical removal of the pituitary tumor, adrenal tumor, or ectopic source (if possible). Cure rates for pituitary microadenomas are very good and the transphenoidal surgery itself has low morbidity and mortality. Transient postoperative diabetes insipidus can occur. Complications after the resection of cortisol-producing adrenal tumors are more frequent and include wound infection, bleeding, pulmonary embolism, and respiratory

Table 31.3 Interference with tests for Cushing's syndrome [42,44].

Test	False positive	False negative
24 hour UFC	High fluid intake (5 liters/day) Carbamazepine Fenofibrate (increase if measured by HPLC) Digoxin (if measured by HPLC) Some synthetic glucocorticoids (immunoassays) Drugs that accelerate dexamethasone metabolism by induction of CYP 3A4: Phenobarbital Phenytoin Carbamazepine Primidone Rifampin Rifapentine Ethosuximide Pioglitazone Alcohol	Drugs that impair dexamethasone metabolism by inhibition of CYP 3A4I Aprepitant/fosaprepitant Itraconazole Ritonavir Fluoxetine Diltiazem Cimetidine
1 mg overnight DST	Depression, anxiety, obsessive compulsive disorder, morbid obesity, alcoholism, and diabetes mellitus can be characterized by overactivation of the HPA axis Drugs that accelerate dexamethasone metabolism by induction of CYP 3A4: Phenobarbital Phenytoin Carbamazepine Primidone Rifampin Rifapentine Ethosuximide Pioglitazone Alcohol Drugs that raise cortisol binding globulin: Estrogens Mitotane	Drugs that impair dexamethasone metabolism by inhibition of CYP 3A4I Aprepitant/fosaprepitant Itraconazole Ritonavir Fluoxetine Diltiazem Cimetidine
Midnight salivary cortisol	Cigarettes, cigars, pipe smoking, chewing tobacco and licorice (both contain 11β-hydroxysteroid dehydrogenase type 2 inhibitor glycyrrhizic acid)	Eating or drinking before the test Improper collection

infections. After surgery, a period of secondary adrenal insufficiency ensues. Unfortunately, adrenal carcinoma is often widely metastatic at the time of presentation and the prognosis is poor [47]. When surgical resection is not possible, medical therapy with ketoconazole, metyrapone, aminoglutethimide, mitotane, or cabergoline may be useful to decrease cortisol levels [48,49].

Patients with Cushing's syndrome have an increased incidence of hypertension, cardiovascular disease, diabetes mellitus, thromboembolism, delayed wound healing, and increased susceptibility to infection. Despite this increased risk of operative complications, emergent surgery can usually be safely performed in the face of hypercortisolism. If surgery can be postponed, the carefully monitored use of one or more of the agents mentioned above to control hypercortisolism may be of benefit in reducing surgical complications. After surgery patients must be observed for evidence of steroid withdrawal symptoms which may require replacement steroids that are then slowly tapered [45].

Primary aldosteronism

Primary aldosteronism (PA) is manifested by hypertension, increased aldosterone levels, low plasma renin levels, metabolic alkalosis, and hypokalemia. In about two-thirds of patients, it results from a unilateral adrenal adenoma. In the remainder of cases idiopathic hyperplasia is the usual cause. Adrenal carcinoma is an extremely rare cause. Adenomas are treated with adrenalectomy of the affected side which cures about three-fourths of patients.

The diagnosis of hyperaldosteronism is made when there is an elevated plasma aldosterone concentration above 20 ng/dL and a plasma aldosterone concentration (PAC) to plasma renin activity (PRA) ratio above 30 (sensitivity and specificity of 90% for the diagnosis of aldosterone-producing adenoma) [50,51]. The testing for elevated aldosterone levels can be difficult due to interfering substances, hypokalemia, and low salt diet [50]. The 2008 Endocrine Society guidelines recommend when the PAC/PRA ratio is being used for case detection of primary aldosteronism the following protocol should be followed [50].

Protocol: The test is performed by measuring the aldosterone to renin ratio (ARR) in the morning:

1. Withdraw agents that markedly affect the ARR for at least 4 weeks: spironolactone, eplerenone, amiloride, and triamterene (potassium wasting diuretics).
2. Encourage the patient to liberalize (rather than restrict) sodium intake.
3. Avoid products derived from licorice root (e.g., confectionery licorice, chewing tobacco).
4. Correct hypokalemia.
5. Collect blood mid-morning, after the patient has been up (sitting, standing, or walking) for at least 2 hours and seated for 5–15 min.

Table 31.4 Confirmatory tests [50].

Test	Test instructions	Interpretation
Oral sodium loading test	Patients should increase their sodium intake to 6 g/day for 3 days, verified by 24-hour urine sodium content. Patients should receive adequate slow-release potassium chloride supplementation to maintain plasma potassium in the normal range Urinary aldosterone is measured in the 24-hour urine collection from the morning of day 3 to the morning of day 4	PA is unlikely if urinary aldosterone is lower than 10 μg/24 hours in the absence of renal disease where PA may coexist with lower measured urinary aldosterone levels Elevated urinary aldosterone excretion [> 12 μg/24 hours at the Mayo Clinic, > 14 μg/24 hours at the Cleveland Clinic] makes PA highly likely
Saline suppression test	Patients stay in the recumbent position for at least 1 hour before and during the infusion of 2 liters of 0.9% saline IV over 4 hours, starting at 0800–0930 hours. Blood samples for renin, aldosterone, cortisol, and plasma potassium are drawn at time zero and after 4 hours, with blood pressure and heart rate monitored throughout the test	Post-infusion plasma aldosterone levels < 5 ng/dL make the diagnosis of PA unlikely, and levels > 10 ng/dL are a very probable sign of PA Values between 5 and 10 ng/dL are indeterminate

If the results of the ARR in the above conditions are not diagnostic, and if hypertension can be controlled with relatively non-interfering medications (see Table 31.4), withdraw other medications that may affect the ARR [48] for at least 2 weeks:

a. Beta-adrenergic blockers, central alpha-2 agonists (e.g., clonidine and alpha-methyldopa), non-steroidal anti-inflammatory drugs.

b. Angiotensin-converting enzyme inhibitors, angiotensin receptor blockers, renin inhibitors, dihydropyridine calcium channel antagonists.

c. This test should not be performed in patients with severe uncontrolled hypertension, renal insufficiency, cardiac insufficiency, cardiac arrhythmia, or severe hypokalemia.

Adrenal venous sampling is done to confirm that the patient has unilateral disease. Venous catheters are inserted via both femoral veins and both adrenal veins are catheterized simultaneously. Blood samples are obtained from each adrenal vein, and a peripheral site at baseline. If the test is done with ACTH, then an intravenous bolus of 0.25 mg of ACTH followed by an infusion of ACTH (0.25 mg in 250 mL normal saline) at a rate of 150 mL/hour is administered. Blood samples are collected at 5 minutes, 10 minutes, and 15 minutes post-ACTH infusion and levels for aldosterone and cortisol if ACTH is used. If ACTH is not used, then levels for aldosterone and cortisol are drawn at baseline and the catheters removed. The ratio of aldosterone-to-cortisol (AC) is calculated [52–54]. Diagnosis of a unilateral hyperfunctioning adrenal gland is made if the AC ratio on one side is at least four times greater than on the contralateral side if ACTH is used and greater than two if ACTH is not used. An AC ratio that was lower than the periphery on the unaffected side especially after stimulation suggests a suppressed gland and therefore, a unilateral hyperfunctioning gland on the contralateral side [52–54].

If the patient has a unilateral adenoma and surgery is planned, preoperative sodium restriction and a potassium-sparing diuretic such as spironolactone are used to correct the electrolyte abnormalities and hypertension. It is preferable to treat medically for 1–2 months before surgery to reduce the incidence of postoperative complications. After surgery electrolyte concentrations and blood pressure must be monitored. Recovery of the renin–aldosterone system may take many months but normal function is the usual outcome.

Hypoaldosteronism

Aldosterone deficiency without concomitant glucocorticoid deficiency is usually hyporeninemic hypoaldosteronism and rarely results from a primary abnormality of the adrenal cortex. Diabetes mellitus and tubulointerstitial renal disease are disorders that can be associated with decreased renin secretion, leading to subsequent hypoangiotensinemia and low aldosterone levels. The mineralocorticoid deficiency is manifested by hyperkalemia, hyperchloremic metabolic acidosis, and occasional sodium depletion. Most patients with hyporeninemic hypoaldosteronism are asymptomatic but hyperkalemia and metabolic acidosis can lead to arrhythmias. Treatment with furosemide, 40–120 mg/day helps relieve hyperkalemia and metabolic acidosis, although hypotension may be induced. This is typically combined with Florinef, which increases renal potassium and hydrogen ion excretion and causes salt retention. Correction of hyporeninemic hypoaldosteronism is desirable before surgery to prevent potential complications [55].

References

1. Chrousos GP. Stress and disorders of the stress system. *Nat Rev Endocrinol* 2009; **5**: 374–81.

2. Bornstein SR, Chrousos GP. Clinical review 104: adrenocorticotropin (ACTH)- and non-ACTH-mediated regulation of the adrenal cortex: neural and immune inputs. *J Clin Endocrinol Metab* 1999; **84**: 1729–36.

3. Elenkov IJ, Chrousos GP. Stress system – organization, physiology and immunoregulation. *Neuroimmunomodulation* 2006; **13**: 257–67.

4. Moore FA, Moore EE. Evolving concepts in the pathogenesis of postinjury multiple organ failure. *Surg Clin North Am* 1995; **75**: 257–77.

5. Hoen S, Asehnoune K, Brailly-Tabard S *et al.* Cortisol response to corticotropin stimulation in trauma patients: influence of hemorrhagic shock. *Anesthesiology* 2002; **97**: 807–13.

6. Young EA, Abelson J, Lightman SL. Cortisol pulsatility and its role in stress regulation and health. *Front Neuroendocrinol* 2004; **25**: 69–76.

7. Grossman AB. Clinical review: the diagnosis and management of central hypoadrenalism. *J Clin Endocrinol Metab* 2010; **95**: 4855–63.

8. Belavý DL, Seibel MJ, Roth HJ *et al.* The effects of bed rest and counter measure exercise on the endocrine system in male adults – evidence for immobilization induced reduction in SHBG levels. *J Endocrinol Invest* 2011; **35**: 54–62.

9. Litinski M, Scheer FA, Shea SA. Influence of the circadian system on disease severity. *Sleep Med Clin* 2009; **4**: 143–63.

10. Al-Damluji S, Cunnah D, Perry L, Grossman A, Besser GM. The effect of alpha adrenergic manipulation on the 24 hour pattern of cortisol secretion in man. *Clin Endocrinol (Oxford)* 1987; **26**: 61–6.

11. Caufriez A, Moreno-Reyes R, Leproult R *et al.* Immediate effects of an 8-h advance shift of the rest-activity cycle on 24-h profiles of cortisol. *Am J Physiol Endocrinol Metab* 2002; **282**: E1147–53.

12. Zoli A, Lizzio MM, Ferlisi EM *et al.* ACTH, cortisol and prolactin in active rheumatoid arthritis. *Clin Rheumatol* 2002; **21**: 289–93.

13. Vgontzas AN, Zoumakis M, Papanicolaou DA *et al.* Chronic insomnia is associated with a shift of interleukin-6 and tumor necrosis factor secretion from nighttime to daytime. *Metabolism* 2002; **51**: 887–92.

14. Fantidis P, Perez De Prada T, Fernandez-Ortiz A *et al.* Morning cortisol production in coronary heart disease patients. *Eur J Clin Invest* 2002; **32**: 304–30.

15. Baylis C, Handa RK, Sorkin, M. Glucocorticoids and control of glomerular filtration rate. *Semin Nephrol* 1990; **10**: 320–9.

16. Riad M, Mogos M, Thangathurai D, Lumb PD. Steroids. *Curr Opin Crit Care* 2002; **8**: 281–4.

17. Offner PJ, Moore EE, Ciesla D. The adrenal response after severe trauma. *Am J Surg* 2002; **184**: 649–53.

18. Marik, PE, Zaloga GP. Adrenal insufficiency in the critically ill: a new look at an old problem. *Chest* 2002; **122**: 1784–96.

19. Lamberts, SW J, Briuning HA, De Jong FH. Corticosteroid therapy in severe illness. *N Engl J Med* 1997; **337**: 1285–92.

20. Ho JT, Al-Musalhi H, Chapman MJ *et al.* Septic shock and sepsis: a comparison of total and free plasma cortisol levels. *J Clin Endocrinol Metab* 2006; **91**: 105–14.

21. Marik PE, Pastores SM, Annane D *et al.* Recommendations for the diagnosis and management of corticosteroid insufficiency in critical ill adult patients: Consensus statements from an international task force by the American College of Critical Care Medicine. *Crit Care Med* 2008; **36**: 1937–49.

22. Fleager K, Yao J. Perioperative steroid dosing in patients receiving chronic oral steroids, undergoing outpatient hand surgery. *J Hand Surg Am* 2010; **35**: 316–18.

23. Axelrod L. Perioperative management of patients treated with glucocorticoids. *Endocrinol Metab Clin North Am* 2003; **32**: 367–83.

24. Arlt W, Allolio B. Adrenal insufficiency. *Lancet* 2003; **361**(9372): 1881–93.

25. Gross AK, Winstead PS. Current controversies in critical illness-related corticosteroid insufficiency and glucocorticoid supplementation. *Orthopedics* 2009; **32**: 652–7.

26. Oelkers W. Adrenal insufficiency. *N Engl J Med* 1996; **335**: 1206–12.

27. Neary N, Nieman L. Adrenal insufficiency: etiology, diagnosis and treatment. *Curr Opin Endocrinol Diabetes Obes.* 2010; **17**: 217–23.

28. Annane D, Maxime V, Ibrahim F *et al.* Diagnosis of adrenal insufficiency in severe sepsis and septic shock. *Am J Respir Crit Care Med* 2006; **174**: 1319–26.

29. Nye EJ, Grice JE, Hockings GI. *et al.* Comparison of adrenocorticotropin (ACTH) stimulation tests and insulin hypoglycemia in normal humans: low dose, standard high dose, and 8-hour ACTH- (1–24) infusion tests. *J Clin Endocrinol Metab* 1999; **84**: 3648–55.

30. Cope CL, Black E. The production rate of cortisol in man. *Br Med J* 1958; **1**: 1020–4.

31. Debono M, Ross RJ, Newell-Price J. Inadequacies of glucocorticoid replacement and improvements by physiological circadian therapy. *Eur J Endocrinol* 2009; **160**: 719–29.

32. Oelkers W, Diederich S, Bah V. Diagnosis and therapy surveillance in Addison's disease: rapid adrenocorticotropin (ACTH) test and measurement of plasma ACTH, renin activity, and aldosterone, *J Clin Endocrinol Metab* 1992; **75**: 259–64.

33. Mah PM, Jenkins RC, Rostami-Hodjegan A *et al.* Weight-related dosing, timing and monitoring hydrocortisone replacement therapy in patients with adrenal insufficiency. *Clin Endocrinol (Oxford)* 2004; **61**: 367–75.

34. Salem M, Tainsh RE, Bromberg J, Loriaux DL, Chernow B. Perioperative glucocorticoid coverage: a reassessment 42 years after emergence of a problem, *Ann Surg* 1994; **219**: 416–25.

35. Glowniak JV, Loriaux DL. A double-blind study of perioperative steroid requirements in secondary adrenal insufficiency. *Surgery* 1997; **121**: 123–9.

36. Graham GW, Unger BP, Coursin DB. Perioperative management of selected endocrine disorders. *Int Anesthesiol Clin* 2000; **38**: 31–67.

37. Salem M, Tainsh RE, Bromberg J, Loriaux DL, Chernow B. Perioperative glucocorticoid coverage; a reassessment 42 years after emergence of a problem. *Ann Surg* 1994; **219**: 416–25.

38. Jabbour SA. Steroids and the surgical patient. *Med Clin North Am* 2001; **85**: 1311–17.

39. Roquilly A, Mahe PJ, Seguin P *et al.* Hydrocortisone therapy for patients with multiple trauma: the randomized controlled HYPOLYTE study. *J Am Med Assoc* 2011; **305**: 1201–9.

40. Carroll TB, Findling JW. The diagnosis of Cushing's syndrome. *Rev Endocr Metab Disord* 2010; **11**: 147–53.

41. Fassnacht M, Libé R, Kroiss M, Allolio B; Medscape. Adrenocortical carcinoma: a clinician's update. *Nat Rev Endocrinol* 2011; **7**: 323–35.

42. Nieman LK, Biller BM, Findling JW *et al.* The diagnosis of Cushing's syndrome: an Endocrine Society Clinical Practice Guideline. *J Clin Endocrinol Metab* 2008;**93**: 1526–40.

43. Findling JW, Raff H. Cushing's Syndrome: important issues in diagnosis and management. *J Clin Endocrinol Metab* 2006; **91**: 3746–53.

44. Zeiger MA, Thompson GB, Duh QY *et al.* American Association of Clinical Endocrinologists and American Association of Endocrine Surgeons Medical Guidelines for the Management of Adrenal Incidentalomas: executive summary of recommendations. *Endocr Pract* 2009; **15**: 450–3.

45. AbdelMannan D, Selman WR, Arafah BM. Peri-operative management of Cushing's disease. *Rev Endocr Metab Disord* 2010; **11**: 127–34.

46. Nieman LK. Approach to the patient with an adrenal incidentaloma. *J Clin Endocrinol Metab* 2010; **95**: 4106–13.

47. Clayton RN. Mortality in Cushing's disease. *Neuroendocrinology* 2010; **92**: 71–6.

48. Owen LJ, Halsall DJ, Keevil BG. Cortisol measurement in patients receiving metyrapone therapy. *Ann Clin Biochem* 2010; **47**: 573–5.

49. Vilar L, Naves LA, Azevedo MF *et al.* Effectiveness of cabergoline in monotherapy and combined with ketoconazole in the management of Cushing's disease. *Pituitary* 2010; **13**: 123–9.

50. Funder JW, Carey RM, Fardella C *et al.* Case detection, diagnosis, and treatment of patients with primary aldosteronism: an Endocrine Society Clinical Practice Guideline. *J Clin Endocrinol Metab* 2008; **93**: 3266–81.

51. Weinberger MH, Fineberg NS. The diagnosis of primary aldosteronism and separation of two major subtypes. *Arch Intern Med* 1993; **153**: 2125–9.

52. Mathur A, Kemp CD, Dutta U *et al.* Consequences of adrenal venous sampling in primary hyperaldosteronism and predictors of unilateral adrenal disease. *J Am Coll Surg* 2010; **211**: 384–90.

53. Mulatero P, Bertello C, Sukor N *et al.* Impact of different diagnostic criteria during adrenal vein sampling on reproducibility of subtype diagnosis in patients with primary aldosteronism. *Hypertension* 2010; **55**: 667–73.

54. Stowasser M, Gordon RD, Gunasekera TG *et al.* High rate of detection of primary aldosteronism, including surgically treatable forms, after 'non-selective' screening of hypertensive patients. *J Hypertens* 2003; **21**: 2149–57.

55. Torpy DJ, Stratakis CA, Chrousos GP. Hyper- and hypoaldosteronism. *Vitam Horm* 1999; **57**: 177–216.

Chapter 32

Disorders of calcium metabolism

Pamela T. Prescott

Calcium is an abundant mineral and has diffuse cellular functions in bone metabolism, cell division, coagulation, enzyme regulation, glycogen metabolism, muscle contraction, neurotransmission, protein synthesis, and degradation. Calcium is ingested in the diet and absorbed in the small intestine. It is distributed throughout the body, but 99% appears in the bone [1–3]. Adult humans contain more than 1 kg of calcium, of which over 99% is skeletal and dental and only 0.1% is in extracellular fluids. About half the calcium in serum is bound to protein, primarily of which is albumin. Decreases in serum albumin are accompanied by decreases in calcium (a drop of 1 g/dL of albumin lowers the calcium by about 0.8 mg/dL). Several calcium determinations and measurement of ionized (physiologically active) calcium levels may be needed to accurately assess calcium status.

Calcium is maintained in a very narrow range by a redundant system of parathyroid hormone (PTH), vitamin D, and calcitonin; all acting at multiple target organs, including bone, kidneys, and the gastrointestinal tract. As ionized (free, metabolically active) calcium levels decrease, the parathyroid glands secrete PTH, which raises calcium levels by stimulating bone resorption, renal calcium reabsorption, phosphate excretion, and renal 1,25-dihydroxycholecalciferol (1,25-$[OH]_2D_3$) synthesis. Vitamin D, in turn, promotes bone resorption, increases intestinal absorption of dietary calcium and phosphate, and inhibits PTH secretion [1,4–14]. Finally, calcitonin, released by parafollicular cells of the thyroid in response to hypercalcemia, has been shown to transiently inhibit bone resorption [5].

Serum calcium exists in three forms: (1) free or ionized calcium, the physiologically active form that accounts for 50% of total serum calcium, (2) calcium complexed to anions, including bicarbonate, lactate, phosphate, and citrate, and (3) calcium bound to plasma proteins, constituting the remaining 40%. Approximately 80% of the protein-bound calcium fraction is associated with albumin. Two gadolinium-based contrast agents (gadodiamide and gadoversetamide) interfere with colorimetric total serum calcium methods, particularly in patients with chronic kidney disease and cause pseudo or spurious hypocalcemia. When giving gadolinium, ionized calcium levels should be followed for 4–5 days after use of the contrast agent if calcium determination is required [10–12].

Measurements of serum calcium, PTH, 25-hydroxyvitamin D, and 1,25-dihydroxyvitamin D3 are used regularly in the diagnosis and treatment of calcium disorders. The normal serum calcium level is 8.5–10.5 mg/dL, with interlaboratory variation in the reference range [10]. Hypocalcemia is defined as total serum calcium lower than 8.5 mg/dL or as ionized serum calcium lower than 4.5 mg/dL [10]. Hypercalcemia is defined as a serum calcium level greater than 10.5 mg/dL. The severity of hypercalcemia may be classified based on total serum and ionized calcium levels (Table 32.1).

Vitamin D is produced in the skin or ingested. In the skin, sun exposure or other forms of ultraviolet light transform 7-dehydrocholesterol to D3 [15]. Vitamin D3 and vitamin D2 (ergocalceferol) are taken in from the diet (cholecalceferol). All the forms of vitamin D are metabolized in the liver to 25-hydroxyvitamin D. 25-hydroxyvitamin D is then metabolized in the kidneys to the active form 1,25-dihydroxyvitamin D3. The renal production of 1,25-dihydroxyvitamin D3 is tightly regulated by plasma PTH levels and serum calcium and phosphorus levels [6,8,13]. The normal value of vitamin D is based on the minimum need to adequately absorb calcium and control the PTH level for adequate bone health [16].

The normal range for 25-hydroxyvitamin D is 30–100 mg/dL [15,17]. The levels of 25-hydroxyvitamin D adequacy are listed in Table 32.2. Vitamin D deficiency and insufficiency have been linked to a wide variety of chronic diseases including common cancers [18], cardiovascular disease [19,20], autoimmune disorders [21,22], and infectious diseases [23].

The normal value for 1,25-dihydroxyvitamin D3 is 16–56 pg/mL [24]. Lab testing for 1,25-dihydroxyvitamin D3 is usually only performed when a patient has hypercalcemia and the cause is being explored [25].

Medical Management of the Surgical Patient, ed. Michael F. Lubin, Thomas F. Dodson, and Neil H. Winawer. Published by Cambridge University Press. © Cambridge University Press 2013.

Table 32.1 Normal and hypercalcemic serum calcium levels.

	Total calcium mg/dL	Ionized calcium mg/dL
Normal	8.5–10.5	4.5–5.6
Mild	10.2–11.9	5.7–8.0
Moderate	12.0–13.9	8.1–9.9
Severe	> 14.0	10.0–12.0

Table 32.2 Levels of 25-hydroxyvitamin D deficiency [17].

	mg/dL
Normal	30–100
Deficient	< 20
Insufficient	21–29

Table 32.3 Medications that alter calcium levels.

Medications that cause hypocalcemia	Medications that cause hypercalemia
Alcohol	Calcium
Bisphosphonates (alendronate, ibandronate, residronate, pamidronate, zoledronic acid)	Calcitriol
Cinnacalcet	Cholecalceferol
Ethylenediaminetetraacetic acid (EDTA)	Ergocalceferol
Estrogen	Hydrochlorothiazide
Furosemide	Lithium
Glucocorticoids	Teraratide
Phosphate-containing enemas	Vitamin A
Proton pump inhibitors	
Raloxifene	
Pseudohypocalcemia: gadolinium	

Parathyroid hormone is synthesized in the parathyroid glands and after cleavage of precursor molecules, is released into the circulation as an 84-amino-acid polypeptide and small fragments [1,4]. The amino-terminal 1–34 amino acids compose the biologically active portion of the molecule. Highly specific immunoradiometric assays are available that measure the intact hormone. Parathyroid concentration depends on many factors such as 25-hydroxyvitamin D levels, dietary calcium and phosphorus intakes, kidney function, physical inactivity, and drug use [23]. Parathyroid hormone release is primarily controlled by serum calcium levels, although modest hypomagnesemia also evokes a PTH response, whereas severe hypomagnesemia impairs release [4]. Parathyroid hormone increases serum calcium by increasing bone resorption, decreasing calciuria, and indirectly increasing gastrointestinal absorption of calcium by its effects on the production of 1,25-dihydroxyvitamin D3 and stimulation of the vitamin D-dependent calcium pump [3,6,26].

The normal PTH range is 15–65 pg/mL [27]. Modifications to PTH assays have allowed for more rapid testing of PTH when an immediate result is needed. Intraoperative monitoring of PTH levels serves as a guide and improves the cure rate of minimally invasive parathyroidectomy (secondary to hyperfunctioning parathyroid glands) [28]. The normal range for the quick test is 12–88 pg/mL. Depending on the protocol, intraoperative PTH samples are collected at 5 min, 10 min, 15 min, 20 min after excision of an abnormal parathyroid gland. A decrease in the PTH level of 50–70% (depending on the criterion) from baseline indicates a successful operation [29–32].

Calcitonin is synthesized in the thyroidal perifollicular cells in response to hypercalcemia. Calcitonin directly inhibits bone resorption and may indirectly increase calciuria. The physiologic importance of calcitonin in humans is questioned [9].

Medications can alter calcium levels (see Table 32.3) [33,34].

Both hypercalcemia and hypocalcemia may be associated with life-threatening cardiac arrhythmias as well as morbidity affecting other organ systems. Effective treatment is available and clinicians should be alert to abnormalities in serum calcium, which are present in more than 2% of hospitalized patients. Furthermore, both hypercalcemia and hypocalcemia suggest significant underlying pathology and efforts to diagnose and treat these conditions should be instituted.

Hypercalcemia

In the ambulatory setting, hypercalcemia is typically mild, asymptomatic, and detected incidentally. Hypercalcemia affects the function of many organs. When it is severe, hypercalcemia can cause arrhythmias and heart block. Gastrointestinal symptoms include anorexia, nausea, vomiting, constipation, and ileus. Prolonged hypercalcemia may be associated with peptic ulcer disease and pancreatitis. Affected patients may exhibit polyuria and polydipsia resulting from reversible nephrogenic diabetes insipidus. Acute and chronic renal failure with nephrolithiasis and nephrocalcinosis may occur. Neuropsychiatric symptoms include poor concentration and memory, weakness, lethargy, depression, coma, and rarely psychosis.

Causes of hypercalcemia are listed in Table 32.4 [35–41]. The three most common causes of hypercalcemia are primary hyperparathyroidism, malignancy, and granulomatous diseases. Hypercalcemia may be discovered when serum calcium is measured as a screening test or as part of the evaluation for fatigue, unexplained weakness, neuromuscular disability, renal stones, or osteopenia [41].

Hyperparathyroidism is diagnosed when there is hypercalcemia and inappropriately normal or elevated levels of PTH. Not all patients have elevated serum or ionized calcium levels at every laboratory draw for calcium. In those with mild hyperparathyroidism, the serum calcium may be at the upper

Table 32.4 Causes of hypercalcemia.

Primary hyperparathyroidism

Familial hypocalciuric hypercalcemia

Malignancy (PTHrP, cytokines, prostaglandin E, 1,25-dihydroxycholecalciferol)

Granulomatous disease (1,25-dihydroxycholecalciferol)
    Sarcoid
    Tuberculosis
    Fungal infections
    Leprosy
    Silicone
    Lymphoma

Hyperthyroidism

Hypothyroidism (rare)

Acromegaly (rare)

Calcium ingestion

Vitamin D intoxication

Vitamin A intoxication

Thiazides

Lithium

Immobilization in association with:
    Adolescence
    Paget's disease
    Any state with increased bone resorption

Renal disease
    Diuretic phase of acute renal failure
    Renal transplantation
    Tertiary hyperparathyroidism

limit of normal, and the ionized calcium normal or slightly elevated [41]. Hyperparathyroidism may present as part of a multiple endocrine neoplasia syndrome. With prolonged hyperparathyroidism, hypophosphatemia and a hyperchloremic acidosis may occur. Immunoradiometric assays for intact PTH (IRMA, PTH-intact) are usually used to confirm the elevation in PTH.

The next most common cause of hypercalcemia is associated with malignancy. This is almost always related to a systemic or local osseous humoral cause. The most common cause of solid tumor hypercalcemia is excessive elaboration of parathyroid hormone-related protein. This protein, which is a product of many normal tissues, has substantial homology with the amino-terminal end of the parathyroid hormone and binds to the same receptor [42,43]. It can be measured by specific assays that do not measure parathyroid hormone, permitting laboratory distinction between these two common causes of hypercalcemia. The hypercalcemia of malignancy may also be mediated by various cytokines, including lymphotoxin, interleukin-1, and tumor necrosis factor, by tumorous production of 1,25-dihydroxyvitamin D3 or prostaglandins that increase osteoclast-mediated resorption [44].

Familial hypocalciuric hypercalcemia may be difficult to discern from hyperparathyroidism. Parathyroid hormone levels are typically not elevated yet are not appropriately suppressed. Lack of tissue damage, onset in childhood, family history, and low urinary calcium levels should help with the diagnosis. Although parathyroidectomy is the usual therapy for primary hyperparathyroidism, it is neither required nor recommended for familial hypocalciuric hypercalcemia.

Granulomatous disease causes hypercalcemia in a few patients and this is typically mediated by 1,25-dihydroxyvitamin D3 hydroxylated in the granuloma [35]. Vitamin D and vitamin A cause bone resorption. Thiazide diuretics, by decreasing calciuria, can cause a transient hypercalcemia. If this persists, even on the drug, a work-up to exclude another causes is appropriate. Lithium alters the set-point for calcium feedback of PTH release, resulting in mild hypercalcemia without appropriate suppression of PTH. Immobilization leads to hypercalcemia in states of increased bone turnover (adolescence, Paget's disease, hyperthyroidism) and aggravates hypercalcemia resulting from other causes. Other, less common, causes are listed.

Therapy for hypercalcemia

Patients with hypercalcemia should discontinue the use of any oral calcium and vitamin D supplements as well as any medications that raise calcium levels (Table 32.3). If possible clinicians should also attempt to increase the weight-bearing mobility of the patient [45].

Therapy for asymptomatic hyperparathyroidism may include bisphosphonates, estrogen, selective estrogen receptor modulators (SERMs), or cinacalcet, although there are insufficient data to recommend them as an alternative [41]. Both estrogen (for selected postmenopausal women) and bisphosphonates may provide skeletal protection, even though hypercalcemia may persist. Cinacalcet has been approved by the US Food and Drug Administration for the treatment of secondary hyperparathyroidism associated with renal failure and hypercalcemia associated with parathyroid cancer [41].

For patients with symptoms or severe side-effects of hyperparathyroidism surgery is recommended. Granulomatous diseases can be treated with corticosteroids [46]. A therapeutic response may take days or weeks to achieve and high doses (5–8 times maintenance doses) are typically required. Chloroquine, hydroxychloroquine, and ketoconazole can be used if the patient fails to respond or develops dangerous side-effects from corticosteroid therapy [47]. Malignancy-associated hypercalcemia is usually severe and normally requires several modalities to lower serum calcium and limit the hypercalcemic effects. Patients with hypercalcemia and thyrotoxicosis may show a hypocalcemic response to beta-blockers. Treatment of the hyperthyroidism usually normalizes the calcium [48]. Selected patients with renal failure and hypercalcemia require dialysis [49].

For severe hypercalcemia, rehydration with intravenous saline and early mobilization are important. Forced saline diuresis with large amounts of normal saline (150–250 mL/hour) together with furosemide may be needed [45]. Cardiovascular and electrolyte status need to be monitored. If further treatment is necessary, salmon calcitonin (4–12 MRC U/kg every 6–12 hours subcutaneously) exhibits a hypocalcemic effect in 2 hours and can be used safely in the presence of hepatic and renal disease. Bisphosphonates, like pamidronate and zoledronic acid, have become the standard. Etidronate was previously used, but pamidronate and zoledronic acid are easier to administer and more effective [50]. Zoledronic is more efficacious than pamidronate, and has a longer duration of action [51]. Pamidronate 60–90 mg is infused intravenously over 4–24 hours. Zoledronic 4 mg is infused over 15 minutes. Pamidronate and zoledronic acid are potent inhibitors of bone resorption but may not affect tubular calcium reabsorption, as seen with some malignancies. In these patients gallium nitrate is infused at a rate of 200 mg/m^2 over 5 days. Care should be taken given the potential for nephrotoxicity [50].

The treatment options and adverse effects for hypercalcemia are listed in Table 32.5 [44,45,50–53].

For patients with hypercalcemia who need surgery, careful evaluation is needed. During anesthesia, several factors may alter the serum ionized calcium level, thus potentiating the adverse effects of hypercalcemia. The duration of nondepolarizing relaxants is likely to be prolonged, especially if muscle weakness coexists. A reduction in the duration of action of atracurium has been reported in a patient whose serum calcium was elevated secondary to hyperparathyroidism [54].

Hypocalcemia

Modest hypocalcemia commonly occurs in critically ill patients but is not clinically significant. When symptoms do occur, they involve multiple organs, and may include tetany, muscle spasms, hyper-reflexia, paresthesias (circumoral, extremities), weakness, irritability, depression, dementia, and, rarely psychosis. The classic symptoms include muscle twitching, spasms, tingling, and numbness. Carpopedal spasm is characteristic but in severe cases can progress to tetany, seizures, and cardiac dysrhythmias [55,56]. In patients without overt signs, underlying neuromuscular excitability can become evident with provocation tapping of the parotid gland over the facial nerve, evoking facial muscle spasm (Chvostek's sign) [56]. However, 10% of normal people have a positive Chvostek's sign. Conversely, a small study of patients with hypoparathyroidism and biochemically confirmed hypocalcemia found that 29% were negative for Chvostek's sign, which makes this test a poor discriminator. Trousseau's sign is more specific, with 94% of hypocalcemic patients displaying a positive sign compared with 1% of normocalcemic people [55]. The Trousseau sign is induced by inflation of a blood pressure cuff; the subsequent muscle hypoxia can precipitate carpopedal spasm [56].

Cardiovascular manifestations include hypotension, bradycardia, arrhythmias, and digitalis and catecholamine

Table 32.5 Treatment options and adverse effects for hypercalcemia.

Treatment	Dose	Adverse effects
Intravenous normal saline	200–500 mg/hour	Volume overload with congestive heart failure and third spacing of fluid
Furosemide	20–40 mg with hydration if volume overload is present	Dehydration and hypokalemia
Bisphosphonates Pamidronate	60–90 mg intravenously over 2–4 hours (mixed in 200–500 mL of normal saline or 5% dextrose and water)	Renal failure Osteonecrosis of jaw Flu-like symptoms (fever, lymphocytopenia, malaise, and myalgias) Hypocalcemia
Zoledronic acid	4 mg intravenously over 15 minutes (mixed in 50 mL of normal saline or 5% dextrose in water)	Renal failure Osteonecrosis of jaw Flu-like symptoms (fever, lymphocytopenia, malaise, and myalgias) Hypocalcemia
Other treatments Salmon calcitonin	4 international units (IU)/kg usually administered intramuscularly or subcutaneously every 12 hours; doses can be increased up to 6 to 8 IU/kg every 6 hours Nasal calcitonin can not be used.	Useful for 48 hours only, tachyphylaxis quickly develops Nausea, diarrhea
Glucocorticoids	40–60 mg oral daily for 10 days	Hypertension, hypokalemia, glucose intolerance, hypertension, immunosuppression
Cinacalcet	30 mg twice daily, increase dose incrementally (60 mg twice daily, 90 mg twice daily, 90 mg 3–4 times/day) as necessary to normalize serum calcium levels. Maximum daily dose: 360 mg daily as 90 mg 4 times/day.	FDA approved for treatment of hypercalcemia and elevated PTH in parathyroid cancer or chronic kidney disease. Nausea, vomiting, diarrhea, dizziness, anorexia

insensitivity. Electrocardiographic QT intervals are prolonged. Laryngospasm and bronchospasm may occur as well [57].

Causes of hypocalcemia are listed in Table 32.6. Hypocalcemia results from a deficiency of parathyroid hormone, impaired parathyroid action, a deficiency of vitamin D, impaired vitamin D action, complexing or precipitation of calcium, increased osteoblastic activity, or drugs that inhibit bone resorption (Table 32.6). Patients with hypoparathyroidism typically have hyperphosphatemia, whereas those with vitamin D deficiency have low serum phosphorus levels. Measurement of serum parathyroid hormone levels distinguishes hypoparathyroidism from pseudohypoparathyroidism because levels are increased in the latter. Levels of 25-hydroxyvitamin D assess renal hydroxylation. Severe hypomagnesemia (less than 1 mg/dL) impairs both parathyroid hormone release and activity [58].

Surgical patients with hypocalcemia require normalization of serum levels to prevent cardiorespiratory and neurologic manifestations. Ionized calcium determinations should be performed in patients with hypoalbuminemia, although the reliability of this measurement is variable. Patients with hyperphosphatemia should be treated with dietary restrictions and phosphate binders (aluminum hydroxide or aluminum carbonate) to lower their serum phosphate levels because vigorous administration of calcium may result in enhanced soft

Table 32.6 Causes of hypocalcemia.

Hypoparathyroidism (subnormal parathyroid hormone release)
  Idiopathic (autoimmune)
  Postsurgical
  Infiltrative (metastatic cancer, hemochromatosis, amyloidosis, granulomatous disease, Wilson's disease)
  Irradiation
  Severe hypomagnesemia

Pseudohypoparathyroidism

Vitamin D deficiency
  Decreased absorption
  Decreased 25-(OH)D$_3$ (severe liver disease)
  Decreased 1,25-(OH)$_2$D$_3$ (renal failure, vitamin D-dependent rickets)

Hyperphosphatemia
  Tumor lysis
  Rhabdomyolysis
  Iatrogenic

Massive blood transfusion (citrate)

Osteoblastic metastases

Parathyroidectomy (hungry bones)

Drugs
  Anticalcemic agents (discussed in text)
  Asparaginase
  Cisplatin
  Cytosine arabinoside
  Foscarnet
  Ketoconazole

tissue precipitation. Patients with hypomagnesemia require normalization of their serum magnesium levels to achieve normal calcium levels.

Symptomatic hypocalcemia should be treated emergently with intravenous calcium [10]. A 100–200 mg bolus of elemental calcium, diluted to minimize venous irritation should be given over a 10-minute period. The advantage of calcium gluconate (90 mg elemental calcium per 10 mL ampule) is that it is less irritating to the veins than calcium chloride (272 mg of elemental calcium per 10 mL ampule). Intravenous calcium therapy only raises the calcium level for 1 to 2 hours. If the hypocalcemia is severe, an infusion of 15 mg/kg elemental calcium (about 100–200 mg of elemental calcium in 500 mL) over 4–6 hours can be given. This will raise the serum calcium by 2–3 mg/dL [59,60]. Serum calcium levels should be monitored every few hours during treatment because hypercalcemia, nausea, arrhythmias, bradycardia, and digitalis toxicity may occur. When the patient is stable, oral calcium should be started, at a dose of 1–4 g elemental calcium per day. If the patient was hypercalcemic prior to neck surgery, subsequent hypocalcemia could be from temporary or permanent damage to the parathyroid glands, or hungry bone syndrome. These patients may require both oral and intravenous calcium therapy along with vitamin D in the form of 1,25-dihydroxyvitamin D3.

For patients with hypocalcemia who need surgery, several surgical factors alter the serum calcium and ionized calcium levels, and may potentiate the adverse effects of the hypocalcemia. These include abnormal acid–base status and electrolytes; transfusion of large volumes of citrated blood; and the use of cardiopulmonary bypass [59]. Acidosis decreases calcium binding to albumin thus increasing ionized calcium, while alkalosis increases calcium binding resulting in lower ionized calcium levels. Massive blood transfusions and cardiopulmonary bypass (which requires massive blood transfusions) expose the patient to a high amount of citrate that can temporarily lower calcium levels. Calcium levels should be monitored closely, so treatment, if needed, can be started immediately. Symptomatic hypocalcemia should be treated emergently with intravenous calcium [10]. A 100–200 mg bolus of elemental calcium, diluted to minimize venous irritation, should be given over a 10-min period. Calcium chloride provides more elemental calcium per gram than does either calcium gluconate or calcium gluceptate but all are acceptable forms of therapy. Subsequent treatment varies according to the cause of the hypocalcemia. A continuous calcium infusion (100–200 mg of elemental calcium in 500 mL over 6 hours) may be adequate in the acute perioperative setting but oral calcium or the addition of vitamin D may be indicated for future long-term therapy. If needed, a short-acting vitamin D preparation such as 1,25-dihydroxyvitamin D3 can be utilized but should be maintained at mildly hypocalcemic levels to stimulate the remaining parathyroid tissue to recover. Serum calcium levels should be monitored every few hours during treatment because hypercalcemia, nausea, arrhythmias, bradycardia, and toxicity from digitalis may occur.

References

1. Bringhurst F. Demay M, Kroenberg H. Hormones and disorders of mineral metabolism. In Wilson JD, Kronenberg KM, Melmed S, Polansky KS, Laresen PR, eds. *Williams Textbook of Endocrinology*. 11th edition. Philadelphia, PA: W. B. Saunders/ Elsevier Health Sciences; 2007, pp. 1155–209.

2. O'Toole JF. Disorders of calcium metabolism. *Nephron Physiol* 2011; **118**: 22–27.

3. Perez AV, Picotto G, Carpentieri AR *et al.* Minireview on regulation of intestinal calcium absorption. Emphasis on molecular mechanisms of transcellular pathway. *Digestion* 2008; **77**: 22–34.

4. Marx SJ. Hyperparathyroid and hypoparathyroid disorders. *N Engl J Med* 2000; **343**: 1863–75.

5. Marcus R. Diagnosis and treatment of hyperparathyroidism. *Rev Endocr Metab Disord* 2000; **1**: 247–52.

6. Holick MF. Vitamin D deficiency. *N Engl J Med* 2007; **357**: 266–81.

7. Baird GS. Ionized calcium. *Clin Chim Acta* 2011; **412**: 696–701.

8. DeLuca HF. Overview of general physiologic features and functions of vitamin D. *Am J Clin Nutr* 2004; **80** (Suppl): 1689S–96S.

9. Wallach S, Rousseau G, Martin L, Azria M. Effects of calcitonin on animal and in vitro models of skeletal metabolism. *Bone* 1999; **25**: 509–16.

10. Khan MI, Waguespack SG, Hu MI. Medical management of postsurgical hypoparathyroidism. *Endocr Pract* 2011; **17** (Suppl 1): 18–25. Erratum in 2011; **17**: 967. Dosage error in article text.

11. Prince MR, Erel HE, Lent RW *et al.* Gadodiamide administration causes spurious hypocalcemia. *Radiology* 2003; **227**: 639–46.

12. Gandhi MJ, Narra VR, Brown JJ *et al.* Clinical and economic impact of falsely decreased calcium values caused by gadoversetamide interference. *Am J Roentgenol* 2008; **190**: W213–17.

13. Christakos S, Ajibade DV, Dhawan P, Fechner AJ, Mady LJ. Vitamin D: metabolism. *Endocrinol Metab Clin North Am* 2010; **39**: 243–53.

14. Takeyama K, Kato S. The vitamin D3 1 alpha-hydroxylase gene and its regulation by active vitamin D3. *Biosci Biotechnol Biochem.* 2011; **75**: 208–13.

15. Holick MF. Vitamin D: a D-Lightful health perspective. *Nutr Rev* 2008; **66** (10 Suppl 2): S182–94.

16. Hollis BW. Assessment and interpretation of circulating 25-hydroxyvitamin D and 1,25-dihydroxyvitamin D in the clinical environment. *Endocrinol Metab Clin North Am* 2010; **39**: 271–86.

17. Hollis BW, Wagner CL. Normal serum vitamin D levels. *N Engl J Med* 2005; **352**: 515–16.

18. Davis CD. Vitamin D and cancer: current dilemmas and future research needs. *Am J Clin Nutr* 2008; **88**: 565S–9S.

19. Agarwal M, Phan A, Willix R Jr, Barber M, Schwarz ER. Is vitamin D deficiency associated with heart failure? A review of current evidence. *J Cardiovasc Pharmacol Ther* 2011; **16**: 354–63.

20. Pilz S, März W, Wellnitz B *et al.* Association of vitamin D deficiency with heart failure and sudden cardiac death in a large cross-sectional study of patients referred for coronary angiography. *J Clin Endocrinol Metab* 2008; **93**: 3927–35.

21. Caramaschi P, Dalla Gassa A, Ruzzenente O *et al.* Vitamin D and autoimmune rheumatic diseases. *Clin Rheumatol.* 2011; **30**: 443–4.

22. Bartley J. Vitamin D: emerging roles in infection and immunity. *Expert Rev Anti Infect Ther* 2010; **8**: 1359–69.

23. Mora JR, Makoto Iwata M, Andrian UH. Vitamin effects on the immune system: vitamins A and D take centre stage. *Nature Reviews Immunology* 2008; **8**: 685–98.

24. Hollis BW. Assessment and interpretation of circulating 25-hydroxyvitamin D and 1,25-dihydroxyvitamin D in the clinical environment. *Endocrinol Metab Clin North Am* 2010; **39**: 271–86.

25. Jones G. Pharmacokinetics of vitamin D toxicity. *Am J Clin Nutr* 2008; **88**: 582S–6S.

26. Potts JT. Parathyroid hormone: Past and present. *J Endocrinol* 2005; **187**: 311–25.

27. Aloia JF, Feuerman M, James MS, Yeh K. Reference range for serum parathyroid hormone. *Endocr Pract* 2006; **12**: 137–44.

28. Sokoll LJ. Measurement of parathyroid hormone and application of parathyroid hormone in intraoperative monitoring. *Clin Lab Med* 2004; **24**: 199–216.

29. Barczynski M, Konturek A, Hubalewska-Dydejczyk A, Cichon S, Nowak W. Evaluation of Halle, Miami, Rome, and Vienna intraoperative iPTH assay criteria in guiding minimally invasive parathyroidectomy. *Langenbecks Arch Surg* 2009; **394**: 843–9.

30. Lupoli GA, Fonderico F, Panico A *et al.* Stricter criteria increase the validity of a quick intraoperative parathyroid hormone assay in primary hyperparathyroidism. *Med Sci Monit* 2009; **15**: CR111–16.

31. Richards ML, Thompson GB, Farley DR, Grant CS. An optimal algorithm for intraoperative parathyroid hormone monitoring. *Arch Surg* 2011; **146**: 280–5.

32. Sugino K, Ito K, Nagahama M *et al.* Minimally invasive surgery for primary hyperparathyroidism with or without intraoperative parathyroid hormone monitoring. *Endocr J* 2010; **57**: 953–8.

33. Liamis G, Milionis HJ, Elisaf M. A review of drug-induced hypocalcemia. *J Bone Miner Metab* 2009; **27**: 635–42.

34. Ruppe MD. Medications that affect calcium. *Endocr Pract* 2011; **17** (Suppl 1): 26–30.

35. Iannuzzi MC, Fontana JR Sarcoidosis: clinical presentation, immunopathogenesis, and therapeutics. *J Am Med Assoc* 2011; **305**: 391–9.

36. Broome JT, Solorzano CC. Lithium use and primary hyperparathyroidism. *Endocr Pract* 2011; **17** (Suppl 1): 31–5.

37. Sharretts JM, Kebebew E, Simonds WF. Parathyroid cancer. *Semin Oncol* 2010; **37**: 580–90.

38. Lameire N, Van Biesen W, Vanholder R. Electrolyte disturbances and acute kidney injury in patients with cancer. *Semin Nephrol* 2010; **30**: 534–47.

39. Pelosof LC, Gerber DE. Paraneoplastic syndromes: an approach to diagnosis and treatment. *Mayo Clin Proc* 2010; **85**: 838–54.

40. De Sanctis V, Fiscina B, Ciccone S. Severe hypercalcemia in a patient

treated for hypoparathyroidism with calcitriol. *Pediatr Endocrinol Rev* 2010; 7: 363–5.

41. Bilezikian JP, Khan AA, Potts JT Jr; Third International Workshop on the Management of Asymptomatic Primary Hyperthyroidism. Guidelines for the management of asymptomatic primary hyperparathyroidism: summary statement from the third international workshop. *J Clin Endocrinol Metab* 2009; **94**: 335–9.

42. Dunne FP, Lee S, Ratcliffe WA *et al.* Parathyroid hormone-related protein (PTHrP) gene expression in solid tumours associated with normocalcaemia and hypercalcaemia. *J Pathol* 1993; **171**: 215–21.

43. Isowa S, Shimo T, Ibaragi S *et al.* PTHrP regulates angiogenesis and bone resorption via VEGF expression. *Anticancer Res* 2010; **30**: 2755–67.

44. Lumachi F, Brunello A, Roma A, Basso U. Cancer-induced hypercalcemia. *Anticancer Res* 2009; **29**: 1551–5.

45. Stewart AF. Clinical practice. Hypercalcemia associated with cancer. *N Engl J Med* 2005; **352**: 373–9.

46. Iannuzzi MC, Fontana JR. Sarcoidosis: clinical presentation, immunopathogenesis, and therapeutics. *J Am Med Assoc* 2011; **305**: 391–9.

47. Sharma OP. Hypercalcemia in granulomatous disorders: a clinical review. *Curr Opin Pulm Med* 2000; **6**: 442–7.

48. Iqbal AA, Burgess EH, Gallina DL, Nanes MS, Cook CB. Hypercalcemia in hyperthyroidism: patterns of serum calcium, parathyroid hormone, and 1,25-dihydroxyvitamin D3 levels during management of thyrotoxicosis. *Endocr Pract* 2003; **9**: 517–21.

49. Lameire N, Van Biesen W, Vanholder R. Electrolyte disturbances and acute kidney injury in patients with cancer. *Semin Nephrol* 2010; **30**: 534–47.

50. McMahan J, Linneman T. A case of resistant hypercalcemia of malignancy with a proposed treatment algorithm. *Ann Pharmacother* 2009; **43**(9): 1532–8.

51. Major P, Lortholary A, Han J *et al.* Zoledronic acid is superior to pamidronate in the treatment of hypercalcemia of malignancy: a pooled analysis of two randomized, controlled clinical trials. *J Clin Oncol* 2001; **19**: 558–67.

52. Deftos LJ. Calcitonin as a drug. *Ann Intern Med* 1981; **95**(2): 192–7.

53. Silverberg SJ, Rubin MR, Faiman C *et al.* Cinacalcet hydrochloride reduces the serum calcium concentration in inoperable parathyroid carcinoma. *J Clin Endocrinol Metab* 2007; **92**(10): 3803–8.

54. Aguilera IM, Vaughan RX. Calcium and the anaesthetist. *Anaesthesia* 2000; **55**: 770–90.

55. Cooper MS, Gittoes NJ. Diagnosis and management of hypocalcaemia. *Br Med J* 2008; **336**: 1298–302.

56. Urbano FL. Signs of hypocalcemia: Chvostek's and Trousseau's. *Hosp Physician* 2000; **36**: 43–5.

57. Mavroudis K, Aloumanis K, Stamatis P *et al.* Irreversible end-stage heart failure in a young patient due to severe chronic hypocalcemia associated with primary hypoparathyroidism and celiac disease. *Clin Cardiol* 2010; **33**(2): E72–5.

58. Swaminathan R. Magnesium metabolism and its disorders. *Clin Biochem Rev* 2003; **24**(2): 47–66.

59. Aguilera IM, Vaughan RX. Calcium and the anaesthetist. *Anaesthesia* 2000; **55**: 770–790.

60. Vasa FR. Endocrine problems in the chronically critically ill patient. *Clin. Chest Med.* 2001; **22**: 193–208.

Chapter

33

Pheochromocytoma

Pamela T. Prescott

Pheochromocytomas are not a common medical/surgical problem. They are estimated to cause only 0.1–0.5% of all cases of hypertension [1,2], and are seen in 4–7% of patients with incidentally found adrenal adenomas [2,3]. That being said, at some time in their careers medical consultants are likely to be asked to evaluate a patient with a suspected pheochromocytoma. Because catecholamines have major regulatory effects on many different body systems, it is vital that these be anticipated and properly managed in the perioperative period. Pheochromocytomas are associated with an increased risk of adverse reactions to many commonly prescribed drugs and clinicians must also be aware of this potential hazard. The removal of a pheochromocytoma has great potential for complications, both during and after surgery because of the release of catecholamines during manipulation or stimulation of the tumor.

Pathophysiology

Pheochromocytomas arise from chromaffin cells of the neural crest that migrate to form the adult adrenal medulla and sympathetic ganglia. These cells synthesize catecholamines through a series of enzymatically controlled steps, starting with the conversion of tyrosine to dihydroxyphenylalanine (dopa) by tyrosine hydroxylase. This is the rate-limiting step in catecholamine synthesis. Dopa is then converted to dopamine, which is subsequently decarboxylated to norepinephrine. The methylation of norepinephrine to epinephrine is accomplished through the action of phenylethanolamine-N-methyl transferase, an enzyme that is induced by glucocorticoids that reach the adrenal medulla in high concentrations through the corticomedullary venous sinuses from the adrenal cortex. Norepinephrine and epinephrine are the major products of most pheochromocytomas [4]. Epinephrine is produced mainly in the adrenal medulla; thus, a pheochromocytoma that produces epinephrine is nearly always located in the adrenal gland. Norepinephrine is produced and secreted in the central nervous system and the sympathetic post-ganglionic nerve endings as well as in the adrenal medulla. Dopamine is also produced and secreted by some pheochromocytomas. The metabolism of catecholamines takes place mostly in the same cells where the catecholamines are synthesized [4]. Once catecholamines reach the plasma, they have a half-life of only 1–2 minutes before they are taken up by cells or enzymatically degraded [5]. Metanephrine, normetanephrine, and vanillylmandelic acid are the major metabolites.

Catecholamines bind to adrenergic and dopaminergic cell-surface receptors, which in turn induce second messengers. Norepinephrine is primarily an alpha-adrenergic agonist that causes vasoconstriction and hypertension with little metabolic activity. Epinephrine, an alpha- and beta-adrenergic agonist, has positive inotropic and chronotropic effects on the heart and causes vasodilation [6]. Its metabolic effects include inhibition of insulin secretion and stimulation of glycogenolysis in the liver. Hypersecretion of catecholamines has many dramatic physiologic effects. In contrast, adrenal medullary hypofunction is not clinically significant because norepinephrine is available from other sources.

Presentation

Pheochromocytoma is a highly treatable endocrine disorder but if misdiagnosed or improperly treated, it can be fatal [7,8]. Nearly 90% of pheochromocytomas in adults occur in the adrenal medulla. Of those that occur outside the adrenal 1% are found in the abdomen, 1% in the chest, and 1% in the urinary bladder. As a general rule, pheochromocytomas are approximately 10% familial, 10% bilateral, and 10% malignant [9]. The incidence of pheochromocytomas is increased in familial conditions such as tuberous sclerosis, Sturge–Weber syndrome, von Recklinghausen's disease, Von Hippel–Lindau disease, neurofibromatosis, familial pheochromocytoma, and multiple endocrine neoplasia (MEN) syndromes. MEN 1 consists of hyperparathyroidism, pituitary adenomas, pancreatic islet cell tumors, and rarely pheochromocytoma. MEN 2 A consists of pheochromocytoma, medullary carcinoma of the thyroid, and hyperthyroidism. MEN 2B consists of medullary thyroid cancer and mucosal neuroma syndrome. In the familial conditions, the incidence of bilateral adrenal tumors increases [10].

Although the presence of pheochromocytoma in pregnancy is extremely rare, the tumor constitutes a very high risk for both mother and fetus. Pheochromocytoma should be considered in any pregnant woman with hypertension, especially if paroxysmal or labile, or with unexplained "spells." Maternal and fetal survival depends on an early diagnosis, correct medical therapy, and correct timing of delivery and surgery [11].

Clinical features

Because nearly all pheochromocytomas are functional and produce high levels of catecholamines, a wide variety of symptoms and signs can occur. Hypertension is the most common feature and despite the emphasis usually placed on the intermittent nature of symptoms, they are more likely to be sustained. Only about half of all patients have the classic paroxysmal symptoms of headache, pallor, palpitations, and sweating associated with hypertension [12–14]. Orthostasis is frequent. The sudden onset of hypertension in a previously normotensive person, especially occurring during the induction of anesthesia, should suggest the possibility of pheochromocytoma. Other reported symptoms include a sense of doom or apprehension, anxiety, trembling, mild abdominal pain, and constipation. Less common presentations include intestinal pseudo-obstruction and ileus, cardiomyopathy, coronary artery spasm, and peripheral vascular spasm. In elderly patients, symptoms may be less marked because of the decline in sensitivity to catecholamines that occurs with advanced age. A serious complication of pheochromocytoma is myocarditis and subsequent congestive heart failure. Infiltrates of histiocytes, plasma cells, and other inflammatory cells are seen in the myocardium on postmortem studies. Severe arrhythmias can be associated with pheochromocytomas, including supraventricular, nodal, and ventricular arrhythmias [14].

Few physical findings suggest pheochromocytoma other than hypertension. In the associated endocrine neoplasias and neuroectodermal disorders, thyroid enlargement, neurofibromas, or café au lait spots may be present [15].

Biochemical evaluation

It is essential to establish the diagnosis of pheochromocytoma preoperatively because intraoperative diagnosis of pheochromocytoma has a mortality approaching 50% [14]. The diagnosis of pheochromocytoma is made by documenting the excess secretion of catecholamines. Biochemical diagnosis can be difficult because of inadequate specificity of biochemical tests and the high rate of false-positive and false-negative results [16]. Biochemical tests include measurements of plasma and urinary catecholamines, plasma and urinary fractionated metanephrines, urinary total metanephrines, and urinary vanillylmandelic acid (VMA). Among all patients with pheochromocytoma, sensitivities for testing are the highest for measurements of plasma free metanephrines at 99%, followed by urinary fractionated metanephrines at 97% [17]. Sensitivities of the other tests are lower with urinary catecholamines at 86%, plasma catecholamines at 84–93%, urinary total metanephrines at 77%, and urinary VMA at 64% [17]. Plasma free

metanephrines and urinary fractionated metanephrines offer the highest sensitivities [16–20] but no one method can absolutely diagnose or exclude the presence of pheochromocytoma.

Plasma levels of catecholamines and free metanephrines must be obtained under carefully controlled conditions with patients in the supine position, with placement of an indwelling catheter, and after an overnight fast. The laboratory draw for plasma catecholamines and free metanephrines must be as stress-free as possible as venipuncture itself can cause levels to be falsely elevated. Interfering substances for plasma catecholamines and free metanephrines include coffee, tricyclic antidepressants, nicotine, and phenoxybenzamine [17]. Urinary collections are also prone to false-positive and false-negative results from numerous interfering substances including: decongestants, several antibiotics (chloramphenicol, nalidixic acid, tetracycline, erythromycin), antihypertensives (reserpine, guanethidine, labetalol, phentolamine, and methyldopa), amphetamines, benzodiazepines, diuretics in doses sufficient to produce sodium depletion, nitrates, bromocriptine, MAO inhibitors, phenothiazines, caffeine, ethanol, and marijuana [20]. Certain clinical situations may increase both plasma catecholamine and urine catecholamine metabolites to levels usually seen in pheochromocytoma. These situations include acute clonidine withdrawal, acute alcohol withdrawal, vasodilator therapy with hydralazine or minoxidil, acute myocardial ischemia or infarction, acute cerebral vascular accident, cocaine abuse, severe congestive heart failure, and hypoglycemia [21].

The oral clonidine test, which suppresses plasma catecholamine secretion in patients with essential hypertension (but not in pheochromocytomas), may be useful. The failure of 0.3 mg of oral clonidine to reduce plasma levels of normetanephrine in patients with hypertension is suggestive of pheochromocytoma [16]. Provocative tests for catecholamine release such as glucagon have high rates of morbidity and mortality and poor sensitivity and have therefore been abandoned [22].

Adrenal imaging

Pheochromocytoma is classically characterized as brightly enhancing on computerized tomography (CT) but has a range of appearances [23]. The sensitivity of CT scanning with use of a contrast agent for the diagnosis of pheochromocytoma is 85–95%, with a specificity of 70–100% [24,25]. High signal intensity on T2-weighted MRI is highly characteristic for pheochromocytoma. The sensitivity of MRI exceeds 95%, with a specificity of 100% [24,26,27]. Either may be used as the definitive imaging study depending on availability, cost, and patient preference [24].

Treatment

Preparation for surgery includes controlling hypertension preoperatively, preventing hypertensive crisis during surgery, control of possible arrhythmias and volume expansion [2,28].

There is no accepted standard for medication for blood pressure control, but most use alpha-adrenergic blockade [24,28,29]. Oral phenoxybenzamine, a selective irreversible alpha-adrenergic blocker (half-life of 24 hours), is used to blunt the vasoconstrictor effects of excess catecholamine secretion and is usually started 7–14 days preoperatively to allow for normalization of blood pressure and heart rate [24,28]. The initial dose of phenoxybenzamine is 10 mg once or twice daily. This is increased by 10–20 mg in divided doses every 2–3 days as needed to control blood pressure. Other more selective alpha-1-blockade medications can also be used (doxazosin, terazosin, or prazosin) [24,28]. Phenoxybenzamine is likely to cause preoperative orthostatic hypotension and volume depletion [30,31]. The change in vascular tone associated with alpha-blockade therapy necessitates fluid administration to prevent considerable hypotension during surgery.

After adequate alpha-adrenergic blockade has been achieved beta-adrenergic blockade is initiated, which typically occurs 2–3 days preoperatively. The beta-adrenergic blocker should not be started first because blockade of vasodilatory peripheral beta-adrenergic receptors with unopposed alpha-adrenergic receptor stimulation can lead to a further elevation in blood pressure [14,30,31]. Calcium channel blockers and angiotensin receptor blockers have also been used [28,32,33].

Phentolamine, an alpha-adrenergic blocker (half-life of 5 minutes) can be used for inpatient treatment of paroxysmal hypertension before or during surgery. It is given intravenously as a frequent bolus, or as a continuous infusion [33,34].

In summary pheochromocytomas are rare tumors that can have significant perioperative risk if unrecognized. These risks can be minimized by appropriate preoperative medical treatment to block the effects of catecholamines for at least 7–14 days before surgery. Adequate preoperative alpha-adrenergic blockade can reduce the number of perioperative complications. All patients with pheochromocytoma should receive appropriate preoperative medical management to block the effects of released catecholamines [24,33].

References

1. Omura M, Saito J, Yamaguchi K, Kakuta Y, Nishikawa T. Prospective study on the prevalence of secondary hypertension among hypertensive patients visiting a general outpatient clinic in Japan. *Hypertens Res* 2004; **27**: 193–202.

2. Streeten DH, Anderson GH, Elias MF. Prevalence of secondary hypertension and unusual aspects of the treatment of hypertension in elderly individuals. *Geriatr Nephrol Urol* 1992; **2**: 91–8.

3. Bernini GP, Vivaldi MS, Argenio GF *et al.* Frequency of pheochromocytoma in adrenal incidentalomas and utility of the glucagon test for the diagnosis. *J Endocrinol Invest* 1997; **20**: 65–71.

4. Eisenhofer G, Huynh TT, Hiroi M, Pacak K. Understanding catecholamine metabolism as a guide to the biochemical diagnosis of pheochromocytoma. *Rev Endocr Metab Disord* 2001; **2**: 297–311.

5. Goldstein DS, Cannon RO 3rd, Quyyumi A *et al.* Regional extraction of circulating norepinephrine, DOPA, and dihydroxyphenylglycol in humans. *J Auton Nerv Syst* 1991; **34**: 17–35.

6. Kantorovich V, Eisenhofer G, Pacak K. Pheochromocytoma: an endocrine stress mimicking disorder. *Ann NY Acad Sci* 2008; **1148**: 462–8.

7. Manger WM. The protean manifestations of pheochromocytoma. *Horm Metab Res* 2009; **41**: 658–63.

8. Manger WM. An overview of pheochromocytoma: history, current concepts, vagaries, and diagnostic challenges. *Ann NY Acad Sci* 2006; **1073**: 1–20.

9. Barron J. Phaeochromocytoma: diagnostic challenges for biochemical screening and diagnosis. *J Clin Pathol* 2010; **63**: 669–74.

10. Eisenhofer G, Lenders JW, Timmers H *et al.* Measurements of plasma methoxytyramine, normetanephrine, and metanephrine as discriminators of different hereditary forms of pheochromocytoma. *Clin Chem* 2011; **57**: 411–20.

11. Oliva R, Angelos P, Kaplan E, Bakris G. Pheochromocytoma in pregnancy: a case series and review. *Hypertension* 2010; **55**: 600–6.

12. Manger W, Gifford RW. Pheochromocytoma: current diagnosis and management. *Cleve Clin J Med* 1993; **60**: 365–78.

13. Kopetschke R, Slisko M, Kilisli A *et al.* Frequent incidental discovery of phaeochromocytoma: data from a German cohort of 201 phaeochromocytoma. *Eur J Endocrinol* 2009; **161**: 355–61.

14. Brouwers FM, Eisenhofer G, Lenders JW, Pacak K. Emergencies caused by pheochromocytoma, neuroblastoma, or ganglioneuroma. *Endocrinol Metab Clin North Am* 2006; **35**: 699–724.

15. Jabbour SA, Davidovici BB, Wolf R. Rare syndromes. *Clin Dermatol* 2006; **24**: 299–316.

16. Eisenhofer G, Goldstein DS, Walther MM *et al.* Biochemical diagnosis of pheochromocytoma: how to distinguish true- from false-positive test results. *J Clin Endocrinol Metab* 2003; **88**: 2656–66.

17. Lenders JW, Pacak K, Walther MM *et al.* Biochemical diagnosis of pheochromocytoma: which test is best? *J Am Med Assoc* 2002; **287**: 1427–34.

18. Grossman A, Pacak K, Sawka A *et al.* Biochemical diagnosis and localization of pheochromocytoma: can we reach a consensus? *Ann NY Acad Sci* 2006; **1073**: 332–47.

19. Unger N, Pitt C, Schmidt IL *et al.* Diagnostic value of various biochemical parameters for the diagnosis of pheochromocytoma in patients with adrenal mass. *Eur J Endocrinol* 2006; **154**: 409–17.

20. Henry JB, ed. Adrenal gland. In *Clinical Diagnosis and Management by Laboratory Methods*. 20th edn. Philadelphia, PA: W. B. Saunders; 2001, p. 313.

21. Bravo EL. Pheochromocytoma. *Cardiol Rev* 2002; **10**: 44–50.

22. Lenders JW, Pacak K, Huynh TT *et al.* Low sensitivity of glucagon provocative testing for diagnosis of

pheochromocytoma. *J Clin Endocrinol Metab* 2010; **95**: 238–45.

23. Johnson PT, Horton KM, Fishman EK. Adrenal mass imaging with multidetector CT: pathologic conditions, pearls, and pitfalls. *Radiographics* 2009; **29**: 1333–51.

24. Zeiger MA, Thompson GB, Duh QY *et al.* The American Association of Clinical Endocrinologists and American Association of Endocrine Surgeons medical guidelines for the management of adrenal incidentalomas. *Endocr Pract* 2009; **15** (Suppl 1): 1–20.

25. Hamrahian AH, Ioachimescu AG, Remer EM *et al.* Clinical utility of noncontrast computed tomography attenuation value (Hounsfield units) to differentiate adrenal adenomas/hyperplasias from nonadenomas: Cleveland Clinic experience. *J Clin Endocrinol Metab.* 2005; **90**: 871–7.

26. Elsayes KM, Menias CO, Siegel CL *et al.* Magnetic resonance characterization of pheochromocytomas in the abdomen and pelvis: imaging findings in 18 surgically proven cases. *J Comput Assist Tomogr* 2010; **34**: 548–53.

27. Jalil ND, Pattou FN, Combemale F *et al.* Effectiveness and limits of preoperative imaging studies for the localization of pheochromocytomas and paragangliomas: a review of 282 cases. *Eur J Surg* 1998; **164**: 23–8.

28. Pacak K, Eisenhofer G, Ahlman H *et al.* Pheochromocytoma: recommendations for clinical practice from the First International Symposium. *Nat Clin Pract Endocrinol Metab* 2007; **3**: 92–102.

29. Weingarten TN, Cata JP, O'Hara JF *et al.* Comparison of two preoperative medical management strategies for laparoscopic resection of pheochromocytoma. *Urology* 2010; **76**: 508.e6–11.

30. Kohl BA, Schwartz S. How to manage perioperative endocrine insufficiency. *Anesthesiol Clin* 2010; **28**: 139–55.

31. Roizen MF, Schreider BD, Hassan SZ. Anesthesia for patients with pheochromocytoma. *Anesthesiol Clin North Am* 1987; **75**: 269–75.

32. van der Horst-Schrivers AN, Kerstens MN, Wolffenbuttel BH. Preoperative pharmacological management of phaeochromocytoma. *Neth J Med* 2006; **64**: 290–5.

33. Chen H, Sippel RS, O'Dorisio MS *et al.* The North American Neuroendocrine Tumor Society consensus guideline for the diagnosis and management of neuroendocrine tumors: pheochromocytoma, paraganglioma, and medullary thyroid cancer. *Pancreas* 2010; **39**: 775–83.

34. McMillian WD, Trombley BJ, Charash WE, Christian RC. Phentolamine continuous infusion in a patient with pheochromocytoma. *Am J Health Syst Pharm* 2011; **68**: 130–4.

Rheumatologic disorders

C. Ronald MacKenzie

The rheumatologic diseases are a disparate group of conditions, often systemic in nature, characterized by multi-system involvement. Due to the predominant involvement of the joints and musculoskeletal system, such patients often require surgery, particularly of an orthopedic nature. The protean clinical manifestations of these diseases, coupled with important medication-related management considerations, present challenges encompassing the span of perioperative medical practice. Indeed such patients are amongst the most challenging encountered in the perioperative setting [1,2].

The rheumatic diseases: a concise primer

Table 34.1 presents a general classification of the rheumatic diseases.

Table 34.1 Classification of the rheumatic diseases.

Osteoarthritis

Disorders of the synovium
  Rheumatoid arthritis

Connective tissue diseases
  Systemic lupus erythematosus
  Systemic sclerosis
  Inflammatory disease of the muscle

Spondylarthropathy
  Ankylosing spondylitis
  Psoriatic arthritis
  Enteropathic arthropathies

Vasculitides
  Temporal arteritis
  Polyarteritis nodosa
  Microscopic polyangitis
  Churg–Strauss
  Wegener's granulomatosis

Metabollic bone disease
  Osteoporosis

Crystal-induced arthropathies
  Gout
  Calcium pyrophosphate associated arthropathy

Osteoarthritis

The most common form of arthritis, osteoarthritis (OA) is a heterogeneous group of common conditions that share similar pathologic and radiographic features (cartilage loss). An age-related disorder, it is uncommon before age 40 but increases in prevalence thereafter; by age 70 most people have pathological changes of OA though may not be symptomatic. Other risk factors include female gender, ethnicity (> blacks), genetic predisposition, obesity (especially the knee), and trauma. A focal disease not affecting all joints equally; even within a given joint its involvement may be patchy. Its primary symptoms are use-related joint pain and stiffness (gelling). Treatment is mainly symptomatic (NSAIDs, analgesics, intra-articular injections). In those with severe disease total joint arthroplasty is a common outcome.

Disorders of the synovium

Rheumatoid arthritis (RA) is the prototypical disorder affecting the synovium. This chronic systemic inflammatory disease affects females more often than males. Its peak onset is in the 4–5th decade. Usually RA presents insidiously over several weeks to months with symmetrical joint pain and swelling, usually in the hands, wrists, and feet, the larger joints becoming affected later. Extra-articular manifestations may arise but have become less common in the modern therapeutic era. Relevant laboratory studies include markers of the inflammatory response (ESR, CRP), rheumatoid factor, and anti-cyclic citrullinated peptide (anti-CCP) antibodies. Treatment involves NSAIDs, corticosteroids, disease-modifying antirheumatic drugs (DMARDs), principally methotrexate, corticosteroids, and an expanding array of new biological agents. Many of these medications increase the risk of postoperative infection and may impair wound healing.

Connective tissue diseases

The most common of these conditions is systemic lupus erythematosus (SLE). A prototypical autoimmune disease, this condition occurs mainly in woman during their reproductive years and disproportionately affects minorities. A hallmark is its diverse clinical expression and undulating course. The most prevalent and severe manifestation of systemic involvement is renal disease (lupus nephritis). Systemic lupus erythematosus-specific autoantibodies (ANA, anti-DNA) are important diagnostic determinants. Pregnancy and certain drugs are known disease precipitants. Corticosteroids remain the mainstay of therapy although a new monoclonal antibody (Belimumab) has recently been approved for the treatment of mild to moderate SLE.

Another important condition of the connective tissue is that commonly known as scleroderma. Scleroderma exists in two major forms: localized (limited) disease confined to the skin and subcutaneous tissues and systemic sclerosis (SSc) which may be limited or diffuse in its distribution. Clinical manifestations arise as a consequence of a small vessel obstructive vasculopathy, the pathological accumulation of collagen in the skin and other organ systems, and autoimmunity as evidenced by a number of associated autoantibodies. Often a severely debilitating disease, pulmonary disease (fibrosis) has become the most common form of death for such patients. There is no effective treatment for this disorder.

A less common but important third form of connective tissue disease are the inflammatory diseases of the muscle – dermatomyositis (DM) and polymyositis (PM). These heterogeneous groups of disorders share the clinical features of a progressive skeletal muscle weakness and fatigue and a decrease in endurance. Disease-specific autoantibodies are also frequently found but ultimately the diagnosis is made by muscle biopsy that demonstrates an inflammatory infiltrate. Treatment includes corticosteroids, intravenous immune globulin (IVIG), and immunosuppressive therapy with medication such as methotrexate.

Spondyloarthropathy

The spondyloarthropathies comprise a group of inflammatory disorders with overlapping clinical manifestations and shared genetic marker (HLA-B27). Ankylosing spondylitis, with its well-known back (axial) involvement, is the prototypical condition but other disorders such as psoriatic arthritis (PsA) and the enteropathic arthropathies are now categorized similarly. Once difficult to treat, new biologic therapies such as tumor necrosis factor (TNF) inhibitors have markedly improved the clinical course and symptomatic experience of patients suffering with these conditions. As these patients frequently develop a peripheral joint inflammatory arthritis, they are frequent candidates for total joint arthroplasty.

Vasculitides

The term vasculitis refers to several diseases involving inflammation of the blood vessels with resultant tissue necrosis and organ failure. The spectrum of disease is broad with overlapping features. While its classification systems had historically relied on eponyms, it is now categorized according to the size of the involved blood vessels. Temporal arteritis is the best known example but also included are such conditions as polyarteritis nodosa, Wegener's granulomatosis, and Churg–Strauss syndrome to name a few. Treatment paradigms rely on corticosteroids and immunosuppressants.

Metabolic bone disease

Osteoporosis is a widely recognized disorder of skeletal muscle characterized by low bone mass and microarchitectural deterioration of bone, increasing its fragility and susceptibility to fracture. Such fractures may have devastating consequences for patients and, with the aging of the population, have become so common as to constitute a threat to public health. Owing to the causal association between this condition and fracture of the hip and the importance of bone quality in osseous healing (spinal fusion) it is one of the most important rheumatic diseases now encountered on orthopedic services.

Crystal-induced arthropathies

Owing to fluid shifts and dehydration, gout (uric acid) and pseudo-gout (Ca^{++} pyrophosphate) deposition in peripheral joints occurs frequently after surgery. As such they are common management problems in the postoperative period.

Perioperative considerations in the rheumatic diseases patient

Given the chronic, inflammatory nature of rheumatic disease, coupled with the involvement of multiple organ systems, these patients may present daunting challenges in the perioperative context. Further, the often complex and expanding pharmacological regimens employed to control the inflammatory disease process heighten the risk of postoperative infection and may threaten the integrity of the surgical wound. However, the holding of such suppressive medication in the setting of surgery may result in flares of the underlying disease, an undesirable development in the postoperative period. As a consequence of this tension, the medical management of the patient's chronic disease has received considerable attention and recommendations concerning drug therapy in the perioperative setting have been developed.

With respect to anesthesiological considerations a number of issues are relevant [3]. These include management of the airway, the site and duration of surgery, and the presence of comorbidities. Each is an important determinant of the type of anesthesia to be used, need for invasive monitoring, and the anticipated period that the patient will spend in the recovery room. General and regional anesthesia techniques are commonly used in the surgical treatment of patients with rheumatic disease, especially in orthopedic surgery. Endotracheal intubation and general anesthesia present a particular danger in patients with rheumatoid arthritis or ankylosing spondylitis (AS). In patients with cervical spine involvement, such as the patient with severe RA (instability) or the converse, the rigid airway in AS, fiberoptic intubation may be required. Regional anesthesia may be employed including local anesthesia for minor procedures, peripheral nerve block for surgery of the upper and lower extremity, and epidural/spinal anesthesia for arthroplasty in the lower extremity. Although the relative merits of regional versus general anesthesiology is still debated, many procedures, particularly orthopedic surgery are well suited for regional anesthetic techniques. Regional anesthesia may reduce the incidence of major postoperative complications. Potential benefits include a reduction in blood loss [4,5], as well as reduced rates of venous thromboembolism, postoperative respiratory events, and death [6,7]. Further postoperative pain management, an important management issue for patients with a painful rheumatic disease, may be best managed with regional anesthetic approaches [8]. An alternative or adjunctive technique is that of peripheral nerve blocks that utilize long-acting anesthetics and infusion methodologies. Such approaches provide excellent intraoperative anesthesia and postoperative pain relief [9,10].

Patients undergoing major surgical procedures should have continuous electrocardiographic and pulse oximeter monitoring intraoperatively. At the discretion of the anesthesiologist, arterial and Swan–Ganz catheter monitoring may be helpful in selected patients. Such monitoring is often employed in patients undergoing bilateral joint replacement surgery and in those with a history of prior cardiac disease.

Postoperative pain control may employ a number of options. These include the intravenous or intramuscular routes (systemic) and/or the administration of epidural analgesia. Patient-controlled analgesia (PCA) via an epidural route is a very effective method of postoperative pain control and facilitates postoperative physical therapy. Such approaches are especially important in the restoration of range of motion in patients undergoing orthopedic procedures such as total knee replacement (TKR). Patient-controlled analgesia reduces the systemic absorption of and need for analgesics, thereby minimizing the problem of narcotic-induced respiratory depression. Parenterally administered non-steroidal anti-inflammatory agents (NSAIDs) are another alternative to traditional analgesia after surgery and can be used to reduce narcotic requirements. Such drugs should be avoided in patients with well-known contraindications to NSAIDs including peptic ulcer, chronic renal disease, ischemic heart disease, and the concomitant use of anticoagulants.

Cardiovascular disease

Patients with rheumatologic disease such as SLE or RA demonstrate increased mortality from cardiovascular disease, especially ischemic heart disease. Not fully explained on the basis of traditional risk factors (hypertension, hyperlipidemia) [11], the increase in cardiac-related mortality is believed a function of the underlying inflammatory response, mediating not only the joint and organ system damage accompanying these conditions but promoting the development of coronary artery disease.

As discussed elsewhere, algorithms have been developed by the American College of Cardiology/American Heart Association to assess perioperative cardiac risk [12,13]. Patients with rheumatologic disease, especially those with severe arthritis, may not be capable of exercise nor provide secure estimates (METS equivalents) of their exercise capacity. Thus the patient's functional status may not provide an adequate screen for the presence of significant cardiac disease. These patients will require clinical judgment about how much invasive testing is needed.

Dysfunction of the cardiac valves is not an uncommon manifestation of the rheumatic diseases [14]. The Libman–Sacks vegetations of SLE and regurgitation of the mitral valve are well described in RA [15]. Aortic valve disease, particularly aortic insufficiency also occurs in the HLA-B27 associated spondyloarthropathies [16]. In these conditions the aortic regurgitation results from aortitis and dilatation of the aorta [17]. Similarly there is a high prevalence of aortic valve involvement in the systemic vasculitides [11]. In these conditions the inflammatory involvement of the great vessels results in aneurysmal dilatation of the aorta and aortic root dilatation with aortic insufficiency and occasionally aortic dissection. Finally, in addition to the prothrombotic considerations, antiphospholipid antibodies in SLE are associated with mitral valve nodules and mitral regurgitation [18].

Surgical risks in patients with valvular heart disease depend on the valve affected as well as the nature and severity of the valvular lesion. The highest perioperative risk is associated with hemodynamically significant aortic stenosis. While a prevalent valvular lesion in the aging population, it is relatively uncommon in the rheumatic diseases. Mitral valve disease and aortic insufficiency, when not severe, are usually well tolerated in the surgical setting. Nonetheless any valvular disease associated with significant left ventricular dysfunction increases the postoperative risk. Therefore rheumatic disease patients with a significant cardiac murmur should undergo an echocardiographic assessment preoperatively, particularly if a major procedure is planned.

While cardiac conduction system disease and arrhythmias are frequently a marker for underlying cardiac disease, pulmonary disease, metabolic abnormalities, or drug toxicity, they are also more frequently seen in patients with connective tissue diseases. Most prevalent in scleroderma, myocardial fibrosis compromises the cardiac conduction system leading to heart block, electrocardiographic abnormalities, and arrhythmias [11]. Therefore, patients with this and other rheumatic diseases may present with conduction system disease problems preoperatively. Thus the perioperative physician should be aware of this association and institute corrective action before surgery.

Pulmonary disease

Asthma and chronic obstructive pulmonary disease are the most common causes of pulmonary disease and raise the likelihood of postoperative atelectasis or pneumonia, particularly when abdominal or thoracic surgery is performed. Smoking history or cardiac disease further increases postoperative risk. Rheumatic disease patients also have a high prevalence of lung disease, most commonly interstitial lung disease and pulmonary artery hypertension (PAH). Interstitial lung disease results in a decrease in lung volumes (restrictive defect) and a reduction in diffusion capacity. Pulmonary artery hypertension arises from an increase in pulmonary vascular resistance with or without intrinsic parenchymal lung disease. Such involvement frequently accompanies certain of the rheumatic diseases, most commonly the systemic connective tissue diseases such as scleroderma, SLE, mixed connective tissue disease (MCTD), and the inflammatory diseases of the muscle (polymyositis (PM) and dermatomyositis (DM)).

Restrictive lung disease may also reflect chest wall pathology. In scleroderma, the skin over the thorax may be thickened and bound down, limiting chest wall excursion. Similarly, DM and PM patients may have impaired inspiratory effort due to chest wall muscle weakness. While surgery performed under regional anesthesia is generally well tolerated, careful assessment of pulmonary function is essential when scalene nerve block is employed such as in upper extremity surgery. Such blocks result in ipsilateral diaphragmatic paralysis which further compromises lung function.

The hallmark of PAH is the elevation of right-sided pressures potentially compromising venous return. Anesthetic agents, with their anti-inotropic effect, may aggravate this situation. In severe PAH, the hypotension and decreased venous return accompanying regional anesthesia may have dire consequences. Therefore careful preoperative assessment and perioperative management for patients with PAH requires a close collaboration between medical consultants and anesthesia to minimize risk [19,20].

Fat emboli syndrome refers to a constellation of signs and symptoms arising as a consequence of the systemic embolization of fat released from the bone marrow [21]. Frequent clinical phenomena include alterations in mental status, petechial rash and hypoxemia due to pulmonary compromise. This complication may precipitate frank respiratory failure in patients with underlying lung disease. It is seen in the setting of total joint arthroplasty, particularly bilateral procedures, as a consequence of the positioning of the prosthesis under pressure.

Upper airway compromise has been reported in patients with RA due to arthritis affecting the cricoarytenoid joints. These joints move with the vocal cords and while patients are usually asymptomatic, such joint involvement may produce hoarseness, a tipoff to the presence of this condition. Trauma at the time of intubation will produce swelling of the vocal cords which can lead to compromise of the airway and respiratory distress. In such circumstances, re-intubation or tracheostomy may be required. Preoperative pulmonary function studies and fiberoptic laryngoscopy can provide the definitive diagnosis and help plan anesthesia strategy.

The evaluation and management of patients with chronic rheumatic disease frequently includes detailed preoperative pulmonary function testing and echocardiography to anticipate these perioperative challenges. Postoperative therapy with bronchodilators and nebulizer therapy and early mobilization can prevent atelectasis. Careful attention to bowel function, an issue often underestimated, is also important. Gastrointestinal problems may contribute to respiratory compromise as the distended abdomen in the bed-bound patient prevents full chest expansion by compromising diaphragmatic excursion.

Renal disease

Renal function may be impaired in rheumatic disease and confers a significant risk to the patient in the perioperative setting. Glomerulonephritis complicating SLE or use of nephrotoxic drugs (NSAIDS) can lead to a loss of renal function. Acute postoperative renal compromise in hip fracture patients is more common in patients with underlying renal disease. Additional risk factors include male sex, hypertension, diabetes, as well as the preoperative use of nephrotoxic agents. Higher complication rates and mortality have been reported postoperatively in hip fracture patients with postoperative renal impairment when compared with patients with stable renal function [22]. Identification of patients at high risk for postoperative renal dysfunction in non-cardiac surgery permits discontinuation of nephrotoxic medications such as NSAIDS and ACE inhibitors and careful monitoring of fluid status.

In rheumatologic patients undergoing lower extremity arthroplasty, hypotensive anesthesia has advantages in reducing blood loss and improved cement fixation. The decrease in renal blood flow seen with hypotensive general anesthesia however may precipitate renal failure [23] in patients with underlying renal disease. Hypotensive epidural anesthesia has been shown to be safe in patients with chronic renal disease who undergo total hip replacement when cardiac output is maintained by judicious fluid management and low-dose epinephrine infusion [24].

Hip implants with metal-on-metal articulations have been very popular with orthopedic surgeons as they were believed to be more durable and wear-resistant when compared with implants composed of metal on ceramic or polyethylene. These metal components however shed metallic ions that accumulate in the presence of chronic kidney disease and thus have been avoided in patients with renal disease [24]. However, recent experience with this implant design has been unfavorable, with some patients developing severe tissue and bony damage, accelerated prosthetic wear, and high rates of failure, such that the use of metal-on-metal implants has been substantially curtailed.

Medication management of patients with rheumatic disease

Patients with RA and SLE are inherently at increased risk for infection as compared with the general population. In addition medications used in the treatment of rheumatic diseases are immunosuppressive, further enhancing this risk. These drugs may also have an impact on wound healing. Although there are few data derived from clinical trials addressing these risks, recommendations have been extrapolated from various studies and clinical experience.

Methotrexate (MTX) is the most rigorously studied in RA patients undergoing total joint arthroplasty. On the basis of several studies, including a prospective clinical trial, MTX appears to be safe in the perioperative period [25]. In this study, patients (388) undergoing orthopedic surgery were randomized to either continue or stop MTX at the time of surgery. Those continuing therapy experienced a 2% postoperative infection rate and developed no RA flares; in contrast, 15% of patients who discontinued MTX developed infections and complications after surgery and 8% experienced flares in their disease. For comparison, a control group not chronically treated with MTX experienced a 10.5% infection/complication rate and 2.6% had RA flares. Additional retrospective studies also support the safety of MTX in the perioperative period, such that the standard of practice should be to continue this medication prior to surgery.

Hydroxychloroquine and sulfasalazine, two medications employed in the treatment of mild RA, have favorable toxicity profiles but have not been studied in the perioperative period. Conflicting results have been published in regard to another frequently prescribed medication, leflunamide. Significant impairment in wound healing has been reported in leflunamide-treated patients (40%) [26]. This observation was not sustained by another study involving patients who discontinued leflunamide one month prior to surgery [27]. Prudent clinical practice appears to support a recommendation to hold leflunamide and sulfasalazine until normal postoperative bowel and renal function has been demonstrated.

With respect to biologic agents, now commonly employed in the treatment of rheumatic diseases, all carry an important risk of immunosuppression and increased risk of infection. Gram-positive organisms are the most commonly reported bacteria complicating such therapy, a microbiology paralleling that seen in early postoperative infection. A small prospective study has addressed this risk. In patients undergoing foot and ankle procedures, no increase in infection was noted in patients continued on anti-TNF therapy [28]. In another (retrospective) study of RA patients undergoing orthopedic surgery [29], 11% (10/91) had a postoperative infection; the majority of patients who acquired infection were receiving TNF inhibitor therapy. Other factors such as age, steroid use, and diabetes were not significantly different between the groups. Conflicting results have been obtained concerning this issue from observations made on patients receiving anti-TNF therapy for inflammatory bowel disease [30]. Nonetheless, consensus opinion supports the discontinuation of these medications in patients with underlying rheumatic disease [31,32].

Rituximab, a monoclonal antibody directed against the CD-20 cell (lymphocyte) surface marker, is increasingly used in the treatment of various rheumatic diseases. The risk of infection with rituximab is comparable to that of other biologic agents employed in RA, but as yet there are no data regarding its use in the perioperative setting. Since the B-cell depletion and the consequent reduction in immunoglobulins induced by this medication may persist for up to a year, perioperative planning to address the risk of infection associated with this therapy is generally not feasible.

Corticosteroids should not be forgotten in this context as they remain a backbone of rheumatologic therapy. Steroids are likewise an established risk factor for postoperative infection and delayed wound healing. Concern relating to potential adrenal suppression in patients chronically receiving such therapy has promoted a time-honored practice of "stress dose" steroid coverage in the perioperative setting. Such treatment generally involves the perioperative administration of augmented steroid dosing in patients who have received low-dose steroid therapy for > 6 months prior to surgery or in those treated with moderate to high doses for a duration of more than 3 weeks. Does the persistence of this practice hold up to close scrutiny?

Arguing for a modification of traditional practice are the observations that the duration and dose of steroid therapy are not reliable predictors of corticosteroid need in the perioperative period. Further, the commonly used tests to assess adrenal function do not accurately predict steroid requirements in this setting [33]. A prospective study of patients on chronic steroid therapy randomized to receive their usual daily dose versus stress doses at the time of surgery [34] showed no difference between the groups, even when adrenal insufficiency was present based on ACTH stimulation. A quantification of the endogenous steroid response in orthopedic surgery has been reported [35]. Patients undergoing knee arthroscopy or total knee replacement showed significant increases in cortisol levels over baseline only in the arthroplasty group.

Thus, while the published record is scant, the available evidence supports limiting the routine use of stress dose steroids in the perioperative setting. A daily dose of 5–7.5 mg of prednisone approximates the normal daily adrenal output of cortisol (30 mg). Patients believed to be at increased risk for adrenal insufficiency include those currently taking > 20 mg prednisone daily for > 3 weeks, those who have taken such doses for more than 2 weeks in the preceding year, and those who are receiving replacement corticosteroid therapy for known adrenal insufficiency. While surgery may produce sufficient "stress" to provoke adrenal insufficiency, surgeries vary in the amount of stress they produce and the circulating cortisol concentration usually normalizes within 24–48 hours in most patients after surgery [36]. Thus the amount of supplementation should depend on the anticipated degree of stress (a function of the duration and severity of the surgical procedure) and the chronic daily steroid dose. Table 34.2 provides recommendations for perioperative glucocorticoid coverage according to the magnitude of the surgery to be performed.

Table 34.2 Recommendations for perioperative glucocorticoid coverage.

Surgical stress	Target hydro-cortisone equivalent	Preoperative steroid dose	Intraoperative steroid dose	Postoperative steroid dose[b]	Postoperative steroid dose day I[b]	Postoperative steroid dose day 2[b]
Minor (e.g., inguinal herniorrhaphy)	25 mg/day for 1 day	Usual daily dose of steroid	None[a]	None[a]	Usual daily dose[a]	
Moderate (e.g., colon resection, total joint replacement, lower extremity revascularization)	50–75 mg/day for 1–2 days	Usual daily dose of steroid	50 mg hydrocortisone	20 mg hydrocortisone every 8 hours	20 mg hydrocortisone every 8 hours	
Major (e.g., pancreatoduodenectomy, esophagectomy)	100–150 mg/day for 2–3 days	Usual daily dose of steroid	50 mg hydrocortisone	50 mg hydrocortisone every 8 hours	50 mg hydrocortisone every 8 hours	50 mg hydrocortisone every 8 hours

[a] If the postoperative course is uncomplicated, patients can resume their usual steroid dose on postoperative day 1.
[b] If postoperative complications occur, continued glucocorticoid administration will be necessary comensurate with the level of stress.

Antiphospholipid syndrome

Antiphospholipid syndrome (APS) is a condition consisting of vascular thrombosis (and/or pregnancy-related morbidity) arising as a consequence of the presence of antiphospholipid antibodies (aPL), most often the lupus anticoagulant or anti-cardiolipin antibodies [37]. This syndrome exists in a primary form, unassociated with an underlying connective tissue disease or is considered secondary when it arises in the setting of such conditions as SLE. As a consequence of their inherent hypercoaguability, patients with APS who require surgery are at significant risk for postoperative thrombosis. Their need for long-term anticoagulation results in challenges in perioperative management, specifically the delicate balance between the propensity to thrombosis versus the risk of postoperative bleeding, a direct consequence of the compelling need for prompt anticoagulation.

Although fraught with risk, surgery may be necessary in these patients and recommendations have been published from which to guide management [38]. First, the important adjunctive role of physical methods in the prevention of venous thrombosis should not be overlooked. Methods such as intermittent venous compression should be aggressively utilized both before and after surgery. Second, the period of time without anticoagulation should be minimized. Thus patients on chronic coumadin therapy should stop this medication 3–4 days before surgery, allowing for a normalization of the international normalized ratio (INR), with concomitant therapy with low molecular weight (LMW) heparin started at therapeutic dosages and not discontinued until the night before surgery. For many procedures, particularly orthopedic surgery, coumadin can be restarted the night of the surgical procedure given the delay in its onset of action. If there is no contraindication, low molecular weight heparin in prophylactic dosages can be re-started simultaneously and maintained until a therapeutic INR has been achieved. Note that conventional dosages of these agents may result in "under coagulation" of patients with APS and larger dosages, if feasible, may be considered necessary postoperatively, irrespective of the bleeding risk conferred by such therapy. Given the frequent use of epidural and spinal anesthesia in patients undergoing orthopedic surgery, the risk of epidural and spinal hematoma as a complication of such anesthesia should be noted. Indeed the avoidance of this serious complication forms the rationale for the omitting of the heparin dose the night before surgery. Heparin is not re-started until at least 4 hours after the removal of the epidural/spinal needle.

Hip fracture

Hundreds of thousands of patients are admitted to hospital in the USA annually for treatment of a fractured hip, resulting in major costs to society, to patients, and to their families [39–41]. Within the first year of fracture, 20% of elderly hip fracture patients die, compared with 9% of age-matched, non-fracture patients. Further, one-sixth of patients who survive 1 year after fracture are confined to long-term care facilities, and another one-third continue to require assistive devices or the help of others to manage their daily activities. Therefore most experience permanent functional impairment and the rates of permanent institutionalization are high. Risk factors believed to increase the need for nursing home placement include living alone prior to the fracture, having no children, and female gender.

The majority of hip fractures occur in frail, elderly women with osteoporosis who have sustained a fall. Risk factors for hip fracture include increasing age, poor general health, maternal history of hip fracture, a history of thyroid disease, poor depth perception, the use of psychoactive medication, sedentary lifestyle, and major live events [42].

Femoral neck and intertrochanteric fractures occur with equal frequency and most require surgical intervention to restore mobility and functional status, Although controversial, more severe (i.e., displaced) intracapsular femoral neck fractures are often treated with joint replacement because this fracture may result in a compromised blood supply to the femoral head, leading to osteonecrosis and secondary osteoarthritis ultimately necessitating total hip replacement [43–46]. Internal fixation is the usual surgical approach to displaced femoral neck fractures. However, in the frail, elderly patient with lower anticipated functional requirements and life expectancy, such fractures may be treated with total joint arthroplasty as well.

Hip, wrist, and vertebral fractures in the elderly arise from low-energy mechanisms and are often called fragility fractures. The initiation of antiresorptive therapy for osteoporosis after such fractures has been shown to substantially reduce the risk of subsequent fracture [47,48]. Despite the importance and effectiveness of therapy, a surprisingly low percentage of patients are prescribed osteoporosis therapy following such fractures [49,50]. Indeed studies investigating the treatment of osteoporosis after hip fracture report treatment rates in the 5–30% range. The reasons for these low rates include the lack of patient and physician education, impediments to follow-up, the addition of new physicians to the patient's treatment team, the cost of treatment, and a lack of consensus as to who is responsible for initiating such treatment. Irrespective of the underlying reasons, it is clear that this is an important missed primary care opportunity [51].

Postoperative crystal-induced arthritis

Crystal-induced acute arthritis is a common complication of acute illness and surgery [52,53]. Dehydration, fluid shifts, the use of diuretics and the inattention to the maintenance of chronic therapy for these disorders, all contribute to its presence in the postoperative setting. Acute episodes may present as a febrile episode mistaken for infection and in the critically ill the problem may be overlooked altogether. Nonetheless, in most instances, acute episodes arise in patients with a history of attacks and the joint involvement tends to mirror earlier episodes. Most attacks are delayed several days after surgery and if recognized quickly, will respond well to the institution of therapy. As these episodes may be clinically indistinguishable from acute septic arthritis, joint aspiration should be performed in order to confirm the diagnosis whenever possible.

Effective resolution of the condition can be achieved with a number of pharmaceutical agents. Non-steroidal anti-inflammatory drugs are the most common form of medication employed in the treatment of crystal-induced arthritis and are often satisfactory in the postoperative setting as long as the usual cautions and contraindications are honored (renal dysfunction, peptic ulcer). Colchicine, a traditional and effective agent, is somewhat problematic after surgery owing to its potential for gastrointestinal side-effects. Further, in the setting of renal and hepatic dysfunction, colchicine is contraindicated. Corticosteroids, orally, intravenously, or by intra-articular injection are very effective and often the most practical way to bring an acute episode to resolution after surgery. Modest dosages usually are sufficient. Prednisone 20 mg and tapering of over 5–7 days or its equivalents by other routes is usually sufficient.

References

1. MacKenzie CR, Paget SA. Perioperative care of the rheumatic disease patient. In Hochberg MC, Silman AJ, Smolen MS, Weinblatt ME, Weiman MH, eds. *Rheumatology*. 5th edn. Philadelphia, PA: Mosby Elsevier; 2010.

2. MacKenzie CR, Sharrock NE. Perioperative medical considerations in patients with rheumatoid arthritis. *Rheum Clin N Am* 1998; **24**: 1–17.

3. Urban MK. Anesthesia for orthopedic surgery. In Miller RD, Eriksson LI, Fleisher LA *et al.*, eds. Miller's Anesthesia. 7th edn. Philadelphia, PA: Elsevier; 2009.

4. Stevens RD, Van Gessel E, Flory N *et al.* Lumbar plexus block reduces pain and blood loss associated with total hip arthroplasty. *Anesthesiology* 2000; **93**: 115–21.

5. Modig J. Regional anesthesia and blood loss. *Acta Anaesthesiol Scand Suppl* 1998; **32**: 44–8.

6. Perka C, Arnold U, Buttergeit F. Influencing factors on perioperative morbidity in knee arthroplasty. *Clin Orthop* 2000; **181**: 191–6.

7. Rodgers A, Walker N, Schug S *et al.* Reduction in postoperative mortality and morbidity with epidural or spinal anesthesia: results from overview of randomized trials. *Br Med J* 2000; **321**: 1–12.

8. Wu CL, Seth R, Cohen BS *et al.* Efficacy of postoperative patient-controlled and continuous infusion epidural analgesia versus intravenous patient-conatrolled analgesia with opioids. *Anesthesiology* 2005; **103**: 1079–88.

9. Richman JM, Liu SS, Courpas G *et al.* Does continuous peripheral nerve block provide superior pain control to opioids? A meta-analysis. *Anesth Analg* 2006; **102**: 248–57.

10. Swenson JD, Bay N. Loose E *et al.* Outpatient management of continuous peripheral nerve catheters placed using ultrasound guidance: an experience in 620 patients. *Anesth Analg* 2006; **103**: 1436–43.

11. Roman MH, Salmon J. Cardiovascular manifestations of rheumatologic disease. *Circulation* 2007; **116**: 2346–55.

12. Fleisher LA, Beckman JA, Brown KA *et al.* ACC/AHA 2007 guidelines on perioperative cardiovascular evaluation and care for noncardiac surgery: a report of the American College of Cardiology/American Heart Association Task Force on Practice Guidelines. *J Am Coll Cardiol* 2007; **50**: 159–242.

13. Kwon E, Fleisher LA, Eagle K. Cardiac risk assessment in noncardiac surgery. In Newman MF, Fleisher LA, Fink MP, eds *Perioperative Medicine: Managing for Outcome*. Philadelphia. PA: Saunders Elsevier; 2008.

14. Coblyn J, O'Gara PT. The heart in rheumatic disease. In Hochberg MC, Silman AJ, Smolen JS, Weinblatt ME, Weisman MH, eds. *Rheumatology*. 3rd edn. Maryland Heights, MO: Mosby Elsevier; 2003.

15. Guedes C, Bianchi-Flor P, Cormier B *et al.* Cardiac manifestation of

rheumatoid arthritis: a case-controlled transesophageal echocardiography study in 30 patients. *Arthritis Care Res* 2001; **45**: 129–35.

16. Bergfeldt L. HLA-B27 associated cardiac disease. *Ann Int Med* 1997; **127**: 621–9.

17. Buckley BH, Roberts WC. Ankylosing spondylitis and aortic regurgitation: description of the characteristic cardiovascular lesion from study of eight necropsy patients. *Circulation* 1973; **48**: 1014–27.

18. Farzaneh-Far A, Roman MJ, Lockshin MD, Devereux RB *et al.* Relationship of antiphospholipid antibodies to cardiovascular manifestations of systemic lupus erythematosus. *Arthritis Rhem* 2006; **54**(12): 3918–25.

19. Ramakrishna G, Sprung J, Ravi BS *et al.* Impact of pulmonary hypertension on the outcome of noncardiac surgery. Predictors of perioperative morbidity and mortality. *J Am Coll Card* 2005; **45**: 1691–9.

20. McGlothlin D, De Marco T. Perioperative risk assessment of pulmonary arterial hypertension patients undergoing general surgery. *Adv Pulmon Hypertens* 2007; **6**(2): 66–73.

21. Parisi MD, Koval K, Egoi K. Fat embolism syndrome. *Am J Ortho* 1990; **31**: 507–12.

22. Bennet SJ, Berry OM, Goddard J *et al.* Acute renal dysfunction following hip fracture. *Injury* 2010; **41**: 335–8.

23. Sharrock NE, Beksac B, Flynn E *et al.* Hypotensive epidural anaesthesia in patients with preoperative renal dysfunction undergoing total hip replacement. *Br J Anaesth* 2006; **96**: 207–12.

24. Grubl A, Marker GA, Brodner W *et al.* Long-term follow-up of metal-on-metal total hip replacement. *J Orthop Res* 2007; **25**: 841–8.

25. Grennan DM, Gray J, Loundon J *et al.* Methotrexate and early postoperative complications in patients with rheumatoid arthritis undergoing elective orthopedic surgery. *Ann Rheum Dis* 2001; **60**: 214–17.

26. Fuerst M, Mohl H, Baumgartel K *et al.* Leflunomide increases the risk of early healing complications in patients with rheumatoid arthritis undergoing elective orthopedic surgery. *Rheum Int* 2006; **26**: 1138–42.

27. Tanaka N, Sakahashi H, Sato E *et al.* Examination of the risk of continuous leflunomide treatment on the incidence of infectious complications after joint arthroplasty in patients with patients with rheumatoid arthritis. *J Clin Rheum* 2003; **9**: 115–18.

28. Bibbo C, Goldberg JW. Infectious and healing complications after elective orthopaedic foot and ankle surgery during tumor necrosis factor-alpha inhibition therapy. *Foot Ankle Int* 2004; **25**: 331–5.

29. Giles JT, Bartlett SJ, Gelber AC *et al.* Tumor necrosis factor inhibitor therapy and risk of serious postoperative orthopedic infection in rheumatoid arthritis. *Arthritis Rheum* 2006; **55**: 333–5.

30. Marchal L, D'Haens G, van Assche G *et al.* The risk of post-operative complications associated with infliximab therapy for Crohn's disease: a controlled cohort study. *Ailment Pharmacol Ther* 1996; **19**: 749–54.

31. Pham T, Claudepierre P, Deprez X *et al.* Anti-TNF alpha therapy and safety monitoring. Clinical tool guide elaborated by the Club Rhumatismes et Inflammations (CRI), section of the French Society of Rheumatology (SFR). *Joint Bone Spine* 2005; **72** (Suppl): 1–58.

32. Ledingham J, Deighton C. British Society for Rheumatology Standards, Guidelines and Audit Working Group (SGWAG) Update on the British Society for Rheumatology guidelines for prescribing TNR-alpha blockers in adults with rheumatoid arthritis (update of previous guidelines of April 2001). *Rheumatol* 2001; **44**: 157–63.

33. Bromberg JS, Alfrey EJ, Barker CF *et al.* Adrenal suppression and steroid supplementation in renal transplant recipients. *Transplant* 1991; **51**: 123–9.

34. Glowniak JV, Loriaux DL. A double-blind study of perioperative steroid requirements in secondary adrenal insufficiency. *Surgery* 1997; **121**: 123–9.

35. Leopold SS, Casnellie MT, Warme WJ *et al.* Endogenous cortisol production in response to knee arthroscopy and total knee arthroplasty. *J Bone Joint Surg Am* 2003; **85**A: 2163–7.

36. Salem M, Tainsh RE, Bromberg J *et al.* Perioperative glucocorticoid coverage. A reassessment 42 years after emergence of a problem. *Ann Surg* 1994; **219**: 416–25.

37. Harris EN, Khamashta MA. Antiphospholipid syndrome: diagnosis and management. In Hochberg MC, Silman AJ, Smolen JS, Wienblatt ME, Weisman MH. *Rheumatology*. 4th edn. Maryland Heights, MO: Mosby Elsevier; 2008.

38. Erkan D, Leibowitz E, Berman J, Lockshin M. Perioperative medical management of antiphospholipid syndrome: hospital for special surgery experience, review of literature, and recommendations. *J Rheum* 2002; **294**: 843–9.

39. Cumming RG, Nevitt MC, Cummings SR. Epidemiology of hip fractures. *Epidemiol Rev* 1997; **19**: 244–57.

40. Praemer A, Furner S, Rice DP. *Musculoskeletal Conditions in the United States*. Park Ridge, IL: American Academy of Orthopedic Surgeons; 1992.

41. Koval KK, Chen AL, Aharonoff GB, Egol KKA, Zuckerman JD. Clinical pathway for hip fracture in the elderly. The Hospital for Joint Disease experience. *Clin Ortho Rel Res* 2004; **425**: 72–81.

42. Peterson MGE, Allegrante JP, Augurt A, Robbins L, MacKenzie CR. Major life events as antecedents to hip fracture. *J Trauma* 2000; **48**: 1096–100.

43. Maccaulay W, Yoon RS, Parsley B, Nellans KW, Teeny SM. Displaced femoral neck fractures: is there a standard of care? 2007; **30**: 748–9.

44. Baker RP, Squires B, Gargan MF, Bannister GC. Total hip arthroplasty and hemiarthroplasty in mobile, independent patients with a displaced intracapusular fracture of the femoral neck. A randomized, controlled trial. *J Bone Joint Surg* 2006; **88**: 2583–9.

45. Blomfeldt R, Tornkvist H, Ponzer S, Soderqvist A, Tidermark J. Comparison of internal fixation with total hip replacement for displaced femoral neck fractures. Randomized, controlled trial performed at four years. *J Bone Joint Surg* 2005; **87**: 1680–8.

46. Blomfeldt R, Tornkvist H, Eriksson K, Soderqvist A, Ponzer S, Tidermark J. A randomized controlled trial comparing bipolar hemiarthroplasty

with total hip replacement for displaced intracapsular fractures of the femoral neck in elderly patients. *J Bone Joint Surg* 2007; **89**: 160–4.

47. Black DM, Cummings SR, Karpg DB *et al.* Randomized trial of effect of alendronate on risk of fracture in woman with existing vertebral fractures. Fracture Intervention Trial Research Group. *Lancet* 1996; **348**: 1535–41.

48. Lyles KW, Colon-Emeric CS, Magaziner JS *et al.* HORIZON Recurrent Fracture Trial. Zolendronic acid and clinical features and mortality after hip fracture. *N Engl J Med* 2007; **357**: 1799–809.

49. Hooven F, Gehlbach SH, Pekow P *et al.* Follow-up treatment for osteoporosis after fracture. *Osteoporosis Int* 2005; **16**: 296–301.

50. Torgerson DJ, Dolan P. Prescribing by general practitioners after an osteoporotic fracture. *Ann Rheum Dis* 1998; **57**: 378–9.

51. Miki RA, Oetgen ME, Kirk J *et al.* Orthopedic management improves the rate of early osteoporosis treatment after hip fracture. A randomized clinical trial. *J Bone Joint Surg Am* 2008; **90**: 2346–53.

52. Shaw M, Mandell BF. Perioperative management of selected problems in patients with rheumatic diseases. *Rheum Dis Clin N Am* 1999; **25**: 623–39.

53. Kang EH, Lee EY, Lee YJ *et al.* Clinical features and risk factors of postoperative gout. *Ann Rheum Dis* 2008; **67**: 1271–5.

Cerebrovascular disease

Kumiko Owada, Duncan Borland, and Michael Frankel

Introduction

Stroke affects 795,000 people each year in the USA and is a leading cause of long-term disability in the adult population. The impact of stroke on society is large not only because of the medical cost of acute care but also due to the cost of long-term disability. Stroke also has a significant impact on individual quality of life. In the past decade there have been considerable advances in treatment and prevention of stroke. Some of the incidence of stroke is associated directly or indirectly with surgical procedures. This chapter will review the mechanisms of stroke associated with surgical procedures and the issues surrounding management of stroke relevant to surgical patients.

Pathophysiology

Stroke can be divided into two types; ischemic and hemorrhagic. Ischemic stroke comprises about 87% of all strokes. Hypoperfusion in the brain tissue associated with either arterial occlusion or decreased blood flow causes ischemia that will progress with time to infarction. The concept of "penumbra" represents brain tissue which suffers from acute hypoperfusion but has yet to suffer cell death. The penumbra represents salvageable brain tissue that may be amenable to reperfusion therapy. Available therapeutic modalities for acute stroke focused on salvaging penumbra are discussed in the section below.

Atherosclerotic disease causing intra- or extracranial arterial stenosis is associated with ischemic stroke. Arterial stenosis, if significant enough, can cause hypoperfusion in the distal tissues especially in the setting of hypotension. When the symptoms are caused by this mechanism, they can fluctuate depending on the systemic blood pressure. Thromboembolism is another mechanism by which atherosclerotic disease leads to stroke. Thrombi can break off from atherosclerotic plaques in the proximal arteries, causing occlusion of distal smaller arteries. Thrombi can originate in the heart especially when atrial fibrillation or left ventricular dilation is present. This type of stroke is called cardio-embolic stroke. Lastly the term lacunar stroke is given to the type of stroke involving small penetrating vessels and strongly associated with chronic hypertension. The less common mechanisms include arterial dissection, hypercoagulability, septic emboli, vasculitis, and venous infarction that all together comprise approximately 5% of ischemic strokes.

Transient ischemic attack (TIA) is an event where the symptoms of stroke are short-lived. By the conventional definition TIA symptoms last less than 24 hours, however, most symptoms last less than one hour. Recently, validity of the definition of TIA based on the arbitrarily chosen time period of 24 hours has been questioned. A newer definition was proposed by several investigators with a focus on the pathophysiologic mechanism of TIA and defined as "a brief episode of neurological dysfunction caused by local brain or retinal ischemia, with clinical symptoms typically lasting less than one hour, and without evidence of acute infarction" [1]. The significance of TIA lies in the fact that many strokes are preceded by TIA. Easton et al. noted the risk of having ischemic stroke is 10–15% in the 3-month period following TIA, with half occurring within 48 hours [1].

Hemorrhagic stroke represents 13% of all strokes and consists of intracerebral hemorrhage (10%) and subarachnoid hemorrhage (3%). Intracerebral hemorrhage is commonly associated with malignant hypertension. Hemorrhagic conversion of ischemic infarct can occur especially with large infarcts and acute reperfusion. Subarachnoid hemorrhage is associated with aneurysmal rupture or rupture of arteriovenous malformation (AVM), however, can also occur without an identified vascular abnormality.

Symptoms

Symptoms of stroke depend on the area of the brain that is affected. The most common symptoms include hemiparesis (weakness in one side of the body), hemi-sensory loss (numbness in one side of the body), facial droop (weakness in one side of the face), dysarthria (slurred speech), aphasia (difficulty with speech production or comprehension), visual changes, and difficulty with balance (vertigo or instability). The characteristic that is common to all the symptoms is acuteness; when the symptoms develop gradually, causes other than vascular etiology should be sought. Hemiparesis is caused by damage to the contralateral brain and usually associated with gaze preference to the side of the lesion. Gaze preference may serve as an important clue in localization of the lesion; if the lesion is above the brainstem, gaze preference is in the direction opposite to the weakness while with the brainstem lesion, it can be toward the side of the weakness. Facial droop and dysarthria can be caused by either cortical or subcortical lesions. On the other hand, aphasia represents a cortical lesion in the language center located in the cortex of the dominant brain, typically on the left side. Lesions in the non-dominant brain can manifest as contralateral neglect (ignoring one side of the body; not recognizing their own hand or dressing only one side of the body). Posterior circulation strokes involve the vertebrobasilar system and cause symptoms associated with lesions in the brainstem, cerebellum, and occipital lobes. These include hemiparesis, quadriparesis (lesion in brainstem), gaze paralysis (cranial nerves), vertigo (vestibular system), imbalance/ataxia (cerebellum), Horner's syndrome (sympathetic system), and visual field cuts (visual cortex).

Diagnosis

The diagnosis of acute stroke is achieved by careful history taking, examination, and imaging. Characterizing the symptoms and delineating the time course are important in guiding the imaging and choice of the treatment to follow. The examination should focus on recognizable patterns of cerebral dysfunction to aid in localization of the suspected pathology. Non-contrast computed tomography (CT) of the brain remains the test of choice in the acute setting. Computed tomography is very sensitive to the presence of hemorrhage, however, early ischemic stroke, especially small infarcts, can be missed. It should also be kept in mind that 5–10% of the patients with subarachnoid hemorrhage have negative CT; therefore when subarachnoid hemorrhage is suspected by history (sudden "worst headache") lumbar puncture and evaluation of cerebrospinal fluid for xanthochromia is necessary. Computed tomography angiography (CTA) and CT perfusion scan (CTP) can provide more information on the location of vascular occlusion and presence of penumbra and can serve as important tools in decision making, however, they are limited by the high radiation dose, IV contrast use, and availability. Magnetic resonance imaging (MRI), and especially diffusion weighted imaging (DWI) sequence, is more sensitive to focal ischemia. Magnetic resonance angiography is believed to be less sensitive in detecting intracranial arterial occlusion than CTA [2], but is the imaging of choice when contraindication to CT contrast (renal failure) is present. Conventional cerebral angiography may be needed to further define the underlying pathology especially when intervention is considered. Emergent cerebral angiography in acute stroke is becoming more widely available at larger stroke centers and has an advantage of providing diagnosis and intra-arterial treatment. Carotid

ultrasound can be used to evaluate for carotid stenosis. Echocardiography should be considered when cardiac or aortic arch evaluation is necessary; for instance when cardio-embolic source of thrombi is suspected.

Treatment

Available thrombolytic treatment for acute ischemic stroke is time-dependent. All patients with symptoms suggestive of acute stroke should be rapidly assessed for suitability for thrombolytic therapy [3]. Currently, intravenous tissue-plasminogen activator (tPA) is recommended for use in acute ischemic stroke within 4.5 hours of symptoms onset [4]. Intra-arterial thrombolysis is another option for acute therapy. A randomized trial (PROACT; Pro-urokinase for Acute Cerebral Thromboembolism) established its efficacy in patients with less than 6 hours of middle cerebral artery occlusion [5]. In August 2004, the FDA approved the Merci Retriever device, a mechanical embolectomy device, after reviewing patient data obtained in the Mechanical Embolus Removal in Cerebral Ischemia (MERCI) trial. In this trial, the device was used for 141 patients at 25 medical centers in the USA who were ineligible for thrombolytic therapy presenting within 8 hours of symptoms onset, and showed 66% of the patients treated only with the device achieved partial or complete reperfusion [6]. In 2008, another mechanical embolectomy device, the Penumbra System, received FDA approval with slightly higher rates of partial or complete recanalization [7]. Mechanical embolectomy may be safely utilized in patients with a contraindication to intravenous thrombolytic therapy such as those with recent surgery.

The medical management of patients who do not receive reperfusion therapy should focus on stabilization and prevention of subsequent events. Antiplatelet therapy should be considered, and aspirin is an effective and cost-efficient treatment to prevent recurrent stroke. In selected patients with high risk of recurrent stroke or the patients in whom aspirin therapy failed, other antiplatelet regimens should be considered. These include clopidogrel (Plavix) and combination therapy with extended release dipyramidole and low-dose aspirin (Aggrenox). The detailed discussion of medical therapy of stroke is in the section below. In the setting of acute stroke, blood pressure is commonly elevated. Lowering of blood pressure may exacerbate tissue ischemia leading to worsening of neurological deficits. It is a general consensus to maintain relatively high blood pressure for 1–2 days after acute ischemic stroke in order to ensure adequate cerebral perfusion to prevent neurological deterioration.

Communication, swallowing, and mobility concerns need to be addressed in all patients. Expert consultation for assessment of safety in swallowing, rehabilitation of speech, and mobility and range of motion exercises should be initiated early in the post-stroke period. Adequate therapy should prevent complications such as falls and development of deep vein thrombosis, pulmonary embolism, contractures, and pressure ulcers. Many patients benefit from a short stay in a rehabilitation facility before they are discharged to their home environment.

Perioperative stroke
Perioperative stroke risk

Physicians are often requested to assess risk in patients awaiting surgery. Guidelines [8] have been published to assist in cardiac evaluation but a similar source for cerebrovascular risk assessment is lacking. This section will summarize some of the important issues in surgical patients at risk for stroke.

Some surgical procedures are associated with higher risk of perioperative stroke such as cardiac and vascular surgeries. Double- or triple-valve surgery carries the highest stroke risk (9.7%) followed by isolated valve surgery (4.8–8.8%), aortic repair (8.7%), combined coronary artery bypass grafting (CABG) and valve surgery (7.4%), carotid endarterectomy (5.5–6.1%), and isolated CABG (1.4–3.8%) [9,10]. The timing of surgery is also an important factor; urgent surgeries carry more risk than elective surgeries. Surgery and anesthesia may contribute to stroke by several mechanisms. Hypotension from hemorrhage, fluid loss, or effect of anesthetic agents may contribute to cerebral ischemia especially in the patients who have arterial stenosis. Dislodged thrombus, fragmented plaque or cholesterol crystals may result in distal embolization. This can occur during angiography or intra-operatively with manipulation of vascular structures (i.e., clamping of the carotid artery or aorta). Hypercoagulability can result from surgical trauma and tissue injuries and is exacerbated by immobility and dehydration during postoperative period.

Identification of perioperative stroke risk factors should be included in the evaluation of risk and benefit of the surgical procedure for each patient. Patient-related risk factors include advanced age, female sex, history of hypertension, diabetes mellitus, renal insufficiency, smoking, chronic obstructive pulmonary disease, peripheral vascular disease, cardiac disease, or systolic dysfunction, history of stroke or TIA, carotid stenosis, atherosclerosis of aorta, and abrupt discontinuation of antithrombotic therapy before surgery [11–14]. Procedure-related risk factors include type and nature of the surgical procedure, type of anesthesia, duration of the surgery (and for cardiac procedures, duration of cardiopulmonary bypass and aortic cross-clamp time), manipulation of proximal aortic atherosclerotic lesions, arrhythmias, hyperglycemia, hypotension, and hypertension. If possible, any elective surgical procedures should be avoided during the 6-month period following stroke or TIA given the high risk of stroke during this period of tenuous brain vascular reserve.

It is reasonable to evaluate patients with symptomatic carotid stenosis with carotid Doppler ultrasound and consider revascularization prior to cardiac or major vascular surgery. Asymptomatic carotid stenosis (often identified by carotid Doppler following discovery of carotid bruit during preoperative examination) requires more careful evaluation of risk and benefit of revascularization. The risk of perioperative stroke in the patients with asymptomatic carotid stenosis, especially with unilateral disease, is lower than once thought. Naylor reported a risk of 1.8%, which increased to 3.2% and 5.2% with unilateral and bilateral significant stenosis (50–99%), respectively [15]. The risk was higher in the patients with unilateral carotid occlusion (7–11%). In addition to the relatively low risk with non-significant stenosis, evidence suggested 60% of perioperative stroke could not be attributed to the carotid disease alone when the correlation between distribution of infarcts and carotid disease was studied. Considering that there is relatively significant risk of death or stroke associated with carotid revascularization procedures themselves (3% with carotid endarterectomy (CEA)), it is the general consensus that revascularization before surgical procedure is unwarranted in the patients with carotid stenosis who are asymptomatic [16]. However, the benefit of revascularization may be greater than the risk if stenosis is high-grade and hemodynamically significant, especially with presence of bilateral disease. When asymptomatic carotid stenosis is identified during preoperative evaluation (i.e., carotid bruit in asymptomatic patients) further evaluation is needed to identify the patient who may benefit from carotid revascularization prior to surgery. These patients should undergo detailed neurological examination and history taking focused on identification of unreported symptoms of TIA or stroke, and CT or MRI of the brain to evaluate for "silent" infarcts [10]. Vascular studies such as carotid Doppler or CT/MR angiography to evaluate degree of stenosis may be considered, however further validation of their clinical usefulness in risk stratification is needed before solid recommendation for preoperative use of such studies can be made.

Evaluation of risk factors related to cardiac function and the status of the aorta can guide modification of surgical strategy in attempt to reduce the risk of perioperative stroke. Preoperative echocardiography can be used in risk stratification and planning of surgical technique by assessing systolic function and looking for cardiac thrombi. Transesophageal echocardiography or intraoperative epi-aortic ultrasound can be used to identify atherosclerotic disease of aorta so that aortic cannulation or clamping of calcified plaques can be avoided [17].

The patients who require anticoagulation with vitamin K antagonist (VKA) because of mechanical heart valve, atrial fibrillation, or venous thromboembolism (VTE) should be managed carefully in the perioperative period (see Figure 35.1). These patients are at higher risk for perioperative stroke since anticoagulation needs to be reversed for surgical procedure to prevent hemorrhagic complications. American College of Chest Physicians recommend stopping VKA 5 days before surgery in patients who require temporary interruption of anticoagulation and normalization of international normalized ratio (INR). It is further recommended to bridge anticoagulation with therapeutic-dose low molecular weight

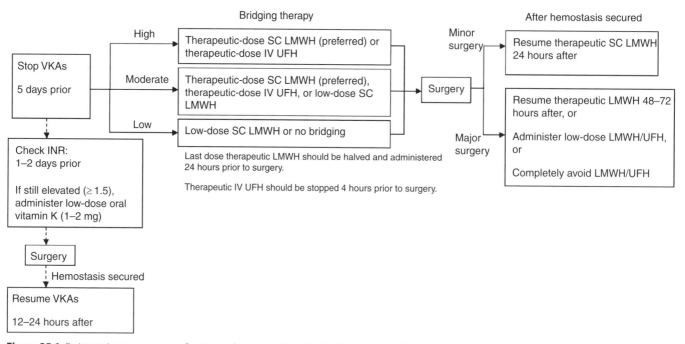

Figure 35.1 Perioperative management of patients who are receiving vitamin K antagonists (VKAs). IV UFH, intravenous unfractionated heparin; SC LMWH, subcutaneous low molecular weight heparin.

heparin (LMWH) or unfractionated heparin (UFH) for patients with mechanical heart valve, atrial fibrillation, or VTE at high risk for thromboembolism. In such patients, the last dose of LMWH should be halved and administered 24 hours prior to surgery and UFH should be stopped 4 hours prior to surgery. For the patients who require antiplatelet therapy with aspirin or clopidogrel, it is recommended to stop these medications 7–10 days prior to surgery except in the patient at high risk for cardiac event for which aspirin should be continued up to and beyond the time of surgery and clopidogrel to be held 5–10 days prior. Separate recommendations for the management of the patient with coronary stents can be found in the guideline published by the American College of Chest Physicians [18].

Mechanisms of perioperative stroke

Evidences suggest that most perioperative strokes are ischemic from embolism. Data from Likosky *et al.* show 63% of all perioperative strokes associated with CABG were embolic or thrombotic while only 9% were due to hypoperfusion [19]. In the same study, only 1% of perioperative stroke was hemorrhagic. Other etiologies were 10% multiple causes, 3% lacunes and 14% were unknown. As noted before, manipulation of large vessels with atherosclerotic disease can cause distal arterial occlusion by dislodging thrombi, fragmenting plaque and generating cholesterol crystals. The use of cardiopulmonary bypass pump is associated with stroke by release of particulate matter that can occlude cerebral arteries. Almost half of all perioperative strokes occur within the first day after surgical procedure [10]. The rest occur after successful recovery from

anesthesia and are likely contributed largely by postoperative atrial fibrillation and coagulopathy.

Coronary artery bypass grafting is associated with a significant risk of stroke. Previous studies noted 1.3–3.6% stroke incidence in post-CABG patients [12]. Increasing evidence suggests that the use of cardiopulmonary bypass pump (simply called "pump") during CABG is associated with higher risk of stroke [20–22]. Suggested mechanisms behind this phenomenon include athero-embolism, air embolism, or other undetermined factors. The risk of stroke was found to be significantly lower when CABG was performed off-pump. Although the exact mechanism of the higher rate of stroke with on-pump CABG remains unclear, it is believed that atherosclerotic disease of aorta and associated thromboembolism subsequent to aorta manipulation play an important role. When the complexity of the procedure requires the use of a pump, intraoperative epi-aortic ultrasonography before aorta manipulation to avoid calcified plaque may significantly reduce the incidence of stroke. Given the significant rate of stroke associated with CABG and the devastating effect of such a complication, the individualized procedural risk should be carefully assessed prior to operation and all available preventive measures, such as avoidance of aortic side-clamping, should be taken especially for high-risk patients [23]. The online risk calculator offered by the Society of Thoracic Surgeons (STS) website (http://www.sts.org/quality-research-patient-safety/quality/risk-calculator-and-models/risk-calculator) that can calculate individualized risk of stroke associated with cardiac surgeries based on demographic and clinical information can be useful in assessment of perioperative stroke risk and planning of surgical procedures.

Carotid endarterectomy is often utilized as a prophylactic procedure to prevent stroke. The North American Symptomatic Carotid Endarterectomy Trial (NASCET) was a landmark study establishing the benefit of surgery for symptomatic patients with carotid stenosis greater than 70% [24]. Similar findings were reported by the European Carotid Surgery Trial [25]. The evidence suggests that CEA can provide an absolute reduction of 11–17% in the risk of stroke within 2–3 years of the procedure in symptomatic patients with severe stenosis [26,27]. In 1995, publication of the Asymptomatic Carotid Atherosclerosis Study (ACAS) was followed by an increase in CEA given the proposed benefit of the procedure in preventing strokes. It demonstrated that selected patients with asymptomatic carotid stenosis of 60% or more would benefit from CEA surgery if the incidence of any stroke and death resulting from angiography and surgery was kept below 3% [28].

The decision to perform prophylactic CEA in asymptomatic patients requires careful and individualized assessment of degree of hemodynamic compromise from the stenosis, medical comorbidities, and risks associated with the procedure. Using a mathematical model of natural history of carotid artery stenosis compatible with major randomized controlled trials and the natural history data in order to quantify the benefit of prophylactic CEA, Nagaki *et al.* concluded that prophylactic CEA for severe carotid stenosis consistently yielded a benefit in patients who experienced symptoms within 6 months before the procedure [27]. The same study concluded that CEA for asymptomatic patients, on the other hand, has only marginal benefit and is not likely to have a large effect in reducing the burden of stroke. In such cases, the risk of the procedure including complication was considered greater than the benefit. Having said that, it is still reasonable to consider CEA in asymptomatic patients with severe carotid stenosis as long as the candidates are carefully evaluated and selected based on their medical comorbidities, expected life expectancy, and the risk of complication associated with the procedures.

Carotid artery stenting (CAS) was introduced in 1994 as an alternative to CEA for carotid revascularization. The Carotid Revascularization Endarterectomy Versus Stenting Trial (CREST) is a landmark study that investigated effectiveness and safety of CAS as compared with CEA in both symptomatic and asymptomatic patients with carotid stenosis. In this randomized trial, a total of 2,502 patients were randomized into CEA or CAS and followed for 4 years for primary end-points; the occurrence of any stroke, myocardial infarction (MI), or death. The study found CAS and CEA had similar net outcomes for symptomatic and asymptomatic patients. However, during the perioperative period (approximately 30 days after procedure) there was a lower incidence of MI with CAS and a lower incidence of stroke with CEA. Younger patients were found to have slightly better outcomes with CAS [29]. The patient's age, other medical comorbidities, and availability of an experienced surgeon should be taken into account when selecting which modality is better for carotid revascularization. Similar to coronary artery stenting, stent thrombosis caused by

intimal damage of the arterial wall triggering platelet activation and aggregation as well as inflammatory response is a serious complication of CAS [30]. Dual antiplatelet therapy with aspirin and clopidogrel has been shown to decrease recurrent ischemic events in post-CAS patients and is recommended for prevention of stent thrombosis [31].

Postoperative management

As noted in the previous section, almost half of strokes associated with surgical procedures occur during the postoperative period. Therefore, it is critical to manage surgical patients appropriately after the procedure and to monitor for and identify the symptoms of stroke if they develop. Risk factors for postoperative stroke include cardiac dysfunction (heart failure, low ejection fraction, myocardial infarction, and arrhythmias), dehydration, blood loss, and hyperglycemia [10,12,32]. Atrial fibrillation is a major etiology of postoperative stroke with reported incidence of 30–50% of those strokes [10,33,34]. Some of the predictors of postoperative atrial fibrillation are advanced age, past history of atrial fibrillation or supraventricular arrhythmias, preexisting heart failure or low ejection fraction, preoperative withdrawal of angiotensin-converting enzyme inhibitor or beta-blockers, history of myocardial infarction, and high postoperative magnesium levels [10,34]. A peak incidence of postoperative atrial fibrillation occurs within 2–4 days of surgery.

To prevent atrial fibrillation and decrease the risk of postoperative stroke, several measures can be taken. The patients should be carefully monitored for arrhythmias as well as for electrolyte abnormality for a minimum of 3 days after cardiac procedures. Their fluid balance should also be closely monitored and corrected if necessary. When postoperative atrial fibrillation does develop, heparin therapy should be considered especially for high-risk patients such as those with a history of stroke or TIA, and these patients should be on anticoagulation therapy for 30 days after the return of a normal sinus rhythm [35]. In many cases postoperative atrial fibrillation resolves spontaneously after 4–6 weeks.

Recommendations for preoperative management of patients who require vitamin K antagonist (VKA) were discussed in the previous section. Postoperatively, VKA should be resumed 12–24 hours after surgery and when there is adequate hemostasis. For the patients who are receiving therapeutic-dose UFH/LMWH prior to major surgery, it is generally recommended to either delay the initiation of therapeutic dose for 48–72 hours after surgery when hemostasis is secured, to administer low-dose heparin when hemostasis is secured, or to completely avoid anticoagulation. Anticipated bleeding risk and adequacy of hemostasis should be considered for individual cases in deciding when to resume anticoagulation postoperatively. For the patient whose anti-platelet therapy with aspirin or clopidogrel was held prior to procedure, these medications should be resumed approximately 24 hours after surgery when there is adequate hemostasis [18].

During the postoperative period, patients should be closely monitored for signs and symptoms of stroke. It is often difficult due to the effect of medications such as anesthetic agents or analgesics and immobilization. It requires particular attention to and understanding of the possible signs of stroke by physicians as well as nursing staff. When there is a sign of stroke, neurologic consultation should be obtained immediately. Intravenous tPA, which can be the first line of thrombolytic treatment for acute ischemic stroke, is contraindicated for patients with a history of major surgery within 14 days due to increased bleeding risk. However, intra-arterial tPA and mechanical embolectomy procedure may be safely administered for the postoperative patients, making immediate neurological assessment critical for the management of postoperative stroke [6,36].

Medical therapy for stroke prevention

Patients with ischemic stroke are at risk for vascular events including recurrent strokes or TIA and myocardial infarction (MI). Patients with history of stroke should be identified and appropriate long-term control of risk factors to prevent vascular events should be initiated prior to discharge from the hospital. The most important aspects include lifestyle modifications (smoking cessation, healthier diet, and regular exercises), treatment of hypertension, treatment of hyperlipidemia, diabetic control, and antithrombotic therapy.

Antiplatelet therapy reduces the risk of recurrent vascular events in patients with recent ischemic stroke or TIA. Currently available oral preparations that have been shown to be effective in clinical trials of patients with ischemic stroke and/or TIA include aspirin, clopidogrel, extended release dipyramidole with aspirin, and ticlopidine. All are effective in preventing recurrent vascular events in patients who have had an ischemic stroke.

Aspirin is a cost-effective method of stroke prevention for most patients, although the optimal effective dose remains unclear. In 1998, the FDA provided a statement recommending doses between 50 mg and 325 mg to prevent recurrent stroke [37]. After endarterectomy, doses between 81 mg and 325 mg have been shown to be more effective than higher doses [38]. In the most recent guidelines from the American College of Chest Physicians, aspirin dose of 50–100 mg/day is recommended over higher dose for patients who had non-cardio-embolic stroke or TIA [39].

Numerous trials have investigated aspirin, newer antiplatelet agents, and combined therapy for their efficacy and safety in prevention of vascular events including ischemic stroke. In the CAPRIE trial, approximately 20,000 patients with recent ischemic stroke, MI, or peripheral arterial disease were randomized to receive clopidogrel or 325 mg of aspirin [40]. For the primary end-point of MI, stroke or vascular death, clopidogrel was more effective than aspirin but the relative benefit (9%) and absolute benefit (0.5%) were small. In 2004, the MATCH trial investigated the effect of adding aspirin to clopidogrel [41]; 7,599 patients with high vascular risk (recent ischemic stroke or TIA and at least one additional vascular risk factor) who were already on clopidogrel were randomized to receive aspirin (75 mg) or placebo, and monitored for primary end-point of a composite of ischemic stroke, MI, vascular death, or rehospitalization for acute ischemia (stroke, TIA, MI, angina), or worsening of peripheral arterial disease. The trial found no significant reduction in risk of vascular events, however there was an increase in life-threatening or major bleeding with addition of aspirin to clopidogrel.

In the ESPS-2 trial, patients with recent ischemic stroke or TIA were studied using combination therapy with extended-release dipyramidole and 50 mg of aspirin [42]. The combination therapy was shown to be more effective in preventing stroke than low-dose aspirin, however, it was not more effective in preventing the primary end-point of stroke or death. The Prevention Regimen for Effectively Avoiding Second Strokes (PRoFESS) trial is a large, multicentered, randomized trial which compared aspirin 25 mg plus extended-release dipyramidole 200 mg given twice daily with clopidogrel 75 mg given once daily [43]. A total of 20,333 subjects were enrolled from 695 centers in 35 countries and randomized into the two treatment groups. Primary outcome was recurrent stroke of any type and the secondary outcome was a composite of stroke, MI, or death from vascular causes. The study shows that, among patients who suffered a non-cardio-embolic ischemic stroke, the risk of recurrent stroke or the composite of stroke, MI, or death from other vascular events are similar between the two treatment groups. There was also no significant difference in the risk of fatal or disabling stroke, although there were more hemorrhagic strokes with aspirin plus extended-release dipyramidole. Although all of the clinical trials can be helpful in choosing the best therapy depending on the individual risk factors and risk for side-effects, it is difficult to clearly determine which regimen is the most effective since each study had different entry criteria, primary end-points and doses of aspirin. Therefore the cost, tolerability, and once-daily dosing make aspirin a logical choice for initial therapy. For patients in whom aspirin therapy fails (i.e., have a recurrent event on aspirin), combination therapy should be considered.

Cilostazol is a newer antiplatelet drug which inhibits phosphodiesterase 3, increases cAMP concentrations and subsequently inhibits platelet aggregation [44]. The CSPS study in Japan established the efficacy of cilostazol and prompted its recommendation for use in secondary prevention of stroke in the Japanese guideline [45,46]. CSPS 2 was designed to investigate the efficacy and safety of cilostazol compared with aspirin in prevention of stroke in patients with non-cardio-embolic ischemic stroke [44]; 2,672 patients (1,337 on cilostazol twice daily and 1,335 on aspirin daily) were enrolled. The study showed cilostazol significantly lowered the risk of stroke compared with aspirin and also had significantly fewer hemorrhagic events. In addition to its antiplatelet ability, cilostazol has other beneficial effects in prevention of vascular events including improvement of endothelial function, dilation of blood vessels by increased production of nitric oxide and reduction of intracellular calcium ion concentrations, and inhibition of smooth muscle proliferation and inflammation. Further studies involving cilostazol use in different ethnic groups and patients with a variety of comorbidities are needed to make a solid recommendation for its use.

Warfarin is an effective antithrombotic agent for prevention of cardio-embolic stroke in the patients with atrial fibrillation or mechanical cardiac valves. In the patients without a cardiac source of embolism, however, warfarin is no better than aspirin in prevention of stroke and is associated with increased risk of minor bleeding (WARSS study) [47]. There is a question whether the lower target INR (1.4–2.8) used in the study affected the outcome. The investigators of WARSS felt that higher target INR would increase the risk of major hemorrhage without having an effect in prevention of stroke. Compared with aspirin, warfarin incurs more cost (medication itself and cost of monitoring); therefore, it would be appropriate to use aspirin instead of warfarin if stroke is not associated with cardio-embolic source.

In recent years, the efficacy and safety of newer oral anticoagulants other than warfarin have been studied in multiple trials. As noted above, warfarin is indicated for prevention of stroke in patients who are at risk for cardio-embolic stroke; however its use is limited by bleeding complications and non-compliance associated with the need for frequent monitoring of INR and food restrictions to avoid interactions. Data from one of the new oral anticoagulants, dabigatran, are promising [48]. Dabigatran is a direct thrombin inhibitor, and unlike ximelagatran which is another drug of its class, dabigatran has no hepatotoxicity. It also requires no monitoring of INR and has few interactions. The RELY study randomized 18,113 patients with non-valvular atrial fibrillation and at least one stroke risk factor and investigated efficacy and safety of dabigatran compared with warfarin [49]. The trial found that the rate of primary outcome, systemic embolism, or stroke (including hemorrhagic stroke) was significantly lower among the patients who received 150 mg twice-daily dose of dabigatran than the patients who received warfarin, while the rate of major bleeding was similar. With 100 mg twice-daily dabigatran, the rate of primary outcome, systemic embolism, or stroke was similar when compared with the warfarin group, while the rate of major bleeding was lower.

Statin medications were designed to limit atherosclerosis but also appear to have additional beneficial effects by promoting plaque stabilization, providing an anti-inflammatory effect (decreased C-Reactive Protein (CRP)) and reducing the risk of thrombosis [50]. The JUPITER trial studied the effect of rosuvastatin in 17,802 apparently healthy men and women without hyperlipidemia but with elevated CRP and found that administration of rosuvastatin 20 mg daily significantly reduced vascular events, including stroke [51]. Based on the results of this study and other evidence, statins

should be considered in all ischemic stroke and TIA patients who have LDL levels higher than 100. Use of statin in the patients with LDL level less than 100 would be an acceptable but unproven approach for prevention of recurrent ischemic stroke or TIA.

Management of hypertension is an important aspect of stroke prevention. As noted above, it is a general practice to allow permissive hypertension for 24–48 hours after acute ischemic stroke in order to prevent cerebral hypoperfusion and extension of ischemia. After the period of permissive hypertension, anti-hypertensive medications should be considered. The most recent guidelines by the Joint National Committee recommend goal blood pressure of 140/90 and a lower level of 130/80 if comorbidity such as diabetes or renal disease exists [52]. This goal blood pressure of 130/80 is probably appropriate for the patients with stroke or TIA. A review of randomized trials of antihypertensive medications by the Blood Pressure Lowering Treatment Trialists' Collaboration published in 2000 found no strong evidence to suggest that any particular drug or class of drugs was more beneficial in preventing stroke [53]. A similar conclusion was reached in another review in 2002 [54]. Angiotensin-converting enzyme inhibitors (ACEI) were designed to treat hypertension. However, they appear to have beneficial effects beyond blood pressure control, including anti-atherogenesis, endothelial cell modulation, and platelet inhibition [55]. Two studies of ACEI showed a reduction in stroke risk (HOPE, PROGRESS) [56,57]. The HOPE trial studied the effects of ramipril in patients with high risk for ischemic events and found a beneficial effect. The combined endpoint of MI, stroke, or vascular death was significantly reduced, and furthermore, the end-point of stroke alone was also reduced. PROGRESS tested the effects of combining perindopril with a diuretic, indapamide, in patients with ischemic stroke, TIA, or intracerebral hemorrhage and found that the combination therapy dramatically reduced the risk of recurrent stroke. Much of the benefit was related to tighter control of blood pressure, and no benefit was found for perindopril therapy alone.

The ALLHAT trial was a randomized trial comparing ACEI (lisinopril) and calcium-channel blocker (amlodipine) for the effects on clinical events in hypertensive patients with high risk of vascular disease [58]. The study found no significant differences between the two medications for the primary outcome (a composite of fatal coronary heart disease or non-fatal MI) and all-cause mortality. However, stroke rates were higher on lisinopril in blacks (RR 1.51, 95% CI 1.22–1.86) but not in non-blacks (RR 1.07, 95% CI 0.89–1.28), and in women (RR 1.45, 95% CI 1.17–1.79), but not in men (RR 1.10, 95% CI 0.92–1.31). Some of the effect may be explained by the less optimal control of blood pressure in the lisinopril group. Further studies are needed to determine the beneficial effects of ACEI or calcium channel blockers in preventing recurrent stroke independent of their effects on lowering blood pressure.

References

1. Easton JD, Saver JL, Albers GW *et al.* Definition and evaluation of transient ischemic attack: a scientific statement for healthcare professionals from the American Heart Association/American Stroke Association Stroke Council; Council on Cardiovascular Surgery and Anesthesia; Council on Cardiovascular Radiology and Intervention; Council on Cardiovascular Nursing; and the Interdisciplinary Council on Peripheral Vascular Disease: The American Academy of Neurology affirms the value of this statement as an educational tool for neurologists. *Stroke* 2009; **40**: 2276–93.

2. Bash S, Villablanca JP, Jahan R *et al.* Intracranial vascular stenosis and occlusive disease: evaluation with CT angiography, MR angiography, and digital subtraction angiography. *AJNR Am J Neuroradiol* 2005; **26**: 1012–21.

3. Frankel MR, Chimowitz M. Acute stroke. In *Emergency Neurology, Principles and Practice*. Cambridge: Cambridge University Press; 1999.

4. Del Zoppo GJ, Saver JL, Jauch EC *et al.* Expansion of the time window for treatment of acute ischemic stroke with intravenous tissue plasminogen activator: a science advisory from the American Heart Association/American Stroke Association. *Stroke* 2009; **40**: 2945–8.

5. Furlan A, Higashida R, Wechsler L *et al.* Intra-arterial prourokinase for acute ischemic stroke. *J Am Med Assoc* 1999; **282**: 2003–11.

6. Smith WS, Sung G, Starkman S *et al.* Safety and efficacy of mechanical embolectomy in acute ischemic stroke: results of the MERCI Trial. *Stroke* 2005; **36**: 1432–8.

7. Bose A, Henkes H, Alfke K *et al.* The Penumbra system: a mechanical device for the treatment of acute stroke due to thromboembolism. *AJNR Am J Neuroradiol* 2008; **29**: 1409–13.

8. Fleisher LA, Beckman JA, Brown KA *et al.* ACC/AHA 2007 Guidelines on Perioperative Cardiovascular Evaluation and Care for Noncardiac Surgery: Executive Summary: A Report of the American College of Cardiology/American Heart Association Task Force on Practice Guidelines (Writing Committee to Revise the 2002 Guidelines on Perioperative Cardiovascular Evaluation for Noncardiac Surgery). *Circulation* 2007; **116**: 1971–96.

9. Bucerius J, Gummert JF, Borger MA *et al.* Stroke after cardiac surgery: a risk factor analysis of 16,184 consecutive adult patients. *Ann Thorac Surg* 2003; **75**: 472–8.

10. Selim M. Perioperative stroke. *N Engl J Med* 2007; **356**: 706–13.

11. Limburg M, Wijdicks EF, Li H. Ischemic stroke after surgical procedures: Clinical features, neuroimaging, and risk factors. *Neurology* 1998; **50**: 895–901.

12. Hogue CW Jr, Murphy SF, Schechtman KB *et al.* Risk factors for early or delayed stroke after cardiac surgery. *Circulation* 1999; **100**: 642–7.

13. Filsoufi F, Rahmanian PB, Castillo JG *et al.* Incidence, imaging analysis, and early and late outcomes of stroke after cardiac valve operation. *Am J Cardiol* 2008; **101**: 1472–8.

14. Kikura M, Oikawa F, Yamamoto K *et al.* Myocardial infarction and cerebrovascular accident following non-cardiac surgery: differences in postoperative temporal distribution and risk factors. *J Thromb Haemostasis* 2008; **6**: 742–8.

15. Naylor AR, Mehta Z, Rothwell PM *et al.* Carotid Artery Disease and Stroke During Coronary Artery Bypass: a Critical Review of the Literature. *Eur J Vasc Endovasc Surg* 2002; **23**: 283–94.

16. Blacker DJ, Flemming KD, Link MJ *et al.* The preoperative cerebrovascular consultation: common cerebrovascular questions before general or cardiac surgery. *Mayo Clinic Proceedings* 2004; **79**: 223–9.

17. Kellermann, K, Jungwirth B. Avoiding stroke during cardiac surgery. *Semin Cardiothorac Vasc Anesth* 2010; **14**: 95–101.

18. Douketis JD, Berger PB, Dunn AS *et al.* The perioperative management of antithrombotic therapy. *Chest* 2008; **133** (6 Suppl): 299S–339S.

19. Likosky DS, Marrin CA, Caplan LR *et al.* Determination of etiologic mechanisms of strokes secondary to coronary artery bypass graft surgery. *Stroke* 2003; **34**: 2830–4.

20. Puskas JD, Williams WH, Duke PG *et al.* Off-pump coronary artery bypass grafting provides complete revascularization with reduced myocardial injury, transfusion requirements, and length of stay: a prospective randomized comparison of two hundred unselected patients undergoing off-pump versus conventional coronary artery bypass grafting. *J Thorac Cardiovasc Surg* 2003; **125**: 797–808.

21. Brizzio ME, Zapolanski A, Shaw RE *et al.* Stroke-related mortality in coronary surgery is reduced by the off-pump approach. *Annal Thorac Surg* 2010; **89**: 19–23.

22. Sedrakyan A, Wu AW, Parashar A *et al.* Off-pump surgery is associated with reduced occurrence of stroke and other morbidity as compared with traditional coronary artery bypass grafting: a meta-analysis of systematically reviewed trials. Supplemental Appendix I. *Stroke* 2006; **37**: 2759–69.

23. Hilker M, Arlt M, Keyser A *et al.* Minimizing the risk of perioperative stroke by clampless off-pump bypass surgery: a retrospective observational analysis. *J Cardiothorac Surg* 2010; **5**: 14.

24. N.A.S.C.E.T. Collaborators. Beneficial effect of carotid endarterectomy in symptomatic patients with high-grade carotid stenosis. *N Engl J Med* 1991; **325**: 445–53.

25. E.C.S.T.C. Group. MRC European Carotid Surgery Trial: interim results for symptomatic patients with severe (70–99%) or with mild (0–29%) carotid stenosis. *Lancet* 1991; **25**, 337 (8752): 1235–43.

26. E.C.S.T.C. Group. Randomised trial of endarterectomy for recently symptomatic carotid stenosis: final results of the MRC European Carotid Surgery Trial (ECST). *Lancet* 1998; **351** (9113): 1379–87.

27. Nagaki T, Sato K, Yoshida T *et al.* Benefit of carotid endarterectomy for symptomatic and asymptomatic severe carotid artery stenosis: a Markov model based on data from randomized controlled trials. *J Neurosurg* 2009; **111**: 970–7.

28. Executive Committee for the Asymptomatic Carotid Atherosclerosis Study. Endarterectomy for asymptomatic carotid artery stenosis. *J Am Med Assoc* 1995; **10**, 273: 1421–8.

29. Mantese VA, Timaran CH, Chiu D et al. The Carotid Revascularization Endarterectomy Versus Stenting Trial (CREST): Stenting versus carotid endarterectomy for carotid disease. *Stroke* 2010; **41** (10 Suppl 1): S31–4.

30. Chaturvedi S, Yadav JS. The role of antiplatelet therapy in carotid stenting for ischemic stroke prevention. *Stroke* 2006; **37**: 1572–7.

31. Bhatt DL, Kapadia SR, Bajzer CT et al. Dual antiplatelet therapy with clopidogrel and aspirin after carotid artery stenting. *J Invasive Cardiol* 2001; **13**: 767–71.

32. Kam PC, Calcroft RM. Peri-operative stroke in general surgical patients. *Anaesthesia* 1997; **52**: 879–83.

33. Almassi GH, Schowalter T, Nicolosi AC et al. Atrial fibrillation after cardiac surgery: a major morbid event? *Ann Surg* 1997; **226**: 501–13.

34. Lahtinen J, Biancari F, Salmela E et al. Postoperative atrial fibrillation is a major cause of stroke after on-pump coronary artery bypass surgery. *Ann Thorac Surg* 2004; **77**: 1241–4.

35. Epstein AE, Alexander JC, Gutterman DD et al. Anticoagulation: American College of Chest Physicians guidelines for the prevention and management of postoperative atrial fibrillation after cardiac surgery. *Chest* 2005; **128** (2 Suppl): 24S–7S.

36. Chalela JA, Katzan I, Liebeskind DS et al. Safety of intra-arterial thrombolysis in the postoperative period. *Stroke* 2001; **32**: 1365–9.

37. Albers GW, Amarenco P, Easton JD et al. Antithrombotic and thrombolytic therapy for ischemic stroke. *Chest* 2001; **119** (1 Suppl): 300S–20S.

38. Taylor DW, Barnett HJ, Haynes RB et al. Low-dose and high-dose acetylsalicylic acid for patients undergoing carotid endarterectomy: a randomised controlled trial. *Lancet* 1999; **353**(9171): 2179–84.

39. Albers GW, Amarenco P, Easton JD et al. Antithrombotic and thrombolytic therapy for ischemic stroke: American College of Chest Physicians Evidence-Based Clinical Practice Guidelines (8th Edition). *Chest* 2008; **133** (6 Suppl): 630S–69S.

40. CAPRIE Steering Committee. A randomised, blinded, trial of clopidogrel versus aspirin in patients at risk of ischaemic events (CAPRIE). *Lancet* 1996; **348**(9038): 1329–39.

41. Diener HC, Bogousslavsky J, Brass LM et al. Aspirin and clopidogrel compared with clopidogrel alone after recent ischaemic stroke or transient ischaemic attack in high-risk patients (MATCH): randomised, double-blind, placebo-controlled trial. *Lancet* 2004; **364** (9431): 331–7.

42. Diener HC, Cunha L, Forbes C et al. European Stroke Prevention Study 2. Dipyridamole and acetylsalicylic acid in the secondary prevention of stroke. *J Neurol Sci* 1996; **143**: 1–13.

43. Diener HC, Sacco RL, Yusuf S et al. Effects of aspirin plus extended-release dipyridamole versus clopidogrel and telmisartan on disability and cognitive function after recurrent stroke in patients with ischaemic stroke in the Prevention Regimen for Effectively Avoiding Second Strokes (PRoFESS) trial: a double-blind, active and placebo-controlled study. *Lancet Neurol* 2008; **7**: 875–84.

44. Shinohara Y, Katayama Y, Uchiyama S et al. Cilostazol for prevention of secondary stroke (CSPS 2): an aspirin-controlled, double-blind, randomised non-inferiority trial. *Lancet Neurol* 2010; **9**: 959–68.

45. Gotoh F, Tohgi H, Hirai S et al. Cilostazol Stroke Prevention Study: a placebo-controlled double-blind trial for secondary prevention of cerebral infarction. *J Stroke Cerebrovasc Dis* 2000; **9**: 147–57.

46. Shinohara Y, Gotoh F, Tohgi H et al. Antiplatelet cilostazol is beneficial in diabetic and/or hypertensive ischemic stroke patients. Subgroup analysis of the cilostazol stroke prevention study. *Cerebrovasc Dis* 2008; **26**: 63–70.

47. Mohr JP, Thompson JL, Lazar RM et al. A comparison of warfarin and aspirin for the prevention of recurrent ischemic stroke. *N Engl J Med* 2001; **345**: 1444–51.

48. Medi C, Hankey GJ, Freedman SB. Stroke risk and antithrombotic strategies in atrial fibrillation. *Stroke* 2010; **41**: 2705–13.

49. Ezekowitz MD, Wallentin L, Connolly SJ et al. Dabigatran and warfarin in vitamin K antagonist-naive and -experienced cohorts with atrial fibrillation. *Circulation* 2010; **122**: 2246–53.

50. Gorelick PB. Stroke prevention therapy beyond antithrombotics: unifying mechanisms in ischemic stroke pathogenesis and implications for therapy: an invited review. *Stroke* 2002; **33**: 862–75.

51. Ridker PM, Danielson E, Fonseca FA et al. Rosuvastatin to prevent vascular events in men and women with elevated C-reactive protein. *N Engl J Med* 2008; **359**: 2195–207.

52. Chobanian AV, Bakris GL, Black HR et al. The Seventh Report of the Joint National Committee on Prevention, Detection, Evaluation, and Treatment of High Blood Pressure: the JNC 7 report. *J Am Med Assoc* 2003; **21**, 289: 2560–72.

53. Neal B, MacMahon S, Chapman N; Blood Pressure Lowering Treatment Trialists' Collaboration. Effects of ACE inhibitors, calcium antagonists, and other blood-pressure-lowering drugs: results of prospectively designed overviews of randomised trials. *Lancet* 2000; **356**(9246): 1955–64.

54. ALLHAT Officers and Coordinators for the ALLHAT Collaborative Research Group. Major outcomes in high-risk hypertensive patients randomized to angiotensin-converting enzyme inhibitor or calcium channel blocker vs diuretic. *J Am Med Assoc* 2002; **288**: 2981–97.

55. Gorelick PB. New horizons for stroke prevention: PROGRESS and HOPE. *Lancet Neurol* 2002; **1**: 149–56.

56. Yusuf S, Sleight P, Pogue J; The Heart Outcomes Prevention Evaluation Study Investigators. Effects of an angiotensin-converting enzyme inhibitor, ramipril, on cardiovascular events in high-risk patients. *N Engl J Med* 2000; **342**: 145–53.

57. PROGRESS Collaborative Group. Randomised trial of a perindopril-based blood-pressure-lowering regimen among 6105 individuals with previous stroke or transient ischaemic attack. *Lancet* 2001; **358**(9287): 1033–41.

58. Leenen FH, Nwachuku CE, Black HR et al. Clinical events in high-risk hypertensive patients randomly assigned to calcium channel blocker versus angiotensin-converting enzyme inhibitor in the Antihypertensive and Lipid-Lowering Treatment to Prevent Heart Attack Trial. *Hypertension* 2006; **48**: 374–84.

Management of the surgical patient with dementia

Monica W. Parker, James J. Lah, and Allan I. Levey

Improvement in medical care and lifestyle practice has resulted in greater life expectancy for American adults. In 2008, 39 million people aged 65 and over lived in the USA, accounting for 13% of the total population. This older population grew from 3 million in 1900 to 39 million in 2008. The "oldest-old" population grew from just over 100,000 in 1900 to 5.7 million in 2008 [1].

Older adults frequently have multiple medical problems that can result in an increased need for hospitalization and utilization of healthcare expenditures. Older age, cognitive impairment, polypharmacy, and functional and sensory impairment are risk factors most likely to result in postoperative delirium [2]. Geriatric patients with dementia are at higher risk for the development of delirium. Delirium costs are $38–$152 billion dollars per year [3]. Management of the surgical dementia patient is geared toward prevention of delirium. Delirium is prevented through the identification of dementia and preoperative management of risk factors. This will improve surgical outcomes, decrease length of hospitalization, and reduce healthcare costs.

We will address the challenges of geriatric patients with dementia who undergo surgical procedures and outline strategies for their management.

The geriatric patient with dementia

Dementia affects more than 5 million people over age 65 [4]. Impaired cognitive status adversely affects postoperative rehabilitation and recovery. Dementia is frequently unrecognized and undiagnosed. The DSM–IV definition of dementia is impairment in short- and long-term memory, impairment in abstract thinking, disturbances of cortical function, and personality change. Dementia is a major risk factor for the development of delirium [5].

Some dementias are "brain related" and others are "medical disorder" related. Brain-related dementias are progressive neurodegenerative dementias that we cannot reverse with specific treatment. Medical disorder dementias include those medical conditions that have a definitive treatment, such as vitamin deficiencies, drug–drug interactions, thyroid hormone abnormalities, trauma (e.g., subdural hematomas), and depression. The most commonly diagnosed progressive dementia is Alzheimer's disease with a prevalence of 60–80%. This is followed by vascular dementia which affects 14–17% [4]. Mild cognitive impairment (MCI) is an intermediate state between normal aging and dementia [6]. Persons with MCI are at higher risk of developing postoperative cognitive disorder (POCD). Symptoms of this disorder are loss of memory and concentration after surgery [7]. Lewy Body and Parkinson's dementia will present with physical and cognitive deficits in the geriatric patient. Bradykinesia, gait instability, tremors, anxiety or depression are some of the symptoms. An assessment of baseline cognitive and physical function should be a part of the preoperative examination.

The initial patient interview should be oriented towards inquiring whether or not the patient has symptoms suggestive of mild cognitive impairment, dementia, delirium, and/or depression. Depression and dementia are associated with poor functional outcomes and death in geriatric persons who undergo hip surgery [8]. A detailed history should be obtained from the family and caregivers about cognitive status [9]. Questions should include whether the patient has the ability to perform activities of daily living (ADLs) independently. Activities of daily living are walking, grooming, toileting, and feeding; and instrumental activities of daily living (IADLs) are cooking, driving, and financial management. Inquiries about substance abuse and alcohol use should also be made. Family and caregivers should be able to explain the type of assistance that the patient requires to accomplish ADLs and IADLs. An inability to be independent with ADLs is indicative of cognitive impairment and further testing is required.

Cognitive screening in the outpatient office is accomplished with a number of tools. Screening tools frequently employed include the Mini-Mental Status Exam (MMSE), the Mini-Cog and the Geriatric Depression Scale (GDS). The MMSE is a screening tool that has been most commonly used for cognitive

Medical Management of the Surgical Patient, ed. Michael F. Lubin, Thomas F. Dodson, and Neil H. Winawer. Published by Cambridge University Press. © Cambridge University Press 2013.

Table 36.1 2002 criteria for potentially inappropriate medication use in older adults: considering diagnoses or conditions.

Disease or condition	Drug	Concern	Severity rating (high or low)
Heart failure	Disopyramide (Norpac), and high sodium content drugs (sodium and sodium salts [alginate bicarbonate, biphosphate, citrate, phosphate, salicylate, and sulfate])	Negative inotropic effect. Potential to promote fluid retention and exacerbation of heart failure	High
Seizures or epilepsy	Clozapine (Clozaril), chlorpromazine (Thorazine), thioridazine (Mellaril), and thiothixene (Navane)	May lower seizure thresholds	High
Blood clotting disorders or receiving anticoagulant therapy	Aspirin, NSAIDs, dipyridamole (Persantin), ticlopidine (Ticlid), and clopidogrel (Plavix)	May prolong clotting time and elevate INR values or inhibit platelet aggregation, resulting in an increased potential for bleeding	High
Bladder outflow obstruction	Anticholinergics and antihistamines, gastrointestinal antispasmodics, muscle relaxants, oxybutynin (Ditropan), flavoxate (Urispas), anticholinergics, antidepressants, decongestants, and tolterodine (Detrol)	May decrease urinary flow, leading to urinary retention	High
Arrhythmias	Tricyclic antidepressants (imipramine hydrochloride, doxepin hydrochloride, and amitriptyline hydrochloride)	Concern due to proarrhythmic effects and ability to produce QT interval changes	High
Parkinson's disease	Metoclopramide (Reglan), conventional antipsychotics, and tacrine (Cognex)	Concern due to their antidopaminergic/cholinergic effects	High
Cognitive impairment	Barbiturates, anticholinergics, antispasmodics, and muscle relaxants. CNS stimulants: dextroamphetamine (Adderall), methylphenidate (Ritalin), methamphetamine (Desoxyn), and pemolin	Concern due to CNS-altering effects	High
Syncope or falls	Short- to intermediate-acting benzodiazepine and tricyclic antidepressants (imipramine hydrochloride, doxepin, hydrochloride, and amitriptyline hydrochloride)	May produce ataxia, impaired psychomotor function, syncope, and additional falls	High
SIADH/hyponatremia	SSRIs: fluoxetine (Prozac), citalopram (Celexa), fluvoxamine (Luvox), paroxetine (Paxil), and sertraline (Zoloft)	May exacerbate or cause SIADH	Low
COPD	Long-acting benzodiazepines: chlordiazepoxide (Librium), chlordiazepoxide-amitriptyline (Limbitrol), clidinium-chlordiazepoxide (Librax), diazepam (Valium), quazepam (Doral), halazepam (Paxipam), and chlorazepate (Tranxene). Beta-blockers: propranolol	CNS adverse effects. May induce respiratory depression. May exacerbate or cause respiratory depression	High
Chronic constipation	Calcium channel blockers, anticholinergics, and tricyclic antidepressants (imipramine hydrochloride, doxepin hydrochloride, and amitriptyline hydrochloride)	May exacerbate constipation	Low

SIADH, syndrome of inappropriate antidiuretic hormone secretion ; COPD, chronic obstructive pulmonary disease; SSRIs, selective serotonin reuptake inhibitors; CNS, central nervous system.

assessment in the USA and abroad. This is a 30-item screening tool that assesses memory, orientation, recall, and visuospatial capability. An MMSE score of 23 or less correlates with a diagnosis of cognitive impairment. It has a sensitivity of 87% and specificity of 89% [10]. Newer more time-efficient screeners have been developed to detect mild cognitive impairment which may progress to Alzheimer's disease. The Mini-Cog/FAQ consists of a three-item recall combined with a clock-drawing test and a rating of functional assessment. It is simple to administer and has a sensitivity of 89% and a specificity of 95% [1]. The Mini-Cog/FAQ can be easily completed in the course of a preoperative visit by a trained assistant. The GDS is a 15-item questionnaire that screens for depression. A score of 5 or more indicates depression. The advantage of this tool is its ease of administration. Depression is amenable to treatment. Treatment of depression will minimize the onset of delirium.

Preoperative evaluation of the geriatric patient with dementia requires that chemical, hormonal, and drug regimen assessments be conducted to manage and correct abnormalities that may result in greater surgical risk. Malnutrition is 12–50% higher among the hospitalized elderly [12]. Malnutrition is defined as a body mass index (BMI) of less than 21 and a serum albumin level less than 3.5 [13]. Patients suffering from malnutrition have higher rates of postoperative mortality. In cardiac surgery, delirium onset can be predicted by the presence of low MMSE score, high GDS score, low albumin, and a history of prior TIA/stroke [14].

The establishment of baseline oxygen, thyroid hormone levels, vitamin B_{12}, folate, hematologic, and renal function is obtained with preoperative laboratory. Patients with undiagnosed endocrinopathies may present with neurocognitive impairment. Thyroid hormone deficiencies may result in diminished memory, attention, and visuospatial organization [15]. Hyperthyroidism frequently results in elevated blood pressure and tachycardia. Hypercalcemia is indicative of hyperparathyroidism. Manifestations of this include confusion and psychosis [16]. Correction of deficiencies and fluid imbalances will minimize the likely onset of delirium and POCD. Postoperative cognitive disorder is currently described as deterioration in cognition associated with surgery. There is an increased association with death [17]. This condition has not been well studied or characterized, but its onset is believed to result from a combination of surgery-induced physiologic stressors such as increased cortisol, hypoxia, and anesthesia that may trigger cellular degeneration and Alzheimer's disease pathogenesis [18].

Geriatric patients with dementia may likely have several chronic diseases. Persons with multiple chronic diseases will frequently take greater than five medications (polypharmacy) for the management of their comorbid illness. Geriatric patients are susceptible to adverse drug events (ADEs) related both to polypharmacy and physiologic changes associated with aging [19]. Polypharmacy is likely to result in anticholinergic

excess and toxicity. Symptoms of anticholinergic excess include restlessness, agitation, disorientation, hallucinations, tremor, arrhythmia, delirium, sedation, seizures, and coma. Drug-induced delirium is a significant risk factor for prolonged hospitalization and poor surgical outcomes [20]. Many of these prescribed medications have adverse side-effects independent of anesthesia administration. The Beers Criteria, a list of medications to avoid using in the elderly, was developed in 1997 and updated in 2003 [21]. This list has not been easy to use. In recent years, two tools have been developed. The Screening Tool of Older Peoples Prescriptions (STOPP) and Screening Tool to Alert Doctors to Right Treatment (START) have wider applicability in the US and internationally [2]. These tools provide an indication of which medications are appropriate for managing specific clinical events. A careful medication review will alert the surgeon to drugs that may cause an ADE (Table 36.1). Some medications must have therapeutic levels assessed to prevent toxicity and interaction with anesthetic compounds.

The importance of physical and neurological examination

The preoperative cardiovascular and physical examinations are particularly important for the assessment of coexisting medical comorbidity. Abnormalities in both can cause or exacerbate cognitive impairment. A baseline ECG to evaluate for arrhythmias will help document cardiac status. Atrial fibrillation is not uncommon in the geriatric patient. It can be treated with electrical or medical cardioversion when indicated [23]. Untreated atrial fibrillation may result in adverse cardiovascular events, delirium, and death [24]. Treatment of congestive heart failure before surgery will decrease the risk of acute cardiac decompensation. Congestive heart failure patients are at higher risk of death from exacerbations. Each of these events may trigger an acute or vascular event and delirium postoperatively.

Stroke is a known risk factor for vascular dementia. Physical signs of vascular compromise are easy to detect and are dependent on the area of the brain involved. Hemiparesis and hemianopia are easy to detect. Other deficits, which are not easily detected, include aphasia (left middle cerebral artery) acute confusional state (right middle cerebral artery), apathy, abulia, or lack of motivation (anterior cerebral artery). Continuous monitoring of heart rhythm and rate during surgery will permit early intervention for arrhythmia.

Neuroimaging with a head CT scan or MRI to look for brain structure abnormalities, specifically hippocampus degeneration, may be obtained preoperatively when physical exam and history indicate cognitive dysfunction. Preoperative management of the patient with dementia has focused on establishing a patient's baseline cognitive function, and managing those problems that may contribute to the onset of delirium and poor post-surgery rehabilitation.

Ethical and legal considerations

The ethical treatment of patients with and without dementia requires that informed consent be obtained. Informed consent means that the patient understands the diagnosis, the treatment for this diagnosis and has the capacity to make a decision regarding treatment. When the capacity to make decisions is absent, a surrogate should be sought whenever possible [25]. Family members usually fill this role [26]. While competence may easily be judged in persons with severe cognitive impairment, the physician may face particular problems in those with mild cognitive impairment. Decision-making capacity can be qualitatively assessed in the presence of mild cognitive impairment to determine patients' wishes [27]. The patient with mild dementia may report a reasonably well-preserved ability to perform most activities of daily living, have a non-focal neurological examination and yet show striking abnormalities in discrete cognitive domains such as executive functioning. In these instances, neuropsychological testing, a formal assessment of mental competence, should be completed by a psychiatrist or neurologist [28].

Decisions regarding prescribed treatment, life-sustaining measures, withholding/withdrawal of treatment should be discussed with the patient and his surrogate decision maker before surgery. In a landmark judgment in 1990, the Supreme Court ruled in Cruzan vs. Director, Missouri Department of Health, that the state could require "clear and convincing" evidence regarding patients' wishes for life-sustaining procedures [29]. Moreover the Court noted that affidavits produced by family members specifying the patient's premorbid verbal directives were considered supportive, but not definitive evidence. The Patient's Self Determination Act passed by Congress in 1990 requires that healthcare providers educate the patient about issues concerning advance directives. Federal law requires all facilities certified by Medicare and Medicaid to furnish information that enables patients to express their wishes regarding the use or refusal of medical care. The *Living Will* is among the oldest mechanisms used to communicate a patient's wishes concerning medical interventions. It details those interventions desired and those not wanted in specific clinical situations. The *Durable Power of Attorney* is a legal document that names surrogates to make decisions on medical care when the patient is unable to do so. This is the most flexible of advance directives, allowing surrogates to receive and process information in a manner identical to the patient. They can make decisions on behalf of the patient, even in the event of unexpected or unusual events in the clinical course [30]. The *Pre-Hospital Advance Directive* (PHAD) is a legal document on a standardized form that is uniform within a state or emergency medical services (EMS) region. It is meant to prevent EMS providers from beginning resuscitative efforts. A common modification of this document is the pre-hospital Do Not Resuscitate (DNR) form. Unlike the PHAD, these forms are usually initiated, and their provisions agreed to, by the patient's physician. They are particularly relevant in the care of patients in nursing homes or hospices [31].

Important issues to address with the patient and family prior to surgery:

1. Increased likelihood of confusion and agitation in the immediate postoperative period.
2. Increased risk of long-term cognitive decline.
3. Ascertain and document the patient's wishes regarding life-sustaining procedures.
4. Provide information to patient and family on advance directives.

The patient with dementia is particularly prone to delirium in the postoperative period. Educating the family about the increased risk of postoperative agitation, its recognition and management is likely to make its occurrence less stressful. Identification of the patient's principal caregivers and providing them with additional information on the signs and delirium may aid in its early diagnosis and management.

Intraoperative management of care

The type and duration of anesthesia used for geriatric patients with dementia will affect surgical recovery. General anesthesia has usually been the anesthesia of choice for the patient with Alzheimer's disease [32]. Light sedation vs deep sedation for hip replacement was shown to decrease the incidence of delirium in geriatric patients [3]. Higher doses of general anesthesia are associated with prolonged mechanical ventilation, delirium onset, and prolonged hospitalization [34]. Sedation with benzodiazepines and significant postoperative pain have been factors cited as etiologic factors for post-anesthesia delirium. Regional anesthesia for hip repair has been associated with faster recovery [35]. In several studies, higher doses of opioid pain medications, and lower fluid administration were associated with prolonged recovery time and emergence from anesthesia and subsequent development of delirium [36]. Regional anesthesia and analgesia use in geriatric patients with dementia may be best for the prevention of postoperative complications and prolonged hospitalization in this patient group [37]. Further study is needed to document the efficacy of this anesthetic practice.

Postoperative care

Delirium and postoperative cognitive impairment commonly occur in the immediate postoperative period in the geriatric patient. Delirium affects both the demented and normal elderly patient and is characterized by restlessness, confusion, and agitation. Distinguishing features include acute onset, altered sleep-wake cycle, fluctuating levels of consciousness, and altered psychomotor activity. Common etiologies of delirium in the postoperative setting include both intoxication and withdrawal of medications, infections, conditions predisposing to hypoxia such as chronic obstructive pulmonary disease (COPD), CHF, and toxic/metabolic causes such as hepatic encephalopathy and electrolyte abnormalities.

There are different types of delirium. Hyperactive delirium is characterized by increased psychomotor activity with the patient exhibiting disruptive behavior, agitation, and psychosis. While this form of delirium may be easily detected, the hypoactive variant is more difficult to recognize and is characterized by withdrawal and apathy. Simple bedside tests of attention and orientation may be useful in the diagnosis of delirium in the postoperative patient. Examples of such tests include digit span forward and backward, naming of the months of the year in reverse order and serial subtraction of 7s from 100 [38].

In addition to these methods, a more formal cognitive assessment of the patient may help in early detection of the delirium and its treatment (Table 36.2). Such evaluation may be especially useful if a formal assessment of mental status was also performed prior to surgery.

Table 36.2 Diagnostic criteria for delirium.

DSM–IV–TR diagnostic criteria
1. Disturbance of consciousness (i.e., reduced clarity of awareness of the environment) with reduced ability to focus, sustain, or shift attention
2. A change in cognition (such as memory deficit, disorientation, language disturbance) or the development of a perceptual disturbance that is not better accounted for by a preexisting, established, or evolving dementia
3. The disturbance develops over a short period of time (usually hours to days) and tends to fluctuate during the course of the day
4. There is evidence from the history, physical examination, or laboratory findings that the disturbance is caused by the direct physiological consequences of a general medical condition
The Confusion Assessment Method (CAM) Diagnostic Algorithm[a]
See the *American Psychiatric Publishing Textbook of Geriatric Psychiatry*, 2009, pp. 222–41 for the complete version of table.

[a] The CAM ratings should be completed following brief cognitive assessment of the patient, for example, with the Mini-Mental State Examination. The diagnosis of delirium by CAM requires the presence of features 1 and 2 and of either 3 or 4.
Source: Diagnostic criteria for delirium reprinted from American Psychiatric Association. *Diagnostic and Statistical Manual of Mental Disorders*, 4th edn, Text Revision. Washington, DC: American Psychiatric Association, 2000. Used with permission.
CAM diagnostic algorithm adapted from Inouye SK, Vandyck CH, Alessi CA et al. Clarifying confusion: The Confusion Assessment Method – a new method for detection of delirium. *Ann Intern Med* 1990; **113**: 941–8. Used with permission. See *The American Psychiatry Publishing Textbook for Geriatric Psychiatry*; 2009, pp. 222–41 for online version of table.

A thorough history obtained from the family or caregiver and physical examination by the physician are invaluable in the diagnosis of delirium. In the hospitalized patient, preoperative evaluation of the patient may already have documented all medications that the patient was taking. Medications to avoid in the geriatric patient have been previously discussed. The avoidance of anticholinergic medications preoperatively and postoperatively remains important. Particular attention must be paid to a history of alcohol abuse as delirium tremens may present a serious, life-threatening complication. Physical examination of the delirious patient must be directed at identifying a source of infection, ascertaining fluid status, source of pain and the management of comorbid conditions such as CHF and COPD. Fecal impaction and urinary retention are common causes of postoperative confusion in the geriatric patient and must be addressed in the physical examination. Patients with cognitive impairment may not be able to verbalize complaints of pain efficiently and may require more frequent assessment of pain/discomfort in the postoperative period. Effective pain control has been shown to reduce the incidence of delirium [39]. Minimizing the use of sedating opioid and other anticholinergic medications may reduce postoperative complications.

Laboratory evaluation that may be useful in the detection of an underlying cause for delirium includes a CBC. Serum electrolytes may help detect acid–base abnormalities or acute renal failure. Pulse oximetry and/or arterial blood gas measurement may be useful in the detection of hypoxia and confirmation of acid–base abnormalities. A chest X-ray may be performed upon suspicion of underlying pneumonia. A urinalysis may be indicated when a urinary tract infection is suspected, particularly with the insertion of Foley catheters.

Postoperative management of patients with dementia will require the monitoring for and consistent management of complications that contribute to delirium. The diagnosis of delirium has been made easier with DSM–IV criteria and use of the Confusion Assessment Method (CAM). The CAM is a tool developed with a 94–100% sensitivity and 95% specificity for diagnosis of delirium [40]. The CAM can be administered at the bedside by a trained technician. Correcting the source of identified delirium will allow quicker postoperative recovery and rehabilitation. The postoperative management of the geriatric patient with dementia is best accomplished with a multidisciplinary team of surgeon, primary care, and nursing specialists to diminish surgical complication occurrence [41].

Delirium management

The prompt treatment of delirium in the postoperative period is of paramount importance and must be instituted even while the search for an underlying cause is in progress. All non-essential medications should be held and the need for centrally acting medication re-evaluated. Whenever possible, these should be replaced with peripherally acting equivalents. Non-pharmacologic measures to reduce the symptoms of delirium include clear and concise communication between the caregivers and patients. Aids to help orientation include providing verbal reminders of date, time, and identity of relatives and members of the treatment team. The provision of a clock or calendar in the room, ensuring adequate lighting and controlling of excessive noise are other examples of simple measures that can help provide an unambiguous environment to delirious patients. Other useful strategies to employ are measures to increase the competence of patients. These include the provision of an interpreter for non-English speakers, ensuring that the patients have their glasses, hearing aids, or dentures. Visits by members of the treatment team should permit maximum periods of uninterrupted sleep. Sleep deprivation is a factor that may exacerbate dementia.

Pharmacologic management of delirium

The decision to use pharmacological interventions in the management of delirium must be made only after careful consideration of the potential adverse effects of such treatment. The delirious patient may require such treatment in order to prevent injury or to allow further diagnostic work-up or treatment. Antipsychotic medications are the most commonly used drugs in the management of delirium. Haloperidol is the most studied medication used in treatment. Doses of haloperidol should be as low as possible and administered as often as every 4 hours via IV, IM, or oral routes [42].

Newer atypical antipsychotic medications, risperidone, olanzapine, and quetiapine are being used for the management of postoperative delirium (Table 36.3). Studies are emerging that show that these medications may be effective with fewer side-effects than haloperidol [43]. When delirium occurs in the setting of seizures or alcohol withdrawal, benzodiazepines are

Table 36.3 Pharmacological treatment of delirium.

Class and drug	Dose	Adverse effects	Comments
Antipsychotic Haloperidol	0.5–1.0 mg twice daily orally, with additional doses every 4 hours as needed (peak effect, 4–6 hours)	Extrapyramidal symptoms, especially if dose is > 3 mg/day	Usually agent of choice
	0.5–1.0 mg intramuscularly; observe after 30–60 min and repeat if needed (peak effect, 20–40 min)	Prolonged corrected QT interval on electrocardiogram	Effectiveness demonstrated in randomized controlled trials
		Avoid in patients with withdrawal syndrome, hepatic insufficiency, neuroleptic malignant syndrome	Avoid intravenous use because of short duration of action
Atypical antipsychotic Risperidone	0.5 mg twice daily	Extrapyramidal effects equivalent to or slightly less than those with haloperidol	Tested only in small uncontrolled studies
Olanzapine	2.5–5.0 mg once daily	Prolonged corrected QT interval on electrocardiogram	Associated with increased mortality rate among older patients with dementia
Quetiapine	25 mg twice daily		
Benzodiazepine Lorazepam	0.5–1.0 mg orally, with additional doses every 4 hours as needed[a]	Paradoxical excitation, respiratory depression, oversedation	Second-line agent
			Associated with prolongation and worsening of delirium symptoms Reserve for use in patients undergoing sedative and alcohol withdrawal, those with Parkinson's disease, and those with neuroleptic malignant syndrome
Antidepressant Trazodone	25–150 mg orally at bedtime	Oversedation	Tested only in uncontrolled studies

[a] Intravenous use of lorazepam should be reserved for emergencies.
Source: Adapted from Inouye SK. Current concepts: delirium in older persons. *N Engl J Med* 2006; **354**: 1157–65. Used with permission.

the preferred choice of pharmacologic agents in treatment. Lorazepam has a rapid onset and short duration of action and can be given by both oral and parenteral routes in dosages ranging from 0.5 mg every 12 hours to 1 mg every 8 hours.

Postoperative care for the geriatric patient with dementia

Postoperative issues for geriatric patients with dementia are centered on pain management, restoration of physical function, delirium prevention, and management. Pain can be effectively managed with non-opioid medications and progressed as needed (Table 36.4). Naproxen sodium immediately after surgery is as effective as narcotics [4]. Regularly administered acetaminophen is as effective as narcotics in managing postoperative pain [45].

Summary

As the geriatric population grows, the number of patients with dementia who will likely undergo major surgery will increase. Dementia and advanced age are significant risk factors for morbidity and mortality. Careful assessment of the geriatric surgical patient is required to both diagnose and further evaluate cognitive impairment. Detection and management of comorbid medical illness will improve cognitive function and surgical outcome. Physicians must be familiar with the ethical and legal issues associated with the care of demented patients. Cognitive function deterioration is a common adverse outcome of surgery in the geriatric patient. Worsening cognitive dysfunction is precipitated by the development of chemical and physiologic abnormalities that cause life-threatening delirium. Increased vigilance, early detection, and prompt treatment can reverse conditions that will ensure better long-term prognosis.

Table 36.4 The WHO 3-step model for pain management.

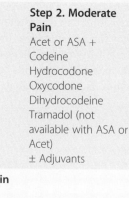

Step 3
Morphine
Hydromorphone
Methadone
Levorphanol
Fentanyl
Oxycodone
± Non-opioid
analgesics
± Adjuvants

Step 2. Moderate Pain
Acet or ASA +
Codeine
Hydrocodone
Oxycodone
Dihydrocodeine
Tramadol (not available with ASA or Acet)
± Adjuvants

Step 1. Mild Pain
Aspirin (ASA)
Acetaminophen (Acet)
Non-steroidal anti-inflammatory drugs (NSAIDs)
± Adjuvants

"Adjuvants" refers either to medications that are co-administered to manage an adverse effect of an opioid, or to so-called adjuvant analgesics that are added to enhance analgesia.
In 1986, the World Health Organization (WHO) developed a 3-step conceptual model to guide the management of cancer pain. It provides a simple, well-tested approach for the rational selection, administration, and titration of a myriad of analgesics. Today, there is wide consensus favoring its use for the medical management of all pain associated with serious illness.

References

1. AgingStats.gov – Federal Interagency Forum on Aging-Related Statistics. *Older Americans 2010: Key Indicators of Well-Being.* www.agingstats.gov/agingstatsdotnet/main_site/default.aspx

2. Dasgupta D, Hillier LM. Factors associated with prolonged delirium: a systematic review. *Int Psychogeriatr* 2010; **22**: 373–94.

3. Leslie DL, Marcantonio ER, Zhang Y *et al.* One-year health care costs associated with delirium in the elderly population. *Arch Intern Med* 2008; **168**: 27–32.

4. Alzheimer's Association. *2010 Alzheimer's Disease Facts and Figures.* www.alz.org/documents_custom/report_alzfactsfigures2010.pdf.

5. Robinson TN, Raeburn CD, Tran AZ *et al.* Postoperative delirium in the elderly: risk factors and outcomes. *Ann Surg* 2009; **249**: 173–8.

6. Reisberg B, Ferris SH, Kluger A *et al.* Mild cognitive impairment (MCI): a historical perspective. *Int Psychogeriatr* 2008; **20**: 18–31.

7. Bekker A, Lee C, de Santi S *et al.* Does mild cognitive impairment increase the risk of developing postoperative cognitive dysfunction? *Am J Surg* 2010; **199**: 782–8.

8. Bellelli G, Frisoni GB, Turco R, Trabucchi M. Depressive symptoms combined with dementia affect 12-months survival in elderly patients after rehabilitation post-hip fracture surgery. *Int J Geriatr Psychiatry* 2008; **23**: 1073–7.

9. Mayeux R, Foster NL, Rossor M *et al.* The clinical evaluation of patients with dementia. In Whitehouse PJ, ed. *Dementia*, Vol. 40. Philadelphia, PA: Davis; 1993, pp. 92–129.

10. Milne AJ, Culverwell A, Guss R *et al.* Screening for dementia in primary care:

a review of the use, efficacy and quality of measures. *Int Psychogeriatr* 2008; **20**: 911–26.

11. Steenland NK, Auman CM, Patel PM *et al.* Development of a rapid screening instrument for mild cognitive impairment and undiagnosed dementia. *J Alzheimer's Dis* 2008; **15**: 419–27.

12. Evans C. Malnutrition in the elderly: a multifactorial failure to thrive. *Permanente J* 2005; **9**: 38–41.

13. Beers MH, Porter RH, Jones TV *et al.*, eds. *The Merck Manual of Diagnosis and Therapy*. 18th edn. Whitehouse Station, NJ: Merck Research Laboratories; Hoboken, NJL John Wiley and Sons; 2006.

14. Rudolph JL, Jones RN, Levkoff SE *et al.* Derivation and validation of a preoperative prediction rule for delirium after cardiac surgery. *Circulation* 2009; **119**: 229–36.

15. Mafrica F, Fodale V. Thyroid function, Alzheimer's disease and postoperative cognitive dysfunction: a tale of dangerous liaisons? *J Alzheimers Dis* 2008; **14**: 95–105.

16. Papageorgiou SG, Christou Y, Kontaxis T *et al.* Dementia as presenting symptom of primary hyperparathyroidism: favourable outcome after surgery. *Clin Neurol Neurosurg* 2008; **110**: 1038–40.

17. Deiner S, Silverstein JH. Postoperative delirium and cognitive dysfunction. *Br J Anaesth* 2009; **103** (Suppl 1): i41–6.

18. Xie Z, Tanzi RE. Alzheimer's disease and post-operative cognitive dysfunction. *Exp Gerontol* 2006; **41**: 346–59.

19. Hayes BD, Klein-Schwartz W, Barrueto F Jr. Polypharmacy and the geriatric patient. *Clin Geriatr Med* 2007; **23**: 371–90.

20. Lin R, Heacock LC, Fogel JF. Drug-induced, dementia-associated and non-dementia, non-drug delirium hospitalizations in the United States, 1998–2005: an analysis of the National Inpatient Sample. *Drugs Aging* 2010; **27**: 51–61.

21. Fick DM, Cooper JW, Wade WE *et al.* Updating the Beers criteria for potentially inappropriate medication use in older adults. *Arch Intern Med* 2003; **163**: 2716–24.

22. Levy HB, Marcus EL, Christen C. Beyond the Beers criteria: a comparative overview of explicit criteria. *Ann Pharmacother* 2010; **44**: 1968–75.

23. Winkel TA, Schouten O, Hoeks SE *et al.* Prognosis of transient new-onset atrial fibrillation during vascular surgery. *Eur J Vasc Endovasc Surg* 2009; **386**: 683–8.

24. Banach M, Kazmierski J, Kowman M *et al.* Atrial fibrillation as a nonpsychiatric predictor of delirium after cardiac surgery: a pilot study. *Med Sci Monit* 2008; **14**: CR286–291.

25. Appelbaum PS. Assessment of patient's competence to consent to treatment. *N Engl J Med* 2007; **357**: 1834–40.

26. Curtis JR, Vincent JL. Ethics and end-of-life care for adults in the intensive care unit. *Lancet* 2010; **376**: 1347–53.

27. Rodin MB, Mohile SG. Assessing decisional capacity in the elderly. *Semin Oncol* 2008; **35**: 625–32.

28. Marson DC, Hawkins L, McInturff B, Harrell LE. Cognitive models that predict physician judgments of capacity to consent in mild Alzheimer's disease. *J Am Geriatr Soc* 1997; **45**: 458–64.

29. Supreme Court of the United States. *Cruzan v. Director, Missouri Department of Health*. http://law2.umkc.edu/faculty/projects/ftrials/conlaw/cruzan.html

30. Hornbostel R. Legal and financial decision making in dementia care. In Whitehouse PJ, ed. *Dementia*, Vol. 40. Philadelphia, PA: Davis; 1993, pp. 417–32.

31. Iserson KV. Nonstandard advance directives: a pseudoethical dilemma. *J Trauma-Injury Infect Crit Care* 1998; **44**(1): 139–42.

32. Williams AS. Perianesthesia care of the Alzheimer's patient. *J Perianesth Nurs* 2009; **24**: 343–7.

33. Sieber FE, Zakriya KJ, Gottschalk A *et al.* Sedation depth during spinal anesthesia and the development of postoperative delirium in elderly patients undergoing hip fracture repair. *Mayo Clinic Proceedings* 2010; **85**: 18–26.

34. Shetty VD, Vowler SL, Villar RN. The role of anaesthesia and the anaesthetist in reducing the length of stay after primary total hip replacement. *J Bone Joint Surg – Br Vol* 2009; **91B** (Suppl 1): 19.

35. DiNino G, Adversi M, Dekel BG *et al.* Peri-operative risk management in patients with Alzheimer's disease. *J Alzheimer's Dis* 2010; **22** (Suppl 3): 121–7.

36. Radtke FM, Franck M, MacGuill M *et al.* Duration of fluid fasting and choice of analgesic are modifiable factors for early postoperative delirium. *Eur J Anaesthesiol* 2010; **27**: 411–16.

37. Halaszyni TM. Pain management in the elderly and cognitively impaired patient: the role of regional anesthesia and analgesia. *Curr Opin Anaesthesiol* 2009; **22**: 594–9.

38. Fayers PM, Hjermstad MJ, Ranhoff AH *et al.* Which Mini-Mental State Exam items can be used to screen for delirium and cognitive impairment? *J Pain Symptom Manage* 2005; **30**: 41–50.

39. Leung JM, Sands LP, Paul S *et al.* Does postoperative delirium limit the use of patient-controlled analgesia in older surgical patients? *Anesthesiology* 2009; **111**: 625–31.

40. Inouye SK, Vandyck CH, Alessi CA *et al.* Clarifying confusion: The Confusion Assessment Method – a new method for detection of delirium. *Ann Intern Med* 1990; **113**: 941–8.

41. Sieber FE. Postoperative delirium in the elderly surgical patient. *Anesthesiol Clin* 2009; **27**: 451–64.

42. Lonergan E, Britton AM, Luxenberg J, Wyller T. Antipsychotics for delirium. *Cochrane Database Syst Rev* 2007; **2**: CD005594.

43. Gleason OC. Delirium. *Am Fam Physician* 2003; **67**: 1027–34.

44. Derry C, Derry S, Moore RA, McQuay HJ. Single dose oral naproxen and naproxen sodium for acute postoperative pain in adults. *Cochrane Database Syst Rev* 2009; **1**: CD004234.

45. Post ZD, Restrepo C, Kahl LK *et al.* A prospective evaluation of 2 different pain management protocols for total hip arthroplasty. *J Arthroplasty* 2010; **25**: 410–15.

37

Neuromuscular disorders

Jaffar Khan and Lilith Judd

Neuromuscular disease in surgical patients can be divided into disorders of the neuromuscular junction, peripheral nerves, and muscle.

Neuromuscular junction

Myasthenia gravis

Of all the neuromuscular diseases, myasthenia gravis probably has the most significant implications for surgical patients [1]. This disorder results from an autoimmune attack on the acetylcholine receptors of the postsynaptic (muscle) side of the neuromuscular junction. Characteristic clinical features include fluctuating weakness and fatigue, usually involving the extraocular muscles and eyelids (producing diplopia and ptosis). Weakness of the limbs can be severe, sometimes resulting in almost total paralysis. Sensation and deep tendon reflexes remain intact. Respiratory muscle weakness is common and can be fatal. The introduction of practical mechanical ventilation has resulted in a dramatic decrease in the mortality rate.

Although the clinical features of myasthenia gravis are sufficiently characteristic in some cases, confirmatory tests are usually necessary [2]. The acetylcholine receptor (AchR)-antibody level is elevated in over 80% of patients with myasthenia gravis. Elevated levels of this antibody are extremely specific for this disease [3]. As a result the AchR-antibody serum test is typically the first step in confirming the diagnosis, and the presence of elevated levels eliminates the need for additional confirmatory testing. In antibody-negative patients or when faced with an acutely symptomatic patient, the edrophonium test is often used. Electrodiagnostic studies (repetitive nerve stimulation and single fiber electromyography) are often useful, particularly in antibody-negative patients or patients with cardiac disease or asthma, in whom edrophonium is relatively contraindicated. The characteristic finding on 2- to 3-Hz repetitive motor nerve stimulation is a progressive decrease in the amplitude of the motor response. Single fiber electromyography may reveal the presence of jitter or blocking (a difference in the timing of activation or a failure of neuromuscular transmission in one of a pair of muscle fibers within a motor unit).

Many effective therapies have been developed for myasthenia gravis [4]. Acetylcholine esterase inhibitors increase the concentration of acetylcholine near the impaired receptors. This provides symptomatic relief of weakness. Pyridostigmine (Mestinon) is used most commonly and is generally given at a dosage of 60 mg every 3–6 hours, depending on the patient's response.

Immunosuppression with prednisone frequently is efficacious. Patients beginning prednisone therapy or undergoing a titration of the dosage should be cautioned that weakness might increase during the first 10–14 days before the beneficial effect becomes apparent. Azathioprine [5,6] and cyclosporine [7,8] are effective and are often used in patients who do not respond to other treatments or are at increased risk for complications from prednisone. Mycophenolate mofetil (CellCept) is used with success in severe refractory myasthenia [9]. The rapid onset of therapeutic effect, safe side-effect profile, and patient tolerability make this drug a desirable candidate for future investigation in the treatment of myasthenia gravis [10].

Thymectomy is recommended as an option for patients with non-thymomatous generalized myasthenia, except at the extremes of age [11]. However, about 10% of patients with myasthenia have a thymoma and their prognosis is worse, even if the tumor is removed. The incidence of thymoma increases with age and the tumor may develop at any time during the course of the illness. Chest computed tomography should be performed at the time of diagnosis. Thymectomy produces permanent remission in about 50% of patients, although remission may not occur for many months after surgery.

Hyperthyroidism is found in 5% of patients with myasthenia gravis. Hypothyroidism also is more common in these patients than in the general population. Treatment of the thyroid abnormality usually improves muscle strength.

The term *myasthenic crisis* refers to progressive respiratory or bulbar weakness. Intubation usually should be done when the vital capacity falls to about 15 mL/kg. Causes of myasthenic crisis include infection, thyroid dysfunction, and medications

---

Medical Management of the Surgical Patient, ed. Michael F. Lubin, Thomas F. Dodson, and Neil H. Winawer. Published by Cambridge University Press. © Cambridge University Press 2013.

that adversely affect neuromuscular transmission. The most common pharmacologic offenders are aminoglycosides, quinine, quinidine, magnesium, and neuromuscular blocking agents. Many medications are reported to exacerbate myasthenia occasionally, including most antiarrhythmic agents. Hypokalemia is a common cause of increased weakness in patients with myasthenia, especially those who are taking prednisone. As a precautionary measure, potassium replacement is advisable in these patients. In addition to correcting any precipitating factor, the most effective treatment for myasthenic crisis is plasma exchange, which almost always has a dramatic effect over a few days. High-dose intravenous immunoglobulin (400 mg/kg daily for 5 days) is also efficacious [12].

Myasthenia gravis in surgical patients

Thymectomy is often performed in patients with myasthenia gravis to remove thymomas, if present, and to attempt to induce remission. Patients should not undergo this surgery until medical management has been used to increase their strength, particularly in the respiratory muscles. If respiratory function remains significantly impaired (vital capacity 20 mL/kg or less) after maximal medical improvement, a course of intravenous immunoglobulin (400 mg/kg daily for 5 days) should be given. Patients who undergo surgery with significant respiratory weakness are more likely to require prolonged postoperative mechanical ventilation. After sternotomy, accurate measurement of the vital capacity usually is not possible because of incisional pain. In general, if the use of medications with neuromuscular blocking potential is avoided during surgery, a normal potassium level is maintained, and preoperative medication regimens are resumed, problems with extubation are unlikely. However, in a large number of cases, neuromuscular agents are used which can increase need for postoperative respiratory support. Recently, a few case reports and case series showed reversal of a rocuronium-induced neuromuscular blockage with sugammadex (Bridion), a cyclodextrin that reverses steroidal neuromuscular relaxants. Sugammadex, which is not currently available in the USA, resulted in decreased need for prolonged intubation in myasthenic patients in Europe [13].

Pre- and postoperatively, intravenous pyridostigmine (Mestinon) can be given, but the dosage used (1–4 mg) should be one-thirtieth to one-fifteenth the oral dosage (60–90 mg every 4–6 hours) because of the lack of first-pass hepatic metabolism. After surgery, remission may occur within a few weeks but can be delayed for several months. Medical therapy can gradually be withdrawn on an outpatient basis according to the patient's clinical status. The prednisone dosage can often be tapered over 6–8 weeks. A dose of pyridostigmine can be omitted during the day to determine whether the drug is still needed.

Patients occasionally develop weakness as a result of unsuspected myasthenia gravis during hospitalization for a surgical procedure. This is most often related to the administration of a medication with neuromuscular blocking activity [14], although hypokalemia, hypermagnesemia, and infection are also capable of unmasking myasthenia gravis [15].

Intravenous magnesium should not be used in patients with myasthenia, except when life-threatening hypomagnesemia exists [16]. The use of aminoglycosides, quinine, quinidine, and intraoperative neuromuscular blocking agents also should be avoided. In addition, lincomycin, clindamycin, polymyxin, and colistin are capable of exacerbating myasthenia. Other antibiotics and antiarrhythmic drugs have been implicated rarely but are not completely contraindicated. These include erythromycin, penicillins, sulfonamides, tetracyclines, ciprofloxacin, vancomycin, procainamide, calcium channel blockers, and beta-blockers. There are anecdotal reports of numerous medications that have been associated with worsening of myasthenia, and it is prudent to suspect any newly added medication in this setting.

Lambert–Eaton syndrome

Lambert–Eaton syndrome is a rare disorder of neuromuscular transmission caused by autoantibodies directed against calcium channels in the presynaptic terminal [17]. This abnormality impairs acetylcholine release. Patients have proximal muscle weakness but it differs from myasthenia gravis in that extraocular muscles are rarely involved and deep tendon reflexes are reduced. About half of patients are eventually found to have small cell carcinoma of the lung. The presence of anti-VGCC antibodies provides laboratory support for diagnosis and may eliminate the need for electrophysiologic testing. However, repetitive nerve stimulation can be utilized to confirm the diagnosis and when supportive of the diagnosis shows a characteristic increase in the electrical response when recorded over a muscle after exercise or rapid repetitive stimulation.

Symptomatic treatment is provided with 3,4-diaminopyridine, an aminopyridine that augments presynaptic acetylcholine release and improves neuromuscular transmission. Although poorly effective when used in isolation, pyridostigmine can be helpful when used in conjunction with 3,4-diaminopyridine. Other possible treatment considerations include plasma exchange, intravenous immunoglobulin, and prednisone. The response to treatment of small cell carcinoma is unpredictable, but when detected cancer should be removed or treated medically. Medications that exacerbate myasthenia gravis may also exacerbate Lambert–Eaton syndrome.

Prolonged neuromuscular blockade

Neuromuscular blocking agents are frequently used to facilitate mechanical ventilation. Although routine use of these agents typically does not result in any complications, some patients may develop persistent weakness for up to 1 week after the drugs are discontinued. This is more common in patients with renal or hepatic dysfunction in which the metabolism of the medications may be reduced or with the concomitant use of drugs that potentiate the action of neuromuscular blocking agents [18]. The diagnosis can be confirmed with repetitive nerve stimulation. A typical decrement of the motor response occurs when neuromuscular blockade is present, although in patients with severe weakness, the motor response may be absent. If the weakness persists beyond 10 days, the repetitive nerve stimulation should be repeated and a diligent search for another etiology of the weakness should be pursued. Otherwise, supportive care should be maintained until the pharmacologic effects of the paralytics have resolved.

Peripheral neuropathy

Peripheral neuropathy may be generalized (polyneuropathy), focal (mononeuropathy), or multifocal (multiple mononeuropathy). All three syndromes may cause clinically significant problems for surgical patients.

Mononeuropathy

Mononeuropathies present as the dysfunction of an individual peripheral nerve and are common in patients undergoing surgical procedures. Mononeuropathies usually result from mechanical forces including compression or direct trauma occurring intraoperatively. Compression neuropathies are probably the most frequent disorders. Patients with diabetes and other conditions associated with polyneuropathy are predisposed to the development of compressive neuropathy [19]. Patients who are undergoing general anesthesia are at risk because they may be positioned in such a way that continuous pressure is applied to a nerve.

One of the most common mononeuropathies seen in postoperative patients is a radial nerve palsy, which is analogous to the well-known "Saturday night palsy" in which a person awakens from alcohol-induced anesthesia with a wristdrop from the arm having been draped over an object [20]. Continuous pressure over the mid-humerus damaging the radial nerve also can occur during surgery or be associated with impaired mobility before or after surgery. There is weakness of wrist extension and the brachioradialis with a normal triceps. Intrinsic hand muscles appear to be weak because they are at a mechanical disadvantage and cannot be effectively activated without adequate wrist extension. There may be loss of sensation over the dorsum of the hand in the web space between the thumb and index finger. The prognosis is good, with recovery usually occurring over weeks to months. A splint should be used to keep the hand in a more functional position and prevent contracture.

Ulnar neuropathy is also seen in postoperative patients, resulting from compression at the elbow [21]. Pressure over the medial elbow is the usual cause when this condition develops during surgery. There is numbness of the fifth and medial portion of the fourth digits and palm. In more severe cases, weakness of abduction and, sometimes, flexion of the ulnar digits may be seen. Recovery is usual when the condition is mild but some permanent disability is seen in severe cases.

Patients should be advised to avoid pressure over the elbow and prolonged elbow flexion (which stretches the nerve across the ulnar groove).

The other common pressure palsy involves the peroneal nerve as it passes behind the head of the fibula [22]. Pressure behind the knee, resulting from prolonged leg crossing or squatting, is the usual cause, and patients who have recently experienced significant weight loss are predisposed. This also can occur during surgery when pressure is applied to that area. There is weakness of ankle dorsiflexion and often eversion, without weakness of ankle inversion. There may be sensory loss in the web space between the first two toes and, sometimes, the anterolateral foot and leg. Prognosis is good, with most patients recovering in 3 to 8 weeks. A brace (ankle–foot orthosis) improves the ability to walk by relieving footdrop.

Infrequently, obturator, lateral femoral cutaneous, peroneal, and sciatic neuropathies may result when a patient is placed in the lithotomy position during surgery. These compression neuropathies are more likely to occur if the position is maintained for more than 2 hours [23]. Numerous neuropathies are reported as a complication of cardiac surgery [24]. These neuropathies are usually a consequence of intraoperative positioning or a direct result of the surgical procedure. The phrenic nerve is at risk for injury during the internal mammary artery dissection and intraoperative hypothermia. Rarely, a recurrent laryngeal neuropathy may develop as a result of intraoperative hypothermia, tracheal intubation, central venous catheter placement, or surgical dissection. Numbness and pain along the medial calf to the great toe can result from an injury to the saphenous nerve during a vein harvest.

In addition to the pressure palsies, mononeuropathies related to the trauma of an invasive procedure are commonly encountered in surgical patients. The femoral nerve is often damaged after femoral artery catheterization [25]. This usually is related to pressure from a hematoma, although inaccurate needle placement also is a potential cause. A hematoma may be evident on physical examination or it may lie proximal to the inguinal ligament and escape detection by physical inspection. Computed tomography or magnetic resonance imaging through the pelvis is necessary in this setting because evacuation of the hematoma can be beneficial. Femoral neuropathy is also a relatively common complication of hysterectomy or other gynecologic surgery, probably because of traction on the nerve. Femoral neuropathy causes weakness of knee extension that often is not recognized until patients begin to walk. The knee jerk is reduced or absent and there may be loss of sensation over the anterior thigh and medial leg (the saphenous branch of the femoral nerve provides sensory innervation to the medial leg). When they are severe, these nerve injuries commonly result in prolonged or permanent disability, although significant recovery is possible even after 1 year.

Damage to the spinal accessory nerve is a common complication of lymph node biopsy. An incision over the lateral neck puts this nerve at risk as it crosses the sternocleidomastoid muscle. Patients often develop insidious shoulder pain that increases with continued use of the shoulder joint. There is weakness of the trapezius, which causes scapular winging and instability of the shoulder joint. The winging is most evident when patients abduct the shoulders to 90 degrees. Testing for weakness of the shoulder shrug is rarely useful because muscles other than the trapezius also serve this action. Depending on the level of injury, there may be weakness of the sternocleidomastoid muscle. This can be recognized by asking patients to turn their heads in the opposite direction against resistance. This injury commonly results in long-term disability because this slender nerve is usually severed and reanastomosis is difficult. Range-of-motion exercises prevent frozen shoulder but strenuous use of the joint should be avoided because it may hasten the development of degenerative arthritis.

Polyneuropathy

Polyneuropathy occasionally requires diagnostic or therapeutic intervention in surgical patients. Typical clinical features include distal numbness, tingling, or burning; weakness of distal muscles; and reduced deep tendon reflexes. Numerous metabolic, toxic, inflammatory, and hereditary causes are known. The most common etiologies are diabetes and alcoholism. Neuropathies can be conveniently divided into two categories: (a) those in which peripheral myelin is the primary target (demyelinating neuropathies), and (b) those in which peripheral axons are primarily damaged (axonal neuropathies). Secondary damage to myelin or axons can occur in either type but they can often be differentiated with nerve conduction studies and electromyography. Demyelinating neuropathies show a greater degree of conduction velocity slowing and conduction block on nerve conduction studies than do axonal neuropathies.

Demyelinating neuropathies are either inflammatory (Guillain–Barré syndrome or chronic inflammatory demyelinating polyneuropathy) or hereditary (most commonly the dominantly inherited Charcot–Marie–Tooth disease). Virtually all toxic and metabolic neuropathies are axonal, as is the neuropathy caused by vasculitis. Additionally, axonal neuropathy may result as a complication of critical illness and sepsis.

One common demyelinating neuropathy seen in the perioperative patient is Guillain–Barré syndrome (GBS), more recently referred to as acute inflammatory demyelinating polyneuropathy. It can occur after an infection but for an unknown reason may also develop during the postoperative period [26,27]. Patients usually first develop tingling or numbness in the feet and hands, followed by weakness of the lower and then the upper extremities, the respiratory muscles, and the facial muscles. Deep tendon reflexes are lost or reduced and mild distal sensory loss is common. There is frequently autonomic nerve involvement, which results in fluctuations in blood pressure and pulse rate. Atypical clinical patterns are fairly common, with asymmetry, greater involvement of upper extremity or facial muscles, and a predilection for the proximal muscles occurring in individual cases. Muscle and back pain

are common and the creatine kinase level is sometimes elevated (although usually less than 1,000 U/L). This sometimes mimics polymyositis. The cerebrospinal fluid cell count is usually normal and the protein level elevated, although the latter is frequently normal during the first week of illness. Progression to maximum weakness usually occurs during the first few weeks but quadriplegia with respiratory paralysis may be seen as early as the first day of illness. Spontaneous recovery is the rule over several weeks to months, although a significant minority of patients retain some permanent disability.

Treatment of GBS involves both modulation of the autoimmune process and supportive measures. Both plasma exchange and intravenous immunoglobulin are proven to be beneficial in the treatment of moderate to severe GBS [28–30]. Although some authorities believe that plasma exchange is still the treatment of choice because it has a longer track record, several randomized control trials and meta-analyses show that plasma exchange and intravenous immunoglobulin are equally efficacious in GBS [30,31]. Furthermore, current evidence also shows that both therapies used in combination are no more effective than each therapy used alone.

Supportive care involves careful treatment of both respiratory and autonomic dysfunction. In patients with actively progressing disease, respiratory function should be monitored at least twice a day. When the vital capacity reaches about 15 mL/kg, elective intubation should usually be performed. Inspiratory force can be estimated by asking patients to forcefully inhale through the nose (sniff) and vital capacity can be approximated by asking them to inhale and forcefully exhale. Patients should be instructed to cough to assess their ability to clear the airway and prevent aspiration. Patients with impending respiratory failure related to neuromuscular disease typically take rapid, shallow breaths and become diaphoretic. Blood gas analysis is usually consistent with hyperventilation initially, with carbon dioxide retention being a late, preterminal finding. Patients frequently develop autonomic dysfunction. Symptoms and signs of cardiac arrhythmias, labile blood pressure, urinary retention, and gastrointestinal dysfunction should be identified and appropriately managed.

More common than Guillain–Barré syndrome in hospitalized patients, critical illness polyneuropathy (CIP) is a condition which occurs in 49–77% of ICU patients with ICU stays greater than 7 days and is associated with critical illness and sepsis [32]. Critical illness polyneuropathy is usually characterized by a relatively symmetric flaccid weakness with sensory loss that can progress to quadriplegia and diaphragmatic weakness. This diagnosis is usually considered when a patient "fails to wean" from the ventilator, as duration of weaning is 2–7 times longer. The facial muscles may be mildly involved, however the ocular muscles are typically spared. The reflexes are often reduced or absent. Compared with the Guillain–Barré syndrome, dysautonomia is not a feature of CIP. Sepsis is the major risk factor for the development of this polyneuropathy, however there is also an association with multi-organ failure and systemic inflammatory response syndrome. Female gender, severity of illness, low serum albumin, duration of ICU stay, use of vasopressors, and hyperglycemia have also been implicated as potential factors in the development of CIP. The pathophysiology of CIP is likely multifactorial involving pro-inflammatory cytokines, microcirculation impairment, and metabolic alterations [32]. Electrophysiologic testing and sural nerve biopsy demonstrates extensive axonal loss, distinguishing this neuropathy from the typical Guillain–Barré syndrome [33–35].

Treatment of CIP is generally primarily supportive including respiratory support, physical therapy, and splints. However there has been some consideration for preventative care, including aggressive management of underlying risk factors such as hyperglycemia and sepsis. Additional care should be given to protecting possible sites of nerve entrapment and thereby preventing superimposed compression neuropathies. The use of immunosuppression, plasma exchange, or intravenous immunoglobulin has not led to a significant improvement in the final outcome. Overall, the prognosis for recovery is good; however, incomplete recovery with permanent neurologic residual is common [32,36].

Multiple mononeuropathy

Multiple mononeuropathy is occasionally encountered after surgery. It is most commonly associated with open heart surgery, and there is a predilection for involvement of the shoulder girdle and other upper extremity nerves. The brachial plexus is susceptible to stretch injury during sternal retraction. Traction on the nerves may be responsible in some instances but the involvement of nerves distant from the incision suggests that embolic occlusion of small vessels with nerve ischemia also may be contributory. A hematoma secondary to a fracture of the first rib may compress the nearby plexus and result in a similar injury [24].

Neuralgic amyotrophy (Parsonage–Turner syndrome) is a form of multiple mononeuropathy involving an upper extremity [37]. Pain in the shoulder region is followed after a few days by weakness resulting from multiple lesions in the brachial plexus or peripheral nerves. It has occurred after viral illness and immunization, and also is seen occasionally during the postoperative period. The prognosis for multiple mononeuropathies after surgery is good, with most patients recovering after several weeks or months.

Median, ulnar, and radial nerve injury may occur in combination after placement of a shunt in the upper extremity for hemodialysis. These patients present with an acute, painful, weak arm soon after the procedure. The distal forearm and hand muscles are usually affected. There is wrist drop with additional weakness of wrist flexion and the intrinsic hand muscles. Sensation of the hand is reduced or absent. Although hematoma formation, the surgical procedure, or anesthetic technique are possible causes, ischemic injury to the peripheral nerve as a result of diversion of blood flow by the shunt is commonly implicated. Diabetic patients with peripheral

neuropathy and small vessel disease appear to be at high risk for this complication. Early recognition of the problem is important because patients may improve after prompt ligation of the shunt [12].

Myopathy

Myopathies are less common than disorders of the neuromuscular junction and neuropathies in the perioperative period, however special attention should be given to malignant hyperthermia given its acuity and critical illness myopathy.

Primary myopathies rarely present clinical problems in patients undergoing surgical procedures, with the notable exception of malignant hyperthermia [38]. This causes life-threatening muscle rigidity and is precipitated by potent inhaled anesthetics and depolarizing neuromuscular blocking agents. Severe episodes are characterized by combined metabolic and respiratory acidosis (inability to ventilate because of rigidity), tachycardia, cardiac arrhythmias, and myoglobinuria. Extreme hyperthermia may be a late sign. The potential for this reaction should be anticipated in anyone with a personal or family history of malignant hyperthermia. This is usually an inherited disorder with a variable pattern of inheritance. The responsible genetic defect occurs in the calcium release channel, known as the ryanodine receptor. When triggered by the anesthetic agent, there is an efflux of calcium through this channel into the sarcoplasm, which results in contraction of the muscle fiber [39]. Although the ryanodine receptor has a major role in muscle contraction, there are multiple genetic alleles and loci where a mutation may result in an increased susceptibility for the development of malignant hyperthermia [40]. Dantrolene is a calcium channel blocker used to treat an episode. Rapid recognition of the syndrome, discontinuation of the inciting medications and treatment with dantrolene has significantly reduced the mortality. It is given at a rate of 2 mg/kg every 5 minutes to a total dose of 10 mg/kg. There appears to be an increased incidence of malignant hyperthermia in patients with other myopathies, most notably central core disease (a congenital myopathy) and Duchenne muscular dystrophy. Patients with myotonic dystrophy occasionally experience transient rigidity after the administration of succinylcholine but the mechanism for this is probably different and treatment usually is not required. Safe anesthetic agents for these patients include nitrous oxide, thiopental, opiates, droperidol, and pancuronium.

Similar to, and often confused with, the polyneuropathy that develops in the context of critical illness and sepsis, critical illness myopathy (CIM) or acute quadriplegic myopathy may result in the surgical patient who has a prolonged course in the ICU. In addition to CIP, CIM should be considered when the patient "fails to wean" from the ventilator. The patient develops weakness of respiration and the extremities with retained sensation. The deep tendon reflexes may be normal or slightly reduced. In severe cases the reflexes may be absent. Important features that distinguish the myopathy (CIM) from the polyneuropathy (CIP), such as retained sensation, may be difficult to identify due to coexisting encephalopathy and mechanical ventilation, however some have proposed that CIM and CIP are interrelated and often coexistent conditions [32].

This myopathy usually occurs in critically ill patients with asthma, chronic obstructive pulmonary disease, organ transplants, the use of corticosteroids, non-depolarizing neuromuscular blocking agents, and amino-glycosides [32,41,42]. The role of medications in CIM is unclear given there are prospective trials that show these agents as independent risk factors and others that find no association. In one trial, there is even suggestion that steroids might even be protective. Currently there is no consensus regarding the extent that these agents contribute to the pathogenesis of CIM. Similar to CIP, CIM likely results from a multifactorial process that includes a combination of pro-inflammatory cytokines in sepsis and metabolic alterations [32]. Additionally, immunological

denervation of muscle and the patient's immobilization due to the critical illness likely contribute [43].

In ideal situations nerve conduction studies reveal low amplitude motor nerve responses with normal sensory nerve responses in patients with CIM. Electromyography may reveal acute denervation potentials and myopathic motor unit potentials with early recruitment. Some investigators convincingly showed that electrical inexcitability of muscle tissue occurs in acute quadriplegic myopathy [44,45]. Steroids and humeral changes that occur during sepsis are theorized to result in the changes in the electrical properties of neural tissue. Overall, the prognosis for the return of neurologic function is good if the concurrent medical illness resolves. Specific treatment for CIM is also largely supportive. Mechanical ventilation, physical therapy, and protection of common sites of nerve compression should be performed as needed.

References

1. Johns TR, Howard JF, eds. Myasthenia gravis. *Semin Neurol* 1982; **2**: 193–280.

2. Phillips LH, Melnick PA. Diagnosis of myasthenia gravis in the 1990s. *Semin Neurol* 1990; **10**: 62–9.

3. Somnier FE. Clinical implementation of anti-acetylcholine receptor antibodies. *J Neurol Neurosurg Psychiatry* 1993; **56**: 496–504.

4. Finley JC, Pascuzzi RM. Rational therapy of myasthenia gravis. *Semin Neurol* 1990; **10**: 70–82.

5. Bromberg MB, Wald JJ, Forshew DA, Feldman EL, Albers JW. Randomized trial of azathioprine or prednisone for initial immunosuppressive treatment of myasthenia gravis. *J Neurol Sci* 1997; **150**: 59–62.

6. Myasthenia Gravis Clinical Study Group. A randomized clinical trial comparing prednisone and azathioprine in myasthenia gravis. Results of the second interim analysis. *J Neurol Neurosurg Psychiatry* 1993; **56**: 1157–63.

7. Tindall RS, Phillips JT, Rollins JA, Wells L, Hall K. A clinical therapeutic trial of cyclosporine in myasthenia gravis. *Ann NY Acad Sci* 1993; **681**: 539–51.

8. Tindall RS, Rollins JA, Phillips JT, Greenlee RG, Wells L, Belendiuk G. Preliminary results of a double-blind, randomized, placebo-controlled trial of cyclosporine in myasthenia gravis. *N Engl J Med* 1987; **316**: 719–24.

9. Hauser RA, Malek AR, Rosen R. Successful treatment of a patient with severe refractory myasthenia gravis using mycophenolate mofetil. *Neurology* 1998; **51**: 912–13.

10. Ciafoloni E, Massey JM, Tucker-Lipscomb B, Sanders DB. Mycophenolate mofetil for myasthenia gravis: an open-label pilot study. *Neurology* 2001; **56**: 97–9.

11. Gronseth GS, Barohn RJ. Practice parameter: thymectomy for autoimmune myasthenia gravis (an evidence-based review). *Neurology* 2000; **55**: 7–15.

12. Arsura EL, Bick A, Brunuer NC et al. High-dose intravenous immunoglobulin in the management of myasthenia gravis. *Arch Intern Med* 1986; **146**: 1365–8.

13. De Boer HD, van Egmond J, Driessen JJ, Booij LH. Sugammadex in patients with myasthenia gravis. *Anaesthesia* 2010; **65**: 653.

14. Wittbrodt ET. Drugs and myasthenia gravis: an update. *Arch Intern Med* 1997; **157**: 399–408.

15. Howard JF. Adverse drug effects on neuromuscular transmission. *Semin Neurol* 1990; **10**: 89–102.

16. Krendel D. Hypermagnesemia and neuromuscular transmission. *Semin Neurol* 1990; **10**: 42–5.

17. Pascuzzi RM, Kim YI. Lambert–Eaton syndrome. *Semin Neurol* 1990; **10**: 35–41.

18. Murray MJ, Cowen J, De Block H et al. Clinical practice guidelines for sustained neuromuscular blockade in the adult critically ill patient. *Crit Care Med* 2002; **30**: 142–56.

19. Upton RM, McComas AJ. The double crush in nerve entrapment syndromes. *Lancet* 1973; **11**: 359–62.

20. Stewart JD, ed. The radial nerve. In *Focal Peripheral Neuropathies*. New York, NY: Elsevier Science Publishing; 1987, pp. 194–210.

21. Stewart JD, ed. The ulnar nerve. In *Focal Peripheral Neuropathies*. New York, NY: Elsevier Science Publishing; 1987, pp. 163–93.

22. Stewart JD, ed. The common peroneal nerve. In *Focal Peripheral Neuropathies*. New York, NY: Elsevier Science Publishing; 1987, pp. 290–306.

23. Warner MA, Warner DO, Harper CM, Schroeder DR, Maxson PM. Lower extremity neuropathies associated with lithotomy positions. *Anesthesiology* 2000; **93**: 938–42.

24. Sharma AD, Parmley CL, Sreeram G, Grocott HP. Peripheral nerve injures during cardiac surgery: risk factors, diagnosis, prognosis and prevention. *Anesth Analg* 2000; **91**: 1358–69.

25. Stewart JD. The femoral and saphenous nerves. In *Focal Peripheral Neuropathies*. New York, NY: Elsevier Science Publishing; 1987, pp. 322–32.

26. Hughes RAC, ed. Epidemiology. In *Guillain–Barré Syndrome*. London: Springer-Verlag; 1990, pp. 101–19.

27. Arnason BG, Asbury AK. Idiopathic polyneuritis after surgery. *Arch Neurol* 1968; **18**: 500–7.

28. Guillain–Barré Syndrome Study Group. Plasmapheresis and acute Guillain–Barré syndrome. *Neurology* 1985; **35**: 1096–104.

29. Van der Meché FGA, Schmitz PIM. A randomized trial comparing intravenous immune globulin and plasma exchange in Guillain-Barré syndrome. *N Engl J Med* 1992; **326**: 1123–9.

30. Hughes RA, Swan AV, van Doorn PA. Intravenous immunoglobulin for Guillain- Barré syndrome. *Cochrane Database Syst Rev*. 2010; **6**: CD002063.

31. Plasma Exchange/Sandoglobulin Guillain–Barré Syndrome Trial Group. Randomized trial of plasma exchange, intravenous immunoglobulin, and combined treatments in Guillain–Barré Syndrome. *Lancet* 1997; **349**: 225–30.

32. Hermans G, De Jonghe B, Bruyninckx F, Van den Berghe G. Clinical review: critical illness polyneuropathy and myopathy. *Crit Care* 2008; **12**: 238–46.

33. Bolton CF. Electrophysiologic studies of critically ill patients. *Muscle Nerve* 1987; **10**: 129–35.

34. Bolton CF, Gilbert JJ, Hahn AF, Sibbald WJ. Polyneuropathy in critically ill patients. *J Neurol Neurosurg Psychiatry* 1984; **47**: 1223–31.

35. Bolton CF, Laverty DA, Brown JD *et al.* Critically ill polyneuropathy: electrophysiological studies and differentiation form Guillain-Barré syndrome. *J Neurol Neurosurg Psychiatry* 1986; **49**: 563–73.

36. Witt NJ, Zochodne DW, Bolton CF *et al.* Peripheral nerve function in sepsis and multiple organ failure. *Chest* 1991; **99**: 176–84.

37. Rubin DI. Neuralgic amyotrophy: clinical features and diagnostic evaluation. *Neurologist* 2001; **7**: 350–6.

38. Gromert GA. Malignant hyperthermia. In Engel AC, Bank BQ, eds. *Myology*. New York, NY: McGraw-Hill; 1986, pp. 1763–84.

39. Baraka AS, Jalbout ML. Anesthesia and myopathy. *Curr Opin Anaesthesiol* 2002; **15**: 371–6.

40. Hogan K. The anesthetic myopathies and malignant hyperthermias. *Curr Opin Neurol* 1998; **11**: 469–76.

41. MacFarlane IA, Rosenthal FD. Severe myopathy after status asthmaticus. *Lancet* 1977; **2**: 615.

42. Latronico N, Fenzi F, Recupero D *et al.* Critical illness myopathy and neuropathy. *Lancet* 1996; **347**: 1570–82.

43. Hund E. Myopathy in critically ill. *Crit Care Med* 1999; **27**: 2544–7.

44. Rich MM, Bird SJ, Raps EC, McCluskey LF, Teener JW. Direct muscle stimulation in acute quadriplegic myopathy. *Muscle Nerve* 1997; **20**: 665–73.

45. Trojaborg W, Weimer LH, Hays AP. Electrophysiologic studies in critical illness associated weakness: myopathy or neuropathy – a reappraisal. *Clin Neurophysiol* 2001; **112**: 1586–93.

Chapter

38 Perioperative management of patients with Parkinson's disease

Christine D. Esper and Jorge L. Juncos

Introduction and overview of Parkinson's disease

Patients with Parkinson's disease (PD) face surgery more often than their age-matched counterparts due in large part to orthopedic and other injuries provoked by the gait and balance difficulties in advanced stages of the illness. General surgical procedures are at least as common in PD as in their age-matched counterparts, but the perioperative management can be complicated given the nature of the illness and its treatments. Recent advances in neurosurgical techniques and an improved understanding of the pathophysiology of motor symptoms in PD has led to a renewed interest and an increase in the number of patients undergoing various neurosurgical procedures for PD. This chapter provides an overview of the principles and preoperative management of patients with PD and other Parkinsonian states.

Parkinson's disease is an adult-onset neurodegenerative disorder characterized by progressive slowness of movement (bradykinesia), muscular rigidity, stooped posture, tremor, postural instability, and varying degrees of cognitive impairment. It affects close to 1 million Americans, with an annual incidence of 20 new cases per 10,000 and a prevalence of 59–187 cases per 100,000 [1–3]. The median age of onset is 60 years and the mean duration of the disease from diagnosis to death is 15 years [4]. Its pathology is concentrated in the brain and consists of selective degeneration of the nigrostriatal dopaminergic pathway and the presence of alpha synuclein pathology including Lewy bodies and Lewy neurites in surviving mesencephalic dopamine neurons, as well as in other brainstem and cortical neurons [5]. Biochemically, the denervation results in striatal dopamine depletion which is linked to the above signs and symptoms [6]. The cause of selective neuronal death, and therefore the etiology of PD is unknown, although hereditary and environmental factors are thought to play a role.

In the past few decades however, it has become clear that the pathology of PD is not limited to the brain. Investigators have demonstrated alpha synuclein and Lewy body pathology in the Meissner and Auerbach plexuses, and in other autonomic fibers that regulate sudomotor responses, salivation, upper and lower gastrointestinal (GI) motility, bladder emptying, and sexual function [7,8]. Associated symptoms are seborrhea, sialorrhea, constipation and impaired bladder emptying, and sexual dysfunction. The same pathology has recently been demonstrated in the cardiac sympathetic system and may contribute to the sensitivity of these patients to postural symptoms and other cardiac symptoms [9].

Given the motor symptoms of PD, it is not surprising that they can interfere in the operative and perioperative management of PD. Tremor can make the electrocardiographic or electroencephalographic monitoring of patients difficult in the awake patient (e.g., regional or spinal anesthesia; stereotactic neurosurgery). General anesthesia will instead suppress tremor. The rigidity of PD can involve the chest wall limiting ventilatory reserve, thereby increasing the risk of hypoventilation and atelectasis during the postoperative period. Although swallowing is usually not affected in the early stages of PD, acute dysphagia can result from abrupt withdrawal of antiparkinsonian medications during the perioperative period. Vasomotor instability and autonomic dysfunction affects many patients with PD. For instance, asymptomatic orthostatic hypotension can become clinically significant under the influence of anesthetics, analgesics, and benzodiazepines, a situation compounded by any unanticipated delay in resuming antiparkinsonian medications after surgery. Other autonomic defects include urinary hesitancy, severe constipation and paroxysmal autonomic discharges with profuse sweating and flushing. Postoperatively these defects can lead to urinary retention, obstipation, ileus, and dehydration.

Parkinsonian symptoms with more severe forms of autonomic failure suggest an atypical Parkinsonian disorder such as multiple systems atrophy (MSA), also known as Shy–Drager syndrome [10]. These patients typically have a history of symptomatic orthostatic syncope [11], are at higher risk of complications, and require special preoperative planning.

Cognitive slowing can parallel the slowing of motor function and make patients with PD particularly sensitive to psychoactive drugs and anesthesia, leading to postoperative confusion and hallucinations. This risk is particularly high in patients with PD and dementia, and dementia can affect up to 80% of patients with advanced PD [12]. The severity of dementia in PD is highly variable. Nonetheless, even mildly demented patients have a significantly increased risk of postoperative delirium. The most common forms of dementia in PD are due to coexisting senile dementia of the Alzheimer type (SDAT), dementia with Lewy bodies, and a combination of both. In addition, up to 50% of patients with PD have comorbid affective illnesses including cyclothymia, major depression, and anxiety disorders with panic [13]. Unrecognized active symptomatology in these domains can impair cognition and increase the risk of perioperative complications in PD.

Symptomatic treatment of PD aims to re-establish dopamine transmission in the striatum. This strategy involves: (a) enhancing the cerebral availability of levodopa, the precursor amino acid of dopamine, (b) using direct dopamine agonists (ropinirole, pramipexole, apomorphine) to stimulate postsynaptic dopamine receptors directly, (c) blocking the peripheral breakdown of levodopa by the enzyme catechol-O-methyltransferase (COMT) using COMT inhibitors like entacapone or tolcapone, and (d) blocking the oxidative breakdown of dopamine at the synapse with the selective monoamine oxidase B (MAO-B) inhibitor selegiline and rasagiline. Adjunctive therapy includes anticholinergic drugs like trihexyphenidyl and benztropine, and amantadine, a weak glutamate (N-methyl-D-aspartate or NMDA) receptor antagonist with anticholinergic properties. These drugs are more likely to contribute to postoperative confusion and delirium in the elderly. Abrupt discontinuation of antiparkinsonian medications in preparation for surgery can also lead to acute confusion. This reaction is more likely with higher doses of antiparkinsonian drugs and appears to be a dose-dependent phenomenon.

Drug-induced increases in Parkinsonian signs and symptoms are not uncommon. This can be due to either antiparkinsonian drugs or Parkinson-promoting drugs such as antipsychotics or other medications. Transient aggravation of symptoms is typified by motor fluctuations that result from the interaction between disease progression and the chronic use and schedule of antiparkinsonian therapy. Motor fluctuations range from the premature or sudden termination of drug effects ("off spells"), to an excessive and aberrant sensitivity to therapy (i.e., "denervation hypersensitivity") that lead to dyskinesias and dystonias ("on" symptomatology). The fluctuations are mediated in part by the progressive loss of dopamine nerve end terminals that destroys the ability of the striatum to buffer fluxes in dopamine availability. In PD, the cerebral availability of dopamine is subject to fluctuations in plasma levodopa levels. These in turn reflect levodopa's short half-life (about 2 hours when given with carbidopa) and its intermittent oral administration. Because levodopa is absorbed primarily in the proximal small intestine, its availability is also subject to the vagaries of gastric emptying, a function of a myriad of other factors including the timing, quantity, and composition of meals.

Antiparkinsonian drug therapy may also involve affective and cognitive functions. These include visual hallucinations, compulsive behavior, sleep disturbances (insomnia and hypersomnia), sleep phenomena such as vivid dreams (rapid eye movement-related behavioral disturbances such as screaming and punching during sleep) and nocturnal myoclonus (leg jerking) [14–16]. It is important to recognize these early signs because their presence suggests a lower threshold for post-anesthetic delirium. In a delirious PD patient, motor symptoms may not respond as well to drug therapy, and increasing drug therapy may only aggravate the delirium.

Preoperative management
General medical considerations

The preoperative medical evaluation of patients with PD, regardless of age, is not unlike that of other elderly patients. Areas that require special attention in PD are outlined below.

In PD mild pharyngeal dysfunction leads to decreased spontaneous swallowing, accumulation of saliva in the posterior pharynx, and sialorrhea. This may worsen acutely with sedation and result in aspiration during the postoperative period. To avoid this, frequent and extended suctioning is needed. In addition, pharyngeal dysfunction may predispose PD patients to severe laryngospasm if all antiparkinsonian therapy is removed abruptly, and the staff should be prepared to provide the extra care necessary. Antiparkinsonian therapy should be resumed as soon as possible after surgery.

Pulmonary status also needs special attention since pulmonary function tests often reveal restrictive pulmonary deficits in PD patients, even if asymptomatic. These abnormalities are partially relieved by levodopa therapy. Their restrictive qualities are due to postural abnormalities (stooping, scoliosis), rigidity of the chest wall musculature, and the advanced spinal osteoarthritis often associated with the illness. If asymptomatic, the patient does not need more than a routine preoperative evaluation consisting of a good history, chest exam, and roentgenogram. If the pulmonary reserve is in doubt, abbreviated pulmonary function tests with arterial blood gases should be considered. In addition, PD patients often do poorly if they develop pneumonia. This is due to easy fatigability, decreased respiratory capacity, and a weak cough reflex [17–19].

As noted above, the possibility of autonomic insufficiency is a particular concern in PD. Even in the absence of overt autonomic failure, patients can have some autonomic instability and special sensitivity to drugs that may cause hypotension, including antiparkinsonian drugs [20]. Constipation is a universal problem and is taken for granted by many patients [21]. Many have a tendency to delay evacuation and rely on suppositories and enemas to do so. Constipation may be a source of abdominal distension, ileus, or obstruction. Distension of the rectosigmoid may be a source of urinary retention, subsequently leading to a urinary tract infection. These problems need to be detected before surgery as they can be compounded by both anesthesia and postoperative opiate analgesic agents.

Neurologic considerations

Parkinson's disease is the most common of a host of neurologic illnesses that look like, but are not idiopathic PD. These disorders present special management problems that need to be anticipated. Perhaps the two most important disorders to differentiate from PD are multiple systems atrophy and progressive supranuclear palsy (PSP). Like PD, they are both progressive neurodegenerative disorders of unknown etiology in which slowness, rigidity, and gait impairment are prominent. In contrast to PD, tremor is often absent, the course is more rapid, and the response to therapy is poor. Multiple systems atrophy features prominent autonomic failure that may influence the surgical decision and strategy of anesthesia. Signs of autonomic failure include impotence, unexplained urinary dysfunction, postural hypotension, abnormal conduction or repolarization on electrocardiography and impaired sweating [11].

Progressive supranuclear palsy features loss of supranuclear gaze control (e.g., decreased vertical and later horizontal gaze) described by patients as "trouble reading" not related to a refraction error. Patients note trouble walking downstairs (failure of down gaze), and when advanced, difficulty looking for items on a table. In addition, patients develop axial dystonia out of proportion to the appendicular rigidity that is the opposite of what is normally encountered in PD [22,23]. Rigidity of the neck may make endotracheal intubation difficult and does not respond well to the usual perioperative muscle relaxants. Patients with MSA and PSP may be more prone to sleep apnea and other respiratory abnormalities than PD patients, making them more sensitive to sedatives and hypnotics. This diagnostic outline is meant to raise an index of suspicion for MSA and PSP when evaluating preoperative Parkinsonian patients. Appropriate neurologic consultation should be sought when these entities are suspected. Of note, the combination of decreased blink rate typical of PSP and MSA and prolonged post-anesthesia unconsciousness can lead to corneal abrasions.

Cervical spondylosis is not infrequent in PD, in part due to the affected age group and the accelerated osteoarthritic changes that stem from axial akinesia and postural abnormalities (e.g., anterocollis). Clinically significant cervical spondylosis may be adversely affected by a difficult intubation. Although not a contraindication to intubation, it may influence the route (nasotracheal versus oral) and preparation. Clinical signs of cervical spondylosis include neck and shoulder pain, pain radiating down the arms, leg and gait spasticity, hyperactive reflexes in the legs, brisk to patchy reflexes in the arms and extensor plantar responses. Of note, in both cervical spondylosis and MSA or PSP, these findings can be due to involvement of the corticospinal track. Involvement of the corticobulbar track can lead to pseudobulbar palsy, which increases the risk of aspiration.

The presence of dementia significantly increases the risk of perioperative confusion and delirium. Dementia is found in approximately 15–20% of patients with PD and remains undetected in its early stages. The Mini Mental State Examination (MMSE) and the Montreal Cognitive Assessment battery are simple, expeditious albeit relatively insensitive tools used to screen for dementia [24]. Early on, a history of ill-defined occupational, personal, and financial difficulties, loss of interest in hobbies, vague memory complaints, and personality changes may be a more sensitive indicator of dementia in all Parkinsonian states than the MMSE. Pseudodementia due to depression is probably a more common cause of these complaints than dementia of the Alzheimer type. Depression affects > 40% of patients with PD at some point in the illness and is usually accompanied by vegetative signs such as poor sleep and appetite, weight loss, apathy, and asthenia.

Pharmacotherapeutic issues

Drug interactions which may have been tolerated preoperatively may become critical postoperatively and thus need to be anticipated during the preoperative evaluation. The following is a brief review of Parkinsonian drug therapy and how it may need to be altered perioperatively. Table 38.1 lists commonly prescribed drugs which may aggravate Parkinsonian signs and which should be avoided in Parkinsonian patients.

The mainstay therapy of PD is still levodopa. It is administered in the form of carbidopa/levodopa to minimize the incidence of peripheral side-effects such as nausea and hypotension. Carbidopa is a peripheral dopa decarboxylase inhibitor that blocks the conversion of levodopa to dopamine. Peripheral conversion of levodopa to dopamine is believed to be responsible for many of levodopa's GI and cardiovascular side-effects. To effectively block peripheral dopa decarboxylase, doses of carbidopa should be 75 mg/day; that is, three tablets of carbidopa/levodopa (25/100) or two tablets of controlled release carbidopa/levodopa (50/200) (Sinemet CR). Dopamine agonists are not as effective at alleviating symptoms, particularly when used as monotherapy (e.g., ropinirole, pramipexole). As noted above, they may be more difficult to use in the immediate perioperative period. Patients on low-dose dopamine agonists prior to surgery who experience postoperative hypotension can be managed on just levodopa for short periods of time. Patients on a high dose of dopamine agonists may experience withdrawal reactions when these doses are abruptly interrupted. This withdrawal reaction may lead to further cardiovascular instability and an acute worsening of Parkinsonian motor and non-motor symptoms. Reintroduction of at least a fraction (e.g., 50% of the original dose) should be considered whenever possible so long as the general medical condition of the patient allows.

The hypotensive effect of levodopa is probably due to a central mechanism and may be more pronounced in patients with high baseline blood pressures. The hypotensive effect of dopamine agonists is caused by several mechanisms:

Table 38.1 Drugs to be used with caution in Parkinson's disease.

Drug category	Generic name
Dopamine antagonists	Haloperidol
Typical antipsychotics	Perphenazine Chlorpromazine Triflouperazine Flufenazine Thiothixene Thioridazine Loxapine
Atypical antipsychotics (can be used with caution)	Risperidone Olanzapine Ziprasidone Quetiapine Aripiprazole
Anti-emetics	Compazine Metoclopramide Thiethylperazine Droperidol
Antidepressants	Combinations of perphenazine and amitriptyline (Triavil™, Etrafon™) Phenelzine (MAO inhibitor) Tranylcypromine (MAO inhibitor)
Narcotics	Meperidine Fentanyl
Antihypertensives and miscellaneous postoperative medications	Reserpine Tetrabenazine Alpha methylparatyrosine Rauwolfia serpentina Rauverid Wolfina Deserpine Rescinnamine Rauwiloid
Drugs with low potential to aggravate symptoms	Alpha-methyldopa Phenytoin Lithium carbonate Buspirone

MAO, monoamine oxidase.

(a) relaxation of vascular smooth muscle in splanchnic and renal circulation, (b) inhibition of noradrenergic nerve endings, and (c) central inhibition of sympathetic activity. Dopamine agonists have a higher incidence of severe hypotension and other side-effects than levodopa. Accordingly, and unlike levodopa, administration of dopamine agonists can be halted the night prior to surgery and resumed as soon as the patient is hemodynamically stable.

As noted, levodopa and dopamine agonists can also precipitate cardiac arrhythmias and delirium. When used in chronic, stable doses and stopped before surgery, these complications tend to be minor and manageable and do not require routine discontinuation of the drugs. If concerns over perioperative hypovolemia exist, dopamine agonists should be reduced over 2–3 weeks before considering reductions in the levodopa dose. If the baseline dose of levodopa is high (e.g., > 800 mg/day), it too may be decreased slowly to approximately 300–400 mg/day. This should be attempted only if the risks of hypovolemia outweigh the postoperative discomfort the patient is likely to experience as a consequence of increased symptoms.

Ancillary antiparkinsonian therapy such as anticholinergics and amantadine may increase the risk of postoperative delirium but should not be stopped abruptly or withheld for extended periods. Abrupt withdrawal of these and other antiparkinsonian medications may result in acute exacerbation and relative unresponsiveness of Parkinsonian symptoms. If the individual is not demented nor exhibits signs of drug-induced delirium, the likelihood of this complication is small and the drugs need not be changed. If dementia or delirium is suspected, these drugs should be tapered or stopped over 2–4 weeks.

Special consideration should be given to the use of selegiline, an MAO-B inhibitor devoid of the hypertensive reactions to tyramine and other amino acids characteristic of non-selective MAO-A or MAO-AB inhibitors (see Table 38.1). Selegiline is used to enhance the efficacy of levodopa but it can also accentuate its side-effects. Because of its long biologic half-life, it can be discontinued without tapering. The concomitant use of meperidine and selegiline should be avoided due to potentially serious adverse reactions (delirium). Based on studies in laboratory animals, selegiline should also be avoided in patients with active peptic ulcer disease. Rasagiline, a more recent MAO-B inhibitor, should be discontinued at least 14 days before an elective surgery that requires anesthesia. The use of selective MAO-B inhibitors in PD can lead to unpredictable cardiovascular interactions with anesthetics and analgesics, mainly hypotension and arrhythmias [25].

Non-selective MAO inhibitors should also be discontinued at least 2 weeks before surgery. Selegiline probably does not need to be stopped preoperatively for the reasons mentioned above. Nonetheless, as a general precaution we recommend stopping selegiline 1 week prior to surgery to minimize the risk of perioperative drug interactions. The symptomatic effect of selegiline on PD symptoms is rather modest compared with that of levodopa and dopamine agonists, thus stopping the drugs over a few days generally does not result in serious motor deterioration.

Given the high incidence of depression in PD, it is not unusual for these patients to be treated with antidepressants. The use of non-selective MAO inhibitors in combination with the selective serotonin reuptake inhibitor (SSRI), fluoxetine, can lead to acute "serotonergic" reactions characterized by delirium, rigidity, and fever [25,26]. Severe symptoms include tachycardia, hypertension, and hyperthermia that can lead to shock. Hyperthermia can also lead to rhabdomyolysis, metabolic acidosis, seizure, renal failure, and disseminated intravascular coagulation [27]. Although these reactions are far less likely with the use of selegiline and rasagiline, it is important to keep them in mind, particularly when patients are likely to be exposed to anesthetics and analgesics during and following surgery [28]. In addition, the use of fluoxetine in PD may aggravate Parkinsonian symptoms, and in combination with selegiline, may lead to acute mania.

One should also avoid the discontinuation of these drugs during the perioperative period. Precipitous elimination of SSRIs and norepinephrine-serotonin reuptake inhibitors (NSRIs) can lead to a "serotonin discontinuation syndrome" characterized by dizziness, electric shock-like sensations, sweating, nausea, insomnia, tremor, confusion, nightmares, and vertigo [29]. Careful tapering of the drug and prompt resumption can avoid this potentially serious complication postoperatively.

In the case of prolonged cerebral stereotactic procedures performed with the patient awake, small doses of carbidopa/levodopa sublingually (Parcopa®) may be needed to maintain patient comfort. Treating the symptoms may limit neurological testing during micro-electrode recordings however.

Anesthesia management

The specific choice of anesthetics is made by the anesthesiologist in consultation with the treating neurologist. The choice of general over regional anesthesia should be determined by the usual considerations. When appropriate, local or regional anesthesia is preferred over general anesthesia because the first two provide less control of Parkinsonian or drug-induced hypoventilation than the latter. Neuroleptanesthesia is not recommended due to the use of agents (e.g., droperidol) that antagonize dopamine transmission in the brain and elsewhere. Experience has shown that the potential arrhythmogenic and myocardial depressant effects of chronic dopamine-induced depletion of myocardial catecholamines is rather small. In brief, the anesthetic strategy should maintain a balance between inadequate anesthesia with its accompanying autonomic nervous system stimulation, and a needlessly deep anesthesia with its concomitant cardiopulmonary depressant effects.

Good anesthetic control of PD patients has been reported using thiopental or diazepam induction followed by enflurane and nitrous oxide for anesthesia/analgesia. Hyman *et al.* reported a favorable experience using nitrous oxide and sufentanil infusion anesthesia and vencuronium for muscle relaxation in patients undergoing autologous transplantation of adrenal medulla to brain [30]. Fentanyl analgesia should be used with caution since it can increase muscle tone, a problem already present in PD patients. General precautions such as anticipating tachycardias in response to pancuronium or hypotension in response to d-tubocurarine are particularly important in patients with PD. Intraoperatively, the appearance of a fine body tremor may be misinterpreted as ventricular fibrillation on the cardiac monitor since the typical Parkinsonian tremor may be absent from the limbs.

Intra- and perioperative nasogastric suction may help reduce the risks and consequences of nausea and vomiting, particularly in PD patients where most anti-emetics are contraindicated. Following surgery competitive muscle relaxants must be fully reversed to avoid compromising ventilatory function. Anti-emetics that may be better tolerated include domperidone (limited availability in the USA), tribemethobenzamide, and serotonin 5-HT$_1$ receptor antagonists such as ondasetron and granisetron.

Postoperative management
General medical considerations

The postoperative care of PD patients is much like that of other elderly patients. Special emphasis should be placed on airway protection, chest physiotherapy with incentive spirometry and postural drainage, early mobilization, and avoiding aspiration [31]. Patients with PD may require more time to wake up from anesthesia but should be awake by the evening of the day of surgery. Surgical and post-surgical complications such as pain, infection, and blood loss can lead to a protracted, poor response to antiparkinsonian medication. This poor response is also seen in ambulatory patients with mild medical problems such as urinary tract infections. The mechanisms in both cases are unknown but attempts to fine-tune symptoms at this time are futile and ill-advised. Patients generally recuperate on their own within days to weeks after surgery without a change in medication.

Postoperative psychosis can develop upon awakening from anesthesia or the onset can be delayed as long as 5–7 days, with many patients exhibiting the first signs after returning home. Immediate postoperative delirium may be caused by the intraoperative use of atropine, acute metabolic derangement, or the withdrawal reactions previously described. Delayed onset delirium does not appear to be related to a particular anesthetic or to the choice of anti-parkinsonian drug therapy and usually clears spontaneously within 3 days.

Parkinsonian motor symptoms, including so-called "off" spells, can be severely debilitating following surgery. Although the symptoms can mimic other postoperative problems, they should not be assumed to be due to parkinsonism until medical and surgical postoperative complications have been ruled out. "Off" symptoms include profound feelings of "weakness," shortness of breath (air hunger), urinary retention, anxiety, and intense tremor. These "adrenergically charged" reactions, if persistent, can be arrhythmogenic. "On" spells consist of abnormal involuntary movements and muscle contractions termed dyskinesias and dystonias. The latter can be particularly painful.

Constipation that should have been dealt with aggressively preoperatively, needs to be managed gingerly postoperatively when vital signs may be unstable. Aggressive treatment of constipation postoperatively with enemas or disimpaction can elicit vagal reflexes with concomitant bradycardia and hypotension. Some articles elaborate on specific interventions that address these and other important nursing issues [32,33].

Postoperative dysphagia or unconsciousness may make oral antiparkinsonian therapy impractical or nearly impossible. With excellent nursing care, patients with mild to moderate PD who were on small doses of medication can probably remain unmedicated for a week or longer if necessary. If unmedicated much longer, patients lose the long duration response to levodopa and may reach levels of disability that may compromise their respiratory function and overall recovery. If the gastrointestinal tract is functional, levodopa can be given directly into the duodenum using a levodopa/carbidopa solution fed through a silastic tube with a weighted mercury tip. This technique is discussed under pharmacologic management below. In patients with a functional gastrointestinal tract, with advanced disease and who require high doses of medication, enteral administration of liquid carbidopa/levodopa should be started as soon as possible after surgery.

Dopamine withdrawal syndrome

Sudden withdrawal of all antiparkinsonian therapy in PD can lead to a dopamine withdrawal syndrome that clinically resembles the better known neuroleptic malignant syndrome (NMS). The onset of this potentially fatal syndrome is usually 24–72 hours following abrupt withdrawal of a dopaminomimetic drug. It is thought to be mediated by acute cerebral dopamine depletion. In contrast, NMS has been linked to an aberrant and acute antagonism (blockage) of cerebral dopamine receptors for which there may be individual (genetic?) predisposition. Fully developed, it is characterized by alterations in mental status (delirium to coma), hyperpyrexia, autonomic instability, muscular rigidity, acidosis, rhabdomyolysis, and renal failure. Prompt resumption of antiparkinsonian therapy is critical [34,35]. Other therapeutic measures are discussed below under pharmacologic management. The differential diagnosis includes malignant hyperthermia from exposure to anesthetics, sepsis, exposure to anti-emetics and drugs used to alleviate gastric paresis (metoclopramide), tricyclic antidepressants with lithium, stimulants (cocaine, amphetamines), and some anticonvulsants.

Pharmacologic management

Liquid levodopa was mentioned above and has been used in numerous patients with PD to treat motor fluctuations. It has been administered either by constant enteral infusion or by intermittent oral bolus. Postoperative PD patients may also benefit from these delivery strategies when intubated or unconscious. The solution can be prepared by pulverizing and dissolving 10 tablets of regular carbidopa/levodopa 10/100 in 1,000 mL of tap water with 1g of ascorbic acid to yield a 1 mg/mL solution of levodopa. Depending on how well the tablet is pulverized, the solution may need to be filtered (using a regular coffee filter) to remove particulate matter.

The solution is stable for at least 24 hours when refrigerated and protected from light. Levodopa is relatively insoluble in a basic medium and will not dissolve at concentration > 2 mg/mL. Ascorbic acid serves to acidify the solution and prevent the oxidation of levodopa and dopamine. Carbidopa is much less soluble than levodopa but apparently enough gets into solution to block nausea and vomiting. Dosing guidelines can be extrapolated from the following example: if the patient uses 100 mg of levodopa every 4 hours, the infusion rate can start at 25 mL/hour and then be adjusted according to the clinical response.

Postoperative patients with a non-functional gastrointestinal tract have few options to treat PD symptoms. Repeated parenteral injection of anticholinergics such as benztropine has been advocated, but their use can lead to a slower recovery of gastrointestinal function, and in the elderly, to delirium. Subcutaneous injections and infusion of a soluble dopamine agonist called apomorphine can be used for this purpose. Of note, its use is limited by the need to orally administer a peripheral dopamine blocker to control the side-effect of nausea [36,37]. Domperidone is the anti-emetic of choice for this purpose. It is a peripheral dopamine blocker which improves gastric emptying. Although it is used routinely in Canada, it has not been approved by the FDA in the USA.

The management of postoperative emesis presents another dilemma in PD patients. In mild cases, nasogastric suctioning and small doses of benadryl or benzodiazepines (weak antiemetics) may work at the expense of sedating the patient [38]. Conventional anti-emetics may aggravate Parkinsonism by virtue of their dopamine antagonisms. Other limiting side-effects include sedation, dysphoria, and hallucinations. In patients with mild PD where nasogastric suctioning fails, and who are not psychotic, the short-term use of these agents in low doses may be tolerated with only modest aggravation of parkinsonian signs. In this case we favor the cautious use of metoclopramide before compazine or droperidol. Patients with advanced disease, or with marked dystonic clinical features may not tolerate even small doses of these agents.

Nausea and vomiting in levodopa-treated patients is thought to be mediated by the stimulation of dopamine receptors in the area postrema of the brainstem. In contrast, perioperative emesis is multifactorial. Ondansetron, a selective 5-HT$_3$ serotonin receptor blocker, is effective in the treatment of perioperative nausea and vomiting in non-parkinsonian patients. Although ondansetron does not block dopamine receptors, it may be effective in treating postoperative emesis in PD through alternative mechanisms. Unlike conventional anti-emetics, ondansetron is less likely to cause extrapyramidal side-effects in PD [39]. Finally domperidone may be another promising candidate to alleviate postoperative nausea in PD without aggravating Parkinsonism.

In PD patients meperidine should be avoided as noted above.

Postoperative situations unique to PD

Transient antiparkinsonian treatment failure

Patients with PD often experience transient periods of poor response to therapy following surgery, as noted above. This phenomenon is poorly understood, but like emesis, is probably also multifactorial. Suspected causes include a lingering depressant effect of general anesthetics and analgesics, and a slowing of gastric emptying which results in delayed and incomplete levodopa absorption. It seems that the stress of anesthesia makes the clinical heterogeneity of the illness more apparent. Patients with Parkinson-like disorders (i.e., MSA, PSP, PD/DAT) tend to do less well than patients with idiopathic PD. Other than good medical care and reassurance, no other specific neurologic measures need to be taken since the patients generally return to baseline within 1–2 months. A few complain that they never return to their preoperative level of Parkinsonian function, an unexplained situation that may be due to unmasking of disease progression.

Postoperative delirium

Delirium is a major concern in the postoperative care of PD patients and the elderly in general. As noted above, antiparkinsonian drugs may act synergistically with the various anesthetics and analgesics to promote a protracted alteration in mental status. The use of intraoperative atropine is another source of delirium. In some patients the delirium is manifested mainly by confusion and hallucinosis without significant agitation. In these cases, observation and supportive care by staff and family may be sufficient. Polypharmacy, particularly antiparkinsonian polypharmacy, should be avoided or simplified using the above guidelines. Although levodopa therapy should not be withdrawn entirely, ancillary therapy such as anticholinergics, amantadine, and selegiline can be withdrawn as the situation warrants. If additional intervention is necessary, dopamine agonists can also be reduced or withdrawn over a few days while remaining vigilant for signs of the dopamine withdrawal syndrome.

If the above actions fail, or if patients are in danger of hurting themselves or others, quetiapine, an atypical antipsychotic with minimal extrapyramidal side-effects, should be considered. If treatment with quetiapine is unsuccessful, another option is clozapine, a second-generation antipsychotic [40]. This is not used as routinely as quetiapine due to the small risk of agranulocytosis. Monitoring of parameters is required, including a baseline white blood cell (WBC) count/

absolute neutrophil count (ANC), then every week thereafter for 6 months, then every 2 weeks for 6 months, then every month thereafter [41]. Other neuroleptics should be avoided as they are more likely to worsen parkinsonian signs, and can also cause a potentially irreversible side-effect known as tardive dyskinesia (TD). Lastly, psychotic PD patients respond poorly or adversely to general sedatives such as benzodiazepines and barbiturates. The onset of action of bupropion is too long (> 5 days) to be useful in an acute situation. Diphenhydramine, in doses of 12.5–25 mg repeated up to every 6 hours may be useful as a general sedative [42].

Dopamine withdrawal syndrome – management

Proper management of the dopamine withdrawal syndrome requires early recognition and transfer to a critical care unit for monitoring. Management involves aggressive cooling measures, vigorous hydration, and stabilization of the cardiovascular and renal systems. Immediate withdrawal of any dopamine antagonists (see Table 38.1 under anti-emetics) and resumption of antiparkinsonian therapy are critical. If a patient does not respond to levodopa within the first few hours, bromocriptine can be considered as it has been shown to be effective in the management of selected non-parkinsonian patients with neuroleptic malignant syndrome. In this setting, doses as high as 100 mg/day have been recommended. In a critically ill PD patient the acute introduction of more than 20–40 mg of bromocriptine cannot be advocated, however. Even at these doses patients face the potential complications of severe nausea, emesis, hypotension, and psychosis. Alternatives to consider include a muscle relaxant such as diazepam (3–5 mg by IV bolus), and dantrolene (1 mg/kg by rapid IV push repeated every 1–3 minutes as needed up to maximum of 10 mg/kg). For patients with severe peripheral vasoconstriction, nitroprusside drip has been recommended (0.5–1 mg/kg/min by constant infusion). Management also requires careful monitoring of renal function, cardiac function, rhabdomyolysis, myoglobinuria, acidosis and the continuing threat of superimposed infection.

The perioperative management of parkinsonian patients undergoing neurosurgical procedures such as stereotactic pallidotomy or deep brain stimulation therapy involves the same principles outlined above, as well as other subspecialty considerations which are beyond the scope of this chapter. For the interested reader, two references are provided that cover the overlapping topic of the perioperative and ICU management of general neurology patients [43,44].

References

1. Rajput AH. Epidemiology of Parkinson's disease. *Can J Neurol Sci* 1984; **11**(1 Suppl): 156–9.

2. Rajput AH, Stern W, Laverty WH. Chronic low-dose levodopa therapy in

Parkinson's disease: an argument for delaying levodopa therapy. *Neurology* 1984; **34**: 991–6.

3. Tanner CM. Epidemiology of Parkinson's disease. *Neurologic Clin* 1992; **10**: 317–27.

4. Lees AJ, Hardy J, Revesz T. Parkinson's disease. *Lancet* 2009; **373**(9680): 2055–66.

5. Forno LS. *Pathology of Parkinson's Disease*. London: Butterworths; 1982.

6. Hornykiewicz O, Kish SJ. Biochemical pathophysiology of Parkinson's disease. *Adv Neurol* 1987; **45**: 19–34.

7. Montastruc JL, Senard JM, Rascol O, Rascol A. Autonomic nervous system dysfunction and adrenoceptor regulation in Parkinson's disease. Clinical and pharmacological consequences. *Lab Pharmacol Med Clin* 1996; **69**: 377–81.

8. Pfeiffer RF. Gastrointestinal, urological, and sexual dysfunction in Parkinson's disease. *Mov Disord* 2010; **25** (Suppl 1): S94–7.

9. Oka T, Yamamoto H, Ohashi N *et al.* Association between epicardial adipose tissue volume and characteristics of non-calcified plaques assessed by coronary computed tomographic angiography. *Int J Cardiol* 2012; **161**: 45–9.

10. Barr A, ed. The Shy–Drager syndrome. In *Handbook of Clinical Neurology*. New York, NY: Elsevier-North Holland; 1979.

11. Esper CD, Factor SA. Current and future treatments in multiple system atrophy. *Curr Treat Options Neurol* 2007; **9**: 210–23.

12. Mayeux RY, Stern Y, Rosenstein R *et al.* An estimate of the prevalence of dementia in idiopathic Parkinson's disease. *Arch Neurol* 1988; **45**: 260–2.

13. Mayeux R, Stern Y, Rosen J, Leventhal J. Depression, intellectual impairment, and Parkinson disease. *Neurology* 1981; **31**: 645–50.

14. Cummings JL. Managing psychosis in patients with Parkinson's disease. *N Engl J Med* 1999; **340**: 801–3.

15. Dewey RB, O'Suilleabhain PE. Treatment of drug-induced psychosis with quetiapine and clozapine in Parkinson's disease. *Neurology* 2000; **55**: 1753–4.

16. Friedman JH, Factor SA. Atypical antipsychotics in the treatment of drug-induced psychosis in Parkinson's disease. *Mov Disord* 2000; **15**: 201–11.

17. Paulson GD, Tafrate RH. Some "minor" aspects of parkinsonism, especially pulmonary function. *Neurology* 1970; **20**: 14–17.

18. Mier M. Mechanisms leading to hypoventilation in extrapyramidal disorders, with special reference to Parkinson's disease. *J Am Geriatr Soc* 1976; **15**: 230–8.

19. Vincken WG, Gauthier SG, Dollfuss RE *et al.* Involvement of upper-airway muscles in extrapyramidal disorders. A cause of airflow limitation. *N Engl J Med* 1984; **311**: 438–42.

20. Irwin RP, Nutt JG, Woodward WR, Gancher ST. Pharmacodynamics of the hypotensive effect of levodopa in parkinsonian patients. *Clin Neuropharmacol* 1992; **15**: 365–74.

21. Pfeiffer RF. Gastrointestinal dysfunction in Parkinson's disease. *Parkinsonism Relat Disord* 2011; **17**: 10–15.

22. Steele JC. Progressive supranuclear palsy. *Brain* 1972; **95**: 693–704.

23. Esper CD, Weiner WJ, Factor SA. Progressive supranuclear palsy. *Rev Neurol Dis* 2007; **4**: 209–16.

24. Folstein MS, Folstein SE, McHugh PR. "Mini-mental state". A practical method for grading the state of patients for the clinician. *J Psychiatr Res* 1975; **12**: 189–98.

25. Brod TM. Fluoxetine and extrapyramidal side effects. *Am J Psychiatry* 1989; **146**: 1352–3.

26. Steur EN. Increase of Parkinson disability after fluoxetine medication. *Neurology* 1993; **43**: 211–13.

27. Sun-Edelstein C, Tepper SJ, Shapiro RE. Drug-induced serotonin syndrome: a review. *Expert Opin Drug Saf* 2008; **7**: 587–96.

28. Fernandes C, Reddy P, Kessel B. Rasagiline-induced serotonin syndrome. *Mov Disord* 2011; **26**: 766–7.

29. Narayan V, Haddad PM. Antidepressant discontinuation manic states: a critical review of the literature and suggested diagnostic criteria. *J Psychopharmacol* 2011; **25**: 306–13.

30. Hyman SA, Rogers WD, Smith DW *et al.* Perioperative management for transplant of autologous adrenal medulla to the brain for parkinsonism. *Anesthesiology* 1988; **69**: 618–22.

31. Lipowski ZJ. Delirium in the elderly patient. *N Engl J Med* 1989; **320**: 578–82.

32. Berry P, Ward-Smith PA. Adrenal medullary transplant as a treatment for Parkinson's disease: perioperative considerations. *J Neurosci Nurs* 1988; **20**: 356–61.

33. Delgado J, Billo JM. Care of the patient with Parkinson's disease: surgical and nursing interventions. *J Neurosci Nurs* 1988; **20**: 142–50.

34. Guze BH, Baxer LR Jr. Neuroleptic malignant syndrome. *N Engl J Med* 1985; **313**: 163.

35. Kaufman CA. Neuroleptic malignant syndrome. In Meltzer H, ed. *Psychopharmacology: The Third Generation of Progress.* New York, NY: Raven Press; 1987.

36. Frankel JP, Lees AJ, Kempster PA, Stern GM. Subcutaneous apomorphine in the treatment of Parkinson's disease. *J Neurol Neurosurg Psychiatry* 1990; **53**: 96–101.

37. Broussolle E, Marion MH, Pollak P. Continuous subcutaneous apomorphine as replacement for levodopa in severe parkinsonian patients after surgery. *Lancet* 1992; **340** (8823): 859–60.

38. Mitchelson F. Pharmacological agents affecting emesis. A review (Part I). *Drugs* 1992; **43**: 295–315.

39. Scuderi P, Wetchler B, Sung YF *et al.* Treatment of postoperative nausea and vomiting after outpatient surgery with the 5-HT3 antagonist ondansetron. *Anesthesiology* 1993; **78**: 15–20.

40. Pfeiffer RF, Kang J, Graber B, Hofman R, Wilson J. Clozapine for psychosis in Parkinson's disease. *Mov Disord* 1990; **5**: 239–42.

41. Alvir JM, Lieberman JA, Safferman AZ, Schwimmer JL, Schaaf JA. Clozapine-induced agranulocytosis: incidence and risk factors in the United States. *N Engl J Med* 1993; **329**: 162–7.

42. Golden WE, Lavender RC, Metzer WS. Acute postoperative confusion and hallucinations in Parkinson disease. *Ann Intern Med* 1989; **111**: 218–22.

43. Ropper AH. *Neurological and Neurosurgical Intensive Care.* New York, NY: Raven Press; 1993.

44. Galvez-Jimenez N, Lang AE. The perioperative management of Parkinson's disease revisited. *Neurol Clin* 2004; **22**: 367–77.

Delirium in the surgical patient

Neil H. Winawer

Introduction

The acute confusional state known as delirium is the most common cause of altered mental status in surgical patients. The cardinal feature of delirium is an alteration in the level of consciousness that fluctuates over time. Despite its common occurrence delirium can often go unrecognized, leading to delays in treatment. This can have significant implications as patients with delirium suffer from higher postoperative complication rates, longer lengths of stay, and delayed functional recovery [1].

Delirium is usually acute in onset but may develop gradually. It can persist for hours to days and can fluctuate throughout the course of a day. A clouding of consciousness is most common but patients can also show hyperalert, irritable, or agitated behavior. The sleep–wake cycle is often markedly disrupted. Sleep is usually fragmented, with restlessness and agitation. Psychomotor abnormalities may range from hyperactivity to lethargy, stupor, obtundation, and catatonia. Most cases of delirium improve or resolve within 1–4 weeks if sufficient attention is given to correcting the underlying disorder causing the cerebral dysfunction. However, the development of delirium, particularly in frail, elderly patients is a marker for progressive decline [2].

Multiple signs and symptoms may accompany delirium. Patients may be grossly psychotic with severe perceptual distortions that can include hallucinations (tactile, auditory, visual, olfactory), paranoia, delusions, thought disorganization and language incoherence resembling schizophrenia. Signs of cognitive dysfunction such as disturbances in memory, attention, concentration, and orientation are usually the first to be recognized. Behavioral abnormalities such as agitation, disinhibition, and combativeness may also occur.

Given the significant morbidity and mortality associated with delirium it is important for the preoperative consultant to identify those patients at increased risk. Advanced age, comorbid medical conditions, and the type of surgery all contribute to the incidence of delirium, which can be highly variable [3].

Pathogenesis

Although much is known about the pathogenesis of delirium, its exact biologic mechanisms remain poorly understood. Delirium is a difficult disorder to study, as it occurs suddenly and characteristically waxes and wanes. Early studies noted that most episodes of delirium were characterized by specific electroencephalographic changes (abnormal slow-wave activity), implying that the disorder was one of global cortical dysfunction [4]. The ability to reverse the process in certain conditions led researchers to suspect that delirium was a disorder of cerebral oxidative metabolism. However, other investigations have supported a role of subcortical structures based on the observation that patients with infarcts in the thalamus and basal ganglia are at increased risk of developing delirium. Nonetheless, most patients who develop delirium have no identifiable abnormalities on imaging studies.

Several examples suggest that cholinergic pathways play a significant role in the pathogenesis of delirium. It has been observed that hypoxia and hypoglycemia are associated with decreased acetylcholine production in the central nervous system, the level of which correlates with the degree of cognitive decline [5]. Medications that decrease the level of acetylcholine in the CNS frequently cause confusion in the elderly. These drugs include neuroleptics, tricyclic antidepressants, benzodiazepines, and opiates. Additionally, Alzheimer's disease, characterized by a loss of cholinergic neurons, increases the risk of developing delirium. Other neurotransmitters such as serotonin and norepinephrine have also been implicated given their effects on arousal and sleep. Cytokine activation may also play a role in specific disorders (e.g., sepsis).

Diagnosis

Although delirium can develop at any time during hospitalization, it typically presents early in the postoperative period. The diagnosis is usually suspected when a patient becomes acutely agitated, uncooperative, and confused but is less apparent when patients are quiet and withdrawn. Social isolation is

Medical Management of the Surgical Patient, ed. Michael F. Lubin, Thomas F. Dodson, and Neil H. Winawer. Published by Cambridge University Press. © Cambridge University Press 2013.

common in patients with a known history of psychiatric illness (e.g., depression, schizophrenia) and delirium in these patients is often erroneously attributed to a worsening of their underlying condition.

Nursing observations often provide the earliest and most helpful clues when suspecting delirium, given the waxing and waning nature of the disorder. If delirium is suspected, initial evaluation should focus on eliciting the elements that characterize the disorder. The hallmark features of delirium as defined in the Diagnostic and Statistical Manual of Mental Disorders (DSM–IV) are as follows [6]:

1. Disturbance of consciousness (i.e., reduced clarity of awareness of the environment) with reduced ability to focus, sustain, or shift attention.
2. A change in cognition (e.g., memory deficit, disorientation, language disturbance) or the development of a perceptual disturbance that is not accounted for better by a preexisting, established, or evolving dementia.
3. Disturbance develops during a short period (usually hours to days) and tends to fluctuate during the course of the day.
4. Varies based on cause (see specific disorders for discussion).

Patients with delirium typically have difficulty with attention. They are unable to focus and have decreased levels of awareness. Often these derangements are subtle and may be overlooked by the treating physician. Delirious patients may exhibit a variety of cognitive defects including disorientation, memory loss and difficulty with language and speech (rambling, incoherent, or difficult to follow). While assessing the patient's degree of cognitive impairment, it is also vital to have established a baseline for comparison. Hence, a thorough preoperative evaluation should include a formal cognitive assessment (e.g., Folstein mini-mental status exam; see Figure 39.1) in those at risk of developing delirium.

Clinicians face two diagnostic challenges in the evaluation of delirium. The first is recognizing the presence of the disorder and the second is looking for medical conditions that may have precipitated the episode. Despite advances in medical technology, the cornerstone in the evaluation of delirium remains the history and physical examination. Initial evaluation should focus on the patient's state of arousal. Patients should be assessed for their level of orientation and questioned on routine items to assess for deficits in memory. Conversation may often reveal a disorganized thought process or be devoid of any real content. If the clinician does not know the patient's baseline mental status, relatives or caregivers can often relay information that may aid in the assessment. After a thorough evaluation, further investigation may be warranted; however, over-reliance of laboratory testing and diagnostic imaging can minimize time spent at the bedside, making the subtleties that characterize the disorder difficult to detect.

Several formal cognitive tests are useful in identifying delirium (see Figures 39.1 and 39.2). While these tests are valuable tools in making the diagnosis it is important to realize that a normal examination does not necessarily rule out delirium as patients can perform relatively well during lucid intervals. Therefore the examination should be repeated periodically. Based on ease of use, test performance, and generalizability, the Confusion Assessment Method (CAM) was identified as the best bedside instrument in a prospective study examining 11 delirium assessment tools. Its sensitivity was 86%, and its specificity was 93% for diagnosing delirium, compared with the gold standard (DSM-based diagnosis made by a geriatrician, psychiatrist, or neurologist) [7]. A modified version of the CAM has been validated in mechanically ventilated patients [8].

Cause

Once the diagnosis of delirium is established, efforts should focus on identifying an underlying cause. The medical history should include a review of the medication administration record (MAR) looking for offending agents (Table 39.1). Age appears to place patients at greatest risk. Elderly patients take the most medications yet have a decreased ability to metabolize drugs. They may often have visual and hearing impairments that predispose to disorientation.

Patients with preexisting central nervous system conditions such as cerbrovascular disease, dementia, and Parkinson disease have higher rates of postoperative delirium. Other central nervous systems abnormalities such as epilepsy and traumatic brain injury can also place patients at increased risk. The association between depression and delirium has been well documented.

The type of surgery can also influence the development of delirium. Lengthy procedures place patients at increased risk for intraoperative hypoxemia. Cardiac surgery can result in hypoperfusion and microemboli formation resulting in cerebral ischemia. Orthopedic procedures, most notably femoral neck fracture repair has been associated with high rates of delirium. These patients are also at higher risk for fat emboli. Patients undergoing cataract surgery often experience delirium due to vision loss and the use of ophthalmic drugs with anticholinergic side-effects.

A variety of metabolic insults can cause delirium. Hypoxia, whether from anesthetics, pulmonary emboli, pneumonia or other underlying respiratory/cardiac disease may cause altered mental status. These include dehydration, hyponatremia, hyperglycemia, hypoglycemia, acid-base disorders, hypercalcemia, hyperphosphatemia, hepatic, renal, and endocrine diseases.

Postoperatively, patients are at increased risk of developing infections. Pneumonia, urinary tract infections, intra-abdominal and wound infections can all cause confusion in susceptible patients. Delirium may be the only clinical clue, as systemic symptoms such as fever, chills, cough, purulent sputum, and leukocytosis may often be absent.

Orientation

1. Ask for year, season, date, day, month. Then ask specifically for parts omitted. One point for each correct. (0–5)
2. Ask in turn for name of state, county, town, hospital or place, floor or street. One point for each correct. (0–5)

Registration

Ask the patient whether you may test his or her memory. Then say the names of three unrelated objects, clearly and slowly, about 1 sec for each. After you have said all three, ask the patient to repeat them. This first repetition determines his or her score (0–3) but keep saying them until he or she can repeat all three up to six trials. If the patient does not eventually learn all three, recall cannot be meaningfully tested.

Attention and Calculation

Ask the patient to begin with 100 and count backward by 7. Stop after five subtractions (93, 86, 79, 72, 65). Score total number of correct answers, one point for each. (0–5)

If the patient can not or will not perform this task, ask him or her to spell the word world backward. The score is the number of letters in correct order, e.g., dlrow = 5. (0–5)

Recall

Ask the patient whether he or she can recall the three words you previously asked him or her to remember. (0–3)

Language

Naming: Show the patient a wrist watch and ask him or her what it is. Repeat for pencil. (0–2)

Repetition: Ask the patient to repeat this phrase after you: "no ifs, ands, or buts." Allow only one trial. (0 or 1)

Three-stage command: "Take a piece of paper in your right hand, fold it in half, and put it on the floor." Give the patient a piece of blank paper and repeat the command. Score 1 point for each part correctly executed. (0–3)

Reading: On a blank piece of paper print the sentence "Close your eyes," in letters large enough for the patient to see clearly. Ask him or her to read it and do what it says. Score 1 point only if the patient actually closes his or her eyes. (0–1)

Writing: Give the patient a blank piece of paper and ask him or her to write a sentence for you. Do not dictate a sentence; it is to be written spontaneously. It must contain a subject and verb and be sensible. Correct grammar and punctuation are not necessary. (0–1)

Copying: On a clean piece of paper, draw intersecting pentagons, each side about 1 inch, and ask him or her to copy it exactly as it is. All 10 angles must be present and 2 must intersect to score 1 point. Tremor and rotation are ignored. (0–1)

Estimate the patient's level of sensorium along a continuum, from alert on the left to coma on the right.

Total possible score is 30 point. Patients with a total of 23 points or less are highly likely to have a cognitive disorder.

Figure 39.1 Mini-Mental Status Examination: Instructions for Administration and Scoring [15].

Postoperative patients, in unfamiliar surroundings, can become disoriented. Additionally, the sensory overload associated with an ICU setting can lead to sleep deprivation. Often patients may have uncontrolled postoperative pain, which, in several studies, has been shown to increase delirium rates [9].

Patients who abuse alcohol are at risk for developing withdrawal symptoms in the postoperative period. If unrecognized, these symptoms may progress to delirium tremens. Chronic alcoholics may also have end organ damage such as cerebral atrophy and liver disease, which can predispose to

Table 39.1 Drugs commonly associated with delirium [16].

Class	Examples
Anticholinergic drugs	Tricyclic antidepressants, neuroleptics, antihistamines, benztropine, belladonna alkaloids
Opioids	Morphine, codeine, meperidine
Benzodiazepines	Diazepam, lorazepam, tenazepam
Antiparkinsonian agents	Levodopa/carbidopa, amantadine, bromocriptine
Histamine-2 receptor blockers	Ranitidine, cimetidine, famotidine, nizatidine
Cardiovascular agents	Beta-blockers, digoxin, diuretics, calcium channel blockers
Antibiotics	Penicillin, cephalosporins, gentamycin
Anticonvulsants	Phenytoin, carbamazepine
Anti-inflammatory agents	Prednisone, non-steroidal agents, cyclosporine, OKT3
Oral hypoglycemics	Glyburide, glipizide, glimepiride

encephalopathy. Patients with anxiety or sleep-related disorders may become dependent upon benzodiazepines. The withdrawal symptoms associated with these agents are similar to those of alcohol withdrawal.

Work-up

Physical examination should address vital signs, fluid status, and the appearance of localizing signs of infection. A focused neurologic examination should assess the patient's level of consciousness and look for the presence of localizing neurologic findings. Routine head computed tomography (CT) or magnetic resonance imaging (MRI) is not recommended. Although neuroimaging may uncover chronic abnormalities that can precipitate delirium it rarely reveals reversible causes [10].

Laboratory analysis should consist of a complete blood count (CBC), looking for evidence of infection, and serum electrolytes looking for evidence of hypernatremia/hyponatremia, acidosis/alkalosis, or acute renal failure. Pulse oximetry can quickly and non-invasively rule out underlying hypoxia but an arterial blood gas should also be performed if acid-base derangements are suspected or if pulse oximetry is unreliable.

Figure 39.2 The Confusion Assessment Method (CAM) Diagnostic Algorithm [6]. The diagnosis of delirium by CAM requires the presence of features 1 and 2 and either 3 or 4.

Feature 1: Acute Onset and Fluctuating Course

This feature is usually obtained from a family member or nurse and is shown by positive responses to the following questions: Is there evidence of an acute change in mental status from the patient's baseline? Did the (abnormal) behavior fluctuate during the day, that is, tend to come and go, or increase and decrease in severity?

Feature 2: Inattention

This feature is shown by a positive response to the following question: Did the patient have difficulty focusing attention, for example, being easily distractible, or having difficulty keeping track of what was being said?

Feature 3: Disorganized Thinking

This feature is shown by a positive response to the following question: Was the patient's thinking disorganized or incoherent, such as rambling or irrelevant conversation, unclear or illogical flow of ideas, or unpredictable switching from subject to subject?

Feature 4: Altered Level of Consciousness

This feature is shown by any answer other than "alert" to the following question: Overall, how would you rate this patient's level of consciousness? (alert [normal], vigilant [hyperalert], lethargic [drowsy, easily aroused], stupor [difficult to arouse], or coma [unarousable])

A chest radiograph and urinalyisis may be indicated to rule out pneumonia or urinary tract infection. Blood and urine cultures should also follow if clinical suspicion warrants. An electrocardiogram should be performed in all patients who are at risk for ischemia.

Treatment

Due to the potential morbidity and mortality associated with delirium, its onset should be treated as a medical emergency. Initial evaluation should focus on identifying and treating the underlying cause. If no cause is readily apparent then supportive care should be provided as preventing iatrogenic functional decline will improve the chances of recovery. Several simple measures if implemented early and often can result in significant benefits. Providing a room with a closed, fixed window can help orient the patient and correct sleep cycles. Large calendars, clocks, or familiar objects (such as family photographs) are useful to help connect patients to the outside world. In this regard family members or sitters should be allowed at the bedside to provide frequent orientation. The use of immobilizing devices, such as bladder catheters and restraints, should be minimized. Although the use of restraints is sometimes necessary to prevent self injury (in the absence of family or a sitter), it can lead to further agitation, social isolation, and increased morbidity [11].

Delirious patients may require pharmacologic treatment to prevent injury or to allow further evaluation or treatment. Antipsychotic medications have traditionally been used as these agents control psychotic symptoms, decrease agitation, and provide sedation. Haloperidol (Haldol) is the most commonly used agent as it is potent and has minimal hemodynamic or respiratory side-effects. It can be given orally for maintenance therapy or intravenously/intramuscularly when a faster onset of action is desired. Because the peak action of intramuscular haloperidol occurs 30 minutes after administration, patients can be re-evaluated within the first hour in emergencies and repeated doses can be given hourly if rapid tranquilizing is desired [12]. Peak action after oral ingestion occurs within 2–4 hours. After patients are adequately sedated, doses can be given orally or intramuscularly every 4–6 hours. Extrapyramidal symptoms (Parkinsonian side-effects, akathisia, dystonic reactions, and tardive dyskinesia) are the main side-effects of treatment. The newer neuroleptics (e.g., olanzapine) appear to have similar efficacy with fewer side-effects, however there is currently less evidence to support their use. Patients receiving antipsychotics in the perioperative period should have their baseline ECG reviewed to assess the duration of the QT interval given the potential for these agents to prolong ventricular repolarization.

Benzodiazepines (e.g., diazepam, lorazepam) are the drugs of choice in alcohol and sedative withdrawal syndromes. Benzodiazepines are useful adjuncts to neuroleptics to help reduce extrapyramidal side-effects. They have a quicker onset of action than the neuroleptics (5 minutes intravenously) but can cause oversedation, hypotension, and respiratory depression, which can be life threatening.

Prevention

Despite the prevalence, adverse medical consequences, and economic impact of delirium few high caliber preventative studies exist. The job of the preoperative consultant is to identify those patients at highest risk and recommend interventions. The United Kingdom's National Institute for Health and Clinical Excellence (NICE) has published guidelines on the prevention of delirium in both surgically and medically managed hospitalized adults [13]. The guidelines are based on a systematic review that ultimately identified eight studies of multicomponent interventions to prevent delirium. The recommendations emphasize a multidisciplinary, team-oriented approach that addresses cognitive impairment, dehydration, hypoxia, infection, immobility, pain, poor nutrition, medication overuse, vision and hearing impairment, and sleep deprivation. This approach has been shown to reduce the incidence of delirium by approximately 30%.

Patients in the ICU frequently experience high rates of delirium. Typically gamma-aminobutyric acid (GABA) agonists such as propofol and benzodiazepines are administered to these patients but they are associated with respiratory depression and delirium. A newer agent, dexmedetomidine (an alpha-2 adrenoceptor agonist), has been shown to reduce the incidence of delirium in the critically ill, however, further study is needed prior to its widespread use [14].

References

1. Inouye SK, Rushing JT, Foreman MD. Does delirium contribute to poor hospital outcomes? A three-site epidemiologic study. *J Gen Int Med* 1998; **12**: 234–42.

2. Francis J, Kapoor WN. Prognosis after discharge of elderly medical patients with delirium. *J Am Geriatr Soc* 1992; **40**: 601–6.

3. Dyer CB, Ashton CM, Teasdale TA. Postoperative delirium. *Arch Intern Med* 1995; **155**: 461–5.

4. Romano J, Engel GL. Delirium: I. Electroencephalographic data. *Arch Neurol Psychiatr* 1944; **149**: 41.

5. Tune LE, Holland A, Folstein MF *et al.* Association of postoperative delirium with raised serum levels of anticholinergic drugs. *Lancet* 1981; **2**: 651–3.

6. American Psychiatric Association. *Diagnostic and Statistical Manual.* 4th edn. Washington, DC: APA Press; 1994.

7. Wong CL, Holroyd-Leduc J, Simel DL, Straus SE. Does this patient have delirium? Value of bedside instruments. *J Am Med Assoc* 2010; **304**: 779–86.

8. Ely EW, Inouye SK, Bernard GR *et al.* Delirium in mechanically ventilated

patients. *J Am Med Assoc* 2001; **286**: 2703–10.

9. Lynch EP, Lazor MA, Gellis JE. The impact of postoperative pain on the development of delirium. *Int Anesth Res Soc* 1998; **86**: 781–5.

10. Koponen H, Hurri L, Stenback U *et al.* Computed tomography findings in delirium. *J Nerv Ment Dis* 1989; **177**: 226.

11. Evans L, Strumpf NE. Tying down the elderly: a review of the literature on physical restraint. *J Am Geriatr Soc* 1989; **36**: 65–74.

12. Stoudemire A. Delirium. In Lubin MF, Walker HK, Smith RB III, eds. *Medical Management of the Surgical Patient*. 3rd edn. Philadelphia, PA: JB Lippincott; 1995, pp. 378–87.

13. O'Mahony R, Murthy L, Akunne A, Young G. Synopsis of the National Institute for Health and Clinical Excellence guideline for prevention of delirium. *Ann Intern Med* 2011; **154**: 746–51.

14. Wunsch H, Kress JP. A new era for sedation in ICU patients. *J Am Med Assoc* 2009; **301**: 542–4.

15. Folstein MF, Folstein SE, McHugh PR. "Mini-mental state": a practical method for grading the cognitive state of patients for the clinician. *J Psychiatr Res* 1975; **12**: 189–98.

16. Winawer N. Postoperative delirium. *Med Clin North Am* 2001; **85**(5): 1229–39.

Surgery in the elderly

Yelena Melyakova and Michael F. Lubin

Introduction

Surgical and anesthetic care have improved markedly in the last half century. It is likely that the greatest benefit of this improvement has been for the elderly population. Older patients can benefit from surgery that would not have been contemplated in the past; thus, patients are living longer and with a better quality of life than ever before.

The literature in surgical care of the elderly patient is extensive and growing rapidly, and indicates that with careful planning and care, the elderly can undergo surgery safely and with approximately the same risk as many younger patients. This section discusses the following topics as they pertain to the elderly population: (a) physiologic decrements of aging; (b) risks of surgery; (c) preoperative evaluation; (d) anesthesia; (e) common surgical procedures; and (f) postoperative care.

Physiologic decrements of aging

Although physicians see many elderly patients who appear old and sick with many underlying health problems, a large percentage of the elderly population is quite well. These people can function entirely normally and have no limitations to their activities. Despite this degree of functional normality, however, all older people experience various decrements in physiologic function that are of importance in planning their care, particularly when they are under stresses such as surgery [1]. These decrements make even healthy older patients more fragile and more likely to suffer postoperative complications and death than their younger counterparts [2–4]. Physicians must take these factors into account in their evaluations.

The cardiovascular system has been studied and reviewed extensively. Although the ability of aging heart muscle to contract is unaffected, diastolic function deteriorates. Other important changes include decreases in maximal heart rate and cardiac output with exercise. The decreases in output are, in great part, the result of increased afterload because of increased stiffness of the arteries and decreased responsiveness to catecholamine stimulation [5]. These changes are important when patients undergo the stresses of surgery.

Although there is evidence in population studies for an increase in blood pressure with age, there is great controversy about its cause. Some feel that this truly is an age-related change; others feel that it is the result of atherosclerotic changes in the vessels, a specific disease process that can be prevented [5].

Age-related decreases in pulmonary function are quite marked and have important physiologic consequences in patients undergoing surgery. The elasticity of the lung tissue decreases and compliance increases. These changes result in an increase in residual volume and uneven ventilation [6].

Because of the uneven ventilation, arterial oxygen tension decreases in a predictable way. Sorbini and colleagues found a linear relationship with age; P_aO_2 of those less than 30 years of age was 94 mmHg, while it was only 74 mmHg for those over 60 [7]. The authors were able to estimate P_aO_2 by using the following equation: P_aO_2 (mmHg) $= 109 - 0.43 \times$ (age).

Other pulmonary changes are measurable on standard pulmonary function testing. There is a linear decrease in vital capacity of approximately 25 mL/year beginning in the third decade [8]. Measurements of airflow decrease as well, with decrements in maximum minute ventilation, FEV1, and maximum mid-expiratory flow rate.

The airway receptors undergo functional changes with age and are less likely to respond to drugs used in younger counterparts to treat the same disorders. Older adults have decreased sensation of dyspnea and diminished ventilatory response to hypoxia and hypercapnia, making them more vulnerable to ventilatory failure during high demand states (i.e., heart failure, pneumonia, etc.) and possible poor outcomes [9]. It is not surprising that pulmonary complications are among the most frequent and important in this population.

The effects of aging on the kidneys are important because of the kidneys' function in maintaining water and salt balance. They also perform a crucial role in the elimination of many drugs [10]. Grossly, the kidneys decrease by 20–30% in weight from age 30 to 80. There is a significant decrease in the number of glomeruli and an increase in interstitial fibrosis [11].

Along with these anatomic changes comes an important decrease in creatinine clearance. Because of concomitant

Medical Management of the Surgical Patient, ed. Michael F. Lubin, Thomas F. Dodson, and Neil H. Winawer. Published by Cambridge University Press. © Cambridge University Press 2013.

decrease in the lean mass of the body, however, there is generally no increase in the serum creatinine, which can be misleading to those unaware of these changes. Two groups have developed estimates of creatinine clearance (C_{Cr}) as a function of age. The following equations can be used [12,13]:

$$C_{Cr}(\text{ml/min}) = \frac{(140 - \text{age}) \times \text{Weight (kg)}}{72 \times S_{Cr}}$$

$$\text{or}$$

$$C_{Cr}(\text{ml/min}) = 135 - 0.84 \times \text{age}$$

These decreases in clearance in the absence of increases in serum creatinine must be taken into account when administering drugs primarily excreted by the kidney.

In addition to decreases in creatinine clearance, tubular function is also affected by age, and there are decreases in concentrating and diluting ability, which can lead to over-hydration, dehydration, hypernatremia, or hyponatremia if careful attention is not paid to fluid administration. Other important physiologic changes affect water balance. These include a decrease in thirst perception so that elderly patients who are volume-depleted drink less and more slowly to replete the deficit. Data suggest that certain disorders in anti-diuretic hormone (ADH) physiology predispose at least some apparently normal elderly patients to excessive ADH secretion, resulting in unexpected hyponatremia.

Although the cardiovascular, pulmonary, and renal systems are vital in the survival of surgical patients, other systems undergo important physiologic changes that affect the patient's recovery as well. Osteoporosis is quite common, most severely in white women. Care must be taken in transferring patients to avoid fracture of brittle bones [14]. Skin changes are equally as important and are often overlooked. The epidermis and dermis undergo degenerative changes, and the possibility for pressure ulcers is quite high if care is not taken to reposition the patient frequently. Repositioning may even need to be done in the operating room if the procedure is long.

Admission to the hospital may be the greatest danger to elderly patients [15]. Bedrest causes deconditioned muscles in all patients and this is particularly problematic in elderly patients with relatively little muscle reserve. Loss of muscle power begins almost immediately and in elderly patients can result in the inability to transfer, toilet, and even walk independently. Loss of these functions will result in the loss of the ability to live independently [16].

The final important areas of altered physiology are the distribution, metabolism, and elimination of drugs. Drug distribution is affected by the alterations in body composition. Lean body mass, plasma volume, and total body water decrease. Extracellular water decreases by 40%, and body fat increases by about 35%. These changes will alter drug action depending on the water and lipid solubility of the agent. For water-soluble drugs, there is a smaller volume of distribution, resulting in a higher concentration at the same dose. For lipid-soluble drugs, there may be relatively larger volume; this often results in prolonged action of the drug.

Drug metabolism in the liver is altered for some drugs. These changes are quite variable and not easily predicted. Some important drugs that have a decreased metabolic clearance in the elderly are the benzodiazepines, warfarin, and phenytoin. Renal clearance is invariably decreased in all older patients because of the changes in renal function already discussed. Thus, drugs such as digoxin, antibiotics, and others cleared primarily by the kidney must be adjusted for this decrease [10,17].

Risks of surgery

The safety of surgery in the elderly has been discussed for over 40 years. In a 1967 lecture entitled, "Is risk of indicated operation too great in the elderly?" Alton Ochsner said, "In 1927 as a young professor of surgery at Tulane Medical School, I practiced and taught that an elective operation for inguinal hernia in a patient over 50 years old was not justified" [18]. Now the literature has titles such as "Surgery for aortic stenosis in severely symptomatic patients older than 80" [19] and "Open heart surgery in the elderly: results for a consecutive series of 100 patients aged 85 years or older" [21,22].

The first reports of the results of surgery in geriatric patients appeared in the late 1930s. These studies reported an overall mortality of about 20%, while the rate for abdominal surgery was over 30%. Recent reviews have reported mortality rates for elective surgery at 0–5.4% and rates for emergency surgery vary from 13–30% [22]. In more recent years there have been reports of surgical series of patients in their 80s and 90s having surgery [3,23]. Reports of mortality range from 10–20% for emergency surgery down to an average of about 3–7% for elective surgery. A paper looked at major surgery in a nursing home population and found a mortality rate of only 4%; all of the deaths occurred in patients undergoing emergency surgery [24]. There have also been a number of papers reporting small series of selected patients over the age of 100 who have successfully had surgical procedures [25,26].

The profusion of reports in the literature prompted Linn and Linn in 1982 to review 108 studies of surgery in the elderly from 1930 to 1980 [27]. They found flaws and omissions in many of the studies. There were differences in lower age limits, methods used to calculate mortality, lengths of follow-up, mixes of emergency vs elective operations, and types of operations. They came to two main conclusions: emergency surgery is much riskier than elective surgery and, since 1941, the trend has been toward increasing mortality for elective, but not emergency, procedures.

It is quite clear that the first conclusion is true; Linn and Linn found an overall mortality of 28% for general emergency surgery and 43% for specialty emergency procedures. Elective surgery mortality rates averaged about 9%. These basic findings have been shown in a large number of papers.

Table 40.1 Mortality rates from a review of 108 studies of surgery in the elderly from 1930 to 1980 [27].

Year	Mortality (%)
1931–1940	11.0
1941–1950	5.0
1951–1960	7.3
1961–1970	9.2
1971–1980	9.5

Their second conclusion is much more controversial and certainly misleading. The authors divided the studies by decade, which yielded the rates shown in Table 40.1.

They proposed two possibilities for explaining this trend toward increasing mortality. The first is that surgical care is deteriorating, and the second is that surgeons are taking patients with greater risks; they did not indicate that one was more likely than another. However, it is clear from Dr. Ochsner's earlier comment, and from the subsequent titles listed, that surgeons are doing more extensive operations on sicker patients.

The extent of the increase in risk for older patients related to age alone is uncertain. There have been many papers that have examined this issue. The first of these papers was by Goldman and colleagues in the *New England Journal of Medicine* [28]. They studied over 1,000 patients, 324 of whom were over 70. They found an independent, statistically significant increase in risk for those over 70. Sikes and Detmer did a study comparing the mortality for different age groups from birth to 94 years [29]. They found that rates increased slowly from 2.6% in those below 64 years of age to 3.5% in those aged 70–74 years. From there, however, the rates increased from 4.4% to 10.3% for those aged 90–94 years. The authors did an adjusted mortality rate for procedure; they did not, however, adjust for comorbidity.

Other studies have separated some important factors in the mortality among elderly patients. Turnbull and associates studied mortality in patients over 70 and found only a 4.8% mortality for procedures [30]. There were 193 deaths in the group; 79 patients died of metastatic disease from the original tumor or from treatment, and 48 were felt to have died of the tumor directly. Therefore, 25% died of cancer even though they were included in the surgical mortality. They then calculated the mortality for procedures if those patients who died of far-advanced cancer and "multiple organ decompensation" were excluded and found a rate of only 2.8%. Only six of 4,050 patients died intraoperatively or in the first 24 hours after surgery – three of cardiorespiratory failure and three of uncontrolled bleeding.

A study done by Turrentine *et al.* in 2006 evaluated 7,696 patients aged 80 years or older, who underwent a surgical procedure. They determined that although several risk factors for postoperative morbidity and mortality increase with age, increasing age itself remains an important risk factor for postoperative morbidity [31].

It should be clear that comparing crude death rates can be very difficult. Seymour and Pringle suggested that, in comparing mortality, "non-viable" cases should be separated from potentially viable patients. In their study, mortality decreased from 12% to 5.8% [32]. This must be done for the younger population as well for proper comparison, but it is clear that the effect on mortality rates in the elderly will be much larger than the effect on younger patients.

Additional studies have concluded that surgery is safe and effective for cardiopulmonary bypass [21,33], resection of abdominal aneurysms [34], lung resection [35,36], abdominal surgery [37], orthopedic procedures [38], and major gynecologic surgery in appropriately selected individuals [39]. Finally, a study in Canada looked at almost 9,000 patients over 65 who had a surgical procedure. Using correlation and multiple regression analysis, they found that the severity of illness was a much better predictor of outcome than age [40]. It is clear that a strong case can be made for the safety of surgery even in the very old if appropriate precautions are taken [2].

Another strong argument in favor of surgery was demonstrated by Andersen and Ostberg [41]. They compared the survival rates of 7,922 surgical patients over age 70 with a matched sample of the general population. They found improved survival over 2–16 years of follow-up study, demonstrating that surgery appears to result in long-term improvement in survival. Another more recent study found the same results in an elderly population followed at the Mayo Clinic [42]. It is certainly clear that there is no negative effect on overall long-term survival as a result of surgical intervention.

Another important question has been raised by a number of authors. Can, could, or should physicians turn some of the emergency surgical cases into elective procedures? It has been shown that the elderly can have emergency surgery and return to their previous living situation [43]. The mortality in emergency procedures, however, is much higher than in elective ones. Seymour and Pringle reviewed this question, using hernias, peptic ulcers, and colorectal carcinomas as pertinent areas of study [44]. They found that 17% of surgical procedures in persons aged 45–64 years were emergencies. In those over age 75, however, emergencies accounted for 37% of the group. Femoral hernias showed a large increase in emergency procedures; inguinal hernias were increased as well. Peptic ulcers showed the same kind of trends as the hernias, although not quite as striking. Finally, the same kind of result is found in colorectal carcinoma, so that the rate of emergency operations for rectal carcinoma is highest in the oldest age group.

From these data, the authors did a prospective study of 74 emergency operations. They felt that the emergency procedure could have been avoided in one-third of the patients. Eight of 10 patients with strangulated hernias had been diagnosed before the emergency. Nine of 36 patients with an acute abdomen had a disease that might have been amenable to surgical therapy, and seven of 22 with cancer had symptoms for

3 months before their emergency operations. Although their conclusions were based on speculation rather than on statistics, it seems fair to say that at least some elderly patients are not having elective surgery for known or diagnosable conditions until they have become emergencies, with much increased mortality.

There are recent studies confirming the increased mortality of emergency surgery in older patients. Keller and colleagues found a 20% mortality in emergency surgery vs a 2% mortality in elective surgery [45]. In another study by Schoon and Arvidsson studying surgery in patients over 80, only one of 43 deaths within 30 days of surgery occurred after elective surgery [46].

One study looked at all the factors affecting morbidity in emergency general surgery and found that age was one of the predictors of postoperative complications [47].

Barriers to early surgery

There are a number of causes for the reticence to take elderly patients for elective surgery. The first is the mistaken belief among physicians that elderly people in general are not good candidates. This can be disproved easily and convincingly as we have shown above. The second problem is that there are sick elderly patients who have higher mortalities, not so much because of their age but because of comorbid conditions; however, this is true in younger patients as well. The most common problems in the elderly are dementia, chronic obstructive pulmonary disease, diabetes, coronary artery disease, heart failure, and hypertension. It is clear that the increased risk from these and other diseases must be evaluated, therapy instituted in those whose condition can be improved, and surgery avoided in those patients who are at a risk that appears to be unacceptable to the medical team and patient.

The last reason is the patient's reluctance to undergo surgery. Many elderly patients are quite frightened of having surgery, feeling that they have little chance of survival. Often, families have the same concerns. This, physicians can assure them, is definitely not true. The elderly are frequently concerned that surgery will not improve their quality of life, will make them more dependent on others, or will cause them to have to live in a care facility [48]. In addition, they often do not want to undergo the anticipated pain, discomfort, and rigors of surgery and the recovery period to treat a process that may not bother them very much, if at all. This obstacle is often difficult, if not impossible, to overcome.

Postoperative mortality

Although it is clear that the elderly can undergo surgery without undue risk, it is still unfortunately true that some patients do die. There are no surprises in the disease processes that cause the mortality, but it is helpful in evaluating patients preoperatively and in caring for them postoperatively to know which complications might be prevented or need to be treated.

Palmberg and Hirsjarvi reviewed a large number of surgical cases in elderly patients to study the mortality statistics [49]. They found that 33% died of pulmonary emboli, 20% died of pneumonia, 11% died of "cardiac collapse" (with no pathologic evidence of myocardial infarction), and 9% of the primary illness. Aspiration, strokes, and gastrointestinal bleeding each contributed 6%, and myocardial infarction contributed only 2%.

Other papers have found similar results, although the rates of myocardial infarction are usually in the 20–30% range. Pneumonia is the cause of death in about 15–30%, while pulmonary emboli contribute 10–20%. Sepsis is also seen regularly [30]. The highest death rates are for those patients having abdominal procedures, particularly those with perforation, obstruction, or bowel infarction.

Statistics for those with comorbid diseases are interesting [49]. Mortality in those with dementia was a surprising 45%. This is likely to be the result of patient selection, since only absolutely necessary or life-threatening surgery is likely to be done in these patients. In addition, demented patients cannot cooperate very well in postoperative care. Those with diabetes had a 26% rate, and those with cardiac disease died 17% of the time. Although the rate for cardiac disease seems relatively low compared with other disease states, unfortunately cardiac disease is very common. For this reason, those with cardiac disease alone, or in combination with diabetes, gangrene, dementia, or pulmonary disease, accounted for 44 of the 54 deaths.

Preoperative evaluation

In many ways, the preoperative evaluation of the elderly differs little from the work-up of younger people. Basically, a good history and physical must be done; but the elderly do present unique problems in preoperative evaluation.

First, physicians must remember all the expected physiologic decrements. Although elderly patients can often withstand the initial stresses of surgery, once a complication ensues, they have less reserve and are less likely to survive. Wilder and Fishbein found the mortality among those with complications was 62% but only 13% among those who appeared to be having a smooth postoperative course [50]. The most important decrements are in cardiac, pulmonary, and renal function as we have seen. These are the systems that sustain the most postoperative problems. Any underlying disease in these organ systems markedly diminishes the patient's ability to survive a complication.

Evaluating an older patient's history is fraught with difficulties. Some elderly patients are less than patient with long, meticulous histories, so history-taking should be to the point. In addition, elderly patients are often hard of hearing, and their memory of and attention to specific symptoms may be less than ideal. The elderly often minimize their symptoms out of fear of the consequences of the disease or because they feel that old age is naturally accompanied by infirmity.

Symptoms may be less apparent and less specific than in younger patients, particularly in regard to infections and pain, which can be especially difficult to document [51]. Often, patients or their families complain of non-specific problems such as confusion, malaise, incontinence, falls, syncope, or refusal to eat.

Even specific complaints may be confusing. The presence of angina may be represented by prominent shortness of breath or epigastric discomfort rather than by classic substernal chest pain. Chest pain may be a manifestation of intra-abdominal processes rather than cardiac in origin. Abdominal pain is often poorly localized and may seem to be less severe than one would expect. Thus this misdirection can delay the diagnosis in such important diseases as appendicitis, mesenteric insufficiency, and perforations of ulcers or diverticuli.

Fever can be absent in many disease states that in younger people are manifest as febrile illness, and these diseases may present in the elderly as malaise or delirium. This is commonly true with pneumonia and urinary tract infection. Many patients complain of dyspnea for which an etiology cannot be found; it is important, however to make the diagnosis of heart failure or coronary disease if either of these is the etiology of the dyspnea. Obstructive sleep apnea is often under-recognized and undertreated in the elderly [52]. A heavy smoking history and symptoms of chronic bronchitis or emphysema are also quite important to elicit. Large numbers of elderly patients present with urinary and bowel complaints, and the physician must be aware of the possibilities of urinary incontinence, urinary outlet obstruction, increased risk of constipation, and colon cancer. A careful history of medications is crucial: substantial numbers of elderly patients go to more than one doctor; they often take a number of over-the-counter drugs; and increasing numbers of patients are taking herbs and other complementary treatments that may have important clinical effects.

Taking note of visual and hearing impairments is important to help to provide sensory stimuli for patients who are at high risk for delirium, which presents great problems in providing postoperative care. Confused and disoriented patients, i.e., those with postoperative delirium, remove nasogastric tubes and intravenous lines, disrupt wounds, fall from beds and break bones. Studies have shown that these people have a much greater in-hospital mortality and decreased quality of life after discharge [49,53]. Patients with underlying dementia are at greater risk of falling and in-hospital delirium. Multiple studies have looked into association between baseline cognitive impairment and postoperative delirium. Most of these studies concluded that reduced preoperative neurocognitive and functional status predict postoperative delirium. However, in the group that developed delirium, there was no clear evidence of cognitive and functional decline from baseline 3–6 months after surgery [54,55].

Physical examination also presents difficult problems. An acutely ill elderly patient may cooperate poorly; the examination should be direct and performed as expeditiously as possible. Nutritional assessment including the state of hydration is a primary area of concern that is often overlooked or addressed in a cursory fashion. Ideally all geriatric patients at risk for malnutrition should receive consultation from a dietician. Lower mortality and moderate improvement in nutritional status were found in patients receiving individualized nutritional treatment during and after acute hospitalization [56].

Chapter 2 provides a good way to assess nutritional status. It can be very difficult to assess fluid status in these patients. The most important pitfalls are found in evaluating skin turgor and peripheral edema. Turgor is hard to assess because of senile skin changes; we believe that the skin over the forehead is the most reliable area to check. Neck veins can be helpful particularly if they are clearly distended or flat. Presence of peripheral edema can be quite misleading since many elderly patients have venous insufficiency and are often sedentary, accumulating dependent fluid. Patients are frequently quite unhappy with edema and wish it to be treated; unfortunately, many physicians are disturbed by edema as well and frequently treat it despite its usual benign nature. Vigorous diuresis to remove the edema may leave the patient significantly intravascularly depleted, predisposing to intraoperative hypotension and renal failure. Blood urea nitrogen : creatinine (BUN/Cr) ratio can be quite helpful in those who are not malnourished. While there are other causes of an increased ratio (e.g., steroid therapy and gastrointestinal bleeding), any BUN/Cr ratio above 10 should result in a careful assessment, looking for intravascular volume depletion.

Protein-calorie malnutrition has been shown to increase postoperative complications and decrease survival; hyperalimentation can decrease complications and increase survival in high-risk groups of patients [57] (see Chapter 2). Even though malnutrition in the geriatric population has declined over the past several decades, it is still relevant today. Elderly patients are often malnourished for a multitude of reasons: underlying disease states such as heart disease, diabetes, or pulmonary disease; drugs that interfere with digestion, absorption, appetite, and taste or smell; inadequate dentition; physical disability causing an inability to shop, cook or feed oneself; and poverty.

The recognition, evaluation, and therapy of protein-calorie malnutrition are therefore a very important part of the preoperative evaluation [58]. Recognition and evaluation can be carried out in the same manner as in younger patients. In addition, it has been shown by Kaminski *et al.* that older patients can tolerate aggressive enteral and parenteral hyperalimentation as well [59]. Decisions regarding hyperalimentation should be made by assessing the patient and the problem, not by looking at age.

Skin changes in elderly patients also add to the risks of hospitalization and surgery. Subcutaneous tissue decreases and the epidermis thins and becomes much more fragile. Pressure ulcers can occur with rather short episodes of bed rest and lack of position change, such as during prolonged surgery. A Swedish study looked into risk factors associated with pressure ulcer development among adult patients undergoing surgery and concluded that those who developed pressure ulcers were significantly older, weighed less, and had a lower BMI and serum albumin [60]. Pressure ulcers are an important cause of increased morbidity and frequently result in institutionalization of patients.

Biochemical deficiencies also occur with increased frequency. Elderly patients have often been shown to be deficient in vitamin A, D, cyanocobalamine, pyridoxine, calcium, and iron. The latter two are absorbed less well in the elderly. Vitamin C and zinc appear to have a role in wound healing, and some studies indicate that at least some patients have decreased levels. Some surgeons routinely supplement both in operative patients.

Cardiac status, particularly in reference to signs of heart failure, needs careful evaluation. Systolic murmurs are quite common, and are frequently benign; significant aortic stenosis, however, is important to identify because it is an important risk factor. Low systolic blood pressure, narrow pulse pressure, enlarged and sustained PMI pulsation, and left ventricular hypertrophy on the electrocardiogram can be helpful in identifying patients who may have significant aortic stenosis. There continues to be a great degree of controversy about the management of carotid bruits. Bruits that are accompanied by ischemic symptoms should be evaluated before surgery. Arterial bruits in the absence of symptoms, on the other hand, are a difficult problem; there are supporters of aggressive intervention and others who are much less aggressive and recommend no intervention without symptoms. This area of evaluation is discussed in detail in Chapter 35.

Evidence of underlying pulmonary disease will help to identify those at risk for atelectasis and pneumonia. Obstructive sleep apnea is a common breathing disorder, with a high prevalence in both the general and surgical populations. Obstructive sleep apnea in the elderly is frequently undiagnosed. Furthermore, adverse respiratory and cardiovascular outcomes are associated with obstructive sleep apnea in the perioperative period; therefore, it is imperative to identify and treat patients at high risk for the disease [52].

Laboratory assessment, as in all other patients, is still controversial. For a detailed discussion of preoperative testing see Chapter 3. Some authors still recommend all the "standard" laboratory tests: complete blood counts, electrolytes, chemistry panels, urinalysis, chest X-ray, and electrocardiogram. Some recommend routine pulmonary function tests, while others recommended routine use of diagnostic Swan–Ganz catheterization. The routine use of Swan–Ganz is not supported by good evidence [61].

For the well elderly, most geriatricians believe that there are few preoperative tests that need to be done. These recommendations include a hematocrit, a test of renal function, usually creatinine, an electrocardiogram, and a chest X-ray. There is increasing evidence that, even in the elderly, only

clinically indicated tests need to be done [62]. Many elderly patients have underlying diseases and take many medications, including over-the-counter drugs and therefore many patients will have indications for a significant number of preoperative tests. For indications for preoperative testing, see Chapter 3.

Seymour et al. did a study of electrocardiograms in 222 surgical patients over 65 [63]. Only 21% had a normal preoperative electrocardiogram, and 53% had a major abnormality. Twenty-seven patients had a postoperative cardiovascular complication, including 22 cases of heart failure, three definite myocardial infarctions, and two suspected myocardial infarctions. Of interest, however, is that, in men, there was no correlation between preoperative abnormalities and postoperative complications, while in women there did seem to be some minor predictive value; they were not, however, clinically helpful. There were a large number of non-specific changes in the electrocardiograms after surgery. The authors suggested that preoperative electrocardiograms should be done as a baseline measure to aid in interpretation of postoperative electrocardiographic changes. A recent study has again shown the lack of predictive value for risk of surgery with an electrocardiogram [64].

A study of chest X-rays was done by Tornebrandt and Fletcher [65]. They studied 100 consecutive patients over 70 for elective surgery. Of 91 chest X-rays, 43 were abnormal: 28 had cardiomegaly, 11 pulmonary hypertension, seven chronic pulmonary disease, and one a pleural effusion. Of the 27 patients without an indication, 10 had abnormal findings: five had cardiomegaly, two atelectasis, and one each had emphysema, pulmonary hypertension, and tracheal deviation. Ten percent of the patients developed a postoperative complication, for which a comparison film was helpful. The authors did not attempt to see if the abnormal findings were predictive of postoperative complications, and it is hard to determine whether the routine use of chest X-rays really makes a difference in care. Because of the high incidence of cardiopulmonary complications, however, a recent chest X-ray is probably useful for comparison when a postoperative chest X-ray is necessary.

Although some authors recommend routine pulmonary function testing [66], there are no definitive studies supporting its routine use. Clinicians should not recommend routine preoperative spirometry before high-risk surgery because it is no more accurate in predicting risk than clinical evaluation. Patients who might benefit from preoperative spirometry include those who have unexplained dyspnea or exercise intolerance and those who have chronic pulmonary obstructive disease or asthma in whom uncertainty exists as to the status of airflow obstruction when compared with baseline. Optimization of chronic pulmonary obstructive disease or asthma, deep-breathing exercises, incentive spirometry, and epidural local anesthetics reduce the risk of postoperative pulmonary complications in elderly surgical patients [67]. It seems reasonable to use the same indications employed for younger patients (see Chapter 12).

Arterial blood gases, however, may be more important. As discussed in the physiology section, P_aO_2 falls progressively from an average P_aO_2 of 94 mmHg for those under 30 to only 74 mmHg for those over 60 in normal non-smoking patients. There is, however, a wide range of normal in elderly patients and it is impossible to know if a given patient's baseline P_aO_2 is 74 or 92 mmHg. Those with a smoking history or evidence of chronic obstructive pulmonary disease are obviously affected even more. Since there is such a high incidence of postoperative cardiopulmonary complications, many patients may benefit from having a baseline P_aO_2 to help with diagnosis and therapy postoperatively.

Although specific management of disease states is beyond the scope of this chapter, some unique points must be emphasized in pulmonary care. Patients should stop smoking before the procedure. It has been shown that stopping smoking for 8 weeks before surgery is important to significantly decrease the incidence of postoperative complications. They should also be educated about incentive spirometry, coughing, and deep breathing. Finally, meticulous attention to pulmonary toilet both before admission and after surgery will help to reduce complications postoperatively.

The indications for invasive monitoring are still debated; most experts, however, do not believe that routine use is beneficial. Del Guercio and Cohn studied 148 consecutive patients who had been "cleared" for surgery by routine assessment [68]. The authors used a staging system that required Swan–Ganz catheterization in all patients and multiple cardiopulmonary function measurements. They reported that many patients had unsuspected abnormalities that put them at increased risk, however they still were able to undergo surgery. They were able to identify a very high-risk group for mortality although these patients had been "cleared" for surgery. Surgery was canceled or modified in some, and all of those who underwent the original procedure died.

The study, however, does not help to decide which patients need this kind of invasive testing. First, it was not controlled. The authors also included a number of young patients who were diseased, whom they called "physiologically old"; about one-third of the patients were under 60 and approximately half were under 70. From the data, it seems clear that some patients can benefit from this type of invasive evaluation; it is not clear from this study which patients do benefit. In addition, complications from procedures must be considered.

A later study by Schrader et al. has shown that routine use is usually unnecessary [69]. They looked at 46 patients, over the age of 90, who had surgery. None of their patients had invasive monitoring and underwent 51 procedures, many of which were major surgery. There were seven major complications; only one of the major complications might have been predicted by the preoperative use of Swan–Ganz catheterization. Most importantly, there were no perioperative deaths in their entire series. While it seems clear that there are patients who need intensive monitoring and evaluation preoperatively, it is also clear that age alone is not a primary indication for these tests.

Anesthesia

Although specifics of anesthetic care are beyond the scope of this chapter, some information is interesting and helpful to the non-anesthesiologist. There is a continuing debate over the choice of regional or general anesthesia. There appear to be arguments both for and against each approach. It seems clear that there is no appreciable difference in mortality [70,71].

General anesthesia has a number of advantages. The patient is unconscious and this prevents unwanted movement. There is no anxiety during the procedure. In addition, control of respiration through endotracheal intubation is felt by some to be helpful in the elderly because of decreased respiratory function. There appear to be some drawbacks, however. It appears that there is an increased incidence of pulmonary complications. There may be an increased incidence of mental disturbances in those who undergo general anesthesia [71]; there have also been some small studies that have not found differences [72].

Regional methods have advantages as well. Some patients prefer being awake for their procedure. Some anesthesiologists believe that there is less suppression of respiration, less hypoxia, and perhaps fewer respiratory complications, but this is unclear [71]. Disadvantages include difficulties with moving of anxious patients and a somewhat higher incidence of intra-operative and postoperative hypotension. In Hole's study of epidural versus general anesthesia in hip surgery, an equal number of patients in each group (four of 29 and four of 31) did not want the same kind of anesthesia if they were to be operated on for the other hip [71]. A recent clinical trial of anesthesia in hip surgery reached similar conclusions about the lack of a significant difference between methods [73].

Evaluation of risk

There have been a number of people who have attempted to find ways to quantify the risks of surgery from the data gleaned from history, physical examination, and laboratory data. As with all other patients assessment of preoperative risk can begin with the Revised Cardiac Risk Index (Chapter 9). The most commonly used system to identify cardiac risk has been that devised by the American Heart Association in conjunction with the American College of Cardiology [76]. Some of the major conclusions of the system are of interest. The most influential conclusion is that evaluation for preoperative revascularization should generally be limited to those patients who have indications for evaluation even without surgery unless the surgery involves major vascular procedures in patients with limited mobility. Another important factor limiting the need for evaluation is the ability of the patient to exercise; most patients who can exercise at the 4 METS level (e.g., walking on level ground at a 4 mph pace) will not need preoperative evaluation.

Common surgical problems in the elderly

Cardiovascular surgery

There is no doubt that cardiovascular surgery is feasible in the elderly patient. Many studies have been done to show that coronary bypass, valve replacement, and vascular surgery can be done in the elderly with acceptable mortality [77,78]. This can be true, even in those with severe cardiovascular disease, since the mortality from the underlying disease is very high. As discussed earlier, however, should these patients require emergency surgery, the mortality is much higher, frequently in the 80% range.

Coronary bypass surgery

There are now many studies of elderly patients who have undergone coronary artery bypass grafting (CABG) procedures. Many of these studies have been done on those between 80 and 90 years of age. One study compared 3-year outcomes of multivessel revascularization in very elderly acute coronary syndrome patients. In very elderly patients with acute coronary syndrome and multivessel coronary artery disease, coronary artery bypass grafting appears to offer an advantage over percutaneous coronary intervention in survival [33]. Optimizing the benefit of coronary artery bypass grafting in very elderly patients requires absence of significant congestive heart failure, lung disease, and peripheral vascular disease. Those with unstable angina, recent myocardial infarction, reduced cardiac function, and left main artery disease are at perhaps higher risk than younger patients because of their decreased reserve.

A number of studies have been done in those who are in New York Heart Association (NYHA) Class IV. Even these patients can be considered for CABG procedures despite mortality rates in the 15–20% range, since the prognosis without surgery is quite bad. Patients with particularly high mortality are those undergoing emergency procedures and those requiring intra-aortic balloon pulsation.

Other very important factors in deciding to do surgery are the long-term survival and functional improvement if surgery is done. Both of these areas have been studied and there are good data to show that a large percentage of the elderly who survive surgery have increased long-term survival and are able to function at a higher level after surgery [78]. Considerable numbers of patients have been shown to go from NYHA Class IV to NYHA Classes I and II. The latest innovation in bypass surgery has improved results even more. Off-pump bypass procedures lead to fewer complications, shorter hospitalizations, and lower costs [79,80]. Mortality and morbidity rates are lower as well [81].

Valvular surgery

There are many elderly patients who have significant valve pathology, particularly aortic stenosis and mitral insufficiency. The results of surgical procedures in these patients are mixed [82,83]. There can be great benefit to these patients if they are properly selected and well cared for.

Aortic valve replacement can be a life-saving and life-sustaining procedure. When found early enough, particularly before the onset of significant myocardial dysfunction, elderly patients can have remarkable results from aortic valve replacement. Studies have shown increases in long-term survival and impressive increases in functional capacity. Operative mortality in those without severe myocardial dysfunction can be as low as a few percent.

Overall mortality for those with aortic valve replacement has been in the 10% range. Patients who do survive have had excellent results from their surgery [83]. Their long-term survival is excellent; in one study 5-year survival was 70% (including operative mortality) compared with a published 5-year survival of about 20% in those without surgery. Additionally, functional improvement is often dramatic with some studies showing almost all patients improving to NYHA Classes I and II.

Patients with severe aortic valve disease who are too ill for surgical aortic valve replacement have an improved prognosis if treated with minimally invasive transcatheter aortic valve implantation rather than continuing on medical management alone [84].

One study documented outcomes in 249 high-risk octogenarians after minimally invasive aortic valve replacement. The mean age at operation was 84 ± 3 (range 80–95) years. Postoperative complications included stroke in 10 patients (4%), pneumonia in 3 patients (1%), renal failure requiring dialysis in two patients (1%), cardiac arrest in two patients (1%), pulmonary embolism in one patient (1%), and sepsis in one patient (1%). Follow-up was available for 238 patients (96%) and extended up to 12 years. Overall, long-term survival after minimally invasive aortic valve replacement at 1, 5, and 10 years was 93%, 77%, and 56%, respectively. There was no significant difference in long-term survival compared with that of a US age- and gender-matched population [85].

Mitral valve replacement is, unfortunately, not as successful [86]. Patients with mitral valve disease often can go for long periods of time without symptoms and, even after symptoms begin, they can be controlled reasonably well with medication. Thus, by the time the usual elderly patient is considered for surgery, there is often a good deal of underlying myocardial dysfunction. Mortality in mitral valve surgery is often in the 20% range and can be as high as 50% in those with significant heart failure, previous mitral procedures (valvulotomy), and pulmonary hypertension. Most patients appear to die of low output states accompanied by multiple organ failure. There is good evidence, however, that if patients survive surgery, their survival is approximately that of the population in general. There is a clear-cut difference in mortality between those with mitral stenosis who do better, and those with mitral regurgitation who do less well.

Results of combined surgical procedures show an increase in mortality. Those who get aortic and mitral valves have a modestly increased mortality. Those who have coronary bypass procedures and mitral valve replacement appear to have a greatly increased risk of death and some authors suggest that this combination of procedures should be avoided if possible.

Vascular surgery

Since atherosclerosis is a disease of aging, many elderly patients may be candidates for vascular surgery. A number of different procedures have been studied, particularly aortic aneurysm repair and carotid endarterectomy.

Many studies have been done for aortic aneurysms [34,87]. It is abundantly clear that emergency aneurysmectomy is a deadly procedure. Mortality ranges from 40–80%, usually in the upper range. Alternatively, mortality for elective procedures generally is in the 5–10% range. Symptomatic aneurysm repair usually falls in the middle of these.

It appears clear that patients who have diagnosed abdominal aneurysms larger than 6 cm should be seriously considered for elective aortic replacement if they do not have a high risk of mortality because of underlying diseases. There is a high risk of rupture in these patients and high mortality from emergency surgery.

Results of surgery in older patients with carotid artery disease are still not clear-cut. Cerebrovascular disease is discussed in detail in Chapter 35. As in younger patients, there are few definitive surgical indications for patients with carotid disease. It is clear that many elderly patients, particularly those with transient hemispheric symptoms can get relief of those symptoms, with acceptable, but somewhat increased, morbidity (perioperative stroke) and mortality. Surgery can be performed with low morbidity and mortality in the right hands, but clear-cut benefits for those without symptoms are not obvious [88]. Most papers indicate that a lot of the morbidity from stroke appears to result from the presence of significant intracranial vascular disease that is obviously more prevalent in this aged population.

Chronic statin therapy was associated with a reduction in all cardiac and vascular outcomes after major vascular surgery [89].

Peripheral arterial reconstructions in the elderly can be helpful procedures that can be done with little increase in morbidity and mortality compared with younger patients. There is still the continued higher risk of perioperative myocardial infarction, since coronary disease is so prevalent in those with peripheral vascular disease. The procedures usually result in increases in functional state and can prevent loss of limbs.

Orthopedic surgery
General considerations

Arthritis, particularly of the hip, is a very important factor limiting the mobility and independence of elderly patients. Fractures are also an important cause of morbidity and

mortality. They are also very important as causes of immobility, dependency, and institutionalization.

Hip fracture

There are approximately 320,000 hospital admissions for hip fractures in the USA each year. Elderly patients account for the vast majority of these fractures. Many of these patients are women who have substantial degrees of osteoporosis.

The care of these patients is clearly operative if at all possible. Morbidity from the procedure in unselected populations is quite low (approximately 5%) considering that significant proportions of these patients have chronic diseases and are debilitated. While mortality is not particularly high for the procedure and perioperative period, these patients often suffer a great loss of mobility and become more dependent on others for a variable length of time. It has been shown that the functional state after surgery depends heavily on the functional state of the patient before the fracture and not on chronological age. About 70% of those who were able to walk before the fracture are able to walk in some way after the operation. While there are some patients who must be admitted to nursing homes after the procedures, most patients who lived independently or with some assistance before the fracture are able to live independently or with some assistance after the procedure as well.

There are a number of important factors in the postoperative morbidity and mortality of femoral fracture patients. The procedures themselves are neither elective nor emergent. It is quite important that patients have adequate preoperative care to assure that they have had appropriate fluid resuscitation and that cardiopulmonary physiology is optimized. On the other hand, there are many studies showing that the sooner the operation is undertaken, the better the results. A recent study in 2011 shows that most of the reason for delay and increased mortality is the care of concomitant illness.

Many patients have some degree of delirium postoperatively and this complication must be anticipated. Rate of delirium is variable and depends on many factors; the major factor is the presence of cognitive impairment preoperatively. Also, selection of proper type of anesthesia is very important. A study was done on 114 geriatric patients without dementia who underwent hip fracture repair under spinal anesthesia with propofol sedation. The use of light propofol sedation decreased the prevalence of postoperative delirium by 50% compared with deep sedation. Limiting depth of sedation during spinal anesthesia is a simple, safe, and cost-effective intervention for preventing postoperative delirium in elderly patients [90].

Many patients suffer postoperative pulmonary complications so that, as much as possible, pre- and postoperative preparation and prophylactic measures should be taken. Another common, difficult and avoidable problem is that of pressure ulcers. These need to be avoided if at all possible since they contribute to increased lengths of stay, perioperative mortality, and admission to nursing homes instead of more independent living arrangements.

Elective joint replacement

The case for elective hip replacement is also strong, particularly since this can be performed with good results in a well-selected population [91]. Most of these selected patients have very painful and disabling joint disease. In one study of 100 hip replacement cases of patients in their 80s, patients returned home within 3 weeks in 92 of the cases. In this population, there were only two deaths, one from myocardial infarction and the other from pulmonary embolism [92]. Deep vein thrombosis and urinary tract infection were the most common postoperative complications, as in most studies of hip repair. The vast majority of the patients had good to excellent results and have been happy to have had the surgery done.

Other elective joint replacement surgery has been done in the elderly population. Knee joints are commonly affected by osteoarthritis. Because the elderly are less mobile than younger patients, they in some ways are better candidates for replacement, since loosening with use is a major problem with this procedure. Ankle, shoulder, and elbow replacements have all been done in selected patients with good results.

The evaluation of rehabilitation units for geriatric patients with orthopedic problems is just beginning [38]. There is some evidence to show that these units can be helpful in getting patients to be more self-sufficient and independent. Units have been developed for rehabilitation of hip fracture and replacement and amputations. The most important obstacle to rehabilitation is alteration in mental status; those with signs of dementia do poorly.

Abdominal surgery

General considerations

A great deal of work has been done to evaluate abdominal surgery in the elderly population since this is a major site for operations. More importantly, the morbidity and mortality from abdominal surgery can be high depending on a number of factors. The following factors are significantly associated with poorer prognosis: increasing age; emergency procedures; malignancy; poor physical status; and the site of surgery in the abdomen. Factors of aging, emergency surgery, malignancy, and poor physical status have been addressed earlier in this chapter; one other factor that appears to be very important in abdominal surgery for these patients is infection. The risks of infection are much higher in abdominal surgery than in most other sites; the elderly seem to have a higher risk of infection than younger patients and they have much more difficulty in handling these infections.

Gall bladder disease

One of the more common problems in the elderly is the question of what to do with the discovery of gallstones. This decision is made more (or less) difficult by the findings of the results of emergency surgery for acute cholecystitis. Patients who must undergo emergency surgery for gall bladder disease have a mortality that ranges from 12–20%. The corresponding mortality for those who have elective surgery is between 3% and 5%. Thus emergency surgery appears to be something to avoid, as we have noted earlier [93,94]. One study has suggested that there is no indication for emergency cholecystectomy in the elderly; it suggests that patients should be stabilized if at all possible with fluids and antibiotics before the patient goes to the operating room. This is not a proven concept, and others believe that the only therapy for symptomatic gall bladder disease is immediate surgery. There is general agreement, however, that medical therapy alone is not an option in these patients.

Many elderly patients who present with symptomatic gall bladder disease already have gangrene and empyema; a significant number have been found to have perforations, which can lead to subphrenic abscesses as well. This is not surprising since these patients often present with fewer and less severe symptoms, despite more severe disease.

Complications of importance in those having surgery for gall bladder disease are not surprising. Many patients have sepsis with common Gram-negative organisms, wound infections, and pulmonary complications as expected in those having upper abdominal surgery.

The advent of laparoscopic procedures for gall bladder disease has been a great boon for elderly patients. The risks of the surgery, particularly pulmonary complications, appear to be lower in this approach and therefore an elective operation can be undertaken with the expectation that there will be a good result. A number of studies have shown better results with this approach [95,96].

Appendicitis

Appendicitis is one of the most frequently missed diagnoses in the elderly population. This can be of great consequence, since the disease can be fatal and, importantly, can be cured if the diagnosis is made in time [97]. The reason that the diagnosis is frequently missed is because it is not considered. Any elderly patient with abdominal pain should have appendicitis in the differential diagnosis. While symptoms are usually less severe than in younger patients, the elderly still most frequently present with the symptoms of abdominal pain, nausea, and fever. They will frequently have abdominal tenderness as well.

A significant number of elderly patients have already perforated the appendix before operation. Although there are often delays in the diagnosis because of non-specific and muted symptoms, there are other factors involved. The appendix atrophies with age and the walls thin. In addition, the blood supply to the organ is also compromised with age. Thus, with infection, and increased pressure in the appendix, blood supply is quickly impeded, and the thinned wall more easily perforates.

Mortality in this disease depends heavily on the state of the patient's underlying health, and even more importantly, on the progression of the disease. In those operated on early, mortality is quite low. If the diagnosis can be made before complications, the laparoscopic approach can be used as well with lower risks [98]. However, as perforation, abscess, and sepsis appear, the mortality rates increase from 5% up to 20–25%.

Colon resection

Elective resection of the colon is a reasonably safe procedure in the elderly. While most resections are for carcinoma which will be addressed later, other indications include diverticular disease, polyps, and other benign disorders. Mortality for elective resections is usually below 5%. The laparoscopic approach has been used for colon resection as well with excellent results [99,100].

Gynecologic surgery

Major gynecologic surgery has been done for many years in elderly women. Elective vaginal hysterectomy for such indications as prolapse has been shown to be very safe with mortality rates in the range of 1% [101]. Major gynecological surgery in women older than 80 had a higher mortality rate, at approximately 3.6% range [102,103]. Studies have shown that elderly women who have surgery for pelvic malignancies have substantial survival after surgery so that age alone should not be considered a contraindication for surgery for pelvic cancers. Laparoscopic procedures have been used for gynecologic disease with good results in properly selected cases.

Cancer surgery

General considerations

Since cancer risk increases with age, the elderly have a disproportionate number of cancers and surgery is still the primary treatment modality for most forms of this disease process. The decision to perform cancer surgery in the elderly patient, however, also rests on a number of factors. The first is the combination of the life expectancy of the patient without surgery and the natural history of the underlying cancer. Radical surgery for a prostate cancer in an ill 90-year-old man is probably not indicated; alternatively, resection of a bowel cancer in a vigorous 70-year-old woman is clearly indicated. The second factor is the availability of non-surgical therapy. The final factor is the risk of the proposed surgery in relation to the chance of cure or life prolongation.

Lung cancer

Most lung cancers occur in the older age group. Since there is no curative non-surgical therapy, resection is the therapy of choice, if possible. Given equivalent levels of pulmonary function, in general, the elderly do quite well in comparison with younger patients with lung resections [104,105]. Mortality from surgery in elderly patients overall is in the 5% range. Five-year survival in a group of patients over 70 years of age in one study was 37%, which is quite good [106]. Some studies of patients treated without operation have had 0% 1-year survival. Video-assisted thoracic surgery for lobectomy for early stage cancer is now available and it carries lower mortality and morbidity rates [107]. A study looking at clinical stage I non-small cell lung cancer treatment with lobectomy utilizing video-assisted thoracic surgery vs thoracotomy was done in 333 patients over the age of 70. It demonstrated decreased morbidity with no perioperative deaths in the video-assisted thoracic surgery patients compared with an in-hospital mortality rate of 3.6% (3 of 82) for thoracotomy patients [108]. Therefore, minimally invasive video-assisted thoracic lobectomy should be considered in older patients for early stages of lung cancer.

Colon cancer

Often colon surgery in the elderly is for cancer. As with lung cancer, there is no curative non-surgical therapy for these patients. A number of studies have been done in the over-75 age group; these studies have shown the mortality for colon resection is between 2% and 9%, most in the lower range since most operations are elective [109,110]. In one study, all nine patients in their 90s survived the surgery. Laparoscopic procedures have been used effectively for colon cancer in properly selected cases with very good results [111]. Most patients who are admitted from home are able to return, and most importantly, postsurgical survival compares well with younger patients with bowel cancer. Because of the relatively long natural history of bowel cancers in general, the survival of older patients may not differ from their normal disease-free cohort, since they often die from other causes.

Other cancers

Esophageal cancer is a deadly disease that cannot be treated without surgery. One study from Japan showed that surgical results are reasonably good in the elderly [112]. This study showed a moderate increase in mortality in the elderly that appeared to result from an increase in pulmonary complications. The survival of the elderly group followed for 5 years is approximately 25%, essentially identical to those less than 60 years of age. A more recent study continues to support operative therapy if possible [113].

Similar results have been found in a number of studies of gastric cancer [114]. Mortality is often somewhat greater in the elderly; however, many of their cancers are found at a later stage of disease. Their survival rates compare favorably with a younger population, and since non-surgical therapy offers nothing, surgical intervention is clearly indicated if the perioperative mortality is deemed to be reasonable.

Studies of the therapy of breast cancer have shown that 5-year survivals have been in the 50% range. Since the risks of curative surgery are quite low in this disease process, operations should be offered to patients [115,116].

Organ transplantation in the elderly population

It is worth noting that in recent years consideration has been given to whole organ transplants to elderly recipients. A recent study has found that due to excellent life expectancy and quality of life in the geriatric population, heart transplantation can be given consideration. The age of 65 is no longer an absolute contraindication to heart transplantation, which can be performed safely in a well-selected geriatric patient. An inherent limitation to transplantation remains in the shortage of organ donors, not patient age [117].

Living donor transplant of the kidney to the properly selected elderly patient has become a safe and viable option for prolonging life. It is important to provide counseling to both donor and recipient and ensure that the donor makes a fully cognizant decision, realizing all of the risks and implications of the donation [118].

Postoperative care of the elderly patient

As with preoperative care, the postoperative management of the elderly patient is basically the same as for the younger patient. However, meticulous attention to detail and awareness of potential problems give these patients a better chance of survival and less opportunity for postoperative complications.

Even in the recovery room, attention to details of care is important. Hypothermia is common because of cool operating rooms, room-temperature intravenous infusions, and cold blood transfusions [119]. Some elderly patients are particularly susceptible because of faulty temperature regulation. Hypothermia itself depresses the heart. In addition, on rewarming, the increased metabolic activity and cardiac output needed puts an added stress on the heart.

Narcotic-induced ventilatory depression can last longer than usual in the elderly. Particularly in patients who have had general anesthesia, there can be a significant drop in P_aO_2 after surgery. This appears to be caused by a combination of shunting and an increase in ventilation–perfusion mismatching; this effect increases with increasing age. Campbell has stated that, in those in whom postoperative complications are expected, the continued use of mechanical ventilation into the postoperative period may help to prevent some of these complications [66]. In this way, adequate ventilation even in the face of narcotic analgesics and good tracheobronchial toilet can be provided. There is no objective evidence to support or refute this method of care.

It is clear, however, that it is quite important for elderly patients to be up in a chair and moving as soon as possible after surgery. This allows for increases in ventilation and easier clearing of secretions and results in less atelectasis. An important factor in avoiding pulmonary complications is adequate pain relief as well. Patients in pain, particularly from thoracic or abdominal surgery, are less likely to cough, breathe deeply, and cooperate with respiratory therapy.

Postoperative delirium is common in elderly patients, and those who manifest these changes have a mortality about twice that of patients who do not have delirium [120]. It has been estimated that 20–30% of elderly patients become delirious following surgery; Bedford reported that 33% of

4,000 patients who exhibited delirium during their hospital admission died within 1 month [120].

Hole et al. feel that this effect may be related to decreased oxygenation of the brain. They argue that there is a decrease in cardiac output with positive pressure ventilation and that hyperventilation with resulting hypocapnia causes a further decrease in blood flow from the resulting cerebral vasoconstriction [71]. Others feel that it may be an effect of the anesthetic agents themselves [90].

Some interesting factors appear to influence these changes. Those who have regional anesthesia appear to be affected to a lesser degree; those who have shorter procedures are often less affected; those who are febrile and are given other drugs are more frequently affected.

The prevention of postoperative delirium has been studied and there are data to support a variety of methods to decrease the incidence of this important complication. Marcantonio et al. looked at a group of patients having hip surgery and intervened in a number of different areas [121]. These included: oxygenation; fluids and electrolyte balances; pain; medications; bowel and bladder functions; nutrition; mobilization; observation for and treatment of complications; and environmental factors like lighting and sensory stimulation. They were able to decrease the incidence of delirium from 50% to 32%. For more detailed information on perioperative delirium see Chapter 39.

Heart failure and myocardial infarction are two important and deadly postoperative complications. Heart failure can be prevented, at least in part, by meticulous attention to intravenous infusions and urine output. At times, it will be essential to use invasive monitoring by Swan–Ganz catheterization. As discussed above, clinical judgment must be used to decide which patients are likely to need this monitoring method.

Although physicians are unable to prevent myocardial infarction, it is possible to anticipate its occurrence and to be able to recognize its unusual presentations in the elderly. The most common atypical presentations of myocardial infarction include sudden dyspnea or exacerbation of heart failure. Other presentations can be acute delirium, strokes, peripheral emboli, and weakness.

Pulmonary embolism is a frequent complication that is theoretically preventable. Chapter 22 covers the discussion of DVT and pulmonary embolism prophylaxis in detail. There is evidence that, for most procedures, low-dose heparin before and after surgery is helpful. This method is not helpful in orthopedic procedures and low molecular weight heparin or coumadin prophylaxis should be used; intermittent compression stockings are used in neurosurgery and open prostatectomy, where anticoagulation is dangerous.

Because of their frailty and decreases in physiologic reserve, older patients who have complications have a greatly increased mortality, so that prevention and early intervention are crucial to their well-being. As in all care of the elderly, careful attention to detail in all aspects of postoperative management will result in lower morbidity and mortality.

References

1. Boss GR, Seegmiller JE. Age-related physiological changes and their clinical significance. *West J Med* 1981; **135**: 434–40.

2. Brown NA, Zenilman ME. The impact of frailty in the elderly on the outcome of surgery in the aged. *Adv Surg* 2010; **44**: 229–49.

3. Polanczyk CA, Marcantonio E, Goldman L *et al.* Impact of age on perioperative complications and length of stay in patients undergoing noncardiac surgery. *Ann Intern Med* 2001; **134**: 637–43.

4. Abrass IB. The biology and physiology of aging. *West J Med* 1990; **153**: 641–5.

5. Safar ME. Arterial aging – hemodynamic changes and therapeutic options. *Nat Rev Cardiol* 2010; **7**: 442–9.

6. Wang L, Green FH, Smiley-Jewell SM, Pinkerton KE. Susceptibility of the aging lung to environmental injury. *Semin Respir Crit Care Med* 2010; **31**: 539–53.

7. Sorbini CA, Grassi V, Solinas E, Muiesan G. Arterial oxygen tension in relation to age in healthy subjects. *Respiration* 1968; **25**: 3–13.

8. Muiesan G, Sorbini CA, Grassi V. Respiratory function in the aged. *Bull Physiopathol Respir (Nancy)* 1971; **7**: 973–1009.

9. Sharma G, Goodwin J. Effect of aging on respiratory system physiology and immunology. *Clin Interv Aging* 2006; **1**: 253–60.

10. Klotz U. Pharmacokinetics and drug metabolism in the elderly. *Drug Metab Rev* 2009; **41**: 67–76.

11. El Nahas M. Cardio-kidney-damage: a unifying concept. *Kidney Int* 2010; **78**: 14–18.

12. Abdelhafiz AH, Brown SH, Bello A, El Nahas M. Chronic kidney disease in older people: physiology, pathology or both? *Nephron Clin Pract* 2010; **116**: c19–24.

13. Cockcroft DW, Gault MH. Prediction of creatinine clearance from serum creatinine. *Nephron* 1976; **16**: 31–41.

14. Syed FA, Ng AC. The pathophysiology of the aging skeleton. *Curr Osteoporos Rep* 2010; **8**: 235–40.

15. Creditor MC. Hazards of hospitalization of the elderly. *Ann Intern Med* 1993; **118**: 219–23.

16. Gill TM, Allore HG, Gahbauer EA, Murphy TE. Change in disability after hospitalization or restricted activity in older persons. *J Am Med Assoc* 2010; **304**: 1919–28.

17. Cusack BJ. Pharmacokinetics in older persons. *Am J Geriatr Pharmacother* 2004; **2**: 274–302.

18. Ochsner A. Is risk of indicated operation too great in the elderly? *Geriatrics* 1967; **22**: 121–30.

19. Gilbert T, Orr W, Banning AP. Surgery for aortic stenosis in severely symptomatic patients older than 80 years: experience in a single UK centre. *Heart* 1999; **82**: 138–42.

20. Rosengart TK, Finnin EB, Kim DY *et al.* Open heart surgery in the elderly: results from a consecutive series of 100 patients aged 85 years or older. *Am J Med* 2002; **112**: 143–7.

21. Alexander KP, Anstrom KJ, Muhlbaier LH *et al.* Outcomes of cardiac surgery in patients > or = 80 years: results from the National Cardiovascular Network. *J Am Coll Cardiol* 2000; **35**: 731–8.

22. Pofahl WE, Pories WJ. Current status and future directions of geriatric general surgery. *J Am Geriatr Soc* 2003; **51** (7 Suppl): S351–4.

23. Liu LL, Leung JM. Predicting adverse postoperative outcomes in patients aged 80 years or older. *J Am Geriatr Soc* 2000; **48**: 405–12.

24. Keating HJ 3rd. Major surgery in nursing home patients: procedures, morbidity, and mortality in the frailest of the frail elderly. *J Am Geriatr Soc* 1992; **40**: 8–11.

25. Katlic MR. Surgery in centenarians. *J Am Med Assoc* 1985; **253**: 3139–41.

26. Bridges CR, Edwards FH, Peterson ED, Coombs LP, Ferguson TB. Cardiac surgery in nonagenarians and centenarians. *J Am Coll Surg* 2003; **197**: 347–56; discussion 356–7.

27. Linn BS, Linn MW, Wallen N. Evaluation of results of surgical procedures in the elderly. *Ann Surg* 1982; **195**: 90–6.

28. Goldman L, Caldera DL, Nussbaum SR *et al.* Multifactorial index of cardiac risk in noncardiac surgical procedures. *N Engl J Med* 1977; **297**: 845–50.

29. Sikes ED Jr, Detmer DE. Aging and surgical risk in older citizens of Wisconsin. *Wis Med J* 1979; **78**: 27–30.

30. Turnbull AD, Gundy E, Howland WS, Beattie EJ Jr. Surgical mortality among the elderly. An analysis of 4,050 operations (1970–1974). *Clin Bull* 1978; **8**: 139–42.

31. Turrentine FE, Wang H, Simpson VB, Jones RS. Surgical risk factors, morbidity, and mortality in elderly patients. *J Am Coll Surg* 2006; **203**: 865–77.

32. Seymour DG, Pringle R. A new method of auditing surgical mortality rates: application to a group of elderly general surgical patients. *Br Med J (Clin Res Ed)* 1982; **284**: 1539–42.

33. Sheridan BC, Stearns SC, Rossi JS *et al.* Three-year outcomes of multivessel revascularization in very elderly acute coronary syndrome patients. *Ann Thorac Surg* 2010; **89**: 1889–94; discussion 1894–5.

34. Alonso-Perez M, Segura R, Pita S, Cal L. Operative results and death predictors for nonruptured abdominal aortic aneurysms in the elderly. *Ann Vasc Surg* 2001; **15**: 306–11.

35. Conti B, Brega Massone PP, Lequaglie C, Magnani B, Cataldo I. Major surgery in lung cancer in elderly patients? Risk factors analysis and long-term results. *Minerva Chir* 2002; **57**: 317–21.

36. Port JL, Kent M, Korst RJ *et al.* Surgical resection for lung cancer in the octogenarian. *Chest* 2004; **126**: 733–8.

37. Reiss R, Deutsch AA, Nudelman I. Abdominal surgery in elderly patients: statistical analysis of clinical factors prognostic of mortality in 1,000 cases. *Mt Sinai J Med* 1987; **54**: 135–40.

38. Beaupre LA, Jones CA, Saunders LD *et al.* Best practices for elderly hip fracture patients. A systematic overview of the evidence. *J Gen Intern Med* 2005; **20**: 1019–25.

39. Susini T, Scambia G, Margariti PA *et al.* Gynecologic oncologic surgery in the elderly: a retrospective analysis of 213 patients. *Gynecol Oncol* 1999; **75**: 437–43.

40. Dunlop WE, Rosenblood L, Lawrason L, Birdsall L, Rusnak CH. Effects of age and severity of illness on outcome and length of stay in geriatric surgical patients. *Am J Surg* 1993; **165**: 577–80.

41. Andersen B, Ostberg J. Long-term prognosis in geriatric surgery: 2–17 year follow-up of 7922 patients. *J Am Geriatr Soc* 1972; **20**: 255–8.

42. Hosking MP, Warner MA, Lobdell CM, Offord KP, Melton LJ 3rd. Outcomes of surgery in patients 90 years of age and older. *J Am Med Assoc* 1989; **261**: 1909–15.

43. Salem R, Devitt P, Johnson J, Firmin R. Emergency geriatric surgical admissions. *Br Med J* 1978; **2**: 416–17.

44. Seymour DG, Pringle R. Surgical emergencies in the elderly: can they be prevented? *Health Bull (Edinb)* 1983; **41**: 112–31.

45. Keller SM, Markovitz LJ, Wilder JR, Aufses AH Jr. Emergency and elective surgery in patients over age 70. *Am Surg* 1987; **53**: 636–40.

46. Schoon IM, Arvidsson S. Surgery in patients aged 80 years and over. A retrospective comparative study from 1981 and 1987. *Eur J Surg* 1991; **157**: 251–5.

47. Akinbami F, Askari R, Steinberg J, Panizales M, Rogers SO Jr. Factors affecting morbidity in emergency general surgery. *Am J Surg* 2011; **201**: 456–62.

48. Reiss R. Moral and ethical issues in geriatric surgery. *J Med Ethics* 1980; **6**: 71–7.

49. Palmberg S, Hirsjarvi E. Mortality in geriatric surgery. With special reference to the type of surgery, anaesthesia, complicating dieeases, and prophylaxis of thrombosis. *Gerontology* 1979; **25**: 103–12.

50. Wilder RJ, Fishbein RH. The widening surgical frontier. *Postgrad Med* 1961; **29**: 548–51.

51. Samiy AH. Clinical manifestations of disease in the elderly. *Med Clin North Am* 1983; **67**: 333–44.

52. Adesanya AO, Lee W, Greilich NB, Joshi GP. Perioperative management of obstructive sleep apnea. *Chest* 2010; **138**: 1489–98.

53. Heijmeriks JA, Dassen W, Prenger K, Wellens HJ. The incidence and consequences of mental disturbances in elderly patients post cardiac surgery – a comparison with younger patients. *Clin Cardiol* 2000; **23**: 540–6.

54. Jankowski CJ, Trenerry MR, Cook DJ *et al.* Cognitive and functional predictors and sequelae of postoperative delirium in elderly patients undergoing elective joint arthroplasty. *Anesth Analg* 2011; **112**: 1186–93.

55. Papon MA, Whittington RA, El-Khoury NB, Planel E. Alzheimer's disease and anesthesia. *Front Neurosci* 2011; **4**: 272.

56. Feldblum I, German L, Castel H, Harman-Boehm I, Shahar DR. Individualized nutritional intervention during and after hospitalization: the nutrition intervention study clinical trial. *J Am Geriatr Soc* 2011; **59**: 10–17.

57. Mullen JL, Buzby GP, Matthews DC, Smale BF, Rosato EF. Reduction of operative morbidity and mortality by combined preoperative and postoperative nutritional support. *Ann Surg* 1980; **192**: 604–13.

58. Corish CA. Pre-operative nutritional assessment in the elderly. *J Nutr Health Aging* 2001; **5**: 49–59.

59. Kaminski MV Jr, Nasr NJ, Freed BA, Sriram K. The efficacy of nutritional support in the elderly. *J Am Coll Nutr* 1982; **1**: 35–40.

60. Lindgren M, Unosson M, Krantz AM, Ek AC. Pressure ulcer risk factors in patients undergoing surgery. *J Adv Nurs* 2005; **50**: 605–12.

61. Harvey S, Harrison DA, Singer M *et al.* Assessment of the clinical effectiveness of pulmonary artery catheters in management of patients in intensive care (PAC-Man): a randomised controlled trial. *Lancet* 2005; **366** (9484): 472–7.

62. Dzankic S, Pastor D, Gonzalez C, Leung JM. The prevalence and predictive value of abnormal preoperative laboratory tests in elderly surgical patients. *Anesth Analg* 2001; **93**: 301–8.

63. Seymour DG, Pringle R, MacLennan WJ. The role of the routine pre-operative electrocardiogram in the elderly surgical patient. *Age Ageing* 1983; **12**: 97–104.

64. Liu LL, Dzankic S, Leung JM. Preoperative electrocardiogram abnormalities do not predict postoperative cardiac complications in geriatric surgical patients. *J Am Geriatr Soc* 2002; **50**: 1186–91.

65. Tornebrandt K, Fletcher R. Pre-operative chest x-rays in elderly patients. *Anaesthesia* 1982; **37**: 901–2.

66. Campbell JC. Detecting and correcting pulmonary risk factors before operation. *Geriatrics* 1977; **32**: 54–7.

67. Smetana GW. Preoperative pulmonary assessment of the older adult. *Clin Geriatr Med* 2003; **19**: 35–55.

68. Del Guercio LR, Cohn JD. Monitoring operative risk in the elderly. *J Am Med Assoc* 1980; **243**: 1350–5.

69. Schrader LL, McMillen MA, Watson CB, MacArthur JD. Is routine preoperative hemodynamic evaluation of nonagenarians necessary? *J Am Geriatr Soc* 1991; **39**: 1–5.

70. Wickstrom I, Holmberg I, Stefansson T. Survival of female geriatric patients after hip fracture surgery. A comparison of 5 anesthetic methods. *Acta Anaesthesiol Scand* 1982; **26**: 607–14.

71. Hole A, Terjesen T, Breivik H. Epidural versus general anaesthesia for total hip arthroplasty in elderly patients. *Acta Anaesthesiol Scand* 1980; **24**: 279–87.

72. Zuo C, Zuo Z. Spine surgery under general anesthesia may not increase the risk of Alzheimer's disease. *Dement Geriatr Cogn Disord* 2010; **29**: 233–9.

73. Lien CA. Regional versus general anesthesia for hip surgery in older patients: does the choice affect patient outcome? *J Am Geriatr Soc* 2002; **50**: 191–4.

74. Detsky AS, Abrams HB, McLaughlin JR *et al.* Predicting cardiac complications in patients undergoing non-cardiac surgery. *J Gen Intern Med* 1986; **1**: 211–19.

75. Gerson MC, Hurst JM, Hertzberg VS *et al.* Prediction of cardiac and pulmonary complications related to elective abdominal and noncardiac thoracic surgery in geriatric patients. *Am J Med* 1990; **88**: 101–7.

76. Eagle KA, Berger PB, Calkins H *et al.* ACC/AHA guideline update for perioperative cardiovascular evaluation for noncardiac surgery – executive summary: a report of the American College of Cardiology/American Heart Association Task Force on Practice Guidelines (Committee to Update the 1996 Guidelines on Perioperative Cardiovascular Evaluation for Noncardiac Surgery). *J Am Coll Cardiol* 2002; **39**: 542–53.

77. Easo J, Holzl PP, Horst M *et al.* Cardiac surgery in nonagenarians: Pushing the

boundary one further decade. *Arch Gerontol Geriatr* 2011; **53**: 229–32.

78. Krane M, Voss B, Hiebinger A *et al.* Twenty years of cardiac surgery in patients aged 80 years and older: risks and benefits. *Ann Thorac Surg* 2011; **91**: 506–13.

79. Hoff SJ, Ball SK, Coltharp WH *et al.* Coronary artery bypass in patients 80 years and over: is off-pump the operation of choice? *Ann Thorac Surg* 2002; **74**: S1340–3.

80. Hoff SJ, Ball SK, Leacche M. Results of completion arteriography after minimally invasive off-pump coronary artery bypass. *Ann Thorac Surg* 2011; **91**: 31–6; discussion 36–7.

81. Demaria RG, Carrier M, Fortier S *et al.* Reduced mortality and strokes with off-pump coronary artery bypass grafting surgery in octogenarians. *Circulation* 2002; **106** (12 Suppl 1): I5–I10.

82. Olsson M, Granstrom L, Lindblom D, Rosenqvist M, Ryden L. Aortic valve replacement in octogenarians with aortic stenosis: a case-control study. *J Am Coll Cardiol* 1992; **20**: 1512–16.

83. Pasic M, Carrel T, Laske A *et al.* Valve replacement in octogenarians: increased early mortality but good long-term result. *Eur Heart J* 1992; **13**: 508–10.

84. Rajani R, Buxton W, Haworth P *et al.* Prognostic benefit of transcatheter aortic valve implantation compared with medical therapy in patients with inoperable aortic stenosis. *Catheter Cardiovasc Interv* 2010; **75**: 1121–6.

85. ElBardissi AW, Shekar P, Couper GS, Cohn LH. Minimally invasive aortic valve replacement in octogenarian, high-risk, transcatheter aortic valve implantation candidates. *J Thorac Cardiovasc Surg* 2011; **141**: 328–35.

86. Goldsmith I, Lip GY, Kaukuntla H, Patel RL. Hospital morbidity and mortality and changes in quality of life following mitral valve surgery in the elderly. *J Heart Valve Dis* 1999; **8**: 702–7.

87. Henebiens M, Vahl A, Koelemay MJ. Elective surgery of abdominal aortic aneurysms in octogenarians: a systematic review. *J Vasc Surg* 2008; **47**: 676–81.

88. Ommer A, Pillny M, Grabitz K, Sandmann W. Reconstructive surgery for carotid artery occlusive disease in the elderly – a high risk operation? *Cardiovasc Surg* 2001; **9**: 552–8.

89. Le Manach Y, Ibanez Esteves C, Bertrand M *et al.* Impact of preoperative statin therapy on adverse postoperative outcomes in patients undergoing vascular surgery. *Anesthesiology* 2011; **114**: 98–104.

90. Sieber FE, Zakriya KJ, Gottschalk A *et al.* Sedation depth during spinal anesthesia and the development of postoperative delirium in elderly patients undergoing hip fracture repair. *Mayo Clin Proc* 2010; **85**: 18–26.

91. Ekelund A, Rydell N, Nilsson OS. Total hip arthroplasty in patients 80 years of age and older. *Clin Orthop Relat Res* 1992; **281**: 101–6.

92. Phillips TW, Grainger RW, Cameron HS, Bruce L. Risks and benefits of elective hip replacement in the octogenarian. *Can Med Assoc J* 1987; **137**: 497–500.

93. Margiotta SJ Jr, Horwitz JR, Willis IH, Wallack MK. Cholecystectomy in the elderly. *Am J Surg* 1988; **156**: 509–12.

94. Harness JK, Strodel WE, Talsma SE. Symptomatic biliary tract disease in the elderly patient. *Am Surg* 1986; **52**: 442–5.

95. Kuwabara K, Matsuda S, Ishikawa KB, Horiguchi H, Fujimori K. Comparative quality of laparoscopic and open cholecystectomy in the elderly using propensity score matching analysis. *Gastroenterol Res Pract.* 2010; 2010: 490147.

96. Pessaux P, Tuech JJ, Derouet N *et al.* Laparoscopic cholecystectomy in the elderly: a prospective study. *Surg Endosc* 2000; **14**: 1067–9.

97. Smithy WB, Wexner SD, Dailey TH. The diagnosis and treatment of acute appendicitis in the aged. *Dis Colon Rectum* 1986; **29**: 170–3.

98. Kirshtein B, Perry ZH, Mizrahi S, Lantsberg L. Value of laparoscopic appendectomy in the elderly patient. *World J Surg* 2009; **33**: 918–22.

99. Faiz O, Warusavitarne J, Bottle A *et al.* Laparoscopically assisted vs. open elective colonic and rectal resection: a comparison of outcomes in English National Health Service Trusts between 1996 and 2006. *Dis Colon Rectum* 2009; **52**: 1695–704.

100. Tei M, Ikeda M, Haraguchi N *et al.* Postoperative complications in elderly patients with colorectal cancer: comparison of open and laparoscopic surgical procedures. *Surg Laparosc Endosc Percutan Tech* 2009; **19**: 488–92.

101. Richter HE, Goode PS, Kenton K *et al.* The effect of age on short-term outcomes after abdominal surgery for pelvic organ prolapse. *J Am Geriatr Soc* 2007; **55**: 857–63.

102. Mains LM, Magnus M, Finan M. Perioperative morbidity and mortality from major gynecologic surgery in the elderly woman. *J Reprod Med* 2007; **52**: 677–84.

103. Toglia MR, Nolan TE. Morbidity and mortality rates of elective gynecologic surgery in the elderly woman. *Am J Obstet Gynecol* 2003; **189**: 1584–7; discussion 1587–9.

104. Dillman RO, Zusman DR, McClure SE. Surgical resection and long-term survival for octogenarians who undergo surgery for non-small-cell lung cancer. *Clin Lung Cancer* 2009; **10**: 130–4.

105. Takamochi K, Oh S, Matsuoka J, Suzuki K. Risk factors for morbidity after pulmonary resection for lung cancer in younger and elderly patients. *Interact Cardiovasc Thorac Surg* 2011; **12**: 739–43.

106. Birim O, Zuydendorp HM, Maat AP *et al.* Lung resection for non-small-cell lung cancer in patients older than 70: mortality, morbidity, and late survival compared with the general population. *Ann Thorac Surg* 2003; **76**: 1796–801.

107. Heerdt PM, Park BJ. The emerging role of minimally invasive surgical techniques for the treatment of lung malignancy in the elderly. *Anesthesiol Clin* 2008; **26**: 315–24, vi–vii.

108. Cattaneo SM, Park BJ, Wilton AS *et al.* Use of video-assisted thoracic surgery for lobectomy in the elderly results in fewer complications. *Ann Thorac Surg* 2008; **85**: 231–5; discussion 235–6.

109. Fitzgerald SD, Longo WE, Daniel GL, Vernava AM 3rd. Advanced colorectal neoplasia in the high-risk elderly patient: is surgical resection justified? *Dis Colon Rectum* 1993; **36**: 161–6.

110. Patel SA, Zenilman ME. Outcomes in older people undergoing operative intervention for colorectal cancer. *J Am Geriatr Soc* 2001; **49**: 1561–4.

111. Law WL, Chu KW, Tung PH. Laparoscopic colorectal resection: a safe

option for elderly patients. *J Am Coll Surg* 2002; **195**: 768–73.

112. Sugimachi K, Inokuchi K, Ueo H *et al.* Surgical treatment for carcinoma of the esophagus in the elderly patient. *Surg Gynecol Obstet* 1985; **160**: 317–19.

113. Xijiang Z, Xizeng Z, Xishan H, Hongjing J. Surgical treatment for carcinoma of the esophagus in the elderly patient. *Ann Thorac Cardiovasc Surg* 1999; **5**: 182–6.

114. Endo S, Yoshikawa Y, Hatanaka N *et al.* Treatment for gastric carcinoma in the oldest old patients. *Gastric Cancer* 2011; **14**: 139–43.

115. Gandhi S, Verma S. Early breast cancer in the older woman. *Oncologist* 2011; **16**: 479–85.

116. Chatzidaki P, Mellos C, Briese V, Mylonas I. Perioperative complications of breast cancer surgery in elderly women (≥80 Years). *Ann Surg Oncol* 2011; **18**: 923–31.

117. Daneshvar DA, Czer LS, Phan A, Trento A, Schwarz ER. Heart transplantation in the elderly: why cardiac transplantation does not need to be limited to younger patients but can be safely performed in patients above 65 years of age. *Ann Transplant* 2010; **15**: 110–19.

118. Cooper M, Forland CL. The elderly as recipients of living donor kidneys, how old is too old? *Curr Opin Organ Transplant* 2011; **16**: 250–5.

119. Heymann AD. The effect of incidental hypothermia on elderly surgical patients. *J Gerontol* 1977; **32**: 46–8.

120. Hodkinson HM. Mental impairment in the elderly. *J R Coll Physicians Lond* 1973; **7**: 305–17.

121. Marcantonio ER, Flacker JM, Wright RJ, Resnick NM. Reducing delirium after hip fracture: a randomized trial. *J Am Geriatr Soc* 2001; **49**: 516–22.

Chapter 41

Perioperative medical management of obese patients

Madhuri Rao and John G. Kral

Introduction

The high prevalence of obesity and its comorbidities requires physicians to recognize obesity as a serious condition affecting all specialties. This is especially true for patients needing operations. New developments in the practice of surgery and new insights into the pathogenesis and pathophysiology of obesity have profound impacts on the perioperative management of these patients.

This chapter incorporates recent advances affecting the medical management of obese patients having surgery.

Prevalence

In 2007–2008, the age-adjusted prevalence of obesity in the USA was 33.8% overall, 32.2% among adult men, and 35.5% among adult women. The corresponding prevalence estimates for overweight and obesity combined (BMI ≥ 25) were 68.0%, 72.3%, and 64.1% [1].

Although the increases in the prevalence of obesity previously observed did not appear to be continuing at the same rate over the past 10 years, the high prevalence is still worrisome because of the unrelenting increases in children and also the dramatic rise in severe obesity, a devastating rapidly increasing form of the disorder (see Figure 41.1). An estimated 17% of children and adolescents aged 2–19 years are obese and Fontaine *et al.* showed that younger adults lose more years of life than older adults [2].

There is a dose–response relationship between body fat and risks of diabetes, coronary artery disease, hypertension, and cancer mortality, resulting in increased prevalence of these associated morbid conditions.

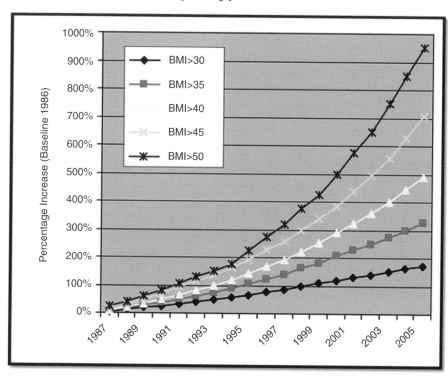

Figure 41.1 Percentage increase in BMI categories since 1986 (source: Behavioral Risk Factor Surveillance Survey; results adjusted for changes in population demographics to be comparable to 2005 demographics). Reprinted with permission from Sturm R. Increases in morbid obesity in the USA: 2000–2005. *Public Health* 2007; **121**: 492–6.

Pathogenesis of obesity

Obesity reflects interactions between genetic disposition and environmental factors attributed to imbalance between energy intake and expenditure. More than 70 gene loci, including those involved in central nervous regulation systems such as leptin, energy expenditure, and adipocyte differentiation have been identified. Obesity influences the pathogenesis of hypertension, type 2 diabetes, dyslipidemia, kidney, heart, and cerebrovascular disease [3,4]. Table 41.1 summarizes the common surgical diseases associated with obesity.

Adipose tissue distribution seems to be more important in the pathogenesis of obesity than "patient size" or body mass index (BMI). Abdominal adiposity through the mechanism of insulin resistance increases the risk of developing type 2 diabetes mellitus and cardiovascular disease [5].

The excess free fatty acids secreted by adipose tissue result in an increased secretion of inflammatory cytokines and adipokines. These have been associated with hyperinsulinemia, hyperglycemia, insulin resistance, diabetes, endothelial dysfunction, and plaque development, progression, and rupture. Adiponectin,

another important adipokine, has protective cardiometabolic actions but levels decline with increasing obesity [6].

The changing practice of surgery
Laparoscopic versus open surgery

There are several fundamental differences between laparoscopic and open surgery including the obvious fact that there is less tissue trauma in the absence of the larger incisions necessary for exposure in obese patients. Compared with access by laparotomy, laparoscopic approaches to major abdominal operations have been shown to reduce organ system impairment resulting in decreased recovery time and perioperative morbidity. The systemic inflammatory response syndrome (SIRS) is attenuated in laparoscopic surgery. Systemic inflammatory response syndrome defines the clinical response of the body to an insult and includes two or more of the SIRS criteria which are:

- Body temperature of more than 38 °C or less than 36 °C.
- Heart rate of more than 90 beats per minute.
- Respiratory rate of more than 20 breaths per minute or a P_aCO_2 level of less than 32 mmHg.
- Abnormal white blood cell count ($> 12,000/\mu L$ or $< 4,000/\mu L$ or $> 10\%$ bands).

The mediators of stress response, such as interleukin-6 and interferon-gamma have shown to be lower in laparoscopic procedures [7,8].

The systemic benefits of a laparoscopic approach include:

- Decreased pulmonary complications owing to improved postoperative ventilation.
- Decreased postoperative ileus. Although some studies note no significant differences in the return of bowel function between laparoscopic and open operations [9,10], most other studies showed a more rapid return of gastrointestinal function allowing for early oral feeding [11–16]. Early oral feeding plays an important role in preventing gut-bacterial translocation and immunity in the postoperative phase.
- Decreased incidence of wound-related complications.
- Reduced formation of postoperative adhesions.

Several studies have compared commonly performed open versus laparoscopic non-bariatric procedures in severely obese patients. Laparoscopic appendectomy in both acute and perforated appendicitis in the morbidly obese was shown to have shorter length of stay and lower morbidity and cost [17,18]. Laparoscopic colorectal surgery has been found to be safe in some small-scale studies [19]. Laparoscopic radical nephrectomy can also be performed safely in obese patients, possibly with decreased respiratory and cardiac morbidity [20,21]. In gynecological surgery, it has been shown that laparoscopic staging can be used even in obese patients.

Table 41.1 Obesity-related surgical diseases.

Weight related	
Orthopedic	*Vascular*
Joint disease	Varicose veins
Disc prolapse	Thromboembolism
Blount's disease	
Fractures	*Dermal*
	Decubitus ulcers
Gastrointestinal	Intertrigo
Esophageal reflux	
Hemorrhoids	*Gynecologic*
Herniae	Urinary incontinence
Metabolic	
Gastrointestinal	*Genitourinary*
Cholelithiasis	Urolithiasis
Neoplasia	Neoplasia
Esophageal	Renal
Colo-rectal	Endometrial
Biliary	Cancer
Pancreatic	Fibroids
Cirrhosis	Prostate
Vascular	*Breast*
Atherosclerotic	Cancer
Gynecologic	Fibroadenoma
Cesarian sections	

Laparoscopic approaches may involve increased operative time, probably due to the learning curve, but have been shown to decrease hospital stay, ileus and febrile morbidity compared with laparotomy [22]. For bariatric procedures, there are extensive data [23] suggesting safety, efficacy, and lower complication rates with laparoscopic approaches.

Most of the above procedures require the patient to be put in reverse Trendelenburg position (head-up) that has been shown to improve respiratory mechanics and oxygenation in obese patients. However, it is important to also remember that this positioning together with the pneumoperitoneum has an additive effect on reducing venous return and promoting stasis and risk of deep vein thrombosis (DVT). Sequential compression devices help reverse this effect and must be used in all unless there is a strong contraindication.

Obesity in the elderly surgical patient

There has always been a hesitancy to operate on older patients particularly above 65 years of age. Obesity decreases the physiologic reserves of individuals who have adapted cardiac, respiratory, renal, and muscular functions to the increased load imposed by increased body mass. This is particularly relevant in older patients placing special demands on preoperative assessment and optimization. The recent advances in diagnostic imaging and minimally invasive surgery have benefitted this population of aging patients and obese patients.

Aging is associated with changes in body composition. After 20–30 years of age, lean body mass progressively decreases and fat mass increases [24]. There is body fat redistribution with increase in intra-abdominal, intramuscular, and intrahepatic fat, and consequent insulin resistance [25]. This decrease in lean body mass associated with aging is termed sarcopenic obesity. Regular exercise can help reduce age-related and weight loss-induced bone loss and resistance exercise training helps in decreasing sarcopenia [26].

Trauma, emergency surgery, and critical care considerations

Although some early studies found conflicting data, recently obesity has been more strongly associated with adverse outcomes in injured patients [27–30]. It is important to recognize that diagnosis may be delayed in obese patients due to the unreliability of physical examination and the poor quality of diagnostic imaging such as ultrasound and X-rays. Not all institutions are equipped with CT scanners that can accommodate severely obese patients. The special airway risks, increased prothrombotic state, and the increased risk of infection in these patients should not be neglected in the acute setting. Medications should be appropriately dosed considering that in the stressed state, obese patients tend to metabolize protein rather than fat stores. This and other differences in the metabolism of obese patients should be factored in while providing nutritional support. The fact that a patient is

obese, counterintuitively does not rule out the existence of deficiencies [31,32].

Obesity severity assessment

For obese patients undergoing elective or emergent surgery there is no standardized severity score although several have been proposed for risk assessment for bariatric surgery [33]. The existing severity assessment tools for critically ill surgical patients or perioperative assessment for general non-bariatric surgery, e.g., POSSUM, ASA, APACHE 2 or 3, and the AHA Criteria do not incorporate obesity as a parameter. Tables 41.2 and 41.3 list some of the existing obesity severity scores.

Clinical assessment

There are specific challenges and limitations in evaluating and examining obese patients due to their physical characteristics, body habitus, and mobility restrictions.

History

- Emphasis on age of onset/chronology of the obesity.
- Dietary history.

Table 41.2 Obesity surgery mortality risk score (OS-MRS). Score designed to predict risk of mortality from bariatric surgery [33].

One point scored for each of five preoperative factors:
1. Body mass index > 50 kg/m^2
2. Male sex
3. Hypertension
4. Risk for pulmonary embolism
5. Age > 45 years
0–1   Class A – Lowest risk (mortality 0.31%)
2–3   Class B – Intermediate risk (mortality 1.90%)
4–5   Class C – High risk (mortality 7.56%)

Table 41.3 Obesity Severity Index: Physiological [82].

Male sex	1[a]	Neck:thigh > 0.70	2
Age > 40 years	1	Cardiomegaly	2
Smoker	2	Uncontrolled blood pressure	2
Sleep apnea history	1	Hemoglobin > 15 g/L	1
Thromboembolism	1	pCO$_2$ > 45 mmHg	1
Diabetes	1	Hyperinsulinemia	2
		BMI 35–40 = 2; BMI > 40 = 3	

[a] Arbitrary units reflecting risk. Maximum 20 points.

- Relevant social, family, and medication history.
- It is important to evaluate for comorbidities such as coronary artery disease, atherosclerotic vascular disease, diabetes mellitus, obstructive sleep apnea and associated syndromes.
- The endocrine or iatrogenic causes of obesity, which are mostly uncommon but need to be ruled out, include:
  - Hypothalamic obesity (uncommon).
  - Cushing's syndrome (uncommon).
  - Polycystic ovarian disease (common).
  - Genetic syndromes with hypogonadism – Prader–Willi syndrome, Bardet–Biedl syndrome, Ahlstrom's syndrome, Cohen syndrome, and Carpenter syndrome (very uncommon).
- Factors that increase obesity risk:
  - Male gender.
  - Age: men > 45 years and women > 55 years.
  - Adult onset.
  - Cigarette smoking.
  - Hypertension.
  - Hypertriglyceridemia, high LDL cholesterol, low HDL cholesterol.
  - Insulin resistance/glucose intolerance: impaired fasting glucose (IFG), HbA1c elevation.
  - Family history of premature coronary artery disease.

General examination

The BMI is a good screening tool for estimating body fat in people with normal muscle mass on a population level. Disease risk for type 2 diabetes, hypertension, and cardiovascular disease can be estimated based on BMI [34]. It is the fat distribution, however, that determines the severity of the health risk posed by obesity. Abdominal fat that has venous drainage through the liver is associated with insulin resistance.

Waist to hip circumference ratio has been shown to be a better indicator of associated comorbidities although most prospective studies have shown BMI, waist circumference, and waist stature ratio in adults to be similar indicators of body fatness [35,36]. The serum triglyceride levels together with waist circumference can be used as a screening tool [37].

Increased neck circumference is another important risk factor that correlates with visceral adipose tissue (VAT) and insulin resistance. Studies suggest that upper-body subcutaneous fat and epicardial adipose tissue may be pathogenically important. Neck circumference [38] was associated with increase in CVD risk factors even after adjustment for VAT and BMI [39,40].

The next section will go on to emphasize the history, examination, investigations, and interventions relevant to each organ system being discussed.

System-wise pathophysiology and perioperative management

Obesity is associated with an increase in intra-abdominal pressure (IAP). It has been demonstrated that chronically elevated IAP contributes to the pathogenesis of several comorbid conditions associated with obesity, such as hypertension, type 2 diabetes, gastroesophageal reflux, urinary stress incontinence, venous stasis, obstructive sleep apnea, etc. It has also been shown that these conditions improve after weight loss resulting in decreased IAP [41,42].

Airway/pulmonary effects

Obesity is associated with increased risk of pre-, intra- and postoperative pulmonary complications. Obese patients have reduced functional residual capacity (FRC) that is exaggerated while recumbent during anesthesia and pharmacological muscle paralysis. There is also increased intrathoracic pressure from the fat load on the chest.

It is important to examine neck fat distribution that could affect positioning during intubation. A thorough ENT examination is recommended, looking for macroglossia, hypertrophic tonsils, poor dentition, and other associated features that could dictate the need for advanced intubation techniques. Fatty infiltration of the glottis may cause airway closure and rapid desaturation.

Increased intra-abdominal pressure of obesity/intra-abdominal hypertension is associated with obesity contributing to the above problems of decreased FRC and increased risk of gastroesophageal reflux disease (GERD) [43,44]. People with GERD could have microaspiration leading to pneumonitis and resultant interstitial fibrosis over a period of time. A strong independent positive association has also been demonstrated between BMI and adult-onset asthma. The pro-inflammatory state of obesity contributes to increased airway reactivity potentiated by GERD [45].

Respiratory syndromes associated with obesity

It is crucial that all patients be screened for obstructive sleep apnea (OSA) and obesity hypoventilation syndrome (OHS) preoperatively. Obstructive sleep apnea and obesity seem to potentiate each other [46–48]. The incidence and severity of OSA is greater in obese patients compared with non-obese patients [49]. The prevalence of OSA in some studies of bariatric surgical patients was up to 70% [50,51].

Sleep apnea is characterized by recurrent episodes of upper airway obstruction during sleep caused by increased upper airway collapsibility during sleep. Obesity increases pharyngeal collapsibility through mechanical effects on pharyngeal soft tissue and lung volume and through CNS acting signal proteins (adipokines) that affect airway neuromuscular control [52]. Obstructive sleep apnea is associated with glucose intolerance and insulin resistance, which in turn lead to diabetes and cardiovascular disease [53,54], hypertension, heart failure, and pulmonary hypertension.

Obesity hypoventilation syndrome, also known as Pickwickian syndrome, is defined as a BMI $> 30 \, kg/m^2$ and an awake $P_aCO_2 > 45$ mmHg in the absence of a known cause for hypoventilation. The pathogenesis is similar to OSA but there is also an element of decreased ventilatory drive.

Several OSA scoring systems can be used for screening obese patients preoperatively. The simplest "test" of all is to observe the patient in the waiting room, drowsy, sleeping, or snoring. Any abnormalities detected could be useful in determining the need for a preoperative consultation with the pulmonologist and the anesthesiologist who can help formulate a perioperative management plan. The practice guidelines published by the American Society of Anesthesiologists recommends considering preoperative initiation of continuous positive airway pressure (CPAP) therapy for severe OSA, or non-invasive positive pressure ventilation if needed [55]. Preoperative weight loss would indeed be the ideal solution but is not always possible (further discussion on this topic is presented later in this chapter). Obstructive sleep apnea patients who gain weight have an increased risk of OSA progression as opposed to those who lose weight and have improvement of symptoms [56].

Upper airway imaging using CT, MRI, or nasopharyngoscopy provides some insight into the mechanism of OSA and is being used to help in guiding its treatment. Uvulopalatopharyngoplasty (UPPP) is a surgical option that can be considered to help enlarge the oropharynx and reduce upper airway collapsibility although its long-term results are poor [57].

Other tests should include a CBC to rule out polycythemia, pulmonary function tests and ECG (to rule out right heart strain). Exercise tolerance should be evaluated. The ability to climb a flight of stairs or blow out a candle at an arm's length are simple tests that can be performed in the office. There should be a low threshold to perform pulmonary function tests. Bear in mind that the quality of routine chest X-rays may be impaired because of inadequate settings that do not penetrate excess chest wall adipose tissue.

Postoperatively, care should be taken to ensure adequate analgesia (yet judiciously avoiding sedating narcotics), appropriate positioning, monitoring, and early ambulation. Plan for early extubation, chest physiotherapy and mandate rigorous use of the incentive spirometer. These are important in preventing atelectasis. Preoperative exercise therapy and smoking cessation also contribute in reducing postoperative pulmonary complications.

Cardiovascular effects

Changes in cardiac hemodynamics alter left ventricular structure and function leading to heart failure. Most severely obese patients have diastolic heart failure.

Diagnosed or occult congenital heart disease (CHD) increases surgical risk in obese patients. Table 41.4 lists some

Table 41.4 Obesity-related cardiac conditions.

Cardiomyopathy of obesity
Atherosclerotic cardiovascular disease
Heart failure
Systemic hypertension
Pulmonary hypertension
Cor pulmonale
Cardiac arrhythmias
Deep vein thrombosis/pulmonary embolism
Poor exercise capacity

of the cardiac conditions associated with obesity. This risk may be compounded by associated diabetes, elevated serum triglycerides, reduced serum HDL, chronic inflammation, and a prothrombotic state. There is higher risk for perioperative adverse cardiac events in obese patients. Load-related myocardial hypertrophy results in arrhythmias that include atrial fibrillation, atrial flutter, ventricular tachycardia, and bradyarrhythmias.

Obese patients react to the stress of anesthesia and surgery with left ventricular dysfunction. Intraoperative depression of cardiac output that persists after surgery and is not followed by a normal elevation predicts poorer outcome in trauma victims not stratified for weight. There are significant decreases in cardiac index and right and left ventricular stroke work during surgery and this continues during the postoperative period [58]. Ventricular hypertrophy is a part of the cardiomyopathy of obesity that predisposes to tachyarrhythmias or prolonged QTc intervals [59]. The cardiomyopathy is virtually totally reversible by weight loss [60]. Untreated obese patients are at risk because of their limited reserves to withstand the operative stresses of pain and hypoxia.

Exercise testing and echocardiography are limited in obese patients, and have been variable in demonstrating cardiac abnormalities. Dipyridamole stress testing and other radionuclide cardiographic techniques might be necessary in these patients to assess myocardial perfusion and ventricular function as they are often unable to physically exercise, although recent development of a weight-bearing treadmill (AlterG®) should facilitate exercise testing. Laboratory investigations should include a complete lipid panel. Ensure usage of appropriate size cuff to measure blood pressure. Figure 41.2 shows the algorithm published by the American Heart Association and gives a stepwise guide to the preoperative cardiac work-up of obese patients.

Renal effects

Obesity has been shown to cause renal damage starting at the cellular level. Table 41.5 lists some of the changes causing renal damage in obesity [61,62]. Here, too IAP contributes by affecting pressure on renal venous and urinary outflow.

Proteinuria has been demonstrated to be a more important indicator than creatinine clearance. The PREVEND Study (Prevention of Renal and Vascular End Stage Disease) [63] documented that progressively higher values of waist to hip ratio were associated with a higher prevalence of microalbuminuria and diminished eGFR. Again, it is the distribution of adipose tissue rather than the actual BMI itself that is implicated in the pathology. Visceral fat secretes oxidized polyunsaturated fatty acids stimulating aldosterone secretion that impairs podocyte function [64]. Elsayed *et al.* showed that a one standard deviation increase in waist to hip ratio implied a 22% increase in risk of end-stage renal disease, but the same did not hold true for increase in BMI [64].

It has also been suggested that obesity is associated with increased incidence of postoperative renal insufficiency or acute kidney injury in obese patients undergoing cardiac surgery [65] and non-cardiac surgery [66].

Gastrointestinal effects

Consider upper endoscopy (EGD)/esophageal pH monitoring for confirmation or diagnosis of GERD that can have implications during intubation and induction of anesthesia. Obesity is

Table 41.5 Renal damage caused by obesity.

Glomerular hyperfiltration
Albuminuria/proteinuria
Glomerulomegaly
Increased mesangial matrix and mesangial cell proliferation
Podocyte hypertrophy
Focal segmental or global glomerulosclerosis
Interstitial fibrosis

a risk factor for cholelithiasis and relevant symptoms warrant a right upper quadrant ultrasound. Due to the high prevalence of non-alcoholic steatohepatitis (NASH), steatosis, and unexpected cirrhosis in obese patients, it is important to include liver tests in the preoperative evaluation as this may influence anesthetic choice [67].

Nasogastric tube placement is indicated for certain procedures and can be difficult owing to the common fat pad at the gastroesophageal junction of patients with compromised lower esophagus due to increased intra-abdominal pressure and GERD, and can lead to perforation. For this reason, whenever possible gastric intubation should be done endoscopically or during open procedures, a guiding finger, and/or inspection.

Infectious complications

Obese patients are at a greater risk for wound infection than patients of normal weight [68]. It is not certain if there is a primary immune defect in obesity. Susceptibility to pneumonia from respiratory compromise and to cellulitis from intertriginous changes under an abdominal panniculus or in the edematous lower legs can be explained even without immune compromise. There is evidence though for impaired immunocompetence in obese patients (Table 41.6).

It is important to pay attention to the routine infection control measures such as showering on the evening before and morning of surgery, use of hair clippers, and the use of the correct dose of weight-adjusted prophylactic antibiotics.

Hypercoagulability

Venous thromboembolism (VTE) is the most dreaded complication of surgery in obese patients. It too is related to the increased intra-abdominal and intrathoracic pressure of obesity and is compounded by operations. Both obesity and

Figure 41.2 Cardiac and pulmonary algorithm assessment for elective non-cardiac surgery in severely obese patients. CAD, coronary artery disease; ECG, electrocardiogram; CVD, cardiovascular disease; RVH, right ventricular hypertrophy; LBBB, left bundle-branch block [86]. Reprinted with permission from *Circulation* 2009; **120**: 86–95; ©2009 American Heart Association, Inc.

Table 41.6 Defects in the immune system of obese patients.

Abnormalities in the leptin-proopiomelanocortin system [83]
Elevated adipose tissue levels of TNFα [84]
Hypercortisolism
Impaired leukocyte function [85]

Table 41.7 Comorbid conditions contributing to thromboembolism in obesity.

Condition	Chemical abnormality
Dyslipidemia	↑ Serum triglycerides ↑ Serum low-density lipoprotein cholesterol ↓ Serum high-density lipoprotein cholesterol ↑ Blood viscosity
Diabetes	↑ Serum antithrombin III ↑ Serum fibrinogen ↑ Serum fibronectin ↓ Tissue plasminogen activity
Hypertension	
Renal failure	

Table 41.8 Increased body fat mass predisposes to thromboembolism in obesity.

↑ Intra-abdominal pressure
Varicose veins
↑ Blood volume/intrathoracic pressure
Cardiopulmonary failure
Polycythemia
↑ Serum-free fatty acids
Glucose intolerance/hyperinsulinemia
Fatty liver
↓ Locomotion
Hypostasis

intra-abdominal and intrathoracic surgery are risk factors for venous thromboembolism. Tables 41.7 and 41.8 outline the factors involved in the pathogenesis of VTE in obese patients. Obese patients have increased levels of fibrinogen, factor VIII, and von Willebrand factor. They also have decreased antithrombin III levels and decreased fibrinolytic activity.

The association between the abdominal obesity component of metabolic syndrome and VTE has been demonstrated in several studies. Obesity is associated with elevated levels of thrombosis promoting factors and decrease in fibrinolysis. Plasminogen activator inhibitor 1 (PAI-1), a prothrombotic peptide, is abundant in adipose tissue and related to insulin resistance and has been linked to obesity-related thromboembolism [69].

Preoperative evaluation should elicit previous history of deep vein thrombosis (DVT) or pulmonary embolism (PE) that could be an indicator for further testing and thrombophilia screening. A baseline duplex ultrasound to detect or document preexisting DVT may be useful. Consider a prophylactic inferior venacaval filter for high-risk patients (history of venous stasis disease, BMI > 60, known hypercoagulable state) [50].

Non-pharmacological strategies for VTE prevention should include pneumatic compression devices fitted before the start of anesthesia and should stay on until full mobilization postoperatively. The importance of early ambulation cannot be over-emphasized and should be mandated. There are quite a few papers that have made recommendations for thromboprophylaxis in obese patients undergoing bariatric surgery that can be extrapolated to obese patients undergoing non-bariatric surgeries [50,45,70].

Pharmacological prophylaxis may include administration of low-dose warfarin before elective surgeries to restore antithrombin III levels, especially in obese patients with a history of prior VTE [71]. Generally, low molecular weight heparin (LMWH) is easy to administer and widely used but the usual 40 mg dose may not be adequate [72]. The LMWH dose should be titrated to a therapeutic anti-Xa level that is 0.1–0.4 IU/mL. The infusion of dextrose solutions in the pre- and postoperative period to suppress free fatty acid release has also been recommended although the antilipolytic effects of insulin may be just as effective.

Fluid and electrolyte abnormalities

Extracellular water increases with expanding fat mass through unknown mechanisms [73]. This influences distribution volumes of medications as well as volume status.

Obese patients often have histories of diuretic use either for treatment of hypertension or for treatment of "swelling" or edema. This together with low-calorie diets and chronic malnutrition may result in low potassium levels [74]. Comorbid conditions such as hyperinsulinemia and hypertension can contribute to electrolyte abnormalities. Fatty liver is associated with decreased protein synthesis and decreased serum albumin that in turn predisposes to fluid and electrolyte abnormalities [75].

Preoperative weight loss

It is logical to recommend nutritionally sound weight loss before elective operations. Preoperative weight loss may reverse some of the pathophysiological changes of obesity but it must be gradual. Some studies have looked at preoperative weight loss with very low energy diet for 2 weeks prior to bariatric surgery and found that there was significant reduction in liver volume and progressive reduction of visceral adipose tissue. The functional benefit was that there was improved operative exposure [70,76,77]. There are no randomized or observational trials to assess the impact of the above on decreasing operative time or complications. Starvation and rapid weight loss may lead to cardiac arrhythmias and sudden death. It is unrealistic to expect full cooperation with preoperative weight-loss programs.

The increasing numbers of severely obese patients and the improved outcomes of anti-obesity surgery, particularly through the laparoscopic approach, have led to a wider adoption of surgical treatment of obesity. Preoperative weight loss has been evaluated as a method for reducing operative complications in several studies. A large study by Benotti *et al.* found that preoperative weight loss was associated with a reduction in complications after gastric bypass [78]. It is logical to assume that the results can be extrapolated to include obese patients undergoing non-bariatric surgeries as well. Surgical weight loss has the same effect as caloric restriction affecting the same molecular pathways and preventing or even curing fatal or non-fatal diseases. Dyslipidemia and type 2 diabetes influence thrombogenesis and atherosclerosis associated with hypertension, stroke, and coronary artery disease all of which are improved by bariatric surgery [79]. Mechanical or physical weight-related conditions improved by surgical weight loss include sleep apnea, pulmonary function, stress urinary incontinence, congestive heart failure, herniae, and osteoarthritis [80,81].

Given all the benefits and relative safety of bariatric surgery, it is important to consider referring candidates for such surgery as a part of a preoperative work-up when other procedures are being considered. The three most commonly performed bariatric procedures are gastric bypass, laparoscopic adjustable gastric banding, and biliopancreatic diversion, all of which can be performed laparoscopically at specialized centers.

Summary

Obesity is a highly prevalent disorder worldwide and is associated with several conditions requiring operations. The surgeon, anesthesiologist, and internist taking care of the obese patient must be aware of potential complications and the ways to recognize and prevent perioperative complications. Obesity in itself should not be a contraindication for surgery but should be an indication for a more thorough work-up and more attentive care. The advances in surgical techniques and laparoscopy together with better understanding of risk factors will improve work-up and preparation of obese patients for surgery thus reducing morbidity and mortality.

References

1. Flegal KM, Carroll MD, Ogden CL, Curtin LR. Prevalence and trends in obesity among US adults, 1999–2008. *J Am Med Assoc* 2010; **303**: 235–41.

2. Fontaine KR, Redden DT, Wang C, Westfall AO, Allison DB. Years of life lost due to obesity. *J Am Med Assoc* 2003; **289**: 187–93.

3. Isono S. Obstructive sleep apnea of obese adults: pathophysiology and perioperative airway management. *Anesthesiology* 2009; **110**: 908–21.

4. Vassallo J. Pathogenesis of obesity. *J Malta Coll Pharm Pract* 2007; **12**: 19–22.

5. Decoda Study Group, Nyamdori R, Qiao Q *et al.* BMI compared with central obesity indicators in relation to diabetes and hypertension in Asians. *Obesity (Silver Spring)* 2008; **16**: 1622–35.

6. Bray GA, Clearfield MB, Fintel DJ. Nelinson DS. Overweight and obesity: the pathogenesis of cardiometabolic risk. *Clin Cornerstone* 2009; **9**: 30–40.

7. Wang SZ, Chen Y, Lin HY, Chen LW. Comparison of surgical stress response to laparoscopic and open radical cystectomy. *World J Urol* 2010; **28**: 451–5.

8. Miyake H, Kawabagta G, Gotoh A *et al.* Comparison of surgical stress between laparoscopy and open surgery in the field or urology by measurement of humoral mediators. *Int J Urol* 2002; **9**: 329–33.

9. Bokey EL, Moore JW, Chapuis PH, Newland RC. Morbidity and mortality following laparoscopic-assisted right hemicolectomy for cancer. *Dis Colon Rectum* 1996; **39**(10 Suppl): S24–8.

10. Ho YH, Tan M, Eu KW, Leong A, Choen FS. Laparoscopic-assisted compared with open total colectomy in treating slow transit constipation. *Aust N Z J Surg* 1997; **67**: 562–65.

11. Young-Fadok TM, HallLong K, McConnell EJ, Gomez RG, Cabanela RL. Advantages of laparoscopic resection for ileocolic Crohn's disease. Improved outcomes and reduced costs. *Surg Endosc* 2001; **15**: 450–4.

12. Young-Fadok TM, Radice E, Nelson H, Harmsen WS. Benefits of laparoscopic-assisted colectomy for colon polyps: a case-matches series. *Mayo Clin Proc* 2000; **75**: 344–8.

13. Muckleroy SK, Ratzer ER, Fenoglio ME. Laparoscopic colon surgery for benign disease: a comparison to open surgery. *J Surg Laparosc Surg* 1999; **3**: 33–7.

14. Kakisako K, Sato K, Adachi Y *et al.* Laparoscopic colectomy for Dukes A colon cancer. *Surg Laparosc Endosc Percutan Tech* 2000; **10**: 66–70.

15. Marubashi S, Yano H, Monden T *et al.* The usefulness, indications, and complications of laparoscopy-assisted colectomy in comparison with those of open colectomy for colorectal carcinoma. *Surg Today* 2000; **30**: 491–6.

16. Marcello PW, Milsom JW, Wong SK *et al.* Laparoscopic restorative proctocolectomy: case-matched comparative study with open restorative proctocolectomy. *Dis Colon Rectum* 2000; **43**: 604–8.

17. Varela JE, Hinojosa MW, Nguyen NT. Laparoscopy should be the approach of choice for acute appendicitis in the morbidly obese. *Am J Surg* 2008; **196**: 218–22.

18. Corneille MG, Steigelman MB, Myers JG *et al.* Laparoscopic appendectomy is superior to open appendectomy in obese patients. *Am J Surg* 2007; **194**: 877–81.

19. Kamoun S, Alves A, Bretagnol F *et al.* Outcomes of laparoscopic colorectal surgery in obese and nonobese patients: a case-matched study of 18 patients. *Am J Surg* 2009; **198**: 450–5.

20. Fugita OEH, Chan DY, Roberts WW, Kavoussi LR, Jarrett TW. Laparoscopic radical nephrectomy in obese patients: outcomes and technical considerations. *Urology* 2004; **63**: 247–52.

21. Kapoor A, Nassir A, Chew B et al. Comparison of laparoscopic radical renal surgery in morbidly obese and non-obese patients. *J Endourol* 2004; **18**: 657–60.

22. Eltabbakh GH, Shamonki MI, Moody JM, Garafano LL. Hysterectomy for obese women with endometrial cancer: laparoscopy or laparotomy: *Gynecol Oncol* 2000; **78**: 329–35.

23. Nguyen NT, Lee SL, Goldman C et al. Comparison of pulmonary function and postoperative pain after laparoscopic versus open gastric bypass: a randomized trial. *J Am Coll Surg* 2001; **192**: 469–76.

24. Baumgartner RN, Stauber PM, McHugh D, Koehler KM, Garry PJ. Cross-sectional age differences in persons 60+ years of age. *J Gerontol A Biol Sci Med Sci* 1995; **50**: M307–16.

25. Carter A, Côté M, Lemieux I et al. Age-related differences in inflammatory markers in men: contribution of visceral adiposity. *Metabolism* 2009; **58**: 1452–8.

26. Ross R, Pedwell H, Rissanen J. Response of total and regional lean tissue and skeletal muscle to a program of energy restriction and resistance exercise. *Int J Obes Relat Metab Disord* 1995; **19**: 781–7.

27. Choban PS, Weireter LJ, Maynes C. Obesity and increased mortality in blunt trauma. *J Trauma* 1991; **31**: 1253–7.

28. Neville A, Brown CV, Weng J, Demetriades D, Velmahos G. Obesity is an independent risk factor for mortality in severely injured blunt trauma patients. *Arch Surg* 2004; **139**: 983–7.

29. Brown CV, Neville AL, Rhee P et al. The impact of obesity on the outcomes of 1,153 critically injured blunt trauma patients. *J Trauma* 2005; **59**: 1048–51.

30. Byrnes MC, McDaniel MD, Moore MB, Helmer SD, Smith RS. The effect of obesity on outcomes among injured patients. *J Trauma* 2005; **58**: 232–7.

31. Xanthakos SA. Nutritional deficiencies in obesity and after bariatric surgery. *Pediatr Clin North Am* 2009; **56**: 1105–21.

32. Kaidar-Person O, Person B, Szomstein S, Rosenthal RJ. Nutritional deficiencies in morbidly obese patients: a new form of malnutrition? Part A: Vitamins. *Obes Surg* 2008; **18**: 870–6.

33. DeMaria EJ, Murr M, Byrne K et al. Validation of the obesity surgery mortality risk score in a multicenter study proves it stratifies mortality risk in patients undergoing gastric bypass for morbid obesity. *Ann Surg* 2007; **246**: 578–84.

34. Greenway F. Clinical evaluation of the obese patient. *Prim Care* 2003; **30**: 341–56.

35. Flegal KM, Shepherd JA, Looker AC et al. Comparisons of percentage body fat, body mass index, waist circumference, and waist-stature ratio in adults. *Am J Clin Nutr* 2009; **89**: 500–5.

36. Qiao Q, Nyamdorj R. Is the association of type II diabetes with waist circumference or waist-to-hip ratio stronger than that with body mass index? *Eur J Clin Nutr* 2010; **64**: 30–4.

37. Kahn HS, Valdez R. Metabolic risks identified by the combination of enlarged waist and elevated triacylglycerol concentration. *Am J Clin Nutr* 2003; **78**: 928–34.

38. Sjöström CD, Håkangärd AC, Lissner L, Sjöström L. Body compartment and subcutaneous adipose tissue distribution – risk factor patterns in obese subjects. *Obes Res* 1995; **3**: 9–22.

39. Yang L. Visceral adiposity is closely correlated with neck circumference and represents a significant indicator of insulin resistance in WHO grade III obesity. *Clin Endocrinol* 2010; **73**: 197–200.

40. Preis SR. Neck circumference as a novel measure of cardiometabolic risk: the Framingham Heart study. *J Clin Endocrinol Metab* 2010; **95**: 3701–10.

41. Varela JE, Hinojosa M, Nguyen N. Correlations between intra-abdominal pressure and obesity-related co-morbidities. *Surg Obes Relat Dis* 2009; **5**: 524–8.

42. Nguyen NT, Lee SL, Anderson JT et al. Evaluation of intra-abdominal pressure after laparoscopic and open gastric bypass. *Obes Surg* 2001; **11**: 40–5.

43. Ayazi S, Hagen JA, Chan LS et al. Obesity and gastroesophageal reflux: quantifying the association between body mass index, esophageal acid exposure, and lower esophageal sphincter status in a large series of patients with reflux symptoms. *J Gastrointest Surg* 2009; **13**: 1440–7.

44. Schneider JH, Küper M, Königsrainer A, Brücher B. Transient lower esophageal sphincter relatation in morbid obesity. *Obes Surg* 2009; **19**: 595–600.

45. Davis G, Patel JA, Gagne DJ. Pulmonary considerations in obesity and the bariatric surgical patient. *Med Clin North Am* 2007; **91**: 433–42.

46. Naimark A, Cherniack RM. Compliance of the respiratory system and its components in health and obesity. *J Appl Physiol* 1960; **15**: 377–82.

47. Phillips BG, Hisel TM, Kato M et al. Recent weight gain in patients with newly diagnosed obstructive sleep apnea. *J Hypertens* 1999; **17**: 1297–300.

48. Phillips BG, Kato M, Narkiewicz K, Choe I, Somers VK. Increases in leptin levels, sympathetic drive, and weight gain in obstructive sleep apenea. *Am J Physiol Heart Circ Physiol* 2000; **279**: H234–7.

49. Kim TH, Chun BS, Lee HW, Kim JS. Differences of upper airway morphology according to obesity: study with cephalometry and dynamic MD-CT. *Clin Exp Otorhinolaryngol* 2010; **3**: 147–52.

50. Kuruba R, Koche LS, Murr MM. Preoperative assessment and perioperative care of patients undergoing bariatric surgery. *Med Clin North Am* 2007; **91**: 339–51.

51. Association of Anaesthetists of Great Britain and Ireland. *Peri-operative Management of the Morbidly Obese Patient*. June 2007. www.docstoc.com/docs/28872663/PERI-OPERATIVE-MANAGEMENT-OF-THE-MORBIDLY-OBESE PATIENT?utm_source=email&utm_medium=email&utm_campaign=2&utm_content=3

52. Schwartz AR. Obesity and obstructive sleep apnea: pathogenic mechanisms and therapeutic approaches. *Proc Am Thorac Soc* 2008; **5**: 185–92.

53. Ip MS, Lam B, Ng MM et al. Obstructive sleep apnea is independently associated with insulin resistance. *Am J Respir Crit Care Med* 2002; **165**: 670–6.

54. Punjabi NM, Shahar E, Redline S *et al.* Sleep-disordered breathing, glucose intolerance, and insulin resistance: the Sleep Heart Health Study. *Am J Epidemiol* 2004; **160**: 521–30.

55. Gross JB, Bachenberg KL, Benumof JL *et al.* Practice guidelines for the perioperative management of patients with obstructive sleep apnea: a report by the American Society of Anesthesiologists Task Force on perioperative management of patients with obstructive sleep apnea. *Anesthesia* 2006; **104**: 1081–93.

56. Peppard PE, Young T, Palta M, Dempsey J, Skatrud J. Longitudinal study of moderate weight change and sleep-disordered breathing. *J Am Med Assoc* 2000; **284**: 3015–21.

57. Fleetham JA. Upper airway imaging in relation to obstructive sleep apnea. *Clin Chest Med* 1992; **13**: 399–416.

58. Agarwal N, Shibutani K, San Filippo JA, Del Guercio LR. Hemodynamic and respiratory changes in surgery in the morbidly obese. *Surgery* 1982; **92**: 226–34.

59. Alpert MA, Terry BE, Cohen MV *et al.* The electrocardiogram in morbid obesity. *Am J Cardiol* 2000; **85**: 908–10.

60. Alpert MA, Terry BE, Hamm CR *et al.* Effect of weight loss on the ECG of normotensive morbidly obese patients. *Chest* 2001; **119**: 507–10.

61. Lastra G, Manrique C, Sowers JR. Obesity, cardiometabolic syndrome, and chronic kidney disease: the weight of the evidence. *Adv Chronic Kidney Dis* 2006; **13**: 365–73.

62. Serra A, Romero R, Lopez D, Navarro M *et al.* Renal injury in the extremely obese patients with normal renal function. *Kidney Int* 2008; **73**: 947–55.

63. Diercks GF, van Boven AJ, Hillege HL *et al.* Microalbuminuria is independently associated with ischaemic electrocardiographic abnormalities in a large non-diabetic population. *Eur Heart J* 2000; **21**: 1922–7.

64. Elsayed EF, Sarnak MJ, Tighiouart H *et al.* Waist-to-hip ratio, body mass index, and subsequent kidney disease and death. *Am J Kidney Dis* 2008; **52**: 29–38.

65. Virani SS, Nambi V, Lee W *et al.* Obesity: an independent predictor of in-hospital postoperative renal insufficiency among patients undergoing cardiac surgery? *Tex Heart Inst J* 2009; **36**: 540–5.

66. Glance LG, Wissler R, Mukamel DB *et al.* Perioperative outcomes among patients with the modified metabolic syndrome who are undergoing noncardiac surgery. *Anesthesiology* 2010; **113**: 859–72.

67. Machado M, Marques-Vidal P, Cortez-Pinto, H. Hepatic histology in obese patients undergoing bariatric surgery. *J Hepatol* 2006; **45**: 600–6.

68. Dindo D, Muller MK, Weber M, Clavien PA. Obesity in general elective surgery. *Lancet* 2003; **361**: 2032–5.

69. Prandoni P, Bilora F, Marchiori A *et al.* An association between atherosclerosis and venous thrombosis. *N Engl J Med* 2003; **348**: 1435–41.

70. Colles SL, Dixon JB, Marks P, Strauss BJ, O'Brien PE. Preoperative weight loss with a very-low-energy diet: quantitation of changes in liver and abdominal fat by serial imaging. *Am J Clin Nutr* 2006; **84**: 304–11.

71. Bern MM, Bothe A Jr, Bistrian B *et al.* Effects of low-dose warfarin on antithrombin III levels in morbidly obese patients. *Surgery* 1983; **94**: 78–83.

72. Simone EP, Madan AK, Tichansky DS, Kuhl DA, Lee MD. Comparison of two low-molecular-weight heparin dosing regimens for patients undergoing laparoscopic bariatric surgery. *Surg Endosc* 2008; **22**: 2392–5.

73. Waki M, Kral JG, Mazariegos M *et al.* Relative expansion of extracellular fluid in obese vs. non-obese women. *Am J Physiol* 1991; **26**: E199–203.

74. Colt EWD, Wang J, Stallone F *et al.* A possible low intra-cellular potassium in obesity. *Am J Clin Nutr* 1981; **34**: 367–72.

75. Kral JG, Lundholm K, Sjöström L *et al.* Hepatic lipid metabolism in severe human obesity. *Metabolism* 1977; **26**: 1025–31.

76. Mechanick JI, Kushner RF, Sugerman HJ *et al.* American Association of Clinical Endocrinologists, The Obesity Society, and American Society for Metabolic and Bariatric Surgery medical guidelines for clinical practice for the perioperative nutritional, metabolic, and nonsurgical support of the bariatric surgery patient. *Endocr Pract* 2008; **14** (Suppl 1): 1–83.

77. Fris RJ. Preoperative low energy diet diminishes liver size. *Obes Surg* 2004; **14**: 1165–70.

78. Benotti PN, Still CD, Wood GC *et al.* Preoperative weight loss before bariatric surgery. *Arch Surg* 2009; **144**: 1150–5.

79. Sugerman HJ, Kral JG. Evidence-based medicine reports on obesity surgery: a critique. *Int J Obes* 2005; **29**: 735–45.

80. Karlsson J, Taft C, Sjöström L, Sullivan M. Ten-year trends in health-related quality of life after surgical and conventional treatment for severe obesity: the SOS intervention study. *Int J Obes* 2007; **31**: 1248–61.

81. Kral JG, Otterbeck P, Touza MG. Preventing and treating the accelerated ageing of obesity. *Maturitas* 2010; **66**: 223–30.

82. Kral JG. Obesity. In Lubin MF, Walker HK, Smith III RB, eds. *Medical Management of the Surgical Patient.* Fourth Edition. Philadelphia, PA: Lippincott; 2006, pp. 467–78.

83. Smith AI, Funder JW. Proopiomelanocortin processing in the pituitary, central nervous system, and peripheral tissues. *Endocr Rev* 1988; **9**: 159–79.

84. Hotamisligil GS, Arner P, Caro JF, Atkinson RL, Spiegelman BM. Increased adipose tissue expression of tumor necrosis factor-a in human obesity and insulin resistance. *J Clin Invest* 1995; **95**: 2409–15.

85. Koltermann OG, Olefsky JM, Kurakara C, Taylor K. A defect in cell-mediated immune function in insulin-resistant diabetic and obese subjects. *J Lab Clin Med* 1980; **96**: 535–43.

86. Poirier P, Alpert MA, Fleisher LA *et al.* Cardiovascular evaluation and management of severely obese patients undergoing surgery. *Circulation* 2009; **120**: 86–95.

Chapter

Transplantation medicine

42

Sudha Tata, Remzi Bag, Ram Subramanian, Kathleen Nilles, and Stephen Pastan

Solid organ transplantation

The field of organ transplantation has been revolutionized over the past decades. Major advances have been made in surgical technique, immunosuppressive management, prevention and treatment of the infections that occur in the immunocompromised host, as well as in the screening and selection of candidates for transplantation. These advances have translated into a steady improvement in organ and patient survival, and have allowed transplantation to be made available to an increasing number of patients. This chapter will review lung, liver, kidney, and pancreas transplantation with a special emphasis on perioperative medical care.

Lung transplantation

Introduction

Lung transplantation (LTx) is the standard of care for end-stage lung diseases that do not respond to conventional medical or surgical treatments. The annual number of lung transplants has significantly increased to approximately 2,800 worldwide due to consistent growth in the number of bilateral lung transplants (BLTx) during the past 15 years [1,2]. Of the 28,664 solid organ transplants performed in the USA in 2010, 1,770 were adult lung transplants [3].

For end-stage lung diseases, LTx offers better survival and quality of life. As the technical difficulties with surgery have been addressed and critical care management improved, the first-month mortality has declined to 5–7% resulting in 3 month-, 1-, 5-, and 10-year survivals of 92.6%, 84%, 53.5%, and 27% respectively [2]. Long-term survival continues to be limited due to chronic rejection (bronchiolitis obliterans syndrome) and ensuing recurrent infections [4].

Candidates should have end-stage lung disease with limited life expectancy of 12–24 months despite optimal medical therapy. Disease-specific selection guidelines can be found in the literature [5]. Since 2005, a new lung allocation algorithm was initiated in the USA based on the diagnosis, severity of illness, and net transplant benefit within 1 year. Diagnostic groups are summarized in Table 42.1. Median time to transplant varies and is less than 35 days for those in the highest quartile [6].

Donor shortage continues to be a limiting factor worldwide. In 2009, lungs from only 1,570 of 14,632 donors were suitable for transplantation in the USA. Attempts to increase the donor pool include living donor lobar donation, donation after cardiac death, ex vivo lung perfusion and donors with extended criteria [6,7]. Use of donors with extended criteria such as reduced arterial oxygenation, donor age between 55–65, unilateral infiltrate, aspiration, trauma or > 20 pack-year smoking history may increase postoperative and long-term complications.

Bilateral lung transplant is the procedure of choice in pulmonary vascular or suppurative diseases. Therefore, almost

Table 42.1 Lung Allocation Score (LAS) primary diagnostic groupings for lung transplant candidates.

LAS lung disease diagnosis grouping	
Group A (Obstructive lung disease)	Chronic obstructive pulmonary disease (COPD) due to chronic bronchitis or emphysema Lymphangioleiomyomatosis (LAM) Bronchiectasis Sarcoidosis with a mean pulmonary artery (PA) pressure ≤ 30 mmHg
Group B (Pulmonary vascular disease)	Idiopathic pulmonary arterial hypertension (iPAH) Eisenmenger's syndrome
Group C (Cystic fibrosis or immunodeficiency disorders)	Cystic fibrosis (CF) Immunodeficiency disorders such as hypogammaglobulinemia
Group D (Restrictive lung disease)	Idiopathic pulmonary fibrosis (IPF) Sarcoidosis with mean PA pressure > 30 mmHg Obliterative bronchiolitis (non-retransplant)

Modified from Organ Procurement and Transplantation Network; http://optn. transplant.hrsa.gov/ar2008/default.htm.

Medical Management of the Surgical Patient, ed. Michael F. Lubin, Thomas F. Dodson, and Neil H. Winawer. Published by Cambridge University Press. © Cambridge University Press 2013.

all of the single lung transplantations (SLTx) are performed in obstructive and restrictive diseases for which BLTx may also be done. Surgical approach for BLTx can be clam shell with sternal transection, anterolateral thoracotomies with sternal sparing, median sternotomy or two separate posterolateral incisions [8]. Hypoxia, progressive hypercapnia, and persistent acidosis (pH < 7.2) with hemodynamic instability are indications for cardiopulmonary bypass (CPB). Other indications for CPB include diagnosis of pulmonary artery hypertension (PAH) and need for cardioplegia for cardiac repair or coronary artery bypass grafting. Some centers utilize CPB routinely to allow better control of reperfusion pressures.

Postoperative management

Postoperative stay and operative mortality

The expected postoperative hospital stay is 7–21 days in the USA. Thirty-day mortality at high-volume centers ($\geq$ 20 LTx/year) is 4.1%. Very low-volume centers have a 30-day mortality of 9.6% [9]. Bronchial dehiscence, severe pulmonary hypertension (PH), cardiopulmonary bypass (CPB), prolonged air leak, and primary graft dysfunction (PGD) are associated with increased risk of postoperative mortality. Although uncommon, preoperative mechanical ventilation and extracorporeal membrane oxygenation (ECMO) are strong risk factors for mortality after LTx. Other risk factors include older recipient age and underlying lung disease (PAH, idiopathic pulmonary fibrosis (IPF)). Comorbidities such as coronary artery disease (CAD), diabetes mellitus, cachexia, obesity, collagen vascular diseases particularly scleroderma, and esophageal dysfunction are also important factors. There are also additional risks in poor pre-transplant functional status, pre-transplant colonization with *Aspergillus* species, re-transplantation, preformed HLA antibodies, lower pre-transplant forced expiratory volume in 1 second, and longer ischemic time.

Ventilator and hemodynamic management, immunosuppression, prevention and treatment of infection, prevention of other organ dysfunction, and detection of early rejection are the focus of perioperative management.

Special monitoring required

All patients are transferred to the ICU for close monitoring. Most patients continue to need invasive mechanical ventilation during the immediate postoperative period. For SLTx split lung ventilation with two ventilators may be required if there is a significant difference in lung compliances. Hemodynamic monitoring consists of continuous measurement of pulmonary arterial pressures, cardiac output, mixed venous oxygenation via pulmonary artery catheter, and arterial pressure measurement. Other monitoring includes continuous ECG, continuous pulse oximetry and occasionally co-oximetry, continuous assessment of urinary output, quality (sanguinous vs serous) and quantity of chest tube drainage. Arterial blood gas, electrolyte and cell counts are performed every 4 to 6 hours

initially. Trough levels of immunosuppressive medications are performed daily. Chest X-ray is done immediately on arrival to ICU and at least daily while intubated. A bronchoscopy is performed in the operating room or immediately after arrival to ICU to assess the bronchial anastomosis and airways, provide pulmonary toilet, and obtain respiratory specimens for culture. All invasive monitoring lines are removed as soon as possible.

Ventilator and hemodynamic management

Occasionally, lung transplant recipients may be extubated in the OR, but most arrive in ICU intubated and sedated. Standard ICU protocols and ventilator bundles with low tidal volume, lowest possible F_iO_2 and settings minimizing peak airway pressures to < 25 cm H_2O are followed. Minimal positive end expiratory pressure (PEEP) is preferred unless significant respiratory failure is present. Efforts are made to extubate patients with standard weaning trials as soon as possible provided there are no signs of PGD. Supplemental oxygen is necessary for most patients after extubation to keep oxyhemoglobin saturation above 90% during ambulation and at rest. Most patients will be oxygenating adequately on room air by the time of discharge.

Particular attention is given to pulmonary toilet with closed circuit endotracheal suction, incentive spirometry, positive expiratory pressure vibratory therapy, and external chest physiotherapy to mobilize secretions, as the cough reflex and bronchial mucociliary transport are impaired due to surgery. Bronchoscopy is performed prior to extubation to reinspect the bronchial anastomoses and clear secretions. Physical therapy is initiated early for patient mobilization and continued through discharge.

The allograft has increased capillary permeability and is prone to pulmonary edema, therefore fluid management focuses on negative fluid balance provided cardiac output is maintained. Colloids are preferred over crystalloids for fluid resuscitation.

Any change in gas exchange, compliance (tidal volume, peak and plateau pressures, auto-PEEP), forced expiratory volume in 1 second (FEV1), or vital signs requires further evaluation.

Alimentation

Oral diet is begun with clear liquids after extubation. Nutritional support using nasoenteric tubes is an option when endotracheal intubation is prolonged.

Immunosuppression

Immunosuppression is mostly center specific. Two-thirds of the centers use induction with an antilymphocyte antibody [3]. Maintenance immunosuppression is started on the day of surgery and is achieved by combination of the following three classes of medications: (1) calcineurin inhibitors (tacrolimus or cyclosporine), (2) antimetabolite cell cycle inhibitors (azathioprine, mycophenolate mofetil, or mycophenolate sodium), and (3) corticosteroids. Sirolimus or everolimus, mammalian target of rapamycin inhibitors may seldom be used, but are contraindicated in the first 6–12 weeks post-transplant due to reports of bronchial dehiscence. Optimal immunosuppression navigates the delicate balance of toxicity, rejection, and infection risk, hence requires monitoring of therapeutic drug levels and side-effects closely.

Antibiotic coverage

Broad-spectrum prophylactic antibiotics are started preoperatively in light of the patient's history of airway organisms and adjusted according to the susceptibilities of donor or recipient specimens. Intravenous ganciclovir or oral valganciclovir are used for cytomegalovirus (CMV) mismatched transplants and occasionally for any CMV positivity in lieu of surveillance. Trimethoprim sulfamethoxazole is used for prophylaxis against *Pneumocystis jiroveci*. Some centers use inhaled amphotericin B, nystatin suspension, or an azole for fungal prophylaxis.

Pain management

Adequate pain control not only ensures patient comfort, but also allows the patient to engage fully in chest physiotherapy and early mobilization. Non-steroid anti-inflammatory drugs are avoided due to potential renal toxicity. Some utilize a thoracic epidural catheter placed either intraoperatively or before extubation. Narcotic analgesics may be used judiciously, but may cause somnolence, hypoventilation, and CO_2 retention.

Deep venous thrombosis prophylaxis

A mechanical prophylactic device, such as compression stockings or an intermittent compression device is started preoperatively until use of heparin is deemed safe by absence of any significant bleeding or sanguinous chest tube drainage.

Postoperative complications
Primary graft dysfunction

Primary graft dysfunction (PGD) is a severe form of ischemia–reperfusion injury with an incidence of 10–25% and 30-day mortality of 50%. Increased P_aO_2/F_iO_2 ratio with infiltrates on CXR without an underlying etiology is typical. The clinical presentation is similar to acute respiratory distress syndrome (ARDS). Patients with IPF and PH are at increased risk of developing PGD. Other risk factors include use of CPB, blood product transfusion, and some donor variables (poor preservation of the graft, prolonged mechanical ventilation, aspiration, hemodynamic instability after brain death, donor age > 45 years) [10]. The diagnosis is established by exclusion of possible alternative processes with similar clinical presentation such as aspiration, pneumonia, volume overload, myocardial dysfunction, hyperacute rejection, or obstruction of pulmonary venous anastomosis. The management is supportive and similar to treatment of ARDS. Inhaled nitric oxide improves hemodynamics and ventilation perfusion matching in this

setting. Extracorporeal membrane oxygenation (ECMO) may be required when hemodynamic instability accompanies PGD. Survivors of PGD have longer ICU and hospital stay with worse long-term lung function, increased risk of chronic rejection, and decreased long-term survival.

Respiratory failure

Respiratory failure due to ARDS, pneumonia, sepsis, transfusion-related lung injury, hemodynamic instability (e.g., perioperative bleeding, volume overload, myocardial dysfunction, arrhythmia, shock with metabolic acidosis, obstruction of pulmonary venous anastomosis) or host–allograft interactions (PGD, hyperacute, acute, antibody-mediated rejection) can ensue and lead to prolonged mechanical ventilation. The management focus is to detect and treat the underlying cause, and to provide ventilator support with a low tidal volume alveolar protective strategy and limited use of PEEP. Inspection of pressure, volume and flow waveforms, adequate pain control and anxiolytics are useful in addressing patient–ventilator dyssynchrony. Paralytics and tracheostomy are seldom needed. Intercurrent infections, postoperative diaphragmatic dysfunction due to phrenic nerve injury, and critical care neuromyopathy may delay liberation from ventilatory support.

Hypotension and shock

Hypotension is very common intra- and postoperatively. Intraoperative clamping of the pulmonary artery leading to right ventricular failure can be treated with inhaled nitric oxide and pulmonary vasodilators. Hypotension during graft reperfusion is due to auto-infusion of residual prostacyclin from procurement, air embolism, or redistribution of blood flow [11]. Tension pneumothorax, pneumopericardium, or pericardial tamponade may result in hemodynamic compromise. Cardiac dysfunction, blood loss, systemic inflammatory response syndrome, and sepsis are other causes of hypotension. Judicious fluid resuscitation maintaining cardiac output while minimizing risk of pulmonary edema are important; inotropic and vasoactive agents guided by serial hemodynamic measurements, mixed venous oxygen saturation, and arterial blood gas (ABG) measurement are usually effective. Severe hypotension unresponsive to fluid and vasopressors, severe hypoxia, and myocardial dysfunction may require CPB intraoperatively; ECMO may be used for the same indications postoperatively.

Postoperative bleeding

Hemorrhage can be seen in up to 25% of cases. Risk factors include severe adhesions (previous thoracic surgery or chest tube, cystic fibrosis, pleurodesis), BLTx, retransplantation, CPB, prolonged procedures, and coagulopathy. Mild to moderate bleeding is managed by observation, hemodynamic support, and blood products. Severe hemorrhage is the most common indication for re-operation.

Cardiac complications

Atrial fibrillation is common with increasing age [12]. Patients with known coronary artery disease (CAD) are closely monitored and may need intraoperative repair or postoperative balloon pumps. Some centers perform intraoperative repair of the aortic or mitral valves. Pericardial tamponade is rare and manifests with hemodynamic compromise. Swan–Ganz catheter and echocardiography are helpful in diagnosis.

Infections

Infection and PGD account for the majority of early 30-day mortality after LTx. In the perioperative period, pathogens arising from either the recipient's or the donor's flora are the greatest threat and include bacteria (*Pseudomonas aeruginosa*, *Staphylococcus aureus* including methicillin-resistant strains), fungi (*Candida*, *Aspergillus* species), and viruses (mostly community respiratory viral pathogens, but also herpes and cytomegalovirus) [13]. The approach to other ICU-associated infections including catheter and wound infections, aspiration, and *Clostridium difficile* colitis is similar to those of non-immunosuppressed patients. Cultures, antigen, and polymerase chain reaction assays from donor and recipient specimens including blood, urine, and bronchoalveolar lavage samples dictate the appropriate therapy.

Rejection

Hyperacute or acute vascular rejection may occur in the early postoperative period. The presentation may mimic other pathologies including PGD. The diagnosis is made by histopathological evaluation of transbronchial biopsies. Treatment is by high-dose pulse steroids (methylprednisolone 10–15 mg/kg IV daily for 3–5 days) and antithymocyte globulin when refractory [14]. Antibody-mediated rejection may require plasma exchange, intravenous immunoglobulin, and rituximab in addition to methylprednisolone.

Airway complications

Airway complications (stenosis, malacia, defects, or dehiscence) requiring stent placement or other interventions occur in 7–18% [15]. Small defects noted on bronchoscopic examination or as persistent air leaks are treated conservatively with reduction in corticosteroids until spontaneous healing occurs and seldom require endoscopic stent placement. Significant dehiscence necessitating operative repair or retransplantation occurs in less than 1%, and carries high risk of mortality. Some bronchial stenoses may respond to dilatation, cryoablation, or laser debridement.

Vascular complications

Pulmonary venous thrombosis may present with hypoxemia, hypotension, pulmonary edema, effusion, or infiltrates on CXR within the first few days of surgery. Absence of flow in the pulmonary vein on transesophageal echocardiogram in the appropriate setting is diagnostic. Risk factors include hypercoagulable states, torsion of the vascular anastomosis, and external compression due to sutures or pericardium. Severe cases require surgical exploration with relief of compression, thrombolysis, or anticoagulation.

Errors in surgical techniques may cause stenosis, kinking and torsion of the pulmonary artery with thrombosis requiring immediate re-operation and revision of the anastomosis [11]. The diagnosis is by Doppler echocardiogram, computerized tomographic angiogram, or magnetic resonance imaging. Occasionally mild to moderate stenosis responds to percutaneous endovascular stent placement.

Gastrointestinal complications

Gastrointestinal (GI) complications may occur with an incidence of 50% and are a significant cause of morbidity and mortality in LTx. Gastroparesis may result from injury to the vagus nerve and from medications. Aspiration due to gastroesophageal reflux disease or intraesophageal reflux may result in chemical pneumonitis and may play a role in acute and chronic rejections. Nausea and diarrhea may be caused by medication (mycophenolate mofetil, tacrolimus) or may be due to opportunistic infections (cytomegalovirus, *C. difficile* colitis), ileus, and less likely to ischemic bowel during the acute postoperative period.

Other organ dysfunction

Derangements in the other organ systems including acute kidney injury, electrolyte imbalances (hypo/hyperkalemia, hypomagnesemia), hematologic disturbances (cytopenias, disseminated intravascular coagulation, and microangiopathic hemolytic anemia), and critical care neuromyopathy are common and management is similar to non-immunosuppressed patients. Phrenic nerve injury at times recovers spontaneously several months after the surgery.

Liver transplantation

Introduction

Liver transplantation provides life-saving therapy in the setting of acute liver failure, decompensated chronic liver disease, and hepatocellular carcinoma. The most common etiology of acute liver failure is drug hepatotoxicity, with acetaminophen toxicity being the leading cause. Common etiologies of chronic liver disease include hepatitis C, non-alcoholic steatohepatitis (NASH), and alcoholic liver disease. The Mayo End Stage Liver Disease (MELD) score, based on the objective parameters of serum bilirubin, INR, and creatinine, has replaced the Child–Pugh classification to define chronic liver disease severity, and to prioritize potential recipients for organ allocation [16]. With advances in surgical technique, pre- and post-transplant management, and immunosuppressive strategies, overall post-transplant outcomes have steadily improved, with average 1-year and 5-year patient survival rates of 90% and 75% respectively.

The medical care of the patient undergoing liver transplantation involves the management of hepatic and extra-hepatic organ dysfunction prior to transplantation, and close monitoring of the post-transplant patient for surgical and medical complications. Critical illness in the pre-transplant setting presents with acute liver failure, or acute on chronic liver failure. The differing pathophysiologic processes underlying the two kinds of liver failure require specific approaches to management [17]. In the immediate post-transplant setting, clinical parameters reflecting hepatic graft function are closely monitored. Specific potential complications in the post-transplant phase include anatomical issues and multi-organ effects of immunosuppressive therapy. The following sections will address the management of the pre-transplant and post-transplant phases of liver transplantation.

Pre-transplant management of acute liver failure

Acute liver failure (ALF) is a clinical syndrome of diverse etiology, characterized by encephalopathy and coagulopathy in the setting of acute liver dysfunction, and in the absence of chronic liver disease. A characteristic specific to the advanced stages of hepatic encephalopathy in ALF is the development of potentially catastrophic cerebral edema and intracranial hypertension that can progress to herniation.

Hepatic encephalopathy

Hepatic encephalopathy is defined by neuropsychiatric symptoms in the setting of liver disease, without the presence of other causes of altered mental status. Impaired hepatic clearance of toxins, and in particular ammonia, results in astrocytic swelling; this cytotoxic edema can induce changes in mental status ranging from mild cognitive impairments to coma. Hepatic encephalopathy is divided into four grades based on the West Haven criteria [18], with grade I representing subtle cognitive changes and attention deficits, grade II lethargy and apathy, grade III confusion and semi-stupor, and grade IV comatose state. In patients with grade III or IV hepatic encephalopathy, elective endotracheal intubation should be performed for airway protection, followed by the maintenance of adequate sedation and analgesia to ensure patient–ventilator synchrony. Following this, neurosurgical placement of an intra-parenchymal monitor should be strongly considered in order to continuously measure and treat intracranial hypertension. Pharmacologic osmotherapy for intracranial hypertension includes mannitol and hypertonic saline. Additional therapeutic measures for refractory intracranial hypertension include therapeutic hypothermia (target core body temperature of 32–33 °C) and barbiturate coma to suppress CNS metabolic demand. Those therapeutic interventions should be targeted to maintain an intracranial pressure (ICP) < 25 mmHg and a cerebral perfusion pressure (CPP = MAP−ICP) > 60 mmHg.

Coagulopathy

In addition to hepatic encephalopathy, a worsening coagulopathy as evidenced by a rising prothrombin time (PT)/international normalized ratio (INR) is a characteristic finding in the setting of worsening acute liver failure (ALF). The INR is the most reliable and sensitive biochemical indicator of hepatic synthetic function; therefore, in the absence of bleeding, the INR should not be corrected with coagulation factors (e.g., FFP), and instead should be used as a prognostic indicator to predict spontaneous recovery or the need for liver transplantation. If transient correction of coagulopathy is required to perform invasive procedures such as ICP monitor placement, Recombinant Factor 7a at a minimum dose of 40 µg/kg can be utilized. The administration of a single dose typically normalizes the INR to less than 1.5 within 30 minutes of administration, and provides a therapeutic window of approximately 90–120 minutes for the performance of invasive procedures.

In addition to the aforementioned neurologic and hematologic issues, the patient with ALF can progress to multi-organ system dysfunction, which necessitates critical care management of cardiopulmonary, metabolic, infectious disease, and renal issues. In particular, the management of acute kidney injury (AKI) in ALF requires careful attention. Acute kidney injury in ALF can result from direct intrarenal injury or shock-related renal hypoperfusion. A diagnosis of hepatorenal syndrome (HRS) should not be invoked in the setting of AKI in ALF, since the pathophysiology of HRS requires the presence of chronic portal hypertension. If renal replacement therapy is necessary, continuous renal replacement therapy (CRRT) is indicated even in hemodynamically stable patients, since conventional hemodialysis can induce sudden dramatic increases in intracranial pressure (ICP).

Additional treatment considerations in acute liver failure

The etiologies of ALF are numerous, and potentially reversible causes should be sought. Certain etiologies require specific management, including treatment of autoimmune hepatitis with high-dose corticosteroids, herpes simplex virus (HSV) hepatitis with acyclovir, and acute fatty liver of pregnancy and HELLP syndrome by delivery of the fetus. Acetaminophen toxicity is treated with N-acetyl-cysteine (NAC). Additionally, NAC has been shown to improve transplant-free survival in ALF of any etiology, and oral or IV NAC is recommended for all patients with ALF [19].

Pre-transplant management of acute on chronic liver failure

Acute on chronic liver failure (ACLF) is characterized by the splanchnic and systemic manifestations of chronic portal hypertension. The pathophysiology of portal hypertension in chronic liver disease involves the combined influences of intrahepatic resistance to portal flow and increased portal inflow due to pathologic splanchnic vasodilation. In addition, the splanchnic vasodilation results in a shunting of the cardiac output to the splanchnic circulation and an associated decrease in effective arterial blood volume perfusing other organ systems. These hemodynamic derangements in the splanchnic and systemic circulation form the basis for current management strategies in decompensated cirrhosis, with a specific focus being the reversal of splanchnic vasodilation with splanchnic vasoconstrictors.

Hepatic encephalopathy

Hepatic encephalopathy in decompensated cirrhosis typically is not associated with intracranial hypertension and cerebral edema, since the chronicity of the process allows for extra neural ammonia fixation mechanisms to develop. Potential precipitants of hepatic encephalopathy include benzodiazepines, narcotics, electrolyte or acid-base imbalances, dehydration, overdiuresis, infection, gastrointestinal bleeding, constipation, or recent transjugular intrahepatic portosystemic shunt (TIPS). Therapeutic pharmacologic approaches aimed at reducing hyperammonemia include enteral administration of lactulose, rifaximin, and flagyl. Additional management is supportive, and patients with stupor or coma warrant elective intubation for airway protection. Successful reversal of hepatic encephalopathy in ACLF is dependent on the reversal of the inciting etiology, and adequate pharmacologic therapy with the agents listed above.

Gastroesophageal variceal bleeding

Gastroesophageal variceal bleeding is a dreaded complication of chronic portal hypertension that requires emergent intervention. Endotracheal intubation for airway protection should be performed to prevent aspiration during massive hematemesis. During resuscitation for hemorrhagic hypotension or shock, intravenous fluids and blood products must be administered carefully, as excess volume increases portal pressure and bleeding risk; a transfusion goal for hemoglobin is 8 g/dL. Intravenous octreotide should be initiated to induce splanchnic vasoconstriction, and prophylactic antibiotics should be administered to prevent infections (including spontaneous bacterial peritonitis (SBP)), decrease the risk of rebleeding, and to improve survival [20]. Following pharmacologic therapy, emergent endoscopic therapy with possible variceal banding should be performed. In the setting of bleeding esophageal varices that are refractory to endoscopic therapy, or in the setting of bleeding gastric varices, urgent TIPS placement should be performed by interventional radiology.

Cardiovascular derangements

Patients with advanced portal hypertension may demonstrate parameters similar to septic shock, with a low mean arterial pressure, wide pulse pressure and a low systemic vascular resistance. In addition, a new concept of "cirrhotic cardiomyopathy" is in the process of being defined [21], which is characterized by both systolic and diastolic heart dysfunction, and decreased response to beta agonist therapy. Given the presence of an immunocompromised state, the cirrhotic patient is very susceptible to an infectious trigger-induced septic hypotension, which can further worsen the baseline low mean arterial pressure. Therapeutic management of new onset shock in a cirrhotic includes an anticipation of a septic insult, and early goal-directed therapy with intravenous fluids and vasoactive agent support. Based on extrapolation from current septic shock guidelines, norepinephrine is the preferred vasoactive agent of choice, with low-dose vasopressin and dopamine being adequate choices as a second agent. In addition, cirrhotic patients may be at risk for relative adrenal insufficiency [22].

Hepatorenal syndrome

Hepatorenal syndrome is defined as renal impairment (Cr > 1.5 g/dL or CrCl < 40 mL/min) in the setting of decompensated cirrhosis. Hepatorenal syndrome results from reduced effective blood volume due to splanchnic vasodilation; it remains a diagnosis of exclusion. In particular, a challenge of volume expansion and diuretic withdrawal is critical to identify reversible hypovolemia. Type 1 HRS progresses rapidly, whereas Type 2 has a protracted course; both types are fatal without liver transplantation. Therapeutic interventions are aimed at splanchnic vasoconstriction in order to re-establish an effective arterial blood volume; current pharmacologic agents include octreotide and terlipressin. In the presence of persistent renal dysfunction associated with metabolic acidosis, and fluid and electrolyte abnormalities, continuous renal replacement therapy is indicated.

Ascites

Ascites is an additional consequence of decompensated cirrhosis, and is associated with the development of SBP. Tense ascites can produce abdominal compartment syndrome, characterized by restrictive lung mechanics, hypotension due to decreased venous return from inferior vena cava compression, and renal and mesenteric vascular compromise. Management includes sodium restriction, and diuretic therapy with spironolactone and furosemide; refractory ascites is managed with serial large-volume paracentesis or TIPS.

Pulmonary complications

Pulmonary complications include hepatopulmonary syndrome, portopulmonary hypertension, and hepatic hydrothorax. In the hepatopulmonary syndrome, excess pulmonary vasodilation limits oxygen diffusion from the alveolus to the pulmonary capillary, thereby inducing hypoxemia. Management includes supplemental oxygen and embolization of arterio-venous malformations if present. Portopulmonary hypertension is a form of pulmonary arterial hypertension (pulmonary artery pressure > 25 mmHg with normal pulmonary capillary wedge pressure) resulting from portal hypertension. Epoprostenol infusion or oral sildenafil may improve hemodynamics and reduce pulmonary pressures, but prognosis is poor if cor pulmonale develops. In both syndromes, liver transplant is the definitive treatment, although severe pulmonary hypertension (mean PA pressure > 35 mmHg) is a contraindication to transplantation. Finally, in hepatic hydrothorax, ascites enters the thoracic cavity, creating pleural effusions. Management of hepatic hydrothorax includes diuretics and therapeutic thoracentesis. Chest tubes are contraindicated, as re-expansion pulmonary edema and hypovolemic shock can occur. A TIPS may reduce the recurrence of refractory hydrothorax.

Postoperative care of the transplant recipient

The liver transplantation operation involves vascular anastomoses involving the portal vein, hepatic artery, hepatic vein, and inferior vena cava, and a biliary anastomosis. Following transplant, careful attention to volume status, surgical drain output, hemodynamic parameters, and neurological status are critical. Intracranial pressure is monitored for 48 hours postoperatively if a monitor was placed in the pre-transplant phase in the setting of ALF. Immunosuppression is started at the time of surgery and tailored to each patient's comorbidities and underlying etiology of liver failure. Improvements in hepatic encephalopathy, coagulopathy, bilirubin, metabolic acidosis, hypoglycemia, and renal failure are evidence of adequate graft function. Postoperative complications can be separated into intra-hepatic and extra-hepatic etiologies [23].

Intrahepatic complications post-transplant

Bleeding

Bleeding is an early postoperative complication with multifactorial etiologies. Technical difficulties with vascular anastomoses are surgical complications that can cause hemorrhage. Additional risk factors for postoperative bleeding include thrombocytopenia, severe coagulopathy, liver biopsy, use of heparin, and poor graft function. Hemorrhage presents with hypotension, tachycardia, renal failure, decrease in mixed venous oxygen saturation, or abdominal distension. Transfusion of blood or fresh frozen plasma and emergent surgical exploration are usually required.

Biliary complications

Biliary leaks are important causes of morbidity and mortality following liver transplantation, and occur most frequently at the anastomoses. Although biliary leaks can be asymptomatic, fever, jaundice, pain, peritonitis, and sepsis may occur. Diagnostic modalities include endoscopic retrograde cholangiopancreatography (ERCP) or percutaneous transhepatic cholangiopancreatography (PTC). Placement of a stent or biliary drain can be performed, although if the anastomotic leak is significant, surgical reconstruction is necessary.

Biliary strictures and stenoses occur in the early or late postoperative phases, and present with severe cholestasis, ascending cholangitis, hepatic abscess, or sepsis. Progression to septic shock and multi-organ failure may occur. Management includes broad-spectrum antibiotics, ERCP with stent placement, and percutaneous drainage if hepatic abscess is present. Late biliary complications include multiple strictures, dilations, and abscesses, and are frequently related to biliary tract ischemia with necrosis due to hepatic artery thrombosis. Although treatment with ERCP can be attempted, if significant intrahepatic biliary disease is present, re-transplantation is usually required.

Vascular complications

Vascular complications are common in the early postoperative period and require prompt recognition and treatment to avoid significant morbidity and mortality. Complications include hepatic artery thrombosis, portal vein thrombosis, hepatic vein thrombosis, and vena cava obstruction. In such cases, Doppler ultrasound is the preferred initial diagnostic modality for evaluation of vascular patency. Confirmation with angiography or MRI is recommended before invasive management is undertaken.

One of the most devastating early complications of liver transplantation is hepatic artery thrombosis (HAT). Graft necrosis induces sharp increases in liver transaminases as well as significant cholestasis, biliary leak, bacteremia, and sepsis. Re-transplantation is often urgently required, but emergent thrombectomy may be helpful if HAT is discovered early. Portal vein thrombosis presents with graft dysfunction or signs of portal hypertension including ascites and variceal bleeding. Thrombectomy, thrombolysis with tissue plasminogen activator, or anatomical bypass with TIPS may be performed for definitive treatment.

Less frequent vascular complications include hepatic vein thrombosis and vena cava obstruction. Hepatic vein thrombosis presents with acute transaminitis, jaundice, abdominal pain, ascites, and hepatomegaly. If fulminant necrosis occurs, re-transplantation is necessary. Chronic anticoagulation with warfarin is recommended to prevent recurrence of hepatic vein thrombosis. Vena cava obstruction has a high mortality without surgical reconstruction. Clinical presentation includes edema, ascites, hepatomegaly, renal failure, and fulminant hepatic necrosis. If the graft damage is severe and surgical intervention fails, re-transplantation may be necessary.

Graft dysfunction

Graft dysfunction occurs from various etiologies, and may improve spontaneously with supportive treatment. Persistent transaminitis and graft dysfunction may represent vascular derangements, rejection, or primary graft non-function. Upon exclusion of vascular complications, percutaneous liver biopsy is recommended for evaluation. Additional etiologies of graft dysfunction include small-for-size syndrome, which occurs when graft size is less than 50% of the recipient's expected liver volume. Treatment is supportive and re-transplantation may be necessary. Large-for-size syndrome results when the graft is larger than the recipient's expected liver volume; treatment is supportive.

Rejection is defined as graft inflammation resulting from antibody or T-cell mediated interactions between the donor liver and the recipient's immune system. Hyperacute rejection occurs in the first 48 hours following transplant; ABO blood incompatibilities are the primary cause. Salvage therapies for hyperacute rejection may include plasma exchange, B-cell depletion, gamma globulin administration, and splenectomy. If acute liver failure results, re-transplantation is necessary. Acute cellular rejection (ACR) is often mild and is rare with appropriate immunosuppression. Transaminitis and cholestasis are observed but many patients are asymptomatic. Mild cases are treated with corticosteroids and adjustment of immunosuppression; severe or refractory cases may require T-cell depletion therapy. Chronic rejection typically occurs 6 months or later after transplantation and may be triggered by prior episodes of ACR. Treatment is supportive and re-transplantation may be necessary.

Primary non-function is the complete, irreversible failure of a new graft. Donor risk factors include age, presence of steatosis >30%, prolonged hospitalization, acidosis, hypernatremia, or donation after cardiac death. Recipient factors include hemodynamic instability and reperfusion injury. Surgical causes include difficulty with donor organ procurement and prolonged warm or cold ischemia time. Primary non-function is fatal, and patients with this condition receive the highest priority for urgent re-transplantation.

Extra-hepatic complications post-transplant

Infectious complications

Infections cause significant morbidity and mortality in the immunosuppressed transplant patient. Common bacterial infections include pneumonia, cholangitis, urinary tract infections, wound infections, antibiotic-associated *C. difficile*, bacteremia, and sepsis. Patients are also at high risk for fungal infections from *Candida albicans*, *Aspergillosis*, *Histoplasma capsulatum*, *Cryptococcus neoformans*, and *Coccidioides immitis*. Additional opportunistic infections include HSV, *Pneumocystis jiroveci* pneumonia, cytomegalovirus, *Toxoplasma gondii*, and *Mycobacterium tuberculosis*. Early recognition of infection and use of appropriate antimicrobial agents are critical in reducing mortality.

Neurological complications

Neurological complications are relatively frequent in the post-transplant period. Hepatic encephalopathy generally resolves with appropriate graft function. Multi-factorial delirium is common; correction of reversible factors and re-orientation are management strategies. If severe behavior problems occur, haloperidol can be used. Seizures may occur from immunosuppressants, particularly calcineurin inhibitors. Central pontine myelinosis can occur if hyponatremia is rapidly corrected with intraoperative crystalloid fluids; this irreversible complication can be avoided by the judicious correction of hyponatremia.

Renal complications

Acute kidney injury may be due to intraoperative hypotension as well as use of nephrotoxic antibiotics and immunosuppressants. Survival is reduced when acute kidney injury occurs in the post-transplant setting. Management includes withdrawal of offending medications, avoidance of further renal insults, and when necessary, renal replacement therapy.

Kidney transplantation

Introduction

Kidney transplantation is the preferred treatment for patients with end-stage renal disease (ESRD). Compared with dialysis, transplantation improves both longevity and quality of life [24]; each year approximately 17,000 patients receive a kidney transplant in the USA. One-year graft survival is over 90% for kidneys from deceased donors, and over 95% for kidneys from living donors; 10-year graft survival now approaches 50% and 60% for deceased donor and living donor kidneys respectively [2].

In addition to clearance for the transplant surgical procedure, the evaluation of a transplant recipient includes an assessment of the impact of the kidney on the patient's long-term survival and quality of life. Because cardiovascular disease is the most common cause of death, special attention is paid to defining a patient's cardiovascular risk. The average duration of a kidney transplant operation is 3 hours, and the average length of stay is 3–5 days. The initial doses of immunosuppressive medications are given at the time of surgery.

Postoperative management

Immunosuppressive management

Immune suppression differs by transplant center. Most centers employ induction therapy with antibodies against T-cell proteins, such as polyclonal rabbit anti-thymocyte globulin, monoclonal anti-CD52 antibodies (alemtuzumab), or antibodies which antagonize IL-2 (basiliximab); studies show patients who receive induction have greater graft survival [25]. Maintenance immune suppression usually combines a calcineurin inhibitor (tacrolimus or cyclosporine) and an antimetabolite (most commonly mycophenolate mofetil) [26]. Many centers still employ long-term corticosteroid therapy. Belatacept is a newly approved monoclonal antibody that inhibits T-cell costimulation; its use may replace calcineurin inhibitor therapy in many kidney transplant patients in the coming years [27].

Perioperative management

Patients should be intensively monitored for the first 12 hours post-transplant. In some hospitals this occurs in an ICU or step-down unit, although the patient may be transferred from the post-anesthesia care unit (PACU) to a regular hospital bed with specialized nursing care. The bedside monitoring includes careful attention to blood pressure, oxygenation, and urine output, which should be recorded hourly. Patients should receive intravenous fluids postoperatively to maintain adequate extracellular fluid volume and to replace urinary losses which may be voluminous. Laboratory studies are done within a few hours of surgery to follow the hemogram and serum creatinine. A renal ultrasound with Doppler should be done routinely postoperatively to confirm adequate arterial and venous blood flow. Pain is managed with a patient-controlled analgesia (PCA) pump for the first 12–24 hours.

Blood-pressure management

Postoperatively the management of blood pressure plays a vital role in preserving organ function. It is important to prevent episodes of hypotension as this may decrease renal perfusion. Similarly, timely management of hypertension can prevent cardiopulmonary complications in the immediate post-transplant period. Management of hypotension and hypertension is discussed below.

Postoperative complications

Hypotension

Hypovolemia is the most common cause of hypotension post-transplant due to bleeding, or to inadequate volume replacement of urine output that may be exacerbated by the use of diuretics. It is important to initially match the urine output with isotonic saline; some living-donor transplant kidneys can produce over 8 liters of urine in the first 24-hour period post transplant. The formation of a perinephric hematoma or retroperitoneal bleeding may occur. Hematocrit and hemoglobin should be monitored frequently, especially in patients deemed to be of high cardiac risk. Immediate restoration of hemodynamic stability should be attempted with intravenous saline-containing fluids or with blood products. Coagulation studies should be obtained as well if bleeding is suspected. Imaging of the transplant kidney with ultrasound or CT scan of the abdomen and pelvis will demonstrate a significant site of bleeding. A perinephric hematoma may cause compression of the ureter resulting in decreased urine output, and may need to be urgently evacuated in the operating room. Although sepsis is unusual immediately postoperatively it may present within the first 24 hours of surgery and cultures should be obtained as appropriate. If an acute cardiac event is suspected of causing hypotension an ECG, cardiac enzymes, and echocardiography should be obtained urgently.

Hypertension

Many factors contribute to hypertension postoperatively. Decreased GFR with slow or delayed allograft function leads to expansion of the extracellular volume. Pain, and reduction or withdrawal of pre-transplant antihypertensive medications occur commonly. In addition, calcineurin inhibitors are potent vasoconstrictors and lead to an increase in systemic vascular resistance [28]. Studies by Paoletti et al. [29] have shown that only 5% of the renal transplant recipients are normotensive. Management of postoperative hypertension includes adequate pain control, volume management and anti-hypertensive medications. It is important to note that mild elevations of postoperative systolic blood pressure may be allowed in the 120 mmHg to 150 mmHg range, to maintain adequate perfusion to the renal allograft. Intravenous beta-blockers and hydralazine can be used to manage perioperative hypertension. Once the patient is able to tolerate them, it is advisable to switch the patient to oral medications that can be continued long term. Diuretics can be used in the perioperative period, as patients frequently have sodium and water retention from intravenous volume replacement. Beta-blockers and calcium antagonists are commonly prescribed and are effective. However, the non-dihydropyridine calcium blockers verapamil and diltiazem must be used with caution as they are potent inhibitors of cytochrome P450 3A4 and can markedly increase trough levels of the calcineurin inhibitors; reduction of the dose of tacrolimus or cyclosporine accompanied by careful monitoring of trough levels is required. Use of angiotensin converting enzyme (ACE) inhibitors or angiotensin receptor blockers (ARB) in the early post-transplant period is not recommended as they may cause an acute rise in creatinine as well as hyperkalemia.

Oliguria

The monitoring of urine output starts immediately as soon as the vascular and ureteral anastamoses have been performed in the operating room. It is important to document the average daily urine output from the patient's diseased native kidneys prior to surgery, so as to estimate the accurate urine volume from the new renal allograft. In the perioperative period, there are multiple causes of decreased urine output (see Table 42.2). If the patient is hypotensive, volume depleted or is at risk for hemorrhaging, aggressive repletion of volume status with saline-containing fluids or blood products should restore the circulation and improve urine volume.

A sudden decrease in a previously good urine output is particularly worrisome, and should be urgently addressed. Renal arterial or venous thrombosis is of paramount concern in the immediate postoperative period; a renal ultrasound with arterial and venous Doppler studies should be performed at the bedside, and the patient emergently returned to the operating room if vascular compromise is suspected. Ureteral obstruction may occur. Early obstruction may be due to a blocked Foley catheter, blood clots, or ureteral edema; routine placement of a ureteral stent can help reduce the incidence of these complications. External ureteral compression can be caused by a large lymphocele due to disruption of the lymphatics of the allograft or of the iliac vessels, or by a perinephric hematoma; imaging will demonstrate evidence of hydroureter, as well as point to the cause of external compression. Hyperacute rejection is rarely seen, due to the success of modern human leukocyte antigen (HLA) typing and antibody screening procedures. Delayed graft function is common and is discussed below. Urine leaks can occur in the early postoperative period. Demonstrating an elevated creatinine level in the surgical drain fluid confirms this diagnosis. Small leaks usually resolve with ureteral stenting and prolonged Foley catheter drainage of the bladder; however, surgical repair may be required.

Electrolyte abnormalities

Postoperative hyperkalemia is usually due to delayed renal allograft function, or to medications which reduce renal potassium secretion; these include calcineurin inhibitors, ACE inhibitors, and trimethoprim. Management includes

Table 42.2 Oliguria post kidney transplant.

Causes	Treatment
Hypotension with volume depletion or bleeding	Volume repletion with intravenous fluids, blood products
Hypotension with sepsis	Volume repletion; broad-spectrum antibiotics; vasopressors
Hypotension with reduced cardiac perfusion	Treat myocardial dysfunction or coronary occlusion; vasopressors
Renal venous or arterial thrombosis	Exploration in operating room
Internal ureteral obstruction	Flush Foley; ureteral stent; percutaneous nephrostomy
External ureteral compression: lymphocele or hematoma	Percutaneous drainage; exploration in operating room
Urine leak	Ureteral stent and Foley catheter; Exploration in operating room
Delayed graft function	Medical management, dialysis, supportive care
Acute rejection	Intravenous steroids or anti-lymphocyte antibodies

dietary potassium restriction, the use of oral sodium polystyrene sulfonate (Kayexalate) and dialysis. Hypokalemia is often due to a high urine output contributed to by the use of diuretics, as well as from low dietary intake, and can be managed with oral potassium chloride supplements. The tubular effects of calcineurin inhibitors post-transplant often results in renal magnesium wasting and hypomagnesemia. Oral magnesium oxide supplementation is often required, but commonly causes diarrhea. While in the hospital, some patients may benefit from intravenous magnesium sulfate to a target serum magnesium level of at least 1.6 mg/dL. Patients may have hypercalcemia due to hyperparathyroidism that persists post-transplant. Hypophosphatemia is also commonly present, and can be treated with an increase in dietary phosphorus or with oral potassium phosphate supplements.

Delayed graft function

Delayed graft function (DGF) is defined as the need for dialysis during the first week post-transplant; it occurs in 20–40% of patients [30]. Acute tubular necrosis (ATN) is the most common reason for DGF. Warm ischemia time during harvesting, cold ischemia time during storage, and reperfusion injury during surgery are all factors which contribute to ATN [31]; kidneys from older donors appear to be more susceptible [30]. Recipient factors which increase the risk of DGF include male gender, African-American race, a history of obesity, prior sensitization to HLA antigens, diabetes, and prolonged time on the transplant waiting list [32]. Patients with DGF are at risk for worse short-term and long-term graft survival. Management of DGF includes continuation of immunosuppressive therapy including calcineurin inhibitors, renal replacement therapy as medically indicated and management of concurrent medical conditions including hypertension and diabetes. Acute rejection is another important cause of allograft dysfunction which must be promptly diagnosed and treated; at our center a transplant kidney biopsy is done one week post-transplant to look for rejection if the patient remains dialysis-dependent without an increase in urine output or decrease in creatinine. Other causes of DGF and oliguria (discussed above) that must be ruled out include vascular thrombosis, ureteral obstruction, and drug-induced nephrotoxicity.

Acute rejection

Rejection of the allograft is a serious complication of renal transplantation [33]. Hyperacute rejection due to preformed antibodies occurs immediately after the vascular anastamosis, and is rarely seen in the current transplant era. Acute cellular rejection occurs in about 10–15% of patients within the first 3 months and is suspected when the serum creatinine plateaus above the normal range, or suddenly rises after an initial decline. Rejection may also be mediated by newly formed antibodies directed against the donated allograft. An allograft biopsy should be performed when acute rejection is suspected; the Banff classification scheme is used to classify the type and extent of the rejection process [34]. Tools for managing acute rejection include intravenous steroids, antibodies directed against lymphocytes, plasmapheresis, and the use of intravenous immune globulin [33].

Diabetes

Diabetes mellitus is the most common cause of ESRD in patients undergoing renal transplantation in the USA. Prior to transplant surgery, diabetic patients maybe on low dose or no insulin due to a decrease in the clearance of endogenous insulin by the failed native kidneys. The use of steroids and calcineurin inhibitors, particularly tacrolimus, impairs glucose tolerance and often result in hyperglycemia post transplant. The requirement for exogenous insulin will increase as renal function improves postoperatively. New-onset diabetes after transplant (NODAT) develops in about 25% of previously non-diabetic patients; Hispanics and African-Americans are at increased risk. In addition to the immunosuppressive medications mentioned above, other risk factors include obesity, older age, hepatitis C, and cytomegalovirus (CMV) infection [35]. The use of a steroid-free regimen is associated with a reduced incidence of NODAT [36]. Reinforcement of diabetic education, close monitoring of blood sugar, dietary consultation, and exercise all play a role in controlling diabetes and in helping to prevent long-term complications. Oral agents as well as insulin may be used safely in kidney transplant recipients.

Post-transplant infections

Kidney transplant patients are at risk for a variety of bacterial, fungal, and viral infections [37]. This risk is highest in the early post-transplant period, when the degree of immunosupression is highest, but persists for the life of the transplant. Bacterial infections that occur early post-transplant include wound infections, which are relatively uncommon, and urinary tract infections (UTI) which are common and may cause pyelonephritis in the transplant kidney with associated acute renal failure, bacteremia, and sepsis. Antibiotics prescribed for several months post-transplant may reduce the risk of UTI; trimethoprim-sulfamethoxazole is commonly used both to lower the incidence of UTI and as prophylaxis against *Pneumocystis jiroveci* pneumonia. The risk of CMV infection varies depending on whether the donor and/or recipient have been previously infected; valgancicovir or valacyclovir are commonly utilized to prevent primary infection or reactivation. Other common viruses that cause post-transplant infections include Epstein–Barr virus, shingles due to varicella-zoster, HSV and BK polyomavirus. In patients with diarrhea *C. difficile* colitis is not infrequent. Patients with a history of hepatitis B or C infections may experience reactivation. Careful history and physical exam should be performed, and bacterial and fungal cultures, as well as appropriate viral specimens should be obtained. Because immunosuppressive medications reduce the signs and symptoms of infection, such as localizing pain and fever, it is appropriate to use broad-spectrum antibiotics in a patient who appears systemically ill until definitive culture data are analyzed.

Pancreas transplantation

Introduction

Over 1000 pancreas transplants are performed yearly in the USA [38]. Deceased-donor kidney and pancreas transplants are usually performed simultaneously for type 1 diabetic patients with end-stage kidney disease. However, a pancreas transplant may be done months or years after a living- or deceased-donor kidney transplant. Pancreas transplant alone is infrequently performed, as the risk of immunosuppressive medications is felt to outweigh the benefits of a pancreas transplant, except in patients with brittle diabetes and severe hypoglycemia unawareness who may otherwise suffer significant hypoglycemic complications.

The current preferred operation utilizes an intraperitoneal approach with the kidney on the left side and the pancreas on the right; venous drainage can be into either the iliac or portal venous systems. The exocrine pancreas is most often anastamosed to the small intestine via a duodenal stump, although some surgeons prefer to drain the pancreas through the recipient's bladder. Immunosuppressive therapy is similar to that utilized in kidney transplantation. One-year patient survival is above 95%; long-term survival of simultaneous kidney and pancreas transplant patients exceeds that of diabetic patients undergoing deceased-donor kidney transplantation alone. The percentage of pancreatic grafts which still function is approximately 85% at 1 year and 50% at 10 years [2].

Postoperative complications

Anastomotic leak

Surgical technical failure remains the most common cause of early graft loss; the need for reoperation can approach 35% [39]. Improved surgical methods have reduced the frequency of anastamotic leaks which may occur postoperatively in pancreases which are enterically drained; the overall rate has been reported to be 2–10% [40]. Because the use of immunosuppressive medications may reduce the inflammatory response and mask the signs and symptoms of intestinal perforation, a high index of suspicion must be maintained. Abdominal pain, nausea, vomiting, fever, leukocytosis, and hypotension may occur, and should prompt the ordering of an abdominal and pelvic CT scan with oral contrast. The CT may show a peripancreatic fluid collection, extra-intestinal air, or extravasation of contrast [41]. Reoperation is usually required to repair the leak. Computerized tomography scanning can also be used to diagnose a urinary anastomotic leak in a bladder-drained pancreas. Small leaks usually resolve with prolonged Foley catheter drainage of the bladder, but large leaks require reoperation [42].

Graft thrombosis

Graft thrombosis remains a common complication of pancreas transplantation with an incidence of 3–10% [39]. Patients present with hyperglycemia, graft tenderness, and elevation of serum amylase and lipase. Computerized tomography angiography with intravenous contrast and MR angiography with gadolinium are both excellent tools with which to evaluate the pancreatic circulation, although Doppler ultrasound may provide a more rapid assessment of pancreatic blood flow; venous thrombosis is most common. Unless the thrombus is of limited extent, attempts to surgically reestablish blood flow are usually unsuccessful and a transplant pancreatectomy is performed. Potentially modifiable risk factors for pancreatic thrombosis include minimization of cold ischemia time, screening for hypercoagulable states prior to transplant [43], avoidance of after cardiac death (DCD) donors, and of donors of advanced age. Rejection may also be a cause of graft thrombosis [44]. Some programs employ postoperative heparinization, but this may lead to clinically significant bleeding.

Infection and pancreatitis

Postoperative pancreatitis occurs commonly; it is important to distinguish this from a wound infection in or around the pancreatic allograft. The incidence of infection is highest in the first 3 months after transplant [45]. Fever, abdominal pain, nausea, vomiting, ileus, leukocytosis, and elevation of the amylase and lipase occur in both settings. Either CT or MRI scanning with intravenous contrast can help establish the correct diagnosis. If a localized abscess is detected it can often be treated with percutaneous drainage. Peripancreatic fluid collections occur in the setting of pancreatitis in addition to a diffusely swollen, hyperemic graft; diagnostic aspiration can rule out infection, blood cultures should also be obtained. Impairment of glucose homeostasis may not occur, even with significant inflammation of the pancreas. Similarly, the degree of elevation of the amylase and lipase does not always correlate with the severity of pancreatic inflammation.

Ideally antimicrobial treatment should be guided by culture results. In addition to gram-positive and gram-negative bacterial pathogens, yeast and fungi as well as viruses such as CMV may cause pancreatic infections; appropriate fungal cultures as well as viral PCR testing should be done [37]. Management of pancreatitis includes aggressive fluid resuscitation and NPO status; parenteral nutrition provides adequate nutrition in prolonged cases. Broad-spectrum antibiotics can be prescribed empirically until culture results are known to be negative. Pancreatitis usually resolves with conservative therapy. Rejection of the pancreatic allograft also presents with elevation of amylase and lipase, although abdominal pain and tenderness are much less prominent and may be absent. Biopsy of the pancreas or the accompanying kidney can determine the presence and degree of rejection.

Bleeding

Bleeding after pancreas transplant surgery is a common reason for reoperation. Early intra-abdominal bleeding often occurs near the superior mesenteric or splenic arteries [40]. If bleeding persists after reversal of any coagulation abnormalities, including discontinuation of prescribed anticoagulants, re-exploration with evacuation of the hematoma should be performed. Postoperative gastrointestinal bleeding is often from the duodenal-ileal anastamotic suture line, and usually resolves with supportive treatment.

References

1. The International Society of Heart and Lung Transplantation.; http://www.ishlt.org/.

2. *Scientific Registry of Transplant Recipients* 2010; http://www.srtr.org/.

3. Christie JD, Edwards LB, Kucheryavaya AY *et al.* The Registry of the International Society for Heart and Lung Transplantation: twenty-seventh official adult lung and heart-lung transplant report – 2010. *J Heart Lung Transplant* 2010; **29**: 1104–18.

4. Yusen RD, Shearon TH, Qian Y *et al.* Lung transplantation in the United States, 1999–2008. *Am J Transplant* 2010; **10**: 1047–68.

5. Orens JB, Estenne M, Arcasoy S *et al.* International guidelines for the selection of lung transplant candidates: 2006 update – a consensus report from the Pulmonary Scientific Council of the International Society for Heart and Lung Transplantation. *J Heart Lung Transplant* 2006; **25**: 745–55.

6. *Organ Procurement and Transplantation Network*; http://optn.transplant.hrsa.gov/ar2008/default.htm.

7. Cypel M, Yeung JC, Liu M *et al.* Normothermic ex vivo lung perfusion in clinical lung transplantation. *N Engl J Med* 2011; **364**: 1431–40.

8. Boasquevisque CH, Yildirim E, Waddel TK, Keshavjee S. Surgical techniques: lung transplant and lung volume reduction. *Proc Am Thoracic Soc* 2009; **6**: 66–78.

9. Weiss ES, Allen JG, Meguid RA *et al.* The impact of center volume on survival in lung transplantation: an analysis of more than 10,000 cases. *Annals Thoracic Surg* 2009; **88**: 1062–70.

10. Lee JC, Christie JD. Primary graft dysfunction. *Proc Am Thoracic Soc* 2009; **6**: 39–46.

11. Hartwig MG, Davis RD. Surgical considerations in lung transplantation: transplant operation and early postoperative management. *Resp Care Clinics North Am* 2004; **10**: 473–504.

12. Mason DP, Marsh DH, Alster JM *et al.* Atrial fibrillation after lung transplantation: timing, risk factors, and treatment. *Annals Thoracic Surg* 2007; **84**: 1878–84.

13. Remund KF, Best M, Egan JJ. Infections relevant to lung transplantation. *Proc Am Thoracic Soc* 2009; **6**: 94–100.

14. Martinu T, Chen DF, Palmer SM. Acute rejection and humoral sensitization in lung transplant recipients. *Proc Am Thoracic Soc* 2009; **6**: 54–65.

15. Santacruz JF, Mehta AC. Airway complications and management after lung transplantation: ischemia, dehiscence, and stenosis. *Proc Am Thoracic Soc* 2009; **6**: 79–93.

16. Murray KF, Carithers RL Jr. AASLD practice guidelines: evaluation of the patient for liver transplantation. *Hepatology* 2005; **41**: 1407–32.

17. Ford RM, Sakaria SS, Subramanian RM. Critical care management of patients before liver transplantation. *Transplant Rev (Orlando)* 2010; **24**: 190–206.

18. Atterbury CE, Maddrey WC, Conn HO. Neomycin-sorbitol and lactulose in the treatment of acute portal-systemic encephalopathy. A controlled, double-blind clinical trial. *Am J Dig Dis* 1978; **23**: 398–406.

19. Lee WM, Hynan LS, Rossaro L *et al.* Intravenous N-acetylcysteine improves transplant-free survival in early stage non-acetaminophen acute liver failure. *Gastroenterology* 2009; **137**: 856–64.

20. Bernard B, Grange JD, Khac EN *et al.* Antibiotic prophylaxis for the prevention of bacterial infections in cirrhotic patients with gastrointestinal bleeding: a meta-analysis. *Hepatology* 1999; **29**: 1655–61.

21. Zardi EM, Abbate A, Zardi DM *et al.* Cirrhotic cardiomyopathy. *J Am Coll Cardiol* 2010; **56**: 539–49.

22. Fernandez J, Escorsell A, Zabalza M *et al.* Adrenal insufficiency in patients with cirrhosis and septic shock: Effect of treatment with hydrocortisone on survival. *Hepatology* 2006; **44**: 1288–95.

23. Mueller AR, Platz KP, Kremer B. Early postoperative complications following liver transplantation. *Best Pract Res Clin Gastroenterol* 2004; **18**: 881–900.

24. Wolfe RA, Ashby VB, Milford EL *et al.* Comparison of mortality in all patients on dialysis, patients on dialysis awaiting transplantation, and recipients of a first cadaveric transplant. *N Engl J Med* 1999; **341**: 1725–30.

25. Hanaway MJ, Woodle ES, Mulgaonkar S et al. Alemtuzumab induction in renal transplantation. *N Engl J Med* 2011; **364**: 1909–19.

26. KDIGO clinical practice guideline for the care of kidney transplant recipients. *Am J Transplant* 2009; **9** (Suppl 3): S1–155.

27. Vincenti F, Charpentier B, Vanrenterghem Y et al. A phase III study of belatacept-based immunosuppression regimens versus cyclosporine in renal transplant recipients (BENEFIT study). *Am J Transplant* 2010; **10**: 535–46.

28. Wadei HM, Textor SC. Hypertension in the kidney transplant recipient. *Transplant Rev (Orlando)* 2010; **24**: 105–20.

29. Paoletti E, Gherzi M, Amidone M, Massarino F, Cannella G. Association of arterial hypertension with renal target organ damage in kidney transplant recipients: the predictive role of ambulatory blood pressure monitoring. *Transplantation* 2009; **87**: 1864–9.

30. Shoskes DA, Cecka JM. Deleterious effects of delayed graft function in cadaveric renal transplant recipients independent of acute rejection. *Transplantation* 1998; **66**: 1697–701.

31. Ojo AO, Wolfe RA, Held PJ, Port FK, Schmouder RL. Delayed graft function: risk factors and implications for renal allograft survival. *Transplantation* 1997; **63**: 968–74.

32. Doshi MD, Garg N, Reese PP, Parikh CR. Recipient risk factors associated with delayed graft function: a paired kidney analysis. *Transplantation* 2011; **91**: 666–71.

33. Nankivell BJ, Alexander SI. Rejection of the kidney allograft. *N Engl J Med* 2010; **363**: 1451–62.

34. Solez K, Colvin RB, Racusen LC et al. Banff 07 classification of renal allograft pathology: updates and future directions. *Am J Transplant* 2008; **8**: 753–60.

35. Rodrigo E, Fernandez-Fresnedo G, Valero R et al. New-onset diabetes after kidney transplantation: risk factors. *J Am Soc Nephrol* 2006; **17** (12 Suppl 3): S291–5.

36. Luan FL, Steffick DE, Ojo AO. New-onset diabetes mellitus in kidney transplant recipients discharged on steroid-free immunosuppression. *Transplantation* 2011; **91**: 334–41.

37. Fishman JA. Infection in solid-organ transplant recipients. *N Engl J Med* 2007; **357**: 2601–14.

38. Axelrod DA, McCullough KP, Brewer ED et al. Kidney and pancreas transplantation in the United States, 1999–2008: the changing face of living donation. *Am J Transplant* 2010; **10** (4 Pt 2): 987–1002.

39. Troppmann C. Complications after pancreas transplantation. *Curr Opin Organ Transplant* 2010; **15**: 112–18.

40. Goodman J, Becker YT. Pancreas surgical complications. *Curr Opin Organ Transplant* 2009; **14**: 85–9.

41. Lall CG, Sandrasegaran K, Maglinte DT, Fridell JA. Bowel complications seen on CT after pancreas transplantation with enteric drainage. *AJR Am J Roentgenol* 2006; **187**: 1288–95.

42. Sollinger HW, Odorico JS, Becker YT, D'Alessandro AM, Pirsch JD. One thousand simultaneous pancreas-kidney transplants at a single center with 22-year follow-up. *Ann Surg* 2009; **250**: 618–30.

43. Adrogue HE, Matas AJ, McGlennon RC et al. Do inherited hypercoagulable states play a role in thrombotic events affecting kidney/pancreas transplant recipients? *Clin Transplant* 2007; **21**: 32–7.

44. Drachenberg CB, Papadimitriou JC, Farney A et al. Pancreas transplantation: the histologic morphology of graft loss and clinical correlations. *Transplantation* 2001; **71**: 1784–91.

45. Rostambeigi N, Kudva YC, John S et al. Epidemiology of infections requiring hospitalization during long-term follow-up of pancreas transplantation. *Transplantation* 2010; **89**: 1126–33.

Chapter 43

Psychological and emotional reactions to illness and surgery

Nisha N. Shah and Charles L. Raison

Few voluntary experiences in life challenge the psychological equilibrium of persons more than hospitalization due to major physical illness and surgery. Not only must patients face the prospect of death, pain, and disability, they must acquiesce to do so with the loss of personal control, identity, and independence. Patients must willingly agree to all of these terms in a foreign environment that is created not to meet their needs per se, but more to cater to the needs of bureaucratic institutions that dictate what the patients' needs are to the hospital staff. Moreover, under these conditions patients must be ready to tolerate a never-ending onslaught of repetitive personal questions and humiliating and invasive examinations and procedures. It is a wonder that most patients do not respond to their physicians and other hospital staff with anxiety, fear, anger, and dependency.

Reactions to the stressors mentioned above can vary among patients. Factors that may influence resilience include preexisting psychological strength, amount of family support available, financial resources, type and extent of illness, surgical procedures involved, and overall prognosis. For example, elderly patients in particular may not have family readily available. Older patients with cognitive impairment may become more confused, disoriented, and agitated without familiar faces to provide a sense of environmental stability. For patients whose prognosis, although improved, may sustain a visible loss of a body part or possible function of a body part, such as women undergoing mastectomy, patients receiving an ostomy, and men undergoing urologic surgery, losing love and sexual desirability or function may lead to a profound experience of grief over the loss. Patients facing financial stressors may suffer from intense anxiety associated with the immediate physical incapacitation after surgery and the fear that they may never be well enough again to deal with their financial obligations.

Despite the stressful nature of illness, hospitalization, and surgery, most patients may be expected to do well. Physicians should, however, be alert for signs and symptoms suggesting that a patient's ability to adapt to the stress of illness is being overwhelmed, indicating some degree of psychological decompensation.

Behavioral regression

While maladaptive and pathologic responses to stressors may be an extension of psychological pathology prior to hospitalization, in most cases these behaviors are out of character for the patient and are likely the result of behavioral regression.

The concept of regression indicates that patients, in reaction to the stress of illness and enforced dependency on others, may resort to more infantile and childlike ways of thinking, feeling, and behaving. Regressive behavior is characterized by withdrawal from interaction with others, helplessness, clinging, excessive dependency, and fear. Regression can be considered akin to a short-term depression with the added problem of staff discomfort during interactions, to which the patients may be oblivious. In most situations, this regression is time limited as patients recover from and adapt to their illnesses.

Under certain circumstances, however, patients may undergo more severe and prolonged regression, particularly those with little or no social support, marginal abilities to cope under severe stress, or preexisting psychiatric disorders. Patients may also whine and complain, and be angry, irritable, and demanding. Serious forms of regression may lead to profound emotional withdrawal, passivity, depression, and occasionally, overtly psychotic behavior. Even the strongest and most psychologically healthy person may at times be overwhelmed emotionally in the context of severe stress, resulting in regressive forms of behavior.

Understanding the concept of behavioral regression under stress and its behavioral manifestations is helpful in the physician's management of these reactions. Because regression involves the display of frightened and childlike behavior, patients' reactions to physicians may resemble those of children to frustrated parents. Physicians, in patients' view, may take on the roles of powerful and authoritative parent figures. Although such dependency may make some patients compliant with treatment and thankful for the physicians' help, other more difficult reactions may occur. Patients may displace their

Medical Management of the Surgical Patient, ed. Michael F. Lubin, Thomas F. Dodson, and Neil H. Winawer. Published by Cambridge University Press. © Cambridge University Press 2013.

anger, fear, and frustration on their physicians and become resistant, difficult, defiant, and critical of the treatment offered; they may even threaten litigation. Reasonable limits should be set for such behavior, and physicians ideally should attempt to help patients understand the feelings that usually underlie such behavior and empathize with those feelings as much as possible rather than responding with anger and defensiveness.

Physicians must give steady and consistent emotional support to patients who are in regressive emotional turmoil by providing information, advice, encouragement, and realistic reassurance. These efforts, termed *ego support* or *shoring-up of the ego*, are directed toward preventing extensive behavioral regression by suppressing anxiety and strengthening patients' psychological defenses and coping mechanisms. Severe regression should be prevented by encouraging patients to pursue rehabilitation efforts, helping them to become as independent as possible, and allowing them to participate as much as is reasonable in decisions regarding their care. The last approach gives patients a sense of control over their treatment.

One of the more common difficulties for physicians is patients who exhibit profound emotional reactions to an illness such as crying or becoming deeply depressed, helpless, and dependant. Physicians who are uncomfortable with these types of intense emotions may actively discourage patients from talking about their feelings, avoid such patients, or offer unrealistic, patronizing reassurance. Such intense emotions, however, are often best handled with carefully titrated brief periods of catharsis that allow patients to ventilate, "blow off steam," or cry, and empathizing with the patients' feelings. Such periods of emotional catharsis are usually transient and provide relief for patients by reassurance that physicians are interested and open to their feelings. Severe regressive behaviors that are persistent or accompanied by evidence of severe depression, anxiety, or significant psychopathologic reactions (especially those that create conflict or tension in the doctor–patient relationship) are indications for psychiatric referral [1].

Identification of high-risk groups

Several characteristics place patients at relatively higher risk for the development of psychiatric complications during illness or surgery. Although no particular patient profile is totally predictive, there are criteria for identifying and monitoring high-risk patients. Groups of psychologically high-risk patients have been delineated by Stoudemire [2]. High-risk groups include the following:

- Patients with histories of psychotic decompensation, delirium, or psychiatric consultation during previous physical illnesses or surgeries.
- Patients who refuse or are resistant to undergo surgery or who threaten to leave the hospital against medical advice or refuse to sign a consent form.

- Patients with histories of difficult or hostile relationships with nursing, medical, or surgical staff.
- Patients with unrealistic or magical expectations of their surgery, including excessive denial.
- Patients who present special diagnostic problems, such as histories of multiple surgeries for questionable or vague indications with negative results (malingering, hysterical, factitious, or hypochondriacal patients).
- Patients who show blasé, apathetic reactions or lack of appropriate concern and anxiety.
- Patients with histories of alcohol and substance abuse or those who are taking multiple psychotropic or analgesic agents.
- Elderly patients with cognitive impairment who are at risk for postoperative delirium.
- Patients with histories of medical litigation or questionable disability suits.
- Patients with histories of chronic pain complaints of obscure cause.

Value of preoperative psychological assessment

Numerous studies have demonstrated the potential value of preoperative preparation of patients to promote increased tolerance to the stresses of the surgical procedure [3]. Education efforts provide patients with information that helps them anticipate surgery, which may diminish uncertainty and alleviate anxiety. Patients who receive information and are familiar with the staff and the medical–surgical routine are better able to anticipate and prepare for whatever discomfort the procedure may entail. Doering *et al.* conducted a study that compared pre- and postoperative anxiety and the need for postoperative pain medications in patients who viewed a videotape of a total-hip replacement surgery the night before surgery and patients who did not [4]. Patients who viewed the videotape the night before surgery were found to have less anxiety, both pre- and postoperatively, and also were found to need less analgesic medication postoperatively. Such preparation is particularly important for children.

Other investigations have reported decreased postoperative delirium in groups of patients who receive preoperative preparation by a psychiatrist or a geriatrician trained in psychological evaluation and testing [5,6]. Several additional studies have reported improved recovery rates in patients who received instruction designed to facilitate coping with the stress of surgery [7,8]. Although surgeons may have a limited amount of time to devote to extensive educational efforts, some programs can be administered by ancillary medical or nursing personnel with the aid of audiovisual guides.

Although significant methodological problems exist for most studies that claim effectiveness of psychiatric and behavioral interventions in improving postoperative outcomes, data suggest that appropriate screening and evaluation of high-risk patients and provision of adequate information to decrease anticipatory anxiety and postoperative confusion will yield therapeutic benefits and perhaps decrease the likelihood of major psychiatric complications.

Acknowledgment

This is an updated version of a chapter by the late Alan Stoudemire, MD.

References

1. Green, SA. Principles of medical psychotherapy. In Stoudemire A, Fogel B, Greenberg D, eds. *Psychiatric Care of the Medical Patient*. 2nd edn. New York, NY: Oxford University Press; 2000, pp. 3–18.

2. Stoudemire, A. Psychologic and emotional reactions to illness and surgery. In Lubin MF, Walker HK, Smith RB, eds. *Medical Management of the Surgical Patient*. Philadelphia, PA: Lippincott Company; 1995, pp. 427–9.

3. Hadj A, Esmore D, Rowland M *et al.* Pre-operative preparation for cardiac surgery utilising a combination of metabolic, physical and mental therapy. *Heart Lung Circ* 2006; **15**: 172–81.

4. Doering S, Katzlberger F, Rumpold G. *et al.* Videotape preparation of patients before hip replacement surgery reduces stress. *Psychosom Med* 2000; **62**: 365–73.

5. Layne OL Jr, Yudofsky SC. Postoperative psychosis in cardiotomy patients. The role of organic and psychiatric factors. *N Engl J Med* 1971; **284**: 518–20.

6. Marcantonio ER, Flacker JM, Wright RJ *et al.* Reducing delirium after hip fracture: a randomized trial. *J Am Geriatr Soc* 2001; **49**: 516–22.

7. Kain ZN, Caldwell-Andrews AA, Mayes LC *et al.* Family-centered preparation for surgery improves perioperative outcomes in children: a randomized controlled trial. *Anesthesiology* 2007; **106**: 65–74.

8. Shelley M, Pakenham KI, Frazer I. Cortisol changes interact with the effects of a cognitive behavioural psychological preparation for surgery on 12-month outcomes for surgical heart patients. *Psychol Health* 2009; **24**: 1139–52.

Chapter 44

Depression and the surgical patient

Nisha N. Shah and Charles L. Raison

During a time when surgeons are under constant scrutiny to have shorter postoperative recovery times as well as better outcomes, depression is often a costly and common comorbidity. The point prevalence for depression in the medically ill is 10–36% for general medical inpatients.

Depression is an omnipresent factor in patient recovery. Depression negatively impacts the ability of patients to care adequately for their wounds and can interfere with optimal behavior choices by promoting activities such as poor nutrition, smoking, and illicit substance use, which can lead to complications in recovery [1]. Furthermore, depression plays a role in how patients perceive their recovery. According to a study looking at three HMO populations by Pearson *et al.* more than half of people in the top 15% of medical resource utilization were suffering from undiagnosed depression [2]. Via these factors, and perhaps also as a result of depression-related pathophysiological changes, depressed and anxious patients have a 5–6 times higher risk for 30-day and in-hospital mortality after surgery when compared with patients with no psychiatric comorbidities [3].

Presentations of depressive symptoms and the *Diagnostic and Statistical Manual of Mental Disorders*

In the surgical setting, patients can present with depressive symptoms during any phase of their treatment. It is of singular importance to establish a time-frame for the onset of depression in relation to the intervention or other illnesses from which the patient may be suffering in order to understand the most likely etiologies for any given patient's presentation (see Figure 44.1). All presentations of depressive symptoms are not necessarily major depressive disorder (MDD). At certain times, depressive symptoms can act as harbingers of other undetected illnesses (see Table 44.1). At other times, depressive symptoms can reflect ongoing treatment with psychoactive medications (Substance Induced Mood Disorder), short-term reactions to acute stressors (Adjustment Disorder with Depressed mood, see Table 44.2) or may be the result of a delirious state (see Table 44.3).

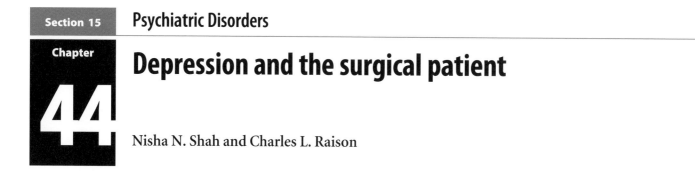

Probable Diagnosis (from high likelihood to low likelihood) given onset of depressive symptoms in relation to surgical intervention

Years**	Months*	Weeks	Days	Hours	Surgical Intervention	Hours	Days	Weeks	Months	Years**
MDD	MDD	MDD	Adjustment Disorder	Delirium		Delirium	Delirium	Adjustment Disorder	MDD	MDD
Medical Condition	Medical Condition	Adjustment Disorder	Delirium	Substance Induced		Subtance Induced	Subtance Induced	MDD	Adjustment Disorder	Medical Condition
Substance Induced	Adjustment Disorder	Medical Condition	Substance Induced	Medical Condition		Medical Condition	Medical Condition	Delirium	Medical Condition	Substance Induced
	Substance Induced	Delirium	Medical Condition	Adjustment Disorder		Adjustment Disorder	Adjustment Disorder	Substance Induced	Susbtance Induced	
			MDD				MDD			

* Adjustment Disorder is usually diagnosed within 3 months of the onset of the stressor
**Delirium can continue for at least a year in the event that it is insufficiently treated

Figure 44.1 This table is a gross generalization of likely common diagnoses associated with depressive symptoms.

Medical Management of the Surgical Patient, ed. Michael F. Lubin, Thomas F. Dodson, and Neil H. Winawer. Published by Cambridge University Press. © Cambridge University Press 2013.

Table 44.1 Medical illnesses and medications associated with the presentation of depressive symptoms.

Neurological disorders	Medications associated with neurological disorders
Meningitis	Antihypertensives (beta-blockers,
Stroke	reserpine, methyldopa)
Epilepsy	Benzodiazepines
Multiple sclerosis	
Dementia	
Parkinson's disease	
Huntington's disease	
Wilson's disease	

Endocrine	Medications associated with endocrine disorders
Thyroid disease (hyper-/hypo-)	Corticosteroids
Adrenal dysfunction	Contraceptives
(Cushing's/Addison's)	
Hyperparathyroidism	
Diabetes mellitus	

Cancer	Medications associated with pain treatment
Pancreatic cancer	Antineoplastics (interferon,
Paraneoplastic syndromes	procarbazine, vincristine,
Brain tumors	vinblastine, tamoxifen)
Lymphomas	

Chronic pain (Metabolic)	Medications associated with pain treatment
Porphyria	Opiates
Renal insufficiency	Corticosteroids
Hepatic encephalopathy	
Metabolic disturbances caused by diabetes mellitus (glucose dysregulation, ketoacidosis)	

Infectious disease	Medications associated with the excess excretion of H2
Lyme disease	Ranitidine
HIV	Cimetidine
Herpes simplex virus	
Syphilis	
Rabies	
Prions	

Table 44.2 Adjustment disorder with depressed mood (summarized from the DSM–IV–TR criteria for adjustment disorder).

1. Emotional and behavioral response to an identifiable stressor within 3 months of onset of the stressor
2. Either is notable about the response:
   (a) It is in excess of what would be expected (with symptoms of depressed mood, hopelessness, and tearfulness)
   (b) Functional impairment in occupational (academic) and social areas
3. No other psychiatric diagnosis or personality disorder can better explain these symptoms
4. These symptoms are not better explained by bereavement
5. The symptoms do not occur beyond an additional 6 months

Table 44.3 Delirium due to a general medical condition (summarized from the DSM–IV–TR criteria for delirium due to a general medical condition).

1. Altered consciousness evidenced by clouded awareness of the environment and loss of concentrative ability – with difficulty in appropriately both sustaining or shifting attention
2. An uncharacteristic change in cognition evidenced by sudden memory deficit, disorientation, speech disturbances, and perceptual disturbances with no precedent that would lead to the diagnosis of dementia
3. These alterations develop within a period of hours to days with a fluctuating course
4. History, physical examination or laboratory findings provide evidence that the disturbance is caused by the direct physiological consequences of a general medical condition

The Diagnostic Statistical Manual of Mental Disorders (DSM–IV) criteria for major depressive disorder are listed in Table 44.4. The DSM–IV is a general road map to guide clinicians in the diagnosis of MDD and therefore can be of particular relevance to patients who present with depressive symptoms prior to a surgical intervention or who have strong personal or familial histories of depression. However, it is important to recognize that too strict an adherence to DSM–IV criteria risks minimizing depressive symptoms following an operation, because by DSM diagnostic rules, MDD cannot be diagnosed if a medical illness or procedure is believed to be causative. Clinicians are required to draw conclusions about whether a patient's mood symptoms have a direct correlation to the condition for which he or she is receiving treatment, and if such a correlation can be made, the patient is said to have a Mood Disorder due to a general medical condition. Caution must be exercised that this diagnosis does not detrimentally "normalize" a patient's depressive suffering or reduce the alacrity with which the depressive symptoms are treated.

Beyond this specific concern, diagnosing depression in the context of medical illness is always a challenge, and the postoperative state is no exception. As with other medical conditions, a number of depressive "somatic" or "neurovegetative" symptoms can be produced by the surgical intervention itself, including decreased appetite, change in weight, sleep disturbance, loss of energy, and diminished capacity to think or concentrate. In the context of medical illness, Endicott suggests replacing these types of somatic symptoms with more psychologically oriented symptoms such as tearfulness, depressed appearance, social withdrawal, decreased talkativeness, brooding, self-pity, pessimism, lack of reactivity, and blunting [4]. In fact, the substitutive criteria of social withdrawal and lack of reactivity were studied by Akechi *et al.* in patients with cancer and were found to be sensitive markers of moderate to severe depression, which would be amenable to therapeutic intervention [5].

Table 44.4 Major depressive disorder (summarized from the DSM–IV criteria for major depressive episode).

(A) A presentation of depressed mood, disinterest, or anhedonia, over a period of 2 weeks or greater, must be subjectively reported or observed by others with five or more of the simultaneously occurring symptoms below

1. Depressed mood, which could be subjectively described as sadness, emptiness or frequent tearfulness as described by observers. The depressed mood occurs daily as well as throughout the day
2. A loss of interest or pleasure in the majority of daily activities, on a daily basis
3. Trouble falling asleep, staying asleep, or sleeping significantly more than baseline, on a daily basis
4. Unintentional changes in weight greater than 5% of the person's total body weight or significantly diminished or excessive appetite
5. Observable changes in psychomotor function (retardation or agitation) by others
6. Report of significant loss of energy and fatigue
7. Daily excessive, inappropriate guilt and feelings of worthlessness, which may appear delusional in presentation. Mere self-reproach or feelings of guilt with regard to sickness are insufficient to meet this criteria
8. Daily marked inability to concentrate, think, or make decisions either noted subjectively or by others
9. Recurring suicidal ideation, with or without a plan, recent suicide attempt, or morbid preoccupation with death

(B) Criteria for a manic, hypomanic, or mixed episode, as associated with bipolar disorder, have never been met
(C) Marked disturbance in social, occupational, and other important areas of functioning are noted as a result of the symptoms of depression
(D) The presentation of these symptoms is not better accounted for by the direct physiological effects of a medication or substance of abuse nor a general medical condition (e.g., anemia or hypothyroidism)
(E) Bereavement, due to the loss of a loved one, does not better account for the symptoms. If after a period of 2 months, bereavement leads to morbid preoccupation with suicidal ideation, a deepening sense of worthlessness, significant disturbance in functionality, and notable psychomotor retardation, a diagnosis of major depressive disorder should be considered

High-risk situations involving depressive symptoms

Evaluating for suicidality

In addition to the increased mortality rate associated with MDD due to postoperative complications, there is the mortality associated with completed suicide. Fifteen percent of patients who suffer from severe affective disorders complete suicide [6]. Thus, any patient presenting with depressive symptoms should be assessed for suicidal thoughts and behaviors.

Table 44.5 Major risk factors (chronic) for suicide.

Predetermined chronic risk factors for suicide	Modifiable chronic risk factors for suicide
Demographic factors	Psychological factors
Gender: Male	Personality variables including aggression, hostility, or impulsivity
Race: White	Bipolar disorder or mood cycling
Age: 24–35 or > 50	More severe depressive symptoms (diminished concentration, insomnia, anhedonia, but not diminished energy level)
Historical factors	
Previous suicidal ideation, and history of being discovered after an attempt	
Family history of suicide	Presence of psychosis
Recent loss of a loved one (or relationship), especially a spouse	Concomitant anxiety or panic attacks
Parental loss at an age before 11	Lack of treatment or inadequate treatment of depressive episode
History of sexual abuse, physical abuse, or corporal punishment during childhood or adolescence	Medical factors
Multiple previous hospitalizations for depression and young age at first hospitalization	Concurrent general medical conditions
Early-onset depression	Social factors
Recent exposure to suicide	Access to means with greater lethality (firearms in particular)
Psychological factors	Social isolation
Diagnosis of depressive episode within a period of 3 months	
Substance dependence and recent intoxication with a substance	
Borderline personality traits or disorder	
Antisocial personality traits or disorder	
Medical factors	
Concurrent general medical conditions	
Chronic physical illness or chronic pain	
Social factors	
Social, familial, or financial instability (familial crisis or unemployment)	
Lack of religious or moral constraints against suicide	
Not living with a child younger than 18	

The evaluation of suicidality should begin with a frank and open discussion about ideas, thoughts, motives, plans, intent, and previous attempts at self-harm. A common misconception about the assessment of suicide risk is that asking about suicidal ideation will bring the idea to patients' minds and increase the

Table 44.6 Criteria for admission of suicidal patients.

1. There is no apparent improvement with the start of medication and therapy between interviews
2. Psychosis is present to such an extent that patients pose a physical threat to themselves or others
3. The presentation of psychosis has exhausted caregivers and all external support
4. Command hallucinations are present
5. Physicians are unclear as to the severity of patients' presentation
6. Patients are intoxicated with medications, alcohol, or illict drugs

Table 44.7 Elaborating the "I WATCH DEATH" mnemonic for delirum.

Infections	Meningitis, encephalitis, urinary tract infections, pneumonia, sepsis, HIV, AIDS defining illnesses, syphilis
Withdrawal	Alcohol, benzodiazepines, barbiturates
Acute metabolic encephalopathy	Acidosis, alkalosis, electrolyte disturbances (e.g., hyponatremia, hypercalcemia, hypoglycemia, hypomagnesemia), renal failure (azotemia), hepatic failure
CNS pathology	Epilepsy, hemorrhage, subdural hematoma, hydrocephalus, abscess, tumor
Trauma	Intracerebral hemorrhage, closed head injury, burn injury
Hypoxia	Pulmonary failure, cardiac failure, hypotension, anemia, carbon monoxide poisoning
Deficiencies	Thiamine, folate, vitamin B_{12}, niacin
Endocrinopathies	Hyper-/hypoglycemia, hyper-/hypothyroidism, hyper-/hypoparathyroidism, hyper-/hypoadrenocorticism
Acute vascular	Shock, stroke, hypertensive encephalopathy, arrhythmia
Toxins or drugs	Illicit drugs, medications, pesticides, and solvents
Heavy metals	Lead, mercury, manganese

risk of suicide. Actually the opposite is true; patients are likely to have been harboring suicidal ideations prior to the discussion and asking them detailed questions about their ideations can actually help the provider conceptualize the risk associated with the ideation. Acute predictors for suicidal behavior and high-risk ideation have multiple similarities [7].

In addition to direct patient information, collateral history obtained from family members often reveals those patients who have already made up their minds to end their lives and want no one to intervene. These patients often set their affairs in order, make out a will, and "get better" suddenly as a result of them perceiving that they have figured a way out of their situation. In questioning potential suicidal patients it is important to ask about the method of suicide and evaluate the chance of rescue. Plans that involve guns, hanging, jumping, or carbon monoxide leave little chance for rescue and are in fact the most frequent methods of completed suicide.

Acute predictors to look for in suicide completion are worsening anxiety, agitation, restless/insomnia, increased inability to concentrate, increased psychotic behavior, and recent intoxication [8]. Chronic risk factors (see Table 44.5), although not specific, should also inform decisions regarding intensive 1 : 1 supervision, admission to an inpatient psychiatric ward, discharge, and the amount of lag time before the patient has mental health follow-up.

If a significant suicide risk exists, immediate psychiatric consultation is needed before patients are discharged from the hospital. Steps should also be taken to protect the patient in the current hospital setting by utilizing family and friends or hospital staff (intensive 1 : 1 supervision) to ensure that the patient is not left alone prior to psychiatric assessment and disposition. Psychiatric hospitalization is often accepted voluntarily by patients who realize that they need additional care. In cases where patients must be hospitalized against their will, the broad grounds for psychiatric commitment usually state that these patients must have a mental illness and be either a danger to themselves or to others, or be unable to care for themselves as a result of a psychiatric condition. Psychiatric commitment varies from state to state and psychiatric consultation is recommended before pursuing this option. Table 44.6 lists criteria for hospital admission for suicidal patients.

Major depressive disorder with psychotic features versus delirium

A delirious presentation is often mistaken for depression in the postoperative patient. This mistake can be a costly one for several reasons. First, and foremost, delirium is a marker for significant ongoing physiological abnormalities, as demonstrated by the fact that the 90-day mortality is as high as 11% for elderly delirious patients versus 3% for patients who are not delirious [9]. Second, the treatment for delirium is quite different from the treatment of depression. Antidepressants do not appear to aid in delirium, and can actually make the condition worse. On the other hand, antipsychotic agents typically resolve delirious symptoms, including anxiety and dysphoria, very rapidly, even without the underlying medical cause having been resolved.

Because both delirium and depression are extremely common in hospitalized patients, it is of utmost importance to be able to tell them apart. The criteria in the DSM–IV for delirium (please see Table 44.3) can help the clinician conceptualize the similarities and differences between delirious and depressed presentations. The similarities shared between the two diagnoses are the reduced ability to concentrate, change in behavior, and sleep disturbances. The two major differentiating factors lie in the apparent disturbance of consciousness ("waxing and waning") and the gross and sudden changes in cognition. In the hyperactive presentation of delirium, patients often show increased arousal and actively respond to hallucinations. Patients with previous history of psychiatric disorders who present with hyperactive delirium are often mistaken as having an acute exacerbation of their psychiatric disorder as opposed to being delirious. It is imperative that an algorithm be employed when addressing the probable causes for a sudden change in behavior in the post-operative patient. I WATCH DEATH is a common mnemonic that can work as a thorough algorithm (please see Table 44.7 for further elaboration on this mnemonic). However, given the associated mortality with delirium, in the event that the surgical team is unsure of the etiological cause of a sudden change in a patient's behavior, a psychiatric consultation is well warranted.

Severe depression can often present with some cognitive dysfunction, psychomotor retardation, worsening sleep–wake cycles, and psychosis. The inherent difference between delirium and severe depression lies in the consistency of symptoms seen in the presentation of depression. Another differentiating factor found in a study conducted by Ohayon and Schatzberg [10], which discusses the high prevalence of psychosis in depression, is that feelings of worthlessness and guilt expressed by the patient are often highly associated with psychosis in depression.

Treatment of depressive symptoms

As detailed above, the etiologies of depressive symptoms are often complex. Therefore, prior to treatment, even after a diagnosis of MDD is established, it is of crucial importance to look at all causative medical and pharmacological factors contributing to the presentation. In many instances treating the illness, removing or decreasing a particular pharmacological agent can be curative. Table 44.1 lists the medical factors and pharmacological agents associated with secondary mood disorders.

Pain and depression

Surgery and pain are intimately connected. Interestingly however, in a recent study conducted by Sommer et al. [11], 41% of 1,490 surgical patients seen in the Netherlands reported moderate to severe pain despite the presence of an acute pain protocol. Another study of 36 UK National Health Service hospitals reported that in a survey of 3,000 postoperative patients 81% reported moderate to severe pain [12]. Evidently, pain is under-treated. Possible reasons that pain medications are under-utilized may include clinicians' over-exaggerated fear of addiction, underestimations of effective doses, and overestimation of the duration of narcotic action. In the event that the clinician has substantiated evidence that the patient has opioid dependence it is still of utmost importance that the patient receive appropriate analgesic treatment.

In fact, in patients who are using methadone, it may be appropriate to restart methadone after surgery and supplement with other analgesic medications to cover the patient's pain appropriately [13]. However, even in those patients who are not using methadone and who may eventually experience withdrawal, if opioids are the only appropriate treatment available they should be used. Dependence should not be a consideration in the terminally ill patient, beyond understanding their level of tolerance.

Patients with acute postoperative and chronic pain (although often under-treated) may be presenting with depression associated with pain or with depression masked under the guise of pain. High rates of pain complaints have been observed in depressed patients, including headaches, abdominal pain, joint pain, back pain, and chest pain [14]. Surprisingly, as opposed to those suffering from pain alone, those suffering from "somatizing" depression or depression and pain, were found to have had significant non-adherence to their opioid prescription, with under-use being twice as likely than over-use [15]. The "somatizing" patient often finds great difficulty with verbalizing feelings and will rarely present to the outpatient clinic with depressive or anxious symptoms [16]. Outside the pain presentation, patients will frequently present with the more neuro-vegetative signs of depression. Therefore, it is imperative that the treating physician not accept patients' denials of depressed mood as reason to exclude the diagnosis.

Indications for the start of treatment for depression

Once recognized through the DSM–IV criteria (Table 44.4) and substitutive criteria discussed earlier in this chapter, the indication to treat MDD is clear. However, in the event that the presentation is not easily distinguished from other diagnoses, collateral corroboration of details with regard to onset, duration, and other neuro-vegetative signs can be helpful.

There are many approaches to the treatment of depression. The appropriate approach for each patient is always determined by the severity of presentation and by the patient's preference. Pharmacological interventions, electroconvulsive therapy, and psychotherapy are some of the modalities currently available for the treatment of MDD in the pre- and postoperative setting. These treatments are often combined into a mix that is uniquely suited to the patient's needs.

Psychopharmacology

Medication is perhaps the most common of the interventions mentioned above. The pharmacy for MDD is ever expanding. Please see Table 44.8 for an organized listing of the categories of different medications available for the treatment of MDD, their dose ranges, their general properties, their common side-effects and potential adverse effects.

With the exception of stimulants, which are only used in extreme cases of treatment-resistant depression, a lag time of 4–6 weeks is typically seen before full symptomatic

Table 44.8 Categories of medications useful for the treatment of major depression.

Classes of antidepressants	Names of antidepressants	Elimination half-life	Considerations	Recommendations
Selective serotonin reuptake inhibitors (SSRIs) Block the reuptake of serotonin	Fluoxetine Paroxetine Sertraline Citalopram Escitalopram Fluvoxamine	2–3 days 1 day 1 day 1 day 27–32 hours 15 hours	1. Benefits a typical depression presentation, if melancholic or atypical symptoms (morning depression, leaden paralysis, loss of reactivity) present, medications in other classes should be considered 2. Caution with concomitant administration of SSRIs and lidocaine, midazolam and fentanyl, due to potential of serotonin syndrome. SSRIs lower the seizure threshold. Serotonin syndrome	1. Continue administering if psychiatrically indicated, up until time of surgery and after surgery resume medication
Tricyclic antidepressants (TCAs) Block the reuptake of serotonin	Amitriptyline Doxepin Imipramine Desipramine Nortriptyline Maprotiline Protriptyline	15–20 hours 15–20 hours 15–20 hours 15–20 hours 1–2 days 1–2 days 3 days	1. Should be considered only after treatment failure with SSRIs in typical depression. However may be appropriate for initial treatment in depression associated with pain and insomnia 2. Interactions with general/regional agents, leading to intraventricular conduction delays. Causes arrhythmia when administered with epinephrine 3. Can act synergistically with other anticholinergic agents, causing toxicity 4. TCAs must be tapered when attempting to stop administration as sudden withdrawal can lead to arrhythmias and cholinergic rebound lowers seizure threshold	1. Continue administering if psychiatrically indicated, up until time of surgery 2. Due to TCA anticholinergic effects an additional anticholinergic may be unnecessary. If an anticholinergic is needed then glycopyrrolate may be needed 3. Enflurance should be avoided as it too decreases the seizure threshold
Monoamine oxidase inhibitors (MAOIs) Prevent degradation of serotonin	Phenelzine Tranylcypromine Isocarboxazid	3 hours, however clinical effect lasts for 10–14 days	1. Benefits those patients with atypical depression. It is often turned to in treatment-resistant depression 2. Due to adrenergic release, blood pressure may be difficult to manage 3. Avoid exogenous pressors as they can make blood pressure lability worse 4. Muscle blockers and opiates are potentiated, with the exception of meperidine 5. Avoid diet with high tryamine content, meperidine, serotonergic antidepressants, and dextromethorphan 6. Avoid abrupt withdrawal as this can lead to delirium and psychosis	1. Taper patient off medication 7–14 days prior to surgery, however, if needed, treatment can continue until surgery 2. Direct vasopressors should be used in place of indirect pressors 3. There must be clear communication with the anesthesiologist about current or previous use of MAOIs 4. The importance of avoiding diet high in tyramine and no meperidine, should be clearly outlined in the chart. Morphine and fentanyl appear to be safe at low doses

Table 44.8 (cont.)

Classes of antidepressants	Names of antidepressants	Elimination half-life	Considerations	Recommendations
Serotonin norepinephrine reuptake inhibitors (SNRIs) Block the reuptake of serotonin, norepinephrine, and dopamine	Venlafaxine Duloxetine Milnacipran	5–11 hours 12 hours	1. Benefits those patients with typical and melancholic presentations of depression who have marked decrease in energy or an anxious component to their presentation. 2. Be aware of dose-dependent increases in blood pressure 3. SIADH or hyponatremia can be caused by this class. Insomnia, dry mouth, constipation and asthenia, sweating and nervousness may occur on initiation	1. Continue administering if psychiatrically indicated, up until time of surgery and after surgery resume medication 2. Monitor metabolites and electrolytes closely prior to start/restart of medication
Atypical antidepressants Noradrenergic and specific serotonergic antidepressant	Mirtazapine	20–40 hours	1. Benefits melancholic presentations of depression and is commonly used as an adjunct medication at low doses (7.5/15 mg) – with well-known appetite stimulation and soporific effects 2. Has rare effects of transient liver enzyme increases and severe neutropenia	1. Continue administering if psychiatrically indicated, up until time of surgery and after surgery resume medication 2. Close monitoring of liver enzymes and monitoring blood counts, on initiation, especially in compromised patients should be practiced

improvement is seen with antidepressants. It is vital to counsel patients prior to medication start that the medications do not usually lead to overnight improvement. That said, there are certain studies that do substantiate immediate clinical benefit, such as improved mood regulation, from just one dose of particular antidepressants [17] as well as from one week of use [18].

Antidepressants should be administered from 6 months to 12 months after their initiation. Gradual tapering of medications after these time periods can be attempted, however, frequent monitoring should occur to observe for depression relapse.

Several general principles enhance safety and compliance:

1. Anticipate with the patient the probable side-effects; include a review of the most common side-effects. Reassure the patient that there are strategies to minimize the adverse effects of medications.
2. Select drugs that have the smallest chance of exacerbating current medical problems. Use the lowest effective dose and gradually titrate the dose. This may minimize side-effects because side-effects are often dose-related.
3. "Start low, go slow," especially in the elderly, neurologically impaired, and medically ill patients.
4. Manage side-effects with adjunctive agents rather than switching to another agent that may delay therapeutic response.

5. Reassure the patient; side-effects frequently improve over time.
6. Educate the patient regularly that psychiatric symptoms often mirror common medication side-effects. Clearly written patient instructions will increase medication compliance. Symptoms that begin after medication initiation or worsen with dose escalation are likely to be medication-related.

Adverse effects of antidepressant medications

There are particular adverse effects associated with antidepressant use that are important to recognize due to their possible deleterious outcomes, as outlined below.

Serotonin syndrome

A potentially fatal adverse effect, serotonin syndrome often presents with a classic triad of symptoms: alterations in mental status, autonomic dysfunction, and neuromuscular excitability. Alterations in mental status can range from delirium to coma. Headaches, hallucinations, agitation, and hypomania are also common in the alterations in mental status associated with serotonin syndrome. Autonomic dysfunction includes hyperthermia, uncontrollable shivering and sweats, hypertension, and tachycardia. Neuromuscular excitability includes myoclonus, seizures, and rigidity.

Serotonin syndrome occurs in any clinical situation where a sudden surge of serotonin occurs due to iatrogenic or organic causes. This surge can either be a result of combining agents that are commonly known to directly increase the bioavailability of serotonin, such as antidepressants, or as a result of agents that are not commonly known to increase serotonin in the system such as opiates and stimulants. The combination of different classes of antidepressants, such as combining monoamine oxidase inhibitors with either tricyclic antidepressants or serotonin reuptake inhibitors is a well-known etiology of serotonin syndrome. Combining serotonin with opiates such as tramadol, meperidine, fentanyl, cyclobenzaprine, buprenorphine, methadone, oxycodone, and pentazocine has also led to serotonin syndrome. Stimulants such as ecstasy (MDMA), dextroamphetamine, methamphetamine, and sibutramine, either in overdose or in combination with other serotonergic agents have also been known to cause the syndrome [19].

The fatal outcomes of serotonin syndrome are related to both the autonomic dysfunction and neuromuscular excitability associated with the syndrome. It is therefore imperative to begin treatment immediately. First: stop the agents responsible; second: treat with $5HT_{2A}$ blockers: cyproheptadine in mild cases, and in extreme cases chlorpromazine, which is the only IV form of a $5HT_{2A}$ blocker available. Chlorpromazine

should be used with caution, given its cardiotoxic and epileptogenic effects. Please see Table 44.9 to learn about appropriate dosing for these medications. Other measures, such as ensuring that the patient is volume repleted and using benzodiazepines as adjunct medications to reduce aspects of the hyperpyrexia associated with serotonin, can be employed [20].

Hypertensive crisis

Hypertensive crisis, another potentially fatal adverse effect, is characterized by marked elevation in blood pressure, severe throbbing headache, stupor, somnolence, confusion, nausea, vomiting, and diaphoresis. Hypertensive crisis is primarily the result of a catecholamine surge in the system. This can occur by two mechanisms. First, when monoamine oxidase inhibitors (MAOI), e.g., phenelzine, isocarboxazid, and tranylcypromine, are taken orally and are irreversibly bound to the monoamine oxidase receptors peripherally (the intestine) as well as centrally, followed by the consumption of tyramine-rich food, causing an acute increase of tyramine in the system [21]. Second, the patient takes a medication with MAOI properties such as linezolid in conjunction with an SSRI or SNRI, increasing the amount of dopamine, serotonin, and norepinephrine in the system leading to a hypertensive crisis [22].

The fatal outcomes associated with hypertensive crisis are associated with the end-organ damage (hypertensive

Table 44.9 Therapeutic options for the serotonin syndrome.

Categories of agents	Agents	Loading dose	Maintenance dose	Precautions
$5HT_{2A}$ (Serotonin) blockers	Cyproheptadine	12–32 mg PO/NGT (crushed)	4–8 mg every 6 hour	1. This agent may cause significant sedation, however, this should not deter the clinician from use
	Chlorpromazine	12.5–25 mg IV/PO	25 mg every 6 hour	1. Fluid load initially due to possible hypotension due to alpha-2 receptor antagonism 2. May cause initial hyperthermia but this quickly resolves to hypothermia
Excessive muscle activity blockers (hyperthermia)	Long-acting benzodiazepines (diazepam)	5–10 mg IV/IM	5–10 mg every 3–4 hour	1. Respiratory depression is common with this class and intubation may be necessary, vigilance with regard to oxygenation is necessary
	Neuromuscular blockade (vercuronium)	0.08–0.1 mg/kg IV	0.8–1.2 μg/kg/min	1. Anesthesiology should be present for intubation and administration
Tachycardia/hypertension	Nitroprusside	0.3 μg/kg/min IV	0.3–10 μg/kg/min	1. May cause significant hypotension, clinician should be ready to fluid bolus patient 2. Slow infusion rate should be employed to avoid cyanide and hepatic/renal impairment
	Esmolol	500 μg/kg over 1 minute	50 μg/kg/min over 4 minutes if optimal pressure is not achieved then repeat bolus dose and increase 4 min infusion to 100 μg/kg/min	1. May cause significant hypotension, clinician should be ready to fluid bolus patient

emergency) via ischemia, infarction, and hemorrhage. Intracerebral hemorrhage has been a documented outcome associated with MAOI and tyramine-rich food consumption [21]. Once a patient's blood pressure reaches accelerated hypertension (a systolic pressure > 180 and a diastolic pressure > 110) with signs or symptoms, pharmacological intervention becomes an immediate necessity. Care should be exercised with regard to which anti-hypertensive medications are given, as some medications could worsen the patient's outcome. Please see Chapter 11 for further guidelines on treatment.

Orthostatic hypotension and sedation

Orthostatic hypotension is defined as a minimum decrease in systolic blood pressure of 20 mmHg or a minimum decrease in diastolic blood pressure of 10 mmHg, within 3 minutes of standing.

Tricyclic antidepressants, SSRIs, SNRIs, and MAOIs are well known to have the adverse effects of orthostatic hypotension and sedation due to their effects on histamine and alpha-adrenoceptors. This is of particular concern in the elderly population, patients who take anti-hypertensive medication, and patients with cardiovascular disease. Fracture and hemorrhage are associated with high morbidity and mortality in the elderly population [23]. Clinicians who place patients on these medications should actively monitor their blood pressures if there is a question of fall risk.

Interestingly, however, in a recent review by Darowski et al. it was found that the risk of fall in patients who suffer from untreated or under-treated depression was equivalent with those who were adequately treated with antidepressants and suffered the adverse effects of sedation or orthostatic hypotension from treatment [24].

Mania

The criteria for a manic episode are listed in Table 44.10. A manic episode represents a psychiatric emergency regardless of cause. Antidepressants can induce a manic episode due to hyperactivation of the limbic system. Manic "switch" can occur within the first week of starting a medication to 3 months after initiation.

Although the presentation of manic switch occurs more frequently in patients who have underlying Bipolar Disorder I and are taking antidepressants, patients with major depressive disorder (or unipolar depression), have also been found to switch to mania when on high doses of antidepressants [25]. For patients who have bipolar disorder, TCAs and MAOIs have been implicated as antidepressant classes that are more likely to cause a switch to mania [26]. In a 15-year follow-up study looking at patients who were admitted for unipolar depression and later found to have bipolar disorder, Goldberg et al. discovered that those patients found to have psychosis associated with their initial depressive presentation were more likely to present with hypomania or mania on their subsequent visits [27].

Table 44.10 Manic episode (summarized from the DSM–IV criteria for manic episode).

1. A period of 1 week of abnormally irritable or expansive/elevated mood.
2. In the event that the mood is primarily expansive/elevated then three of the criteria below must be met. If the mood is irritable then four of the criteria must be met. The symptoms must be present such as to noticeably affect social/occupational functioning:
   (a) Little to no need for sleep
   (b) Shows inability to stay on topic, due to easy distraction in thought process to irrelevant/unrelated subject matter
   (c) Speaks highly of self to the point of grandiosity
   (d) Is excessively talkative, and it appears at times that there is a pressure to continue to speak
   (e) Increase in goal-oriented tasks in occupational or social realms or apparent physical and psychological agitation
   (f) Hedonistic activities (hypersexuality, excessive shopping, illogical business decisions, etc.) are excessively indulged to the point self-detriment
   (g) A subjective sense that the patient's thoughts are racing
3. There are psychotic features present, or the patient must be hospitalized to prevent harm to self and others

When patients present with manic symptoms, efforts should be focused on stopping all plausible pharmacologic culprits, which include but are not exclusively antidepressants. Corticosteroids, withdrawal from benzodiazepines, anticholinergic medications, stimulants and antibiotics, are also known to induce manic switch. Addressing the causal medications may be insufficient in treating the manic symptoms. Interruptions in recovery (e.g., dehydration, sleep deprivation, and fatigue) may require supplemental treatment with mood stabilizers (lithium, valproic acid, and carbamazepine). When deciding which mood stabilizer is most appropriate for the patient, the side-effect profiles of these medications should drive treatment choice (see Table 44.11, for appropriate dosing of mood stabilizers). Furthermore, if the patient also presents with psychotic symptoms, antipsychotic medications (which also have mood-stabilizing properties) should be employed. In the event that there is difficulty in discerning these symptoms, a psychiatric consultation is well warranted. Also, drug interactions are common with particular mood stabilizers, and pharmacy should be consulted to address any possible interaction concerns.

Priapism

Although sexual dysfunction (anorgasmia, erectile dysfunction, etc.) is a common side-effect of antidepressants, it rarely presents as an emergency. Priapism is an emergency, with estimates of prevalence ranging from one case in 6,000–8,000 patients [28]. Defined as a persistent engorgement of the corpora cavernosa lasting for longer than 2 hours, with no precipitant stimulation, priapism can be painful and cause lasting erectile dysfunction and scarring. There is a 4-hour

Table 44.11 Dosing strategies and other information relevant to the use of mood stabilizers.

Antimanic medications	Starting dose	Maintenance dose	Half-life	Peak serum concentration	Therapeutic serum level	Considerations
Lithium	300 mg PO, 2–3 times, daily	900–1200 mg PO, daily	18–30 hours	1–2 hours	0.6–1.2 µg/mL	1. Lithium is the only antimanic agent with proven suicide prevention when maintained 2. Patients on thiazides, NSAIDS, ACE inhibitors, metronidazole, acetazolamide, and methyldopa start at lower doses initially and titrate slowly as they increase the plasma concentration of lithium 3. Lithium should be used with caution in patients with renal, cardiac, or thyroid impairment 4. Although rare, there is an increased risk in pregnancy for Ebstein's anomaly and hypotonia if lithium is taken in the first trimester
Valproate	1,000 mg, PO, daily	No FDA indication for maintenance. For mania management over multiple days 1,200–1,500 mg daily	9–16 hours	3–8 hours	45–125 µg/mL	1. May be more appropriate where psychosis or mixed mania is the predominant presentation 2. Use with caution in patients who have hepatic impairment 3. When taken in the first trimester of pregnancy neural tube defects, death, and coma are known outcomes
Olanzapine	10–15 mg, PO or IM, daily	Continue to titrate to 20 mg, until desired effect is reached and maintain at that dose	36 hours	4–6 hours with oral administration and 15–45 minutes with IM administration	N/A	1. Intramuscular and dissolving tablet formulation are particularly helpful in psychotic or agitated manic patients 2. Patients with hepatic and cardiac impairments, should be started on lower dose and monitored carefully for dyslipidemia and orthostatic hypotension 3. Class C category for pregnant females
Risperidone	2–8 mg, PO, daily	No FDA indication for maintenance. For mania management over multiple	3 hours	1 hour	N/A	1. Can be used as monotherapy in acute mania however, can easily function as an adjunct to lithium or valproate should psychosis be present. Also

Table 44.11 (cont.)

Antimanic medications	Starting dose	Maintenance dose	Half-life	Peak serum concentration	Therapeutic serum level	Considerations
		days continue most efficacious dose				in situations where rapid titration of mood stabilizers is not possible 2. Young African American males may be more prone to EPS than other populations 3. Class C category for pregnant females
Carbamazepine	200 mg, PO, twice daily	Increase dose by 200 mg weekly, with final dose between 800–1,200 mg	24–56 hours	4–8 hours	4–12 µg/mL	1. This medication should only be used in the event that lithium, valproate, olanzapine, and risperidone fail. This medicine is notorious for drug–drug interactions and neurotoxicity such as sedation, ataxia, diplopia, and nystagmus (especially in rapid titration) 2. This medication is an autoinducer and therefore requires increasing doses if used over multiple days 3. Stevens–Johnson syndrome, syndrome of inappropriate antidiuretic hormone secretion (SIADH), aplastic anemia, and agranulocytosis can occur 4. Neural tube defects and other fetal complications can be present when administering during the first trimester of pregnancy
Ziprasidone	40 mg, PO or IM, daily	Increase to 60–80 mg daily, depending on presentation	6.6 hours	6–8 hours with oral administration and 30 minutes with IM administration	N/A	1. Does not share the same metabolic effects with risperidone and olanzapine 2. Known to cause QTc prolongation, patients with cardiac impairments should be monitored closely 3. Can be used as adjunct to lithium or valproate 4. Class C category for pregnant females

time window, from the time of onset, in which treatment should be initiated to avoid damage.

The antidepressant classes known to have effects on alpha-adrenergic receptors and hence erection are the most commonly implicated in priapism. SSRIs and SNRIs such as trazodone, nefazodone (although less than trazodone, due to its more selective alpha-1 receptor selective binding), and venlafaxine are examples of medications with increased risk for priapism. The risk for priapism is often highest during the first month of taking these medications.

All antidepressants or other medications having effects on alpha-adrenergic receptors should be immediately stopped in the presence of priapism. Simultaneously, asking for an urgent urology consult is advised. Depending on the duration of the priapism, aspiration of the cavernous body and an intracavernous injection of a sympathomimetic agent, such as phenylephrine, may be in order [29].

Electroconvulsive therapy

The modern pharmacopeia of antidepressants has afforded clinicians with the ability to treat some of the most complex medical and comorbid depressive presentations with medications. However, in the event that pre- or postoperative patients cannot tolerate the side-effects of antidepressants, electroconvulsive therapy (ECT) may be the best solution. In addition, the results of ECT appear at most within 4 weeks and show a greater than 55–86% remission rate (even in severe cases of melancholia or those with associated psychosis), which is better than the improvement rates associated with antidepressants and antipsychotics used in the treatment of depression [30,31]. Acute suicide risk also substantially decreases, as the Relief of Expressed Suicidal Intent: A Consortium for Research in ECT Study by Kellner et al. points out [32]. Hence, patients who are suffering from depression with melancholic, psychotic, and delusional features or who are acutely suicidal do benefit from this intervention.

The exact mechanism of ECT is unclear; it is thought that perhaps ECT, through seizure activity, affects the levels of neurotransmitters in the brain (especially gamma-aminobutyric acid) and improves the stress regulatory mechanisms in the brain for sleep, appetite, and mood [33]. Some contraindications for the use of ECT are central nervous mass lesions, recent myocardial infarction, or history of unstable ventricular arrhythmia.

During the course of ECT, the patient may experience fluctuations in heart rate (initial bradycardia followed by tachycardia) and blood pressure; these fluctuations, however, can be safely managed with the use of beta-blockers. In fact, due to the implementation of anesthesia given to induce sedation and muscle relaxation, serious immediate side-effects from ECT are rare. Over the normal course of ECT (6–12 treatments) patients may complain of antero-retrograde amnesia, forgetting those moments immediately before and after treatments.

Psychotherapy

In the immediate pre- or postoperative setting, psychotherapy may not seem like a viable option for the treatment of depression. However, in the pre-transplant setting or in the recovery phase of surgery, it may be imperative that patients have appropriate psychotherapeutic intervention to assure a favorable outcome. In a study by Hadj et al., which looked at quality of life scores for cardiac surgery candidates pre- and postoperatively, it was found that those patients who received both psychotherapeutic and physical preparation prior to surgery, had considerably higher quality of life scores than those who did not [34]. Numerous studies speak to the increased mortality after transplant surgery in the event that a patient's depression remains untreated and discuss the capacity of frequent psychotherapeutic follow-up as being invaluable in preventing poor outcomes [35].

A patient's capacity to adapt to psychosocial stressors is indicative of their capacity to handle stressors associated with surgery. Symptoms of depression may be temporarily alleviated by pharmacological therapy or ECT. If a patient, however, is unable to cope with persistent psychosocial stressors these improvements may be shortlived. Many studies show that psychotherapy and medications affect the neurobiology of the brain in different ways, each method helping the brain to process neural stimuli in a manner that may be less deleterious to the patient's functionality [36].

References

1. Wisely JA, Wilson E, Duncan RT et al. Pre-existing psychiatric disorders, psychological reactions to stress and the recovery of burn survivors. Burns 2010; 36: 183–91.

2. Pearson SD, Katzelnick DJ, Simon GE et al. Depression among high utilizers of medical care. J Gen Intern Med 1999; 14: 461–8.

3. Abrams TE, Vaughan-Sarrazin M, Rosenthal GE. Influence of psychiatric comorbidity on surgical mortality. Arch Surg 2010; 145: 947–53.

4. Endicott J. Measurement of depression in patients with cancer. Cancer 1984; 53 (10 Suppl): 2243–9.

5. Akechi T, Ietsugu T, Sukigara M et al. Symptom indicator of severity of depression in cancer patients: a comparison of the DSM–IV criteria with alternative diagnostic criteria. Gen Hosp Psychiatry 2009; 31: 225–32.

6. Nemeroff CB, Compton MT, Berger J. The depressed suicidal patient. Assessment and treatment. Ann NY Acad Sci 2001; 932: 1–23.

7. ten Have M, de Graaf R, van Dorsselaer S et al. Incidence and course of suicidal ideation and suicide attempts in the general population. Can J Psychiatry 2009; 54: 824–33.

8. Busch KA, Fawcett J, Jacobs DG. Clinical correlates of inpatient suicide. J Clin Psychiatry 2003; 64: 14–19.

9. Pompei P, Foreman M, Rudberg MA et al. Delirium in hospitalized older persons: outcomes and predictors. J Am Geriatr Soc 1994; 42: 809–15.

10. Ohayon MM, Schatzberg AF. Prevalence of depressive episodes with psychotic features in the general population. Am J Psychiatry 2002; 159: 1855–61.

11. Sommer M, de Rijke DM, van Kleef M et al. The prevalence of postoperative pain in a sample of 1490 surgical inpatients. Eur J Anaesthesiol 2008; 25: 267–74.

12. Bruster S, Jarman B, Bosanquet N et al. National survey of hospital patients. Br Med J 1994; 309: 1542–6.

13. Richebe P, Beaulieu P. Perioperative pain management in the patient treated with opioids: continuing professional development. *Can J Anaesth* 2009; **56**: 969–81.

14. Katon W, Sullivan M, Walker E. Medical symptoms without identified pathology: relationship to psychiatric disorders, childhood and adult trauma, and personality traits. *Ann Intern Med* 2001; **134**: 917–25.

15. Trafton JA, Cucciare MA, Lewis E *et al.* Somatization is associated with non-adherence to opioid prescriptions. *J Pain* 2011; **12**: 573–80.

16. Kirmayer LJ, Robbins JM. Patients who somatize in primary care: a longitudinal study of cognitive and social characteristics. *Psychol Med* 1996; **26**: 937–51.

17. Murphy SE, Norbury R, O'Sullivan U *et al.* Effect of a single dose of citalopram on amygdala response to emotional faces. *Br J Psychiatry* 2009; **194**: 535–40.

18. Norbury R, Taylor MJ, Selvaraj S *et al.* Short-term antidepressant treatment modulates amygdala response to happy faces. *Psychopharmacology (Berl)* 2009; **206**: 197–204.

19. Boyer EW, Shannon M. The serotonin syndrome. *N Engl J Med* 2005; **352**: 1112–20.

20. Gillman PK. Monoamine oxidase inhibitors, opioid analgesics and serotonin toxicity. *Br J Anaesth* 2005; **95**: 434–41.

21. Krishnan KR. Revisiting monoamine oxidase inhibitors. *J Clin Psychiatry* 2007; **68** (Suppl 8): 35–41.

22. Sola CL, Bostwick JM, Hart DA *et al.* Anticipating potential linezolid-SSRI interactions in the general hospital setting: an MAOI in disguise. *Mayo Clin Proc* 2006; **81**: 330–4.

23. Clement ND, Aitken SA, Duckworth AD *et al.* The outcome of fractures in very elderly patients. *J Bone Joint Surg Br* 2011; **93**: 806–10.

24. Darowski A, Chambers SA, Chambers DJ. Antidepressants and falls in the elderly. *Drugs Aging* 2009; **26**: 381–94.

25. Parker G, Parker K. Which antidepressants flick the switch? *Aust N Z J Psychiatry* 2003; **37**: 464–8.

26. Wada K, Sasaki T, Jitsuiki H *et al.* Manic/hypomanic switch during acute antidepressant treatment for unipolar depression. *J Clin Psychopharmacol* 2006; **26**: 512–15.

27. Goldberg JF, Harrow M, Whiteside JE. Risk for bipolar illness in patients initially hospitalized for unipolar depression. *Am J Psychiatry* 2001; **158**: 1265–70.

28. Nierenberg AA, Adler LA, Peselow E *et al.* Trazodone for antidepressant-associated insomnia. *Am J Psychiatry* 1994; **151**: 1069–72.

29. Broderick GA, Kadioglu A, Bivalacqua TJ *et al.* Priapism: pathogenesis, epidemiology, and management. *J Sex Med* 2010; 7: 476–500.

30. Sackeim HA, Haskett RF, Mulsant BH *et al.* Continuation pharmacotherapy in the prevention of relapse following electroconvulsive therapy: a randomized controlled trial. *J Am Med Assoc* 2001; **285**: 1299–307.

31. Kellner CH, Fink M, Knapp R *et al.* Continuation electroconvulsive therapy vs pharmacotherapy for relapse prevention in major depression: a multisite study from the Consortium for Research in Electroconvulsive Therapy (CORE). *Arch Gen Psychiatry* 2006; **63**: 1337–44.

32. Kellner CH, Fink M, Knapp R *et al.* Relief of expressed suicidal intent by ECT: a consortium for research in ECT study. *Am J Psychiatry* 2005; **162**: 977–82.

33. Sanacora G, Mason GF, Rothman DL *et al.* Increased cortical GABA concentrations in depressed patients receiving ECT. *Am J Psychiatry* 2003; **160**: 577–9.

34. Hadj A, Esmore D, Rowland M *et al.* Pre-operative preparation for cardiac surgery utilising a combination of metabolic, physical and mental therapy. *Heart Lung Circ* 2006; **15**: 172–81.

35. Corruble E, Barry C, Varescon I *et al.* Depressive symptoms predict long-term mortality after liver transplantation. *J Psychosom Res* 2011; **71**: 32–7.

36. Brody AL, Saxena S, Stoessel P *et al.* Regional brain metabolic changes in patients with major depression treated with either paroxetine or interpersonal therapy: preliminary findings. *Arch Gen Psychiatry* 2001; **58**: 631–40.

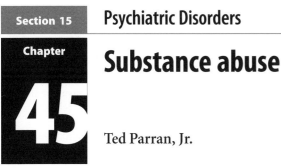

Substance abuse

Ted Parran, Jr.

Problems of drug and alcohol abuse are ubiquitous in hospitalized patient populations. A prevalence study at Johns Hopkins Hospital in 1986 demonstrated active alcoholism in 23% of surgical patients, with subgroup rates ranging from 14% in patients on the urology service, 28% in those on the orthopedic service, to 43% in those on the otorhinolaryngology service [1]. Although this study did not evaluate the prevalence of drug abuse, consideration of the abuse of drugs other than alcohol could only increase the overall rate of affected patients on surgical services. Detection rates by physician staff of patients with substance abuse problems are low in general and lowest on surgery and obstetrics-gynecology services. Data indicate that under 25% of affected patients are identified on these specialty services. In addition, less than half the substance-abusing patients who are identified receive any form of intervention, counseling, or even a medical treatment plan that addresses the substance abuse issues. Therefore, only about 10% of surgical patients with substance abuse problems have their abuse addressed in any way by their physicians or other members of the surgical team.

In a few special populations of surgical patients, problems of substance abuse are of even greater magnitude. Trauma service data indicate that between 30% and 75% of all injured patients have positive results on toxicology testing for legal levels of alcohol intoxication or for drugs of abuse at the time of hospital admission [2–6]. Our experience after a year of testing each consecutive level 1 trauma admission indicated an alcohol intoxication rate of 63%, an illicit drug use rate of 48%, and a combined rate of 78%. Follow-up interviews with these patients revealed that most (92%) had serious drug and alcohol abuse or dependence, with only 8% being substance users who happened to suffer a major trauma [7].

A significant literature is emerging that examines the potential for increased morbidity, mortality, and hospitalization costs associated with drug and alcohol abuse in surgical patients. Although there are some conflicting reports and a vast diversity of research design, a consensus has clearly emerged that substance-abusing patients do carry an increased burden of morbidity, mortality, postoperative complications, and cost associated with their treatment. These include increased intraoperative and postoperative complication rates (i.e., neurosurgical patients with alcoholism and subdural hematoma, patients with alcoholism who undergo transurethral prostatectomy, patients with alcoholism and drug dependency who undergo plastic surgery and burn treatment, and patients with alcoholism who undergo bowel resection or hysterectomy) [8–12]. They have also been shown to have increased postoperative morbidity and, in many studies, increased mortality [13]. Theoretic and actual increased anesthesia risks in surgical patients who abuse drugs and alcohol have been described [14]. Finally, a recent large VA cohort study indicated that as levels of preoperative alcohol abuse increased, the risk of postoperative complications went from 5.6% in low-use patients to 14.0% in the heaviest using patients [15].

Clinically important issues involved in the treatment of substance abuse in surgical patients are considered further in the following order: screening and diagnosis strategies, medical therapy considerations by drug class, brief intervention and treatment planning, and postoperative pain management issues.

Screening approaches

The need for better and more widespread screening for substance abuse problems in hospitalized patients is obvious [16–28]. Because the prevalence of these patients is between

Table 45.1 The CAGE questionnaire[*].

Have you ever felt the need to *Cut* down on your drinking?
Have people *Annoyed* you by criticizing your drinking?[*]
Have you ever felt bad or *Guilty* about your drinking?[*]
Have you ever had a drink first thing in the morning to steady your nerves or to get rid of a hangover (*Eye* opener)?
The family CAGE (f-CAGE) involves asking if "anyone in your family" has felt the need to …

[*] Many clinicians substitute "drinking or drug use" when using the CAGE questionnaire.

Medical Management of the Surgical Patient, ed. Michael F. Lubin, Thomas F. Dodson, and Neil H. Winawer. Published by Cambridge University Press. © Cambridge University Press 2013.

Table 45.2 The Alcohol Use Disorders Identification Test: Self-Report Version (AUDIT).
PATIENT: Because alcohol use can affect your health and can interfere with certain medications and treatments, it is important that we ask some questions about your use of alcohol. Your answers will remain confidential so please be honest.
Place an X in the box that best describes your answer to each question.

Questions	0	1	2	3	4
1. How often do you have a drink containing alcohol?	Never	Monthly or less	2–4 times a month	2–3 times a week	4 or more times a week
2. How many drinks containing alcohol do you have on a typical day when you are drinking?	1 or 2	3 or 4	5 or 6	7 to 9	10 or more
3. How often do you have six or more drinks on one occasion?	Never	Less than monthly	Monthly	Weekly	Daily or almost daily
4. How often during the last year have you found that you were not able to stop drinking once you had started?	Never	Less than monthly	Monthly	Weekly	Daily or almost daily
5. How often during the last year have you failed to do what was normally expected of you because of drinking?	Never	Less than monthly	Monthly	Weekly	Daily or almost daily
6. How often during the last year have you needed a first drink in the morning to get yourself going after a heavy drinking session?	Never	Less than monthly	Monthly	Weekly	Daily or almost daily
7. How often during the last year have you had a feeling of guilt or remorse after drinking?	Never	Less than monthly	Monthly	Weekly	Daily or almost daily
8. How often during the last year have you been unable to remember what happened the night before because of your drinking?	Never	Less than monthly	Monthly	Weekly	Daily or almost daily
9. Have you or someone else been injured because of your drinking?	No		Yes, but not in the last year		Yes, during the last year
10. Has a relative, friend, doctor, or other healthcare worker been concerned about your drinking or suggested you cut down?	No		Yes, but not in the last year		Yes, during the last year
					Total

20% and 40% on surgical services, and because the diagnosis is overlooked in 50–80% of cases, the need for active screening at the time of admission of all surgical patients is indisputable. A good screening test should be clinically powerful (with high sensitivity and an acceptable level of specificity), simple to use, and easy to master and remember, and should have a high degree of patient and physician acceptability. Several good approaches have been developed and tested over the past 20 years, and four are perhaps most appropriate to surgical settings: the AUDIT-C, the CAGE questionnaire, the Trauma Survey, and urine toxicology testing [15,16,19,20].

Much screening for alcohol problems has been focused on the use of the AUDIT or AUDIT-C in recent years. The AUDIT is an alcohol use screening tool that has been validated by the WHO in eight different countries on five continents, and provides an assessment of the relative risk of a patient's alcohol use. As such it can classify patients as low risk (score 1–4), risky (score 5–8), hazardous (score 9–10), and harmful (score > 10). The AUDIT is the optimal alcohol-use disorder screening tool at present, but it is long and does not apply to drug use [29]. The CAGE questions have been widely studied in various patient populations (Table 45.1) and can be used for both alcohol and drug use. Both the AUDIT (Table 45.2) and CAGE consist of questions that are easy to remember and simple to ask, tend not to engender defensiveness and discomfort in patients or physicians, and are far more sensitive and specific in identifying clinically important substance abuse problems than are typical questions regarding amount and frequency of use. Perhaps even more importantly, the CAGE questionnaire can be adapted (f-CAGE) for use in asking family members about the patient's

Table 45.3 Trauma Scale Questionnaire

Since your 18th birthday,

Have you had any fractures or dislocations of your bones or joints?

Have you been injured in a road traffic accident?

Have you injured your head?

Have you been injured in a non-sports-related assault or fight?

Have you been injured after drinking?

use of alcohol or drugs, especially when patients are unable to be meaningfully interviewed or when the surgical team needs corroboration of the patient's self-report [30]. In hospitalized patients, each positive response to a CAGE question indicates a 30–40% likelihood of a substance abuse problem, and two positive responses indicate an 80% sensitivity and specificity for substance abuse.

It is thought that young men tend to produce false-negative results when they are tested with the CAGE questionnaire but not necessarily with the AUDIT Skinner *et al.* observed that young men with substance abuse problems often suffer repetitive traumatic injury [20]. They developed the Trauma Survey (Table 45.3) for use in this population, and positive responses to two of its five categories indicate the likelihood of a substance abuse problem. The Trauma Survey is more clinically useful than are the results of laboratory tests (i.e., liver tests or the mean corpuscular volume) or standard questions regarding the amount and frequency of use, especially in populations of young men.

"For cause" rather than random or universal toxicology testing is one accepted strategy to screen for and assess addictive disease in hospitalized patients. "For cause" is a term that relates to toxicology testing which is prompted by clinical data indicating a significant chance of the presence of a substance abuse disorder. These clinical data can either be epidemiological data indicating a high prevalence rate in certain patient populations (i.e., all level 1 trauma patients), or other screening information indicating a potential diagnosis (i.e., 1 or more on the CAGE and 5 or more on the AUDIT). This "for cause" toxicology testing is widely accepted as justified even without special informed written consent by patients. The prevalence of positive results on toxicology testing at the time of hospital admission is startlingly high in some surgical patient populations, especially trauma patients. A consensus has emerged among trauma services that the use of routine admission toxicology testing is a reasonable part of any standard trauma protocol. Toxicology testing is the single most clinically useful laboratory test after positive results are obtained with an AUDIT, CAGE questionnaire, or Trauma Survey.

Substance abuse screening tools are available and are practical, clinically powerful, and easy to use. Their use should be extended into patient care in general and into surgical populations in particular. Once the use of effective screening is more widespread, detoxification management, referral for counseling and treatment, and management of special considerations such as postoperative pain become critical for the surgical team and its medical consultants.

Medical considerations by drug class

The medical considerations involved in caring for surgical patients with substance abuse problems are vast. The primary areas addressed here are basic pharmacology, management of intoxication and toxicity, management of withdrawal, and other considerations (e.g., nutritional, metabolic) [21]. The various drugs are discussed by class: alcohol and sedative-hypnotics, cocaine and stimulants, and opiates.

Alcohol and sedative-hypnotics

Alcohol and sedative-hypnotic agents (e.g., benzodiazepines, barbiturates) are involved in most of the substance abuse that is encountered in surgical patients [22]. Intoxication with these agents is associated with dose-related and tolerance-related disinhibition, loss of judgment, delay in psychomotor coordination, decrease in cognitive ability, and impairment of short-term memory formation. At high levels of intoxication, consciousness, the gag reflex, respiratory drive, and cardiovascular function are all depressed [21]. Signs of acute toxicity are altered mental status, lethargy and stupor, dilated pupils, slowed respiration, and decreased reflexes. The mixing of different types of sedative-hypnotics can markedly potentiate their toxicity, resulting in a dramatically narrowed toxic/therapeutic ratio and even death. This should be considered in the management of agitated behavior, the treatment of withdrawal, or the consideration of anesthesia or analgesia. The necessity of obtaining accurate blood alcohol content and urine toxicology screening for drugs of abuse for use in perioperative management decisions cannot be overemphasized. The treatment of toxicity involves cardiovascular and respiratory monitoring and support, the cessation of gastrointestinal absorption, and attempts to increase drug excretion. Some investigators have used high doses of naloxone (Narcan) in these patients, with mixed results.

The alcohol and sedative-hypnotic withdrawal syndromes are similar and can be considered in terms of four categories of symptoms and signs (Table 45.4). Category 1 withdrawal involves increases in heart rate, blood pressure, and reflexes accompanied by tremors, diaphoresis, headache, nausea or diarrhea, insomnia, and anxiety. Category 2 withdrawal is benign alcohol hallucinosis, a clinical picture of visual or tactile hallucinations coupled with a clear sensorium. Category 3 withdrawal is withdrawal seizures. These grand mal seizures can be single or multiple discrete seizures, can progress to status epilepticus in the case of barbiturate and perhaps short-acting benzodiazepine (aprazolam) withdrawal, and tend to be of short duration with accordingly short post-ictal

Table 45.4 Alcohol and sedative-hypnotic withdrawal.[*]

Class	Signs and symptoms	Time of onset[+]	Course duration
Class 1	Increased heart rate, blood pressure, and reflexes Diarrhea, nausea, and vomiting Tremor, anxiety, and insomnia	12–24 hours	72–96 hours
Class 2	Visual > auditory > tactile hallucinations	12–24 hours	72–96 hours
Class 3	Grand mal seizures	12–96 hours	6–24 hours
Class 4	Class I signs with delirium disorientation, confusion, hallucinations, agitation, anxiety, insomnia	3–6 days	72–96 hours

* Applies to alcohol and short-acting sedative-hypnotics. See text for time course differences with long-acting sedative-hypnotics.
+ Onset relates to initiation of syndrome after last use of the involved drug.

Table 45.5 Strategies for alcohol withdrawal management. Protocols are described in Table 45.5.

Withdrawal symptoms	Pulmonary or Hepatic Function	
	Impaired	**Not Impaired**
Mild class I symptoms	Low-dose short-acting benzodiazepine: protocol A	Low-dose, long-acting benzodiazepine: protocol C
Severe Class I, class II, III, or class IV symptoms	Intensive short-acting benzodiazepine: protocol B	Intensive long-acting benzodiazepine: protocol D

Table 45.6 Alcohol withdrawal protocols.

Protocol A: Lorazepam 0.5 mg PO, IM, or IV each 4–8 hours per specific signs or symptoms of withdrawal. Discontinue after 72–96 hours

Protocol B: Lorazepam 0.5 to 2 mg PO/IM or IV each 1–4 hours until specific signs or symptoms of withdrawal are suppressed or patient is sleepy. Restart protocol if withdrawal re-emerges

Protocol C: Diazepam 5 mg PO or IV each 4–8 hours per specific sign or symptom of withdrawal. Discontinue after 72–96 hours

Protocol D: Diazepam 10 mg PO or IV each 1 hours until specific sign of withdrawal is suppressed or patient is sleepy. Restart protocol if withdrawal re-emerges

Protocol E: Sedative-hypnotic withdrawal protocol. Phenobarbital 90 mg PO or IM each 2–4 hours until therapeutic (antiseizure) blood level is achieved. Then titrate daily phenobarbital dose to maintain a therapeutic blood level

periods. Category 4 withdrawal is a delayed-type withdrawal that is also known as delirium tremens, or DTs. This is characterized by the hyper-autonomic signs and symptoms of category 1 withdrawal coupled with a state of delirium consisting of global confusion, auditory visual and tactile hallucinations, and agitation.

The first three categories of withdrawal tend to begin within 12–24 hours of the last drink or sedative hypnotic drug ingestion, rapidly escalate to peak symptoms in another 12–24 hours, and ease over an additional 48–72 hours. Delayed withdrawal or DTs begin 3–5 days after the last use and then follow a similar time frame. The only significant exceptions to this involve the long-acting benzodiazepine medications such as diazepam, chlordiazepoxide, clorazepate (Tranxene), and clonazepam (Klonopin). Because of their extended half-lives or active metabolites, the onset of withdrawal from these agents can be delayed for 3–5 days after cessation of use, and symptoms often persist for an additional 7–10 days.

The likelihood that patients will experience one or more categories of withdrawal symptoms is dependent on their previous withdrawal experience. Patients who have not had previous withdrawal symptoms upon abrupt discontinuation of alcohol or sedative hypnotic drug use, are unlikely to go through withdrawal during their hospitalization for surgery. Patients who have had category 3 withdrawal seizures in the past have as much as a 30% risk for recurrent seizures during each subsequent withdrawal episode. The easiest way to predict which patients are at risk for significant withdrawal (and hence which patients require moderate to vigorous withdrawal prophylaxis while they are hospitalized on a surgical service) is to closely interview patients and their families and to review the medical records for data regarding the presence or absence of previous withdrawal symptoms.

The treatment of alcohol withdrawal varies among hospital services. One approach that we recommend for surgical patients is to first evaluate pulmonary function, liver function, and previous withdrawal symptomatology. If patients have reasonable liver function (i.e., the prothrombin time is less than 1.3 times control) and pulmonary function (i.e., the FEV1, is greater than 1.5 L), we suggest the use of long-acting benzodiazepines to treat withdrawal symptoms (Table 45.5). If either hepatic or pulmonary function is impaired beyond the above parameters, the use of short-acting benzodiazepines is urged. It also is useful to assess the intensity of withdrawal signs and symptoms. In patients with mild category 1 or 2 symptoms, the low-dose intermittent use of "as needed" or prn benzodiazepines is reasonable. If the symptoms are intense or severe in any category a higher-dose intensive benzodiazepine regimen is strongly suggested (Table 45.6). There is no role for the use of alcohol in the management of surgical patients experiencing alcohol withdrawal.

Periodically, patients are seen who have been chronically prescribed large doses of benzodiazepines or barbiturates as outpatients. In this case, therapy with these medications either should be maintained without change during the surgical hospitalization, or discontinued and replaced with phenobarbital. The mixing of acute doses of benzodiazepines and phenobarbital is strongly discouraged because of the risk of iatrogenic overdose and respiratory depression. One phenobarbital dosing schedule is outlined in Table 45.6, and can be applied to the treatment of alcohol or sedative-hypnotic withdrawal.

Several electrolyte and nutritional issues must be considered when patients with alcoholism are treated on the surgical service. Thiamine deficiency is seen in this population and can have catastrophic and permanent neurologic consequences. Thiamine should be given intramuscularly or by mouth at a dosage of 100 mg immediately, and then 100 mg/day for 3 days. In addition, patients with alcoholism frequently have vitamin C, vitamin B complex, and folic acid deficiencies. These should be supplemented by the oral, IV, or IM route. Multiple electrolyte abnormalities occur in this population and careful evaluation and management of the serum sodium, potassium, phosphorus, glucose, and magnesium levels is essential. Abnormalities in each of these electrolytes as well as elevated serum ammonia levels can lead to altered mental status, seizures, or cardiac arrhythmias.

A review of all the medical complications of alcohol abuse and dependence is beyond the scope of this chapter but a few problems deserve special mention. Hematologic problems include alcohol-associated anemias, thrombocytopenia, and clotting factor abnormalities. Alcohol-associated liver disease can complicate the selection and dosage of anesthetics. Infectious diseases including especially tuberculosis, but also viral hepatitis B and C, and HIV can be encountered more commonly in alcoholic patients than the general population. Finally, it is important to screen for congestive heart failure symptoms related to alcoholic cardiomyopathy before surgery is undertaken [23].

Cocaine and other stimulants

Cocaine is the most commonly abused stimulant, although the various schedule II and IV amphetamines are still abused by some patient populations and methamphetamine (known as Crystal, Crystal-meth, Meth, or Ice) continues to be heavily abused in some regions of the country. Common properties of stimulants involve inhibition of the reuptake of norepinephrine systemically and dopamine centrally [21]. This produces systemic effects of markedly elevated heart rate, blood pressure, reflexes, and level of smooth muscle spasticity [24]. Cardiac arrhythmias; brain, heart, intestinal, uterine, and muscular ischemia; and seizures are common during stimulant binges and are thought to be caused by norepinephrine surges. Of special medical significance in patients who abuse stimulants is the markedly increased risk for trauma, sexually transmitted diseases,

tuberculosis (including resistant strains), and HIV as a result of intravenous drug use or multiple sexual encounters [25].

Centrally, the excess levels of dopamine and norepinephrine associated with cocaine and other stimulant use produce intense feelings of euphoria, stamina, power, and control associated with sleeplessness, loss of appetite, and physical restlessness [24]. These effects rapidly abate and are replaced by dysphoric and depressive feelings. The evanescent nature of the "high" associated with stimulant use results in frequent repeated administration of the drugs, and the typical binge/crash pattern of stimulant addiction. Urine toxicology testing for cocaine and metabolites remains positive in proportion to the duration and intensity of use. Toxicology often reveals casual use for 18 to 24 hours, whereas serial screenings (i.e., every 12 hours) after a several-day binge can remain positive for as long as 4 days. Toxicology testing for amphetamine use often produces false-positive results in patients who are taking non-prescription cold preparations. These results should be confirmed with gas chromatography.

Toward the end of a binge, which can last from 12 to 72 hours, patients typically report more and more intense feelings of agitation, depression, and even paranoia that may last for several hours. It is during this unstable, agitated phase that much of the violence associated with stimulant abuse occurs. It is these agitated hypervigilant and paranoid patients who are often seen in emergency rooms with trauma, and who need urgent sedation to avoid violent episodes. Following this "post-binge" agitated period or "cocaine psychosis," patients then crash and begin a period of several hours to a few days of hypersomnia and hyperphagia (Table 45.7). This has been called phase 1 withdrawal. Phase 2 withdrawal is characterized by restlessness, edginess, mood swings, sleep disturbance, and stimulant cravings. These phase 2 withdrawal symptoms can affect patients intermittently for a few to several weeks.

The symptoms of category 2 withdrawal are thought to be mediated on the basis of dopamine depletion. Therefore, the

Table 45.7 Stimulant withdrawal.

	Symptoms and signs	Duration
Binge	Repetitive compulsive self-administration of cocaine; dilated pupils; increased pulse, increased blood pressure, decreased sleep, decreased eating; restlessness, grandiosity, pressured thoughts	Hours to several days
Agitated phase	Intense dysphoria, excitement, agitation, paranoia, rare cardiovascular instability	Up to several hours
Phase 1 ("crash")	Restlessness, anxiety, mood lability	12 to 72 hours
Phase 2 ("cravings")	Mood swings, concentration difficulties, strong urges regarding cocaine	Weeks to months

primary interventions include the administration of dopaminergic agents such as amantadine or antidepressant drugs such as desipramine. Although each of these medications has been studied for efficacy in cocaine withdrawal and shown to produce statistically significant decreases in symptoms, none has been demonstrated to clinically decrease relapse rates. One report indicates that propranolol 20 mg twice a day for several weeks may decrease relapse rates to a clinically significant degree. Cocaine-associated symptoms that must be urgently medicated are those seen during the period of agitated paranoia at the end of a binge. At this point, patients tend to respond to intramuscular sedatives, ranging from 100 mg of hydroxyzine for relatively mild cases to 2 mg of lorazepam and/or 5 mg of haloperidol for more agitated patients as a one-time dose.

Finally, the implications of a stimulant binge should be considered in planning anesthesia. Patients with recent stimulant binging and major trauma often have not had much to eat or drink for several hours to days. Their urinalyses commonly show maximally concentrated specimens with ketones, traces of protein, and much sediment. Serum creatinine and blood urea nitrogen determinations frequently do not reflect the true degree of volume depletion secondary to starvation effects. Therefore, accurate assessment of volume status with orthostatic checks or even a central line prior to induction of anesthesia is important. Another concern in undertaking surgery in these patients is the possible existence of a catecholamine-depleted state following a prolonged cocaine or amphetamine binge. Although no empiric evidence exists on this subject, catecholamine-stimulating pressors may not be as effective in these patients. Ruling out severe volume depletion, binge-associated cardiac ischemia, arrhythmia, pneumothorax, and rhabdomyolysis is important before surgery [25]. Other than taking these precautions into account, there is no indication to routinely cancel surgery in cocaine-using patients purely on the basis of a positive toxicology screen.

Opiates

All opiates are abused by some patients, including codeine, hydrocodone, oxycodone, meperidine, methadone, hydromorphone, morphine, heroin, opium, pentazocine, butorphanol, nalbuphine, and buprenorphine (Table 45.8). All opiates (except for methadone and perhaps buprenorphine) are rapidly metabolized and cleared, so their presence is rarely identified by urine toxicology testing performed more than 24 hours after the last use. Based on their observed actions, opiates are classified into two categories: mu-agonists and kappa-agonists [26]. The mu-agonists produce supraspinal anesthesia; euphoria; myosis; sedation; dose-related respiration, pulse, and blood-pressure depression; tolerance; physiologic dependence; and a withdrawal syndrome associated with drug cravings. The kappa-agonists produce spinal anesthesia and physiologic tolerance. These drugs cause significantly less euphoria, myosis, and sedation. Respiratory depression, bradycardia, and hypotension are also less frequent with kappa-agonists. Withdrawal

Table 45.8 Strategies for opiate withdrawal management.

Receptors	Actions	Agonists	Antagonists
mu	Supraspinal analgesia, euphoria, sedation, respiratory depression, physical withdrawal with drug cravings, myosis, constipation	Morphine Meperidol Methadone Oxycodone Codeine Propoxyphene Hydromorphone Buprenorphine* Heroin	Naloxone Naltrexone Pentazocine Nalbuphine
kappa	Spinal analgesia, miosis, sedation, physical withdrawal without drug cravings	Pentazocine Nalbuphine* Butorphanol	Naloxone Naltrexone

* Partial agonist for indicated receptor.

syndromes from mu-agonists are associated with much more drug craving. The kappa-agonists also act as mu-receptor antagonists, precipitating withdrawal in mu-agonist-dependent patients. At higher therapeutic doses, kappa-agonists tend to demonstrate more dysphoric symptoms, which limits their usefulness in the treatment of severe pain.

Opiate intoxication produces a clinical picture of transient nausea; dry mouth; constipation; sleepiness; euphoria; a feeling of tranquility; constricted pupils; warm, dry skin; and depressed respirations, heart rate, and blood pressure. Opiate toxicity presents as depressed mentation ranging from obtundation to coma, with myotic pinpoint pupils, bradycardia, hypotension, and depressed respirations that can progress to apnea and death [21]. This toxic state can be easily reversed by the administration of naloxone (Narcan). The intravenous administration of 0.4 mg usually produces a response in vital signs and pupillary dilation, although patients with greater degrees of intoxication sometimes require multiple doses. The duration of intoxication with most opiates is 1–3 hours, and the duration of naloxone's antagonistic effect is 20–40 minutes, so close patient observation and repeated dosing is important. Methadone has a much longer duration of intoxication and toxicity, and patients who have overdosed on this drug must be monitored for at least 12–24 hours. Naltrexone (Trexan) is an oral form of naloxone that has a half-life of 18 to 24 hours. It occasionally is useful in patients with toxicity, especially if methadone is involved. Because naloxone and naltrexone are mu-receptor and kappa-receptor antagonists, their administration in the proper dosage not only reverses opiate toxicity but can also precipitate opiate withdrawal in patients who are physically dependent. This withdrawal syndrome lasts for only 20 or 30 minutes in the case of naloxone but can last for as long as 24 hours after the administration of naltrexone.

By stage, the signs and symptoms of opiate withdrawal are as follows:

1. Lacrimation, rhinorrhea, diaphoresis, yawning, restlessness, insomnia.
2. Mydriasis, piloerection, muscular fasciculation, myalgia, arthralgia, abdominal pain.
3. Tachycardia, hypertension, tachypnea, anorexia, nausea, extreme restlessness.
4. Diarrhea, emesis, dehydration, hyperactive bowel sounds, orthostatic-hypotension, fetal position.

These withdrawal symptoms vary in intensity depending on the type of opiate used, the dose taken, and the duration of use. The symptoms of craving, restlessness, and insomnia tend to be especially long-lasting [27]. Non-methadone opiate withdrawal generally begins 6–12 hours after the last use, progresses to a peak within 36 hours of initiation, and resolves over an additional 72 hours. Thus most non-methadone opiate withdrawal symptoms resolve within 4–5 days of the last drug use. Methadone withdrawal begins about 48 hours after the last use, gradually builds for a week or so, and then abates over another 7–14 days.

The treatment of opiate withdrawal can involve the use of clonidine, methadone, buprenorphine, or tramadol [27,28,31–33]. All opioid withdrawal protocols involve the off-label use of these medications. The following clonidine protocol has been used extensively in patients with mild to moderate opioid physical dependence who are hospitalized in detoxification units:

Administer clonidine, 0.1 mg orally every 4 hours for 36 hours.
Administer clonidine, 0.1 mg orally every 6 hours for 24 hours.
Administer clonidine, 0.1 mg orally every 8 hours for 24 hours.
Administer clonidine, 0.1 mg orally every 12 hours for 24 hours.
Discontinue clonidine therapy.

Do not administer clonidine if the systolic blood pressure is less than 90 mmHg. Adjunct medications are often helpful, including ibuprofen and acetaminophen for myalgia, dicyclomine for abdominal symptoms, hydroxyzine for anxiety, and amitriptyline with diphenhydramine for sleep. Patients with hemodynamic instability, advanced age, or acute or chronic pain syndromes often do not tolerate this clonidine regimen.

It is in these patients that methadone has historically been used [27]. Difficulties with methadone therapy include the need to first stabilize patients on it and then taper them off relatively slowly, legal issues surrounding the outpatient prescription of methadone for the management of addiction, and the challenge of referral to methadone maintenance programs

– with historically very long waiting lists – for patients who have begun such treatment in the hospital. Methadone has 30% more bioavailability when it is given intramuscularly than when it is given orally. Therefore, patients who cannot take oral methadone should be given two-thirds of their usual daily oral dose in two divided intramuscular injections every 12 hours. Methadone is administered as follows:

Administer 5–10 mg of methadone orally every 12 hours.
Monitor for ablation of withdrawal symptoms. Increase the dose by 5–10 mg until symptoms are suppressed (stabilization dose).
Taper the methadone over 5–20 days by decreasing the dose by 5–20% per day.
Treat re-emergent withdrawal symptoms with oral or transdermal clonidine.

The advent of short-term, inpatient buprenorphine tapering protocols has markedly decreased the number of patients in whom methadone therapy must be initiated during their hospitalization [31,34].

1. Administer buprenorphine, 0.2–0.5 mg subcutaneously every 4 hours for 48 hours.
2. Administer buprenorphine, half the above dose every 4 hours for 48 hours.
3. Administer buprenorphine, one half the second dose every 4 hours for 48 hours.
4. Discontinue buprenorphine administration.

It appears that the withdrawal syndrome from buprenorphine, especially when it is given in this short-term, low-dose tapering method, is mild and often clinically trivial. Therapy is begun at a dosage designed to relieve withdrawal symptoms (and pain if appropriate) without making patients sleepy or sedated. Because 0.3 mg of buprenorphine is equivalent to 10 mg of morphine, we usually start with doses between 0.2 and 0.4 mg. Once this initial therapeutic dose is identified, it is relatively easy to taper drug treatment gradually over 5 or 6 days, often mirroring the decrease in acute pain experienced by the postoperative surgical patient. The administration of buprenorphine, formerly a schedule V and now a schedule III opioid, for the sole purpose of opioid detoxification for longer than 72 hours is problematic given the 1970 Federal Controlled Substances Act. Fortunately, in the postoperative surgical patient there is nearly always acute pain diagnosis present, making this short-term prescribing for pain relief and withdrawal management consistent with both the spirit and letter of the law. Some addiction medicine consultants have switched from using injectable buprenorphine to using sublingual buprenorphine compounded with naloxone (Suboxone) to manage withdrawal in the hospitalized opioid addict. This should only be done by physicians who have a special federal waiver to prescribe the buprenorphine-naloxone product.

Tramadol has also been used for the management of acute opioid withdrawal [32,33]. The protocol reported in the literature involves the administration of tramadol 100 mg PO every 4 hours for 24 hours, then 100 mg every 6 hours for 24 hours, then 100 mg every 8 hours for 24 hours, then 50 mg every 6 hours for 24 hours, and finally 50 mg every 8 hours for 24 hours. This regimen is supplemented with the above-mentioned adjunctive medications, and even occasional "rescue" doses of buprenorphine for severe breakthrough of withdrawal symptoms. With surgical patients it is perhaps optimal to initially treat with buprenorphine, providing acute pain relief and opioid withdrawal management. This buprenorphine can be continued until any similar postoperative surgical patient would be switched to oral analgesics. At this point the switch from buprenorphine to tramadol can occur and the tramadol taper can be carried out in the outpatient setting [32,33].

Common medical complications in patients who are dependent on opiates are related to the degree of opiate tolerance and the delivery system used. The degree of tolerance that patients have for opiate effects can markedly affect decisions relating to anesthesia and analgesia management (see later discussion). A significant proportion of the estimated 1.1 million opiate-dependent persons in North America use, at least intermittently, the intravenous route. Careful observation for track marks, abscesses, and cellulitis is critical. Viral hepatitis is a ubiquitous problem, with seropositivity for hepatitis B and especially for hepatitis C being the rule rather than the exception. Current "best practices" suggest withholding interferon therapy for hepatitis C positive patients with drug addiction, until the patient has documentation of 6 months of sobriety. Human immunodeficiency virus seropositivity also is high, ranging from 6% to 60% depending on the metropolitan area being studied. Other infectious problems include endocarditis, osteomyelitis, bacterial pneumonia, and tuberculosis. In some urban areas, patients who abuse intravenous drugs have a 35% positive rate on PPD testing. All intravenous drug users who are hospitalized require hepatitis testing, HIV testing (with consent), and PPD testing with an anergy panel. Finally, many opiate-dependent patients have ignored or self-treated many symptoms before coming to the hospital. As they come out from under their self-induced opiate anesthetic, serious and at times far-advanced illnesses often emerge. It is important to perform a thorough baseline evaluation and to investigate all emerging symptom complexes.

Presenting the diagnosis and forming a treatment plan

After detoxification has been accomplished, physicians are often reluctant to address important issues in patients with substance abuse problems [35]. There are many reasons for this, including discomfort with this disease in general, lack of training in dealing with these types of patients, lack of institutional and departmental support, and a prevailing sense of therapeutic futility. This feeling of hopelessness and of being overwhelmed by the magnitude of skills needed to treat chemically dependent patients is not supported by recent research.

Data from brief intervention studies indicate that traditional skills used in presenting other difficult diagnoses to patients (i.e., cancer, AIDS) are also effective when presenting the diagnosis of substance abuse [36].

Simple and effective strategies for presenting the diagnosis of alcohol or drug dependence are being taught in most medical schools and many residency programs. Two such strategies are the Eight Basic Actions outlined by Barker and Whitfield [37], and the SOAPE mnemonic by Clark [38]. The primary points of these and other strategies include the need to be clear, concise, and specific about the diagnosis; to appear comfortable during the discussion; to avoid blaming patients; to show support for their present or future willingness to work toward sobriety; to be optimistic about eventual success; and to urge a treatment plan based on abstinence with close follow-up and reinforcement [39].

Several specific pitfalls should be avoided when presenting the diagnosis and forming a treatment plan. The discussion should be kept extremely brief if patients are intoxicated and followed up at a later date. Patients often try to direct the discussion into various reasons or explanations for their problems. Efforts should be made to keep the discussion focused on the diagnosis itself and to avoid speculations about the cause or origin of substance abuse. Because arguments tend to be fruitless, an attempt should be made to defuse them with empathy, respect, and a thorough explanation of the disease as a chronic, progressive illness. Outpatient prescribing of controlled anxiolytics is strongly discouraged in all substance abusing populations and outpatient prescribing of opiate analgesics should be for a specific, self-limited period. Finally, physicians should strive to be clear, comfortable, and caring [39].

In many cases, this simple approach is unsuccessful. Consultation is often needed for these more complicated situations. Given the prevalence of substance abuse problems in surgical patients, it is reasonable for departments of surgery to insist that chemical dependency consultation services be provided by their hospital systems. With the prevalence exceeding 50% on some trauma services, substance abuse consultation is essential for adequate patient care at any level I or level II trauma center in North America [5].

Pain management strategies

The management of acute and chronic pain is a difficult and complicated area of patient care that cannot be summarized in this chapter, but some areas of special attention and concern regarding the surgical patient can be identified. Physicians have varying philosophies and beliefs about pain management, the prescription of opiate analgesics, and the use of pain management consultants. In contrast, the commonalities of addictions are strong, and patients who develop difficulties with the use of one mood-altering drug very commonly develop problems with other mood-altering drugs to which they are longitudinally exposed. Therefore patients with substance abuse problems who are prescribed controlled drugs on a chronic basis create significant problems for physicians in general, and this is certainly true of postoperative surgical situations. Issues concerning the long-term over-prescribing of controlled drugs are one of the leading causes for state medical boards to investigate and take action against physicians, and accidental fatal overdose on prescription opioids is one of the leading causes of accidental death in the nation [40–42]. Therefore the long-term prescribing of opioid analgesics for the management of short-term postoperative surgical acute pain syndromes is strongly discouraged.

Despite the current state of concern nationally regarding indications for the long-term prescribing of chronic opioids, most experts strongly encourage the prescribing of short-term opioids for the short-term management of moderate to severe self-limited pain syndromes, even in patients with addiction histories [43]. This certainly can apply to the majority of postoperative surgical patients. Several basic management principles can be outlined to help guide these short-term prescribing practices: (1) Before opiate analgesics are prescribed for all patients, and especially for patients with substance abuse problems, a clear diagnosis must be identified. (2) A therapeutic plan with specific treatment goals, methods of monitoring symptoms, and expected time course must be outlined and documented in the chart [40,43,44]. (3) The provision of reasonable relief for acute, self-limited pain is a justifiable expectation for all patients, regardless of their chemical dependency status, as long as it can be safely done. (4) Patients who have misused mood-altering chemicals in the past may have higher medication tolerance than other patients, and thus may require higher doses of medication. (5) Even in short-term prescribing situations, patients with substance abuse problems may misuse their prescription analgesics. (6) Physicians should always avoid the use of polypharmacy with controlled drugs if at all possible – in other words the concomitant prescribing of multiple different classes of controlled drugs to a patient with an addiction history increases the danger even in the short term. (7) It is important to prescribe adequate dosages of analgesics while at the same time limiting the amount of drug dispensed, providing no early refills on any controlled prescription, and refusing to prescribe more medication than originally intended unless the diagnosis changes. (8) Frequent brief visits to renew the prescription, monitor the response to treatment, and maintain patient commitment to discontinuing opiate therapy at the predetermined time is an appropriate pattern of management. The more common practice of providing large prescriptions and rare follow-up appointments is dangerous and can increase the chance that the patient will abuse the medication and thus attempt to obtain early refills. (9) When opiate analgesics are prescribed for patients with previous opiate dependence, physicians should attempt to use medications from a different class than the one previously abused. For example, a former heroin (mu-agonist) user who requires opiate-type analgesia should be treated with local or regional anesthesia and kappa-agonists if at all possible. This can provide adequate pain relief with less risk of rekindling the former addiction.

In cases in which opiate therapy has evolved from short-term self-limited to long-term duration, and where the physician has determined that the reason for the prescribing has resolved, it is necessary to gradually taper the medication at a rate of 5–10% per week or to refer the patient elsewhere for medical withdrawal management. Many practitioners ask their patients to sign a treatment plan or informed consent in which they agree to be admitted to the hospital for detoxification if this type of medication-tapering regimen is not completed successfully. Patients who refuse such interventions present very difficult choices: they can be referred to methadone maintenance programs, or can be referred to a physician licensed to provide office-based buprenorphine-naloxone maintenance, or can be abruptly discontinued from opioids and referred to detoxification if withdrawal symptoms emerge. These management decisions are extremely difficult and influenced by many factors, including the personalities and philosophies of patients and physicians, and the rules and regulations of medical boards and state legislatures. What is clear, is that a physician who is uncomfortable about further prescribing of controlled drugs must alter the prescribing to a pattern that is consistent with her or his expertise and clinical comfort. This can involve tapering, referring, medically withdrawing, or discontinuing the controlled drug prescription, and especially when controlled drugs are involved this must be the decision of the physician and not of the patient. Although treatment approaches are never clearcut, the considerations outlined above can help guide this difficult decision-making process.

References

1. Moore RD, Levine DM. Prevalence, detection, and treatment of alcoholism in hospitalized patients. *J Am Med Assoc* 1989; **261**: 403–7.

2. Clark DE, McCarthy E, Robinson E. Trauma as a symptom of alcoholism. *Ann Emerg Med* 1985; **14**: 274–7.

3. Antti-Poika I. Heavy drinking and accidents. *Br J Accident Surg* 1988; **19**: 198–204.

4. Anda RH. Alcohol and fatal injuries among U.S. adults. *J Am Med Assoc* 1988; **260**: 2529–32.

5. Soderstrom CS. A National Alcohol and Trauma Center survey. *Arch Surg* 1987; **122**: 1067–71.

6. Blondel RD, Looney SW. Characteristics of intoxicated trauma patients. *J Addict Dis* 2002, **21**: 1–12.

7. Parran T, Tasse J, Adelman C, Weber E. Toxicology testing and trauma services: the need for a chemical dependence consult service. *J Trauma* 1995; **12**: 236–41.

8. Sonne NM, Tonnesen H. The influence of alcoholism on outcome after

evaluation of subdural hematoma. *Br J Neurosurg* 1992; **6**: 125–30.

9. Tonnesen H. Influence of alcoholism on morbidity after transurethral prostatectomy. *Scand J Urol Nephrol* 1988; **22**: 175–7.

10. Brezel BS, Stein JM. Burns in substance abusers. *J Burn Care Rehabil* 1988; **9**: 169–71.

11. Felding CF, Jensen LM, Ronnesen H. Influence of alcohol intake on postoperative morbidity after hysterectomy. *Am J Obstet Gynecol* 1992; **166**: 667–70.

12. Tonnesen H, Petersen KR. Postoperative morbidity among symptom-free alcohol misusers. *Lancet* 1992; **340**: 334–7.

13. Tonnesen H, Kehlet H. Preoperative alcoholism and postoperative morbidity. *Br J Surg* 1999; **86**: 869–74.

14. Wood PR, Soni N. Anaesthesia and substance abuse. *Anaesthesia* 1989; **44**: 672–80.

15. Bradley K, Rubinsky A, Sun H *et al.* Alcohol screening and risk or postoperative complications in male VA patients undergoing major non-cardiac surgery. *J Gen Intern Med* 2010; **26**: 162–9.

16. Hays JT, Spickard WA. Alcoholism: early diagnosis and treatment. *J Gen Intern Med* 1987; **2**: 420–7.

17. Rydon P, Reid A. Detection of alcohol related problems in general practice. *J Stud Alcohol* 1992; **53**: 197–202.

18. Lewis CM. Perioperative screening for alcoholism. *Ann Plast Surg* 1992; **28**: 207–9.

19. Ewing JA. Detecting alcoholism. *J Am Med Assoc* 1984; **252**: 1905–7.

20. Skinner HA. Identification of alcohol abuse using a history of trauma. *Ann Intern Med* 1984; **101**: 847–51.

21. Kantzian EJ, McKenna GJ. Acute toxic and withdrawal reactions associated with drug abuse. *Ann Intern Med* 1979; **40**: 361–72.

22. Turner RC, Lichstein PR. Alcohol withdrawal syndromes. *J Gen Intern Med* 1989; **4**: 432–44.

23. Eckardt MJ, Hartford TC, Kaelber CT. Health hazards associated with alcohol consumption. *J Am Med Assoc* 1981; **246**: 648–66.

24. Gavin FH, Ellinwood EH. Cocaine and other stimulants. *N Engl J Med* 1988; **318**: 1173–82.

25. Cregler LL, Marck H. Medical complications of cocaine abuse. *N Engl J Med* 1988; **315**: 1495–500.

26. Jaffe JH, Martin WR. Opioid analgesics and antagonists. In Gilman AG, Goodman LS, Rall TW, Murad F, eds. *Pharmacological Basis of Therapeutics.* New York, NY: Macmillan; 1985, pp. 491–531.

27. Fultz JM, Senay EC. Guidelines for the management of hospitalized narcotic addicts. *Ann Intern Med* 1975; **82**: 815–18.

28. Gold MS, Pottash CA, Kleber HD. Opiate withdrawal using clonidine. *J Am Med Assoc* 1980; **243**: 343–6.

29. Bush K, Kivlahan D, Brady K. The Audit alcohol consumption questionnaire. *Archiv Intern Med* 1998, **158**: 1789–95.

30. Frank S, Graham A, Zyzanski S *et al.* Use of the Family CAGE in screening for alcohol problems in primary care. *Archiv Family Med* 1992; **1**: 209–16.

31. Parran TV, Jasinski DR. Buprenorphine detoxification of medically unstable narcotic dependent patients. *Subst Abuse* 1990; **11**: 197–202.

32. Tamaskar R, Parran TV Jr, Heggi A *et al.* Tramadol versus buprenorphine for the treatment of opiate withdrawal: a retrospective cohort control study. *J Addict Dis* 2003; **22**: 5–12.

33. Sobey P, Parran T, Grey SF, Adelman CL, Yu J. The use of tramadol for acute heroin withdrawal: a comparison to clonidine. *J Addict Dis* 2003; **22**: 13–25.

34. Bickel WK, Johnson RE. Clinical trial of buprenorphine. *Clin Pharmacol Ther* 1989; **43**: 72–8.

35. Clark WD. Alcoholism: blocks to diagnosis and treatment. *Am J Med* 1981; **71**: 275–86.

36. Babor TF, Good SP. Screening and early intervention. *Aust Drug Alcohol Rev* 1987; **6**: 325–39.

37. Barker LR, Whitfield CL. Alcoholism. In Barker LIZ, Burton JR, Zieve PD, eds. *Principles of Ambulatory Medicine.* Baltimore, MD: Williams & Wilkins; 2002, pp. 258–9.

38. Clark WD. The medical interview: focus on alcohol problems. *Hosp Pract* 1985; **20**: 59–68.

39. Parran TV. Developing a treatment plan for the chemically dependent primary care patient. In Bigby JA, ed. *Substance Abuse Education in General Internal Medicine: A Manual for Faculty.* Society of General Internal Medicine and the Ambulatory Pediatric Association, Bureau of Health Professions HRSA; 1993, pp. 1–11.

40. Parran T. Prescription drug abuse: a question of balance. *Med Clin North Am* 1997; **81**: 967–78.

41. Dunn K, Saunders KW, Rutter CM *et al.* Opioid prescriptions for chronic pain and overdose. *Ann Intern Med* 2010; **152**: 85–92.

42. Hall A, Logan JE, Toblin RL *et al.* Patterns of abuse among unintentional pharmaceutical overdose fatalities. *J Am Med Assoc* 2008; **300**: 2613–20.

43. Longo L, Parran T. Addiction: Part II. Identification and management of the drug seeking patient. *Am Family Physician* 2000; **61**: 2121–8.

44. Parran TV, Bigby JA. Prescription drug abuse. In Bigby JA, ed. *Substance Abuse Education in General Internal Medicine: A Manual for Faculty.* Society of General Internal Medicine and the Ambulatory Pediatric Association, Bureau of Health Professions HRSA; 1993, pp. 1–35.

Care of the peripartum patient

Stacy Higgins

Introduction

Advances in medical care have led to increasing numbers of complex, high-risk, obstetric patients. With assisted reproductive technology, women at older maternal ages with medical comorbidities are able to conceive. Internists are often consulted to assist or even primarily manage pregnant women with preexisting medical disease or conditions that develop during pregnancy. This chapter will focus on several of the most common conditions that are unique to pregnancy or that occur due to the physiologic changes during the gestational period.

Normal physiologic changes in pregnancy

Cardiovascular

Cardiovascular changes in pregnancy occur predominantly in the first trimester, plateau in the second trimester, and then peak again around the time of labor and delivery. One of the earliest changes seen is a fall in systemic vascular resistance (SVR), reaching its nadir at 14–24 weeks of gestation, and then rising at term [1]. The early fall in SVR relates to peripheral arterial vasodilation, mediated by progesterone and perhaps nitric oxide [2]. In response to falling SVR, the heart rate rises, up to 20% by the third trimester [3]. An increase in heart rate leads to decreased time for diastolic filling and can lead to reduced cardiac output (CO) and perfusion pressures. In the first trimester CO rises and peaks by the end of the second trimester at approximately 30–50% over non-pregnant values. It rises again at the onset of labor, and declines rapidly after delivery [1]. Finally, blood pressure (a product of CO and SVR) falls by approximately 10% in early pregnancy, returning to normal pre-pregnancy values around term [4].

Hematologic

Plasma volume increases up to 10% by 7 weeks' gestation, and plateaus by 32 weeks at 45–50% above baseline. Red cell mass expansion occurs as well, but to a lesser degree, accounting for the dilutional anemia of pregnancy [5]. The increase in red cell mass provides for the increased oxygen demands of the mother and fetus.

Pregnancy is a pro-coagulable state, likely to reduce the amount of blood loss at delivery and the risk of postpartum hemorrhage. This accounts for a four- to six-fold increase in risk of venous thromboembolism compared with non-pregnant matched controls [6].

Respiratory

With the higher metabolic state of pregnancy, oxygen consumption increases. Stimulated by progesterone, there is a 40% rise in minute ventilation secondary to a progressive rise in tidal volume, with a stable respiratory rate of 14–15 breaths/minute [7]. Forced expiratory volume in 1 second (FEV1) and peak expiratory flow rate (PEFR) are unchanged with pregnancy. The rise in tidal volume also decreases maternal carbon dioxide levels, resulting in the excretion of bicarbonate from the kidneys. The result is a chronic respiratory alkalosis with a compensatory metabolic acidosis [8].

There are minimal mechanical changes seen with expansion of the uterus upwards. The lower ribs flare and thoracic circumference increases by 8%, and there is a 5 cm elevation of the diaphragm.

Hepatic

Serum albumin levels decrease during pregnancy because of hemodilution and decreased synthesis, but total cholesterol levels increase markedly secondary to increased synthesis under the stimulation of estrogen. Serum alanine (ALT) and aspartate (AST) aminotransferase levels are comparable to the non-pregnant states, while serum gamma glutamyl transpeptidase levels decrease in the third trimester and total, direct, and indirect bilirubin levels are decreased throughout pregnancy. Placental and bone alkaline phosphatase levels increase in the third trimester, increasing total maternal serum levels [9].

Hypertension in pregnancy

Hypertensive disorders complicate about 10% of all pregnancies, making it the most common medical disorder during pregnancy. Hypertension has been defined as a sustained increase

Medical Management of the Surgical Patient, ed. Michael F. Lubin, Thomas F. Dodson, and Neil H. Winawer. Published by Cambridge University Press. © Cambridge University Press 2013.

in blood pressure > 140/90mmHg [10]. Because of the significant fall in systemic vascular resistance with pregnancy, the diagnosis of preexisting mild hypertension may be obscured. The American College of Obstetrics and Gynecology and the National High Blood Pressure Education Program Working Group on High Blood Pressure in Pregnancy has classified hypertension during pregnancy into four groups: chronic hypertension, gestational hypertension, preeclampsia–eclampsia, and preeclampsia superimposed upon chronic hypertension [11].

Chronic hypertension

Chronic hypertension is defined as hypertension prior to pregnancy or before 20 weeks of gestation, or hypertension that persists for more than 12 weeks postpartum. It is estimated that 3% of pregnant women in the USA have chronic hypertension, with higher prevalence in African-American women and older women [12]. With the trend toward pregnancies later in life, and increased rates of obesity, this diagnosis has become more common during pregnancy. Complications include superimposed preeclampsia, perinatal mortality, abruptio placentae, low birth weight, and intrauterine growth restriction (IUGR) [13].

The optimal blood pressure during pregnancy is still unknown and remains controversial. There is no convincing evidence that medical treatment of mild hypertension (140–159/90–99) improves maternal outcomes during pregnancy, and treatment has potential adverse outcomes to the fetus [14]. Therefore recommendations are that pregnant women with newly diagnosed mild hypertension in the first trimester should be educated on lifestyle and dietary changes, closely observed off medications, and medications not be initiated unless blood pressure persists > 159/99, or end-organ damage is present [15].

Methyldopa is the drug of choice based on long-term data revealing no adverse effects on the neonate or infant [16]. Beta-blockers labetalol and extended-release metoprolol, as well as the calcium channel agent nifedipine, are preferred agents as alternatives or additions. This is in contrast to other beta-blockers which are associated with IUGR, premature labor, and neonatal apnea. The use of diuretics is controversial as they may cause volume depletion and electrolyte abnormalities, although studies have shown no increased evidence of adverse fetal effects [17]. Current recommendations are that women already on diuretics prior to pregnancy may continue these medications unless they develop superimposed preeclampsia, in which case the diuretic should be discontinued. Angiotensin converting enzyme inhibitors, angiotensin receptor blockers, and renin inhibitors are contraindicated in pregnancy [18].

In accelerated hypertension of pregnancy, intravenous (IV) or intramuscular (IM) hydralazine is the most commonly used drug, although other effective parenteral treatments include labetalol, nicardipine, metoprolol, and methyldopa.

Intravenous nitroprusside is only to be used as a last resort because of risk of fetal cyanide toxicity [19].

Gestational hypertension

Gestational hypertension (previously known as pregnancy-induced hypertension) is defined as hypertension without proteinuria after 20 weeks of pregnancy. The etiology is unclear, although it appears to identify women destined to develop essential hypertension later in life. Blood pressure returns to normal immediately after delivery, but may relapse in subsequent pregnancies. Gestational hypertension is a provisional diagnosis that includes women eventually diagnosed with preeclampsia or chronic hypertension.

Preeclampsia–eclampsia

Preeclampsia is exclusively a disease of pregnancy characterized by new-onset hypertension and proteinuria, usually after 20 weeks' gestation, and is commonly associated with edema, hyperuricemia, and proteinuria. A multi-organ disease process that affects about 5% of all pregnancies, it is twice as common in first pregnancies as in subsequent. However, it is also seen in multigravidas who have new partners, suggesting that prior exposure to paternal antigens may be protective [17]. In about 30% of cases, the disease may cause enough placental insufficiency to cause IUGR or fetal death [18]. When new-onset seizures occur in the setting of preeclampsia, it is called eclampsia. Surprisingly, seizures may occur in up to one-third of women with no history of preeclampsia.

Risk factors for preeclampsia are preexisting hypertension, chronic renal disease, obesity, diabetes mellitus, multiple gestations, maternal age over 40, nulliparity, preeclampsia in a previous pregnancy, hydatidiform mole, and thrombophilias.

There are several theories behind the pathogenesis of preeclampsia, but the most prevalent is defective remodeling of the spiral arteries at the time of trophoblast invasion. Because the spiral arteries fail to undergo the normal thinning out of the muscular walls that permit enhanced perfusion of the placenta, perfusion of the intervillous space is impaired, leading to placental hypoxia. Other theories include immunologic intolerance between fetoplacental and maternal tissue, and angiogenic factors [20].

In preeclampsia, there is a paradoxical increase in SVR and a decrease in the physiologic hypervolemia of pregnancy. The amount of plasma volume reduction and hemoconcentration are proportional to the severity of the disease. Pulmonary edema, the most common cardiopulmonary complication of preeclampsia, results from decreased oncotic pressure, increased hydrostatic pressure, and a change in capillary permeability [21]. Older age, multigravidity, and preexisting hypertension favor the development of pulmonary edema. Medical therapy includes furosemide, oxygen, morphine, and restriction of salt and fluid intake.

Glomerular filtration rate and renal plasma flow are uniformly decreased in preeclampsia. Glomerular damage resulting in significant non-selective proteinuria is an important feature of preeclampsia. There is a decreased clearance of uric acid as well, and the degree of serum uric acid elevation correlates with the severity of proteinuria, renal pathologic changes, and fetal demise [22].

Central nervous system complications are most commonly due to cerebral hemorrhage, brain edema, thrombotic microangiopathy, and cerebral vasoconstriction. This results in the sudden development of seizures (eclampsia), along with headache, blurred vision, scotoma, and cortical blindness. The seizures are usually grand mal, and if they occur earlier than 32 weeks of gestation are associated with a worse prognosis. There appears to be no correlation between the magnitudes of blood pressure increase or the degree of proteinuria, making seizure onset difficult to predict [23].

The coagulation system is activated in preeclampsia, and can range from mild thrombocytopenia, escalating to the HELLP syndrome (hemolysis, elevated liver enzymes, and low platelets) [24].

Early recognition of preeclampsia with screening tests before the classic symptoms appear has proven to be difficult and is an area of ongoing research. Identifying targets for prevention has also proven to be difficult. Calcium supplementation (1500 mg daily) reduces the risk of developing preeclampsia in high-risk women and those with low dietary calcium intake [25]. Low-dose aspirin (75–81 mg daily) is effective for prevention in women at increased risk of preeclampsia [26].

The most reliable treatment of preeclampsia is delivery, but this decision needs to balance the risks of worsening preeclampsia against those of fetal immaturity. Women with mild preeclampsia should be monitored for signs of rapid deterioration. If clinical signs or laboratory values worsen, then the patient should be admitted to hospital [27]. The goals of treatment are to prevent seizures, lower blood pressure to avoid maternal end-organ damage, while aiming to prolong the pregnancy for fetal maturity as long as possible. When eclampsia occurs at any time during gestation, termination of the pregnancy is indicated, irrespective of the stage of pregnancy [28].

Similar to hypertension, there is no indication to administer antihypertensive medication to patients with mild preeclampsia. Recommendations are that antihypertensive therapy should be given for a systolic blood pressure > 160 or diastolic > 110 mmHg, with a goal treatment blood pressure of 140–155/90–105 mmHg [29]. Magnesium sulfate is used to prevent seizures in these patients, and has the additional benefit of reducing the incidence of placental abruption [30].

Venous thromboembolic disease

Venous thromboembolic disease (VTE), encompassing both deep venous thrombosis (DVT) and pulmonary embolism (PE), is the leading cause of maternal mortality in the USA,

and complicates anywhere from 0.5–3% of pregnancies [31]. Virchow's triad of hypercoagulation, vascular damage, and venous stasis occurs during pregnancy, resulting in a relative risk of 4.3 for VTE compared with non-pregnant women [32]. Other risk factors related to pregnancy include age > 35, obesity, grand multiparity, bed rest, hyperemesis, preeclampsia, and delivery via cesarean section [33].

During pregnancy 78–90% of DVTs occur in the left leg, and 72% in the iliofemoral vein, where they are more likely to embolize [34]. Typical symptoms are the same as DVT in the non-pregnant state (unilateral leg pain and swelling) as compared with the bilateral leg swelling that can occur with normal pregnancy. Pulmonary embolism occurs more commonly in the postpartum period than during pregnancy, and 64% of postpartum VTEs occur after cesarean delivery [29]. Symptoms of PE are non-specific in pregnancy as many women complain of both shortness of breath and palpitations at some point during the gestational period.

In non-pregnant women, a negative D-dimer test combined with a low clinical probability score has a negative predictive value higher than 99% for ruling out PE. During pregnancy however, ordering a D-dimer is of limited yield as its value increases progressively throughout pregnancy. Ultrasound is the initial test of choice for diagnosing DVT because it is non-invasive, safe, and relatively inexpensive. It also is the best initial test for PE because if positive, anticoagulant treatment will be the same, avoiding fetal and maternal radiation exposure. If inconclusive, spiral computed tomography (CT) is the next test of choice for PE [35]. This test has lower fetal exposure to radiation as compared with ventilation-perfusion (V/Q) scanning, and has positive and negative predictive values comparable with pulmonary angiography. However, in women with a personal or family history of breast cancer, V/Q scan may be preferred as spiral CT does expose the maternal breast to higher doses of radiation as compared with the V/Q scan [36].

Anticoagulation options include low molecular weight heparins (LMWHs), unfractionated heparin (UFH), and warfarin (in the postpartum period only). LMWHs have replaced UFH as first-choice medications for both VTE treatment and prophylaxis in pregnancy. Studies have shown that LMWH is safe and effective, with minimal excretion in breast milk. As compared with UFH, LMWHs have lower rates of adverse effects, including heparin-induced thrombocytopenia, osteoporosis, bleeding, and allergic reactions [37,38]. Therapeutic anticoagulation for a VTE incurred during pregnancy should continue for 3–6 months after diagnosis, including 6 weeks postpartum, unless there is an underlying thrombophilia, in which case prolonged therapy may be needed [39].

Asthma in pregnancy

Asthma is the most common chronic condition seen in pregnancy, affecting 4–8% of pregnant women [40]. It typically follows an unpredictable course during pregnancy, and generally the rule of thirds is seen: one-third of patients improve, one-third worsen, and one-third are unchanged [41]. For multiparous women, their asthma history in previous pregnancies can help predict the course of illness during their subsequent pregnancy.

Exacerbations are more commonly seen in women with severe asthma than in those with mild asthma, and are most likely to occur between 24 and 36 weeks of pregnancy. The most common precipitant of exacerbations are respiratory viral infections, followed by non-adherence to inhaled corticosteroid (ICS) medications [42]. Asthma exacerbations during pregnancy significantly increase the risk of low birthweight babies compared with non-asthmatic women and women without exacerbations [43].

The management of asthma in pregnancy is the same as in non-pregnant women. Education on triggers, the use of devices, medication, and a personal action plan should be reviewed. Long-term control medications are used for maintenance therapy to prevent asthma manifestations and include ICS, cromolyn, long-acting beta-agonists, and theophylline. Particular emphasis on the safety of ICS in pregnancy and adherence to their use should be emphasized as pregnant women have been shown to decrease use by 23% [44]. Rescue therapy includes short-acting beta-agonists. Both budesonide and albuterol have been studied most extensively in pregnancy and have reassuring safety data. Oral steroids can be used as rescue therapy to treat an asthma exacerbation or as long-term control therapy for patients with severe persistent asthma [45].

Patients whose symptoms are not optimally responding to treatment should receive a step up in treatment to more intensive medical therapy. Once control is achieved and sustained for several months, a step-down approach can be considered cautiously, but consider postponing medication tapering until after birth to avoid compromising the stability of control [46]. Most women who experience worsening of their asthma during pregnancy revert back to their pre-pregnancy state several months after birth.

Liver disease in pregnancy

This section will focus on the liver diseases that are unique to pregnancy. These entities generally resolve with termination of pregnancy and include: intrahepatic cholestasis of pregnancy, acute fatty liver of pregnancy, and the HELLP syndrome.

Intrahepatic cholestasis of pregnancy

Intrahepatic cholestasis of pregnancy (ICP) is characterized by pruritis and elevated serum bile acid levels, occurring in the second and third trimester of pregnancy. Its incidence varies significantly around the world, with clear ethnic and racial differences [47]. The etiology is unknown, but a genetic component is postulated given the ethnic association. One theory is a defect in the coding for the multidrug-resistance P-glycoprotein 3 (MDR 3) which is a hepatocellular phospholipid transporter [48]. Mutations may result in loss of function

and increased bile acid levels as a secondary effect. In addition sex hormones such as estrogen and progesterone are thought to play a role as they have cholestatic effects, and can impair the function of bile transporters (such as MDR 3), saturating the hepatic transport systems in some genetically predisposed women [49]. A new hypothesis centers around the fact that women with ICP have increased intestinal permeability, and that a leaky gut can increase the intestinal absorption of endotoxins and contribute to the pathogenesis of the disease [50].

Clinically, patients report generalized pruritus that starts peripherally and spreads centrally, becoming more intense at night. There is no rash, but excoriations may be present. Jaundice occurs in less than 15% of patients, but when it does, appears 2–4 weeks after the onset of pruritus. Patients may also develop diarrhea or steatorrhea. On laboratory exam, elevated fasting levels of total bile acids (TBAs) may be the first or only laboratory abnormality seen, and are the most sensitive and specific markers of the disease. There is mild, predominantly conjugated hyperbilirubinemia; transaminase levels are usually 2–10-fold above normal; alkaline phosphatase level is modestly elevated; and GGT level is normal. If prothrombin time is prolonged, it is because of vitamin K deficiency secondary to decreased absorption of fat-soluble vitamins [51].

Liver biopsy is usually not necessary to confirm diagnosis. On ultrasound, the liver and biliary ducts appear normal.

While there is no associated maternal mortality with ICP, there may be significant fetal morbidity and mortality including prematurity, meconium-stained amniotic fluid (a marker of fetal distress), intrauterine demise (1%), and increased risk of fetal respiratory distress syndrome [52]. Treatment is focused on relief of maternal symptoms. Ursodeoxycholic acid (UDCA) has shown in multiple trials to be efficacious, improving symptoms, bile flow, and biochemical test results without significant adverse maternal or fetal effects reported [53]. It is considered first-line therapy, and is usually dosed at 10–15 mg/kg/day divided twice daily. Other drugs used include cholestyramine which decreases ileal absorption of bile salts and increases fecal elimination. It is not superior to UDCA, and may lead to significant steatorrhea and exacerbate vitamin K deficiency [54]. S-adenosylmethionine (SAMe) is a glutathione precursor used in combination with UDCA for synergistic effect, and dual therapy is recommended at the start until the labs are stabilized [55]. Cholestasis can lead to deficiency of fat-soluble vitamins, so vitamin K should be given to all patients with jaundice to decrease postpartum bleeding.

Long-term maternal prognosis is good, but patients should be warned of the high risk of recurrence in subsequent pregnancies.

Acute fatty liver of pregnancy

Acute fatty liver of pregnancy (AFLP) is a rare disorder occurring in approximately 1 out of 10,000 pregnancies. It is a catastrophic illness appearing in or around the third trimester

Table 46.1 HELLP syndrome.

Hemolysis	• Abnormal peripheral blood smear (schistocytes and/or burr cells) • Serum bilirubin > 1.1 mg/dL • LDH > 600 U/L
Elevated liver enzymes	• AST elevated at least twice normal • ALT elevated at least twice normal
Low platelet count	< 100 K/mm^3

characterized by microvesicular steatosis associated with mitochondrial dysfunction. About half of patients are nulliparous, with an increased incidence in twin pregnancies and preeclamptic patients [56].

Presentation may range anywhere from asymptomatic elevation of aminotransferases to fulminant hepatic failure. Symptoms are generally non-specific for 1–2 weeks and include anorexia, nausea and vomiting, headache and right upper quadrant pain. Laboratory abnormalities may be numerous and include: elevated bilirubin (> 5 mg/dL), elevated aminotransferases ranging from near normal to 1,000s, normochromic normocytic anemia, leukocytosis, normal to low platelet levels, coagulopathy with or without disseminated intravascular coagulation (DIC), metabolic acidosis, renal dysfunction, hypoglycemia, hyperammonemia, and biochemical pancreatitis with elevated amylase and lipase.

Definitive diagnosis is made via biopsy, but is not always required and may prove to be hazardous in a pregnant patient. Features of AFLP may overlap with HELLP syndrome (see below), but the degree of hepatic impairment is much more significant.

Early recognition and diagnosis with immediate delivery of the fetus and aggressive supportive care is the key to management. Patients generally improve clinically and biochemically shortly after delivery; however on occasion there is transient worsening followed by definitive improvement. There are no reports of improvement before delivery. Fetal mortality is currently reported at < 15% [57].

HELLP syndrome

HELLP (**h**emolytic anemia, **el**evated liver enzymes, **l**ow **p**latelets) syndrome (Table 46.1) occurs in up to 20% of pregnancies complicated by severe preeclampsia. Its clinical presentation is variable: 12–18% of patients are normotensive, 13% do not have proteinuria, and 30% are postpartum at diagnosis [58]. This leads many experts to believe that HELLP is a separate entity from preeclampsia.

Clinical symptoms on presentation include right upper quadrant or epigastric pain, nausea, and vomiting. Patients afflicted with the syndrome are more likely to be multiparous and tend to be older than the average woman with preeclampsia. Evaluation should include a CBC, platelet count, and liver enzyme determination. Diagnostic results are listed in Table 46.1 [59]. Liver enzyme levels may be elevated 10–20-fold. Imaging studies such as CT and MRI are useful in detecting the hepatic complications of HELLP, including infarct, hematoma, and rupture.

Delivery is recommended for women with HELLP syndrome if the fetus is older than 28 weeks, and they are routinely delivered 24–48 hours after steroids are administered for fetal lung maturation. Mortality is as high as 3%, and serious morbidity can include DIC, abruption placenta, acute renal failure, pulmonary edema, subcapsular liver hematoma, and retinal detachment [60]. Temporizing medical measures include magnesium sulfate for seizure prophylaxis, and administration of vasodilators such as IV hydralazine, labetalol, or nifedipine. Administration of these medications may improve fetal, neonatal, and maternal outcomes, however, perinatal mortality remains high [61]. Prognosis is primarily dependent on gestational age and the severity at presentation, or secondary to the consequences of severe maternal complications.

Women with a history of the HELLP syndrome carry an increased risk of gestational hypertension in subsequent pregnancies. For those who developed HELLP before 28 weeks' gestation, with future pregnancies they are at increased risk for several obstetric complications, including preterm birth, pregnancy-induced hypertension, and increased neonatal mortality [62].

References

1. Clark SL, Cotton DB, Lee W et al. Central hemodynamic assessment of normal term pregnancy. Am J Obstet Gynecol 1989; **161**: 1439–42.

2. Weiner CP, Knowles RG, Moncada S. Induction of nitric oxide synthases early in pregnancy. Am J Obstet Gynecol 1994; **171**: 838–43.

3. Duvekot JJ, Cheriex EC, Pieters FA et al. Early pregnancy changes in hemodynamics and volume homeostasis are consecutive adjustments triggered by a primary fall in systemic vascular tone. Am J Obstet Gynecol 1993; **169**: 1382–92.

4. Clapp JF 3rd, Seaward BL, Sleamaker RH et al. Maternal physiologic adaptations to early human pregnancy. Am J Obstet Gynecol 1988; **159**: 1456–60.

5. Cavill I. Iron and erythropoiesis in normal subjects and in pregnancy. J Perinat Med 1995; **23**: 47–50.

6. Heit JA, Kobbervig CE, James AH et al. Trends in the incidence of venous thromboembolism during pregnancy or postpartum: a 30-year population-based study. Ann Intern Med 2005; **143**: 697–706.

7. Pernoll ML, Metcalfe J, Kovach PA et al. Ventilation during rest and exercise in pregnancy and postpartum. Respir Physiol 1975; **25**: 295–310.

8. Carlin A, Alferevic Z. Physiologic changes of pregnancy and monitoring. Clin Obstet Gyn 2008; **22**: 801–23.

9. Valenzuela GJ, Munson LA, Tarbaux NM et al. Time-dependent changes in bone, placental, intestinal, and hepatic alkaline phosphatase activities in

serum during human pregnancy. *Clin Chem* 1987; **33**: 1801–6.

10. Chobanian AV, Bakris GL, Black HR *et al*; Joint National Committee on Prevention, Detection, Evaluation, and Treatment of High Blood Pressure. National Heart, Lung, and Blood Institute; National High Blood Pressure Education Program Coordinating Committee. Seventh report of the Joint National Committee on Prevention, Detection, Evaluation, and Treatment of High Blood Pressure. *Hypertension* 2003; **42**: 1206–52.

11. Report of the National High Blood Pressure Education Program Working Group on High Blood Pressure in Pregnancy. *Am J Obstet Gynecol.* 2000; **1831**: S1–22.

12. Wolz M, Cutler J, Roccella EJ *et al*. Statement from the National High Blood Pressure Education Program: prevalence of hypertension. *Am J Hypertens* 2000; **13**: 103–4.

13. Gilbert WM, Young AL, Danielsen B. Pregnancy outcomes in women with chronic hypertension: a population based study. *J Reprod Med* 2007; **52**: 1046–51.

14. Von Dadelszen P, Ornstein MP, Bull SB *et al*. Fall in mean arterial pressure and fetal growth restriction in pregnancy hypertension: a meta analysis. *Lancet* 2000; **355**: 87–92.

15. Ferrer RL, Sibai BM, Mulrow CD *et al*. Management of mild chronic hypertension during pregnancy: a review. *Obstet Gynecol* 2000; **96**: 849–60.

16. Lindheimer MD, Taler SJ, Cunningham FG. ASH position paper: hypertension in pregnancy. *J Clin Hypertens* 2009; **11**: 214–25.

17. Collins R, Yusuf S, Peto R. Overview of randomized trials of diuretics in pregnancy. *Br Med J (Clin Res Ed)* 1985; **290**: 17–23.

18. Redman CW. Controlled trials of antihypertensive drugs in pregnancy. *Am J Kidney Dis* 1991; **17**: 149–53.

19. Duley L, Henderson-Smart DJ, Meher S. Drugs for treatment of very high blood pressure during pregnancy. *Cochrane Database Syst Rev* 2006; **3**: CD001449.

20. Redman CW, Sargent IL. Latest advances in understanding preeclampsia. *Science* 2005; **308**: 1592–4.

21. Hayes PM, Cruikshank DP, Dunn LJ. Plasma volume determination in normal and preeclamptic pregnancies. *Am J Obstet Gynecol* 1985; **151**: 958–66.

22. Karumanchi SA, Maynard SE, Stillman IE *et al*. Preeclampsia: a renal perspective. *Kidney Int* 2005; **67**: 2101–13.

23. Sibai BM. Diagnosis, prevention, and management of eclampsia. *Obstet Gynecol* 2005; **105**: 402–10.

24. Weinstein L. Syndrome of hemolysis, elevated liver enzymes, and low platelet count: a severe consequence of hypertension in pregnancy. *Am J Obstet Gynecol* 1982; **142**: 159–67.

25. Villar J, Abdel-Aleem H, Merialdi M *et al*. World Health Organization randomized trial of calcium supplementation among low calcium intake pregnant women. *Am J Obstet Gynecol* 2006; **194**: 639–49.

26. CLASP (Collaborative Low-dose Aspirin Study in Pregnancy) Collaborative Group. Clasp: a randomized trial of low-dose aspirin for the prevention and treatment of pre-eclampsia among 9364 pregnant women. *Lancet* 1994; **343**: 619–29.

27. Jim B, Sharma S, Kebede T *et al*. Hypertension in pregnancy: a comprehensive update. *Cardiol Rev* 2010; **18**: 178–89.

28. Karumanchi SA, Lindheimer MD. Advances in the understanding of eclampsia. *Curr Hypertens Rep* 2008; **10**: 305–12.

29. Sibai BM. Diagnosis and management of gestational hypertension and preeclampsia. *Obstet Gynecol* 2003; **102**: 181–92.

30. Which anticonvulsant for women with eclampsia? Evidence from the Collaborative Eclampsia Trial. *Lancet* 1995; **345**: 1455–63.

31. Chang J, Elam-Evans LD, Berg CJ *et al*. Pregnancy-related mortality surveillance – United States, 1991–1999. *Morb Mortal Wkly Rep MMWR Surveill Summ* 2003; **52**: 1–8.

32. Heit JA, Kobbervig CE, James AH *et al*. Trends in the incidence of venous thromboembolism during pregnancy or postpartum: a 30-year population based study. *Ann Intern Med* 2005; **143**: 697–706.

33. Deneux-Tharaux C, Carmona E, Bouvier-Colle MH *et al*. Postpartum maternal mortality and cesarean delivery. *Obstet Gynecol* 2006; **108**: 541–8.

34. Zotz RB, Gerhardt A, Scharf RE. Prediction, prevention and treatment of venous thromboembolic disease in pregnancy, *Semin Thromb Hemost* 2003; **29**: 143–54.

35. Snow V, Qaseem A, Barry P *et al*., for the American College of Physicians, American Academy of Family Physicians Panel on Deep Venous Thrombosis/Pulmonary Embolism. Management of venous thromboembolism: a clinical practice guideline from the American College of Physicians and the American Academy of Family Physicians. *Ann Intern Med* 2007; **146**: 204–10.

36. Winer-Muram HT, Boone JM, Brown HL *et al*. Pulmonary embolism in pregnant patients: fetal radiation dose with helical CT. *Radiology* 2002; **224**: 487–92.

37. Greer IA, Nelson-Piercy C. Low molecular weight heparins for thromboprophylaxis and treatment of venous thromboembolism in pregnancy: a systematic review of safety and efficacy. *Blood* 2005; **106**: 401–7.

38. Van Dongen CJ, van den Belt AA, Prins MH *et al*. Fixed dose subcutaneous low molecular weight heparins versus adjusted dose unfractionated heparin for venous thromboembolism. *Cochrane Database Syst Rev* 2004; **4**: CD001100.

39. Buller HR, Agnelli G, Hull RD *et al*. Antithrombotic therapy for venous thromboembolic disease: the Seventh ACCP Conference on Antithrombotic and Thrombolytic Therapy. *Chest* 2004; **126**: 401S–28S.

40. Kwon HL, Triche EW, Belanger K *et al*. The epidemiology of asthma during pregnancy: prevalence, diagnosis and symptoms. *Immunol Allergy Clin North Am* 2006; **26**: 29–62.

41. Hardy-Fairbanks AJ, Baker ER. Asthma in pregnancy: pathophysiology, diagnosis and management. *Obstet Gynecol Clin North Am* 2010; **37**: 159–72.

42. Murphy VE, Gibson P, Talbot PI *et al*. Severe asthma exacerbations during pregnancy. *Obstet Gynecol* 2005; **106**: 1046–54.

43. Murphy VE, Clifton VL, Gibson PG. Asthma exacerbations during pregnancy: incidence and association

with adverse pregnancy outcomes. *Thorax* 2006; **61**: 169–76.

44. Enriquez R, Wu P, Griffin MR *et al.* Cessation of asthma medication in early pregnancy. *Am J Obstet Gynecol* 2006: **195**: 149–53.

45. National Heart, Lung, and Blood Institute, National Asthma Education and Prevention Program. Working group report on managing asthma during pregnancy: recommendations for pharmacologic treatment – update 2004. NIH Publication No. 05-5236.

46. ACOG Practice Bulletin. Asthma in Pregnancy. *Obstet Gynecol* 2009; **111**: 457–64.

47. Lee RH, Goodwin TM, Greenspoon J *et al.* The prevalence of intrahepatic cholestasis of pregnancy in a primarily Latina Los Angeles population. *J Perinatol* 2006; **26**: 527–32.

48. Schneider G, Paus TC, Kullak-Ublick GA *et al.* Linkage between a new splicing site mutation in the MDR3 alias ABCB4 gene and intrahepatic cholestasis of pregnancy. *Hepatology* 2007; **45**: 150–8.

49. Beuers U, Pusl T. Intrahepatic cholestasis of pregnancy – a heterogeneous group of pregnancy-related disorders? *Hepatology* 2006; **43**: 647–9.

50. Reyes H, Zapata R, Hernandez I *et al.* Is a leaky gut involved in the pathogenesis of intrahepatic cholestasis of pregnancy? *Hepatology* 2006; **43**: 715–22.

51. Matin A, Sass DA. Liver disease in pregnancy. *Gastroenterol Clin North Am* 2011; **40**: 335–53.

52. Rioseco AJ, Ivankovic MB, Manzur A *et al.* Intrahepatic cholestasis of pregnancy: a retrospective case-control study of perinatal outcome. *Am J Obstet Gynecol* 1994; **170**: 890–5.

53. Palma J, Reyes H, Ribalta J *et al.* Ursodeoxycholic acid in the treatment of cholestasis of pregnancy: a randomized, double-blind study controlled with placebo. *J Hepatol* 1997; **27**: 1022–8.

54. Kondrackiene J, Beuers U, Kupcinskas L. Efficacy and safety of ursodeoxycholic acid versus cholestyramine in intrahepatic cholestasis of pregnancy. *Gastroenterology* 2005; **129**: 894–901.

55. Binder T, Salaj P, Zima T *et al.* Randomized prospective comparative study of ursodeoxycholic acid and S-adenosyl-L-methionine in the treatment of intrahepatic cholestasis of pregnancy. *J Perinat Med* 2006; **34**(5): 383–91.

56. Ibdah JA. Acute fatty liver of pregnancy: an update on pathogenesis and clinical implications. *World J Gastroenterol* 2006; **12**: 7397–404.

57. Knight M, Nelson-Piercy C, Kurinczuk JJ *et al.* A prospective national study of acute fatty liver of pregnancy in the UK. *Gut* 2008; **57**: 951–6.

58. Cappell MS. Hepatic disorders severely affected by pregnancy: medical and obstetric management. *Med Clin North Am* 2008; **92**: 739–60, vii–viii.

59. Leeman L, Fontaine P. Hypertensive disorders of pregnancy. *Am Fam Phys* 2008; **78**: 93–100.

60. Sibai BM, Ramadan MK, Usta I *et al.* Maternal morbidity and mortality in 442 pregnancies with hemolysis, elevated liver enzymes, and low platelets (HELLP syndrome). *Am J Obstet Gynecol* 1993; **169**: 1000–6.

61. Visser W, Wallenburg HC. Temporizing management of severe pre-eclampsia with and without the HELLP syndrome. *Br J Obstet Gynaecol* 1995; **102**: 111–17.

62. Haram K, Svendsen E, Abildgaard U. The HELLP syndrome: clinical issues and management. A review. *BMC Pregn Childbirth* 2009; **9**: 8.

Part

2

Surgical Procedures and their Complications

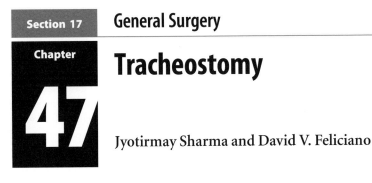

Chapter

47

Tracheostomy

Jyotirmay Sharma and David V. Feliciano

Historically, tracheostomy has been performed for relief of obstruction of the upper airway (trauma, epiglottitis); when prolonged ventilatory support for respiratory failure is likely; for control of secretions in patients with bulbar lesions or closed head injuries; or for sleep apnea. In many centers, open surgical tracheostomy has been replaced with bedside percutaneous dilational tracheostomy. In patients with acute airway obstruction, cricothyroidotomy ("high tracheostomy") is a better choice than tracheostomy, especially if the individual performing the procedure has little or no surgical training; if the procedure is being performed under less than ideal conditions in the emergency center or ICU; or if there is impending asphyxiation. The delay until tracheostomy is performed in patients with prolonged endotracheal intubation varies from center to center, but prospective data demonstrate the advantage of doing the procedure after 7–10 days. In patients with a head injury and poor neurological outcome a tracheostomy should be considered early in their care as this allows for improved oral care and optimal ventilator support. Recent evidence also indicates that patients who cannot be weaned with endotracheal tubes in place can often be weaned rapidly after a tracheostomy is performed. Finally, newer devices are available that enable patients with sleep apnea to be managed without tracheostomies.

Open tracheostomy is best performed in the operating room under local anesthesia supplemented by intravenous sedation after delivery of 100% oxygen by mask, endotracheal tube, or ventilating bronchoscope has been instituted. The patient's neck is hyperextended and a transverse incision is made over the second tracheal cartilage. The strap muscles are separated in the midline and the anterior trachea from the cricoid cartilage to the fourth tracheal cartilage is cleared, which often necessitates division of the thyroid isthmus between sutures. In many cases the posterior border of the thyroid isthmus can be mobilized without division and then retracted superiorly to provide adequate space for a tracheostomy. Either a vertical incision through the second and third cartilages or a three-sided, superiorly based flap (Bjork flap) between the second and third cartilages is made. It is imperative that notification of the tracheal incision be given to the anesthesiologist, as this is the time to deflate the balloon of the endotracheal tube, decrease oxygenation, and also avoid unnecessary cautery. The tracheostomy tube is then inserted as the anesthesiologist removes the endotracheal tube. The tracheostomy tube is secured to the skin with permanent sutures to avoid accidental decannulation.

Percutaneous tracheostomy is performed in the ICU or in the operating room. After infiltration of the pretracheal skin with local anesthetic, a 1–2 cm superficial transverse incision is made midway between the cricoid cartilage and the sternal notch. The subcutaneous tissue over the trachea is spread with a hemostat and the trachea can then be palpated. After the anesthesiologist pulls the endotracheal tube cuff back to just below the vocal cords, a 16-gauge needle is directed posteriorly and inferiorly into the trachea. A flexible bronchoscope passed through the endotracheal tube confirms entry into the trachea. A plastic cannula over the needle is advanced into the trachea, the needle is removed, a guidewire is inserted through the cannula, and the cannula is then removed. After passage of a small dilator over the guidewire and dilatation of the anterior hole in the trachea, the dilator is removed and a plastic guiding catheter is placed over the guidewire. Progressively larger dilators are passed over the wire and guiding catheter. A tracheostomy tube fitted snugly over a 24-French dilator is then passed into the trachea. After removal of the dilator, guidewire, guiding catheter, and endotracheal tube, the airway is secure. The stress of tracheostomy can be considerable if it is performed as an emergent procedure or if there is poor coordination between the operating surgeon and the anesthesiologist. Tracheostomy can be performed in 3–5 minutes by an experienced surgeon in a sedated patient, but elective tracheostomy performed meticulously in the operating room often requires 20–25 minutes. Blood transfusions are almost never required.

Medical Management of the Surgical Patient, ed. Michael F. Lubin, Thomas F. Dodson, and Neil H. Winawer. Published by Cambridge University Press. © Cambridge University Press 2013.

Usual postoperative course

Expected postoperative hospital stay

The duration depends on the reason for the tracheostomy. In patients who are converted to tracheostomies to enhance weaning, ventilatory support often is no longer necessary within 1–2 weeks.

Operative mortality

The hospital mortality rate for patients undergoing tracheostomy is 50% in some series. The mortality rate related directly to the procedure is under 1% and is always associated with hypoxia or hypoxia-induced cardiac arrhythmias.

Special monitoring required

Both oxygen saturation and end-tidal carbon dioxide monitoring are indicated when intubated and ventilated patients undergo tracheostomy.

Patient activity and positioning

The ventilator tubing should be positioned to prevent undue traction or angling of the tracheostomy tube.

Alimentation

Some patients have difficulty swallowing with a tracheostomy tube in place, presumably because of esophageal compression at the site of the balloon. Passage of a feeding tube with the balloon of the tracheostomy tube partially deflated is appropriate in such a situation. Many patients will get a combined tracheostomy and enteric access with nasoenteric tubes or percutaneous endoscopic gastrostomy tubes as part of the same procedure.

Antibiotic coverage

Antibiotics are indicated only if the tracheostomy is performed for respiratory failure caused by pneumonia. The appropriate perioperative antibiotic would be a second-generation cephalosporin or equivalent antibiotic providing gram-positive bacterial prophylaxis. If an enteric procedure is expected, gram-negative bacterial prophylaxis is also indicated.

Procedural complications

Loss of airway

Failure to pass the tracheostomy tube into the distal trachea during open tracheostomy can occur due to poor visualization in the obese patient with a short, deep neck.

Damage to posterior or lateral trachea

Overaggressive passage of or misplacement of dilators during percutaneous dilational tracheostomy may cause perforations of the posterior or lateral trachea mandating open repair.

Postoperative complications

In the hospital

Hemorrhage

Early bleeding from the soft tissues and thyroid gland near the tracheostomy site results from inadequate surgical hemostasis during open tracheostomy and can usually be controlled with packing around the stoma. However if bleeding is persistent, re-exploration of the tracheostomy is required in the operating room with a possibility of endotracheal cannulation to allow for adequate visualization. Late transient arterial bleeding in the presence of a pulsating tracheal cannula is suggestive of a tracheal–innominate artery fistula, an extraordinarily rare event since the introduction of large volume–low pressure balloons on tracheostomy tubes. Hyperinflation of the cuff of the tube occludes the fistula and compresses the artery in most patients. The aspirated blood should be suctioned vigorously as the surgical team is mobilized. Operative therapy is mandatory and involves resection of the innominate artery and repair of the trachea.

Obstruction

Progressive hypoxia despite passage of a suction catheter through the tube suggests that the remainder of the lumen is occluded or there are thick secretions acting as a ball valve at the tip. If equal breath sounds are present and a tension pneumothorax is unlikely, the tracheostomy tube should be changed over a suction catheter.

Infection

Tracheitis, mediastinitis, and pneumonia have all been reported. Frequent suctioning through the tracheostomy tube using meticulous sterile technique should decrease the incidence of infection in the tracheobronchial tree. Loose closure of the skin wound and frequent suctioning around the tracheostomy tube should reduce the incidence of soft tissue infection.

Tracheoesophageal fistula

Increased secretions and tube feedings in the airway associated with severe coughing related to swallowing suggests the presence of a fistula. Once bronchoscopy and esophagoscopy have confirmed the diagnosis, operative repair involves closure of the holes in both organs and the interposition of a bulky vascularized muscle flap.

After discharge

Tracheal stenosis

The late development of stridor, wheezing, dyspnea on effort, or airway obstruction from secretions in patients with histories of prolonged tracheostomy placement mandates bronchoscopy. These strictures are often related to hyperinflation of the balloon and poor surgical technique with resultant devascularization, tracheomalacia, or granulation tissue. Strictures may occur at the level of the previous stoma, at the balloon site, or at the tip of the tracheostomy tube. Resection of the stricture and end-to-end anastomosis of the trachea is indicated although many strictures can be managed with serial dilation, lasers, and tracheal stents.

Further reading

Berrouschot J, Oeken J, Steiniger L et al. Perioperative complications of percutaneous dilational tracheostomy. *Laryngoscope* 1997; **107**: 1538–44.

Engels P, Bagshaw S, Meier M, Brindley PG. Tracheostomy: from insertion to decannulation. *Can J Surg* 2009; **52**(5): 427–33.

Friedman Y, Fildes J, Mizock B et al. Comparison of percutaneous and surgical tracheostomies. *Chest* 1996; **110**: 480–5.

Kilic D, Fındıkcıoglu A, Akin S et al. When is surgical tracheostomy indicated? Surgical "U-shaped" versus percutaneous tracheostomy. *Ann Thorac Cardiovasc Surg* 2011; **17**(1): 29–32.

Marx WH, Ciaglia P, Graniero KD. Some important details in the technique of percutaneous dilatational tracheostomy via the modified Seldinger technique. *Chest* 1996; **110**: 762–6.

Massick DD, Yao S, Powell DM et al. Bedside tracheostomy in the intensive care unit: a prospective randomized trial comparing open surgical tracheostomy with endoscopically guided percutaneous dilational tracheotomy. *Laryngoscope* 2001; **111**: 494–500.

Petros S, Engelmann L. Percutaneous dilatational tracheostomy in a medical ICU. *Intens Care Med* 1997; **23**: 630–4.

Chapter

48

Thyroidectomy

Jyotirmay Sharma and David V. Feliciano

Surgical resection remains the treatment of choice for most thyroid tumors. Goiters and thyroid nodules are problems of enormous magnitude, present in more than 7% of the world's population. Tracheal compression from goiter may respond only to thyroidectomy, and thyroid nodules may harbor carcinoma, occurring in approximately 15% of solitary thyroid nodules and 5% of multinodular goiters.

Thyroid nodules have an annual incidence of 90 per million (approximately 29,000 new cases of thyroid carcinoma occur each year in the USA). The overall mortality is low, four per million per year (approximately 1,000 deaths per year in the USA). In patients with thyrotoxicosis a thyroidectomy can result in an expedient return to a euthyroid state. Included among these are children and women of childbearing age with Graves' disease, those who have failed medical or radioiodine therapy for Graves' disease, those with toxic multinodular goiter (Plummer's disease), and those with toxic adenomas. For the most part, goiter is a benign process, responsive to iodine repletion therapy. However, subtotal or total thyroidectomy is conventional therapy for hyperthyroidism and symptomatic goiter, particularly for patients with ophthalmopathy, or when airway compromise is present. Thyroid lobectomy is generally reserved for benign thyroid nodules or other, appropriately selected clinical circumstances.

Preoperative preparation with antithyroid drugs, propranolol, and potassium iodide (SSKI) or propranolol alone is indicated in patients with thyrotoxicosis to prevent thyroid storm in the postoperative period. Vocal cord function is checked before the administration of paralytic agents by the anesthesiologist, and many surgeons choose to examine vocal cords routinely in all patients in the preoperative setting. In any patient with history of neck surgery or voice changes a preoperative laryngoscopy is required.

Open thyroidectomy is usually performed under general anesthesia through a low collar incision, yielding excellent cosmetic results. Endoscopic thyroidectomy is also performed under general anesthesia with 3 mm and 5 mm instruments and an endoscope. The bilateral parathyroid glands, recurrent laryngeal nerves, and external branches of the superior laryngeal nerves are identified and preserved in both open and endoscopic thyroidectomies. Intraoperative laryngeal nerve monitoring is an available modality for nerve identification and validation of function. Although its routine use is not mandatory and it has not demonstrated improved outcomes, it can be a useful adjunct for inexperienced surgeons and in complex cases. Application of total thyroidectomy for this disease requires that the surgeon have detailed knowledge of the anatomy of the thyroid and parathyroid glands and the recurrent and superior laryngeal nerves.

Thyroidectomy imposes only a modest stress on patients, most procedures are completed in 1.5–2.5 hours, and transfusion is extremely uncommon.

Usual postoperative course

Expected postoperative hospital stay

Outpatient procedures are appropriate for solitary benign nodules and have been performed for thyrotoxicosis and thyroid cancer in some centers; otherwise, the hospital stay is 1 or 2 days.

Operative mortality

Operative mortality is under 0.1%.

Special monitoring required

Respiratory status should be carefully monitored if early postoperative stridor or difficulty in clearing secretions occurs. Patients with thyrotoxicosis who receive appropriate preoperative preparation should undergo routine monitoring.

Patient activity and positioning

The head should be elevated 30–45 degrees to minimize edema and venous oozing. Full activity is resumed the morning after operation.

Medical Management of the Surgical Patient, ed. Michael F. Lubin, Thomas F. Dodson, and Neil H. Winawer. Published by Cambridge University Press. © Cambridge University Press 2013.

Alimentation

A regular diet is resumed the day of surgery.

Antibiotic coverage

None indicated.

Drains

Closed suction drains are removed on the first postoperative day.

Postoperative complications

In the hospital

Hemorrhage

Although it is extremely rare (less than 0.5%), a hematoma in the area of resection may cause airway obstruction early in the postoperative period; 80% of hematomas occur within 6 hours of surgery. In cases of airway compromise, immediate removal of the skin and strap muscle sutures and evacuation of the hematoma in the recovery room or hospital room is necessary. Patients are then returned to the operating room for irrigation of the operative site, control of hemorrhage, and repeat closure of the wound.

Hypoparathyroidism

Transient hypoparathyroidism is seen in 2–4% of all patients after thyroidectomy, and in 15–25% of those who undergo total or repeated thyroidectomy. In patients undergoing central neck dissections the rates for hypoparathyroidism are increased. Permanent hypoparathyroidism occurs in under 0.6% of patients. Symptomatic hypocalcemia (less than 7.5 mg/dL) is characterized by anxiety, perioral or finger tingling, and a positive Chvostek's sign, usually developing 16–24 hours after surgery. Intravenous calcium is given to relieve acute symptoms in the hospital, and oral calcium therapy is prescribed at the time of discharge. A postoperative parathyroid hormone measurement can assess the extent of hypoparathyroidism. In patients with low parathyroid hormone an aggressive oral calcium supplementation of 4–5 g daily can often avoid the need for intravenous supplementation and decrease hospital stay.

Recurrent laryngeal nerve injury

In most cases the recurrent laryngeal nerve is reliably and quickly identified during thyroidectomy. Great care must be taken to avoid traction or cautery injuries to the nerve throughout the remainder of the procedure. Paralysis of one vocal cord causes hoarseness and difficulty in clearing secretions but rarely will cause airway issues. Depending upon the cause of injury, most patients have improvement in symptoms; even with permanent unilateral vocal cord dysfunction, most continue to have a normal voice. A bilateral recurrent nerve injury/palsy can be an airway emergency and may require a tracheostomy. Any suspicion for recurrent laryngeal nerve dysfunction should be evaluated with direct laryngoscopy. In cases of bilateral nerve complications the patient should be monitored in the ICU with an airway cart and tracheostomy tray at the bedside.

Thyroid storm

In adequately prepared patients, thyroid storm should not occur after surgery for thyrotoxicosis, but it may be seen in patients with untreated thyrotoxicosis who are undergoing other operations. Symptoms of tremor, agitation, tachycardia, and hyperthermia are treated with intravenous fluids, propranolol, potassium iodide, and steroids.

After discharge

Recurrent benign nodule or goiter

Recurrence of a benign nodule or goiter can be avoided by performing a total thyroid lobectomy and thus not leaving residual tissue. In patients with hypothyroidism, thyroxine supplementation has been reported to decrease growth of residual contralateral thyroid tissue. In euthyroid patients, routine use of thyroxine to suppress thyroid growth provides minimal benefit and can have serious complications associated with hyperthyroidism.

Late or recurrent hyperthyroidism

Annual thyroid function tests are indicated in patients who are receiving thyroid hormone after operation for goiter or cancer and in those who are originally euthyroid after operation for Graves' disease.

"Permanent" hypoparathyroidism

Permanent hypoparathyroidism is a rare and avoidable complication of thyroidectomy. Careful surveillance of the viability of remaining parathyroids and an autograft of non-viable parathyroids prevents this complication. A postoperative parathyroid hormone level measurement helps assess this state, and immediate intravenous calcium supplementation is necessary. Vitamin D is added to oral calcium replacement to enhance absorption. If serial parathyroid hormone levels begin to rise, first the vitamin D and then the calcium supplement should be tapered.

Further reading

Bilimoria KY, Bentrem DJ, Ko CY *et al.* Extent of surgery affects survival for papillary thyroid cancer. *Ann Surg* 2007; **246**: 375–81; discussion 381–4.

Cooper DS, Doherty GM, Haugen BR *et al.* The American Thyroid Association Guidelines Taskforce. Management guidelines for patients with thyroid nodules and differentiated thyroid cancer. *Thyroid* 2006; **16**: 109–42.

Feliciano DV. Everything you wanted to know about Graves' disease. *Am J Surg* 1992; **164**: 404–11.

Halsted WS. The operative story of goiter. *Johns Hopkins Hosp Rep* 1920; **19**: 171–257.

Inabnet WB, Gagner M. How I do it: endoscopic thyroidectomy. *J Otolaryngol* 2001; **30**: 41–2.

Lowery AJ, Kerin MJ. Graves' ophthalmopathy: the case for thyroid surgery. *Surgeon* 2009; 7(5): 290–6.

Pitt SC, Moley JF. Medullary, anaplastic, and metastatic cancers of the thyroid. *Semin Oncol* 2010; **37**(6): 567–79.

Chapter
49

Parathyroidectomy

Jyotirmay Sharma

Parathyroidectomy is performed most commonly in patients with primary hyperparathyroidism and those who are dialysis-dependent and have symptomatic secondary hyperparathyroidism. In patients who have hypercalcemia on dialysis or after renal transplantation (tertiary hyperparathyroidism), operation is also indicated. A physical examination, chest radiograph, and intact parathormone assay distinguish between primary hyperparathyroidism and the hypercalcemia of sarcoidosis, metastases, or a paraneoplastic syndrome. A 24-hour urinary calcium test is occasionally indicated to rule out familial hypocalciuric hypercalcemia. Currently, virtually all preoperative patients undergo localization studies such as cervical ultrasonography, computed tomography with intravenous contrast or radionuclide scanning after the intravenous injection of ^{99m}technetium-labeled sestamibi in order to allow for shortened operations through limited incisions. A curative parathyroidectomy not only results in improvements in serum calcium but also improvements in bone density, neuropsychiatric symptoms, calciphylaxis, nephrocalcinosis, nephrolithiasis, and cardiovascular risk.

Preoperative therapy to lower extraordinarily elevated serum calcium levels in patients with parathyroid comas or suspected carcinomas should include saline infusions, furosemide, bisphosphonates and, occasionally, calcitonin. Parathyroidectomy is usually performed under general anesthesia through a low collar incision, although local anesthesia is appropriate for elderly and high-risk patients as well as those undergoing minimally radio-guided parathyroidectomy or image-guided focal exploration.

There has been a rapid evolution in parathyroid surgery over the past 15 years. At present, many different operative approaches are being utilized. Conventional parathyroid exploration performed through the standard low collar incision, in which the size and histology of all four glands is assessed, is now accompanied by measurement of intraoperative intact parathyroid hormone (IOPTH) levels. If this measurement shows a drop to normal from the highest preincision intact parathormone level 5 minutes after excision of a suspected adenoma on the immunochemiluminescent assay,

it signifies that all hypersecreting tissue has been removed. Limited or focal or minimally invasive parathyroid exploration followed by measurement of IOPTH levels is appropriate when a preoperative sestamibi scan definitely localizes the enlarged adenoma. With the use of IOPTH and parathyroid localization, a less extensive dissection can be performed with equivalent results in approximately 60–70% of patients. In the remaining 30% of patients, the preoperative localization studies are inconclusive or IOPTH dynamics identifies multigland pathology. With addition of IOPTH, criteria for classification of abnormal parathyroid glands not only include size, histology, and morphology but also function. IOPTH allows the surgeon to determine if the localized tumor is the only functioning tumor in the patient. In our series, IOPTH remained elevated in 22% of patients after a limited neck exploration, and after conversion to a bilateral neck exploration another tumor was identified in all patients. Minimally invasive radio-guided parathyroidectomy (MIRP) involves the injection of intravenous ^{99m}technetium-labeled sestamibi 1.5–2.5 hours before operation. Guided by a gamma probe, the enlarged gland is removed and absence of multigland disease is confirmed with IOPTH measurements. Failure of this limited approach as documented on the IOPTH mandates a conventional cervical exploration. Finally, use of minimal access techniques such as robotic or video-assisted parathyroidectomy, which involve the insertion of an endoscope or a trocar for insufflation of CO_2 and several small-sized operating ports for 2 mm instruments, is available in selected centers.

A solitary parathyroid adenoma is present in 75–85% of patients and should be excised. Double adenomas are present in 2–4% of patients, and excision is appropriate along with biopsy of a normal gland. Sporadic primary hyperplasia is best treated with subtotal parathyroidectomy (excision of 3.5 glands) leaving a small vascularized remnant. IOPTH levels can help guide the extent of surgery in patients with hyperplasia; and an extremely low final IOPTH (< 5 pg/dL) can help ascertain the need for a parathyroid autograft and help avoid permanent hypoparathyroidism. Patients with secondary or tertiary hyperparathyroidism who are unlikely to be candidates for renal transplantation and also unlikely to have familial hyperparathyroidism or a multiple endocrine neoplasia (MEN) syndrome should undergo total parathyroidectomy with an autograft or a near-total parathyroidectomy with a small vascularized remnant. The surgical stress of parathyroidectomy is low and blood transfusions are almost never given.

Usual postoperative course

Expected postoperative hospital stay

Outpatient facilities are appropriate for focal neck explorations and for the excision of solitary and double adenomas and, in some centers, for all less than near-total or total parathyroidectomies. Otherwise, the hospital stay is 1 day.

Operative mortality

Operative mortality is essentially 0%.

Special monitoring required

The serum calcium level should be measured every 12 hours until discharge. An intact parathyroid hormone measurement within 8–12 hours of surgery can predict hypocalcemia (although even with normal parathyroid hormone levels many patients require supplemental calcium due to bone hunger).

Patient activity and positioning

The head should be elevated 30–45° to minimize edema and venous oozing. Patients are out of bed on the day of the operation.

Alimentation

A regular diet is resumed after surgery.

Antibiotic coverage

None indicated.

Drains

Many surgeons no longer place drains. If a closed suction drain is inserted, it is removed on the first postoperative day.

Postoperative complications

In the hospital

Hypoparathyroidism

Early postoperative hypocalcemia may occur in patients who have significant bone resorption or in those who undergo excision of large adenomas or subtotal or total parathyroidectomy. Symptomatic hypocalcemia (< 7.5 mg/dL) is characterized by anxiety, perioral or finger tingling, and a Chvostek sign; it usually develops 12–24 hours after surgery. Intravenous calcium is given to relieve symptoms in the hospital, and oral calcium therapy may be necessary at the time of discharge in patients with dysfunction of a parathyroid remnant, severe bone hunger, or total parathyroidectomy with autotransplantation. In many centers in which patients are discharged shortly after operation, calcium supplementation is given at the time of discharge and continued until the patient returns to the clinic. If patients are supplemented with 4–5 g of oral calcium daily and it is initiated early in the postoperative period, often intravenous calcium can be avoided. Intact parathyroid hormone can be measured to assess the level of hypoparathyroidism.

Hemorrhage and recurrent laryngeal nerve injury

Hemorrhage and recurrent laryngeal nerve injury occur in less than 0.3% of initial operations performed by experienced parathyroid surgeons.

After discharge

"Permanent" hypoparathyroidism

"Permanent" hypoparathyroidism occurs in only 0.6–2% of patients after subtotal or total parathyroidectomy or a second cervical exploration for persistent or recurrent hyperparathyroidism. Vitamin D is added to the calcium replacement to enhance absorption. If serial parathyroid hormone levels begin to rise, first the vitamin D and then the calcium supplement should be tapered. In patients with multigland (> 2) parathyroid resection or reoperative neck exploration, cryopreservation of parathyroid fragments should be considered and is routinely done in many endocrine surgery centers. This allows for a future autotransplantation of parathyroid fragments in the rare setting of permanent hypoparathyroidism.

Persistent or recurrent hyperparathyroidism

Persistent disease (failure of operation) or retrospective misdiagnosis occurs in only 2.5–5% of patients. The rate of recurrence after excision of an adenoma is under 1% but increases to 5–15% in patients with sporadic hyperplasia who undergo subtotal parathyroidectomy. In some series, the recurrence rate for hyperparathyroidism is 10–30% in patients with renal, familial, or MEN-associated disease. Symptomatic persistent or recurrent hyperparathyroidism should be evaluated first by a careful review of the original operative note and pathology report. Preoperative localization studies before reoperation include ultrasound of the neck, computed tomography with angiography or magnetic resonance imaging of the mediastinum, and sestamibi scanning. Ectopic cervical or mediastinal parathyroids account for up to 30% of missed glands and can be challenging. Reoperation by an experienced parathyroid surgeon, particularly after positive localization and concordance of two or more localization studies, results in an 85–90% cure rate.

Further reading

Augustine MM, Bravo PE, Zeiger MA. Surgical treatment of primary hyperparathyroidism. *Endocrine Pract* 2011; **17**: S75–82.

Bauer W, Federman DD. Hyperparathyroidism epitomized: the case of Captain Charles E. Martell. *Metabolism* 1962; **11**: 21–9.

Edis AJ, Beahrs OH, van Heerden JA. "Conservative" versus "liberal" approach to parathyroid neck exploration. *Surgery* 1977; **82**: 466–73.

Irwin GL, Molinari AS, Carneiro DM *et al.* Parathyroidectomy: new criteria for evaluating outcome. *Am Surg* 1999; **65**: 1186–9.

Milas M, Wagner K, Easley KA, Siperstein A, Weber CJ. Double adenomas revisited: nonuniform distribution favors enlarged superior parathyroids (fourth pouch disease). *Surgery* 2003; **134**: 995–1003; discussion 1003–4.

Monchik JM, Barellini L, Langer P *et al.* Minimally invasive parathyroid surgery in 103 patients with local/regional anesthesia, without exclusion criteria. *Surgery* 2002: **131**: 502–8.

Sharma J, Milas M, Berber E *et al.* Value of intraoperative parathyroid hormone monitoring. *Ann Surg Oncol* 2008; **15**(2): 493–8.

Udelsman R, Pasieka JL, Sturgeon C, Young EM, Clark OH. Surgery for asysmptomatic primary hyperparathyroidism: proceeding of the third international workshop. *J Clin Endocrinol Metab* 2009; **94**: 366–72.

Lumpectomy and mastectomy

Jahnavi K. Srinivasan

Patients who develop ductal carcinoma or carcinoma of the breast generally require operative treatment of their disease process in conjunction with chemotherapy and/or radiation therapy. Ductal carcinoma in situ (DCIS) is a non-invasive process that most commonly presents as microcalcifications on screening mammography, and accordingly the incidence has increased substantially from the time that screening mammography became widespread. The rates at which DCIS progresses to an invasive process vary, but it is associated with an elevated risk of developing carcinoma and, accordingly, surgical treatment is the current standard of care. Diagnosis is made by an image-guided biopsy in which a core of tissue is interpreted by a histopathologist. DCIS represents a heterogeneous group of pathologic subtypes, with comedo-type necrosis representing cellular features that are associated with aggressive behavior and higher risk of progression to invasive cancer.

While standard treatment of DCIS formerly was mastectomy secondary to a high incidence of multicentric disease, current care for patients with DCIS largely allows for breast conservation techniques in appropriately selected patients. The Van Nuys Prognostic Index (VNPI) looks at three statistically significant predictors of local recurrence: tumor size, margin width, and pathologic classification. Patients who have increased predictors of recurrence undergo lumpectomy followed by radiation treatment rather than mastectomy, while patients with a low VNPI can undergo lumpectomy alone. Of note, a margin less than 1 cm is an independent predictor of recurrence and, accordingly, re-resection rather than radiation treatment is recommended. Although the recommendation for evaluation of the axilla with sentinel node biopsy in patients with DCIS is controversial, those patients with diffuse DCIS or pathologically aggressive features are generally considered appropriate candidates for sentinel lymph node biopsy. Additional adjuvant treatment with tamoxifen, an anti-estrogen drug, should also be considered on an individual basis as it has been shown to reduce both ipsilateral and contralateral breast cancer events.

Epithelial breast cancers (i.e., non-sarcoma, lymphoma, melanoma) represent the most common form of breast cancers. Carcinoma of the breast is the most common invasive cancer in women and occurs with a 2.5 times greater incidence than either colorectal or lung cancer. It is the second leading cause of death in women next to lung cancer, and leading cause of death in women between the ages of 40 and 50. Factors associated with increased risk in the development of breast cancer include early age of menarch, nulliparity, family history, personal history of breast cancer, advanced age, and late age of first childbirth. Two specific germ-line mutations, BRCA1 and BRCA2, have been implicated in a substantially increased risk of the development of breast cancer (lifetime risk of 40–85%). Therefore, patients with a substantial family history of breast cancer at an early age are offered genetic testing.

Evaluation of patients generally requires a thorough history that looks specifically for factors associated with increased risk of breast cancer, physical examination (focusing on the nipple, full extent of breast tissue, and axilla), and mammography. For non-palpable lesions, the Breast Image Reporting and Data System (BIRADS) categorizes the characteristics of mammographic findings to determine if image-guided biopsy is required as opposed to routine surveillance. Palpable lesions are evaluated with fine needle aspiration (FNA) for further pathologic delineation with axillary FNA of suspicious lymph nodes under ultrasound guidance. Non-palpable lesions are evaluated with image-guided core biopsy versus placement of an image-placed wire for guidance of operative excisional biopsy. Diagnosis of carcinoma is then followed by evaluation of extent of disease through laboratory tests (liver function to assess for metastatic disease) and bone density scans for stage III and IV cancers.

The surgical treatment of breast cancer has changed considerably over the last couple of decades, with a much greater emphasis on breast conservation therapy. Contraindications to breast conservation therapy include small size breast that would be cosmetically deformed by lumpectomy, inability to receive radiotherapy (restrictive pulmonary disease, first or second trimester pregnancy, or recurrence in a previously irradiated field), persistently positive margins, two or more

Medical Management of the Surgical Patient, ed. Michael F. Lubin, Thomas F. Dodson, and Neil H. Winawer. Published by Cambridge University Press. © Cambridge University Press 2013.

tumors in separate breast quadrants, and diffuse/malignant-appearing calcification. In general, patients with a lower stage tumor of I (less than 2 cm plus or minus micro-metastases) or II (2–4 cm plus or minus non-fixed ipsilateral nodal metastasis) are treated with lumpectomy (if breast size will accommodate and patient is radiation candidate), sentinel lymph node biopsy (or axillary dissection if lymph node is positive), and radiation treatment to the breast. In lower stage cancers, mastectomy and sentinel lymph node biopsy (or axillary dissection for a positive sentinel node) is employed if a patient cannot tolerate radiation treatment or if lumpectomy would result in cosmetic deformity to the breast. Locally advanced (stage III) breast cancers and inflammatory breast cancers are treated with neoadjuvant chemoradiation for local control followed by surgery (lumpectomy if able to adequately resect tumor with negative margins, versus total mastectomy). All breast malignancies are tested for estrogen receptor status as well as for the HER2/neu oncogene. Patients with a positive estrogen receptor are generally treated with tamoxifen. Systemic chemotherapy is reserved for patients with large tumors and metastases to the axilla, depending on age and ability to tolerate chemotherapy. For metastatic disease, treatment is generally palliative.

Women requiring mastectomy are generally offered immediate reconstruction if postoperative radiation treatment is not required. When radiation treatment is known to be required postoperatively, physicians will often counsel patients to delay reconstruction in order to improve healing and cosmetic outcomes.

Multiple studies have demonstrated equivalence between breast conservation treatment and radical/modified radical mastectomy in terms of local control, disease-free survival, and overall survival rates. Cancers discovered during pregnancy can be safely treated with breast conservation therapy in the third trimester and radiation treatment can be delayed until after delivery. However, cancers discovered earlier than the third trimester will require mastectomy, as radiation treatment cannot safely be administered during pregnancy and a long delay would be inadvisable. Cytotoxic adjuvant chemotherapy can be administered without risk to the fetus during the second and third trimesters, but not during the first trimester.

Lumpectomy with sentinel lymph node biopsy/axillary dissection, or mastectomy is performed under general anesthesia with minimal stress to the body. Additional breast reconstruction usually doubles the operative time under anesthesia.

Usual postoperative course

Expected postoperative hospital stay

The majority of patients undergoing lumpectomy with axillary lymph node dissection remain in the hospital for an overnight stay. Modified radical mastectomy patients generally remain in the hospital for 2 days, with an addition of 1–2 days if immediate cosmetic reconstruction is undertaken.

Operative mortality

The operative mortality for breast operations is under 1%.

Special monitoring required

Minimal specific monitoring is required for patients. Patients who have closed suction drains in place will be monitored for the amount of blood in the drains. Development of a substantial hematoma or significant sanguinous output from drains is an indication for return to the operating room for operative wound exploration.

Patient activity and positioning

Patients are mobilized out of bed the day of surgery. Supervised upper extremity exercises are performed on the side of surgery to maintain mobility and strength in the shoulder and arm.

Alimentation

Patient diet is advanced as tolerated.

Antibiotic coverage

Patients receive antibiotics for skin prophylaxis (a first-generation cephalosporin or clindamycin) within 30 minutes of operative incision as per standard of care guidelines.

Drains

A closed suction drain is placed in the axilla of patients undergoing full axillary dissection with one to two drains placed under mastectomy flaps to prevent the development of a hematoma.

Postoperative complications

In the hospital

Wound infection

Obesity and older age are risk factors for infection after mastectomy. Infection rates vary from 2–5%, with the majority of infections being gram positive in nature. Infection rates are higher when an implant is placed at the time of surgery. Substantial infection requires evacuation and drainage in the operating room.

Necrosis of the edge of the skin flap

Skin flap necrosis may occur if the overlying skin is devascularized during operative dissection. This occurs most frequently when dissection thins out the overlying skin, but smokers and diabetics are also predisposed to this problem secondary to poor peripheral blood supply.

After discharge

Wound seroma

Wound seroma is one of the most common complications to occur after mastectomy. Premature removal of drains promotes the development of seroma, and should this occur, intermittent aspiration of the site may be required (versus percutaneous bedside replacement of the drain).

Edema of the upper extremity

Patients who require extensive axillary dissection are at much greater risk of developing upper extremity edema. Other predisposing risk factors for development of lymphedema include obesity, extent of local surgery, local radiation, delayed wound healing, and lymphatic obstruction by tumor. A well-fitted compression garment should be worn during the day and particularly during exercise of the limb. Elevation and slow progressive exercise of the affected limb is encouraged in patients who are symptomatic, as there is evidence to show that restriction of limb use does not minimize the development of lymphedema in patients.

Recurrent cancer

About 5–15% of patients who received radiotherapy after breast conservation therapy will have locally recurrent disease within 8 years of their initial treatment. These patients require salvage mastectomy, which has 50–60% 5-year disease-free survival. Patients who undergo mastectomy as initial treatment may also develop local chest wall recurrence, and this often occurs within the first 2–3 years after operation. Unfortunately, up to two-thirds of these patients have metastatic disease, and they have a 5-year disease-free survival of only 25% or less.

Further reading

Goldberg JI, Riedel ER, Morrow M. Morbidity of sentinel lymph node biopsy: relationship between number of excised lymph nodes and patient perceptions about lymphedema. *Ann Surg Oncol* 2011; **18**: 2866–72.

Greenberg S, Stopeck A, Rugo HS. Systemic treatment of early breast cancer-a biological perspective. *J Surg Oncol* 2011; **103**: 619–26.

Kumar S, Sacchini V. The surgical management of ductal carcinoma in situ. *Breast J* 2010; **16**: S49–52.

Sanchez C, Brem RF, McSwain AP *et al.* Factors associated with re-excision in patients with early-stage breast cancer treated with breast conservation therapy. *Am Surg* 2010; **76**: 331–4.

Wood WC. Breast surgery in advanced breast cancer: local control in the presence of metastases. *Breast* 2007; **16**: S63–6.

Chapter 51

Gastric procedures (including laparoscopic antireflux, gastric bypass, and gastric banding)

Jahnavi K. Srinivasan and David V. Feliciano

In the current era, elective gastric procedures performed under general anesthesia are primarily performed for benign lesions (wedge resection and proximal or distal gastrectomy), malignant neoplasm (subtotal or total gastrectomy with lymph node dissection), antireflux wrap procedures (Nissen and Toupet fundoplications), and antiobesity procedures (gastric bypass, sleeve gastrectomy, and banding). The medical treatment of peptic ulcer disease (proton pump inhibitors and *Helicobacter pylori* treatment) has resulted in a significant reduction in the amount of surgery done for complications of peptic ulcer disease. Nevertheless, these procedures are still performed in patients whose disease is undiagnosed at the time of operation or remains refractory to medical treatment. These procedures include parietal cell vagotomy (PCV), vagotomy and pyloroplasty (VP), vagotomy and antrectomy (VA), and hemigastrectomy alone. All of these procedures can be achieved through open or laparoscopic means.

Denervation of the fundus and body of the stomach or PCV is still occasionally necessary for patients with life-threatening complications of duodenal ulcers (hemorrhage, perforation, or obstruction). Such patients usually have untreated *Helicobacter pylori* infections or a virulent ulcer diathesis of unknown cause. Vagotomy and pyloroplasty and VA involve cutting the vagal nerve trunks at the esophageal hiatus and resecting the pylorus or performing a pyloroplasty, where the pylorus is opened longitudinally and closed transversely. With antrectomy, all the gastrin-secreting cells are removed as well and reanastomosis of the remaining stomach to the duodenum (Billroth I) or jejunum (Billroth II) is performed.

Preoperative decompression of the stomach for 5–7 days is indicated in patients with gastric dilation from pyloric obstruction. Parenteral nutrition can be preoperatively considered in patients for 1–2 weeks preoperatively to reverse their catabolic state if chronic obstruction has resulted in significant weight loss or protein calorie malnutrition. Hemigastrectomy (removal of the ulcer and the distal stomach) is 96% curative for patients with both uncomplicated and complicated gastric ulcers and 100% curative for those with benign tumors (leiomyomas). The stress of these procedures is moderate; they take 1.5–2 hours to perform; and blood transfusion is required only in patients with anemia or active bleeding. Reconstruction is achieved via gastroduodenostomy (Billroth I), gastrojejunostomy (Billroth II), or transected proximal jejunum (Roux-en-Y).

Extended subtotal gastrectomy (additional removal of the greater and lesser omentum, the celiac nodes, and occasionally the spleen) or total gastrectomy is reserved for patients with mid-stomach or proximal adenocarcinomas. With a leiomyosarcoma, only the gastrectomy is performed. Reconstruction is by a Roux limb of proximal jejunum. The stress of surgery is moderate; the procedure is performed in 3 hours; and blood transfusion may be necessary if neoplasms are adherent to the pancreas, liver, or retroperitoneum. Utilization of a supplemental jejunal feeding tube (placed at the time of operation) is dependent on the preoperative nutritional status of the patient.

Open or laparoscopic antireflux procedures are performed in symptomatic patients who undergo extensive preoperative testing with esophagogastroduodenoscopy, 24-hour pH testing, and esophageal motility studies. In patients with normal esophageal motility, a laparoscopic Nissen fundoplication (to reinforce the incompetent lower esophageal sphincter) is the procedure of choice. Through five trocars placed in the upper abdomen, the fundus of the stomach is mobilized by division of the short gastric vessels. At least 2 cm of mobilized gastroesophageal junction is then encircled with a short fundal wrap while a 52–60 French dilator is present in the esophagus to prevent narrowing. The stress of surgery is modest, the procedure is performed in less than 2 hours, and blood transfusion is unnecessary.

Open or laparoscopic gastric bariatric procedures are indicated in patients with a body mass index (BMI = weight in kilograms/height in meters^2) of 40 kg/m^2 or higher. This standard, however, is currently under review. Some authorities recommend operative intervention at even lower levels of BMI. Hence, these procedures are also performed in patients with a BMI between 35 and 40 kg/m^2 if associated obesity conditions such as sleep apnea, Pickwickian syndrome, type 1 and 2 diabetes mellitus, or severe hypertension exist. Laparoscopic gastric bypass is performed by creation of a 15–30 mL proximal gastric pouch based on the lesser curve of the stomach. A Roux jejunal limb with a length of 75–150 cm is then passed posterior (retrocolic) or anterior (antecolic) to the transverse colon and stapled to the small gastric pouch. Care is taken to close all mesenteric defects to prevent the development of an internal hernia. At bariatric centers of excellence, the incidence of complications is often quoted to be a 1–2% leak rate, 3% internal hernia rate, and 1% mortality. The necessity of a conversion to an open operation is less than 5% in experienced hands, and failure to achieve adequate weight loss is 4%. Weight loss is achieved through a combination of malabsorption and restriction, with approximately 75% of excess body weight lost 1 year out from surgery. Improvement in glycemic control often occurs independent of weight loss, making this an operation of significant benefit to the diabetic patient.

The laparoscopic insertion of an adjustable gastric band to produce a calibrated outlet below a proximal gastric pouch of 15–30 mL has been performed for over 10 years. The advantages of this operation are that it is easier to perform than gastric bypass and that it preserves the normal gastrointestinal stream and absorption. Weight loss is purely restrictive, and there is less weight loss and more long-term regaining of weight with this procedure as compared with the gastric bypass. The stress of surgery is modest; the procedure is performed in 1–2 hours; and blood transfusion is unnecessary. Approximately 45–55% of excess body weight is lost after 3 years, with a failure to achieve adequate weight loss of about 15%. Complications of surgery include a 3% rate of band slippage requiring operative repositioning, a 1% erosion rate requiring band removal, and a 5% rate of port access site complications.

Recently, the laparoscopic or open lateral (sleeve) gastrectomy has joined the ranks of the more commonly performed bariatric operations. This operation involves resection of 80–85% of the greater curvature of the stomach, thereby making the stomach into a narrow tube. The procedure is generally performed with an endoscope or bougie in place to prevent stenosis of the gastric conduit. Weight loss is achieved purely through restrictive means, but the operation avoids the placement of a foreign body in the abdomen (unlike gastric banding). There is no malabsorption or dumping, and anatomic intestinal continuity is maintained (unlike the gastric bypass). The stress of surgery is moderate, the procedure takes 1.5–2 hours, and blood transfusion is unnecessary. Approximately 60% of excess body weight is lost after 2 years, with a failure to achieve adequate weight loss of about 10%. Complications of surgery include less than 1% staple line leak, 2% gastroesophageal junction stenosis and dysphagia requiring subsequent dilation, and less than 1% mortality.

Usual postoperative course
Expected postoperative hospital stay
The expected postoperative hospital stay is 7–10 days for VP, VA, or subtotal gastrectomy, 12–14 days for total gastrectomy, 1 day for laparoscopic antireflux procedure, and 2 days for gastric bypass or sleeve gastrectomy. The adjustable gastric band procedure is generally an outpatient operation.

Operative mortality
Operative mortality is 1–2% for elective VP, VA, and gastrectomy; 5–15% for emergency VP, VA, and gastrectomy; and 3–8% for elective total gastrectomy. Mortality is less than 1% for laparoscopic antireflux procedure, gastric bypass, or adjustable gastric band.

Special monitoring required
Nasogastric or nasojejunal tube drainage is monitored and replaced intravenously if it is in excess of 750 mL. Serum electrolytes also are measured and replaced as needed.

Patient activity and positioning
Patients are encouraged to be out of bed and to sit in a chair on the day of the operation, and to be ambulatory by postoperative day 1.

Alimentation
After operations for ulcer or neoplasm, patients are permitted clear liquids with the return of bowel function; food intake is advanced as tolerated. As they adjust to the new size of their stomachs and to the loss of the pylorus, patients in the early postoperative period after VAs or gastrectomies of any type are advised to eat slowly, drink less with meals, and avoid milk products. They are also advised to avoid large amounts of foods that are difficult to digest, including oranges, broccoli, and asparagus (post-gastrectomy diet). Patients who have undergone total gastrectomies remain on distal enteral feedings or hyperalimentation until anastomoses are healed (discussed later).

Patients are permitted clear liquids on the first postoperative morning after laparoscopic antireflux procedures. After gastric bypass and sleeve gastrectomy, low-carbohydrate liquids are started on postoperative day 1.

Antibiotic coverage
A second-generation cephalosporin is administered within 30 minutes of any incisions and for two doses postoperatively, as per standard of care. If perforation of a duodenal or gastric ulcer with gross intra-abdominal contamination is noted at surgery, the antibiotic is continued for 5–7 days postoperatively. Antifungal coverage can be added to the treatment of patients with significant contamination from an upper gastrointestinal source.

Anti-emetics
Because of the risk of disruption of the fundoplication due to earlier postoperative vomiting, liberal use of anti-emetics is encouraged.

Drains

After gastrectomy and reconstruction with a gastrojejunostomy, the duodenal stump is drained with a closed suction drain for 5–7 days. Many surgeons recommend that, following a total gastrectomy, the esophagojejunal anastomosis should be drained until a healed anastomosis is demonstrated. The gastric anastomotic staple line is drained for 1–2 days for gastric bypass and sleeve gastrectomy, until oral intake confirms that there is no evidence of leak.

Upper gastrointestinal radiography

Upper gastrointestinal radiography is performed with water-soluble contrast 7–10 days after total gastrectomy to check for healing of the esophagojejunal anastomosis. If a small leak is present, patients remain on distal enteral feedings or hyperalimentation until a repeat study is performed 5–7 days thereafter. The use of radiographic fluoroscopic studies for gastric bypass has been largely abandoned, as it has been demonstrated that these studies have very poor sensitivity in detecting early leakage; most centers of excellence utilize intraoperative endoscopy instead. For sleeve gastrectomy patients, gastrograffin evaluation is performed on postoperative day 1, largely to gauge the capacity of the remnant stomach.

Postoperative complications after open procedures

In the hospital

Wound infection

In patients with bleeding or perforated ulcers, gastric acid is neutralized by blood or food; this allows for overgrowth of bacteria. Open packing or delayed primary closure of the subcutaneous tissue and skin is appropriate after many emergency gastric procedures. If a wound infection does occur, treatment requires drainage and appropriate antibiotics.

The incidence of trocar site infections in laparoscopic surgery is less than 1%. In the case of laparoscopic gastric banding, access port site infection is often related to erosion; therefore, these cases need to be investigated with either radiographic evaluation or endoscopy to rule out more extensive complications. In the presence of erosion, the entire band requires removal. In cases of simple access port site infection, the access port alone requires removal until the infection is cleared.

Duodenal stump leak

Duodenal stump leak occurs in 1–2% of patients after gastric resection with gastrojejunostomy. The presence of right upper quadrant pain, fever, tachycardia, and bilious drainage out of the suction drain placed beneath the stump suggests the diagnosis. The leak is treated with prohibition of oral intake, insertion of a sump drain (if needed) under fluoroscopy, use of intravenous hyperalimentation, and administration of antibiotics and a somatostatin analog (Sandostatin). Re-exploration is indicated only if sepsis does not resolve with insertion of the sump drain. Low-output duodenal stump leaks generally heal non-operatively, provided drainage is adequate. On rare occasions, the patient develops a persistent duodenal fistula that requires subsequent operative intervention months later.

Stomal dysfunction

After gastrectomy, slow gastric emptying occurs in less than 5% of patients, particularly if gastrojejunostomy has been performed. If output through the nasogastric tube is excessive at 7 days after surgery, upper gastrointestinal radiography with water-soluble contrast is performed. If the agent does not pass through the anastomosis, a second study with barium is performed the following day. Passage of the barium is reassuring, and nasogastric tube decompression and hyperalimentation are continued as needed for 2–3 more weeks. Failure of the barium to pass mandates endoscopy to rule out a mechanical obstruction.

After discharge

Nutritional disturbances

Megaloblastic anemia from loss of intrinsic factor and iron-deficiency anemia from unknown causes occur over time in many patients with previous gastrectomies. Lifelong annual monitoring of hemoglobin levels is appropriate, with replacement therapy administered as needed. Occurrences of calcium deficiency and steatorrhea have also been reported. Patients who have had gastric bypass develop iron and B_{12} deficiencies; therefore, exogenous supplementation is necessary.

Dumping syndrome

Early dumping syndrome occurs with the passage of a hypertonic food bolus directly into the duodenum or jejunum after an antrectomy. Sweating, weakness, palpitations, nausea, vomiting, and diarrhea may be precipitated due to hormonal changes; an outpouring of extracellular fluid into the upper gastrointestinal tract may occur as well. Similar symptoms occurring 1–2 hours after a meal are classified as late dumping, and are thought to be precipitated by hypoglycemia secondary to an excessive release of insulin. Symptomatic dumping occurs in less than 15% of patients. Only 1% of patients may require remedial operations after failing to respond to a change in dietary habits (restriction of fluids, carbohydrates, and extra salt with meals). Dumping is commonly seen after consumption of carbohydrate loads by the patient who has undergone gastric bypass. The symptomatic effects from dumping syndrome therefore serve as a negative feedback mechanism to reinforce behavioral modification in this postsurgical population.

515

Diarrhea

About 10–25% of patients have altered bowel movements after truncal vagotomy. This process is thought to be related to a rapid transit time between the stomach and colon, and is characterized by frequent, watery, and explosive bowel movements. Only 1–2% of patients have diarrhea severe enough to require remedial operations after a failure to respond to a change in dietary habits (see earlier) or to the use of common medications such as codeine, diphenoxylate, or cholestyramine.

Gastric atony

Delayed gastric emptying, a persistent problem in 1–2% of patients, is one of the most common post-gastrectomy syndromes they face. Gastroparesis may respond to the administration of metoclopramide or erythromycin lactobionate. The remedial operation consists of near-total gastrectomy with Roux-en-Y gastrojejunostomy.

Marginal or recurrent ulcer

When vagotomy is performed with an ulcer operation, ulcers at the gastrointestinal anastomosis (marginal ulcer) are an uncommon occurrence (less than 1%). Up to 30% of patients with gastroenterostomy without vagotomy, however, develop marginal ulcers. After antral resection, a significantly elevated gastrin level is indicative of a previously undiagnosed Zollinger–Ellison syndrome or retained antrum syndrome.

Other postgastrectomy complications

The afferent loop syndrome, efferent loop syndrome, and alkaline reflux gastritis occur infrequently, but remedial operations are available for correction. In total, 25% of patients with gastrectomy develop a postgastrectomy syndrome.

Gastric stump carcinoma

Carcinomas of the gastric pouch develop in as many as 5% of patients who survive 10–15 years after gastrectomy. Late-developing symptoms of pain and anemia in patients who have previously done well after gastrectomy should be evaluated by endoscopy with biopsy.

Postoperative complications after laparoscopic procedures

In the hospital

Slippage of fundoplication

This very rare complication is most often due to early postoperative vomiting, failure to divide the short gastric vessels, or improper fixation of the wrap to the crura of the diaphragm.

Wound infection

After laparoscopic gastric bypass, infection at port sites occurs in less than 2% of patients. Opening of the port site, irrigation, and open packing are appropriate treatment.

Leakage from gastrointestinal tract

While leak rates vary significantly in the literature, in experienced hands the incidence of anastomotic leakage with laparoscopic operations ranges from 1–5%. If asymptomatic, they can be observed. When there is excessive drainage through a Jackson–Pratt drain placed at surgery or if peritonitis develops, laparoscopic reoperation is indicated.

After discharge

Late failure of fundoplication

In approximately 10% of patients, esophageal reflux recurs due to disruption of the hiatal repair, disruption of the fundoplication, or herniation of the fundoplication. Recurrences are particularly noted in patients with a BMI greater than 30. Reoperative laparoscopic fundoplication is indicated and has an 80% success rate.

Prolonged nausea or vomiting after gastric bypass

Prolonged nausea or vomiting occurs in approximately 10% of gastric bypass patients. These symptoms spontaneously resolve in most patients. Persistent inability to tolerate oral intake requires placement of a feeding tube in the patient's gastric remnant. In severe cases, reversal of gastric bypass can be undertaken.

Stricture of gastrojejunostomy after gastric bypass

Late strictures of the stapled gastrojejunostomy suture line occur in approximately 5–25% of patients (depending on technique utilized for stapling) and are treated with endoscopic balloon dilation. The risk of perforation with balloon dilation is less than 1%.

Iron deficiency anemia after gastric bypass

Because the majority of the stomach is bypassed in the gastric bypass procedure, iron deficiency anemia occurs in 20% of patients. Oral replacement of iron is the preferred therapy.

Need to reposition or remove laparoscopic adjustable gastric band

Because of migration of the band, obstruction in patients with unrecognized esophageal dysmotility, gastric erosions, or patient non-compliance, the band will have to be moved or removed laparoscopically in 10–20% of patients.

Further reading

Donahue PE. Early postoperative and postgastrectomy syndromes. Diagnosis, management, and prevention. *Gastroenterol Clin North Am* 1994; **23**: 215–16.

Feliciano DV. Surgical options and results of treatment of perforated ulcers. *Curr Probl Surg* 1987; **4**: 301–7.

Fontana MA, Wohlgemuth SD. The surgical treatment of metabolic disease and morbid obesity. *Gastroenterol Clin North Am* 2010; **39**: 125–33.

Himpens J, Dobbeleir J, Peeters G. Long-term results of laparoscopic sleeve gastrectomy for obesity. *Ann Surg* 2010; **252**: 319–24.

Hunter JG, Swanstrom L, Waring JP. Dysphagia after laparoscopic antireflux surgery. The impact of operative technique. *Ann Surg* 1996; **224**: 51–7.

Stefanidis D, Hope WWW, Kohn GP *et al.* Guidelines for surgical treatment of gastroesophageal reflux disease. *Surg Endosc* 2010; **24**: 2647–69.

Chapter

52

Small bowel resection

Jahnavi K. Srinivasan and David V. Feliciano

Small bowel resection is performed in a variety of settings, the most common of which are traumatic perforation, thrombotic or embolic infarction, Crohn's disease, and concomitant colectomy. Less common indications for resection include benign or malignant neoplasms (leiomyoma, hemangioma, carcinoid, lymphoma, adenocarcinoma, sarcoma), fistula resulting from a previous repair or resection, symptomatic Meckel's diverticulum, neutropenic enterocolitis, and spontaneous perforation in immunosuppressed patients.

The most significant change in the operative management of small bowel disease in recent years has been the increasing use of laparoscopic approaches. In patients with inflammatory small bowel disease, laparoscopic operations now include diversion for complex fistula, take-down of end or loop stoma, segmental resection, stricturoplasty, and lysis of adhesions. Conversion rates to an open approach have ranged from 2–40% in series published since 1993, with the majority of conversions being secondary to dense adhesive disease or excessive intra-abdominal inflammation.

Open segmental resection and end-to-end anastomosis with suture or staples usually can be performed in 20 minutes. Simple laparoscopic segmental small bowel resection can be accomplished in under an hour. Major laparoscopic resections, particularly those involving the colon in addition to the small bowel, generally take 2–5 hours. Resection of a wide section of accompanying mesentery is only required for malignant neoplasm and not in cases of benign disease. With the exception of resections performed for a neoplasm in the adjacent right colon, most resections of the small bowel for trauma, infarction, or inflammatory bowel disease cause moderate to severe stress. General anesthesia is used, the duration of the procedure depends on the indication, and blood transfusions are necessary only in patients with trauma, extensive inflammation, or infiltrating neoplasms.

Usual postoperative course

Expected postoperative hospital stay

Depending on the indication for surgery and length of operative intervention, hospital stay varies. Generally, for open small bowel resection, a 5–7 day postoperative course is reasonable. Fascial incisions of less than 6 cm have been associated with decreased postoperative pain and ileus; therefore, laparoscopic and "mini-laparotomy" incisions are associated with a decreased postoperative length of stay, generally ranging from 3–5 days.

Operative mortality

Operative mortality is 2–3% for elective resection, 12% for penetrating trauma with two other organ injuries, 25% for superior mesenteric artery embolism, and as high as 60% for superior mesenteric artery thrombosis.

Special monitoring required

Many patients with major abdominal trauma or midgut infarction require postoperative hemodynamic monitoring with an arterial and central venous line. The use of a pulmonary artery catheter is generally reserved for patients whose intravascular volume status cannot be assessed accurately secondary to significant preexisting cardiac or renal insufficiency. Serial measurements of arterial pH are also worthwhile if bowel with borderline viability is left in the abdomen at the first operation. Patients with borderline intestinal viability at the first operation should be strongly considered for a "second-look" operation 24–48 hours after the initial procedure to confirm persistent intestinal viability.

Patient activity and positioning

Patients may be out of bed on the day after the operation and ambulating by postoperative day 1, depending on hemodynamic stability.

Alimentation

For routine procedures, clear liquids are started the day after surgery. Further advancement of diet progresses with the return of bowel function. In cases involving multiple intra-abdominal injuries, extensive adhesiolysis, or major resection of the midgut secondary to infarction, intravenous hyperalimentation is initiated as soon as patients are hemodynamically stable.

Medical Management of the Surgical Patient, ed. Michael F. Lubin, Thomas F. Dodson, and Neil H. Winawer. Published by Cambridge University Press. © Cambridge University Press 2013.

Antibiotic coverage

All patients receive cephalosporin within 30 minutes of operative incision and for two doses postoperatively as per standard of care. In the presence of established peritonitis from infarction or perforation, the antibiotic is continued for 5–7 days postoperatively.

Postoperative complications

In the hospital

Wound infection

See Chapter 63.

Breakdown of enterotomy repair or small bowel anastomosis

See Chapter 63.

Recurrent infarction

If bowel with questionable viability is left in the abdomen or if a borderline stoma is brought to the skin at the first operation, further ischemic changes may occur and necessitate reoperation. Many surgeons choose to close only the skin of the abdominal incision at the first operation and to perform a second operation 12–36 hours later to reassess the questionably viable bowel, particularly in cases of small bowel ischemia from thrombus or emboli. Others monitor the color of a stoma or the serial arterial pH levels to assist in determining whether reoperation is necessary.

Prolonged ileus

Peristalsis may return slowly in patients with multiple intra-abdominal injuries, a superior mesenteric artery embolus or thrombus, chronic obstruction from enteritis or a neo-plasm, or diffuse peritonitis from a perforation. Continuous nasogastric suction, intravenous hyperalimentation, and patience are indicated. If there is serious concern about a possible early mechanical small bowel obstruction instead of an ileus, the use of an oral colon-cleaning agent or barium is indicated, as described in Chapter 63 "Lysis of adhesions." Return to the operating room for failure to demonstrate a return of bowel function should be discouraged (particularly between postoperative days 9 and 21), as the chance of encountering an abdomen that is hostile to re-enter during this period of time is substantially increased.

After discharge

Obstruction

Early in-hospital adhesive small bowel obstruction occurs in 2–3% of patients who undergo small bowel resection. Late episodes of adhesive obstruction occur in 10–25% of patients.

Nutritional deficiency

Massive resection of the midgut may lead to chronic diarrhea and nutritional deficiencies, particularly if the ileocecal valve has been sacrificed. In general, patients require 150 cm of small bowel anastomosed to colon, or 100 cm of small bowel with an intact ileocecal valve anastomosed to colon to prevent the complications of short gut syndrome. In-hospital and subsequent home hyperalimentation is indicated in patients who have short gut syndrome. Progressive hyperplasia of the lining of the remaining midgut may allow for resumption of enteral feedings over time. Patients who have lost a substantial amount of terminal ileum often require iron and B_{12} supplementation.

Further reading

Crohn BB, Ginzburg L, Oppenheimer GD. Regional ileitis: a pathologic and clinical entity. *J Am Med Assoc* 1932; **251**: 73–81.

Edwards MS, Cherr GS, Craven TE *et al.* Acute occlusive mesenteric ischemia: surgical management and outcomes. *Ann Vasc Surg* 2003; **17**: 72–9.

Fazio VW, Marchetti F, Church JM *et al.* Effect of resection margins on the recurrence of Crohn's disease in the small bowel. A randomized controlled trial. *Ann Surg* 1996; **224**: 563–71.

Michelassi F, Hurst RD, Melis M *et al.* Side-to-side isoperistaltic strictureplasty in extensive Crohn's disease: a prospective longitudinal study. *Ann Surg* 2000; **232**: 401–8.

Paski SC, Semrad CE. Small bowel tumors. *Gastrointest Endosc Clin North Am* 2009; **19**: 461–79.

Rosenthal RJ, Bashankaev B, Wexner SD. Laparoscopic management of inflammatory bowel disease. *Dig Dis* 2009; **27**: 560–4.

Schmidt CM, Talamini MA, Kaufman HS *et al.* Laparoscopic surgery for Crohn's disease: reasons for conversion. *Ann Surg* 2001; **233**: 733–9.

Appendectomy

Jahnavi K. Srinivasan and David V. Feliciano

Appendectomy is performed for acute appendicitis (simple, suppurative, gangrenous, gangrenous with perforation); chronic or recurrent appendicitis; as an interval procedure after recovery from an appendiceal abscess; for small (< 2 cm) carcinoid tumors or benign mucoceles not involving the appendiceal orifice; and prophylactically during laparotomy for other conditions. The accuracy of diagnosis in acute appendicitis has increased to over 90% in several series using diagnostic adjuncts such as graded-compression ultrasound and special CT protocols. With graded-compression ultrasound, a uniform pressure is applied to the right lower quadrant of the abdomen by a hand-held transducer. Normal loops of intestine are either displaced or compressed between the anterior and posterior abdominal walls. An inflamed appendix, however, is aperistaltic and non-compressible. In addition, percutaneous drainage of periappendiceal abscesses may allow for a subsequent single laparoscopic operation to remove the remnant of the perforated appendix (interval appendectomy). Interval appendectomy is generally performed 6–8 weeks after the initial abscess drainage.

With the patient under general anesthesia, appendectomy may be performed through a right lower quadrant muscle-splitting incision or by a laparoscopic approach using three ports. The laparoscopic operation affords an operative advantage in morbidly obese patients and patients with a retrocecal appendix, allowing for anatomy to be more easily visualized by virtue of the laparoscope. With simple, suppurative, or gangrenous appendicitis, the stress of operation is minimal. For patients with perforated gangrenous appendicitis and diffuse peritonitis or with a large intra-abdominal abscess, stress can be moderate or major. The duration of a simple appendectomy is 45 minutes, but this increases to 60 to 75 minutes in obese patients with retrocecal appendicitis and rupture. In some of these patients, the usual 6- to 7-cm incision must be extended to gain exposure of the posterior cecum and ascending colon. Blood transfusion is generally not required.

Usual postoperative course

Expected postoperative hospital stay

One to 2 days for simple, suppurative, or gangrenous (without rupture) appendicitis; 7–10 days for perforated appendicitis with diffuse peritonitis or an intra-abdominal abscess.

Operative mortality

Operative mortality is 0.1% for simple or suppurative appendicitis, 0.6% for gangrenous appendicitis, and 5% for perforated appendicitis. The very young patients and the very old patients have the highest mortality after ruptured appendicitis.

Special monitoring required

Patients with sepsis syndrome or shock secondary to perforated appendicitis require postoperative hemodynamic monitoring in a unit with critical care capacity.

Patient activity and positioning

Patients with appendicitis may be out of bed on the day of the operation and resume activity gradually during the first 2 weeks after hospital discharge.

Alimentation

Clear liquids are given on the day of operation, and food intake is advanced as tolerated in patients with non-perforated appendicitis. In those with perforated appendicitis, clear liquids are permitted with the return of bowel function; intake is advanced as tolerated. Patients with perforated appendicitis will often have an ileus for 5–7 days after surgery. Prolonged ileus greater than a week merits postoperative axial imaging to rule out the development of an intra-abdominal abscess.

Medical Management of the Surgical Patient, ed. Michael F. Lubin, Thomas F. Dodson, and Neil H. Winawer. Published by Cambridge University Press. © Cambridge University Press 2013.

Antibiotic coverage

All patients with suspected appendicitis receive a cephalosporin within 30 minutes of any incisions. Those with simple or suppurative appendicitis require no further antibiotic coverage. All patients with gangrenous appendicitis receive antibiotics for 24 hours postoperatively. Patients with perforated appendicitis and secondary peritonitis or intra-abdominal abscess continue to receive antibiotics for 5–7 days postoperatively.

Drains

For 5–7 days postoperatively, closed suction drains are placed in well-defined abscess cavities in the pericecal or pelvic area. The decision for drain removal is based on clinical findings, postoperative computed tomographic scan, or a sinogram performed through the drains.

Wound closure

In adult patients with extensive gangrenous or perforated appendicitis, open packing of the subcutaneous tissue and skin is indicated to avoid the development of a wound infection. Delayed primary closure of the wound can be performed on the postoperative day 6 and has a 10–20% risk of infection.

Postoperative complications
In the hospital
Diffuse peritonitis

Diffuse peritonitis that is present at the time of appendectomy may lead to systemic inflammatory response syndrome or septic shock in the early postoperative period or to intra-abdominal abscess in the late postoperative period.

Postoperative adhesions may also be more problematic in this group of patients.

Wound infection

Wound infection occurs primarily when attempts are made to close the subcutaneous tissue and skin in patients with gangrenous or perforated appendicitis. Treatment includes the administration of antibiotics based on Gram stain results, the opening of a portion of the incision, and daily packing changes until healing by secondary intention occurs.

Intra-abdominal abscess

Intra-abdominal abscess may develop in up to 5–15% of patients with gangrenous or perforated appendicitis. Diagnosis and treatment are aided by computed tomography followed by percutaneous drainage, transrectal drainage for pelvic abscess, or reoperation for large abscesses that are not amenable to percutaneous drainage.

Fecal fistula

Less than 1% of patients experience blow-out of the appendiceal stump that leads to a cecocutaneous fistula through the incision or a drain. Spontaneous closure usually occurs within 2–3 weeks.

After discharge
Late diagnosis of a carcinoid tumor or appendiceal carcinoma

A late pathology report may describe the presence of a carcinoid tumor larger than 2 cm or of an appendiceal carcinoma in the resected specimen. Reoperation with a formal right hemicolectomy and mesenteric resection is indicated in these cases, as well as for involvement of the appendiceal base or the presence of aggressive pathologic elements.

Further reading

Bass J, Rubin S, Hummadi A. Interval appendectomy: an old new operation. *J Laparoendosc Adv Surg Tech A* 2006; **16**: 67–9.

Fitz RH. Perforating inflammation of the vermiform appendix, with special reference to its early diagnosis and treatment. *Trans Assoc Am Phys* 1886; **1**: 107–44.

Frazee RC, Roberts JW, Symmonds RE *et al.* A prospective randomized trial comparing open versus laparoscopic appendectomy. *Ann Surg* 1994; **219**: 725–8.

Lopez PP, Cohn SM. CT scanning in management of acute appendicitis. *J Am Coll Surg* 2010; **211**: 567.

Mattei P, Sola JE, Yeo CJ. Chronic and recurrent appendicitis are uncommon entities often misdiagnosed. *J Am Coll Surg* 1994; **178**: 385–9.

Page AJ, Pollock JD, Perez S *et al.* Laproscopic versus open appendectomy: an analysis of outcomes in 17 199 patients using ACS/NSQIP. *J Gastrointest Surg* 2010; **14**: 1955–62.

Puylaert JB, Rutgers PH, Lalisang RI *et al.* A prospective study of ultrasonography in the diagnosis of appendicitis. *N Engl J Med* 1987; **317**: 666–9.

Open or laparoscopic colon resection is performed for a variety of conditions, the most common of which are benign or malignant neoplasms (tubular or villoglandular adenoma, adenocarcinoma, carcinoid, lymphoma); complications of diverticular disease (perforation with peritonitis or abscess, stricture, bleeding); extensive traumatic perforations; angiodysplasia or arteriovenous malformation with lower gastrointestinal bleeding; and inflammatory bowel disease (ulcerative colitis, segmental colonic Crohn's disease, toxic megacolon). Less common indications for resection include volvulus of the sigmoid colon or cecum; thrombotic, embolic, or low-flow infarction; and premalignant conditions (familial polyposis, Gardner's syndrome).

Hemicolectomy for malignant neoplasms involves excision of the area of the tumor, at least 10 cm of normal proximal colon or small bowel, and 5 cm of normal distal colon as well as excision of the regional lymphatics that accompany the major vessels in the mesentery. In contrast, segmental resection for complications of diverticular disease, Crohn's disease, colonic volvulus, or infarction involves only grossly diseased bowel without excision of the regional lymphatics. Subtotal abdominal colectomy with ileorectostomy is performed for patients with non-familial synchronous scattered benign or malignant neoplasms. It is also used in some patients with megacolon secondary to obstructing neoplasms of the sigmoid or rectosigmoid colon or of the upper rectum, and for patients with non-localized diverticular bleeding. For patients with severe medically refractory ulcerative colitis, familial polyposis, or Gardner's syndrome, a near-total abdominal colectomy is preferred. This involves preservation of a seromuscular short rectal cuff and the sphincter muscles to preserve anal continence and the creation of an ileal pouch–anal anastomosis.

In the last several years, the need for a full preoperative colon preparation prior to surgery has been called into question. Original studies regarding the use of a combination of a cathartic agent along with oral antibiotics (Nichols–Condon preparation) for preoperative colonic cleansing were performed before the era of preoperative intravenous antibiotic administration. Several studies have indicated that the Nichols–Condon prep does not necessarily decrease wound infection rates and may increase colonic bacterial overgrowth. The use of a preoperative cleansing colon preparation is therefore now surgeon-dependent, with some surgeons choosing to use the Nichols–Condon prep, some choosing the cathartic preparation only, and others using no preoperative preparation at all. Cleansing preparations such as polyethylene glycol electrolyte solution (GoLYTELY) are designed to minimize electrolyte shifts and dehydration. Other cathartic agents such as magnesium citrate and Fleet Phospho Soda minimize the volume of agent consumed, but result in greater electrolyte and fluid shifts. These agents should be avoided in patients with delicate cardiac status or renal insufficiency.

After colon resection as described above, a sutured or stapled anastomosis is performed (multiple studies have demonstrated equivalent leak rates of less than 2% between the two techniques). A difficult laparoscopic colectomy may become easier with a 4–8 cm incision to allow for insertion of one hand (hand-assisted) via a port that maintains pneumoperitoneum. The anastomosis for a laparoscopic procedure can be completed within the abdomen (intracorporeal) via a laparoscopic stapling device, or the open ends of intestine can be exteriorized (extracorporeal) for stapled or handsewn anastomosis. Emergency operations involving the right colon are often reconstructed with ileocolostomy. Similarly, when the entire colon is resected, immediate reconstruction with ileorectal anastomosis is often performed as well. However, emergency operations involving the left half of the colon have been traditionally managed by creation of a proximal end colostomy with closure of the distal end of bowel (Hartmann's pouch). There is a belief that the difference in bacteriology in the left colon from that of the right results in increased leaks and abscesses when surgery is urgently performed. Some authors have suggested primary repair or resection with anastomosis when the left colon is involved as well. More recent trauma literature has expanded the use of primary repair or resection with anastomosis in left colon injury when there is minimal tissue damage, little intra-abdominal contamination,

Medical Management of the Surgical Patient, ed. Michael F. Lubin, Thomas F. Dodson, and Neil H. Winawer. Published by Cambridge University Press. © Cambridge University Press 2013.

and favorable anatomic location of the injury (i.e., the injury is not located in a watershed blood supply area such as the splenic flexure). Patients who are in shock, regardless of the area of injury, are generally treated by either resection and stapling of the injury with planned return to the operating room when the patient is stable, or by exteriorization of the injury via ileostomy or colostomy.

Elective colon resection, even near-total colectomy, is a controlled operation with little blood loss and only moderate stress to the patient. Multiple studies have demonstrated that elective laparoscopic colectomies performed for complications of diverticulitis or for cancer result in less blood loss, less postoperative morbidity, shorter hospital stays (on average by 2–4 days), and earlier return to normal activities than open operations. In addition, the 5-year survival after elective resection for colon cancer is improved when the procedure is performed laparoscopically as well. Emergency colon resection for perforated sigmoid diverticulitis, bleeding angiodysplasia, extensive traumatic perforation, toxic megacolon, or infarction from volvulus or low flow may be associated with moderate blood loss and is a significant stress, particularly in elderly patients.

Usual postoperative course
Expected postoperative hospital stay

The expected postoperative hospital stay is 3–5 days after laparoscopic procedures and 4–9 days after open procedures, depending on protocol used and extent of patient's illness prior to surgery.

Operative mortality

Operative mortality is less than 1% for patients with elective resection under the age of 60 and 10% over the age of 60 for both benign and oncologic indications. Reviews of urgent colectomy for toxic megacolon show mortality rates ranging from 15–30%, with increased mortality with advanced age and degree of illness.

Special monitoring required

Postoperative hemodynamic monitoring with an arterial line, central venous line, or pulmonary artery catheter is considered for many elderly patients with emergency resection of the colon, and for younger patients with major abdominal trauma (e.g., injury to the colon).

Patient activity and positioning

Depending on hemodynamic stability and the presence of other injuries, patients may be out of bed on the day after the operation.

Alimentation

Most studies have shown that surgeons advance the diets of patients undergoing laparoscopic procedures more readily than they do for open-surgery patients. In routine cases of both open and laparoscopic surgery, patients can be started safely on clear liquids the day after surgery; diet is then advanced accordingly with return of bowel function. In cases where the patient has had chronic severe obstruction, advancement of diet is delayed until the return of bowel function. If, after 5 days, the patient cannot be started on an enteral diet, initiation of intravenous hyperalimentation is considered. If the patient is critically ill or severely weakened and unable to swallow safely, enteral feeds can be initiated via a temporary nasogastric or operative feeding tube.

Antibiotic coverage

Within 30 minutes of any incisions, all patients receive intravenous cephalosporin (usually second generation), metronidazole, or a combination of antibiotics, at a maximum of two doses postoperatively as per current standard of care. In patients with gross intra-abdominal contamination from perforated sigmoid or cecal diverticulitis, perforated toxic megacolon, gangrenous colon from volvulus or vascular catastrophe, or delayed operation for traumatic perforation, antibiotics are continued for 5–7 days.

Delayed wound closure

Open packing of the skin and subcutaneous tissue of the incision is indicated with gangrenous or perforated colon. Delayed primary closure has been used in some instances at days 5–6 in patients with clean, deep wounds that would otherwise require 6–12 weeks of dressing changes at home. Alternatively, the closed suction devices commonly known as "wound vacs" have been used successfully with increasing frequency to accelerate the rate of wound healing in clean, deep wound beds. These devices have been shown to decrease the time needed for healing by up to 50% for wounds left open for closure by secondary intention.

Drains

Unless a well-defined abscess cavity from a perforation is present, colectomies above the peritoneal reflection are not drained. However, because of a risk of postoperative pelvic sepsis, many surgeons drain the deep pelvis after low anterior resection of the rectosigmoid colon or upper rectum.

Postoperative complications
In the hospital
Wound infection

See Chapter 63.

Breakdown of anastomosis

Disruption of an ileocolostomy or colocolostomy in the early postoperative period is a rare but potentially lethal complication. Leaks are most commonly seen 7–14 days after surgery; patients with obvious fecal peritonitis require early reoperation. In such cases, treatment often requires not only drainage of intra-abdominal contamination, but exteriorization of the leak via temporary ileostomy or colostomy. A partial leak may lead to a contained perianastomotic or pelvic abscess or a colocutaneous fistula through a drainage site or the abdominal incision. Percutaneous drainage of an intraperitoneal abscess may be a worthwhile first step, although a fecal fistula is an obvious risk. Operative transrectal drainage is appropriate for a pelvic abscess that is palpable on rectal examination. Ileocolocutaneous or colocutaneous fistulas are treated with prohibition of oral intake, intravenous hyperalimentation, administration of a somatostatin analog, and protection of the surrounding skin. In the absence of a foreign body, intra-abdominal infection, a short tract (epithelialization), residual neoplasm, or distal obstruction ("FIEND"), the fistula can be expected to close without reoperation if it remains low output (< 300 mL daily).

Pseudomembranous enterocolitis

A sudden onset of tenderness over the remaining colon in association with diarrhea and systemic toxicity is strongly suggestive of pseudomembranous enterocolitis. A specimen of stool is sent for *Clostridium difficile* enterotoxin, and the causative antibiotic responsible for development of the disease is discontinued. In cases of systemic toxicity, patients receive not only enteral flagyl (or enteral vancomycin if treatment is refractory to the use of flagyl), but intravenous flagyl as well. Supportive therapy with appropriate intravenous hydration must also be maintained. If the disease remains refractory to this treatment, operative intervention is then entertained.

After discharge

Change in bowel movements

Patients who have undergone resection of the ileocecal valve or an extensive portion of the left colon (left hemicolectomy, subtotal or total colectomy with anastomosis) have an increased number of bowel movements. These usually decrease over time; the average number of bowel movements in one series of patients with subtotal colectomy and ileorectostomy was two per day after 6 months.

Patients with total colectomy, creation of an ileal pouch, and an ileal pouch–anal anastomosis average five or six bowel movements in 24 hours. Complete daytime continence is present in 90%, even on long-term follow-up. Night-time continence is present in 75% on long-term follow-up 1 year out from surgical intervention.

Treatment in the short and long term often requires the use of soluble fiber supplements such as Metamucil with meals and anti-diarrheal agents that contain atropine to help to reduce intestinal transit time to the rectum.

Recurrent tumor

For 2 years after resection for colorectal carcinoma, the patient is monitored by colonoscopy every 6 months; carcinoembryonic antigen (CEA) levels are obtained every 2 months. After this period, follow-up intervals may be lengthened. Reoperation is indicated if colonoscopy reveals recurrent tumor or the carcinoembryonic antigen level becomes elevated after it has normalized, and if no distant metastases are seen with positron emission tomography. Carcinoembryonic antigen levels that fail to normalize 4–6 weeks postoperatively generally indicate incomplete resection or recurrence (though false positives can occur). It should be noted that some poorly differentiated tumors do not produce CEA, and therefore CEA is most valuable as a surveillance tool when it was noted to be elevated preoperatively. Early detection of recurrent disease is associated with a higher rate of resectability. Carcinoembryonic antigen levels greater than 10 mg/mL are more often associated with liver and lung metastases. Notably, when the CEA elevates above 10 mg/mL, the chances of curative resection of recurrent disease drops substantially. In instances where the tumor burden cannot be completely resected, chemotherapy remains the primary modality of treatment. The use as a surveillance tool of radio-labeled monoclonal antibody directed against tumor-associated antigens is being studied. Incisional or laparoscopic port site recurrences occur in 1–2% of patients with resection for cancer.

Further reading

Dente CJ, Tyburski J, Wilson RF *et al*. Ostomy as a risk factor for posttraumatic infection in penetration colonic injuries: univariate and multivariate analyses. *J Trauma* 2000; **49**: 628–34; discussion 634–7.

Guller D, Jain N, Hervey S *et al*. Laparoscopic vs. open colectomy: outcomes comparison based on large nationwide databases. *Arch Surg* 2003; **138**: 1179–86.

Kemp JA, Finlayson SRG. Outcomes of laparoscopic and open colectomy: a national population-based comparison. *Surg Innov* 2008; **15**: 277–83.

Lacy AM, Garcia-Valdecasas JC, Delgado S *et al*. Laparoscopy-assisted colectomy versus open colectomy for treatment of non-metastatic colon cancer: a randomized trial. *Lancet* 2002; **359**: 2224–9.

Luglio G, Nelson H. Laparoscopy for colon cancer: state of the art. *Surg Oncol Clin N Am* 2010; **19**: 777–91.

Pahlman L. Treatment of colorectal cancer. *Ann Chir Gynaecol* 2000; **89**: 216–20.

Senagore AJ, Duepree HJ, Delaney CP *et al*. Results of a standardized technique and postoperative care plan for laparoscopic sigmoid colectomy: a 30-month experience. *Dis Colon Rectum* 2003; **46**: 503–9.

Weeks JC, Nelson H, Gelber S *et al*. Clinical Outcomes of Surgical Therapy (COST) Study Group. Short-term quality-of-life outcomes following laparoscopic assisted colectomy vs. open colectomy for colon cancer: a randomized trial. *J Am Med Assoc* 2002; **287**: 321–8.

Chapter 55

Abdominoperineal resection/coloanal or ileoanal anastomoses

Jahnavi K. Srinivasan and David V. Feliciano

Abdominoperineal resection (APR, Miles' operation), with excision of the rectum, anus, and sphincter muscles and the creation of a permanent end colostomy, is performed to remove malignant neoplasms of the distal one-third of the rectum or the anus. The most common indication for resection is adenocarcinoma of the rectum or anus that cannot be removed with adequate margins at the time of primary resection, or recurrent disease. Less common indications for APR include residual squamous cell carcinoma of the anus after chemo-radiation treatment, carcinoid, cloacogenic carcinoma, basal cell carcinoma, and malignant melanoma. Abdominoperineal resection is most commonly performed for nonmalignant disease in the setting of medically refractory Crohn's disease with severe perianal fistulae.

The operation is conducted with a transabdominal laparoscopic approach or through a low midline laparotomy incision and a circumferential perianal incision. Included in the excision are the rectosigmoid colon, the rectum, the pelvic mesocolon, the lymph nodes associated with the three sets of hemorrhoidal vessels, the levator muscles out to the ischial tuberosities, the anus, and the perianal skin. The resection of the levator and anal complex necessitates an end-descending colostomy. In instances when the surgeon is able to excise a 2 cm margin of normal bowel beyond the rectal tumor, a Miles' procedure with a permanent colostomy can be avoided by performing a low hand-sewn or stapled coloanal anastomosis accompanied by a temporary diverting ostomy while the anastomosis heals.

A related approach is excision of the colon and most of the rectum alone (without the mesocolon or lymph nodes) and preservation of a seromuscular short rectal cuff to maintain anal continence. An ileal pouch–anal anastomosis is then created and stapled or sewn to the short rectal cuff. In the absence of a known low rectal oncologic diagnosis, this operation is appropriate for patients with severe chronic ulcerative colitis that remains medically refractory, familial polyposis, or Gardener's syndrome in the absence of a known low rectal malignancy. Any instance where a known malignant tumor exists in the low rectum requires mesorectal excision for evaluation of the associated lymph nodes. Ileal pouch–anal anastomosis is generally not considered appropriate in patients with Crohn's disease, given the high incidence (> 60%) of pouch complications such as inflammation of the pouch and severe perianal fistulae.

In an effort to minimize the risk of locoregional recurrence, preoperative neoadjuvant external-beam radiotherapy and radio-sensitizing chemotherapy have been used to shrink large rectal cancers invading into or beyond the muscularis propria (> T2) or those with metastatic perirectal nodes. When neoadjuvant treatment is employed, surgical resection is usually delayed by 4–6 weeks after radiation has been completed. Preoperative colon preparation varies depending on surgeon preference, ranging from the consumption of an oral cathartic, rectal mechanical cathartic, and non-absorbable antibiotics (usually neomycin and erythromycin base), to an oral and/or mechanical rectal cathartic alone, to no preparation at all (see Chapter 49). On the night before operation, the ideal site for the permanent end colostomy in the left lower quadrant is marked by the surgeon or enterostomal therapy nurse. This site selection will avoid colostomy placement at a location that may be inappropriate for the patient (cannot be seen by the patient, too close to incisions or to the pelvis).

The procedure is performed from both a transabdominal and transperineal approach, sometimes with two surgeons operating simultaneously. The surgical team performing the laparoscopic approach (or laparotomy) mobilizes the rectosigmoid colon, rectum, and mesorectum with vessels and lymph nodes off the sacrum. This team then divides the colon with a stapler and creates a proximal end sigmoid colostomy. The second team excises the perianal skin, anus, and levator muscles out to the ischial tuberosities and removes the entire specimen through the perineum.

Extensive resection of a mid-rectal tumor may remove the pelvic peritoneum. Some surgeons leave the pelvis open and allow the small bowel to fall into the hollow of the sacrum; others suture a sheet of absorbable mesh to replace the pelvic peritoneum and support the small bowel above the deep pelvic space, with the hope of keeping it from becoming adherent

Medical Management of the Surgical Patient, ed. Michael F. Lubin, Thomas F. Dodson, and Neil H. Winawer. Published by Cambridge University Press. © Cambridge University Press 2013.

deep in the now-empty pelvic space. This maneuver is particularly useful to keep small bowel out of the radiation field when further postoperative adjuvant treatment is necessary, secondary to significant local invasion. Before the subcutaneous tissue and the skin of the perineal incision are closed, closed suction drains are inserted through the upper medial buttocks into the deep pelvic space for postoperative drainage. In rare cases, the perineal wound must be left open because of sacral bleeding that requires the insertion of pelvic packing, or because of extensive contamination associated with Crohn's disease of the anorectum.

In experienced hands, conversion from a laparoscopic to an open approach ranges from 3–13%, with a diminished conversion rate correlating to case experience over 100 cases. Again, in experienced hands, operative time is only modestly increased (by an average of approximately 30 minutes). Moderate blood loss can occur with either approach, particularly when a neoplasm is affixed to the sacrum or prostate gland. Because the procedure involves two incisions and creates a large dead space in the posterior pelvis that takes time to heal, the stress is moderate to severe in all patients.

Usual postoperative course
Expected postoperative hospital stay
The expected postoperative hospital stay averages 5 days for the laparoscopic approach and 7 days for the open approach.

Operative mortality
Operative mortality is less than 2% in laparoscopic and open cases.

Special monitoring required
In general, reliable peripheral access is all that is necessary. During a difficult procedure, postoperative hemodynamic monitoring with a pulmonary artery catheter may occasionally be necessary in elderly patients with excessive blood loss.

Patient activity and positioning
Patients may be out of bed on the day after the operation, depending on hemodynamic stability.

Alimentation
For routine procedures, patients are permitted clear liquids with the return of bowel function. Food intake is advanced as tolerated.

Antibiotic coverage
At our institution, all patients receive intravenous cephalosporin (typically second generation), metronidazole, or a combination of antibiotics preoperatively within 30 minutes of incision; the Surgical Care Improvement Project (SCIP)

national guideline is 60 minutes. Antibiotics are administered for no more than two doses postoperatively, unless the patient has evidence of infection related to the pelvic wound.

Delayed closure if the perineal wound has been left open
Delayed primary closure of the skin (or transposition of gracilis muscle flaps into the pelvic space, with closure of the skin by the plastic surgery service) can be performed once the pelvic packing has been removed or after perineal cellulitis (from previously resected Crohn's disease) has resolved. While awaiting definitive closure of the skin, a closed-suction wound drainage device is sometimes used during the interim period, provided that the underlying muscular layers are completely closed (to avoid closed suction on intra-abdominal visceral contents).

Drains
Closed suction drains are usually placed in the deep pelvis to prevent fluid and blood from accumulating in the postoperative period. These drains are discontinued when output drops to less than 100 mL per day.

Bladder catheter
Mesorectal excision often results in a disruption of nerves in the sacral plexus. An indwelling Foley catheter is left in place for 3 days after surgery to avoid the significant rate of urinary retention. Attempts to remove the bladder catheter are begun 3 days after operation. Urinary retention is managed with reinsertion of the catheter for another 2–3 days.

Colostomy care
An enterostomal therapist will instruct the patient on the care of the permanent end colostomy.

Postoperative complications
In the hospital
Wound infection
See Chapter 63.

Urinary tract complications
Operative injury to or deliberate excision of a portion of the ureter occasionally occurs during secondary pelvic surgery, or when a large, bulky, or inflamed rectal neoplasm is excised. Repair of the ureter or reimplantation into the dome of the bladder is best performed by a urologist. An unrecognized injury may present as a postoperative ureterocutaneous or cystocutaneous fistula, with fluid containing high levels of creatinine leaking through the perineal wound or through drains. A retrograde cystoureterogram is necessary

to localize the injury. The need for reoperation is determined by the urologist.

Urinary retention after removal of the catheter occurs more commonly in men than in women. Conservative treatment with reinsertion of the catheter succeeds in 70% of patients. Transurethral resection of the prostate may be necessary in the remainder, after 2–3 weeks of outpatient observation with a catheter in place.

Intestinal obstruction

Even with insertion of an absorbable mesh to replace the pelvic peritoneum, adhesive obstruction of the small bowel in the pelvis may occur in the early postoperative period. Conservative management (nasogastric tube placement and parenteral nutrition) should be employed to avoid re-entering a hostile abdomen and inadvertently injuring fused intestinal loops. If conservative management fails, operative intervention should be delayed until the patient is at least 3–4 weeks out from surgery unless clinical status (peritonitis or sepsis from an intra-abdominal source) mandates urgent intervention.

Colostomy complications

Necrosis, retraction, prolapse, and parastomal abscess occur in 5–10% of patients; reoperation is mandatory for these patients.

Pelvic abscess/sepsis

Pelvic abscess is a rare complication that is diagnosed by pelvic computed tomography and treated by reopening the perineal incision. The incidence of pelvic sepsis is generally 5–15%; this complication occurs more often in patients who undergo ileal pouch–anal anastomosis than with patients who have undergone an end colostomy. Treatment in these cases requires broad-spectrum antibiotic coverage and wound exploration to address any undrained sources of infection.

After discharge

Impotence

Impotence develops in 5–40% of men, depending on the level of the tumor, operative technique, and the extent of the resection.

Colostomy complications

Retraction, stricture, or fistula formation occurs in 7–8% of patients. Late parastomal hernia occurs in 10–12%.

Tumor recurrence in the pelvis

Carcinoma recurs in as many as 30% of patients, though 75–90% of node negative cancers are cured by radical resection. Local recurrence is predicted by higher staging of initial presentation and close proximity of the tumor to the anal verge. High histologic grade of the original tumor, local spread of the tumor, and metastases to pelvic nodes are ominous prognostic signs. Positron-emission tomography is used to determine the extent of the recurrence. Repeated transperineal excision, abdominosacral resection, pelvic exenteration, and further radiotherapy all have been used with moderate success to relieve pelvic pain and lengthen survival. Median survival after the initial potentially curative and subsequent palliative resection of recurrent rectal cancer has been demonstrated to be approximately 16 months, with proven survival benefit when compared with non-surgical treatment alone.

Further reading

Barlehner E, Benhidjeb T, Anders S. Laparoscopic resection for rectal cancer: outcomes in 194 patients and review of the literature. *Surg Endosc* 2005; **19**: 757–66.

Greenblatt DY, Rajamanickman V, Pugely AJ. Short term outcomes after laparoscopic-assisted proctectomy for rectal cancer: results from the ACS NSQIP. *J Am Coll Surg* 2011; **212**: 844–54.

Grumann MM, Noack EM, Hoffman IA *et al.* Comparison of quality of life in patients undergoing abdominoperineal extirpation or anterior resection for rectal cancer. *Ann Surg* 2001; **233**: 149–56.

Hiotis SP, Weber SM, Cohen AM *et al.* Assessing the predictive value of clinical complete response to neoadjuvant therapy for rectal cancer: an analysis of 488 patients. *J Am Coll Surg* 2002; **194**: 131–5.

Kakuda JT, Lamont JP, Chu DZJ, Paz IB. The role of pelvic exenteration in the management of recurrent rectal cancer. *Am J Surg* 2003; **186**: 660–4.

Miles WE. A method of performing abdominoperineal excision for carcinoma of the rectum and of the terminal portion of the pelvic colon. *Lancet* 1908; **2**: 1812–13.

Murrell ZA, Dixon MR, Vargas H. Contemporary indications for and early outcomes of abdominoperineal resection. *Am Surg* 2005; **71**: 837–40.

Ng SS, Leung KL, Lee JF. Laparoscopic-assisted versus open abdominoperineal resection for low rectal cancer: a prospective randomized trial. *Ann Surg Oncol* 2008; **15**: 2418–25.

Chapter

Anal operations

56

Jahnavi K. Srinivasan

Anal operations are among the most common operations performed by general surgeons. The procedures include hemorrhoidectomy, incision and drainage of perirectal or ischiorectal abscess, excision and fulguration of anal condylomata, identification of perianal fistula with drainage and seton placement, and partial lateral internal sphincterotomy. Hemorrhoids are caused by increased pressure in the venous plexus of the rectum, resulting in pathologic stretching and dilation of these veins. They are classified according to their position relative to the dentate line because of the variations between the upper two-thirds and lower third of the rectum in regard to innervation, perfusion, and drainage. External hemorrhoids are below the dentate line while internal hemorrhoids are above the dentate line. Accordingly, internal hemorrhoids have a greater tendency to produce bleeding while external hemorrhoids are often sensitive and painful to patients. In general, if symptoms are minimal, management is non-operative. Patients are counseled to avoid constipation and straining during bowel movements and to utilize stool softeners. Small hemorrhoids can be treated with topical anesthetics, warm water (sitz) baths and, if necessary, topical steroids. In general, surgical intervention is indicated when patients have uncontrollable pain, persistent severe bleeding, or prolapse, provided the patient does not have a medical contraindication such as portal hypertension or hematologic dyscrasia. For patients who are poor operative candidates, internal hemorrhoids can be treated in the office via rubber band ligation. In these patients, a rubber band is placed at the base of the hemorrhoid to induce ischemia and sloughing. Band ligation is relatively contraindicated in patients on anticoagulation, as it can result in severe anal bleeding. Operation involves open excision (external and internal) or stapled hemorrhoidectomy (internal hemorrhoids only).

Anal fissures are typically posterior acute or chronic ulcers that result from continued tearing and hypertrophy of the internal sphincter in patients with constipation. This results in painful defecation. Initial treatment is to minimize constipation via diet change and stool softeners. Medical treatment focuses on the use of topical agents that relax the internal sphincter, such as topical nitroglycerin, oral or topical calcium channel blockers, or local Botox injections. If the fissure fails to heal with medical management, operative intervention requires identification of the internal sphincter and partial transection. Generally, the fissure is then cauterized, or in cases of large chronic ulcers, excised and repaired via a local mucosal advancement flap.

Perianal and ischiorectal abscesses are purulent collections that arise from extension of infection in an anal crypt. Individuals who are immunosuppressed (e.g., those with HIV or diabetes) or who have a predisposition toward the development of perianal fistulae (e.g., Crohn's disease) are at greater risk of developing these infections. Perianal abscesses are painful when the patient sits or walks, and prior to defecation. Superficial abscesses present with erythema, swelling, induration, warmth, and tenderness to palpation, whereas deeper abscesses may cause rectal pressure and signs of sepsis. The bacteria most often implicated in these abscesses are those commonly found in the gastrointestinal tract (anaerobic and gram-negative bacteria). However, the last decade has seen a significant increase in community-acquired methicillin-resistant *Staphylococcus aureus* as an etiologic agent. Ischiorectal abscesses generally require some form of multiplanar imaging (CT or MRI) to evaluate the full extent of the abscess because they are located deeply and are not always detectable on physical exam. Prompt incision and drainage is the treatment of choice for these lesions, although fistulas also occur in 25–50% of patients in some series. In cases where a fistula is identified, fistula treatment is required at the time of abscess drainage.

Anal fistulas are openings in the perianal skin that drain purulent or feculent material, secondary to surgical drainage or spontaneous perforation of a crypt abscess into the rectal or sphincteric space. Fistulae in ano heal spontaneously in some patients; however, chronic or extensive fistulae are treated by unroofing the fistula tract via incision of the anoderm and subcutaneous tissues (fistulotomy). If only

---

Medical Management of the Surgical Patient, ed. Michael F. Lubin, Thomas F. Dodson, and Neil H. Winawer. Published by Cambridge University Press. © Cambridge University Press 2013.

part of the internal sphincter is involved, fistulotomy can still be achieved by partial transection of the internal sphincter without the development of incontinence. Involvement of more than two-thirds of the internal sphincter or the external sphincter requires placement of a vessel loop or thread (seton) in the fistula tract. At intervals, the seton is tightened as a means of promoting the body to slowly extrude the foreign body and allow for gradual obliteration of the fistula tract.

Condylomata acuminata or anal warts are caused by the human papilloma virus types 6 and 11. Symptomatic condylomata cause anal pain, soil underclothes, and may undergo degeneration into a squamous cell carcinoma if a giant condyloma is present (Buschke–Löwenstein tumor). For a small condylomata, initial treatment is with topical agents with varying mechanisms of action such as podophyllotoxin, imiquimod, sinecatechins, or trichloroacetic acid. Additional non-excisional treatments include laser ablation or cryotherapy. Treatment of more extensive condylomata is by excision with reconstruction of the anal margin. Though recurrence rates are lower in these cases, patients often still require further treatment with topical agents to suppress recurrent disease. Moreover, tissue pathology should be evaluated for squamous cell carcinoma, as this may require further oncologic treatment. Preventative vaccines such as Gardasil (Merck & Co.), which protects against HPV 6, 11, 16, 18, are being investigated for use in patients, but the vaccine is only preventative and not therapeutic. Moreover, effective preventative use requires its administration prior to exposure to the HPV virus.

Anal operations are performed under local, caudal, spinal, or general anesthesia, with the patient in the high lithotomy or prone, jackknife position, with the hips flexed at the waist in a 90° angle for exposure of the perineum. If local anesthesia is used, many surgeons add epinephrine to decrease blood loss. Most anal operations are performed in 30–60 minutes, blood loss is modest, and there is minimal stress to the patient. Postoperative control of pain is critical.

Usual postoperative course
Expected postoperative hospital stay

Ambulatory procedures are routinely performed on patients undergoing sphincterotomy for anal fissures, drainage of perianal abscesses, and fistulotomies for fistulas in ano, as long as they are able to return to the surgeon's office on a regular basis in the early postoperative period. After an extensive hemorrhoidectomy, the hospital stay is 2–3 days.

Operative mortality

Mortality is less than 0.1% in patients without portal hypertension.

Special monitoring required

The dressing is checked for bleeding every 4 hours during the immediate postoperative period. Patients should also be monitored for urinary retention, as inability to void within 8 hours of surgery generally requires catheterization. Although pelvic sepsis is rare after anal procedures, patients should be counseled to contact their physician if they develop fevers greater than 38.5 °C, rigors, or severe pelvic pain.

Patient activity and positioning

Patients may be out of bed on the day of surgery. After removal of the pressure dressing on the first postoperative day, sitz baths of lukewarm water are permitted.

Alimentation

Clear liquids are permitted on the day of operation, and food intake is advanced as tolerated. Docusate sodium is often administered to soften stools.

Antibiotic coverage

Antibiotics that provide adequate gram-negative and anaerobic coverage (third-generation cephalosporin or fluoroquinolone combined with metronidazole) are administered to patients with perianal or ischiorectal abscesses or fistulas in ano. Antibiotics are administered until the woody cellulitis surrounding the abscess or fistula tract resolves. All patients with valvular heart disease, prosthetic valves, or vascular grafts receive perioperative antibiotics because of the risk of infection from bacteremia.

Analgesia

Use of long-acting local anesthesia such as bupivacaine for a postoperative pudendal nerve block can ease initial postoperative discomfort substantially. For 1–2 weeks after surgery, patients generally require oral narcotic medication as well.

Postoperative complications
In the hospital
Bleeding

Incomplete surgical hemostasis, particularly at the base of a resected hemorrhoid, may lead to postoperative bleeding. Ligation of the bleeding vessel is generally possible only by reoperation because exposure at the bedside is too painful. On rare occasions, postoperative bleeding in a patient with cirrhosis may necessitate the use of balloon catheter tamponade followed by the injection of a sclerosing agent. Prior to surgical intervention, patients with known portal hypertension should be evaluated with consideration for a transjugular intrahepatic portosystemic shunt (TIPS) procedure to decompress their high-pressure rectal varices.

Urinary retention

Failure to void in the first 6–8 hours after operation delays discharge from the ambulatory surgical suite, and has a 2–3% incidence. In-and-out catheter insertion is usually all that is needed in the early postoperative period, although men with enlarged prostates may require indwelling Foley catheter placement for 1–3 days after surgery.

Pelvic sepsis

The incidence of pelvic sepsis is low after anal surgery ($< 1\%$) but can be fatal if not promptly detected. It is most commonly seen in patients who are not adequately drained after an anal procedure has been performed. Stapled hemorrhoidectomy is associated with a higher rate of pelvic sepsis because the tissues are not left open for drainage. Treatment requires broad antibiotic coverage and identification and drainage of any abscesses. In patients who have had an open hemorrhoidectomy, the suture can be divided to allow for adequate drainage.

After discharge

Anal stricture

Excessive excision of anal skin during a hemorrhoidectomy or fissurectomy or suture closure of the remaining skin may cause an anal stricture as healing occurs. Published rates of stenosis are generally less than 1%, although the stenosis rate 1 year postoperatively is thought to be higher. There is a higher rate of stenosis with stapled hemorrhoidectomy as compared with open hemorrhoidectomy. Progressive anal dilation usually solves the problem, although operative release of the stricture may be necessary.

Anal incontinence

A fistula in ano extending into the high intermuscular or supralevator area should not be opened completely at the first operation because damage to the sphincters causes anal incontinence. If this has occurred, a late reoperation with reconstruction of the sphincter mechanism may be necessary.

Further reading

Brisinda G, Vanella S, Cadeddu F. Surgical treatment of anal stenosis. *World J Gastroenterol* 2009; **15**: 1921–8.

Hyman N, O'Brien S, Osler T. Outcomes after fistulotomy: results of a prospective, multicenter regional study. *Dis Colon Rectum* 2009; **52**: 2022–7.

Subhas G, Gupta A, Balaraman S. Non-cutting setons for progressive migration of complex fistula tracts: a new spin on an old technique. *Int J Colorectal Dis* 2011; **26**; 793–8.

Tjandra JJ, Chan MK. Systematic review on the procedure for prolapse and hemorrhoids (stapled hemorrhoidopexy). *Dis Colon Rectum* 2007; **50**; 878–92.

Trombeta LJ, Place RJ. Giant condyloma acuminatum of the anorectum: trends in epidemiology and management: report of a case and review of the literature. *Dis Colon Rectum* 2001; **44**: 1878–86.

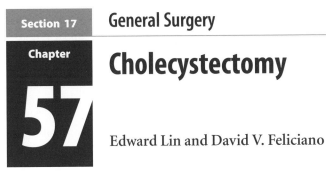

Chapter

57

Cholecystectomy

Edward Lin and David V. Feliciano

Cholecystectomy is indicated for symptomatic calculous cholecystitis (acute or chronic); acalculous acute cholecystitis; a gallbladder that releases stones into the common bile duct (obstructive jaundice, gallstone pancreatitis, cholangitis); carcinoma of the gallbladder; traumatic perforation of the gallbladder; and biliary dyskinesia (low gallbladder ejection fraction). It is also performed after right hepatic artery ligation for hepatic trauma and in preparation for infusion of the hepatic artery with chemotherapeutic agents for metastases. It is included as part of a pancreatoduodenectomy and may be necessary for exposure of the porta hepatis in some patients undergoing portacaval shunt procedures.

Cholecystectomy can best be performed within 48 hours of admission for patients with acute cholecystitis documented on ultrasonography or radionuclide scanning (i.e., HIDA scan) unless general anesthesia is contraindicated. In patients with acute cholecystitis of longer duration, the extent of inflammation may make a laparoscopic approach difficult. If cholecystectomy is to be scheduled electively for acute cholecystitis, it is appropriate to give antibiotics until the time of surgery to help the inflammation subside. Patients with obstructive jaundice, gallstone pancreatitis, or cholangitis undergo cholecystectomy after observation to determine whether the bilirubin level will fall, when the amylase level returns to normal, and when hemodynamic stability has been restored, respectively.

General anesthesia is used for both open and laparoscopic cholecystectomy. Open procedures are completed in 1–1.5 hours and the stress of the routine procedure is moderate. If gangrenous cholecystitis with perforation is present, the underlying disease causes severe stress during the perioperative period. Most patients are discharged from the hospital 2–4 days after operation and return to work in 4–6 weeks.

A laparoscopic approach is used in 90–95% of the more than 750,000 patients who undergo cholecystectomy in the USA each year. Rates of conversion to an open procedure are 5–10% for experienced laparoscopic general surgeons, with most conversions necessitated by adhesions, severe inflammation, unclear anatomy, or, rarely, bleeding. Laparoscopic procedures are completed in 1–1.5 hours; blood transfusions are rarely necessary, and the stress of the routine procedure is modest. Most patients are discharged from hospital the day after the laparoscopic operation and return to work in 1 week. The major concern about the laparoscopic procedure has been the 0.2–0.5% incidence of injuries to the common bile duct, a figure slightly greater than that historically reported for open cholecystectomy. Intraoperative cystic duct cholangiography may be used to delineate anatomy or identify common bile duct injury. While common bile duct injury is sometimes unavoidable, early recognition and referral for treatment is the most appropriate course of action.

Usual postoperative course

Expected postoperative hospital stay

The expected postoperative hospital stay is 2–4 days for open cholecystectomy; 1 day for laparoscopic cholecystectomy.

Operative mortality

Under 0.1% for routine open or laparoscopic cholecystectomy and 10–15% for cholecystectomy performed for empyema or gangrene of the gallbladder, emphysematous cholecystitis, or acalculous cholecystitis in a patient with recent major abdominal surgery or multisystem trauma.

Special monitoring required

Postoperative intensive care monitoring is necessary only in patients with severe sepsis or associated hemorrhagic or necrotizing pancreatitis.

Patient activity and positioning

Patients may be out of bed on the day of surgery, depending on hemodynamic stability.

Alimentation

For patients undergoing routine open or laparoscopic cholecystectomy, clear liquids are allowed the evening after operation or the first postoperative morning. Patients with more

Medical Management of the Surgical Patient, ed. Michael F. Lubin, Thomas F. Dodson, and Neil H. Winawer. Published by Cambridge University Press. © Cambridge University Press 2013.

complicated indications for cholecystectomy are permitted clear liquids with the return of bowel function and food intake is advanced as tolerated. Patients with associated hemorrhagic or necrotizing pancreatitis receive jejunal feedings or intravenous hyperalimentation as soon as they are hemodynamically stable.

Antibiotic coverage

Perioperative antibiotics such as a cephalosporin or broad-spectrum antibiotics are administered to patients who are undergoing cholecystectomy for cholelithiasis with chronic cholecystitis, acute cholecystitis, resolving acute cholecystitis, obstructive jaundice, known choledocholithiasis, or ascending cholangitis. The duration of postoperative antibiotic administration depends on the underlying condition.

Postoperative complications

In the hospital

Wound infection

Subcutaneous wound infections occur in 1–5% of all patients undergoing open cholecystectomy, but in only 1% of those undergoing laparoscopic cholecystectomy.

Subhepatic biloma or abscess

A biloma that occurs from necrosis of the cystic duct stump or unrecognized division of a duct of Luschka (gallbladder–liver connection) is treated with percutaneous drainage. Subhepatic abscesses are extraordinarily rare but their occurrence is almost always related to performance of cholecystectomy in conjunction with another intra-abdominal procedure. When difficult anatomy is encountered, or when the cystic duct cannot be ligated, placement of drains is appropriate to minimize contamination of the surgical bed.

Bile duct injury

Not all biliary injuries require surgical repair. Partial duct disruption, or small tributary leaks are routinely treated with biliary stent placement and decompression of the bile duct.

An injury recognized during open or laparoscopic cholecystectomy is repaired with absorbable sutures, and a T-tube is inserted if an end-to-end anastomosis is required. An unrecognized injury during laparoscopic cholecystectomy leads to postoperative ileus and abnormal liver function test results. With early recognition (< 48 hours) in the postoperative period, immediate laparotomy is performed with biliary reconstruction as indicated. With delayed recognition in the presence of bile peritonitis, an endoscopic retrograde cholangiopancreatogram (ERCP) for diagnosis, biliary stent placement for decompression, and subhepatic drainage are performed before biliary reconstruction approximately 6 weeks later. Late reconstruction of the biliary system is best performed at experienced hepatobiliary centers.

Whether injuries, bile leaks, or inflamed anatomy are encountered during cholecystectomy, placement of drains is highly encouraged to minimize contamination at the surgical site.

Bowel injury

Injury to either the duodenum or the jejunum occurred in 0.3% of patients undergoing laparoscopic cholecystectomy in one series. Sepsis and ileus are usually present within 24 hours, and a laparotomy is performed with closure as indicated.

Bleeding

In one series, bleeding from the bed of the gallbladder or a branch of the cystic artery occurred in 0.3% of patients undergoing laparoscopic cholecystectomy. Either an open or a laparoscopic approach can be used to control the source of hemorrhage.

Retained or residual common bile duct stone

Retained common bile duct stones after either open or laparoscopic cholecystectomy occur less than 5% of the time, and generally present within the first 2 years following surgery (see Chapter 63).

Further reading

Banz V, Gsponer T, Candinas D, Güller U. Population-based analysis of 4113 patients with acute cholecystitis: defining the optimal time-point for laparoscopic cholecystectomy. *Ann Surg* 2011; **254**: 964–70.

Csikesz NG, Tseng JF, Shah SA. Trends in surgical management for acute cholecystitis. *Surgery* 2008; **144**(2): 283–9.

Flum DR, Cheadle A, Prela C *et al.* Bile duct injury during cholecystectomy and survival in Medicare beneficiaries. *J Am Med Assoc* 2003; **290**: 2168–73.

Flum DR, Dellinger EP, Cheadle A *et al.* Intraoperative cholangiography and risk of common bile duct injury during cholecystectomy. *J Am Med Assoc* 2003; **289**: 1639–44.

Kaafarani HM, Smith TS, Neumayer L *et al.* Trends, outcomes, and predictors of open and conversion to open cholecystectomy in Veterans Health Administration

hospitals. *Am J Surg* 2010; **200**: 32–40.

Pfluke JM, Parker M, Stauffer JA *et al.* Laparoscopic surgery performed through a single incision: a systematic review of the current literature. *J Am Coll Surg* 2011; **212**: 113–18.

Sakpal SV, Bindra SS, Chamberlain RS. Laparoscopic cholecystectomy conversion rates two decades later. *J Soc Laparoendosc Surg* 2010; **14**: 476–83.

Chapter

58

Common bile duct exploration

Edward Lin and David V. Feliciano

Common bile duct exploration is indicated for radiologically confirmed or manually palpable gallstones in the common bile duct (choledocholithiasis). These stones can be asymptomatic or causing obstructive jaundice, gallstone pancreatitis, or ascending cholangitis. It is also indicated to diagnose and treat obstructive jaundice from a benign or malignant stricture; to diagnose and treat stenosis of the sphincter of Oddi; or to repair an injury caused by operation or trauma. Choledochotomy is also appropriate when there are no other alternatives to decompress the common bile duct.

When a stone is identified preoperatively, it is most effective to perform a preoperative ERCP (endoscopic retrograde cholangiopancreatogram) with sphincterotomy to allow extraction of, or access to, common bile duct stones. Patients with resolved cholangitis, persistent jaundice, unresolving pancreatitis, or common bile duct stones documented by other tests are ideal candidates for preoperative ERCP. For stable patients, ERCP may also be performed after cholecystectomy is performed. With the availability of ERCP, the need for open or laparoscopic exploration of the common bile duct has decreased significantly in recent years.

Similarly, if the patient is too ill to proceed to the operating room for common bile duct exploration, interventional radiology can be consulted to decompress the biliary tree with a percutaneous transhepatic cholangiocatheter.

Common bile duct exploration, open or laparoscopic, is not a simple task. General anesthesia is used for both open and laparoscopic common bile duct exploration. The procedure adds at least 60 minutes to a routine open cholecystectomy because of the need to expose and open the duct (choledochotomy), extract the stones and perform choledochoscopy, insert a T-tube, close the duct around the T-tube, and perform a completion T-tube cholangiogram. Laparoscopic common bile duct exploration can take as long as the open method. The ideal approach involves balloon dilation of the cystic duct, passage of a flexible fiberoptic endoscope (outer diameter = 3 mm) through the cystic duct, and basket extraction under direct vision of common duct stones. The major disadvantage of the transcystic approach is that the choledochoscope cannot be manipulated to retrieve stones from the hepatic ducts (further up in the liver). Laparoscopic choledochotomy rather than transcystic exploration requires advanced laparoscopic fine suture skills, which are necessary to sew a T-tube into the common bile duct after removal of the stones. Success rates in removing stones with either laparoscopic or open approach are 90–97%. There is growing experience of closing the bile duct after a common bile duct exploration with an internal stent placement, or nothing at all. Blood transfusion is essentially unnecessary with routine open or laparoscopic choledochotomy. In contrast, common bile duct exploration to diagnose and treat obstructive jaundice from a benign (i.e., previous operative injury) or malignant stricture often is associated with moderate blood loss that requires transfusion. Routine exploration creates modest stress for patients who also are undergoing cholecystectomy, whereas exploration for a benign or malignant stricture may cause severe stress from blood loss and extended duration of the procedure. In operations to manage strictures, a plan should be in place for definitive management at the same operation.

Usual postoperative course

Expected postoperative hospital stay

The expected postoperative hospital stay is 5–10 days.

Operative mortality

Operative mortality is 2–3% in elective operations. For procedures to relieve ascending cholangitis, the rates are 15% (urgent operation) and 30% (emergency operation). Operative mortality is 10–20% in patients undergoing exploration and biliary bypass to relieve obstructive jaundice from an unresectable malignant stricture.

Special monitoring required

Postoperative intensive care monitoring is necessary only for patients with severe sepsis or anticipated difficulties from complex biliary surgery.

Medical Management of the Surgical Patient, ed. Michael F. Lubin, Thomas F. Dodson, and Neil H. Winawer. Published by Cambridge University Press. © Cambridge University Press 2013.

Patient activity and positioning

Patients may be out of bed on the day after operation, depending on hemodynamic stability.

Alimentation

For patients undergoing laparoscopic choledochotomy, clear liquids are permitted on the evening after operation or on the first postoperative morning. For those with open procedures, clear liquids are given with the return of bowel function and food intake is advanced as tolerated.

Antibiotic coverage

All patients undergoing common bile duct exploration receive a perioperative cephalosporin or broader-spectrum antibiotics. Patients with ascending cholangitis are maintained on the appropriate antibiotic (determined by bile culture) until sepsis resolves and fever has been absent for 48 hours.

T-tube

The T-tube left in the common bile duct after an open choledochotomy is connected to gravity drainage. A T-tube cholangiogram can be performed as early as postoperative day 6 or 7 to document the absence of retained stones and the free flow of contrast into the duodenum. About 12 hours after a normal cholangiogram, the portion of the T-tube outside the body is clamped off. The clamp is released only if patients develop cholangitis, right upper quadrant pain, or a bile leak around the T-tube. A T-tube inserted at the time of a routine choledochotomy is removed in an outpatient setting 2 weeks after the exploration. Patients are warned to expect a small amount of bile leakage from the T-tube site for 2 or 3 days.

Postoperative complications

In the hospital
Wound infection

See Chapter 57.

Subhepatic abscess

See Chapter 57.

T-tube displacement

Early displacement of the T-tube may precipitate bile peritonitis that is not responsive to percutaneous drainage; reoperation may be necessary. Late displacement when adhesions are present may be treated with insertion of a percutaneous drain near the choledochotomy site.

Retained or residual common bile duct stone

A retained stone is one which appears on a postoperative T-tube cholangiogram and is unexpected; a residual stone is one that the surgeon cannot remove at operation. A postoperative ERCP with sphincterotomy is indicated to allow for passage of the retained or residual stone if no T-tube has been left in the common bile duct at the first operation. If a T-tube is in place, and ERCP is not possible, interventional radiology can establish access to the stone(s) by passing wires through the existing T-tube; antegrade stone removal is achieved via percutaneous transhepatic cholangiography. Interventional radiologists usually require the T-tube tract to mature over 2–4 weeks before attempting stone retrieval.

Pancreatitis

Operative manipulation of the distal common bile duct may precipitate transient, mild postoperative pancreatitis. Pancreatitis is usually self-limited if the common bile duct has been cleared of stones.

After discharge
Stricture

Attacks of cholangitis manifested by pain, fever, jaundice, and elevation of the alkaline phosphatase level in the absence of choledocholithiasis are strongly suggestive of biliary stricture. The diagnosis is confirmed by ultrasound, CT, or MRI to rule out a neoplasm, and by a transhepatic cholangiogram or ERCP to localize the area of obstruction. Transhepatic balloon dilation of the area of stricture may obviate the need for reoperation with biliary reconstruction.

Common bile duct stone

Late cholangitis caused by a common bile duct stone is almost always the result of failure to clear stones from the common bile duct during the first operation. Either endoscopic sphincterotomy or transhepatic extraction is indicated. Patients of Asian descent have a much higher incidence of spontaneously formed intrahepatic ductal stones, which may migrate into the common bile duct long after operation. In addition to endoscopic sphincterotomy, a variety of radiologic procedures for irrigation and extraction of impacted stones are usually attempted, although reoperation with a biliary–enteric bypass may be necessary.

Further reading

Poulose BK, Kummerow KL, Nealon WH *et al.* Biliary obstruction during cholecystectomy: endoscopic retrograde cholangiopancreatography, evade, or explore? *Am Surg* 2011; 77: 985–91.

Rogers SJ, Cello JP, Horn JK *et al.* Prospective randomized trial of LC+LCBDE vs ERCP/S+LC for common bile duct stone disease. *Arch Surg* 2010; **145**: 28–33.

Stromberg C, Nilsson M. Nationwide study of the treatment of common bile duct stones in Sweden between 1965 and 2009. *Br J Surg* 2011; **98**: 1766–74.

Urbach DR, Khajanchee YS, Jobe BA *et al.* Cost-effective management of common bile duct stones: a decision analysis of the use of endoscopic retrograde cholangiopancreatography (ERCP), intraoperative cholangiography, and laparoscopic bile duct exploration. *Surg Endosc* 2001; **15**: 4–13.

Chapter

59

Major hepatic resection

Edward Lin and David V. Feliciano

In addition to treating critical injuries, major hepatic resection is performed to remove malignant neoplasms (hepatoma, cholangiocarcinoma, metastases, carcinoid tumor), benign neoplasms (liver cell adenoma, focal nodular hyperplasia, cavernous hemangioma), cysts (congenital, multicystic disease, echinococcal), and certain abscesses. If the remaining hepatic tissue is normal, as much as 80–90% of the liver can be removed in children and adults.

The availability of MRI and CT scans is leading to earlier detection of hepatocellular carcinoma or hepatic metastases from colorectal cancer. Other biochemical measurements such as elevated alpha-fetoprotein (AFP) and carcinoembryonic antigen (CEA) may prompt earlier imaging.

Preoperative screening with MRI for major hepatic resections is very sensitive in detecting small nodules, showing the relationship between tumor nodules and major intrahepatic and retrohepatic blood vessels, and determining resectability. MRI can also be used to assess volume reserve in patients with cirrhosis who need major hepatic resection.

Major hepatic resection is performed under general anesthesia through an upper abdominal incision for left lobe resection, and a right subcostal resection for right lobe resection. In skilled centers, minimally invasive techniques have been used successfully for major resections. The general stages of major lobectomy include either vascular inflow occlusion (Pringle maneuver or clamping of the porta hepatis) or individual ligation of the lobar hepatic artery, portal vein, and right or left branch of the hepatic duct. Division of the hepatic parenchyma is accomplished using finger fracture techniques, blunt knife handle dissection, cutting staplers, and ultrasonic vibrating-suction device or ultrasonic shears. Blood loss depends on the extent of the resection and involvement of the retrohepatic vena cava. The median blood loss was 600 mL in one recent large series, and only 49% of patients were transfused at any time. In general, intraoperative fluid restriction reduces back-pressure bleeding during major hepatic resection. The operative time is 3–4 hours in experienced hands, and the stress of a major hepatic resection is moderate to severe.

Usual postoperative course

Expected postoperative hospital stay

Typically, 4 to 12 days.

Operative mortality

Small segment resections are associated with low morbidity and mortality. Mortality increases with larger resections primarily due to the functional reserve of the remaining liver.

Special monitoring required

Patients with known cardiac or pulmonary compromise and those who have undergone difficult resections associated with extensive blood loss require postoperative hemodynamic monitoring. The need for arterial or pulmonary catheter monitoring is on an individual basis. During the preoperative and intraoperative period, fluids are administered judiciously to minimize venous bleeding in the surgical bed.

Patient activity and positioning

Patients may be out of bed on the day after the operation.

Alimentation

In most major resections that do not involve the bowel for reconstruction, early oral intake can be started. Hypoglycemia can usually be prevented by the infusion of a 5–10% glucose solution after extensive resection. Early nutritional support through the gastrointestinal tract is preferred. In addition to the theoretical benefit of lowering the incidence of gut-origin sepsis, use of the gastrointestinal tract appears to generate hepatotrophic factors that maintain the integrity of the liver. This is in contrast to the cholestasis and fatty infiltration that occurs in patients who are maintained on intravenous hyper-alimentation for prolonged periods.

Medical Management of the Surgical Patient, ed. Michael F. Lubin, Thomas F. Dodson, and Neil H. Winawer. Published by Cambridge University Press. © Cambridge University Press 2013.

Antibiotic coverage

Perioperative coverage for 24 hours with cephalosporin or broader-spectrum antibiotics is routine.

Drains

It is acceptable not to leave drains in standard hepatic resections. Some surgeons prefer drain placement in the subphrenic and subhepatic spaces for 5–7 days or until drainage decreases to 30–50 mL/day. Initial light bilious output may be expected, which clears over several days. In cases where the surgical bed may be contaminated due to abscess or concomitant bowel surgery, drain placement may be used.

Postoperative complications

In the hospital

Perihepatic abscess

Sterile perihepatic fluid collections or abscesses in the subphrenic or subhepatic area occur in 10–11% of patients. Sterile collections may be observed. Alternatively, fluid collections may be treated with CT-guided percutaneous drainage.

Pleural effusion

Sympathetic pleural effusions occur in 8–10% of patients and are treated conservatively unless pulmonary compromise results.

Prolonged postoperative fever

This is a common problem in patients undergoing emergency resection in which mass ligation techniques are used. A CT scan with contrast or MRI can be used to monitor the viability of the remaining liver and rule out the presence of a perihepatic abscess. Prolonged fever after uncomplicated resections is uncommon.

Postoperative bleeding

A second laparotomy for bleeding from the raw edge of the remaining liver is necessary in only 1–2% of patients after elective operation and 5–7% of patients after emergency resection for severe hepatic injuries. In most instances, a second exploration for bleeding only serves to evacuate blood clots, and a clear source of bleeding may be elusive.

Hepatic failure

Progressive elevation of the transaminases, bilirubin, alkaline phosphatase and the international normalized ratio (INR) occurs in 5% of patients after extensive resection and is usually reversible with enteral nutrition and supportive management. This temporary hepatic insufficiency may result from poor functional reserves of the remaining liver and extent of resection resulting in small-for-size syndrome. While a cause of consternation for the team, supportive care and observation are the only course of action.

After discharge

Prognosis

The median survival for patients without cirrhosis who undergo curative resection for hepatocellular carcinoma is about 24 months; this decreases by 11–12 months for patients with cirrhosis. The overall 5-year survival for elective resection of hepatocellular carcinoma is now nearly 45% in Asia. The overall 5-year survival of patients undergoing hepatic resection for colorectal metastases ranges from 30–45%. Patients with recurrent carcinoma usually have weight loss, abdominal distension, an abdominal mass, and progressive jaundice.

Further reading

Hammond JS, Guha IN, Beckingham IJ, Lobo DN. Prediction, prevention and management of postresection liver failure. *Br J Surg* 2011; **98**: 1188–200.

Lee KF, Chong CN, Wong J *et al*. Long-term results of laparoscopic hepatectomy versus open hepatectomy for hepatocellular carcinoma: a case-matched analysis. *World J Surg* 2011; **35**: 2268–74.

Que FG, Sarmiento JM, Nagorney DM. Hepatic surgery for metastatic gastrointestinal neuroendocrine tumors. *Adv Exp Med Biol* 2006; **574**: 43–56.

Reddy SK, Barbas AS, Turley RS *et al*. A standard definition of major hepatectomy: resection of four or more liver segments. *HPB (Oxford)* 2011; **13**: 494–502.

Swan PJ, Welsh FK, Chandrakumaran K, Rees M. Long-term survival following delayed presentation and resection of colorectal liver metastases. *Br J Surg* 2011; **98**: 1309–17.

Chapter 60

Splenectomy

John F. Sweeney and David V. Feliciano

Benign hematologic diseases are second only to trauma as the most common indication for splenectomy. Immune thrombocytopenic purpura (ITP) is the most common indication for splenectomy and comprises greater than 70% of patients undergoing splenectomy for benign disease. Additional benign hematologic conditions that are indications for splenectomy include patients with congenital hemolytic anemia; metabolism abnormalities; hemoglobinopathies and erythrocyte structure abnormalities (e.g., hereditary spherocytosis and elliptocytosis).

Splenectomy may be indicated as a diagnostic tool or for palliation in patients with malignant hematologic disease. Surgical staging is utilized most often in Hodgkin's disease, resulting in a change in diagnosis and subsequent impact on therapy and prognosis in up to 30–40% of patients. Splenectomy can also provide relief to patients with symptomatic splenomegaly, which may or may not be accompanied by hypersplenism. Patients with malignant hematologic diseases are more likely to have massively enlarged spleens (> 1,000 g), resulting in significant discomfort and pain as well as early satiety. When splenomegaly is accompanied by cytopenias (hypersplenism), the cytopenia often improves or sometimes is even cured by removal of the spleen.

Laparoscopic splenectomy (LS) has become the standard approach in many institutions when splenectomy is indicated for benign hematologic disease and has gained acceptance for patients with malignant hematologic disease and splenomegaly. Although initial reports suggested that LS was associated with longer operative times than those of open splenectomy, increased surgeon experience and technical advancements such as hand-assist devices have improved outcomes in patients with both benign and malignant hematologic disease processes. While there have been no prospective randomized trials, there are numerous retrospective and prospective studies to support the use of LS as a safe and effective alternative to open splenectomy.

The patient's preoperative preparation includes administration of polyvalent pneumococcal vaccine at least 2 weeks before surgery. The evening before surgery, patients commence a clear liquid diet and take a mild laxative several hours before bedtime to decompress the colon and facilitate laparoscopic visualization of the left upper quadrant and spleen. Several units of packed red blood cells should be cross matched, and in patients with ITP, platelets are cross matched for administration if there is evidence of bleeding after the splenic artery has been ligated.

Sequential compression boots are applied for prevention of deep venous thrombosis and a preoperative antibiotic (1 g cephazolin) is given for prevention of surgical site infections. Patients who have been receiving corticosteroids within 6 months of surgery are given stress doses of intravenous corticosteroids. Before transport to the operating room, a beanbag is placed on the operating table to enable subsequent patient positioning and stabilization. After induction of general anesthesia, the patient is positioned in the incomplete right lateral decubitus position at an angle of 45°. The skin is prepared and draped so that either laparoscopy or open surgery can be performed.

We prefer to obtain intra-abdominal access approximately 3–4 cm below the costal margin in the left mid-clavicular line. The abdomen is then insufflated to a pressure of 15 mmHg with carbon dioxide. Two 5-mm trochars are placed in the upper midline or to the left of the midline along the costal margin. The abdomen is inspected with special attention to the greater omentum and splenocolic regions, which are common locations for accessory splenic tissue. Accessory spleens are found in 10–15% of patients with hematologic disease and have been associated with disease recurrence in patients with ITP when they are not removed.

An additional 12-mm trochar is placed in the left anterior axillary line, below the costal margin. The patient is then placed in steep reverse Trendelenburg position and the table rolled to the patient's right giving a true left lateral decubitus position. Ultrasonic shears are used to divide the gastrosplenic ligament and short gastric blood vessels, allowing the stomach to fall to the patient's right and providing excellent exposure to the splenic hilum. The splenic artery can then be easily identified and ligated with hemoclips if desired. Attention is then

Medical Management of the Surgical Patient, ed. Michael F. Lubin, Thomas F. Dodson, and Neil H. Winawer. Published by Cambridge University Press. © Cambridge University Press 2013.

turned toward mobilization of the lower pole of the spleen. The splenophrenic and splenorenal ligaments are divided using ultrasonic shears. If a lower pole vessel is encountered it is divided using an endoscopic stapling device with a vascular cartridge. This approach allows for visualization of the splenic hilum and the tail of the pancreas by retracting the spleen toward the abdominal wall. The superior splenophrenic attachments to the upper pole of the spleen are left intact to prevent torsion of the spleen during division of the hilum. The endoscopic stapling device with a vascular cartridge is then used to divide the well-exposed splenic hilum.

Following division of the remaining upper pole attachments, the spleen is placed into a specimen retrieval bag. The mouth of the bag is brought through the 12 mm Hasson trochar site and the spleen is then morcellated with sponge forceps and removed in pieces. Special care must be taken to avoid ripping the endoscopic bag during this process in order to prevent spillage of splenic tissue in the abdomen. The left upper quadrant is irrigated and inspected for hemostasis. A second search for accessory splenic tissue is undertaken before the 12-mm fascial openings are securely closed with absorbable suture and the skin incisions are closed. The orogastric tube is removed in the operating room, and the patient is taken to the recovery room.

Usual postoperative course

Expected postoperative hospital stay

Five to 7 days for routine open splenectomy; 10–21 days for complex open splenectomy; 1–2 days for laparoscopic splenectomy.

Operative mortality

Operative mortality is 0% to 2% for elective routine splenectomy; 0% to 40% for trauma splenectomy, depending on associated injuries.

Special monitoring required

Platelet counts are monitored after splenectomy for thrombocytopenia and a complete blood count is obtained as necessary in patients with preoperative anemia or pancytopenia.

Patient activity and positioning

Depending on hemodynamic stability, patients may be out of bed on the day after the operation.

Alimentation

For routine or complex procedures, clear liquids are permitted with the return of bowel function and food intake is advanced as tolerated. For trauma patients with multiple associated injuries (usually Injury Severity Score is over 15), early institution of enteral or intravenous hyperalimentation is appropriate.

Antibiotic coverage

A cephalosporin antibiotic is administered for routine elective splenectomy. For trauma splenectomy, antibiotics are given for at least 24 hours after surgery in patients with associated perforations of the gastrointestinal tract.

Drains

Drains are not placed after elective routine or trauma splenectomy. If a trauma splenectomy is performed as part of a distal pancreatectomy, a closed suction drain is usually left in place for 7–10 days.

Postoperative complications

In the hospital

Left lower lobe atelectasis

This occurs in 15–20% of patients after open splenectomy and usually responds to nasotracheal suctioning and chest physiotherapy.

Postoperative pancreatitis or pancreatic fistula

Injury to the tail of the pancreas leads to pancreatic leak, with resulting pancreatitis or pancreatic fistula. This can occur in up to 7% of open splenectomies (especially after trauma) and is seen at a rate of 1–2% after laparoscopic splenectomy.

Left subphrenic abscess

Occurs in only 2–3% of patients who have elective routine or complex open splenectomy, but in 5–7% of those who have trauma splenectomy. Only 2–3% of patients who undergo open splenorrhaphy (splenic repair) after trauma or iatrogenic injury develop this complication.

Rebound thrombocytosis

Aspirin therapy is suggested if the platelet count exceeds 1 million, but this complication is extremely rare.

Persistent thrombocytopenia

Thrombocytopenia persists in 10–30% of patients who undergo splenectomy for ITP. If a radionuclide scan with indium-111-labeled autogenous platelets was not performed before surgery, this study is used occasionally in the postoperative period to rule out residual accessory spleens not detected at the time of splenectomy. Positive results mandate reoperation if thrombocytopenia persists; patients with normal results should remain on immunosuppressive therapy. Splenectomy as a salvage procedure in patients with thrombotic thrombocytopenic purpura had a remarkable success rate of 88% in one recent laparoscopic series.

After discharge

Persistent thrombocytopenia

See earlier discussion.

Overwhelming postsplenectomy infection

Splenectomy usually is not performed in children younger than 2 years and is performed infrequently in children younger than 10 years because of the risk of overwhelming postsplenectomy infection (OPSI) with encapsulated pneumococci, meningococci, or *Hemophilus* organisms. Most episodes of OPSI occur in the first several years after splenectomy. The relative risk of developing OPSI is lowest when splenectomy is performed for trauma and increases progressively as splenectomy is performed for primary splenic disease, hematologic disease, incidental injury at other operation, and incidental injury at operation for malignancy. The long-term risk in adults is thought to be about 0.5–1.45%, and the mortality has decreased to 20–30% with earlier recognition of the overwhelming bacteremias in patients with previous splenectomy. Neither the administration of antipneumococcal vaccine nor the development of antipneumococcal antibodies is uniformly protective against the development of OPSI.

Further reading

Feldman LS. Laparoscopic splenectomy: standardized approach. *World J Surg* 2011; **35**: 1487–95.

Kercher KW, Matthews BD, Walsh RM *et al.* Laparoscopic splenectomy for massive splenomegaly. *Am J Surg* 2002; **183**: 192–6.

Mikhael J, Northridge K, Lindquist K *et al.* Short-term and long-term failure of laparoscopic splenectomy in adult immune thrombocytopenic purpura patients: a systematic review. *Am J Hematol* 2009; **84**: 743–8.

Rosen M, Brody F, Walsh RM *et al.* Hand-assisted laparoscopic splenectomy vs. conventional laparoscopic splenectomy in cases of splenomegaly. *Arch Surg* 2002; **137**: 1348–52.

Schwartz J, Eldor A, Szold A. Laparoscopic splenectomy in patients with refractory or relapsing thrombotic thrombocytopenic purpura. *Arch Surg* 2001; **136**: 1236–8.

Sharma D, Shukla VK. Laparoscopic splenectomy: 16 years since Delaitre with review of current literature. *Surg Laparosc Endosc Percutan Tech* 2009; **19**: 190–4.

Chapter

61

Pancreatoduodenal resection

Edward Lin and David V. Feliciano

Pancreatoduodenal resection (Whipple procedure) is performed for attempted cure of periampullary carcinomas (head of pancreas, ampulla of Vater, duodenal wall, or distal common bile duct); malignant islet cell neoplasms in the head of the pancreas; mucinous cystic neoplasms or mucinous cystadenocarcinoma of the head of the pancreas; intraductal papillary mucinous neoplasms; benign masses from chronic pancreatitis in the head of the pancreas with secondary pancreatic duct, common bile duct, or duodenal obstruction; and, rarely, major trauma to the pancreatoduodenal complex.

Patients with obstructive jaundice (dilated hepatic ductal system) and no evidence of gallstones on ultrasound or computed tomography (CT) should undergo abdominal helical CT or MRI to determine whether there is a mass in the periampullary area and whether hepatic metastases or regional invasion has occurred. Further work-up to localize the area of obstruction in patients without a periampullary mass should include an MRCP (magnetic resonance cholangiopancreatogram) and, if necessary, ERCP (endoscopic retrograde cholangiopancreatogram) or transhepatic cholangiogram. In patients in whom there is the need to differentiate between chronic pancreatitis and ductal carcinoma of the pancreas, PET scanning may be useful. Percutaneous preoperative pancreatic biopsy may yield false negative results: it is not indicated in patients who are at low operative risk and who may have resectable tumors. In patients with suspected islet cell neoplasms, transduodenal ultrasound is helpful for localization.

Percutaneous transhepatic drainage of the obstructed biliary ductal system in the preoperative period is less commonly performed because prospective trials have not demonstrated improvement in postoperative survival. The preoperative administration of parenteral vitamin K and the institution of intravenous or supplemental enteral alimentation are appropriate in patients with 10% loss of body weight, albumin levels less than 2.5 mg/dL, or anergy on delayed hypersensitivity skin testing.

Pancreatic masses can be staged quite accurately before resection by current imaging modalities (primarily MRI) to verify the absence of hepatic, celiac nodal, and pelvic metastases or regional invasion into the portal vein, superior mesenteric vessels, inferior vena cava, or aorta. Traditional resection for cure includes the head, neck, and, sometimes, a portion of the body of the pancreas; the entire duodenum; the distal common bile duct; cholecystectomy, and the antrum of the stomach. A popular approach is the pylorus-preserving pancreatoduodenectomy in which the stomach and a 2 cm cuff of proximal duodenum are preserved to mitigate dumping syndrome and improve the patient's long-term nutritional status. Reconstruction is accomplished by anastomosis of the jejunum to the ends of the remaining pancreas, common bile duct, and stomach.

Experienced surgical teams perform pancreatoduodenectomy in 3–7 hours with a blood replacement of 0–4 units. The procedure is complex because of the underlying disease, the duration of the operation, the complications that are encountered in 40–50% of patients, and the nutritional problems that are associated with reconstruction of the upper digestive tract.

Usual postoperative course
Expected postoperative hospital stay
The expected postoperative hospital stay is 7–20 days, with a median of 17 days in one large series.

Operative mortality
Most modern series report mortalities no higher than 5%.

Special monitoring required
Patients with known cardiac or pulmonary compromise and those who have undergone difficult procedures associated with excessive blood loss require postoperative hemodynamic monitoring.

Patient activity and positioning
Depending on hemodynamic stability, patients may be out of bed on the day after operation.

Medical Management of the Surgical Patient, ed. Michael F. Lubin, Thomas F. Dodson, and Neil H. Winawer. Published by Cambridge University Press. © Cambridge University Press 2013.

Alimentation

Because of the magnitude of the procedure and the compromised nutritional state of many patients, enteral feedings are administered routinely distal to the pancreatic and biliary anastomoses. Clear liquids are permitted with the return of bowel function, and food intake is advanced as tolerated. Ten percent of patients may have delayed gastric emptying after surgery; insertion of a gastrojejunal feeding tube may be beneficial in some instances.

Antibiotic coverage

All patients receive intravenous second-generation cephalosporin preoperatively and for at least 24 hours postoperatively.

Drains

Closed suction drains are usually placed posterior to the pancreatojejunostomy and choledochojejunostomy; they are removed within 5–7 days if no fistula occurs. Some surgeons leave a small plastic stent through the pancreatojejunostomy or a T-tube through the choledochojejunostomy; both are generally removed 2 weeks after surgery.

Postoperative complications

In the hospital

Delayed gastric emptying

Delayed gastric emptying occurs in about 10–15% of patients after either standard or pylorus-preserving pancreatoduodenectomy. Intravenous erythromycin appears to decrease the incidence of this complication. Nasogastric suction and intravenous hyperalimentation are indicated when delayed gastric emptying occurs.

Pancreatic fistula

A leak from the pancreatojejunostomy occurs in 8–15% of patients. Pancreatic fistula is treated by prohibiting oral intake and continuing suction drainage. The administration of 100–150 μg of somatostatin analog (Octreotide) every 8 hours is sometimes used to reduce fistula output.

Intra-abdominal abscess

An abscess caused by leakage from the pancreatojejunostomy or the choledochojejunostomy occurs in 5–10% of cases. The diagnosis is suggested by spiking temperatures, ileus, and leukocytosis, and CT-guided percutaneous drainage is the appropriate treatment.

Wound infections

Wound infections are a reflection of the patient's general condition, but the occurrence is in the range of clean-contaminated cases.

Hyperglycemia

Elevated glucose levels are frequently noted, particularly in elderly patients receiving hyperalimentation. Intravenous insulin is administered as necessary until an enteral diet is resumed.

After discharge

Recurrent carcinoma

The median survival for patients with positive lymph nodes in the resected specimen of ductal adenocarcinoma of the pancreas is about 12–15 months. Patients with recurrent carcinoma usually have back pain, weight loss, an abdominal mass, and hepatic metastases. Pain control is often the most important palliation that can be offered.

Marginal ulcer

The incidence of an ulcer in the gastrojejunostomy generally ranges from 5–10% in long-term survivors. Patients who are *Helicobacter*-negative and who survive long enough for a marginal ulcer to develop are best treated with H_2 blockers or proton-pump inhibitors.

Pancreatic insufficiency

Even with a successful pancreatojejunostomy, pancreatic insufficiency may occur. It is treated with exocrine replacement.

Further reading

Hornick JR, Johnston FM, Simon PO *et al.* A single-institution review of 157 patients presenting with benign and malignant tumors of the ampulla of Vater: management and outcomes. *Surgery* 2011; **150**: 169–76.

Sakamoto Y, Yamamoto Y, Hata S *et al.* Analysis of risk factors for delayed gastric emptying (DGE) after 387 pancreaticoduodenectomies with usage of 70 stapled reconstructions. *J Gastrointest Surg* 2011; **15**: 1789–97.

Samra JS, Bachmann RA, Choi J *et al.* One hundred and seventy-eight consecutive pancreatoduodenectomies without mortality: role of the multidisciplinary approach. *Hepatobiliary Pancreat Dis Int* 2011; **10**: 415–21.

Subhedar PD, Patel SH, Kneuertz PJ *et al.* Risk factors for pancreatic fistula after stapled gland transaction. *Am Surg* 2001; **77**: 965–70.

Tapper E, Kalb B, Martin DR *et al.* Staging laparoscopy for proximal pancreatic cancer in a magnetic resonance imaging-driven practice: what's it worth? *HPB (Oxford)* 2011; **13**: 732–7.

Chapter

62

Adrenal surgery

Jyotirmay Sharma and David V. Feliciano

Adrenalectomy is performed to remove functional masses such as adrenocortical hyperplasia (Cushing's disease), cortisol-secreting adenoma or adenocarcinoma (Cushing's syndrome), aldosterone-secreting adenoma (Conn's syndrome), pheochromocytoma, and adrenal causes of feminizing or virilizing syndromes. Non-functional masses that are also treated with adrenalectomy include adrenal adenocarcinoma, symptomatic adrenal cysts or angiomyolipomas, adrenal incidentalomas > 4 cm discovered on imaging studies, and isolated adrenal metastases with a favorable tumor biology.

With functioning tumors confirmed biochemically, a CT or MRI is performed to determine the side location of the neoplasm as well as its size, local invasion, and hepatic metastases. Patients with a diagnosis of pheochromocytoma receive a ^{131}I-MIBG scan to localize occult second tumors or metastatic disease to the liver, lung, or bone. Selective venous sampling from the adrenal veins and inferior vena cava is useful to confirm the diagnosis of an aldosterone-secreting adenoma versus bilateral adrenal adenomas or micronodular hyperplasia of the zona glomerulosa. When metastases are being evaluated and resection is under consideration, FDG–PET scan is a useful adjunct.

Preoperative alpha and, occasionally, beta blockade is necessary before all adrenalectomies performed for pheochromocytomas. Metyrosine is also a useful adjunct for perioperative blockade of a pheochromocytoma. In patients with aldosterone-secreting adenomas, preoperative administration of spironolactone may help reverse persistent hypokalemia. Perioperative glucocorticoid supplementation is used in patients undergoing adrenalectomies for Cushing's disease or syndrome.

A laparoscopic approach with or without hand-assist under general anesthesia is used when non-malignant adrenal lesions under 10–12 cm are to be excised. An open anterior transabdominal, flank extraperitoneal, or posterior (with resection of the 12th rib) retroperitoneal approach under general anesthesia is used when adrenal adenocarcinoma, a mass > 10–12 cm,

extensive adhesions, or portal hypertension is present. Intermittent compression stockings are applied to the lower extremities before the operation begins. For patients with large vasoactive tumors, arterial blood pressure monitoring and central venous catheterization is often necessary.

For a right adrenalectomy, the patient is placed in the left lateral decubitus position. Four laparoscopic trocars are placed, extending from the epigastrium around and inferior to the right costal margin. The approach involves separation of the right lobe of the liver and the underlying adrenal gland, mobilization of the hepatic flexure of the colon, identification of the right lateral edge of the inferior vena cava, and double clipping and division of the right adrenal vein at the inferior vena cava before removal of the adrenal gland. For a left adrenalectomy, the "open book" approach involves separation of the spleen and the underlying left kidney; medial mobilization of the spleen/distal pancreas; lateral and medial exposure of the adrenal gland; and double clipping and division of the left adrenal vein before removal of the gland.

For a large carcinoma, an open anterior transabdominal approach is performed through an extended subcostal incision on the side of the mass, through a midline incision, or via a thoracoabdominal incision and exposure.

For lesions less than 6–8 cm in size, laparoscopic adrenalectomies performed by experienced surgeons are associated with minimal blood loss. The conversion rate to an open procedure is less than 5%; operating time is 1–2 hours; and stress is modest. An open adrenalectomy performed for adrenocortical carcinoma may be associated with moderate blood loss, a 3–4 hour operating time, and moderate stress.

Usual postoperative course

Expected postoperative hospital stay

The expected postoperative hospital stay is 1–2 days after a laparoscopic approach or open posterior approach and 7–10 days after an open anterior approach.

Medical Management of the Surgical Patient, ed. Michael F. Lubin, Thomas F. Dodson, and Neil H. Winawer. Published by Cambridge University Press. © Cambridge University Press 2013.

Operative mortality

Operative mortality is 0.3% for a laparoscopic approach and less than 5% for an open anterior approach.

Special monitoring required

Patients undergoing bilateral adrenalectomy for Cushing's disease or for familial pheochromocytoma (MEN IIA or B) will require continued postoperative supplementation with glucocorticoids and mineralocorticoids and careful hemodynamic monitoring. Patients undergoing a unilateral adrenalectomy for a pheochromocytoma will need careful hemodynamic monitoring postoperatively, even with appropriate preoperative blockade; these patients may often require vasopressor support for a few hours after resection.

Patient activity and positioning

Depending on their hemodynamic stability, patients who have undergone laparoscopic surgery may be out of bed on the day of the operation.

Alimentation

For routine procedures, patients are permitted clear liquids with the return of bowel function. After a laparoscopic approach, patients usually tolerate oral liquids on the evening after surgery.

Antibiotic coverage

A second-generation cephalosporin is administered preoperatively for prophylaxis.

Drains

Drains are not used.

Postoperative complications

In the hospital

Addisonian crisis

An Addisonian crisis may occur in patients receiving inadequate glucocorticoid replacement or supplementation after bilateral or unilateral adrenalectomy for Cushing's disease or syndrome, respectively. Patients with Addisonian crisis present with hyponatremia, hypoglycemia, hyperkalemia, and refractory hypotension to fluids and vasopressors.

Early postoperative hypotension

Patients who have undergone adrenalectomy for a pheochromocytoma may experience early postoperative hypotension if they have received inadequate preoperative alpha blockade and inadequate intraoperative fluid resuscitation. Treatment is with fluid resuscitation based on central hemodynamic monitoring and administration of vasopressors. Postoperatively, the anti-hypertensives that were administered preoperatively are usually not repeated. A reassessment of the need for anti-hypertensive medications is necessary prior to discharge. Over 70% of patients with pheochromocytomas and 40–50% of patients with aldosteronomas do not require anti-hypertensive medications in the month after surgery.

Wound infections or breakdown

Wound complications are common in patients undergoing open adrenalectomy for Cushing's disease or syndrome. In the past, the loss of bulk of abdominal wall muscles, thinning of the skin, and high glucose levels have been associated with both infections in the incision and dehiscence of closures of the anterior abdominal wall. Poor healing has also been noted with some posterior incisions. In all cases, surgical consultation is necessary.

After discharge
Recurrent tumor

Patients with MEN IIA or B syndrome who have undergone unilateral adrenalectomy for a pheochromocytoma face a greater than 30–50% risk of developing a contralateral pheochromocytoma. If an adrenalectomy has been performed for adrenocortical cancer, the optimistic 5-year survival has been reported to be 20–25%; however, mean survival for most victims is only 24 months.

Further reading

Balasubramaniam S. Practical considerations in the evaluation and management of adrenocortical cancer. *Semin Oncol* 2010; **37**: 619–26.

Brunt LM. The positive impact of laparoscopic adrenalectomy on complications of adrenal surgery. *Surg Endosc* 2002; **16**: 252–7.

Cushing H. The basophil adenomas of the pituitary body and their clinical manifestations (pituitary basophilism). *Bull Johns Hopkins Hosp* 1932; **50**: 137–95.

Henry JF, Defechereux T, Raffaelli M *et al.* Complications of laparoscopic adrenalectomy: results of 169 consecutive causes. *World J Surg* 2000; **24**: 1342–6.

Siren J, Tervahartiala P, Sivula A, Haapiainen R. Natural course of adrenal incidentalomas: seven-year follow-up study. *World J Surg* 2000; **24**: 579–82.

Thompson GB, Grant CS, van Heeden JA *et al.* Laparoscopic versus open posterior adrenalectomy: a case-control study of 100 patients. *Surgery* 1997; **122**: 1132–6.

Webb R, Mathur A, Chang R *et al.* What is the best criterion for the interpretation of adrenal vein sample results in patients with primary hyperaldosteronism? *Ann Surg Oncol* 2012; **19**: 1881–6.

Lysis of adhesions

63

Kevin W. McConnell

Intra-abdominal adhesions are the most common reason for mechanical small bowel obstruction (SBO) and are implicated in infertility and complex abdominal and pelvic pain. Recent studies suggest that 10% of patients who have undergone colectomy will be re-admitted for SBO within 3 years. The annual cost of managing this condition is well over 1 billion dollars.

Hyaluronate/carboxymethyl cellulose (Seprafilm), oxidized regenerated cellulose (Intercede), and other agents are available to attempt to limit postoperative adhesion formation. These agents have been shown to reduce adhesion formation, but have not been proven to decrease the incidence of SBO. Furthermore, there is a possible link to an increased incidence of anastamotic leak. Thus, utilization of these products varies by institution and surgeon. Other techniques that have been shown to decrease postoperative adhesion include a laparoscopic approach, minimization of foreign material (sutures/mesh), and use of powder-free gloves.

Patients usually present with nausea and emesis if the obstruction is complete. If the obstruction is only partial, patients may have less severe symptoms and may still be passing flatus. Many patients are profoundly dehydrated and hypokalemic and require significant resuscitation and electrolyte repletion. Patients with limited cramping and abdominal distension, and no signs of peritonitis, often benefit from fluid and electrolyte repletion, nasogastric tube decompression and observation. This approach may allow laparotomy to be avoided, but mandates close observation for signs of threatened bowel. Patients with a rising white blood cell count, fever, peritonitis, and persistent or increasing pain (possible closed loop obstruction) will likely need surgical exploration. Obstructed small bowel may become ischemic or necrotic without classical signs and symptoms; when a non-operative approach is taken, serial evaluations and a high index of suspicion are necessary.

Patients who fail to improve with nasogastric (NG) decompression or who have signs of threatened bowel require surgical exploration. A midline laparotomy remains the most common approach; however, laparotomy itself is an independent risk factor for SBO. Thus, there has been an increasing acceptance of laparoscopy for adhesiolysis. Laparoscopy requires identifying safe locations for port placement away from the original scar

and potentially adherent bowel. The procedure is technically challenging in the presence of distended bowel, but it offers potential benefits such as a reduction in postoperative pain, decreased pulmonary complications, earlier mobilization, decreased ileus, lower wound infection rate, shorter length of stay, and overall lower costs. Approximately 15–20% of patients cannot be safely managed with laparoscopy and require conversion to an open approach. The most common risks associated with the procedure include iatrogenic enterotomy, bleeding, wound infection, and postoperative ileus. The complexity of the open approach can vary from a simple division of a single obstructing band to multiple-hour extensive lysis in patients with diffuse dense adhesions. Patients with ischemic intestine may have instability and multi-organ dysfunction if this condition is not recognized and treated promptly. Older patients are particularly vulnerable; one recent series reported a 30% mortality rate in elderly patients who have undergone adhesiolysis for SBO within 3 years following a colectomy.

Usual postoperative course
Expected postoperative hospital stay

The expected postoperative hospital stay varies, and depends on the extent of adhesiolysis, indication for surgery, and operative approach. Six to 9 days in the hospital is common.

Operative mortality

Operative mortality varies with indication for operation and age. Patients with adhesiolysis for chronic pain or partial SBO have a mortality rate of less than 1% in some series; however, patients with ischemic bowel and older patients have published mortality rates as high as 30%.

Special monitoring required

Patients with profound dehydration or electrolyte depletion may require ICU monitoring for arrhythmias and for serial electrolyte evaluations and repletion. Close monitoring of the urine output is a key aspect of adequate resuscitation. Patients with prolonged adhesiolyis or resection of ischemic bowel

Medical Management of the Surgical Patient, ed. Michael F. Lubin, Thomas F. Dodson, and Neil H. Winawer. Published by Cambridge University Press. © Cambridge University Press 2013.

should be monitored carefully for adequate fluid and electrolyte repletion and signs of sepsis.

Patient activity and positioning

Early ambulation is important to minimize risk of prolonged ileus, pneumonia, deep venous thrombosis (DVT), and deconditioning. Elevating the head of the bed may assist with ventilation and minimize risk of aspiration.

Alimentation

Prolonged nasogastric tube decompression may be required for some patients. Electrolyte repletion should be followed closely. Total parenteral nutrition should be considered for malnourished patients and those with a prolonged period of NPO status. Enteral nutrition should be used preferentially, as soon as the obstruction is removed and ileus begins to resolve.

Antibiotic coverage

All patients should receive antibiotics within 1 hour of incision and perioperatively for 24 hours. If gangrenous bowel is found at the time of surgery, antibiotic administration may be continued for 4–7 days postoperatively. A detailed discussion of appropriate coverage is beyond the scope of this chapter, but can be found at the Surgical Infection Society website at http://sisna.org/Position-Papers.cgi.

Postoperative complications

In the hospital
Prolonged ileus

Patients may require 7 days or more for peristalsis to return. Early ambulation and minimal utilization of narcotics shorten the period until bowel function resumes. Peripheral mu-receptor antagonists may decrease the duration of ileus, but data are limited. A prolonged ileus may be indicative of an anastomotic leak or recurrent obstruction; this condition is most commonly evaluated using a CT scan with water-soluble oral contrast.

Wound infection

Enterotomies made during a lysis of adhesions and malnutrition from prolonged obstruction increase the risk of postoperative wound infection. The wound is often packed open to allow drainage and prevent infection.

Leak/fistula

The most dreaded risk of adhesiolysis is a leak from an enterotomy or anastomosis. The leak may be contained in the abdomen or may decompress via fistulization into another cavity. Abscesses are generally managed with percutaneous drainage. Enterocutaneous fistulas are treated with bowel rest and total parenteral nutrition (TPN). Low-output fistulas (< 500 mL/24 hour) often close without further surgical management. High output leaks may require reoperation.

After discharge
Recurrent obstruction

Recurrent obstructions or partial obstructions occur in up to one-third of patients, with some requiring multiple operations. Given that prior laparotomy is the most predictive factor of adhesion formation and obstruction, this can create a dangerous cycle of adhesion formation and surgical lysis.

Further reading

McClain GD, Redan JA, McCarus SD *et al.* Diagnostic laparoscopy and adhesiolysis: does it help with complex abdominal and pelvic pain syndrome in general surgery? *J Soc Laparoendosc Surg* 2011; **15**: 1–5.

Parikh JA, Ko CY, Maggard MA *et al.* What is the rate of small bowel obstruction after colectomy? *Am Surg* 2008; **74**: 1001–5.

Schnuriger B, Bamparas G, Bernardino C *et al.* Prevention of postoperative peritoneal adhesions: a review of the literature. *Am J Surg* 2011; **201**: 111–21.

Solomkin JS, Mazuski JE, Bradley JS *et al.* Diagnosis and management of complicated intra-abdominal infection in adults and children: guidelines by the Surgical Infection Society and the Infectious Diseases Society of America. *Surg Infect* 2010; **11**: 79–109.

Zerey M, Sechrist CW, Kercher KW *et al.* Laparoscopic management of adhesive small bowel obstruction. *Am Surg* 2007; **73**: 773–9.

Chapter

64

Ventral hernia repair

S. Scott Davis, Jr. and David V. Feliciano

Ventral hernias encompass a wide variety of abdominal wall defects, including incisional, epigastric, umbilical, and spigelian types; for the purposes of this chapter, the term ventral hernia is restricted to the incisional type. A ventral hernia with a small ring predisposes patients to incarceration and possible strangulation of a segment of small or large intestine. Patients with significant ascites are at risk for rupture of a ventral hernia if there is only skin covering the defect. Patients with large ventral hernias have difficulty wearing regular clothing and are often embarrassed by their appearance. Not infrequently, these hernias can be associated with abdominal pain; however this is not universally true. It is also possible for patients to suffer obstructive symptoms such as abdominal distension, nausea, or vomiting if there is involvement of the intestinal loops in the hernia defect. In patients with very large incisional hernias, there is lateral displacement of the abdominal wall muscles which leads to very poor function of the abdominal wall and resultant issues with back pain, difficulty with mobility, and loss of intra-abdominal domain. For these reasons, elective repair of ventral hernias is indicated in patients who are healthy enough to undergo mechanical bowel cleaning and general anesthesia.

Over 100,000 ventral hernia repairs are performed in the USA each year. Hernias are a complication that can occur in up to 5% of patients undergoing abdominal surgery; these rates are potentially much higher in obese patients, those taking steroids, or smokers. Patients who suffer a wound infection at the time of the initial operation are also at greatly increased risk of developing incisional hernias since the entire fascial closure often heals improperly and, in many cases, the hernia can be quite large. The finding of an incisional hernia is one of the most common reasons for consultation in general surgical clinics.

Ventral herniorrhaphy performed through an open approach involves excision of the thinned-out skin covering the hernia sac itself and all scar tissue (back to normal-appearing rectus muscle or other muscles of the abdominal wall). Once the true size of the hernia defect is seen, a decision is made regarding primary repair versus insertion of a prosthetic patch. Primary repair is possible even with defects as wide as 5–6 cm using lateral divisions of the external oblique muscles from within the incision or the "components separation" technique.

Because of the size of many ventral hernias after debridement, patches made of polyester (porous), polypropylene (porous), or polytetrafluoroethylenes (non-porous) are frequently inserted to fill the musculofascial defect. There are several techniques used to place prosthetic material, but the guiding principle is that the mesh should overlap the normal abdominal wall for 4–5 cm in each direction. Overlapping will provide a good platform for ingrowth that will produce a strong repair. The most effective way to place the mesh is as an "underlay" where the mesh extends beneath the abdominal wall in all directions such that this overlap is achieved.

Surgical stress is moderate because extensive lysis of adhesions and debridement of the sac are necessary when much of the linea alba has been chronically separated. General anesthesia is used in patients with defects exceeding 4–5 cm in diameter. The procedure may last as long as 4–5 hours but blood transfusion is usually unnecessary. Very large incisional hernias associated with loss of domain are an extreme challenge. These procedures often require extensive lysis of adhesions. Even with the component separation technique, a very large hernia defect often cannot be reapproximated. The operation can take several hours to complete, with greatly increased risk of complications when compared with smaller hernia repairs.

Laparoscopic ventral herniorrhaphy is an alternative approach for the repair of ventral hernias. Using the laparoscope, the surgeon has the advantage of complete visualization of the entire abdominal wall, as well as all parts of the previous incision. This advantage is most apparent in patients who have only one small clinical defect residing in a larger incision. In many cases, other small hernias will be discovered during laparoscopy and can also be repaired, avoiding recurrence. Several articles suggest that this approach thus may lead to lower recurrence rates when compared with open hernia repair. The introduction of the laparoscopic trocars is done

Medical Management of the Surgical Patient, ed. Michael F. Lubin, Thomas F. Dodson, and Neil H. Winawer. Published by Cambridge University Press. © Cambridge University Press 2013.

at a location that avoids the hernia site or prior incisions. Dissection is then performed to divide adhesions, reduce the contents of the peritoneal sac, and determine the number of defects or the size of the one large defect. Once the hernia defect is measured, a tailored polypropylene (porous) or polytetrafluoroethylene (non-porous) synthetic mesh sized 3 cm greater than the edge of the defect is inserted through a trocar or trocar site. This mesh is usually of a "composite" nature, in that the inner surface has a barrier to adhesion development between the mesh and the bowel. The outer surface of the mesh then grows into the abdominal wall. The intraperitoneal mesh is anchored to the abdominal wall at 1 cm intervals with sutures or tacks. As noted above, general anesthesia is used for the laparoscopic approach. The procedure may last as long as 2–4 hours and blood transfusion is generally unnecessary.

Usual postoperative course
Expected postoperative hospital stay

The expected postoperative hospital stay is 3–7 days for open procedures and 1–3 days for laparoscopic procedures. Despite being minimally invasive, the laparoscopic approach still is associated with significant narcotic requirements; most of the procedure involves the abdominal wall, which is innervated. It is important to communicate this information to patients preoperatively so they know what to expect.

Operative mortality

Operative mortality is under 1% for elective procedures not involving strangulated or gangrenous bowel.

Special monitoring required

Placement of a preoperative epidural catheter may be a good consideration in patients undergoing larger open hernia repairs. Nasogastric tubes are not placed as a routine. They may be placed intraoperatively by the surgeon during repair of very large ventral hernias which require extensive lysis of adhesions. They may also be placed if the closure of the abdomen is felt to increase the intra-abdominal pressure, in order to keep the gastrointestinal tract as decompressed as possible until return of bowel function occurs. Nasogastric tube drainage is monitored and replaced intravenously if it is excessive. Serial electrolytes are measured and replaced as needed. The volume of postoperative serum drainage through suction drains placed under the skin flaps in open procedures is monitored daily to aid in determining when the drains should be removed.

Patient activity and positioning

Patients may be out of bed on the day after the operation. Because of the risk of recurrence, heavy lifting is discouraged for 6–8 weeks.

Alimentation

Clear liquids are permitted with the return of bowel function. Food intake is advanced as tolerated.

Antibiotic coverage

All patients receive anti-staphylococcal antibiotics preoperatively to prepare for the insertion of a prosthetic mesh. If mesh is inserted, the antibiotics are continued for 1 day after surgery, and discontinued after 24 hours.

Drains

At the conclusion of open procedures, two large-bore closed suction drains are placed under the skin flaps to prevent fluid accumulation and encourage adherence of the flaps to the primary or mesh repair. Drainage is monitored as described earlier.

Postoperative complications
In the hospital
Wound infection

The incidence of wound infection is under 2% in patients undergoing elective open procedures. Wound infection rates with laparoscopic repair should be even rarer, indicating another potential advantage. If the procedure requires concomitant resection of gangrenous small bowel or colon at the first operation, then wound infection rates will be significantly higher. In such a situation, the surgeon should attempt a primary repair without prosthetic. The surgeon may also consider the use of a "biologic mesh" in this situation. Biologic meshes are derived from a variety of materials, including human cadaver dermis, porcine dermis, or porcine pericardium. They may provide additional reinforcement of a primarily closed abdominal wall, leading to potentially decreased recurrence rates. These meshes do not prevent hernias if they are used to bridge hernia defects that are not closed. If a prosthetic patch of polypropylene or polytetrafluoroethylene has been used at the first operation, a postoperative wound infection may necessitate patch removal and result in failure of the repair. Treatment of a wound infection includes the administration of antibiotics based on Gram stain and the opening of a portion of the incision over the repair.

Wound seroma

If the subcutaneous tissue has been dissected extensively during an open repair or a large defect has been repaired laparoscopically, seromas often occur above the prosthetic patch. Even when closed suction drains have been placed above the patch in open repairs as described above, seromas can occur as well. Seromas are observed unless the patient is symptomatic or has an elevated temperature associated with a leukocytosis. Aspiration of a seroma should only be performed in the operating room under sterile conditions. If patients have had biologic mesh repair, then more aggressive percutaneous drainage of the seromas is indicated.

After discharge

Hernia recurrence

Historically, open ventral herniorrhaphy with mesh has been associated with a 10–15% recurrence rate on short-term follow-up. In one very recent disheartening study from the Netherlands, the 10-year cumulative rate of recurrence was 63% after suture repair and 32% after mesh repair. Currently, laparoscopic ventral herniorrhaphies performed by experienced surgeons have a 1–4% recurrence rate, on short-term follow-up.

Further reading

Burger JWA, Luijendijk RW, Hop WCJ et al. Long-term follow-up of a randomized controlled trial of suture versus mesh repair of incisional hernia. *Ann Surg* 2004; **240**: 578–85.

Dumanian GA, Denham W. Comparison of repair techniques for major incisional hernias. *Am J Surg* 2003; **185**: 1–7.

Heniford BT, Park A, Ramshaw BJ, Voeller G. Laparoscopic repair of ventral hernias: nine year's experience with 850 consecutive hernias. *Ann Surg* 2003; **238**: 391–400.

Reitter DR. Five year experience with the "four-before" laparoscopic ventral hernia. *Am Surg* 2002; **66**: 465–8.

Rosen M, Brody F, Ponsky J et al. Recurrence after laparoscopic ventral hernia repair: a five-year experience. *Surg Endosc* 2003; **17**: 123–8.

Chapter

Inguinal hernia repair

Rebecca L. Coefield and David V. Feliciano

Groin hernias are a common surgical problem. They can be indirect (lateral to the inferior epigastric vessels) or direct (medial to the inferior epigastric vessels in Hesselbach's triangle). Inguinal herniorrhaphy is performed for these hernias in over a million patients in the USA each year. Elective procedures for symptomatic reducible hernias are preferred, but urgent and emergency operations are still required for irreducible hernias and strangulated (ischemic bowel) hernias, respectively.

Routine open inguinal herniorrhaphy through a transverse inguinal incision is performed under general, regional, or local anesthesia in an outpatient setting. Rectangular or oval pieces of permanent mesh are inserted in all adult patients to prevent recurrent hernias. Mesh can be placed as an overlay, as a combined over/underlay in the preperitoneal space or as a combination of a shuttlecock-shaped second prosthesis (plug) inserted under the flat sheet mentioned above. Patients are discharged home when they can void. General anesthesia is appropriate for patients with large hernias that are difficult to reduce; for patients with multiple recurrent hernias in whom orchiectomy is a consideration; and for patients who prefer to be asleep. The stress of a routine open inguinal herniorrhaphy is minimal, and blood transfusions are essentially never required. In contrast, an emergent repair of a strangulated inguinal hernia in elderly patients may become life threatening. This is due to severe stress and possible perioperative sepsis of ischemic bowel in such patients.

Laparoscopic inguinal herniorrhaphy can also be performed under general anesthesia in an outpatient setting. The three main operative approaches include intraperitoneal onlay of mesh, transabdominal preperitoneal approach (TAP), and the totally extraperitoneal approach (TEP). There is a steep learning curve for each of these procedures; operative time is slightly longer than with open repairs; and the operation is more expensive to perform because of the additional equipment. However, recovery time is significantly shorter.

Usual postoperative course

Expected postoperative hospital stay

Patients who undergo routine inguinal herniorrhaphy under local, regional, or general anesthesia are discharged on the day of operation after voiding. If gangrenous bowel was resected through a separate midline laparotomy incision, a longer hospitalization is likely.

Operative mortality

Operative mortality is under 0.1% for elective procedures. It increases to 5–10% for emergency procedures.

Special monitoring required

Postoperative hemodynamic monitoring may be required in elderly patients who have undergone emergency resection of gangrenous small bowel in a hernia sac.

Patient activity and positioning

Patients are ambulatory on the day of surgery. Most surgeons discourage the lifting of heavy objects for 4–8 weeks after nonprosthetic repair. When a prosthetic patch is used, most patients return to normal daily activities (modest lifting) within 7–14 days.

Alimentation

Patients receive a regular diet on the day of operation. If incarceration or strangulation was present preoperatively or bowel resection was necessary during the operation, alimentation is begun when bowel function returns.

Antibiotic coverage

For routine repairs with a prosthetic mesh, a perioperative dose of a first-generation cephalosporin antibiotic is administered. If strangulated bowel is present or if there is a need for

Medical Management of the Surgical Patient, ed. Michael F. Lubin, Thomas F. Dodson, and Neil H. Winawer. Published by Cambridge University Press. © Cambridge University Press 2013.

bowel resection during the herniorrhaphy, postoperative antibiotics with further gram-negative coverage are continued for 24 hours postoperatively when a controlled resection has been performed, or for 5–7 days if peritonitis is present.

Special care

A pressure dressing on the wound minimizes pain. A scrotal support and ice bag to the scrotum may decrease edema.

Postoperative complications

In the hospital

Urinary retention

Some men may be unable to void initially or later at home after the operation. Voiding prior to discharge is imperative. Bladder catheterization may be necessary. Elderly patients with prostate enlargement may occasionally require treatment of this condition before normal urination can resume.

Scrotal hematoma

Extensive dissection of a large or recurrent hernia may lead to the slow development of a scrotal hematoma. Local treatment with ice and elevation is indicated but the need for surgical decompression is rare.

Wound infection

Less than 1% of patients undergoing elective procedures develop wound infections. The number is much higher in patients undergoing concomitant resection of gangrenous small bowel. If a synthetic prosthetic patch has been used to complete the repair, a wound infection may result in removal of the patch and failure of the repair.

Delayed intestinal perforation

If strangulated bowel appears to recover intraoperatively after it is removed from the internal inguinal ring, it is returned to the abdominal cavity. On rare occasions, part of the wall of the returned bowel undergoes necrosis, leading to peritonitis. Immediate laparotomy with segmental resection of the involved loop is indicated.

Urinary leak

Unrecognized injury to the bladder has occurred occasionally after repair of a direct inguinal hernia. Leakage of clear fluid from the incision is pathognomonic and demands immediate operative repair.

After discharge

Hernia recurrence

Open repairs performed with insertion of a synthetic prosthetic mesh have a recurrence rate of only 0.5–1.0%. Laparoscopic repairs performed with insertion of a synthetic prosthetic mesh have a recurrence rate of 0.35–5%, depending on the surgeon's experience.

Migration of mesh plug

Rarely, a mesh plug may migrate into the peritoneal cavity. The plug will need to be removed laparoscopically if it causes symptoms.

Testicular atrophy

Inadvertent ligation of the spermatic vessels or a significant scrotal hematoma may cause ipsilateral testicular atrophy. No treatment is possible.

Further reading

Dulucq JL, Wintringer P, Mahajna A. Laparoscopic totally extraperitoneal inguinal hernia repair: lessons learned from 3,100 hernia repairs over 15 years. *Surg Endosc* 2009; **23**: 482–6.

EU Hernia Trialists Collaboration, Grant A. Laparoscopic compared with open methods of groin hernia repair: systematic review of randomized controlled trials. *Br J Surg* 2000; **87**: 860–7.

Eklund AS, Montgomery AK, Rasmussen IC *et al*. Low recurrence rate after laparoscopic (TEP) and open (Lichtenstein) inguinal hernia repair. *Ann Surg* 2009; **249**: 33–8.

Neumayer L, Giobbie-Hurder A, Jonasson O *et al*. Open mesh versus laparoscopic mesh repair of inguinal hernia. *N Engl J Med* 2004; **350**: 1819–27.

Ramshaw B, Shuler FW, Jones HB *et al*. Laparoscopic inguinal hernia repair: lessons learned after 1224 consecutive cases. *Surg Endosc* 2001; **15**: 50–4.

Stylopoulos N. A cost-utility analysis of treatment options for inguinal hernia in 1,513,008 adult patients. *Surg Endosc* 2003; **17**: 180–9.

Chapter

66

Laparotomy in patients with human immunodeficiency virus infection

Jahnavi K. Srinivasan

Early detection and advances in the medical treatment of patients infected with the human immunodeficiency virus (HIV) has moved the care for many patients from acute to chronic care over the last decade. Accordingly, as in any other immunosuppressed patient, there is no strict contraindication to major abdominal surgery in HIV-positive patients. In general, patients with undetected viral load and CD4 T-cell count greater than 200 mm^3 undergo emergent laparotomy for the same indications as any other individual (gastrointestinal perforation, refractory hemorrhage, ischemia, and complete bowel obstruction). CD4 count less than 200 mm^3 is a predictor for postoperative sepsis and, therefore, additional judgment should be exercised before performing laparotomy because several opportunistic medical infections can mimic peritonitis and potentially can prompt unwarranted exploration. These infections most commonly include mycobacterium avium complex (MAC), cytomegalovirus (CMV), and microsporidia. HIV-positive patients who are immunocompromised are also at increased risk for more uncommon malignancies (non-Hodgkin's lymphoma and Kaposi's sarcoma). HIV-positive patients experience frequent diarrhea (30–60%). Therefore, infectious etiologies for patients with abdominal pain and diarrhea must be investigated to rule them out as causes of acute abdominal pain. Organomegaly may also be a cause of pain in these patients.

One retrospective study has shown that 8% of patients presenting to the emergency room with acute abdominal pain and HIV required abdominal surgery. In the same study, acute abdominal pain in patients with advanced HIV was found to be secondary to opportunistic infections in 10% of the patients. The most common cause of emergency laparotomy in AIDS patients is perforated viscous from CMV. In the absence of a working diagnosis, diagnostic laparoscopy can be considered as an initial means of abdominal exploration to avoid a large laparotomy incision. Common acute abdominal conditions such as appendicitis and cholecystitis should be treated accordingly. In patients with a negative laparotomy result, culture and biopsy of mesenteric lymph nodes is indicated in order to help determine rare infectious etiologies for the development of acute pain.

Both appendicitis and biliary disease remain common causes necessitating acute surgical intervention in patients who are HIV-positive. It is worthwhile to keep in mind that patients with acute appendicitis who are HIV-positive are less likely to manifest a leukocytosis. Accordingly, the delay in diagnosis may result in an increased morbidity for these patients if this is not taken into account. HIV-infected patients also have opportunistic infections of the biliary tree, but these patients generally still have cholelithiasis, and despite the unusual etiology of infectious agents causing cholecystitis or cholangitis, they require cholecystectomy (with preoperative endoscopic retrograde cholangiopancreatography (ERCP) and sphincterotomy if cholangitis is involved).

Usual postoperative course

After operative intervention, patients should undergo continued treatment for any opportunistic infections that were present at the time of surgery. Prophylaxis should be continued for all patients with low CD4 counts, and treatment for hospital-acquired infections should be tailored to culture results. Resumption of antiretroviral treatment should be based upon recommendations of the consulting infectious disease service, and is largely dependent on the ability of the GI tract to tolerate oral medications.

Postoperative complications

There is an inverse relationship between the patient CD4 count and the postoperative complication rate: the lower the patient CD4 count below 200 mm^3, the higher the postoperative complication rate (particularly for wound healing, infection, and sepsis). Depending on the CD4 count, wound healing can be substantially delayed in HIV-positive patients. Mortality, particularly as related to patients with low CD4 counts, has been shown to be substantially higher in HIV-positive patients when compared with non-infected patients receiving the same operative procedure. The most common postoperative complication in the HIV-positive patient is pneumonia.

Further reading

Chambers AJ, Lord RS. Incidence of acquired immune deficiency syndrome (AIDS)-related disorders at laparotomy in patients with AIDS. *Br J Surg* 2001; **88**: 294–7.

Dua RS, Wajed SA, Winslet MC. Impact of HIV and AIDS on surgical practice.
Ann R Coll Surg Engl 2007; **89**: 354–8.

Horberg MA, Hurley LB, Klein DB. Surgical outcomes in human immunodeficiency virus-infected patients in era of highly active antiretroviral therapy. *Arch Surg* 2006: **141**: 1238–45.

Saltzman DJ, Williams RA, Gelfand DV. The surgeon and AIDS: twenty years later. *Arch Surg* 2005; **140**: 961–7.

Yoshida D, Caruso JM. Abdominal pain in the HIV infected patient. *J Emerg Med* 2002; **23**: 111–16.

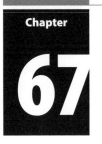

Chapter

67

Abdominal trauma

Jahnavi K. Srinivasan and David V. Feliciano

In patients with blunt abdominal trauma, emergent or urgent laparotomy is performed for hypotension and abdominal hemorrhage (frequently confirmed by diagnostic peritoneal lavage or surgeon-performed ultrasound), overt peritonitis, or obvious signs of abdominal visceral injury without the need for further advanced diagnostic studies. Included are patients with significant blood per rectum after pelvic fracture, evidence of air in the peritoneal cavity or retroperitoneum, intraperitoneal bladder rupture, or renal artery/kidney injury on contrast-enhanced radiographs. All other stable patients whose abdominal examinations are compromised by an abnormal sensorium (related to alcohol, drugs, brain injury), abnormal sensation (due to spinal cord injury), or adjacent injuries are best evaluated by contrasted abdominal helical computed tomography. The use of surgeon-performed ultrasound known as FAST (focused assessment for the sonographic evaluation of the trauma patient) is now routinely performed in all high-volume trauma centers as an adjunct to the secondary survey. The FAST exam has contributed substantially to streamlined algorithms for care of patients assessed after multi-system trauma.

In patients with stab wounds to the abdomen, emergent or urgent laparotomy is performed for abdominal distension and hypotension, overt peritonitis, significant evisceration, or obvious signs of abdominal visceral injury without the need for further advanced diagnostic studies. The last group of patients includes individuals with hematemesis, blood per rectum, or hematuria, patients with a palpable diaphragmatic defect prior to chest tube insertion, and patients with genitourinary injuries detected on contrast-enhanced studies. All other stable and reasonably cooperative patients undergo local exploration of the stab wound to verify peritoneal penetration. Asymptomatic patients with peritoneal penetration can either be watched for 24 hours, undergo a diagnostic peritoneal lavage, or undergo diagnostic laparoscopy to make certain that there is no underlying visceral injury. The diagnosis of intra-abdominal injury is rarely delayed more than 10–12 hours in patients with false-negative results on initial physical examination. Patients who undergo wound exploration that confirms absence of peritoneal penetration can be discharged from the emergency room.

In the past, gunshot wounds thought to traverse the abdominal cavity or visceral/vascular compartment of the retroperitoneum on either physical examination or plain radiograph of the trunk were documented to cause visceral or vascular injuries 96–98% of the time. Several studies, however, have demonstrated safety with observation of a highly selected group of patients who are hemodynamically stable, without peritonitis, and without a clear transabdominal trajectory to the wound. This is presumably due to a broadening of the definition of the abdomen (flanks often included) and to the ever-increasing thickness of the subcutaneous tissue in obese Americans. Therefore, the indications for emergent or urgent laparotomies listed above for stab wounds now apply to gunshot wounds, as well. In asymptomatic patients with gunshot wounds in proximity to the abdomen, either contrast-enhanced helical CT to document the track of the missile or identify actual abdominal injuries or diagnostic laparoscopy to document peritoneal penetration are used at times, especially in obese patients.

General anesthesia is used for trauma laparotomy. After evacuation of blood and clot from the peritoneal cavity, areas of hemorrhage are controlled by manual compression, packing with laparotomy pads, or vascular clamps. Perforations in the gastrointestinal tract are then sealed with non-crushing clamps. The sequence of operative repairs or resections depends on the combination of injuries. Laparotomies for trauma are usually completed in 3 hours or less because longer procedures in previously hypotensive patients can lead to hypothermia, persistent metabolic acidosis, and coagulopathies. These complications can be minimized by performing a "damage control" operation in which shocked patients have control of hemorrhage and gastrointestinal contamination initially, leaving the abdominal incision open with plan for re-exploration once the patient is stabilized. When the patient is adequately resuscitated, visceral reconstructions and closure of the abdominal wall are performed in a series of operations. The need for transfusion is extremely variable, ranging from less than 25% of patients with stab wounds to 50% of patients with gunshot wounds. The stress of the operative procedure depends on the number of organs injured

---

Medical Management of the Surgical Patient, ed. Michael F. Lubin, Thomas F. Dodson, and Neil H. Winawer. Published by Cambridge University Press. © Cambridge University Press 2013.

and the magnitude of blood loss in the perioperative period. Over the last 5 years, the majority of high-volume civilian trauma centers have developed a massive transfusion protocol to guide transfusion in patients arriving in the emergency room with exsanguinating hemorrhage from their injuries. This has helped to minimize trauma-related coagulopathy with demonstration of an improvement in early mortality in some studies.

Usual postoperative course

Expected postoperative hospital stay

Length of stay is variable depending on the injury complex detected at the time of surgery.

Operative mortality

In patients undergoing laparotomy for stab wounds of the abdomen, the mortality rate is 1–2%. The mortality is increased to 3% in patients with routine gunshot wounds, to 25% in patients with major isolated vascular injuries, and to 48% in patients with multiple vascular injuries. Therefore, overall mortality for patients undergoing laparotomy for an abdominal gunshot wound is currently 15% to 17%. In patients requiring an emergency "damage control" laparotomy at a first operation because of profound shock, the mortality is 25–27%.

The mortality after laparotomy for blunt trauma is related to the presence of associated injuries to the brain and chest and to the magnitude of intra-abdominal visceral injuries. For example, the mortality after laparotomy for major blunt hepatic injuries in referral trauma centers ranges from 14–31%.

In all cases of abdominal trauma, mortality is increased in patients with hypothermia, base deficit greater than −15 at presentation to the emergency room, and core body temperature less than 35 °C. Mortality rates from penetrating abdominal trauma have remained somewhat stable over the last decade, with death largely resulting from irreversible shock within the first 24 hours of presentation.

Special monitoring required

Patients with known cardiac or pulmonary compromise and those who undergo difficult procedures associated with excessive blood loss require postoperative hemodynamic monitoring with a pulmonary artery catheter or central venous monitoring in an ICU.

Patient activity and positioning

Patients may be out of bed the day after the operation, depending on hemodynamic stability.

Alimentation

Early enteral feeding through a nasojejunal tube or catheter jejunostomy placed at laparotomy is the standard of care in many centers for patients with major abdominal injury (Penetrating Abdominal Trauma Index 15 to 40 or Injury Severity Score greater than 25 for blunt trauma). Full caloric requirements can be met at 2.5–3 days in properly selected patients, provided there is not a prolonged postoperative ileus or complication requiring the use of pressors. Early enteral feeding has reduced septic morbidity after laparotomy for abdominal trauma in several studies, and has been shown to decrease the incidence of ventilator-associated pneumonia.

In patients with extensive resection of the midgut, marked abdominal distension, or exposure of the midgut under a plastic silo (abdominal wall not closed), early intravenous hyperalimentation may be used in place of enteral feeding. Full caloric requirements can be met at 2–2.5 days in properly selected patients. Disadvantages of intravenous feeding include the fixed rate of long-term catheter infection (3–10%), a higher overall rate of postoperative infection exclusive of catheter infection (possible gut-origin sepsis), and the development of hepatic cholestasis and fatty infiltration.

Antibiotic coverage

Postoperative antibiotics are not routinely administered to patients with blunt abdominal trauma unless rupture of the gastrointestinal tract is found at laparotomy. A second-generation cephalosporin with aerobic and anaerobic coverage is continued for 24 hours in patients who have undergone laparotomy for a penetrating abdominal wound within 8–12 hours of injury. Patients with a long delay between injury and laparotomy and those with extensive fecal contamination are treated for 5–7 days for established peritonitis.

Drains/temporary abdominal wall closure

Suction drains are placed by most surgeons in patients who have undergone repair or resection of a major hepatic injury, repair of a major duodenal or renal injury, or distal pancreatectomy. The duration of drain placement depends on the injury, but typically ranges from 5–7 days in most centers. Patients with initial damage-control laparotomy undergo temporary abdominal wound coverage with a plastic "silo" bag or closed suction abdominal vacuum device until they can be stabilized and returned to the operating room for more definitive closure of the abdominal wall. Prolonged need for an "open abdomen" carries a higher risk of developing an entero-atmospheric fistula and an inability to utilize the enteral tract for nutrition.

Postoperative complications

In the hospital

Wound infection

Infection occurs in 2–3% of patients without colon injuries. If the colon is perforated and moderate to extensive contamination is present, the subcutaneous tissue and skin are packed open in the majority of patients. This substantially decreases the wound infection rate in these high-risk patients.

Intra-abdominal abscess

Abscesses occur in 2.5–3% of patients undergoing laparotomy for abdominal trauma, usually in those with perforation of the stomach (3.9–4%) or small intestine (1–1.5%). When a pancreatic injury occurs in association with an injury to the colon, postoperative abscesses have occurred in up to 58% of patients. Percutaneous drainage by an interventional radiologist is an appropriate first step, followed by reopening of an old drain tract or extraperitoneal surgical drainage if the percutaneous approach fails. Reopening of the midline incision is rarely necessary and carries the highest mortality.

Postoperative hemorrhage

Hemorrhage requiring reoperation occurs in 2–2.5% of patients, almost all of whom had a severe hepatic injury or an intraoperative coagulopathy at the first procedure.

After discharge
Adhesive small bowel obstruction

Similar to those patients who have undergone elective abdominal procedures, late adhesive obstruction occurs in 10–25% of patients.

Incisional hernia

In patients who have undergone only skin closure of the abdominal wall or who have split-thickness skin grafts applied to the open abdomen before discharge, a significant ventral hernia results. Many such patients choose to have reconstruction of the abdominal wall 6–12 months after their original "damage control" procedure. This often requires bilateral myofascial flap mobilization via a "component separation" to allow for primary midline closure without the need for synthetic mesh to close the defect.

Further reading

Chiu WC, Shanmuganathan K, Mirvis SE et al. Determining the need for laparotomy in penetrating torso trauma: a prospective study using triple-contrast enhanced abdominopelvic computed tomography. *J Trauma* 2001; **51**: 860–8.

Davis TP, Feliciano DV, Rozycki GS et al. Results with abdominal vascular trauma in the modern era. *Am Surg* 2001; **67**: 565–70.

Demetriades D, Velmahos G, Cornwell E III et al. Selective nonoperative management of gunshot wounds of the anterior abdomen. *Arch Surg* 1997; **132**: 178–83.

Dente CJ, Shaz BH, Nicholas JM et al. Improvements in early mortality and coagulopathy are sustained better in patients with blunt trauma after institution of a massive transfusion protocol in a civilian trauma center. *J Trauma* 2009; **66**: 1616–24.

Diaz JJ, Cullinane DC, Dutton WD et al. The management of the open abdomen in trauma and emergency general surgery: part 1-damage control. *J Trauma* 2010; **68**: 1425–38.

Kozar RA, Feliciano DV, Moore EE et al. Western Trauma Association/critical decisions in trauma: operative management of adult blunt hepatic injury. *J Trauma* 2011; **71**: 1–5.

Rozycki GS, Ballard RB, Feliciano DV et al. Surgeon-performed ultrasound for assessment of trauma injuries. Lessons learned from 1540 patients. *Ann Surg* 1998; **228**: 557–67.

Tremblay LN, Feliciano DV, Schmidt J et al. Skin only or silo closure in the critically ill patient with an open abdomen. *Am J Surg* 2001; **182**: 670–5.

Chapter

68

Coronary artery bypass procedures

W. Brent Keeling and Vinod H. Thourani

Coronary artery disease (CAD) is a common condition in the USA, but the majority of patients are treated conservatively with pharmacologic and percutaneous coronary interventions (PCI) by interventional cardiologists. However, approximately 150,000 patients in the USA undergo surgical revascularization for treatment of CAD annually. Coronary artery bypass grafting (CABG) is performed for the relief of anginal symptoms and to prolong life. Extended relief of angina can be expected in approximately 90% of those with reasonable distal vessel targets. Coronary artery bypass surgery is indicated in patients with angiographically proven CAD with unstable angina refractory to medical therapy or to percutaneous trans-luminal coronary angioplasty (PTCA), positive results on exercise or thallium stress testing, significant left main coronary artery disease, or complex double or triple-vessel CAD. Coronary artery bypass, when compared with medical therapy, has been shown to provide a survival advantage in patients with left main coronary artery stenosis, triple-vessel disease, double-vessel disease with proximal left anterior descending (LAD) artery stenosis, and in patients with depressed left ventricular function. The recently published results of the multi-institutional randomized SYNTAX (Synergy between Percutaneous Coronary Intervention with Taxus and Cardiac Surgery) trial confirmed that CABG remained the preferred method over PCI for treatment of patients with three-vessel or left main coronary artery disease. In those patients presenting with chest pain and an evolving myocardial infarction of less than 6 hours duration, either percutaneous or surgical revascularization are plausible treatment modalities. Intractable ventricular arrhythmias may be an additional indication for emergent surgical intervention since control of arrhythmias and ultimate survival may result despite the grave prognosis.

Besides routine preoperative laboratory assessment for non-emergent cases, other necessary specific tests include: (1) pulmonary function testing for patients with severe chronic obstructive pulmonary disease; (2) carotid duplex ultrasonography in those patients greater than 65 years of age who have either left main coronary artery disease, symptomatic cerebrovascular disease or carotid bruits, or a previous history of cerebrovascular accident or carotid endarterectomy. Patients with poor left ventricular (LV) function (an ejection fraction (EF) less than 30%) and signs or symptoms of congestive heart failure (CHF) should have hypocontractile areas evaluated for viability utilizing positron-emission tomographic scanning with FDG (fluorodeoxyglucose) imaging or a cardiac MRI. A transthoracic echocardiograph should be obtained in those patients with a cardiac murmur on physical examination or with evidence of structural heart disease on the cardiac catheterization. Smooth induction of general anesthesia with opiates and inhalational agents is necessary to minimize the stress of intubation. The patient can undergo CABG either with the traditional on-pump approach utilizing cardiopulmonary bypass or by the off-pump (OPCAB) technique, the difference being in the use or avoidance of cardiopulmonary bypass in the completion of coronary anastomoses. In OPCAB, the utilization of the latest generation of coronary stabilizing and positioning devices allows a motionless coronary anastomosis with exact precision, while the remaining portions of the heart continue to beat. This procedure has been shown to avoid the inherent adverse consequences of cardiopulmonary bypass.

Following sterile preparation of the skin and draping from the chin to ankles, a median sternotomy is performed. While the left or both internal mammary arteries are harvested, the greater saphenous vein (SVG) and/or radial artery(s) is/are removed utilizing either open or endoscopic harvesting techniques. In those patients undergoing endoscopic conduit harvest, 5,000 IU of intravenous heparin is administered prior to the tunneling process. Following completion of all conduit harvesting, an additional 300 IU/kg is administered for systemic heparization to maintain an active clotting time (ACT) > 300 seconds. Epivascular ultrasound is performed in all patients to rule out a heavily calcified or severely atheromatous ascending aorta. In the conventional on-pump operation (CABG), the ascending aorta and right atrium are cannulated after the patient is systemically heparinized. The patient is then placed on cardiopulmonary bypass and systemically cooled to a core temperature of 34 °C. An aortic crossclamp is placed

Medical Management of the Surgical Patient, ed. Michael F. Lubin, Thomas F. Dodson, and Neil H. Winawer. Published by Cambridge University Press. © Cambridge University Press 2013.

proximal to the aortic cannulation site and myocardial arrest is achieved by utilizing antegrade aortic warm and then cold blood potassium cardioplegia and topical cooling. Myocardial preservation is maintained by redosing cardioplegia via the aortic root every 20 minutes throughout the cross-clamp period (antegrade cardioplegia) or via intermittent or continuous infusion of cardioplegia into the coronary sinus (retrograde cardioplegia). During OPCAB, cardioplegia is not required, since the bypass operation is performed on the beating heart. Blood autotransfusion techniques are utilized to minimize transfusion of banked blood products. Reversed saphenous vein grafts, free radial grafts, or free or in situ internal mammary artery grafts are anastomosed distal to the coronary artery stenoses; while proximal anastomoses of the free grafts are performed to the ascending aorta. The operative strategy for first-time revascularization patients consists of a single left or bilateral internal mammary artery in situ graft(s) (LIMA and/or RIMA) to the LAD and most important lateral wall coronary target, as well as segments of reversed saphenous vein for the remaining required grafts. The radial artery free graft is routinely used in patients with > 75% coronary artery stenosis. Ten-year patency rates may exceed 90% for the LIMA graft, 50–70% for the reverse saphenous vein grafts, and 80% for radial artery grafts.

Patients undergoing on-pump CABG are warmed to normothermia and disconnected from cardiopulmonary bypass following completion of the grafts; during OPCAB, patients are maintained at normothermia. Following restoration of an autogenous heart rate, all cannulae are removed and systemic heparinization is reversed with protamine sulfate. In those patients who require hemodynamic support, inotropic agents or a transcutaneous intra-aortic balloon pump may be necessary. Temporary epicardial pacing wires are placed in patients undergoing isolated CABG only if they require pacing support prior to chest closure. Eighteen French pliable silastic thoracostomy tubes are used in the mediastinum and pleural spaces as necessary for drainage. Following meticulous hemostasis, the patient's sternum is closed with interrupted stainless steel wires and the fascia and skin re-approximated. The operation usually takes 2–4 hours. Patients are either extubated at the conclusion of the procedure or transported to the ICU until extubation occurs some 2–6 hours later.

With the advent of minimally invasive and robotic technology in surgery, coronary revascularization has increasingly been performed using small incisions and minimally invasive means. Most commonly, the left internal mammary artery is harvested from the chest wall using either thoracoscopic or robotic instruments. A small, non-rib spreading anterior thoracotomy is made, and the internal mammary artery is anastomosed to the left anterior descending artery under direct vision. Anastomotic systems including pneumatic-fired clips and individual stainless steel clips can also be used to complete the anastomosis.

Usual postoperative course
Expected postoperative hospital stay
The expected postoperative hospital stay is 3–5 days.

Operative mortality
Operative mortality is from 1–3% for primary CABG. Statistically significant independent predictors of poorer outcome include advanced age, female gender, prior heart surgery, low body mass index, diminished left ventricular ejection fraction, percent stenosis of the left main coronary artery, number of coronary arteries with greater than 70% stenosis, and urgency of operation.

Special monitoring required
In the absence of complications, patients remain in the ICU for 8–24 hours after operation. Healthy, young patients may be transferred to a monitored private room 4–6 hours after OPCAB in selected cases. Arterial blood pressure, electrocardiographic signs, central venous pressure or cardiac index (via Swan–Ganz catheter), urinary output, and chest tube drainage are monitored. Serum potassium and magnesium and hematocrit levels are obtained once on the day of surgery and on postoperative day 1. Arterial blood gases are monitored for extubation criteria. On postoperative day 1, the patient is transferred to a telemetry ward and most invasive monitoring devices are discontinued. The chest tubes are removed when chest drainage is less than 100 mL/tube per 8 hours. Bedside glucose monitoring is performed periodically and subcutaneous or intravenous insulin administered to maintain a glucose level between 100 and 140 mg/dL.

Patient activity and positioning
On the day of operation and while intubated, patients remain on bedrest with the head elevated 30°. After extubation, aggressive pulmonary toilet is performed, including having the patient turn (or turning the patient) from side-to-side every 2 hours and administering bronchodilators and chest physiotherapy. The patient sits at the bedside with assistance as necessary to allow dependent chest tube drainage. On postoperative day 1, the patient is out of bed at mealtime and encouraged to ambulate in the hallway as tolerated.

Alimentation
Clear liquids are permitted after extubation, and food intake is advanced to a low-fat, low-cholesterol, 4 g sodium diet as tolerated. A diabetic diet is provided when appropriate. Mild constipation or nausea are common and are treated with stool softeners and mild anti-emetics.

Antibiotic coverage

Preoperative prophylaxis with a second-generation cephalosporin (cefuroxime), or vancomycin in penicillin-allergic patients, is initiated within 1 hour prior to skin incision and continued for 24 hours after surgery.

Routine postoperative medications

All patients are transferred to the telemetry ward with beta-blockers (metoprolol 25 mg by mouth every 8 hours), enteric-coated aspirin (162 mg by mouth every 24 hours), 2% mupirocin topical nasal gel every 12 hours, chlorhexidine mouthwash (15 mL swish and spit every 12 hours), and simvastatin (40 mg by mouth every evening). Those patients undergoing OPCAB receive clopidogrel 150 mg on the day of surgery when the chest tube output is less than 150 mL per hour for 2 contiguous hours. Thereafter, the patients receive 75 mg by mouth every day for 3–6 months. In those patients undergoing on-pump CABG, clopidogrel (75 mg by mouth every day) is administered starting on postoperative day 1 for 3–6 months.

Pulmonary toilet

Intensive pulmonary toilet post-extubation is performed to prevent atelectasis and pneumonia, including chest physical therapy every 4 hours, incentive spirometry every 1 hour, bronchodilators every 4 hours, and cough and deep breathe exercises every 2 hours while awake.

Postoperative complications

In the hospital

Perioperative myocardial infarction

Advances in intraoperative myocardial protection, including antegrade and retrograde cardioplegic protection, have significantly reduced the incidence of perioperative myocardial infarction (MI) over the last 20 years to a current rate well under 5%. Acute postoperative myocardial ischemia occurs infrequently, but may be seen in patients with acute coronary occlusion, early graft failure, or incomplete revascularization. New-onset acute changes of the patient's electrocardiogram warrant immediate attention and investigation. Serial troponin levels are not generally warranted postoperatively unless the patient has significant EKG changes.

Low cardiac output

A cardiac index (CI) below 2.0 L/min per m^2 or a mixed venous oxygen saturation (SvO$_2$) from the pulmonary artery catheter less than 65% requires therapeutic interventions. Common causes of postoperative low CI include decreased LV preload, preexisting poor LV function, or acute right or left ventricular dysfunction. Other less common causes include postoperative myocardial ischemia or cardiac tamponade. Therapeutic interventions include administration of fluid or red blood cells, optimization of the heart rate to 90–100 beats/min (utilizing epicardial pacing or pharmacologic means), or the administration of inotropic agents (epinephrine, dobutamine, milrinone, dopamine). If the initial therapeutic maneuvers are unsuccessful, transthoracic or transesophageal echocardiography should be performed to exclude the presence of cardiac tamponade. A final therapeutic step is the deployment of a transcutaneous intra-aortic balloon pump via the femoral artery to decrease afterload and to augment diastolic coronary perfusion and cardiac index.

Arrhythmias

Transient conduction abnormalities are frequent following cardiac surgery. The most common aberrations are sustained tachycardia, atrial fibrillation or flutter, and various degrees of atrioventricular blockade, as well as premature ventricular beats, sustained or non-sustained ventricular tachycardia and, less frequently, ventricular fibrillation. Contributing factors include the severity of CAD, duration of aortic cross-clamping and cardiopulmonary bypass, adequacy of myocardial protection, depth of myocardial hypothermia, patient age, severe left ventricular dysfunction (ejection fraction less than 30%), and complex valvular or multiple valvular operations. The most common conduction abnormality is sustained sinus tachycardia, which is treated by correcting the underlying cause (pain, anxiety, low cardiac output, anemia, fever, or beta-blocker withdrawal). Postoperative ventricular arrhythmias range from occasional premature beats to bigeminy, trigeminy, sustained ventricular tachycardia, and ventricular fibrillation. Prophylactic correction of hypoxemia, acidosis, hypokalemia, and hypomagnesemia is particularly important in the immediate postoperative period. Ventricular tachycardia generally responds to beta-blockers and/or intravenous amiodarone. Immediate cardioversion followed by resuscitation and antiarrhythmic therapy is essential for treatment of sustained ventricular tachycardia and ventricular fibrillation. Rarely, patients may require an implanted automatic internal cardiac defibrillator prior to discharge.

Atrial fibrillation and atrial flutter occur in 10–30% of patients following cardiac surgery; these conditions are most commonly seen on the second postoperative day. Acidosis, hypokalemia, hypomagnesemia, or hypoxemia may contribute to the onset of this arrhythmia and should be corrected. The prophylactic use of beta-blockers or amiodarone has been shown to have a protective effect against the development of atrial fibrillation or flutter. Treatment in stable patients involves control of the ventricular rate and conversion to sinus rhythm utilizing beta-blocker therapy combined with intravenous infusions of sotalol, diltiazem, or amiodarone. Immediate electrical cardioversion is recommended for unstable, symptomatic patients. Within 1–3 days, 80% of patients who develop postoperative atrial fibrillation will return to sinus rhythm with beta-blocker therapy alone; only approximately 10% require electrical cardioversion. Among those who do not convert to sinus rhythm prior to hospital discharge, most will revert to sinus rhythm during the next 1–3 months on coumadin and anti-arrhythmic therapy. Patients who remain in atrial fibrillation require anticoagulation since there is a two- or threefold increase in the risk of stroke with long-term atrial fibrillation.

Pulmonary embolism

The incidence of pulmonary embolism following open heart surgery is low and ranges from 0.56% to 2%. The incidence of deep vein thrombosis is equally distributed between the donor leg for saphenous vein harvest and the opposite limb. Significant risk factors include prolonged pre- or postoperative bedrest, previous venous thromboembolism, obesity, and hyperlipidemia. To prevent a preoperative deep venous thrombosis, patients who are bedridden for a prolonged period of time and are not on an intravenous anti-coagulant should be administered bilateral lower extremity sequential compression devices and SQ low molecular weight heparins. Patients who are bedridden postoperatively secondary to mechanical ventilation should have weekly duplex scanning. Hospital mortality in patients who experience pulmonary emboli ranges between 19% and 34%.

Pleural effusion

Blood or serous fluid may accumulate in the pleural cavities following thoracostomy tube removal prior to discharge from the hospital. Significant effusions should be treated by thoracentesis or thoracostomy tube in order to allow the lung to completely expand and to reduce the risk of infection in the compressed lung. Undrained pleural effusions may become organized and require thoracoscopic decortication.

Pneumonia/bronchitis

While 70% of patients undergoing cardiac surgery may develop postoperative atelectasis, pneumonia occurs in only 4%. The most important preoperative predictors for pneumonia include underlying pulmonary disease, COPD, ongoing smoking, and advanced age. Pain associated with sternotomy or the presence of chest tubes interferes with normal respiratory function and thus impairs deep breathing, possibly contributing to the development of atelectasis and/or pneumonia. The diagnosis is suspected in patients with postoperative fever, leukocytosis, and purulent sputum. Identification of pathogenic organisms by gram stain or culture of the sputum or blood and presence of an infiltrate on chest X-ray confirm the diagnosis. Immediate treatment with intravenous broad-spectrum antibiotics is followed by organism-specific antibiotic therapy. Chest physiotherapy and pulmonary toilet are performed to facilitate clearance of pulmonary secretions. Preventative measures include incentive spirometry, antibiotic prophylaxis, bronchodilators (in patients with chronic bronchitis), and preoperative cessation of smoking.

Neurologic complications

Cognitive dysfunction, atypical behavior, and delirium occur in up to 75% of patients in the immediate postoperative period, but nearly all patients regain full cognitive function within 6 months. However, 7% of patients may demonstrate moderate to severe psychometric abnormalities at late follow-up, and approximately 1% are unable to return to work and normal daily activities. Disabling stroke occurs in about 2% of patients while 3% experience transient ischemic events. The mechanisms associated with neurologic complications following open heart surgery include macroembolization of debris from aortic atheroma or left ventricular thrombus; microembolization of aggregates of granulocytes, platelets, and fibrin; air embolism; and cerebral hypoperfusion. Radiologic evaluation utilizing head CT scan or magnetic resonance imaging is used to make the diagnosis. Focal neurologic deficits resulting from intraoperative events are usually noted within the first 24–48 hours and are treated with measures to decrease intracerebral pressure, along with expectant, supportive care. Massive intra-operative air embolism may be effectively treated with emergency hyperbaric therapy.

Phrenic nerve injury

Although the exact incidence of phrenic nerve injuries following coronary surgery is difficult to quantify, approximately 2% of patients appear to be affected. The etiology may include stretch injuries from prolonged, extreme opening of the chest retractor, direct injury during harvest of the internal mammary artery, or cold injury from topical ice slush. The diagnosis is usually suspected by a high diaphragmatic shadow on chest roentogram. Nerve conduction and fluoroscopic studies are used to confirm the diagnosis. Clinical sequelae of unilateral phrenic nerve paralysis include atelectasis, dyspnea on exertion, and pneumonia. Bilateral phrenic paralysis may lead to prolonged respiratory dependence and may require tracheostomy. Most phrenic nerve injuries resolve over a 6- to 18-month period.

Gastrointestinal symptoms

Following CABG, gastrointestinal (GI) complications range from 0.41–2%. These are generally thought to be a consequence of an overall low flow state resulting from decreased cardiac output, and are often associated with respiratory and renal failure. Macroembolism or thrombosis of mesenteric vessels may also be an important etiology. The severity of symptoms is masked by metabolic disturbances and the inability of the sedated, intubated patient to complain, thus leading to a delay in diagnosis. Early recognition and treatment is imperative for treatment of GI complications.

Gastrointestinal hemorrhage

The incidence of GI hemorrhage following CABG ranges from 0.35–3% and usually occurs during the first postoperative month. Although gastritis or peptic ulcers are the most common sources, other causes include esophagitis, ischemic bowel disease, diverticulitis, and arteriovenous malformations. Advanced age and a prior history of GI hemorrhage are the most reliable preoperative predictors of postoperative bleeding. While melena is the most common symptom, hematemesis may also occur. Upper GI hemorrhage sources present more commonly; therefore upper GI endoscopy should be initially performed to guide therapy. GI hemorrhage following CABG is associated with a high mortality rate, ranging up to 75%.

Perforated ulcer

A perforated duodenal or gastric ulcer following CABG occurs in 0.02–0.08% of patients and is usually diagnosed by free intra-abdominal air on a routine upright chest X-ray. Some patients complain of upper abdominal pain and many patients have a previous history of ulcer disease. Most patients with a perforated ulcer are treated with prompt surgical intervention consisting of an omental patch surgical repair. Mortality ranges from 30–50%, reflecting a frequent delay in diagnosis and the subsequent development of sepsis.

Biliary complications

The incidence of cholecystitis following CABG ranges from 0.2–0.5%. Affected patients usually develop symptoms 5–15 days after the procedure and report fever, nausea, and vague, diffuse abdominal pain. Abdominal ultrasonography and cholescintigraphy (HIDA scanning) are the most common diagnostic tests utilized. If the patient is stable, cholecystectomy often is necessary. Percutaneous cholecystostomy and broad-spectrum antibiotics may be more appropriate in severely unstable, septic patients.

Pancreatitis

Although 25–30% of patients undergoing coronary artery bypass procedures may have asymptomatic hyperamylasemia, only 1–2% develop clinical pancreatitis. Even fewer of these patients (0.13–0.6%) develop necrotizing pancreatitis. Pancreatitis generally occurs within a few days after operation; symptoms include fever, nausea, epigastric pain, and leukocytosis with elevated serum amylase and lipase levels. The diagnosis is largely based on clinical grounds, but abdominal computed tomography may assist in evaluating pancreatic morphology and areas of necrosis. Patients with mild pancreatitis receive supportive treatment with intravenous fluids and bowel rest until clinical symptoms resolve. Necrotizing pancreatitis requires enteral feeding and immediate surgical debridement of the pancreas with wide drainage. The mortality rate of necrotizing pancreatitis usually exceeds 50%.

Ischemic colitis

The incidence of ischemic colitis after CABG is estimated to be 0.02–0.3%. The condition typically presents 6 or more days after operation. Advanced age, generalized peripheral vascular disease, the need for emergency surgery, and a period of perioperative hypotension may contribute to the development of ischemic colitis. Signs and symptoms include abdominal distension (often abrupt), severe abdominal pain, vomiting, extreme leukocytosis, and melena. Sigmoidoscopy, computed tomography, laparoscopy, and arteriography may be used for diagnosis and/or treatment. If surgical intervention is performed, the necrotic bowel is excised. The overall mortality for this population ranges between 50% and 95%. Early diagnosis and surgical intervention are essential for a successful outcome.

Diverticulitis

Following open-heart surgery, the incidence of diverticulitis is 0.13–0.25%. The majority of patients have a prior history of diverticulosis or diverticulitis; perioperative splanchnic hypoperfusion is believed to be an inciting factor. Clinical symptoms include fever, leukocytosis, left lower quadrant pain, and abdominal distension. Endoscopy or computed tomography aid in the diagnosis. Intravenous antibiotics and bowel rest are recommended for treatment of non-perforated diverticulitis; segmental colectomy and diverting colostomy are performed for perforated diverticulitis. The overall mortality for those with perforated diverticulitis is approximately 25%.

Hepatic derangements

In approximately 15–20% of cardiopulmonary bypass patients, serum levels of hepatic enzymes are transiently elevated between the second and fourth postoperative days. This rise in enzymes is plausibly related to mechanical blood trauma, hepatic congestion, and hypoperfusion during bypass. Despite this rise in hepatic enzymes, less than 0.5% of patients develop significant hepatic dysfunction as a feature of multisystem organ failure.

Postoperative renal insufficiency

Approximately 15% of patients develop evidence of renal dysfunction following cardiac surgery. Renal blood flow and glomerular filtration rate may be reduced by 25–75% during cardiopulmonary bypass, with partial recovery in the first postoperative day. While many patients suffer mild, transient renal dysfunction, severe renal failure requiring dialysis occurs in 1.5–3.0% of patients. This complication is intimately related to preoperative renal function, postoperative cardiac output, ischemic periods during operation, preoperative administration of radiographic contrast materials, and nephrotoxic medicines. Treatment requires optimization of cardiac output, management of fluid balance, avoidance of nephrotoxic drugs, and prevention of infection. Venovenous hemofiltration may be used to correct fluid and electrolyte imbalances and is not dependent on cardiac output. Renoprotective agents used to prevent or treat renal ischemia include mannitol, lasix, and sodium bicarbonate. The mortality rate among patients who develop severe, acute renal failure is approximately 45%.

Postoperative metabolic disorders

Hypokalemia

Hypokalemia commonly occurs following cardiac surgery and has important effects on the electrical activity of the heart. The large and rapid fluid shifts during and after cardiac surgery are in part responsible for aberrations in serum potassium levels. Hypokalemia is treated with intravenous KCl at a rate of no more than 20 Meq/hour to maintain a serum level of at least 4.0 Meq/L.

Hypomagnesemia

Hypomagnesemia, which mimics potassium in its effects on the electrical activity of the heart, generally occurs following cardiac surgery. Preoperative use of loop diuretics, thiazides, digoxin, or alcohol may also be causes of hypomagnesemia. Affected patients have an increased risk of atrial and ventricular dysrhythmias, which may lead to decreased stroke volume and cardiac index. Intravenous magnesium sulfate should be administered to raise the serum levels to 2 Meq/L.

Hyperglycemia

The inherent surgical stress associated with CABG leads to a rise in blood glucose levels due to increased glucose mobilization related to elevations in cortisol, catecholamine, and growth hormone levels and to the apparent failure of insulin secretion during hypothermia. These mechanisms are present in non-diabetic patients, and are exaggerated in patients with diabetes. A strict protocol utilizing continuous intravenous insulin and sliding scale supplementation is utilized to maintain blood glucose between 100–140 mg/dL. Administration of oral anti-hyperglycemic agents is delayed until the patient is on the telemetry ward, preparing to leave the hospital.

Mediastinal hemorrhage

Two to 3% of patients undergoing open-heart surgery require re-exploration for bleeding. Thoracostomy tubes are placed in the pleural space(s) and mediastinum and are monitored carefully after the procedure for output volumes. When moderate postoperative mediastinal hemorrhage occurs, the platelet count, partial thromboplastin time, prothrombin time, INR (international normalized ratio), and fibrinogen levels are measured. An elevated prothrombin time or INR indicates a defect in the extrinsic coagulation pathway, which is treated with fresh frozen plasma to maintain an INR < 1.5. Secondary to the functional deficit in most of the circulating platelets following cardiopulmonary bypass, platelet transfusions are prescribed in bleeding patients for counts under 100,000/μL. Supplemental cryoprecipitate is administered if the fibrinogen is below 200 mg/dL. Additional maneuvers include warming the patient, increasing the positive end expiratory pressure (PEEP) on the ventilator to 10–15 cm H_2O in an attempt to tamponade venous bleeding sites, and aggressive control of hypertension. Although it may be expensive, recombinant Factor VIIa acts on both the intrinsic and extrinsic pathways to promptly restore normal coagulation in cases of severe coagulopathy unresponsive to more conventional therapy. Re-exploration is indicated if sudden massive bleeding occurs or if excessive chest tube drainage persists during the first few hours after operation. In approximately two-thirds of patients who are re-explored no surgical bleeding source is found, and the hemorrhage is secondary to coagulopathy.

Infection

Sternal wound complications represent a serious morbidity associated with coronary surgery. They occur in 0.5–4% of cases; multiple risk factors include pneumonia, emphysema/chronic obstructive pulmonary disease, prolonged mechanical ventilation (especially with tracheostomy), emergency operations, postoperative hemorrhage with mediastinal hematoma, early re-exploration, obesity, diabetes mellitus, and use of bilateral internal mammary grafts.

Deep sternal wound infections include acute mediastinitis with sternal dehiscence and osteomyelitis of the sternum. The incidence of deep wound infection following sternotomy ranges from 0.4–4% and is usually apparent 2–4 weeks postoperatively. Presenting signs and symptoms include wound drainage, fever, sternal instability, excessive wound pain, leukocytosis, and dehiscence. Any drainage from the wound should be cultured. The clinical signs and character of wound drainage usually suffice for both the diagnosis and localization of the infected tissues; thoracic computed tomography, while unnecessary to make the diagnosis, can be helpful in determining the extent of infection and the proximity of underlying cardiac structures should additional surgery be warranted. Appropriate antibiotics are given intravenously before and up to 4 or 6 weeks after the wound is opened and drained. Although debate continues regarding the most appropriate initial treatment, our institution prefers plastic surgical closure with an immediate pectoralis myocutaneous advancement flap.

Patients who have undergone CABG rarely experience leg wound infections that necessitate extra care. Leg infections seem to occur more frequently in obese women, especially if the thigh veins are harvested. The routine use of endoscopic vein harvest has been associated with a significant reduction in the incidence of this complication.

After discharge
Constrictive pericarditis

Following cardiac surgery, constrictive pericarditis complicates approximately 0.2–0.3% of all operations. While the etiology of the process remains unclear, the disease may progress to a fibrotic, pericardial shell around the heart. Patients complain of dyspnea with minimal exertion, fatigue, and peripheral edema, which may present from 2 weeks to years after surgery. Symptoms and signs are non-specific, and the ECG often shows non-specific ST segment changes. The chest X-ray may show cardiomegaly. Echocardiography, MRI, and CT scan all demonstrate pericardial thickening and occasional pericardial calcium. The most common echocardiographic findings show biatrial dilation, small to normal ventricular size, and a shell of pericardium. Right heart catheterization with elevated atrial and ventricular pressures can be diagnostic.

Corticosteroids and non-steroid anti-inflammatory agents generally are ineffective in preventing constrictive pericarditis in patients with the postpericardiotomy syndrome, but a tapered dose of corticosteroids is recommended in patients with constrictive pericarditis presenting within 2 months of operation. Persistent symptoms after 2 weeks of steroids, presentation after 2 months, or compromised hemodynamic condition are indications for surgical pericardiectomy. In the majority of cases, immediate improvement in performance occurs after subtotal pericardiectomy.

Incisional pain

Postoperative pain is usually transient and can be controlled with oral analgesics. Parasternal numbness may persist for up to 12 months after inferior mesenteric artery harvesting.

Sternal problems

Sternal mobility (clicking) is increased with exertion and coughing. This complication generally resolves in 6–12 weeks as the sternum heals. Infrequently, a sterile non-union may develop and the sternum may need to be rewired. Occasionally, patients complain of a painful sternal wire in the absence of inflammation or infection. This condition can be treated during brief general anesthesia by removal of the wire (or all wires), using small skin incision(s) over each offending wire. If purulent discharge is encountered, proper evaluation for deep sternal wound infection is performed.

Leg edema

The majority of coronary artery bypass patients are discharged from the hospital with some degree of lower leg edema either from the saphenous vein harvest and/or from fluid retention. Excess fluid is controlled with leg elevation, support hose, and diuresis, and generally resolves within a few months.

Peripheral nerve injuries

The reported incidence of upper extremity peripheral nerve injuries ranges from 2–18%. Most of these injuries are attributed to stretching or compression during sternal retraction and involve brachial plexus roots C8 and T1. Other causes include injury from the fractured end of a first rib or injury by needle trauma from a jugular vein cannulation. Ulnar or, more rarely, radial neuropathies may occur after general anesthesia,

even when appropriate precautions are taken with arm positioning, padding, and protection. Most of these injuries become apparent in the first postoperative week when the patient complains of numbness, decreased sensation, or motor strength of the affected part. Such deficits usually resolve spontaneously over 6 weeks to 6 months. Injuries that are slow to resolve require further evaluation by a neurologist.

Peripheral nerve injuries in the lower extremities may occur from saphenous vein harvest trauma and are often attributed to injury of the saphenous nerve. The sensory deficit includes diminished sensation to the medial fore-foot and ankle and usually improves within 1 to 3 months. Injuries to the sciatic, femoral, or common peroneal nerves may occur from needle puncture, compression, or lack of protection over the head of the fibula; these injuries may result in considerable disability.

Recurrent angina

Recurrent angina may be caused by incomplete revascularization, graft closure, or progression of native coronary disease. Unless it is contraindicated, all patients who have undergone CABG are administered daily aspirin to prolong graft patency. Repeat coronary angiography may be necessary to evaluate the source of angina. Repeat angioplasty or bypass surgery is rarely required in the period immediately after the initial procedure.

Postcardiotomy syndrome

The incidence of the postcardiotomy or postpericardiotomy syndrome is approximately 18% and decreases with advancing age. Although it is not well understood, the etiology appears to be an autoimmune inflammatory phenomenon. Symptoms usually develop within the first month after operation; the most common presentation includes fever, pleuritic pain, malaise, and a pericardial friction rub. Some patients develop pleural or pericardial effusions or painful swallowing. The disease may progress to pericardial effusion and, infrequently, to constrictive pericarditis. The differential diagnosis includes atelectasis, pneumonia, endocarditis, and wound infection. A mild leukocytosis may be present, and the ECG may show diffuse non-specific ST segment elevation. The disease is self-limited, with a mean duration of symptoms lasting 1 month; up to 20% of patients develop a recurrence. Patients are encouraged to limit activity and are prescribed analgesics for pain and NSAIDs for anti-inflammatory effects. Severe symptoms may require a tapered dose of corticosteroids.

Further reading

Brown WM, Jones EL. First operation for myocardial revascularization. In Edmunds LH Jr, ed. *Cardiac Surgery in the Adult*. 1st edn. New York: McGraw-Hill; 1997, p. 535.

Eagle KA, Guyton RA, Davidoff R *et al*. ACC/AHA 2004 guideline update for coronary artery bypass graft surgery: summary article. A report of the American College of Cardiology/ American Heart Association Task Force on Practice Guidelines

(Committee to Update the 1999 Guidelines for Coronary Artery Bypass Graft Surgery). *J Am Coll Cardiol* 2004; **44**: e213–e310.

Guyton RA. Coronary artery bypass. In Morris PJ, Wood WC, eds. *Oxford*

Textbook of Surgery. 2nd edn. Oxford: Oxford University Press; 2000, **40.8.3**.

Lattouf OM, Thourani VH, Kilgo PD *et al*. Influence of on-pump versus off-pump techniques and completeness of revascularization on long-term survival after coronary artery bypass. *Ann Thorac Surg* 2008; **86**: 797–805.

Lytle BW. Coronary bypass surgery. In Fuster V, Alexander RW, O'Rourke RA, eds. *Hurst's The Heart*. 10th edn. New York, NY: McGraw-Hill; 2001, p. 1507.

Puskas JD, Thourani VH, Marshall JJ *et al*. Clinical outcomes, angiographic patency, and resource utilization in 200 consecutive off-pump coronary bypass patients. *Ann Thorac Surg* 2001; **71**: 1477–83; discussion 1483–4.

Puskas JD, Thourani VH, Kilgo P *et al*. Off-pump coronary artery bypass disproportionately benefits high-risk patients. *Ann Thorac Surg* 2009; **88**: 1142–7.

Chapter

69

Cardiac rhythm management

Omar M. Lattouf

Therapeutic, device-aided cardiac rhythm management is useful in patients with a variety of rhythm- and rate-related abnormalities, leading to reduction of symptoms of cardiac dysfunction and improvement in quality of life. Single-chamber atrial pacing has been commonly utilized in the treatment of patients with sinus pauses, sick sinus syndrome (sinus node dysfunction), and bradycardia–tachycardia syndrome. As long as AV (atrioventricular) synchrony is maintained and there is no AV block, this method has been noted to be efficacious and safe. If AV block does develop, atrial pacing will not prevent bradycardia. In such cases, ventricular pacing would be required as part of dual chamber pacing (i.e., atrioventricular pacing) or as standalone ventricular pacing. For prevention of atrial fibrillation, dual-site atrial pacing has been shown to be valuable as an adjunct to drug therapy in reducing the incidence of paroxysmal atrial fibrillation.

Single-chamber ventricular pacing has been utilized in patients with high-grade AV block, Mobitz type II, or third-degree heart block. It is usually reserved for patients who are not candidates for dual chamber AV pacing due to other comorbid factors that significantly reduce life expectancy or physical abilities. A major limiting factor for the utilization of this method is the occasional development of pacemaker syndrome, which occurs due to retrograde electrical current conduction through the AV node to the atria. This syndrome causes discordant premature contraction of the atria during the closed phase of the AV valve, with resultant decreased cardiac output. Weakness, dizziness, or even frank syncope are symptoms of this condition.

Currently, dual-chamber pacing is the most commonly applied therapeutic method. In dual chamber pacing, native atrial activity is sensed and transmitted through the atrial lead into the pacemaker unit, initiating an appropriate ventricular stimulating signal down the ventricular wire into the right ventricle in accordance with a preprogrammed time interval. In the absence of a sensed atrial signal, the dual chamber pacer will initiate coordinated timed signals to the atrium and subsequently to the ventricle, resulting in coordinated and specifically timed atrial ventricular contraction.

Right ventricular pacing has also been reported to benefit patients with hypertrophic obstructive cardiomyopathy and documented left ventricular outflow tract gradient.

Cardiac resynchronization therapy

An atrial–biventricular resynchronization technique with optimization of AV delay has been shown to improve systolic function, overall cardiac function, and to reduce mitral regurgitation. Biventricular resynchronization has become acceptable therapy for patients with symptomatic or asymptomatic congestive heart failure (CHF) if the ejection fraction on echocardiography is < 35%, irrespective of the underlying etiology whether ischemic or idiopathic. Biventricular resynchronization is often part of a biventricular pacing–defibrillation implantable technology.

Automatic implantable cardiac defibrillator

Implantable cardiac defibrillators are indicated and increasingly utilized in the management of patients with sudden cardiac death and other serious ventricular dysrhythmias. Patients who are acceptable candidates for automatic implantable cardiac defibrillator (AICD) implantation are those at high risk of ventricular arrhythmia, indicated by the following conditions: non-sustained ventricular tachycardia with decreased left ventricular (LV) function due to coronary artery disease, valvular dysfunction or idiopathic cardiomyopathy; poor LV function and an ejection fraction less than 30% due to prior myocardial infarction; prior history of aborted sudden death due to cardiac dysrhythmias.

Operative technique for implantation of cardiac rhythm management devices

Percutaneous transvenous radiographic-guided lead placement has essentially replaced the more invasive surgical thoracotomy-based epicardiac lead implantation. Nevertheless, a surgical incision to create a subcutaneous pocket for the battery implantation is still required. In some cases surgical access and epicardiac lead implantation via a mini-thoracotomy, thoracoscopic

Medical Management of the Surgical Patient, ed. Michael F. Lubin, Thomas F. Dodson, and Neil H. Winawer. Published by Cambridge University Press. © Cambridge University Press 2013.

technique, or a sub-xyphoidal approach is required, particularly in cases where the transvenous route is inaccessible due to unfavorable anatomy, thrombosed subclavian vein, or persistent left superior vena cava. More recently, electrophysiology (EP) cardiologists have become hesitant to insert percutaneous transvenous pacing hardware in patients with renal failure who are hemodialysis dependent. These patients are thought to be at high risk for bacterial colonization of their indwelling transvenous devices and subsequent development of intravascular or intra-cardiac device endocarditis, due to frequent instrumentation of their venous circulatory system during hemodialysis. Device-related endocarditis is a life-threatening problem that does not respond to intravenous antibiotic therapy; invariably, it will require complex extraction of all of the implanted pacing-defibrillating hardware. Removal of percutaneous transvenous pacing hardware is complex and expensive. There are inherent risks of tearing vascular or cardiac structures during extraction; if the patient is device-dependent, replacement would still be required. For these reasons, epicardiac lead and device implantation has become the procedure of choice at our institution for patients who are hemodialysis-dependent, since these devices would not come in direct contact with the bloodstream and are therefore less likely to become sites for hematogenously introduced bacterial inoculation.

The energy source is usually implanted in the left infra-clavicular area either subcutaneously or in the subpectoral region. For atrial sensing and pacing, an atrial lead is typically positioned in the right atrial appendage. The right ventricular lead is positioned in the ventricular apex. In cases of biventricular resynchronization, the aforementioned two leads are combined with a third lead that is inserted transvenously into the coronary sinus for pacing the left ventricle. With the impulse delivered at the lateral left ventricular wall, this third lead paces the left ventricle.

In surgical epicardiac lead placement, the energy source commonly is placed in the left upper quadrant of the abdomen, away from the rib cage. In cases where the patient has had a prior unsuccessful attempt for endocardiac LV lead placement but successful placement of right-sided leads, the pacemaker energy source is usually placed in the left infra-clavicular position. Occasionally (and for various reasons), the energy source may be in the right infra-clavicular area or in the right upper abdominal area. Pacemaker energy sources should not be placed against the rib cage; this placement would cause pain and discomfort to the patient, particularly in the recumbent position.

An AICD placement has likewise become technically straightforward, and is similar to pacemaker implantation. As with pacemaker implantation, the procedure is carried out under strict antiseptic technique, employing local anesthesia with additional intravenous sedation. The right ventricular lead (sensing, pacing, and defibrillation) is inserted via the subclavian or cephalic vein and directed toward the apex. A right atrial lead is inserted as needed in the usual fashion.

Prior to the completion of the procedure, the device is tested for sensing, defibrillation, and pacing. In rare situations, external defibrillation patches are applied on the epicardiac surface of the heart in candidate patients. Patients with an occluded superior vena cava, patients in need of replacement defibrillators after removal of infected endocardiac defibrillation hardware, or patients at high risk of developing intracardiac hardware endocarditis (i.e., dialysis dependent renal failure patients) may require the placement of patches.

Local anesthesia and intravenous sedation are commonly used for percutaneously performed procedures. General anesthesia with double lumen intubation is required if thoracotomy or thoracoscopic approaches are utilized for lead placement. Subxyphoid surgical approaches and, often, mini thoracotomy procedures may be performed with the use of single lumen intubation.

Usual postoperative course
Expected postoperative hospital stay

Patients undergoing percutaneous device insertion may be observed for several hours. After ensuring for hemodynamic stability and the absence of hemo- or pneumothorax, they can be discharged to reliable family. Patients with other comorbid factors are often kept overnight in the hospital to ensure their hemodynamic stability, pain control, and ability to cope with the operative stress.

Operative mortality

Operative or procedure-related mortality after pacemaker or defibrillator lead implantation is exceedingly rare.

Special monitoring required

Postoperative chest X-ray and ECG are routinely performed. Occasionally a transthoracic echocardiogram is performed to document the absence of pericardial fluid collection. Prior to patient discharge from the hospital the pacemaker/defibrillator is interrogated to ensure its appropriate sensing/pacing/defibrillation programming as the case may be.

Patient activity and positioning

The patient undergoing percutaneous lead placement is placed in the supine position in the operating room. Oxygen is provided to the awake patient via nasal prongs or facial mask. Full vital sign monitoring with oxygen saturation is ensured during awake–sedation procedures. The patient's head and face should be easily accessible to the anesthetist in case the patient experiences respiratory or hemodynamic challenges requiring intubation.

Post-procedure, patients are always encouraged to ambulate on the same day of surgery to improve ventilation and to reduce the risk of deep vein thromboses and the potential for pulmonary emboli.

Alimentation

As in all cases where anesthetic is used, patients should refrain from food and liquid intake until they are fully awake and alert. Avoidance of aspiration is crucial following an operative procedure because it can substantially complicate postoperative care and put the patient's health and life at risk. A fully awake patient may start with sips of liquid as tolerated and advance to the usual diet.

Antibiotic coverage

One of the biggest and most dreaded potential problems complicating device insertion is surgical site infection. In our practice we have regularly utilized meticulous prepping of the incision site and attentive sterile draping with only the immediate surgical field exposed. The surgical field should be covered by transparent antiseptic eluting drape. To ensure adequate tissue levels prior to incision, antibiotics are administered within 1 hour of incision. We routinely continue perioperative antibiotic coverage for 24 hours. Patients are given cephalosporin or, in case of penicillin allergy, Vancomycin as the prophylactic antibiotic.

Postoperative visits

Prior to discharge, patients are instructed on methods of wound care and are asked to immediately call or report to the nearest emergency department should they develop fever, wound infection, respiratory difficulty, or hypotension. Patients are routinely seen in the surgeon's office within 1 month of discharge and are followed up by the referring cardiologist for outpatient device interrogation to ensure continued device function as intended.

Postoperative complications

In the hospital

Infection

Infection remains as the biggest concern in device implantation, although it is increasingly rare due to the aggressive attention to aseptic techniques, the use of prophylactic antibiotics and the avoidance of undue tissue trauma (as well as attention to homeostasis). Any device infection is fraught with complications, prolonged morbidity, added cost, and the need for additional complex procedures to extirpate the device and its components. Every effort should be made to pay extreme attention to avoid wound-related problems. When surgical site infection manifests, early intervention is mandatory.

Perforation

Bleeding, hemothorax, or pericardial tamponade secondary to vascular, right atrial, or right ventricular perforation during lead insertion may occur; this complication should be watched for and avoided. If perforation is suspected, serial echocardiogram should be obtained immediately to ensure that no pericardial effusion has developed. Perforation-related pericardial effusion can create life-threatening situations, and should be a cause for immediate surgical consultations. Occasionally, a percutaneously placed pericardial drain is sufficient to drain the accumulating blood until the perforation self-seals. Our recommended approach is to initiate surgical consultation. Serial echocardiograms should be obtained; if there are any hemodynamic changes secondary to pericardial fluid accumulation, or if the echocardiogram reveals an expanding hematoma or evidence of pericardial tamponade, then surgical evacuation with closure of the point of perforation is best done under controlled circumstances.

Occasionally, a hemothorax may develop secondary to a perforation or tear in the subclavian vein or superior vena cava. Injury to the subclavian artery or aortic valve may develop if the catheter is misplaced into the arterial circulation. Such cases are rare but could add a significant level of complexity and risk to the patient and would require highly specialized attention and surgical strategy. Missing a tear in subclavian vessels with secondary hemothorax could be fatal, unless immediately corrected.

Pneumothorax

Percutaneous access to the subclavian vein requires a Seldinger technique to access and cannulate the subclavian vein. Occasionally, pleural perforation and lung injury may occur, leading to the development of a pneumothorax due to the escape of inhaled air into the pleural space and its entrapment between the lung and the parietal pleura. Such an event could cause respiratory difficulty due to a reduction of the effective lung volume. If the pneumothorax is left untreated and the perforation and air leak is significant, the condition could deteriorate into a tension pneumothorax or subcutaneous emphysema, dissecting in tissue planes and expanding outside of the chest cavity into the neck, face, and soft tissue surrounding vital structures such as the larynx. To avert potential airway obstruction, thorocostomy tube decompression creates an avenue for decompression of the entrapped air. Occasionally if the air leak does not resolve, surgical intervention is necessary to repair the lung tear.

After discharge

Lead erosion

Leads should be tunneled deep in the muscular layer of the chest or abdominal wall in order to avoid the potential for erosion of the overlying skin and exposure of the lead. Once there is exposure, it is difficult, if not impossible, to preserve the lead or the rest of the device components. Invariably, the entire system will require removal.

Lead fracture with conduction abnormality

Lead fractures are typically diagnosed at the time of device interrogation; replacement is mandatory. It is not always possible to remove the fractured lead; therefore, a fractured lead may be left in place as the new lead is inserted and connected to the energy source.

Lead displacement

Lead displacement or lead dislodgement, be it an epicardiac active fixations lead or an endocardiac lead, may occur due to improper location, fixation or due to cardiac movement. Displacement typically manifests with loss of capture and can be fixed by repositioning the lead under sterile conditions.

Diaphragmatic stimulation

Diaphragmatic stimulation by an implanted lead is an avoidable problem. At the time of lead implantation, the lead should be tested at high voltage (i.e., 10 volts), with attention to assess if diaphragmatic pacing occurs. If stimulation occurs, replacing the lead position to an alternative location away from the phrenic nerve will solve the problem.

Other complications

A pacemaker may sense non-cardiac electrical activities, leading to device inhibition or activation. Over- and under-sensing is less commonly encountered with newer-generation pacemakers, AICD-inappropriate shock for atrial fibrillation or sinus tachycardia rarely occurs in newer-generation devices, which are programmed to monitor and track cardiac rate, rhythm, and QRS morphology.

A generator may fail after its finite energy supply is exhausted. Battery life is dependent on the rate of energy consumption. Patients who are paced 100% of the time and/or at higher pacing thresholds are more likely to need earlier pacemaker battery change than a patient who has demand pacing only. Likewise patients who have frequent discharges of an AICD are more likely to consume the battery energy supply and require earlier device replacement.

Subclavian vein thrombosis and superior vena cava thromboses in association with lead insertion have been reported. Their presence is more common in patients with multiple leads inserted in the vein, rendering the subclavian vein unsuitable as an access point for further intervention. If thromboses extend into the superior vena cava, signs and symptoms of superior vena cava syndrome may develop.

Further reading

Abraham W, Fisher WG, Smith AL *et al.* Cardiac resynchronization in chronic heart failure. *N Engl J Med* 2002; **346**: 1945–53.

Corvera JS, Puskas JD, Thourani VH *et al.* Minimally invasive surgical cardiac resynchronization therapy: an intermediate-term follow-up study. *Innov Technol Tech Cardiothorac Vasc Surg* 2007; **2**: 40–7.

El-Chami MF, Hanna IR, Bush H *et al.* Impact of race and gender on cardiac device implantations. *Heart Rhythm* 2007; **4**: 1420–6.

Enzler MJ, Berbari E, Osmon DR. Antimicrobial prophylaxis in adults. *Mayo Clin Proc* 2011; **86**: 686–701.

Kass D. Pathophysiology of physiologic cardiac pains: advantages of leaving well enough alone. *J Am Med Assoc* 2002; **288**: 3159–61.

Kenny RA, Richardson DA, Steen N *et al.* Carotid sinus syndromes: a modified risk factor for non-accidental falls in older adults. *J Am Coll Cardiol* 2001; **38**: 1491–6.

Kusumoto F, Goldschlager N. Device therapy for cardiac arrhythmias. *J Am Med Assoc* 2002; **287**: 1848–52.

Lau CP. Pacing for atrial fibrillation. *Br Med J Heart* 2003; **89**: 106–12.

Moss AJ, Zareba W, Hall WJ *et al.* Prophylactic manipulation of a defibrillator in patients with myocardial infarctions and reduced ejection fraction. *N Engl J Med* 2002; **346**: 877–83.

Sohail MR, Uslan DZ, Khan AH *et al.* Management and outcome of permanent pacemaker and implantable cardioverter-defibrillator infections. *J Am Coll Cardiol* 2007; **49**: 1851–9.

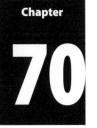

Chapter

70

Aortic valve surgery

Bryon J. Boulton and William A. Cooper

Aortic stenosis

The most common etiology of aortic stenosis (AS) in adults is calcific degeneration of the normal trileaflet valve or bicuspid valve. This degeneration begins at the base of the leaflets and progresses onto the cusps, ultimately leading to decreased leaflet motion. Characteristically this degeneration is without commissural fusion, as opposed to the next leading cause of AS in the adult, rheumatic fever. Rheumatic AS begins with fusion of the commissures and fibrotic changes leading to decreased movement of the cusps. This condition is usually accompanied by similar pathology on the mitral valve as well. Congenital malformations of the aortic valve can accelerate calcific degeneration of the valve, which presents in early adulthood.

Patients with rheumatic disease usually develop symptoms in the fifth or sixth decades of life, while patients with calcific degeneration develop symptoms in the seventh through ninth decades. The classic triad of symptoms in AS includes angina, syncope, and congestive heart failure (CHF). The natural history of each of these symptoms may independently predict a limited life expectancy: 5 years, 3 years, and 2 years respectively. This adverse prognosis is related to the rapid progression of aortic stenosis: a predicted decrease in valve area of 0.1 cm per year and an increase in mean pressure gradient of 7 mmHg per year. There is significant variability among individuals in the progression of disease; therefore, close follow-up is mandatory for all patients with asymptomatic mild and moderate AS. Sudden death may occur in 15–20% of cases; the onset of symptoms, particularly near the age of 60, usually heralds precipitous decline leading to death. Twenty percent of patients with severe AS will develop an acquired von Willebrand syndrome. These patients will demonstrate clinically evident bleeding, which resolves after valve replacement.

Because of the magnitude of the prognosis once patients develop symptoms, operative replacement is indicated at the onset of these symptoms. Operative replacement is also recommended for asymptomatic patients with estimated mean transvalvular gradients exceeding 50 mmHg, or whose valve orifice areas measure less than 0.8 cm (orifice area is calculated using the Gorlin equation, which takes into account the cardiac output and square root of the transvalvular gradient). Operative intervention is also indicated for patients with moderate AS who will undergo another concomitant cardiac procedure.

Aortic regurgitation

Aortic regurgitation (AR) has a number of common causes such as rheumatic fever, infective endocarditis, myxomatous changes, rheumatoid arthritis, lupus, and a host of causes of aortic root dilatation (tertiary syphilis, Marfan syndrome, Ehlers–Danlos syndrome, osteogenesis imperfecta, aortic dissection). Acute aortic regurgitation resulting from aortic dissection is seen primarily in patients with uncontrolled hypertension, ascending aortic aneurysms, annuloaortic ectasia, and Marfan's syndrome. In this setting, an emergent operation may be indicated.

Symptoms of acute aortic regurgitation include tachycardia, pulmonary edema, and cardiogenic shock. Due to increasing left ventricular end diastolic pressure, there are decreasing coronary artery pressures, leading to myocardial ischemia and its constellation of symptoms. Acute AR is also seen in patients with infective endocarditis or ascending aortic dissection involving the aortic valve, and in patients who have undergone balloon valvotomy.

Chronic aortic regurgitation is typically asymptomatic and can be difficult to diagnose by history and physical examination alone; over time the heart compensates via elevated end-diastolic pressure (EDP), ventricular dilatation, and decreased wall tension. The net effect of these compensatory changes allows for a positive aortic gradient and forward aortic ejection. Heart failure negatively impacts patient mortality and long-term outcomes. Therefore, operation is indicated at the earliest sign of the development of failure – seen clinically by congestive heart failure symptoms, S3 gallop, or left ventricular EDD (end diastolic diameter) of 70 mm or more. Unfortunately, statistics still indicate that 40% of patients referred for surgery are in CHF – with 53% in New York Heart Association (NYHA) Functional Classification Classes III or IV, rather than significantly earlier in the disease course.

Medical Management of the Surgical Patient, ed. Michael F. Lubin, Thomas F. Dodson, and Neil H. Winawer. Published by Cambridge University Press. © Cambridge University Press 2013.

Endocarditis

Indications for operation in endocarditis include failure to eradicate infection, severe regurgitation, evidence of perivalvular extension, large (> 10 mm) or hypermobile vegetations, and repeated significant embolic episodes. Emergent surgical intervention is indicated in patients with decompensated CHF unresponsive to medical therapy. Preoperative preparation includes coronary angiography for patients over 50 years of age and for patients with angina. Periodontal evaluation is necessary for patients with poor oral hygiene. Therapeutic antibiotics are administered prior to skin incision.

Diagnosis

Echocardiography is the gold standard in the diagnosis of aortic valve pathology. For patients with aortic stenosis, it can demonstrate whether the valve is bi- or trileaflet, or has calcific or fibrotic disease processes. Continuous wave Doppler ultrasound is used to calculate valve gradients and valve area. In aortic insufficiency, the degree of regurgitation can also be accessed with echocardiography. In patients with either disease processes, left ventricle (LV) wall thickness, size, and ejection fraction are important aspects to be evaluated. Because valve gradient calculations are dependent on flow across the valve, dobutamine stress echocardiography can be used to screen for low-flow/low-gradient aortic stenosis, a condition in which the degree of stenosis is underestimated because of a lower flow state.

To evaluate the extent of coronary atherosclerosis in the asymptomatic aortic stenosis patient, exercise stress testing provides little diagnostic accuracy; therefore, cardiac catheterization should be performed in all patients preoperatively. However, exercise stress testing is useful when evaluating the AS (asymptomatic) patients with no reported symptoms, such as decreased exercise tolerance, angina, or near-syncopal episodes, for the presence of actual symptoms. All patients should also receive carotid duplex scans as part of their preoperative work-up to evaluate for significant stenoses. In symptomatic AS patients, exercise testing should not be performed.

In patients with AR, echocardiography is useful to determine the cause and severity of the aortic regurgitation, along with the access valve morphology. In addition, echocardiography can access the left ventricular wall thickness, chamber dimensions, ejection fraction, and aortic root size. Serial echocardiography is helpful to identify the onset of symptoms in asymptomatic patients and to evaluate for increasing left ventricular size and/or decreasing function, which are all characteristics that indicate worsening heart failure. This scenario should prompt an evaluation of the patient for possible operative intervention.

Aortic valve repair

Isolated aortic valve repair is rarely performed. It is reserved for a select group of patients with limited cuspal prolapse or an enlarged annulus, and few to no calcium deposits. It is performed increasingly in patients with aortic root enlargement: the valve is spared and coaptation is recreated at the time of root repair. The incidence of post-repair persistent regurgitation has been reported to be as high as 17%. The condition is evaluated by intraoperative transesophageal echocardiography (TEE); reoperation is required in half of these patients if this complication has not been addressed before the patient leaves the operating room. Direct repair may be suitable for children or patients who cannot be anticoagulated or who have an exceedingly small annulus or outflow tract, and minimal calcium deposition.

Aortic valve replacement

The issues of anticoagulation and durability are of paramount importance in the decision-making process for aortic valve replacement surgery. The majority (60%) of replacement valves in the aortic position are bioprosthetic and require only 6–12 weeks of postoperative anticoagulation or no anticoagulation at all. Reoperation for valve degeneration occurs in 15% of patients at 10 years and in 35% at 15 years, primarily due to structural valve deterioration. Mechanical valves (36%) are more durable, but require permanent coumadin therapy and increase the incidence of hemolysis, which is typically subclinical and manifested by mild anemia. The bileaflet-disc valve demonstrates the least shear stress but has the highest regurgitant fractions. The optimal candidates for mechanical valves are young adults and patients with small aortic roots, although patients with smaller annula may also benefit from the improved durability of newer-generation bioprosthetic valves designed for supra-annular seating. Cryopreserved homografts (human allograft) (2.6%) represent a very attractive option due to superior valve performance without the need for anticoagulation. However, they are limited in use by scarce supply, rigorous preservation and thawing protocols, and by the technical demands of implantation. The use of an autologous pulmonic valve in the aortic position ("Ross procedure") represents the maximization of flow dynamics, durability (15% reoperative rate at 24 years), and resistance to infection and thrombosis; it also affords for valve growth in children. The main obstacles have been difficulties with sizing and explantation, and opposition to the creation of new right-sided valve disease, although freedom from reoperation due to pulmonic regurgitation has been as high as 81% at 20 years.

Perioperative monitoring includes pulmonary arterial and upper extremity arterial lines as well as large-bore venous access. Operative exposure is via median sternotomy. Cardioplegic techniques are customary and depend upon institutional and surgeon preference; however, in cases of surgery for AR, the ostia of the coronary arteries require direct cannulation, with meticulous attention to avoid obstruction or calcific embolization. The valve is accessed via transverse aortotomy followed by valve excision and debridement of calcifications from the annulus (the usual site for replacement valve seating). Aortic cross-clamp time averages 80 minutes;

total bypass time, 112 minutes; and total operative time, 180–240 minutes. Great attention is paid to de-airing of the patient, accomplished by left ventricular and aortic venting, slow side-to-side rocking of the table, and real-time surveillance of air bubbles via transesophageal echocardiography.

Transcatheter aortic valve implantation

Transcatheter aortic valve implantation (TAVI) has been performed in both the USA and Europe with increasing frequency over the last five years. It is currently pending FDA approval in the USA. The use of TAVI is currently limited to multi-center trials; however, once it is approved by the FDA, it is anticipated that it will be employed across the USA at cardiac centers outside of those involved in the trials. The use of this emerging technology is currently limited to patients who are determined to be 'inoperable' surgical candidates by two surgeons and a cardiologist, and have a Society of Thoracic Surgeons (STS) risk mortality score > 10. Depending on the patient's characteristics, TAVI may be carried out with either a transfemoral or a transapical approach.

Patients who have undergone transapical TAVI have some unique postoperative constraints. Because the apex of the heart is instrumented the patients are prone to ventricular arrhythmias; therefore, they are frequently placed on prophylactic lidocaine or amiodarone drips for 24–48 hours. Since the closure of the muscular apex is prone to tearing aggressive measures are used to prevent tachycardia in the first 24–28 hours postoperatively. Also, because the pleural space is opened, drains are left in place to prevent pleural effusions.

Both transapical and transfemoral approaches require that introducer needles be placed into the femoral arteries. Therefore, patients are at risk for bleeding complications and pseudoaneurysm formation at these sites.

Usual postoperative course

Expected postoperative hospital stay

On average, the expected postoperative hospital stay is approximately 5–7 days. The stay may be shorter if anticoagulation is not required.

Operative mortality

The average mortality rate for primary aortic surgery (with an accounting for significant risk factors) is 2%. After an adjustment for risk factors, it is below 5% for patients greater than 80 years of age. Outcomes for AS are generally better than for AR. Reoperation increases mortality to 5–7%, and depressed left ventricular function can increase the 5-year mortality by 50%.

Special monitoring required

Intraoperative transesophageal echocardiography is used routinely to evaluate cardiac function and anatomy; special attention is paid to the aortic valve before and after replacement.

A Swan–Ganz catheter is usually placed for intraoperative hemodynamic monitoring and postoperative management. Postoperatively, until the patient is no longer maintained on ventilation, mental status is near normal, and inotropic, pressors, and antiarrhythmic drips are no longer required, the patient remains in the ICU. Routine ward care includes 24–48 hours of telemetry monitoring, early ambulation, diuresis, and aggressive pulmonary toilet.

Patient activity and positioning

After extubation, the patient is allowed to sit erect in a chair. Early ambulation is encouraged.

Alimentation

The patient's diet is advanced as tolerated, with no need to delay diet to wait for demonstration of bowel function.

Antibiotic coverage

Routine perioperative antibiotics are necessary. They are administered within 30 minutes of skin incision and continued for 24 hours postoperatively. Antibiotic selection is usually a second-generation cephalosporin or vancomycin for patients allergic to penicillin.

Postoperative complications

In the hospital

Cardiac rhythm disturbances

Perioperative complications include atrial arrhythmias in 40% of patients. The incidence of atrial fibrillation, which usually resolves spontaneously in patients with preoperative sinus rhythm, is 24.6%. Bradyarrhythmias are common. Up to 10% of patients experience postoperative heart block; half of these require permanent pacing.

Bleeding

Postoperative bleeding may be related to several factors: early elevated partial thromboplastin time from residual heparin, thrombasthenia from the extracorporeal bypass circuit, or other surgically correctible factors (e.g., intercostal vessel hemorrhage, bleeding from a disrupted aortotomy suture line or other surgical site). Re-exploration for bleeding occurs in 3.7% of patients, and should be considered if the hourly chest tube output is greater than 500 mL in the first hour, 400 mL/hour for 2 hours, 300 mL/hour for 3 hours, or 200 mL/hour for 4 hours. Factors weighed into the decision for re-exploration include the timing of administration of corrective measures and responsiveness to these measures. Also, increasing hemodynamic compromise, a need for cardiotonic or vasoconstrictive agents, and falling hemoglobin levels should factor into a decision to re-explore the patient. Pericardial tamponade is life threatening; it requires formal operative or bedside emergent re-exploration.

Cerebrovascular accident

Stroke is reported in 3.5% of patients, half of whom will experience permanent deficit. Aortic atherosclerotic debris is the frequent source of embolic stroke; however, ventricular and mural thrombi, and, less commonly, valve thrombus should be considered as well. Carotid atherosclerotic disease is a significant risk factor for stroke; however, it should have been properly assessed and treated as indicated in the preoperative period.

Impaired ejection fraction

Low cardiac output is generally reported as the most common cause of death in the early postoperative period. Work-up starts with optimization of preload – which may need to be higher than usual, with pulmonary capillary wedge pressure of 16–18 mmHg in the hypertrophied ventricle of aortic stenosis – and of rate and rhythm, using external pacing if necessary. Placement of an intra-aortic balloon pump is required in 2.8% of patients, with only 0.5% placed preoperatively and 0.5% placed postoperatively. Perioperative myocardial infarction has a reported incidence of 0.3%.

Wound infection

Deep sternal wound infection is a costly, morbid, and often fatal complication that nearly doubles mortality. Fortunately, it occurs in only 0.4% of isolated aortic valve surgeries. Preoperative Hibiclens scrub to the chest, surgeon double-gloving, perioperative prophylactic antibiotics, and adhesive surgical draping (serving to block contact of skin flora with the wound) have all contributed to low infection rates. Treatment includes tailored antibiotic regimens, early operative drainage and debridement, and coverage of the tissue defect with pectoral muscle and omental flaps.

Postoperative renal insufficiency

Roughly 15% of patients develop evidence of renal impairment after aortic valve surgery. In most patients it is only a mild and transient level of renal dysfunction, which can be attributed to low postoperative cardiac output, periods of ischemia during the operation, nephrotoxic drug exposure, or preoperative renal dysfunction.

Other complications

There are a number of complications that occur relatively infrequently, but are not minor in their impact on the patient. These can be related to being placed on cardiopulmonary bypass, underlying patient risk factors, or no identifiable causes. These include gastrointestinal bleeding, pancreatitis, diverticulitis, ischemic colitis, electrolyte disturbances, pneumonia, pleural effusion, and hepatic dysfunction.

After discharge

Endocarditis

Endocarditis is a valve-related complication that is best treated with aggressive surgical management, which can halve the high (50–75%) mortality rate. Its appearance within several months after discharge typically represents initial surgical contamination or residual infection. Infection beyond 3 months usually results from an invasive procedure-related bacteremia; the importance of lifelong antibiotic prophylaxis must be emphasized. Mechanical and bioprosthetic valves demonstrate nearly equal reinfection rates (between 6% and 8% rate at 10 years, with the peak at 1 month). These rates are approximately 1/50th as common in homografts. Autograft infections are usually reported as zero in larger studies.

Thromboembolism and bleeding

Thromboembolism and bleeding are the most commonly documented complications encountered with prosthetic valves. In mechanical valves in the aortic position, thromboembolism is reported at 0.7–4.7 events per patient-year, and anticoagulant-related bleeding at 0.7–7.9 events. In bioprosthetics, the values are 0.7–1.2 and 0.3–0.8, respectively. Patient selection and education are most effective in preventing these problems; however, after repeated and significant episodes of hemorrhage in anticoagulated patients, consideration may be given to re-replacement of mechanical with bioprosthetic material.

Mechanical failure

Regurgitation or periprosthetic leaks can occur in all valves for many reasons; these include annuloprosthetic size mismatch, suture error, calcification, infection, and inadequate fibrous ingrowth. Structural deterioration in bioprosthetic valves occurs at an expected rate (usually 0.4–1 event per year); 20–25% of these valves need replacement at 20 years. Calcification of tissues, which is often followed by cusp rupture, is the predominant mechanism; it is accentuated in patients less than 30 years of age. Failure of mechanical valves has a much lower incidence and is typically attributable to thrombus, pannus ingrowth, or the presence of long chordal tissue or unraveled sutures, all of which may interfere with disc closure. Homografts have demonstrated nearly equivalent endurance rates to bioprosthetic porcine grafts, which are greatly augmented by the increased cell viability of the implanted graft. Autograft pulmonic valves require reoperation at about half this rate.

Antithrombotic therapy

After aortic valve replacement with a mechanical valve, all patients require lifelong anticoagulation to prevent thromboembolic events. According to the 2008 American Heart Association (AHA) guidelines, all patients with a bileaflet or Medtronic Hall prosthesis should be anticoagulated with warfarin to a goal INR of 2.0–3.0. If a Starr–Edwards or mechanical disc valve has been selected to replace the aortic valve, an INR of 2.5–3.5 should be targeted. If the patient also has a mechanical valve in the mitral position, warfarin dosing should be adjusted for a goal INR of 2.5 to 3.5. This should also be the goal INR. An INR of 2.5–3.5 is also the goal for patients with other comorbidities that require anticoagulation, such as atrial fibrillation.

If a bioprosthetic valve has been placed in the aortic position, all patients should be placed on lifelong aspirin therapy. It is reasonable to place patients with a bioprosthetic valve on temporary postsurgical warfarin therapy for 3 months, with a target INR of 2.0–3.0; the decision is largely left to surgeon preference.

All patients should be discharged from the hospital with a plan for reliable anticoagulation follow-up and INR level monitoring.

Further reading

Bonow RO, Carabello BA, Chatterjee K *et al.* Focused update incorporated into the ACC/AHA 2006 Guidelines for the management of patients with valvular heart disease. *J Am Coll Cardiol* 2008; **52**: e1–142.

Gott JP, Thourani VH, Wright CE *et al.* Risk neutralization in cardiac operations: detection and treatment of associated carotid disease. *Ann Thorac Surg* 1999; **68**: 850–6.

McGiffin DC, Galbraith AJ, McLachlan GJ *et al.* Risk factors for death and recurrent endocarditis after aortic valve replacement. *J Thorac Cardiovasc Surg* 1992; **104**: 511–20.

Moon MR, Miller DC, Moore KA *et al.* Treatment of endocarditis with valve replacement: the question of tissue versus mechanical prosthesis. *Ann Thorac Surg* 2001; **71**: 1164–71.

Sellke F, del Nido PJ, Swanson SJ. *Sabiston and Spencer's Surgery of the Chest*. 8th edn. Philadelphia, PA: Saunders; 2010.

Smith CR, Leon MB, Mack MJ. Transcatheter versus surgical aortic-valve replacement in high-risk patients. *N Engl J Med* 2011; **364**: 2187–96.

Society of Thoracic Surgeons Database, Spring 2011.

Yuh DD, Vricella LA, Baumgartner W. *The Johns Hopkins Manual of Cardiothoracic Surgery*. New York, NY: McGraw-Hill Professional; 2007.

Chapter

71

Mitral valve surgery

Bryon J. Boulton and William A. Cooper

Both in the USA and worldwide, the most common cause of mitral valve pathology in adults is rheumatic fever (RF). Postrheumatic structural changes to the mitral valve typically occur over the 2–10 years following infection, with symptoms appearing over the subsequent 5–10 years. In descending order, secondary etiologies include myxomatous degeneration, endocarditis, idiopathic annular calcification, connective tissue disorders (Marfan syndrome and Ehlers–Danlos syndrome), and hypertrophic cardiomyopathy; however, mitral stenosis (MS) is almost exclusively attributable to rheumatic fever. The onset of decompensated heart failure in MS patients is typically presaged by decreased exercise tolerance with progressive dyspnea secondary to low cardiac output, pulmonary hypertension, and decreased lung compliance. Timely operative intervention early in the symptomatic period can completely reverse heart failure. Mitral regurgitation (MR), where the valve is almost purely regurgitant, is also caused by RF. Ischemic MR is present in up to 20% of patients with coronary artery disease (CAD) requiring operative coronary artery bypass (CAB), and infrequently involves the catastrophic event of ruptured papillary muscle.

Indications for operation depend upon the pathophysiologic condition present. In severe MS, symptoms and signs of worsening heart failure indicate the need for surgery. Angiographic or echocardiographic estimation of a mitral orifice area of 2 cm^2 denotes mild to moderate disease, while 1 cm^2 denotes severe levels. Intervention should be undertaken prior to the appearance of heart failure, which significantly worsens outcome. Operative candidates with mitral regurgitation may be divided into two categories: those for whom acute regurgitation is caused by either abrupt endocarditic cuspal tear or ischemic papillary rupture, resulting in an uncompensated heart that demands immediate surgery; and those with chronic MR who have a well-compensated heart and can be stably situated in New York Heart Association (NYHA) Functional Classification class I or II. Patients in the latter category may best be managed with medical therapy, especially if they are of advanced age and have significant comorbidities. On the other hand, healthy young patients with mild to moderate disease

and low expected risk should be strongly considered for surgery before the development of left ventricular failure. For patients with chronic mitral regurgitation, operation is indicated mainly for NYHA class II or greater, pulmonary pathophysiology such as hemoptysis and hypertension, or signs of right heart failure. Female patients of childbearing age with mild to moderate chronic MR who want to become pregnant are also candidates for operation, because increased flow across the valve during gestation could increase their symptoms. For MS or MR patients, the operation should be performed either before or shortly after the onset of atrial fibrillation (AF), a time when left atrial architecture is sufficiently preserved and reversion to normal sinus rhythm can be reasonably expected. For native valve endocarditis, operation is indicated for failed eradication of infection, grade 4 angiographic regurgitation (independent of failure), repeated significant embolic episodes, and infection with resistant organisms (fungus, *Pseudomonas*, *Serratia*, *Staphylococcus aureus*, *Herellia*). The threshold for operation should be lowered with valve vegetations larger than 1 cm. Evidence of progression to perivalvular abscess, or the ominous finding of AV block (signifying destruction of the AV node) should be considered a failure of non-operative management and operation undertaken immediately.

The choice of surgical repair or replacement is a complex decision that requires that the valve be examined by the surgeon. Mitral commissurotomy is a somewhat outdated technique indicated for rheumatic fusion of commissures in cases of MR, MS, or a combination of both. Commissurotomy is typically performed with mitral annuloplasty and achieves an acceptable reoperative rate of 13% at 10 years. Formal repair is indicated for more extensive structural damage, such as chordal rupture, cuspal tear, or limited cuspal perforation that encompasses well below 50% of the valve mechanism. For MR, repair is generally more feasible than replacement, and can be accomplished with decreased bypass and crossclamp times, hospital stays, and reoperative and mortality rates. However, patients with preoperative shock or serious comorbidities typically will not be considered for repair; therefore, improved

Medical Management of the Surgical Patient, ed. Michael F. Lubin, Thomas F. Dodson, and Neil H. Winawer. Published by Cambridge University Press. © Cambridge University Press 2013.

outcomes with repair may not only reflect technical advantage over replacement, but also less extensive disease and better preoperative conditions.

Mitral valve replacement is chosen for "sicker" patients and those with more extensive valvular destruction. Replacement should include preservation of the posterior leaflet and chordal mechanism; this will preserve ventricular systolic shortening and limit ventricular stress. The choice to use a mechanical or a bioprosthetic valve relies essentially upon the risks of anticoagulation with mechanical valves versus the decreased durability of bioprosthetics. In the former (58% of replacements), mean valve longevity is approximately 20 years and anticoagulation is absolutely required. As for bioprosthetic valves (37% of mitral valve replacements), the most common type is the stented porcine xenograft, which has a mean durability of 10–15 years. Bioprosthetics show decreased shear stress compared with mechanical valves, but are more stenotic at smaller sizes, making them an inferior choice for patients with a diminutive annulus. Bioprosthetics are ideal when anticoagulation is contraindicated or unfeasible (gastrointestinal or central nervous system hemorrhagic potential), when pregnancy is desired (due to the teratogenicity and perinatal complications of Coumadin), and for patients over 30 years of age, after which the strong propensity towards calcification and structural failure begins to decrease. Promising new technologies such as valve treatment with alpha-amino oleic acid (Mosaic valve) seek to stem the process of calcific degeneration; the Mosaic valve has shown favorable 4-year performance data and may change the algorithm of valve choice. Anticoagulation with bioprosthetics is favored by most surgeons postoperatively for 6–12 weeks during the process of valve incorporation.

The choice of a replacement valve for endocarditis depends mainly upon the site of infection. An isolated cuspal infection may be completely resected, allowing for antibiotic penetration and, thus, the use of a mechanical valve. The finding of a deep perivalvular extension may contraindicate the placement of any synthetic material. Finally, the use of "minimally invasive" robotic techniques, for both repair and replacement of mitral valves, has proven cardioplegic arrest. In the USA and in other countries, these procedures have resulted in reduced bypass and crossclamp times and acceptable short-term morbidity and mortality; therefore, robotic methods may become more standard in the future.

Coronary angiography is a routine part of preoperative preparation for patients older than 50 years of age; it is mandatory for any patient with angina or anginal equivalent. Periodontal evaluation is also indicated; patients with endocarditis should receive therapeutic levels of appropriate antibiotics. In non-endocarditic surgery, a standard antistaphylococcal antibiotic regimen (cefazolin, or vancomycin for the penicillin-allergic) should be administered 30 minutes prior to skin incision.

The mitral valve is best accessed via a standard left atrial incision parallel to the interatrial groove. A right atrial incision

and transseptal access are used for reoperative surgery (with scarred tissue) or for calcified left atria, or if tricuspid surgery is planned. Although a median sternotomy affords the least postoperative pain and pulmonary embarrassment, a right anterolateral thoracotomy provides for optimal exposure. Intraoperative transesophageal echocardiography (TEE) is standard and essential for real-time feedback regarding valve mechanics. Perioperative monitoring has been greatly simplified in recent years: thermister tip pulmonary artery (PA) catheters are standard. The use of left atrial catheters has been found to provide no advantage; they are seldom used. Myocardial preservation is customary; great care is taken to avoid harming the conduction system, left circumflex coronary artery, aortic valve apparatus, and particularly the atrioventricular groove, especially during debridement of infected or calcified annuli. Total operative time is typically 150–300 minutes and is generally shorter for mitral repair.

Minimally invasive approaches

Recent advances in surgical technique and equipment have allowed for the popularization of minimally invasive approaches. These utilize a small anterior-lateral thoracotomy; alternative sites of cannulation (e.g., the femoral artery and vein) are frequently used for cardiopulmonary bypass. The same repair and replacement techniques are employed once the left atrium is opened after dissecting out the intra-atrial groove. The risk profile for minimally invasive approaches is similar to that of a traditional median sternotomy approach. However, the risk of stroke is increased from 1% to 2% because of the challenges in the de-airing process; in addition, the aorta is exposed to retrograde flow while the patient is on cardiopulmonary bypass, which allows for embolization of atheromatous material from the aorta into the cerebral circulation.

The advantages of the surgical robot include improved visualization and dexterity. In the repair of the mitral valve, only small port access incisions are required. No spreading of the ribs is necessary, thus decreasing postoperative pain. Studies have shown that the minimally invasive approach offers decreased hospital length of stay and more rapid return to work/physical activity. The postoperative care for mitral valve surgery patients who have undergone minimally invasive operations is the same as that for patients who have received the standard sternotomy approach.

Usual postoperative course
Expected postoperative hospital stay

An average postoperative hospital stay of 5–7 days is required. If a mechanical valve has been placed, a portion of this time is needed for anticoagulation. If a bioprosthetic valve has been used, the surgeon may decide to temporarily anticoagulate the patient.

Operative mortality

The rate of operative mortality is 1% for isolated mitral valve repair or replacement in patients with preserved left ventricular function. Mortality may increase to 10–20% or higher in emergent operations, ischemic mitral regurgitation, or cardiogenic shock. Predictors of a poor outcome include a higher NYHA functional class, an increased ventricular chamber size, the presence of mitral regurgitation (as opposed to mitral stenosis), and a longer duration of cross-clamp time. All told, the rate of early major complication plus operative mortality is 10% for isolated mitral valve surgery; this rate increases with the addition of one or more of the above-mentioned risk factors.

Special monitoring required

Though most patients leave the operating room on one or more cardiotonic or vasotonic intravenous drips, most will have the drips discontinued later the same postoperative day; many patients will also be extubated. Most patients not already taking beta-blocking medications are administered low-dose metoprolol for antiarrhythmic prophylaxis. If the heart maintains a stable rhythm, epicardial pacing wires and telemetry monitoring are discontinued 48 hours postoperatively.

Patient activity and positioning

Patients may be erect and can stand on the day of extubation. Ambulation is encouraged early on, and incentive spirometry and other methods of pulmonary toilet are instituted.

Alimentation

Diet is advanced as tolerated.

Antibiotic coverage

Standard perioperative prophylactic antibiotic regimens can be utilized, with exceptions made for those with underlying comorbidities or endocarditis.

Postoperative complications

In the hospital

Cardiac rhythm disturbances

Transitory atrial arrhythmias are the most common perioperative rhythm disturbance, occurring in 70% of mitral cases, with atrial fibrillation occurring in 20% of all patients with mitral valve replacement. Most patients in sinus rhythm preoperatively will ultimately revert spontaneously; until then, ventricular rate control is accomplished with short-acting beta blockade, calcium channel blockade, and digoxin therapy. Surgical ablation of chronic AF achieves lasting conversion to sinus rhythm in 70% of patients at up to 5 years. This procedure can be performed at the time of mitral surgery, and is frequently performed in patients with mitral disease and AF.

Bradyarrhythmias and AV nodal block are common, usually transient and best managed with pacing or occasionally with oral theophylline. Premature ventricular contractions (PVCs) are also typical and may be suppressed with atrial or atrioventricular pacing to a rate of 90–100 beats/minute, or simply corrected with electrolyte repletion. Ultimately, only 4% of patients without preoperative rhythm disturbances require pacemaker placement (due to persistent rhythm issues) after mitral valve surgery.

Cerebrovascular accident

Perioperative stroke occurs in 5% of patients with isolated mitral valve repair or replacement, and is permanent in less than 1%. An intraoperative embolism (consisting of thrombus or particles, or air) may be responsible; for air embolism, the use of hyperbaric oxygen may reverse the neurologic deficit up to 24 hours postoperatively.

Impaired ejection fraction

Postoperative low cardiac output, characterized by a measured cardiac index of less than 2 L/min per m^2 and low mixed venous saturations, is initially treated by optimizing preload and heart rate (often requiring pacing to greater than, or equal to, 90 beats/min) and with pharmacologic inotropy (contractility) agents (calcium, phosphodiesterase inhibitors such as milrinone, and catecholamines such as epinephrine). Intra-aortic balloon pumps are used in less than 5% of patients.

Severe cardiac dysfunction

Myocardial infarct is reported in 0.3% of mitral operations, and cardiogenic shock in 3%. A sudden development of low ventricular output combined with equalizing chamber pressures as measured by PA catheter should raise suspicion of cardiac tamponade, and prompt either repeat TEE or, in the presence of overwhelming evidence, emergent re-exploration.

Wound infection

Deep sternal wound infections occur in 0.1% of patients and present a particularly precarious problem with a high mortality, especially in the setting of infected prosthetic valves.

Minor complications

There are a number of complications that occur relatively infrequently, but are not minor in their impact on the patient. These can be related to being placed on cardiopulmonary bypass, underlying patient risk factors, or no identifiable causes. These complications include gastrointestinal bleeding, pancreatitis, diverticulitis, ischemic colitis, electrolyte disturbances, pneumonia, pleural effusion, and hepatic dysfunction.

Because the right pleural space is opened in the minimally invasive approach, there is risk for lung damage and a persistent air leak postoperatively, as well as the risk of a persistent or recurrent right pleural effusion. Also, because of the use of the femoral vessels for cannulation, there is a risk of bleeding from these sites, including retroperitoneal hematoma.

After discharge

Bleeding and thrombosis

Late postoperative thromboembolism is reported in up to 1.7% of mitral operations. It is most frequent in ball-in-cage type mechanical valves and, to a lesser degree, in tilting-disc valves. There are no data to suggest any advantage with the maintenance of prothrombin times greater than 1.5–2 times normal. Bleeding occurs at 3% per patient-year, with 0.2% patient-year mortality. Thorough patient education may reduce this rate; however, repeated significant bleeding episodes may prompt consideration of replacing the mechanical valve with a bioprosthetic valve.

Infection

Prosthetic valve endocarditis may be stratified into early and late cases. Infections occurring less than 6 months postoperatively are typically due to intraoperative contamination and are better managed operatively (mortality rate 22–46%) than nonoperatively (65%). Earlier operation is crucial, especially to prevent new perivalvular abscess. Therefore, initial postoperative antibiotics should be immediately initiated, tailored to positive intraoperative cultures, and continued for 6 weeks. Late infections are usually related to dental or other procedures and can be successfully treated medically in the absence of perivalvular extension of infection.

Valve failure

The need for reoperation is uncommon after mitral repair (around 2%), and is usually determined. Valve failure is usually noted during the initial operation, after separation from the bypass, and during physiologic reassessment with TEE. Mitral re-replacement is most common with the use of bioprosthetics – 20–25% at 10 years, higher in patients less than 35 years of age – and is typically due to calcific degeneration with later cuspal tear. Malfunction of mechanical valves seldom occurs, though when it does, it is chiefly due to pannus formation over time; reintervention is required in only 0.5% of patients. Acute appearance of mechanical valve dysfunction, often symptomatic, should raise suspicion of a thrombotic cause, and indicates the need for urgent therapy, either surgical thrombectomy or re-replacement.

Antithrombotic therapy

All patients should receive lifelong antithrombotic therapy with warfarin after mechanical valve replacement of the mitral valve. A goal INR of 2.5–3.5 should be targeted for a patient with any mechanical valve in the mitral position. All patients should be discharged with established follow-up for warfarin therapy adjustment and INR monitoring.

All patients with a bioprosthetic valve placed in the mitral position should be placed on lifelong aspirin therapy prior to discharge from the hospital. Many surgeons will place a patient on temporary warfarin for 3 months postoperatively after bioprosthetic valve placement, targeting an INR of 2.0–3.0.

Some surgeons elect to place low-risk patients who have had a mitral valve repair with an annuloplasty ring on warfarin therapy for 3 months postoperatively, targeting an INR of 2.0–3.0. However, there is mixed evidence supporting the need for this regimen for the prevention of thromboembolic events.

Further reading

Bonow RO, Carabello BA, Chatterjee K et al. 2008 focused update incorporated into the ACC/AHA 2006 guidelines for the management of patients with valvular heart disease. *J Am Coll Cardiol* 2008; **52**: e1–42.

Carpentier A, Adams DH, Filsoufi F. *Carpentier's Reconstructive Valve Surgery*. 1st edn. Philadelphia, PA: Saunders; 2010.

Choudhary SK, Dhareshwar J, Govil A et al. Open mitral commissurotomy in the current era: indications, technique, and results. *Ann Thorac Surg* 2003; **75**: 41–6.

Cohn LH. *Cardiac Surgery in the Adult*. 3rd edn. New York, NY: McGraw-Hill Professional; 2007.

Cox JL. Atrial transport function after the maze procedure for atrial fibrillation: a 10-year clinical experience. *Am Heart J* 1998; **136**: 934–6.

Duarte IG, MacDonald MJ, Cooper WA et al. In vivo hemo-dynamic, histologic, and antimineralization characteristics of the Mosaic bioprosthesis. *Ann Thorac Surg* 2001; **71**: 92–9.

Nifong LW, Chu VF, Bailey BM et al. Robotic mitral valve repair: experience with the da Vinci system. *Ann Thorac Surg* 2003; **75**: 438–42.

Sellke F, del Nido PJ, Swanson SJ. *Sabiston and Spencer's Surgery of the Chest*. 8th edn. Philadelphia, PA: Saunders; 2010.

Society of Thoracic Surgeons Database, Spring 2011.

Thomson DJ, Jamieson EJ, Dumesnil JG et al. Medtronic mosaic porcine bioprosthesis: midterm investigational trial results. *Ann Thorac Surg* 2001; **71**: S269–72.

Trehan N, Mishra YK, Sharma M. Robotically controlled video-assisted port-access mitral valve surgery. *Asian CV Thorac Ann* 2002; **10**: 133–6.

Yuh DD, Vricella LA, Baumgartner W. *The Johns Hopkins Manual of Cardiothoracic Surgery*. New York, NY: McGraw-Hill Professional; 2007.

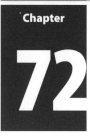

Ventricular assist devices and cardiac transplantation

Duc Q. Nguyen and J. David Vega

Cardiac transplantation and ventricular assist device therapy have become effective therapeutic options for patients with end-stage heart failure. Unfortunately, due to the shortage of organ donors, the annual number of heart transplants in the USA has remained relatively constant, between 2,200 and 2,400.

The development of implantable left ventricular assist devices (LVADs) for use as mechanical circulatory support also spanned several decades, dating back to the 1960s. However, LVADs were only applied for clinical use on a more routine basis in the mid 1980s. Since then, research and development of VAD technology continues to advance as the clinical experience with LVADs evolves over time. The number of LVADs being implanted in the USA continues to grow, with more than 1,000 devices implanted annually.

Heart transplantation and VAD therapy are complementary forms of therapy. Patient selection for both requires extensive evaluation by a multidisciplinary team. Transplantation is reserved for a group of patients with end-stage heart disease not amenable to optimal medical or surgical therapies. The indications for heart transplantation include patients with symptomatic New York Heart Association (NYHA) class III to IV heart failure despite optimal medical therapy, inability to wean from inotropic therapy, poor functional status on exercise testing, refractory ventricular arrhythmia, severe coronary artery disease with poor short-term prognosis, or complications of congenital heart disease that are refractory to medical and surgical intervention.

For transplant candidates who will not survive waiting until an organ is available, an LVAD may be implanted as a bridge to transplantation. Specific criteria for LVAD therapy include: NYHA class IV symptoms that failed to respond to optimal medical management; left ventricular ejection fraction < 25%; functional capacity limited to peak oxygen consumption of < 12 mL/kg per minute; intolerance to weaning of intravenous inotropic therapy; life expectancy < 2 years; and appropriate body size. Lastly, for the patients who are not transplant candidates, LVADs may be implanted as permanent or destination therapy.

Relative and absolute contraindications exist for both heart transplantation and LVAD therapy. Typical exclusion criteria for both types of therapy include advanced age (upper limit varies according to the institution), severe peripheral arterial or cerebrovascular disease, irreversible pulmonary hypertension, active sepsis, chronic renal failure, advanced lung or liver disease, and psychological or social barriers that would preclude successful outcome. Additional contraindications to transplantation include active or recent malignancy, active smoking, drug dependency, diabetes with end-organ disease, and morbid obesity.

Usual postoperative course
Expected postoperative hospital stay

For uncomplicated procedures, the length of hospital stay is generally 1–2 weeks for heart transplant and 2–4 weeks for an LVAD implant. However, several factors may significantly increase the duration of hospitalization for either procedure, including postoperative complications, preoperative clinical status, and comorbidities.

Operative mortality

The operative mortality is about 2–4% for heart transplantation. For LVAD implantation, it is highly variable, depending on several factors, particularly the patient's preoperative severity of illness. Operative mortality rates of 10–20% have been reported with first-generation devices. With increasing clinical experience and the prevalent use of second- and third-generation pumps, 30-day mortality rates have decreased (4–11%).

Special monitoring required

Patients remain in the ICU typically for 3–5 days following heart transplant and up to 1 week after an LVAD implant. These patients require invasive monitoring, including a pulmonary artery catheter and an arterial line. Other parameters to be monitored include electrocardiography, continuous

Medical Management of the Surgical Patient, ed. Michael F. Lubin, Thomas F. Dodson, and Neil H. Winawer. Published by Cambridge University Press. © Cambridge University Press 2013.

pulse oximetry, indwelling urinary catheter, and chest tube drainage. Chest radiography and laboratory assays, including arterial blood gases, electrolytes, and cell counts, are obtained on a daily basis. Patients are usually on inotropic and vasopressor agents that can be weaned over several days. Temporary epicardial pacing wires are routinely inserted for heart transplant. Efforts are made to remove all invasive monitoring lines and indwelling catheters and tubes as soon as possible to reduce the risk of infection.

For transplant recipients, immunosuppressive drug levels are obtained daily. Routine endomyocardial biopsy to evaluate for rejection is performed on a weekly basis for the first 4 weeks. In LVAD patients, once perioperative bleeding is controlled, anticoagulation therapy is initiated, usually on the second or third postoperative day. Pump parameters are monitored to assess for appropriate device function. With continuous-flow LVADs, the flow is non-pulsatile. Therefore, the arterial pulse is greatly diminished and is reflected as a near-flat tracing with an invasive arterial line recording. Once the arterial line is removed, pressure monitoring is greatly enhanced with the use of a Doppler device.

Patient activity and positioning

Patients arrive at the ICU intubated and sedated. Standard ICU protocols regarding mobilization are followed with side-to-side turning. Efforts are made to extubate patients at the earliest possible opportunity and to mobilize them as soon as possible. Incentive spirometry, aggressive pulmonary hygiene, and ambulation with assistance of physical therapy are initiated early and continued throughout the hospital course. With LVAD patients, it is important to immobilize the driveline with a belt-restraining device to avoid trauma to the exit site.

Alimentation

Oral diet is initiated at the earliest opportunity with clear liquids and advanced to a low-sodium diet. Postoperative nausea is common, while ileus occurs less frequently. Speech therapy with swallowing evaluation may be needed if risk of aspiration exists. In patients who remain on prolonged ventilator support, enteral feeding is preferred to hyperalimentation. Adequate nutritional support is critical to the overall recovery of these patients.

Antibiotic coverage

For the heart transplant procedure, the usual cardiac surgery prophylaxis (second-generation cephalosporin or vancomycin for penicillin-allergic patients) suffices. For an LVAD implant using the smaller continuous flow pumps, a similar regimen can also be used. However, because of the risk of device infections, some centers still employ broad-spectrum antimicrobial perioperative prophylaxis to cover Gram positive, Gram negative, and fungal organisms, and may even extend the duration of therapy until all chest tubes are removed.

Postoperative complications

In the hospital

Low cardiac output

The cause for acute graft dysfunction in transplant patients may be multi-factorial, but is often due to hypothermic ischemic injury during preservation, myocardial dysfunction owing to donor instability, and pulmonary hypertension. Acute rejection as the etiology of acute graft dysfunction is rare. Supportive management with inotropic agents (milrinone, epinephrine, and dobutamine) usually suffices. In severe cases, insertion of an intra-aortic balloon pump and/or temporary short-term VAD may be required. In most instances, cardiac function will recover.

Low cardiac output following an LVAD implant may be due to right ventricular (RV) dysfunction, hypovolemia, or inadequate pump flow. Manifestations of RV failure include increased central venous pressure, decreased pulmonary artery and left atrial pressures, and low LVAD flow. Low cardiac output secondary to hypovolemia can be treated with judicious use of crystalloids and/or blood products. Adjustment of pump parameters may be necessary if pump speed is too low. Echocardiography can be very helpful in identifying the cause of the low cardiac output state.

Bleeding

Mediastinal bleeding is a relatively common postoperative complication in both transplant and LVAD patients. Up to 30% of LVAD patients may require surgical re-exploration. Predisposing factors include preoperative anticoagulation, reoperative procedures, prolonged cardiopulmonary bypass, hepatic congestion and dysfunction related to chronic heart failure, and compromised nutritional status. The transition away from the bulkier first-generation LVADs, which normally require extensive surgical dissection to create abdominal pockets, to smaller continuous-flow devices, has decreased the incidence of VAD-associated perioperative bleeding. In both groups of patients, perioperative use of blood product transfusions is common. When bleeding persists or leads to extensive mediastinal collection of clot-causing tamponade physiology, re-exploration is indicated.

Arrhythmias

Arrhythmias occur in 5–30% of heart transplant patients, and include sinus or junctional bradycardia, atrial fibrillation, atrial flutter, and other supraventricular arrhythmias. Both atrial and ventricular dysrhythmias may have already been present preoperatively in the LVAD patients. In these circumstances, anti-arrhythmic agents may need to be continued in the postoperative period.

Neurological events

Neurological complications, such as strokes, can be devastating. The incidence of neurological complications in the heart transplant population is low. For LVAD patients, the incidence varies with the types of device used. First-generation pumps had higher rates of neurological events, although it was lower with the HeartMate XVE device. Reported rates of strokes for second-generation devices range from 2.2 to 17% (HeartMate II). These complications can occur not only early during the hospitalization, but also as late events throughout the duration of LVAD support.

Infections

Infection is a leading cause of mortality and morbidity in the heart transplant recipient. The greatest risk of life-threatening infections occurs in the first 3 months following transplant and with increases in immunosuppression for acute rejection episodes. Bacterial infections are common early infections; they include pneumonia, mediastinitis/sternal wound infections, catheter-related bacteremia, and urinary tract infections. Late infections are usually opportunistic infections. Cytomegalovirus (CMV) remains the most common cause of mortality and morbidity in transplant patients. Fungal infections include *Candida* and *Aspergillus* infections. Aspergillosis is highly lethal in the immunocompromised host. Two protozoal organisms found in heart transplant patients are *Pneumocystis carinii* (diffuse interstitial pneumonia) and *Toxoplasma gondii* (central nervous system infections).

Infectious complications are also frequent in LVAD patients. These include not only the typical postoperative infections associated with cardiac surgery, but VAD-specific infections as well (e.g., driveline exit site and pump pocket infections). These device-related infections may occur early during the perioperative period or late after hospital discharge.

Pleural effusions

Pleural effusions may occur in 5–15% of patients, often within 30 days of the operation. Patients usually present with shortness of breath. Not uncommonly, the effusions are detected on routine chest radiography. In most cases, aggressive diuresis usually leads to improvement. For larger effusions, thoracentesis or catheter-drainage may be required.

After discharge

Acute rejection

The average transplant recipient experiences 1.3 rejection episodes in the first year. The vast majority of cases are mediated by the cellular limb of the immune response. Antibody-mediated rejection is less common. An RV endomyocardial biopsy remains the standard for the diagnosis of acute rejection. Biopsy schedule varies among institutions, but reflects the greater risk of rejection during the first 6 months following transplant. Evaluation of the biopsy sample is graded against a standard scale. Although symptoms of rejection may include fever, dysrhythmias, or signs of heart failure, most episodes of rejection characteristically are insidious. Patients can remain asymptomatic even with

late stages of rejection. Corticosteroid pulse therapy is the mainstay of anti-rejection therapy. Modulation of other immunosuppressive agents may also be indicated. The use of cytolytic therapy generally is reserved for severe rejection with hemodynamic compromise. Antibody-mediated rejection, unlike cellular rejection, more commonly causes hemodynamic compromise, which often necessitates inotropic support.

Cardiac allograft vasculopathy

Cardiac allograft vasculopathy (CAV) is a unique, rapidly progressive form of atherosclerosis in heart transplant patients that remains the leading cause of death after the first year post-transplant. The exact underlying pathogenesis is unknown but likely is related to immunologic mechanisms that are regulated by non-immunologic risk factors. Clinical diagnosis of CAV is difficult. Ventricular arrhythmias, heart failure, and sudden death are commonly the initial presentation of severe CAV. Annual coronary angiograms are performed for CAV surveillance. The process is diffuse and therefore difficult to treat. Percutaneous coronary interventions or surgical revascularization may have palliative therapeutic roles. Immunosuppressive drugs, such as sirolimus, may be useful in reducing the incidence and severity of CAV and slowing the disease progression. Re-transplantation is the only definitive treatment for advanced CAV.

Malignancy

Chronic immunosuppression is associated with an increased incidence of malignancy, about 4–18%. Along with CAV, malignancies have become a significant factor limiting long-term survival of heart transplant recipients. The most common malignancies in this population are lymphoproliferative disorders and carcinoma of the skin.

Driveline and pump pocket infections

Percutaneous driveline exit site infections occur in 12–35% of LVAD patients. These infections are potentially serious adverse events, and are the leading reasons for hospital re-admission. Many of these events are preventable through meticulous care and protection of the driveline. It is imperative that the driveline be adequately immobilized to prevent disruption of subcutaneous tissue ingrowth. Sterile techniques must be employed during exit site care. Any signs of infection should be reported promptly. When a driveline infection is diagnosed, a culture of the site is obtained and adequate antimicrobial treatment is initiated. Unfortunately, once these infections occur, they frequently tend to recur and then become chronic infections. In such circumstances, chronic suppressive antibiotic therapy is required.

Driveline infections may lead to pump pocket infections, which are difficult to treat. An LVAD explantation, with or without heart transplantation, may be the only definitive way to eradicate the infection.

Pump thrombus/thrombosis

In patients with continuous-flow LVAD support, clinically relevant pump thrombus is rare (1.4–4%). Thrombus within the pump usually leads to abnormal pump parameters and hemolysis. Treatment usually requires administration of intravenous heparin to prevent progression of the thrombus. Thrombolytic therapy should be initiated with caution. Surgical pump replacement may be necessary if other modalities are unsuccessful.

Gastrointestinal bleeding

Gastrointestinal (GI) bleeding is a complication of continuous-flow LVADs. Gastrointestinal bleeding may become so severe that anticoagulation therapy must be reduced or discontinued. A patient with a documented history of GI bleeding requires thorough investigation for the source prior to undergoing LVAD implantation.

Further reading

Aggarwal S, Cheema F, Oz MC, Naka Y. Long-term mechanical circulatory support. In Cohn LH, ed. *Cardiac Surgery in the Adult*. 3rd edn. New York, NY: McGraw-Hill Medical; 2008, pp. 1609–27.

Boyle AJ, Russell SD, Teuteberg JJ *et al.* Low thromboembolism and pump thrombosis with the HeartMate II left ventricular assist device: analysis of outpatient anticoagulation. *J Heart Lung Transplant* 2009; **28**: 881–7.

Miller LW, Pagani FD, Russell SD *et al.* Use of a continuous-flow device in patients awaiting heart transplantation. *N Engl J Med* 2007; **357**: 885–96.

Nwakanma LU, Shah AS, Conte JV, Baumgartner WA. Heart transplantation. In Cohn LH, ed. *Cardiac Surgery in the Adult*. 3rd edn. New York, NY: McGraw-Hill Medical; 2008, pp. 1539–77.

Slaughter MS, Pagani FD, Rogers JG *et al.* Clinical management of continuous-flow left ventricular assist devices in advanced heart failure. *J Heart Lung Transpl* 2010; **29**: S1–S39.

Slaughter MS, Rogers JG, Milano CA *et al.* Advanced heart failure treated with continuous-flow left ventricular assist device. *N Engl J Med* 2009; **361**: 2241–51.

Starling RC, Naka Y, Boyle AJ *et al.* Results of the Post-U.S. Food and Drug Administration approval study with a continuous flow left ventricular assist device as a bridge to heart transplantation. *J Am Coll Cardiol* 2011; **57**: 1890–8.

Chapter

73

Thoracic aortic disease

Bradley G. Leshnower and Edward P. Chen

The management of thoracic aortic disease is based upon the aortic pathology and anatomy. The thoracic aorta is evaluated in four separate segments: the aortic root, ascending aorta, transverse arch, and descending aorta. In addition to the aortic disease, factors that affect the timing and extent of surgical replacement of the thoracic aorta include the presence of aortic valve pathology, concomitant cardiac disease, and the patient's age and comorbidities. This chapter will review the most common indications for treatment of diseases of the thoracic aorta and the perioperative care of patients undergoing aortic surgery.

The most common indications for surgery on the thoracic aorta, in descending order, are aneurysmal disease, acute aortic syndromes, trauma, and infection. The incidence of thoracic aortic aneurysms is estimated to be 5.9 cases per 100,000 person-years, and replacement of the ascending aorta accounts for the majority of thoracic aorta procedures. The most common causes of thoracic aortic aneurysms (TAAs) are cystic medial necrosis; atherosclerosis; heritable connective tissue disorders (e.g., Marfan syndrome); familial, bicuspid aortic valve disease; and chronic aortic dissection. The presence or absence of symptoms is the most important factor in the management of patients with thoracic aortic aneurysms. Patients with symptomatic TAAs typically experience chest or back pain, depending upon the location of the aneurysm. The sudden onset of pain is considered an ominous warning sign of imminent rupture or dissection, and surgery is indicated for all patients with symptomatic TAAs.

Operative therapy for asymptomatic TAAs is performed for prophylactic replacement of the aorta in order to prevent rupture or dissection, and thereby improve patient survival. Elective repair of aneurysmal disease of the aortic root and/or ascending aorta is recommended at a diameter of ≥ 5.5 cm or a growth rate of ≥ 0.5 cm/year. Patients with genetic disorders such as Marfan syndrome, Ehlers–Danlos syndrome, Turner syndrome, bicuspid aortic valve disease, or with a familial history of aneurysm and dissection should undergo elective ascending aortic replacement at a diameter ≥ 4.5 cm. In patients undergoing aortic valve replacement, concomitant

ascending aorta replacement for aneurysmal disease is recommended at a size of 4.5 cm. Particular scrutiny should be given to women of childbearing age desiring to become pregnant if they present with TAAs, whether or not they have a significant family history or genetic disorders. In these situations, prophylactic ascending replacement may be indicated at a diameter of > 4 cm.

Isolated aortic arch aneurysms are much less common than ascending TAAs. Total aortic arch replacement for an isolated arch aneurysm should be performed at sizes ≥ 5.5 cm. Aortic replacement for descending and thoracoabdominal aneurysms is recommended at a size of ≥ 5.5 cm. It should be noted that the diameter for intervention on all aortic segments can be adjusted for body size based upon published nomograms correlating the aortic rupture/dissection risk to aortic diameter and body surface area.

Acute aortic syndromes are diseases that require emergent aortic surgery. The most common diagnosis in this group is acute aortic dissection (AAD). Acute aortic dissection is caused by a tear in the aortic intima, which allows blood to flow into the media and split the aortic wall into a true and false lumen. Type A AAD is defined by involvement of the ascending aorta and is considered a lethal disease because of its potential to cause aortic free-wall rupture, cardiac tamponade, coronary malperfusion, and severe aortic insufficiency leading to acute LV failure. Variants of AAD are intramural hematoma and penetrating aortic ulcer. Intramural hematoma occurs when the vaso vasorum of the aorta ruptures and hemorrhages into the aortic media forming a hematoma. Penetrating aortic ulcers occur when atherosclerotic lesions of the aortic intima rupture through the internal elastic lamina and hemorrhage into the media. Both intramural hematoma and penetrating aortic ulcers can evolve into an aortic dissection. Type B AAD is defined by aortic dissection distal to the left subclavian artery which does not involve the ascending aorta.

Emergent surgery is indicated for Type A AAD and all cases of intramural hematoma and penetrating aortic ulcers involving the ascending aorta. Surgical treatment of Type A AAD requires resection of the primary tear, restoration of

Medical Management of the Surgical Patient, ed. Michael F. Lubin, Thomas F. Dodson, and Neil H. Winawer. Published by Cambridge University Press. © Cambridge University Press 2013.

aortic valve competency, aortic replacement, and obliteration of the false lumen at the proximal and distal anastomoses. The management of uncomplicated Type B AAD is aggressive blood-pressure control with intravenous anti-hypertensive beta-blockers and/or calcium channel blockers. A complicated Type B AAD is defined by the presence of visceral or peripheral malperfusion, contained or free rupture, rapid aortic growth, intractable pain, or refractory hypertension despite aggressive intravenous anti-hypertensive medications. Surgical intervention is indicated for patients with complicated Type B AAD with either open aortic replacement or thoracic endovascular aortic repair (TEVAR). Patients with Type B AAD can dissect retrograde into the ascending aorta, which mandates emergent surgical intervention. Therefore Type B AAD patients require serial imaging of the entire thoracic and abdominal aorta; Type A AAD must be excluded at the time of the initial evaluation by computed tomography or transesophageal echocardiography.

Blunt aortic injury is the second-leading cause of death from motor vehicle accidents. The actual incidence of aortic rupture is unknown because many trauma victims die at the scene of the accident; however, autopsy series list the incidence at 12–23%. The most common site of aortic injury is the isthmus, located just distal to the left subclavian artery. The majority of these injuries are considered to be deceleration injuries in which the aorta is transected at the isthmus due to its fixation at that site by the ligamentum arteriosum. The periadventitial tissue around the aorta prevents free rupture in survivors of aortic transection. Once the diagnosis is made, immediate aortic repair is recommended, unless there are significant hemorrhagic thoracic, abdominal, retroperitoneal, or pelvic injuries which would take priority over a contained aortic injury. Surgical options are open repair with segmental replacement of the transected aorta, or TEVAR if the anatomy is amenable. If aortic repair is delayed due to other injuries or hemodynamic instability, treatment with beta-blockers is mandatory.

Infectious aortitis or mycotic endarteritis is a term used to describe an infected aortic aneurysm. Infected aneurysms are typically saccular and are most commonly due to bacterial infections with *Staphylococcus aureus* and *Salmonella*. In the era prior to penicillin, syphilitic aortitis was a common cause of ascending thoracic aortic aneurysms infected by *Treponema pallidum*. All patients presenting with infectious aortitis should be evaluated for impaired immunity. The presence of infectious aortitis is an indication for aortic replacement, ideally with aortic homograft. Infection can also present as a late complication of prior cardiac or aortic surgery. Postoperative mediastinitis can initiate the formation of infected pseudoaneurysms at cannulation sites and anastomotic suture lines. Infected prosthetic aortic grafts and endografts are also indications for aortic replacement with homograft.

Patients who are discovered to have atheromatous disease of the aortic arch are at risk for ischemic stroke. High-risk features include plaques ≥ 4 mm in thickness, mobile plaques, and plaques located proximal to the left subclavian artery.

Patients with high-risk plaques should be anticoagulated with warfarin for a goal international normalized ratio (INR) of 2–3. There is also strong evidence that statin therapy can reduce the risk of stroke in patients with arch atheromas. Only in rare situations, such as persistent TIAs despite adequate anticoagulation, is aortic replacement indicated for the treatment of aortic atheromatous disease.

Preoperative evaluation of the patient undergoing thoracic aortic surgery consists of standard laboratory evaluation, electrocardiogram, non-invasive coronary artery stress or imaging tests, computed tomography of the chest with contrast, transthoracic echocardiography, and carotid duplex for patients > 70 years with left main coronary artery disease, cervical bruits or a history of a prior cerebrovascular accident or carotid endarterectomy. All concomitant coronary artery or valvular heart disease requiring surgical intervention is addressed during the aortic replacement operation. Surgical replacement of the aortic root, ascending aorta, and arch is performed through a median sternotomy with the use of cardiopulmonary bypass, while replacement of the descending thoracic aorta is performed through a left thoracotomy. Procedures involving replacement of the aortic arch require periods of circulatory arrest with advanced circulation management strategies for cerebral protection. The aorta is replaced with a tubular prosthetic Dacron graft which is made from polyester and coated with either gelatin or collagen.

Postoperative course

The average postoperative hospital course for a patient who undergoes proximal (root, ascending, arch) aortic replacement is 7–10 days. Patients undergoing open descending or open thoracoabdominal aortic replacement have a longer average hospital course of 10–14 days.

Operative mortality

At our institution, the mortality for primary, elective replacement of the proximal aorta (root, ascending, arch) aorta is 2–4%, depending upon the amount of aorta replaced. The mortality for emergent repair of acute Type A aortic dissection is 14%. The overall mortality (elective and emergent) for descending or thoracoabdominal aortic replacement is 13%.

Special monitoring required

Patients undergoing proximal aortic surgery (root, ascending, arch) typically stay in the ICU for 1–3 days, depending upon the extent of aortic replacement. Patients undergoing descending or thoracoabdominal aortic replacement have longer ICU stays of 2–5 days. Aortic surgery patients have standard invasive monitoring consisting of a pulmonary artery catheter and a radial or femoral arterial line. Patients undergoing descending or thoracoabdominal aortic replacement will often have a lumbar spinal drain, and cerebrospinal fluid pressures will be measured for an average of 2 days.

Patient activity

After patients are extubated, early ambulation (postoperative day 2–3) and sitting in a chair is strongly encouraged.

Alimentation

Diet is advanced as tolerated.

Antibiotic coverage

Preoperative prophylaxis with a second-generation cephalosporin (cefuroxime), or Vancomycin in penicillin-allergic patients, is continued for 24 hours after surgery.

Major postoperative complications

Mediastinal hemorrhage

Postoperative bleeding following aortic surgery is always a major concern. Meticulous technique when performing aortic anastomoses combined with a careful inspection of all the surgical sites prior to closing the chest in the operating room can reduce postoperative bleeding. Drainage tubes are placed in the mediastinum and pleural spaces, and the amount of bleeding is measured hourly in the ICU. The platelet count, partial thromboplastin time, prothrombin time, INR, and fibrinogen levels are routinely measured and corrected accordingly. Additional maneuvers include warming the patient to reduce coagulopathy, increasing the positive end-expiratory pressure (PEEP) on the ventilator to 10–15 cm H_2O in an attempt to tamponade venous bleeding sites, and aggressive control of hypertension. In cases of severe coagulopathy that are unresponsive to transfusions of platelets, cryoprecipitate and fresh frozen plasma, recombinant Factor VII, is administered. Significant postoperative mediastinal hemorrhage with normal coagulation parameters requires emergent re-exploration in the operating room.

Neurologic injury

All cardiac surgery carries the risk of perioperative adverse neurologic outcomes. There is an increased risk of adverse neurologic outcomes due to a mandatory period of alteration of cerebral blood flow when patients undergo aortic arch replacement. There are two well-described forms of adverse neurologic outcomes associated with aortic arch surgery: permanent neurologic deficit (PND) and transient neurologic deficit (TND). Permanent neurologic deficit appears as a focal neurologic deficit or stroke, which is thought to be the result of embolic phenomena. Transient neurologic deficit is defined as postoperative confusion, delirium, obtundation, or transient focal deficits (resolution within 24 hours) with negative brain computed tomography or magnetic resonance imaging scans. Transient neurologic deficit is a reversible, diffuse, subtle injury which is an indicator of global cerebral injury due to inadequate cerebral protection. At Emory, the incidence of PND and TND following arch replacement is 1.9% and 4.4% respectively. In descending and thoracoabdominal aortic replacement, there is an additional risk of paraplegia from perioperative spinal cord ischemia. At Emory the overall risk of permanent paraplegia following either descending or thoracoabdominal aortic replacement is 3.6%.

Renal failure

Mild, postoperative transient renal dysfunction in aortic surgery patients is not uncommon, as renal blood flow and glomerular filtration rate may be reduced by 25–75% during cardiopulmonary bypass. In patients undergoing arch replacement requiring circulatory arrest, renal function is closely monitored in the postoperative period. At Emory, the incidence of patients undergoing circulatory arrest procedures who develop postoperative renal failure requiring dialysis is 4%.

Aortic surveillance

Patients who have undergone aortic replacement for aneurysmal disease or dissection require lifelong aortic surveillance. It is important to follow the size of the remaining native aorta with annual CT scans because a large percentage of these patients will eventually require a subsequent operation to replace a different section of their aorta. Annual echocardiograms are also crucial in monitoring both the size of the aortic root and the function of the aortic valve.

Further reading

Coady MA, Rizzo JA, Hammond GL *et al.* Surgical intervention criteria for thoracic aortic aneurysms: a study of growth rates and complications. *Ann Thorac Surg* 1999; **67**: 1922–6.

Elefteriades JA. Indications for aortic replacement. *J Thorac Cardiovasc Surg* 2010; **140**: S5–9.

Gleason TG, Bavaria JE. Trauma to great vessels. In Cohn LH, Edmunds LH Jr, ed. *Cardiac Surgery in the Adult*. New York, NY: McGraw-Hill; 2007, pp. 1229–49.

Hiratzka LF, Bakris GL, Beckman JA *et al.* 2010 ACCF/AHA /AATS/ACR/ASA/ SCA/SCAI/SIR/STS/SVM Guidelines for the diagnosis and management of patients with thoracic aortic disease: a report of the American College of Cardiology Foundation/American Heart Association Task Force on Practice Guidelines, American Association for Thoracic Surgery, American College of Radiology, American Stroke Association, Society of Cardiovascular Anesthesiologists, Society for Cardiovascular Angiography and Interventions, Society of Interventional Radiology, Society of Thoracic Surgeons, and Society for Vascular Medicine. *Circulation* 2010; **121**: e266–369.

Leshnower BG, Myung RJ, Kilgo PD *et al.* Moderate hypothermia and unilateral selective antegrade cerebral perfusion: a contemporary cerebral protection strategy for aortic arch surgery. *Ann Thorac Surg* 2010; **90**: 547–54.

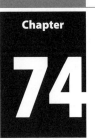

Chapter 74

Pulmonary lobectomy

Adil Sadiq and Felix G. Fernandez

Pulmonary lobectomy is most often performed for neoplasms of the lung, both benign and malignant. It may also be performed for residual bronchiectasis, pulmonary sequestration, refractory lung abscess, pulmonary tuberculosis, and other infectious processes.

Although a reasonable assessment of a patient's pulmonary function may be obtained by noting their exercise tolerance to commonly performed activities like climbing a flight of stairs, more objective assessment of their cardiac status is carried out as per the American College of Cardiology/American Heart Association guidelines. Evaluation of the pulmonary status includes pulmonary function tests, and in marginal cases quantitative ventilation/perfusion scans and cardiopulmonary exercise testing.

The use of Video-Assisted Thoracic Surgery (VATS) in recent years has produced similar or better results when compared with the traditional thoracotomy approach, along with a reduction in the mortality, morbidity, and in-hospital stay. The operation is performed under general anesthesia administered via a double-lumen endotracheal tube. The patient is placed in the lateral decubitus position with the operated side superior; the table is flexed maximally at the level of the patient's hips; and contralateral single lung ventilation is started. Continuous intraoperative monitoring of vital parameters has increased the safety of these procedures. A second-generation cephalosporin is administered preoperatively and continued for two postoperative doses. Intraoperative intercostal blocks help in postoperative pain management. Almost all patients are extubated in the operating suite following surgery.

Usual postoperative course
Expected postoperative hospital stay

The median duration of hospital stay is around 4 days, and is getting shorter with the use of a VATS approach. A protracted course in hospital is seen in patients with preoperative comorbidities or with subsequent postoperative complications.

Operative mortality

The operative mortality for elective surgery is between 1 and 1.5%.

Special monitoring required

Patients are usually observed in a monitored bed for the first 24 hours, where vital signs, pulse oximetry, chest tube drainage, and urine output are followed. Immediate portable upright chest X-rays should be obtained to assure both the presence of lung expansion and the absence of fluid collection. Daily portable upright chest X-rays help the surgeon to monitor lung expansion and pulmonary parenchymal changes. Chest physical therapy, ultrasonic nebulization, deep breathing exercises, and incentive spirometry are initiated in the immediate postoperative period and are continued until recovery. Pulmonary embolism is prevented perioperatively by the use of anti-embolism stockings, unless contraindicated.

Patient activity and positioning

Patients are nursed in the semi-Fowler position. To prevent pulmonary complications, early ambulation is emphasized.

Alimentation

Patients are allowed clear liquids 6 hours after extubation. Diet is advanced to a regular diet as tolerated.

Antibiotic coverage

Pulmonary embolism is prevented postoperatively by the administration of subcutaneous heparin, unless contraindicated.

Chest tubes

Chest tubes are connected to suction at 20 cm water. To prevent pulmonary complications, vigorous pulmonary toilet is emphasized. We favor early chest tube removal to reduce pain and promote pulmonary toilet and ambulation. Our criteria for chest tube removal are cessation of air leak and

Medical Management of the Surgical Patient, ed. Michael F. Lubin, Thomas F. Dodson, and Neil H. Winawer. Published by Cambridge University Press. © Cambridge University Press 2013.

drainage less than 300 mL per 24 hours. In the presence of an air leak, chest tubes are connected to suction for 48 hours to promote pleural apposition, after which they are placed on underwater seal drainage. Suction to the chest tubes beyond 48 hours is infrequently required in cases with large air leaks and when there is an increasing amount of subcutaneous emphysema or when unexpanded lung is associated with the air leak.

Pain management

Pain management strategy includes a patient-controlled analgesia pump for VATS and a thoracic epidural for patients requiring a thoracotomy.

Postoperative complications

In the hospital

Arrhythmias

Arrhythmias are some of the most commonly encountered complications, with an incidence of around 5–10%. The most frequent postoperative arrhythmias are atrial tachycardia, atrial fibrillation, and atrial flutter; they are usually controlled with anti-arrhythmic agents and by correction of any underlying electrolyte abnormalities.

Prolonged air leak

Air leak post surgery is commonly encountered, but is usually self-limiting by the third postoperative day. Prolonged air leak is defined as one persisting beyond a period of 7 days and is seen in 3–10% of cases. Suction to the chest tubes beyond 72 hours is required in cases with large air leaks with associated increasing subcutaneous emphysema or unexpanded lung. Management of prolonged air leaks includes bronchoscopy to rule out a bronchopleural fistula, followed by expectant management. Some patients may be discharged home with Heimlich valves, with a plan for chest tube removal after cessation of air leaks. However, if the air leak is large, especially in the presence of lung collapse or residual ipsilateral pleural space, reintervention should be considered by 1–2 weeks. The intraoperative use of various surgical sealants has been reported to decrease the incidence and duration of postoperative air leaks in various studies.

Persistent intrapleural space

A persistent intrapleural space may be seen in 5–15% of patients after a lobectomy, and may result from technical problems or from disease in the residual lung that prevents it from filling in the ensuing cavity. These cavities rarely become infected nor are they often a source of major morbidity.

Empyema

The incidence of post-lobectomy empyema is 0.01–2%. Unlike a post-pneumonectomy empyema, post-lobectomy empyema is rarely associated with a bronchopleural fistula; instead, the empyema is the result of the combination of a prolonged air leak and a persistent intrapleural space. Management is directed towards re-expansion of the remaining lung into the residual space along with tube drainage of the space and antibiotic therapy.

Bronchopleural fistula

Bronchial stump dehiscence can be either early or late and has an incidence of 1.5–3% following a lobectomy. Risk factors include chronic obstructive pulmonary disease, diabetes, hypoalbuminemia, previous steroid therapy, low preoperative predicted Forced Expiratory Volume in 1 second (FEV1), and postoperative positive pressure ventilation.

Early failure is seen within a few days to a few weeks following surgery and is usually due to technical reasons. Patients typically present with a large air leak and increasing subcutaneous emphysema. On occasion they have a fever and cough up copious amount of clear or purulent secretions. Principles of management include definitive drainage of the pleural space, revision of the bronchial stump and management of the contaminated residual pleural space.

Bleeding

Excessive bleeding is encountered in less than 1% of patients postoperatively, and is suggested by increased chest tube output. Management includes blood transfusion and a re-operation to achieve hemostasis, especially if blood loss has been greater than 300 mL/hour for 2 consecutive hours, or there has been hemodynamic compromise.

Miscellaneous

Other early complications are infrequent and include pulmonary embolism, respiratory failure, recurrent laryngeal nerve palsy, wound infection, and delirium.

After discharge

Bronchopleural fistulas

Patients with bronchopleural fistulas typically present with fever and with a history of coughing up copious amounts of clear or purulent secretions, usually 2 weeks beyond surgery. Late bronchial stump dehiscence is usually secondary to infection and weakened bronchial tissue. Principles of management are the same as that for early fistulas, and include the use of an open drainage with the Eloesser flap, especially in debilitated patients. An Eloesser flap is a single-stage procedure that involves a U-shaped incision and the resection of a number of subjacent posterolateral ribs. The U-shaped flap is then folded into the pleural space creating a permanent communication.

Miscellaneous

Other late complications are uncommon and include arrhythmias and a persistent intrapleural space.

Further reading

Cerfolio RJ. Recent advances in the treatment of air leaks. *Curr Opin Pulmon Med* 2005; **11**: 319–23.

Deslauriers J, Mehran RJ, eds. *Handbook of Perioperative Care in General Thoracic Surgery*. Philadelphia, PA: Elsevier Health Sciences; 2005, pp. 303–91.

Fleisher LA, Beckman JA, Brown KA et al. ACC/AHA 2007 Guidelines on Perioperative Cardiovascular Evaluation and Care for Noncardiac Surgery. *J Am Coll Cardiol* 2007; **50**: e159–242.

Gharagozloo F, Margolis M, Facktor M, Tempesta B, Najam F. Postpneumonectomy and postlobectomy empyema. *Thorac Surg Clin* 2006; **16**: 215–22.

Kozower BD, Sheng S, O'Brien SM et al. STS database risk models: predictors of mortality and major morbidity for lung cancer resection. *Ann Thorac Surg* 2010; **90**: 875–83.

Malapert G, Hanna HA, Pages PB, Bernard A. Surgical sealant for the prevention of prolonged air leak after lung resection: meta-analysis. *Ann Thorac Surg* 2010; **90**: 1779–85.

McKenna RJ Jr, Houck W, Fuller CB. Video-assisted thoracic surgery lobectomy. Experience with 1100 cases. *Ann Thorac Surg* 2006; **81**: 421–6.

Murthy SC. Air leak and pleural space management. *Thorac Surg Clin* 2006; **16**: 261–5.

Shaw JP, Dembitzer FR, Wisnivesky JP et al. Video-assisted thoracoscopic lobectomy: state of the art and future directions. *Ann Thorac Surg* 2008; **85**: S705–9.

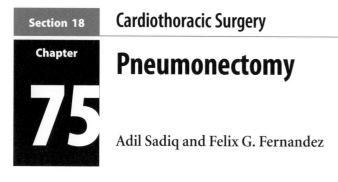

Chapter

75

Pneumonectomy

Adil Sadiq and Felix G. Fernandez

Currently, pneumonectomy is often performed for a bulky and centrally located carcinoma of the lung. Occasionally it is indicated for a destroyed lung secondary to chronic infectious disease such as tuberculosis, bronchiectasis, or fungal disease. In general, we favor preservation of pulmonary parenchyma and avoidance of pneumonectomy through the use of bronchial and/or vascular sleeve resections when possible.

All patients require a thorough evaluation to rule out metastatic disease as well as to ascertain their ability to tolerate the operation. Assessment of their cardiac status is carried out as per the American College of Cardiology/American Heart Association guidelines. Evaluation of the pulmonary status includes pulmonary function tests and, in marginal cases, quantitative ventilation/perfusion scans and cardiopulmonary exercise testing.

The operation is performed under general anesthesia administered via a double-lumen endotracheal tube. Although potentially feasible thoracoscopically for some tumors, our current approach for a pneumonectomy is through a posterolateral thoracotomy. A thoracic epidural is the cornerstone of pain management in patients undergoing a thoracotomy. The patient is placed in the lateral decubitus position with the operated side superior; the table is flexed maximally at the level of the patient's hips; and contralateral single lung ventilation is started. Fiberoptic bronchoscopy allows confirmation of tube position and helps to rule out endobronchial disease. Continuous intraoperative monitoring of vital parameters has increased the safety of these procedures. A second-generation cephalosporin is administered preoperatively and continued for two postoperative doses. Almost all patients are extubated in the operating suite following surgery.

There is variability with respect to the use of a thoracostomy tube after a pneumonectomy. Those surgeons not placing chest tubes typically aspirate 500–1,000 cc of air from the pneumonectomy space to balance the mediastinum. We prefer to leave a 28 Fr chest tube for 24 hours, with the admonition to place it either to water seal or a balanced drainage system. *The chest tube should never be attached to a suction device.*

Usual postoperative course
Expected postoperative hospital stay

The median duration of hospital stay is around 6 days, with a protracted course seen in patients with preoperative comorbidities or with postoperative complications.

Operative mortality

The operative mortality for elective surgery is between 5 and 8%. A right pneumonectomy is associated with approximately twice the operative mortality as a left pneumonectomy.

Special monitoring required

Patients are usually observed in a monitored bed for the first 24 hours, where vital signs, pulse oximetry, chest tube drainage, and urine output are followed. Chest tubes, if present, are connected to a balanced drainage system. The chest tube is removed within 24 hours to remove a potential portal for entry of infection into the pneumonectomy space. Immediate portable upright chest X-rays should be obtained to assure both the presence of contralateral lung expansion and the absence of fluid collections, and to evaluate the possibility of mediastinal shift. To help the surgeon observe lung expansion and monitor parenchymal changes on the non-operative side, daily portable upright chest X-rays are taken. The clinician will also note the gradual rise of fluid in the pneumonectomy space. Chest physical therapy, ultrasonic nebulization, deep breathing exercises, and incentive spirometry are initiated in the immediate postoperative period and are continued until recovery. To prevent pulmonary complications, vigorous pulmonary toilet is emphasized.

Patient activity and positioning

Patients are nursed in the semi-Fowler position. To prevent pulmonary complications, early ambulation is emphasized. Pulmonary embolism is also prevented perioperatively by the use of anti-embolism stockings.

Medical Management of the Surgical Patient, ed. Michael F. Lubin, Thomas F. Dodson, and Neil H. Winawer. Published by Cambridge University Press. © Cambridge University Press 2013.

Alimentation

Patients are kept NPO until the morning of postoperative day 1, at which time clear liquids are initiated. The diet is advanced to a regular diet, as tolerated by the patient.

Antibiotic coverage

Pulmonary embolism is prevented postoperatively by the administration of subcutaneous heparin, unless contraindicated.

Pain management

Administration of thoracic epidural analgesia aids pain management and helps in recovery.

Postoperative complications

In the hospital

Arrhythmias

Arrhythmias are some of the most commonly encountered complications, with an incidence of around 12–18%; these conditions include atrial fibrillation, atrial tachycardia, and atrial flutter. They are usually controlled with anti-arrhythmic or rate-control agents and by correction of any underlying electrolyte abnormalities.

Early post-pneumonectomy empyema and bronchopleural fistula

The overall incidence of empyema is 2–16%. It is associated with a bronchopleural fistula in 75–80% of cases, and the combination has a mortality rate of 30–40%. Empyema without a fistula has a 5% mortality rate. Patients often present coughing up copious serosanguinous secretions.

Bronchial stump dehiscence can be either early or late and is more common after a right pneumonectomy (9–14%) than a left pneumonectomy (2.3%). Risk factors include chronic obstructive pulmonary disease, diabetes, hypoalbuminemia, previous steroid therapy, low preoperative predicted Forced Expiratory Volume in 1 second (FEV1), and postoperative positive pressure ventilation. Early failure is seen within a few days to a few weeks following surgery and is usually due to technical reasons. Patients typically present with a large air leak and increasing subcutaneous emphysema.

In either case, initial management is directed toward prevention of aspiration into the contralateral lung by placing the patient in a reverse Trendelenburg position with the pneumonectomy side down, along with tube drainage of the space. Bronchoscopy is performed to document the presence of a fistula. Definitive treatment includes debridement of the bronchial stump and closure under antibiotic coverage.

Post-pneumonectomy pulmonary edema

Although the incidence of post-pneumonectomy pulmonary edema (PPE) varies between 4 and 7%, it is associated with mortality rates as high as 50%. Post-pneumonectomy pulmonary edema is most common after a right pneumonectomy, and

signs usually manifest within the first 72 hours. Post-pneumonectomy pulmonary edema can progress rapidly, and within a few hours patients need intubation and mechanical ventilation. Preventive strategies are aimed at minimizing the use of blood and blood products along with avoidance of intraoperative pressure and volume trauma to the normal lung. Management is targeted at ventilatory, hemodynamic, and nutritional support. Inhaled nitric oxide has been shown to improve oxygenation in selected cases.

Bleeding

Excessive bleeding is encountered in less than 1% of patients postoperatively, and is suggested by increased chest tube output or a significant fall in serial hematocrit. Management includes blood transfusion or a reoperation to achieve hemostasis, especially if blood loss has been greater than 200 mL/hour for 3 consecutive hours; or if, in the absence of a chest drain, there has been hemodynamic compromise.

Miscellaneous

Other early complications are infrequent and include pulmonary embolism, respiratory failure, recurrent laryngeal nerve palsy, post-pneumonectomy syndrome, wound infection, delirium, and cardiac herniation (the latter especially after an intra-pericardial pneumonectomy).

After discharge

Late post-pneumonectomy empyema

The occurrence of late post-pneumonectomy empyema is less frequently associated with a bronchopleural fistula, but it is often associated with mediastinal induration and extensive pleural space contamination. Principles of management include open window thoracostomy drainage, debridement of the pleural space, closure of a bronchopleural fistula (if present), and obliteration of the pleural cavity.

Late bronchopleural fistulas

Patients with late bronchopleural fistulas typically present with fever and with a history of coughing up copious amounts of clear or purulent secretions, usually 2 weeks beyond surgery. Sometimes minor fistulas are diagnosed radiologically by virtue of a decreasing air-fluid level or the appearance of a new air bubble on the side of the pneumonectomy. Late bronchial stump dehiscence is usually secondary to infection and weakened bronchial tissue. The modified Clagett procedure is the mainstay of management and includes open drainage and thorough debridement, bronchial stump closure, successive antibiotic irrigation and packing, and watertight closure of the chest cavity 7–10 days later, when healthy granulation tissue lines the chest cavity.

Miscellaneous

Other late complications are uncommon and include arrhythmias and respiratory insufficiency, especially in patients with borderline residual pulmonary reserve.

References

Deslauriers J, Grégoire J. Techniques of pneumonectomy. Drainage after pneumonectomy. *Chest Surg Clin North Am* 1999; **9**: 437–48.

Deslauriers J, Mehran RJ, eds. *Handbook of Perioperative Care in General Thoracic Surgery*. Philadelphia, PA: Elsevier Health Sciences; 2005, pp. 303–91.

Fernandez FG, Force SF, Pickens A *et al.* Impact of laterality on early and late outcomes after pneumonectomy. *Ann Thorac Surg* 2011; **92**: 244–9.

Fleisher LA, Beckman JA, Brown KA *et al.* ACC/AHA 2007 Guidelines on Perioperative Cardiovascular Evaluation and Care for Noncardiac Surgery. *J Am Coll Cardiol* 2007; **50**: e159–242.

Gharagozloo F, Margolis M, Facktor M, Tempesta B, Najam F. Postpneumonectomy and postlobectomy empyema. *Thorac Surg Clin* 2006; **16**: 215–22.

Kozower BD, Sheng S, O'Brien SM *et al.* STS Database Risk Models: predictors of mortality and major morbidity for lung cancer resection. *Ann Thorac Surg* 2010; **90**: 875–83.

Liberman M, Cassivi SD. Bronchial stump dehiscence: update on prevention and management. *Semin Thorac Cardiovasc Surg* 2007; **19**: 366–73.

Nwogu CE, Glinianski M, Demmy TL. Minimally invasive pneumonectomy. *Ann Thorac Surg* 2006; **82**: e3–4.

Villeneuve PJ, Sundaresan S. Complications of pulmonary resection: postpneumonectomy pulmonary edema and postpneumonectomy syndrome. *Thorac Surg Clin* 2006; **16**: 223–34.

Chapter

76

Lung transplantation

Radu F. Neamu, David C. Neujahr, and Seth D. Force

Over the course of almost 50 years, lung transplantation has evolved from an experimental project to a significant means to prolong life and its quality in carefully selected patients with end-stage lung diseases. The introduction of cyclosporine as an immunosuppressive agent in the 1980s allowed for sufficient graft survival to make clinical lung transplantation a reality. Since then, more than 32,000 lung transplants have been performed.

Usual postoperative course
Expected postoperative hospital stay

Lung transplantation is a very complex surgical procedure. Usually the hospital stay is lengthy, close to 2 weeks if no complications occur. There is also an association between more severe disease, as determined by high lung allocation scores, and longer durations of hospital stay, averaging 5–6 weeks.

Operative mortality

Advances in surgical technique have lowered the rate of surgical complications and overall mortality. However, the rate of medical complications (usually a consequence of immunosuppression needed to ensure the survivability of the graft) still remains high. The inescapable constant exposure of the lungs to the environment also contributes to the significantly decreased survival rates of lung transplant recipients when compared with other solid organ recipients. Hence, in spite of relatively good 30-day and 1-year survival, the 5-year survival post lung transplant remains at 50%.

Special monitoring required

Routine ICU care plays an important role in a successful transplantation and decreased length of stay; it should be employed conscientiously by the treatment teams. After surgical intervention is performed, the patient remains intubated with a single lumen endotracheal tube and is transferred to the ICU for close hemodynamic monitoring and continuation of mechanical ventilation support. Hemodynamic support comes from the use of vasopressors, inotropes and judicious use of intravenous fluids. Close attention is paid to ensure hemodynamic stability and adequate ventilatory and oxygenation parameters, in parallel with prevention and early recognition of possible early complications. A strong collaboration between all the teams involved in the care of the post-transplant patient is essential for achieving these goals. Expedited management of early complications is critical.

Patient activity and positioning

Lung transplantation will significantly impact multiple organs and systems, impairing the recipient's ability to function independently in the immediate postoperative period. Therefore, physical therapists play an important role in identifying and correcting these impairments in a steady but rapid progression. Early mobilization and frequent changes of position after cessation of mechanical ventilation improves ventilation, lung perfusion, oxygenation, clearance of pulmonary secretions, and drainage from chest tubes. Postural drainage with shaking, vibration, and percussion, or flutter valve use can also facilitate clearance of secretions.

Alimentation

It is well known that malnutrition has a significant detrimental effect on transplant outcomes. Severe gastrointestinal (GI) complications like gastroesophageal reflux, gastroparesis, and distal intestinal obstruction can occur after lung transplantation and alter the ability to provide adequate nutrition. The risk of aspiration is also increased in the acute post-transplant phase. For these reasons, early aggressive measures must be taken to identify and manage these complications. Nutritionists and speech therapists are integral members of the multiteam approach for the lung transplant recipients. Early oral intake and use of the GI tract, if tolerated, are emphasized. If the GI tract is non-functional, then parenteral nutrition can be implemented.

Medical Management of the Surgical Patient, ed. Michael F. Lubin, Thomas F. Dodson, and Neil H. Winawer. Published by Cambridge University Press. © Cambridge University Press 2013.

Immunosuppressive and prophylactic coverage

Immunosuppressive and prophylactic medications to prevent rejection and infection, respectively, are initiated at the time of transplantation. Various regimens are used by each center. Familiarity with the multiple side-effects and drug interactions of these agents is crucial to providing adequate care to lung transplant recipients.

Immunosuppressive induction therapy depletes the T-cell populations and consists of rabbit or equine antithymocyte globulin, murine monoclonal anti-CD3 antibody (OKT3), targeted interleukin-2 (IL-2) receptor antibodies (daclizumab and basiliximab), and wide-scale depletion of multiple immune lineages with Campath 1-H. It is estimated that only about half of the centers use this approach for the initiation of immunosuppression.

Postoperative ventilation

Different modes of ventilation can be applied as long as peak airway pressure ($<$ 30 cm H_2O) is monitored to prevent airway barotrauma. Pressure-controlled modes are preferred to avoid this complication. Weaning from mechanical ventilation should be achieved as soon as feasible. A bronchoscopy to document the integrity of the anastomoses and the lack of significant amount of secretions usually precedes extubation.

After discharge

Routine care

Once the lung transplant recipient is discharged, an intense surveillance schedule is employed for the first year to monitor for allograft dysfunction and correct administration of medications, to allow for prevention or rapid management of complications. The patient should be instructed about the signs and symptoms of rejection or infection. Close contact with a transplant coordinator should be established. Routine clinic visits usually include at least a chest X-ray, pulmonary function tests, chemistry panels, and hemograms. Other tests are obtained at the physician's discretion. The frequency of clinic visits decreases as the patient's clinical status improves. The large majority of centers will also perform scheduled surveillance bronchoscopies to detect clinically silent acute rejection in a timely manner. This procedure involves random transbronchial lung biopsies of the transplanted allografts; results are read by a pathologist experienced in grading rejection. Finally, pulmonary rehabilitation is instrumental in achieving good physiological results.

Postoperative complications

In the hospital

Primary graft dysfunction

Primary graft dysfunction (PGD), the clinical term for ischemia-reperfusion injury of lung transplantation, is a serious complication in the first 72 hours post-surgery. Its grading is based on the presence of bilateral lung infiltrates and the P_aO_2/F_iO_2 ratio, in the absence of other possible etiologies like hyperacute rejection, volume overload, or pneumonia. Once PGD is established, management includes lung protective ventilatory strategies similar to the ARDS protocol, conservative fluid management, and inhaled nitric oxide.

Rejection

Acute rejection, the most common form of rejection in the first year, is an important source of morbidity. A strong association exists between episodes of acute rejection and later development of chronic rejection. Patients present with non-specific complaints and signs like shortness of breath, fevers, cough, and hypoxemia that can also mimic infections. Transbronchial biopsies are usually helpful in establishing the diagnosis and the grade of severity, based on the presence of perivascular infiltrates. Therapy includes augmentation of immunosuppression, ordinarily starting with a pulse dose of intravenous steroids for 3 days, which is then followed by tapering of oral steroids.

The most common form of chronic allograft rejection manifests clinically as bronchiolitis obliterans syndrome (BOS), a cicatricial process of the small airways leading to complete obliteration of the lumen. It is a major cause of late morbidity and mortality in lung transplant recipients. The onset of BOS can be insidious or abrupt with weight loss, dyspnea, cough and recurrent episodes of tracheobronchitis, with *Pseudomonas aeruginosa* being the most common culprit. It is estimated that up to 40% of patients with BOS will succumb within 2 years of onset.

Infections

Lung transplant recipients have an increased propensity to develop infections because of heightened immunosuppression, blunted cough reflex, decreased mucociliary clearance, and constant exposure to the environment.

Bacterial infections of the lower respiratory tract are more frequent within the first month after transplant or can occur later, more often as a harbinger of bronchiolitis obliterans. *Pseudomonas aeruginosa* and *Staphyloccocus* species are among the most common isolates. A common practice is to administer broad-spectrum antibiotics immediately after transplant to cover for all the possible pathogens from the donor lungs until the cultures are finalized.

Cytomegalovirus (CMV) infection is the most common viral infection, especially in seronegative recipients who acquire lungs from a donor exposed to CMV. Prophylaxis with intravenous ganciclovir or oral vanganciclovir has reduced its incidence and impact.

Fungal infections with *Aspergillus* and *Candida* spp. have significant morbidity and mortality in lung transplant recipients. Differentiating between colonization and invasive infection can be difficult. However, with the current use of postoperative prophylactic antifungal therapies, invasive infections occur more rarely.

Prophylaxis against *Pneumocystis jirovecii* is a standard lifelong measure for all lung transplant patients. Treatment options include sulfa-based therapy, atovoquone, dapsone, or monthly inhaled pentamidine.

After discharge

Airway complications

Airway complications consist of bronchial stenosis or dehiscence, granulation tissue overgrowth and tracheobronchomalacia. In general, a specific endoscopic or surgical intervention can be employed for each situation. Extensive use of vasopressors, especially beyond their main purpose, can predispose to later development of airway complications like anastomotic dehiscence or bronchial stenosis.

Pleural effusions are common immediately post-transplant, a consequence of the injury to the pulmonary lymphatics. Beyond the immediate period, a new pleural effusion needs to have adequate diagnostic studies to establish the cause, followed by specific management afterwards.

Other complications

A plethora of complications affecting practically almost every organ and system in the body can occur in a lung transplant recipient. Post-surgical complications are usually a consequence of the administration of immunosuppressive medications. However, most of these complications are common to the entire solid organ transplant patient population.

Lung transplant recipients are more prone to develop skin cancers, lymphoproliferative disorders and other malignancies when compared with the general population. More specific to the lung transplant population, lung cancer seems to have a higher incidence in the native lung of a single lung recipient with underlying COPD or pulmonary fibrosis.

Underscoring the protean effects of immunosuppressive agents, almost 86% of the 5-year survivors will have hypertension and 91% will develop different stages of chronic renal failure. Hyperlipidemia, diabetes mellitus, osteoporosis, and bone marrow failure are all very common complications in the majority of lung transplant recipients, re-emphasizing the need for close follow-up of these patients throughout the rest of their lives.

Further reading

Ahmad S, Shlobin OA, Nathan SD. Pulmonary complications of lung transplantation. *Chest* 2011; **139**: 402–11.

Christie JD, Carby M, Bag R *et al.* Report of the ISHLT Working Group on Primary Lung Graft Dysfunction. Part II: definition. A consensus statement of the International Society for Heart and Lung Transplantation. *J Heart Lung Transpl* 2005; **24**: 1454–9.

Christie JD, Edwards LB, Kucheryavaya AY *et al.* The Registry of the International Society for Heart and Lung Transplantation: Twenty-seventh official adult lung and heart-lung transplant report – 2010. *J Heart Lung Transpl* 2010; **29**: 1104–18.

Collins J, Kazerooni EA, Lacomis J *et al.* Bronchogenic carcinoma after lung transplantation: frequency, clinical characteristics, and imaging findings. *Radiology* 2002; **224**: 131–8.

Date H, Lynch JP, Sundaresan S *et al.* The impact of cytolytic therapy on bronchiolitis obliterans syndrome. *J Heart Lung Transpl* 1998; **17**: 869–75.

Kirk AD. Induction immunosuppression. *Transplantation* 2006; **82**: 593–602.

Lyu DM, Zamora MR. Medical complications of lung transplantation. *Proc Am Thorac Soc* 2009; **6**: 101–7.

Pierre AF, Keshavjee S. Lung transplantation: donor and recipient critical care aspects. *Curr Opin Crit Care* 2005; **11**: 339–44.

Sims KD, Blumberg EA. Common infections in the lung transplant recipient. *Clin Chest Med* 2011; **32**: 327–41.

Stewart S, Fishbein MC, Snell GI *et al.* Revision of the 1996 working formulation for the standardization of nomenclature in the diagnosis of lung rejection. *J Heart Lung Transpl* 2007; **26**: 1229–42.

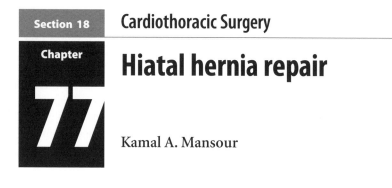

Hiatal hernia repair

Chapter

77

Kamal A. Mansour

Indications for surgical repair of hiatal hernia include failure of strict medical management (intractability); reflux esophagitis with ulcerations, stricture, or bleeding; recurrent aspiration pneumonia; large sliding hernias; and all paraesophageal hernias. The purpose of surgery is twofold: to reposition the stomach below the diaphragm and to re-establish gastroesophageal competence. Three approaches (transabdominal, transthoracic and laparoscopic) and three primary techniques (Belsey, Hill, and Nissen) are used, depending on the preference of the surgeon. The advent of minimally invasive techniques has brought about a shift in the operative approach of patients with hiatal hernia. Today the laparoscopic repair of a hiatal hernia has almost completely replaced the open approach through either a laparotomy or a left thoracotomy. If either procedure is performed well, the magnitude of surgical stress is low. General endotracheal anesthesia is typically used and the operative time is 2–3 hours, depending on the skills of the surgeon. Intraoperative blood transfusions are rarely required.

Usual postoperative course
Expected postoperative hospital stay

The expected postoperative hospital stay ranges from 7–10 days for open procedures and 2–5 days for the minimally invasive approach. Length of stay is also influenced by the age and associated medical condition of the patient.

Operative mortality

Operative mortality is under 1%.

Special monitoring required

Intraoperative assessment of the lower esophageal sphincter zone is performed by pressure manometric studies.

Patient activity and positioning

If a transthoracic approach is used, a chest tube is inserted and removed after 24 hours, after which ambulation is allowed.

Alimentation

A nasogastric tube is usually left in place for the first 24 hours. Patients are then given clear liquids and food intake is advanced to a soft diet, which is maintained until hospital discharge.

Antibiotic coverage

A second-generation cephalosporin is given during the 24-hour perioperative period.

Chest physiotherapy

Chest physiotherapy is stressed, especially when the transthoracic approach is used, to minimize pulmonary complications.

Barium swallow

A barium or gastrografin swallow is performed on the seventh postoperative day to assess the status of the surgical repair and to provide a baseline study for follow-up.

Postoperative complications
In the hospital
Pulmonary complications

Pulmonary complications are caused by retained secretions, which are less frequent following the laparoscopic approach. Pneumothorax is the most common complication of laparoscopic fundoplication.

Medical Management of the Surgical Patient, ed. Michael F. Lubin, Thomas F. Dodson, and Neil H. Winawer. Published by Cambridge University Press. © Cambridge University Press 2013.

Temporary dysphagia

Edema at the cardia may result in temporary dysphagia, which should improve with observation. The patient is maintained on a soft diet until this complication resolves.

Rupture of the stomach

This has been reported in cases in which a Nissen fundoplication was left in the chest or herniated into the chest postoperatively.

Ulceration

Some instances of bleeding peptic ulcer have occurred along the lesser curvature in association with a Nissen repair; their cause is not definitely known.

Splenic injury

Intraoperative splenic injury requiring splenorrhaphy or splenectomy may occur in association with Nissen fundoplication.

After discharge

Recurrence

Hernia recurrence is reported in 8% (Nissen) to 18% (Belsey) of patients following primary open repair. Results after laparoscopic repair compare favorably with open techniques. In the presence of symptomatic, radiologic, and endoscopic evidence of recurrent gastroesophageal reflux, another surgical repair is indicated.

Gas-bloat syndrome

Gas-bloat syndrome occurs in 15% of patients after Nissen fundoplication. It results from over-distension of the stomach that is not relieved by belching or vomiting. Repeated esophageal dilatation or reoperation may be required.

Further reading

Fenton KN, Miller JI Jr, Lee RB, Mansour KA. Belsey Mark IV antireflux procedure for complicated gastroesophageal reflux disease. *Ann Thorac Surg* 1997; **64**: 790–4.

Fisichella PM, Patti MG. Laparoscopic repair of paraesophageal hiatal hernias. *J Laparoendosc Adv Surg Tech* 2008; **18**: 629–34.

Mansour KA, Burton HG, Miller JI Jr, Hatcher CR Jr. Complications of intrathoracic Nissen fundoplication. *Ann Thorac Surg* 1981; **32**: 173–8.

Waring JP. Surgical and endoscopic treatment of gastroesophageal reflux disease. *Gastroenterol Clin North Am* 2002; **31**: S89–109.

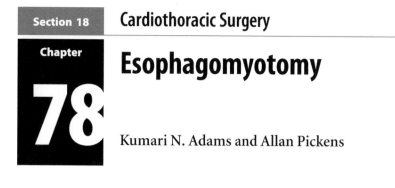

Esophagomyotomy

Kumari N. Adams and Allan Pickens

Esophagomyotomy involves splitting the muscular layers of the distal esophagus and proximal stomach while leaving the mucosa intact. Esophagomyotomy is primarily performed for esophageal diverticula and achalasia. When used to treat esophageal diverticula, the esophagomyotomy is performed in conjunction with a diverticulopexy or diverticulectomy. The most common indication for esophagomyotomy is the treatment of achalasia. This procedure is also known as the Heller myotomy, named after Ernest Heller who introduced the technique in 1913 to originally include a double cardio-esophagomyotomy of the anterior and posterior esophagus. The operation was modified in 1923 by Zaaiger with the primary objective being to adequately divide the two muscle layers (longitudinal and circular) to create an anterior myotomy only.

Four approaches for esophagomyotomy have been described: transabdominal, transthoracic, minimally invasive thoracoscopic, and laparoscopic. The principle tenets of the operation are shared by all four techniques. The tenets are adequate exposure of the esophagus and gastric cardia, identification of the gastroesophageal junction by resection of epiphrenic fat pad, identification of the vagus nerves, and sufficient division of the esophageal muscle layers. Division of the muscle layers involves proximal extension onto the esophagus for 6–8 cm and distal extension onto the gastric cardia for 2–3 cm. Currently, the laparoscopic approach is favored because of technical advantages that include a shorter recovery period. The laparoscopic approach is considered the gold standard.

Reflux is a well-documented side-effect of esophagomyotomy; thus, the myotomy is often accompanied by an anti-reflux procedure. Partial fundoplication is usually done since there may be some esophageal motility dysfunction. The benefit of adding a partial fundoplication is no longer debated; however, the type of partial fundoplication (posterior/Toupet or anterior/Dor) remains controversial.

General anesthesia is utilized for all approaches. For the transabdominal and laparoscopic approaches, most surgeons place the patient in a supine position; however, some prefer the low lithotomy position. If performed transthoracically, the patient is placed in the right lateral decubitus position for a left thoracotomy or left video-assisted thoracoscopic (VATS) approach with a double-lumen endotracheal tube to allow single-lung ventilation. Technical difficulty depends on the patient's surgical history, severity of disease, and technique utilized. Blood transfusions are rarely necessary. Intraoperative endoscopy has become a popular and useful adjunct to the procedure. This allows for both the testing of adequacy and extent of muscle splitting. Some operators have incorporated both endoscopy and manometry intraoperatively. Nasogastric tubes are carefully advanced across myotomies into the stomach to reduce postoperative distension and regurgitation; both can cause esophageal perforation.

Usual postoperative course
Expected postoperative hospital stay

A faster recovery and shorter hospital stay with minimally invasive esophagomyotomy is facilitated by its smaller incisions and less pain. The postoperative stay typically ranges from 1–3 days. Open approaches can extend hospital stay up to 10 days.

Operative mortality

Regardless of approach, operative mortality is low for esophagomyotomy; it ranges from 0–0.7%.

Special monitoring required

Intraoperative manometry, which assesses the accuracy of the myotomy by measuring the residual pressures across the GE junction, can be a useful adjunct; typically, though, it is not available. Intraoperative endoscopy is more commonly used to visually assess the completeness of the esophagocardiomyotomy and test for mucosal perforation. Endoscopy allows the surgeon to check for leaks by insufflating air while submerging the myotomy site under irrigation.

Medical Management of the Surgical Patient, ed. Michael F. Lubin, Thomas F. Dodson, and Neil H. Winawer. Published by Cambridge University Press. © Cambridge University Press 2013.

Patient activity and positioning

When a minimally invasive approach is used, patients may be out of bed on the day of surgery. If a transthoracic (open or VATS) approach is used, a left chest tube is placed at the time of surgery and usually removed within 48 hours. Chest tubes can cause discomfort with activity; thus, patient-controlled anesthesia (PCA) and epidurals are often used with transthoracic approaches.

Alimentation

Immediately after the procedure, esophagomyotomy patients remain NPO with intravenous fluids. Routinely, a contrast swallow study is performed on the first postoperative day. If the contrast study reveals no leak or obstruction, oral feeding can begin. Typically a liquid diet is started and advanced to a soft diet as tolerated. Most patients are discharged on a soft diet with instructions to avoid bulky foods and foods with sharp edges because the myotomy site must be allowed to heal before consuming a regular diet.

Postoperative radiographs

If a transthoracic approach is utilized, postoperative chest X-rays are obtained to detect residual pneumothorax, effusion, and atelectasis. Pneumomediastinum from a perforation also can be detected on a postoperative chest X-ray. Contrast studies are performed on the first postoperative day to assess for leakage. Initially, most radiologists will perform a water-soluble contrast (gastrografin) swallow because extravasation of water-soluble contrast into the mediastinum from a leak has fewer complications than barium. However, if there is no obvious leak, water-soluble contrast should always be followed by barium contrast because barium coats the mucosa more diffusely and has the ability to detect smaller mucosal defects.

Antibiotic coverage

Preoperative prophylaxis with a second-generation cephalosporin (e.g., cefotetan or cefoxitin) is given intravenously 30 minutes prior to the incision and continued for 2 doses postoperatively. If there is a mucosal perforation, broad-spectrum antibiotics and antifungal therapy will be needed.

Drains

For the transabdominal approaches (open or laparoscopic), drains are not routinely used. If a leak is found intraoperatively, an abdominal drain may be placed. During transthoracic approaches, a chest tube is placed. The chest tube is connected to wall suction at 20 cm H_2O. In the absence of an air leak, mucosal perforation, or large pneumothorax, the chest tube is placed to water seal on postoperative day 1 and subsequently to be removed on postoperative day 2.

Postoperative complications

In the hospital

Mucosal perforation

One of the most feared complications is an unrecognized mucosal perforation. Most series report a 1–7% occurrence. Perforation is often recognized intraoperatively. Small microperforations can be detected when endoscopy is utilized. The esophagus is distended with air from the endoscope, and the mucosal surface is then submerged under irrigation to assess for the presence of bubbles. If a leak is found, it should be repaired promptly. Primary suture repair of the perforation is often feasible; the repair site should be covered with the gastric fundus or omentum for reinforcement.

Incomplete myotomy

This, too, can be recognized at the time of operation with the use of intraoperative endoscopy. It is seen as a non-uniform mucosal bulge when the esophagus is distended with air. This characteristic mucosal appearance is due to residual muscle bands that were not adequately transected. These muscle bands must be carefully disrupted.

Pulmonary complications

Rarely pneumothorax after laparoscopic esophagomyotomy occurs; it usually does not require tube thoracostomy because the carbon dioxide is readily absorbed. Aspiration also is rare, but it can occur on induction of general anesthesia. Aspiration is more likely when the esophagus is dilated, making it prone to retain food and liquid; this often occurs with achalasia and esophageal diverticula. Consequently, steps should be taken to avoid aspiration. A nasogastric tube can be inserted if the patient can tolerate it. Rapid sequence intubation is performed on the assumption that residual debris can be present in the aperistaltic dilated esophagus. Lastly, to aspirate any retained esophageal debris, intraoperative endoscopy can be performed with minimal insufflation.

Temporary dysphagia

Patients may initially report postoperative dysphagia as a result of the edema of the surrounding tissues. This usually resolves within 4–6 weeks. Patients are counseled on a post-fundoplication-type diet, with gradual advancement and consumption of small, frequent meals. If the dysphagia does not resolve, it may be due to scarring or an incomplete myotomy. Scarring will respond to careful endoscopic balloon dilation, but an incomplete myotomy will eventually require reoperation.

After discharge
Persistent dysphagia

While 80–98% of patients achieve good outcomes and report complete resolution of dysphagia symptoms, the persistence of dysphagia has been reported in 14–30%. This can be due to the presence of a large, dilated, aperistaltic esophagus despite disruption of the lower esophageal sphincter. Incomplete myotomy and tight fundoplication are other causes of persistent dysphagia. Up to 25% of these patients require intervention.

Gastroesophageal reflux

While the majority of patients report resolution of dysphagia after esophagomyotomy, this procedure alone can result in up to a 48% incidence of gastroesophageal reflux. Consequently, many series have demonstrated that a concurrent anti-reflux procedure with partial fundoplication (Dor or Toupet) significantly decreases the risk of postoperative reflux to 2–9%. Patients are usually followed long-term with esophagoscopy, manometry and 24-hour pH testing, depending on the presenting symptoms. Postoperative reflux can often be controlled with medical therapy.

Further reading

Campos GM, Vittinghoff E, Rabl C et al. Endoscopic and surgical treatments for achalasia: a systematic review and meta-analysis. *Ann Surg* 2009; **249**: 45–57.

Chang AC. Management of distal esophageal pulsion diverticula. In Ferguson MK, ed. *Difficult Decisions in Thoracic Surgery: An Evidence-Based Approach*. 2nd edn. London: Springer-Verlag, 2011, Part 3, pp. 303–11.

Deb S, Deschamps C, Allen MS et al. Laparoscopic esophageal myotomy for achalasia: factors affecting functional results. *Ann Thorac Surg* 2005; **80**: 1191–5.

Eldaif SM, Mutrie CJ, Rutledge WC et al. The risk of esophageal resection after esophagomyotomy for achalasia. *Ann Thorac Surg* 2009; **87**: 1558–63.

Jeansonne LO, White BC, Pilger KE. Ten-year follow-up of laparoscopic Heller myotomy for achalasia shows durability. *Surg Endosc* 2007; **21**: 1498–502.

Kaufman JA, Oelschlager BK. Esophagocardiomyotomy for achalasia (Heller). In Sugarbaker DJ, Bueno R,

Krasna MJ et al., eds. *Adult Chest Surgery*. New York, NY: McGraw-Hill; 2009.

Litle VR. Laparoscopic Heller myotomy for achalasia: a review of the controversies. *Ann Thorac Surg* 2008; **85**: S743–6.

Patti MG, Herbella FA. Fundoplication after laparoscopic Heller myotomy for esophageal achalasia: what type. *J Gastrointest Surg* 2010; **14**: 1453–8.

Patti MG, Pellegrini CA, Horgan S et al. Minimally invasive surgery for achalasia: an 8-year experience with 168 patients. *Ann Surg* 1999; **230**: 587–94.

Rawlings A, Soper NJ, Oelschlager B et al. Laparoscopic Dor versus Toupet fundoplication following Heller myotomy for achalasia: results of a multicenter, prospective, randomized-controlled trial. *Surg Endosc* 2012; **26**: 18–26.

Richter JE, Boeckxstaens GE. Management of achalasia: surgery or pneumatic dilation. *Gut* 2011; **60**: 869–76.

Richter JE. Achalasia – an update. *J Neurogastroenterol Motil* 2010; **16**: 232–42.

Rosemurgy AS, Morton CA, Rosas MA et al. A single institution's experience with

more than 500 laparoscopic Heller myotomies for achalasia. *J Am Coll Surg* 2010; **210**: 637–47.

Schuchert MJ, Luketich JD, Landreneau RJ et al. Minimally-invasive esophagomyotomy in 200 consecutive patients: factors influencing postoperative outcomes. *Ann Thorac Surg* 2008; **85**: 1729–34.

Soares R, Herbella FA, Prachand VN et al. Epiphrenic diverticulum of the esophagus. From pathophysiology to treatment. *J Gastrointest Surg* 2010; **14**: 2009–15.

Tieu BH, Hunter JG. Management of cricopharyngeal dysphagia with and without Zenker's diverticulum. *Thorac Surg Clin* 2011; **21**: 511–17.

Varghese TK, Marshall B, Chang AC et al. Surgical treatment of epiphrenic diverticula: a 30-year experience. *Ann Thorac Surg* 2007; **84**: 1801–9.

Zaninotto G, Portale G, Costantini M et al. Therapeutic strategies for epiphrenic diverticula: systematic review. *World J Surg* 2011; **35**: 1447–53.

Chapter

79

Esophagogastrectomy

Harrell Lightfoot and Allan Pickens

The most common indication for an esophagogastrectomy is esophageal cancer. Other indications include Barrett's esophagus with high-grade dysplasia, non-dilatable esophageal stricture, and irreparable esophageal rupture. There are multiple surgical techniques that present specific advantages and disadvantages. However, the postoperative management and complications associated with any esophagogastrectomy are very similar. The two most common methods for removing the esophagus are the transhiatal esophagectomy (THE), which consists of incisions on the neck and abdomen, and the Ivor Lewis esophagectomy (ILE) which consists of a laparotomy and a right lateral thoracotomy. Both approaches allow resection of the esophagus and mobilization of the gastric conduit. The stomach is the typical conduit used for the neo-esophagus; however, the colon and jejunum may also be used if the stomach is not ideal. Preoperative gastrostomy tubes should be avoided since they can damage the stomach and prohibit its use as the preferred replacement conduit.

The esophagus must be carefully dissected away from other mediastinal structures. Esophageal blood supply originates from small branches off the aorta. Vasoconstriction often controls these small vessels when bluntly transected; otherwise, simple electrocautery suffices. To mobilize the stomach as a conduit, the short gastric, left gastroepiploic, and left gastric arteries are sacrificed. The stomach blood supply is maintained by the carefully preserved right gastroepiploic and right gastric arteries. The stomach is fashioned into a gastric conduit by stapling along the lesser curve of the stomach to create a tubularized gastric conduit. Oversewing the gastric staple line is theorized to reduce gastric conduit leak. Since the gastric conduit is denervated, a gastric emptying procedure should be considered. Either a pyloromyotomy or pylorplasty is most commonly done. Botox injection of the pylorus has also been used to facilitate conduit emptying during early healing. The duodenum is often mobilized with a Kocher maneuver to provide additional conduit length and reduce tension. The gastric conduit is passed through the esophageal hiatus into the native esophageal bed in the posterior mediastinum. Alternate routes for the conduit include the chest hilum and subxyphoid pathways. An esophagogastric anastamosis is performed in the chest for ILE; in the neck for THE. Hand sewn, stapled, and combination anastomoses have been described.

Regardless of the anastamotic technique, there is always a risk of anastamotic leak. Consequently, a drain is routinely placed. Studies have shown that ILE has significantly higher in-hospital mortality, operative blood loss, pulmonary complications, chylothorax and hospital stay when compared to THE; however, THE has a higher incidence of anastomotic leaks and vocal cord paralysis. McKeown and minimally invasive esophagogastrectomies (MIE) are also performed, but to a lesser extent than the previous two approaches. The McKeown, also called three-hole esophagogastrectomy, involves placing incisions on the abdomen, chest, and neck to achieve the conduit mobilization, esophageal dissection, and anastamosis respectively. Minimally invasive esophagogastrectomy utilizes laparoscopy and thoracoscopy to perform the same tasks. The requirement of advanced laparoscopic and thoracoscopic skills has limited the generalized adoption of MIE.

Usual postoperative course
Expected postoperative hospital stay

The expected postoperative hospital stay is typically 7–10 days following a routine esophagogastrectomy. None of the various techniques mentioned previously have reduced the hospital stay for patients requiring removal of the esophagus.

Operative mortality

Overall operative mortality is around 5% for esophagogastrectomy. Comparative studies of transhiatal and transthoracic esophagectomies show no significant difference in the overall morbidity and mortality of both approaches, nor in long-term survival. It is, therefore, a matter for the surgeon to decide as to the best approach to esophageal resection for each patient depending on the patient's specific condition. Survival is highly dependent upon the underlying indication for the esophageal resection. A surgeon who is adept at all of these approaches is

Medical Management of the Surgical Patient, ed. Michael F. Lubin, Thomas F. Dodson, and Neil H. Winawer. Published by Cambridge University Press. © Cambridge University Press 2013.

better able to individualize the surgical procedure to best fit the particular needs of the patient.

Special monitoring required

Depending on the institution, esophagogastrectomy patients will go to the ICU if they require ventilatory support, or directly to the ward if they are extubated and hemodynamically stable. Most patients can be monitored on a regular ward in the immediate postoperative period. Monitoring with telemetry and pulse oximetry should be utilized. Successful ward care is dependent upon both patient comorbidities and nursing diligence.

Alimentation

A nasogastric (NG) tube is typically placed during the operation and can be removed by postoperative day 3 if the patient has not demonstrated clinical signs of an ileus. If the NG tube is inadvertently removed prior to this, replacement is ill-advised as any manipulation could injure the cervical anastamosis. By postoperative day 4, a clear liquid diet can be initiated and slowly advanced to a soft mechanical diet. Aspiration precautions should be employed until the patient becomes comfortable with the new swallowing mechanics. On postoperative day 7 a barium swallow can be performed to document an intact cervical anastomosis and lack of obstruction.

In most cases, a feeding jejunostomy tube is placed during the operation to assist with nutritional needs during recovery. Whether during the immediate postoperative period or weeks after the surgery, the feeding tube can be used to provide supplemental nutrition. It is started at a low rate, typically 10 mL/hour, and advanced to a goal rate based on the patient's caloric needs and nutritional value of the specific tube feed. Please note that jejunostomy feeds are not well tolerated if bolused, and that routine flushing should consist of normal saline, as opposed to free water.

Antibiotic coverage

Standard broad-spectrum antibiotics are required for the perioperative period.

Patient activity and positioning

Early postoperative ambulation and incentive spirometry are vital to patient recovery. Preoperative consultation with acute pain services for epidural placement and postoperative pain management should be considered. Good pain control facilitates early mobilization. Patients who ambulate have less risk of respiratory complications, and fewer have deep venous thrombosis.

Postoperative complications
Early postoperative complications

Most complications occur within the first 1–2 weeks.

Anastomotic leak

Anastomotic leak has been reported in the modern literature to range from 0.8% to over 20%. Typically cervical anastomoses have a leak rate between 5% and 15%; whereas intrathoracic anastomoses have a leak rate between 1% and 4%. Leaks typically occur around postoperative day 5, and are heralded by fevers, tachycardia and leukocytosis. Clinical suspicion based on physical findings and basic laboratory investigations is the initial method of detection. Bile exiting from a chest tube after transthoracic esophagogastrectomy or saliva exuding from the cervical incision after transhiatal esophagectomy are pathognomonic signs requiring no further testing. When there is doubt, the anastomosis is evaluated with a contrast study. Water-soluble contrast (Gastrografin) is used first. If this study is inconclusive, then dilute barium is used for better anatomical definition. Thorough drainage is imperative. Cervical anastamotic leaks can be drained by opening the cervical incision; intrathoracic anastomotic leaks require properly placed drains.

Chylothorax

Injury to the thoracic duct is a known complication associated with esophagogastrectomies. It typically is not appreciated until the patient begins to consume fat in their diet. If a chest tube is still in place, increased or milky output will be seen. Diagnosis is confirmed by quantifying the triglyceride level or identifying chylomicrons within the drainage. Initially, conservative management should be employed by either eliminating dietary fat or starting intravenous hyperalimentation. If high volume persists (> 500 mL/day) or chyle leak continues for 7–14 days, then surgical ligation of the duct will be required. Occasionally a chyle leak can be identified with a lymphangiogram; it should then be embolized.

Hoarseness

Injury to the recurrent laryngeal nerve places the patient at risk of aspiration and dysphagia. If bilateral nerves are injured, then a permanent tracheostomy will be required. Laryngoscopy and evaluation by an otolaryngologist is recommended if the hoarseness persists prior to discharge. Injection of the paralyzed vocal cord may be necessary to allow better vocal cord apposition to facilitate airway protection and improve voice quality.

Late postoperative complications
Dysphagia

Dysphagia is a general expectation following the surgery. It will take several weeks for the patient to become accustomed to their new swallowing mechanics. Most esophageal replacement conduits have no propulsion, thus gravity moves food distally. Changes in diet behavior are typically effective; behavior changes include thorough chewing and frequent small meals.

Reflux

During esophagogastrectomy, the lower esophageal sphincter is removed. This allows positive abdominal pressure to easily force gastric and bile acid into the intrathoracic conduit and residual esophagus. Patients are encouraged to refrain from eating prior to lying supine. Antacids and motility agents can be used in severe cases of reflux.

Dumping syndrome

During the mobilization of the stomach, a vagotomy is performed; consequently, a gastric emptying procedure is necessary. Gastric emptying procedures place the patient at risk of developing dumping syndrome after meals that have high sugar and fat content. The high osmotic load of such foods is believed to contribute to the dumping. Dumping syndrome includes abdominal cramping and diarrhea. It is recommended that such foods be avoided. Anti-motility agents may also be used as needed.

Strictures

Strictures at the esophagogastric anastomosis are common, and some report strictures in up to 50% of cases. Strictures are often associated with leaks. Some resolve with a single dilation and others require regular dilations. Any persistent stricture should be evaluated for malignancy. These dilations can be performed under general anesthetic; however, some appropriately selected patients can be taught to self-dilate with physician-provided Bougie dilators.

Further reading

Boshier PR, Anderson O, Hanna GB. Transthoracic versus transhiatal esophagectomy for the treatment of esophagogastric cancer: a meta-analysis. *Ann Surg* 2011; **254**: 894–906.

Cooke DT, Lin GC, Lau CL *et al.* Analysis of cervical esophagogastric anastomotic leaks after transhiatal esophagectomy: risk factors presentation and detection. *Ann Thorac Surg* 2009; **88**: 177–84.

Donohoe CL, O'Farrell NJ, Ravi N, Reynolds JV. Evidence-based selective application of transhiatal esophagectomy in a high-volume esophageal center. *World J Surg* 2012; **36**: 98–103.

Hulscher JB, Tijssen JG, Obertop H, van Lanschot JJ. Transthoracic versus transhiatal resection for carcinoma of the esophagus: a meta-analysis. *Ann Thorac Surg* 2001; **72**: 306–13.

Luketich JD, Alvelo-Rivera M, Buenaventura PO *et al.* Minimally invasive approach to esophagectomy. *J Soc Laparoendosc Surg* 1998; **2**: 243–7.

Orringer MB. Current status of transhiatal esophagectomy. *Adv Surg* 2000; **34**: 193–236.

Orringer MB, Marshall BM, Iannettoni MD. Transhiatal esophagectomy for treatment of benign and malignant esophageal disease. *World J Surg* 2001; **25**: 196–203.

Orringer MB, Marshall B, Chang AC, Pickens A, Lau CL. Two thousand transhiatal esophagectomies: changing trends, lessons learned. *Ann Surg* 2007; **246**: 363–74.

Sugarbaker D, Bueno R, Krasna M, Mentzer S, Zellos L. *Adult Chest Surgery*. New York, NY: McGraw-Hill; 2009.

Urshel JD. Esophagogastrostomy anastomotic leaks complicating esophagectomy: a review. *Am J Surg* 1995; **169**: 634–40.

Colon interposition for esophageal bypass

Kamal A. Mansour

Indications for colon replacement of the esophagus include gastroesophageal malignancy; benign non-dilatable distal esophageal strictures caused by reflux esophagitis; extensive chemical strictures; benign tumors of the esophagus that are extensive or multiple and are not amenable to simpler measures; congenital atresia of the esophagus for which a primary anastamosis is impossible or impractical; rare cases of achalasia (megaesophagus) in which Heller myotomy fails or is complicated by malignancy; bleeding varices for which shunting fails or stricture formation follows disconnection operation; and rupture of the esophagus for which conservative repair fails or is impossible.

The right or left colon may be used, based on the right or left branch of the middle colic artery. Depending upon the surgeon's preference, the prepared colonic segment is passed through a retrosternal tunnel or brought into the posterior mediastinum through the right or left pleural cavity. An anastomosis is then constructed to the cervical esophagus. Regardless of the approach used, the procedure is of great magnitude. A general endotracheal anesthetic is administered and the procedure usually lasts 4 to 6 hours. Two to four units of blood are frequently required. Intensive preoperative preparation, including correction of fluid, caloric, and protein deficiencies, substantially improves outcome, particularly for elderly or debilitated patients. Careful mechanical bowel preparation is also required.

Usual postoperative course
Expected postoperative hospital stay
The expected postoperative hospital stay is approximately 2 weeks.

Operative mortality
Operative mortality is approximately 12%, depending on the age and condition of the patient and the vascularity of the interposed colonic segment.

Special monitoring required
Standard thoracotomy intensive care is provided for the first 2 or 3 days, including daily chest radiographs, electrolyte and arterial blood gas determinations, urinary output monitoring, and central venous pressure measurement.

Patient activity and positioning
Patients are ambulatory 24–48 hours after operation.

Alimentation
A nasogastric tube is left in the interposed colon and a feeding jejunostomy is performed at operation. Patients are supported by intravenous fluids for the first 2–4 days until bowel sounds are audible, at which time tube feedings are provided. On the ninth or tenth day, a barium swallow is performed to assess the colonic implant for any evidence of leakage. If the reconstruction is intact, patients are allowed oral liquid feedings and food intake is progressively advanced to a soft diet over several days.

Antibiotic coverage
Cephalosporin is given for the first 24 hours postoperatively.

Physiotherapy
Chest physical therapy and vigorous pulmonary toilet are indicated.

Postoperative complications
In the hospital
Pulmonary complications
Pulmonary complications are often relatively minor but may become life-threatening in elderly patients or those with poor respiratory reserve.

Colonic necrosis

Massive necrosis of the colon must be diagnosed early and the involved bowel removed before the patient becomes moribund. The nasocolonic tube aspirate is carefully observed for its color and odor; foul or blood-stained fluid continuing after 48 hours may be the earliest sign of bowel necrosis.

Minor leaks at the cervical anastomosis

This complication occurs in 14.8% of patients but usually resolves with simple drainage. A prolonged delay in oral feeding may be necessary. Patients may require a feeding gastrostomy or, ideally, a feeding jejunostomy (usually performed at the time of operation).

After discharge

Fibrous stricture of the cologastric anastomosis

May require dilation or surgical revision.

Gastric ulceration

Usually occurs just proximal to the cologastric anastomosis on the lesser curvature. Medical therapy generally suffices but vagotomy and drainage may become necessary.

Redundancy of the colon above the diaphragm

Colonic stasis and a prolonged transit time may result from this condition, which may require surgical revision if it is severe.

Further reading

Davis PA, Law S, Wong J. Colonic interposition after esophagectomy for cancer. *Arch Surg* 2003; **138**: 303–8.

De Delva PE, Morse CR, Austen WG *et al.* Surgical management of failed colon interposition. *Eur J Cardiothorac Surg* 2008; **34**: 432–7.

Mansour KA, Bryan FC, Carlson GW. Bowel interposition for esophageal replacement: twenty-five-year experience. *Ann Thorac Surg* 1997; **64**: 752–6.

Thomas PA, Gilardoni A, Trousse D *et al.* Colon interposition for oesophageal replacement. *Multimedia Man Cardio-Thorac Surg MMCTS* 2009; (**0603**): mmcts.2007.002956. doi: 10.1510/mmcts.2007.002956.

Section 19   **Vascular Surgery**

Chapter

81

Carotid endarterectomy

Jayer Chung and Thomas F. Dodson

Carotid endarterectomy (CEA) is the most commonly performed procedure to prevent stroke, with approximately 99,000 operations performed nationally in 2006. Over the last decade, carotid artery stenting (CAS) has emerged as a minimally invasive alternative to CEA. Recent results from the CREST trial suggest that stroke and death occur less frequently with CEA; however, myocardial infarction occurs more frequently with CEA. While CEA remains the gold-standard therapy, many interventionalists continue to reserve CAS for "high-risk" patients, as defined by anatomic and/or medical criteria.

Usual postoperative course

Expected postoperative hospital stay

Since complications from either procedure typically occur within the first 12–24 hours, patients are usually discharged within the first 1–2 days following the operation.

Operative mortality

Mortality following CAS or CEA is less than 1%, and is mostly due to complications of stroke or myocardial infarction.

Special monitoring required

Patients in the post-anesthesia care unit are monitored with an arterial line for a period of 2–4 hours to assess for wide fluctuations in blood pressure. Ideally, the patient's postoperative blood pressure should be similar to the preoperative blood pressure. If medications are required to maintain a patient's blood pressure, he/she is then transferred to the ICU for 24 hour monitoring and appropriate anti-hypertensive or vasopressor medication administration.

Patient activity and positioning

Patients are usually kept on bed rest on the day of operation and are encouraged to ambulate the next day. For CAS patients, the duration of bed rest depends upon whether a mechanical closure device has been placed, in which case the patient must lie flat for 2 hours. If no closure device has been placed, then the patient must lie flat for 6 hours. In addition, frequent pulse examination of the punctured limb is required every 15–30 minutes for the first 2 hours. Afterwards, the pulse examination should occur every 8 hours.

Alimentation

Clear liquids are usually allowed in the postoperative period, keeping in mind the unlikely event of a postoperative complication requiring an urgent return to the operating room. Patients are allowed to resume a regular diet the following day.

Antibiotic coverage

One dose of a cephalosporin is given before the operation and continued for a maximum of 24 hours. If the patient is allergic to cephalosporin antibiotics, vancomycin or clindamycin is administered in the same fashion.

Antiplatelet therapy

After CEA, patients typically resume their preoperative antiplatelet regimen postoperatively. If the patient was not prescribed anti-platelet agents preoperatively, then postoperative aspirin alone is sufficient. However, for CAS procedures, clopidogrel administration is required. At our institution, patients receive 300 mg of clopidogrel prior to the procedure, and 75 mg each day for at least 1 month afterwards. Aspirin regimens are continued as they were preoperatively.

Drain management

Drains after carotid endarterectomy are typically removed on the first postoperative day, unless the patient develops a hematoma, or sanguineous drainage exceeds 30 mL during a 24-hour period.

Pain management

Discomfort from either the neck incision or groin puncture is usually minimal, with patients frequently requiring narcotics for brief periods of time. Many patients prefer over-the-counter analgesics after the first postoperative day.

Medical Management of the Surgical Patient, ed. Michael F. Lubin, Thomas F. Dodson, and Neil H. Winawer. Published by Cambridge University Press. © Cambridge University Press 2013.

Postoperative complications

In the hospital

Nerve injury

Cranial nerve injury occurs in approximately 4–5% of patients after CEA. Deviation of the tongue toward the side of operation may result from injury or traction on the hypoglossal nerve. Transection of the hypoglossal is rare and may require urgent repair. Similarly, damage to the vagus nerve may result in either temporary or permanent hoarseness. Injury to the marginal mandibular branch of the facial nerve results in drooping at the ipsilateral corner of the mouth. Damage to the superior laryngeal nerve may cause the patient's voice to fatigue easily and impair phonation. Trauma to the spinal accessory nerve is an uncommon complication of CEA, but the resulting shoulder dysfunction is troublesome. Fortunately, most cranial nerve injuries are transient and recovery can be expected in 6–12 months.

Bradycardia

Bradycardia is a common complication during or after the operation that can be attributed to manipulation of the carotid sinus. Postoperatively after CEA, atropine is administered in the unlikely event that bradycardia is associated with hypotension. During CAS, atropine is routinely administered, especially when the lesion is treated with balloon angioplasty, after which profound symptomatic bradycardia can ensue.

Hematoma

Postoperative neck hematomas occur in approximately 5% of patients. Of these, a small fraction require return to the operating room for evacuation. An expanding hematoma in the neck must be treated expeditiously to avoid airway compromise.

Cardiac complications

Patients with carotid artery stenosis have a higher risk of cardiac ischemic events than of stroke, illustrating that vascular disease involves the entire vascular tree. With improved perioperative management of risk factors (aspirin, beta-blockers, statin therapy), risk stratification, and modern anesthetic and critical care management, the incidence of cardiac complications has been decreasing. However, the CREST trial shows that the risk of myocardial infarction is twice as high for patients undergoing CEA (2.3%) as for those undergoing CAS (1.1%).

Limb ischemia

The incidence of limb ischemia is low after carotid artery stenting. Monitoring is necessary, particularly if larger sheaths are used. Typically, pulse examinations are performed with Doppler ultrasound probes, and checked every 15 minutes for the first hour, every 30 minutes for the next hour, and then every 4–8 hours thereafter until discharge.

Cerebrovascular accident (CVA)

Thirty-day stroke rates are higher after CAS than after CEA by the most recent randomized data. Stroke rates are approximately 2% following endarterectomy, and lowest among asymptomatic patients. Symptomatic patients who have undergone CAS have elevated stroke rates of 5–8%; conversely, CEA carries a 3–4% risk of stroke among symptomatic patients.

Cerebral hyperperfusion syndrome

This most feared complication of carotid surgery occurs in 0.2–19% of patients, with a higher risk among patients undergoing CAS. Hyperperfusion syndrome can cause severe ipsilateral frontal headaches, seizures, neurologic deficits, and ultimately death from cerebral hemorrhage. Risk factors include a high-grade ipsilateral stenosis (> 90%), contralateral carotid occlusion, recent history of CVA, recent contralateral CEA, diabetes mellitus, advanced age, and severe postoperative or intraoperative hypertension. Of these risk factors, only blood pressure can be controlled; therefore, it is imperative to continuously monitor the patient's blood pressure in the immediate postoperative period. Large fluctuations in blood pressure can be treated in the ICU with the appropriate vasopressors or vasodilators, with patients being ideally maintained at or slightly below their baseline blood pressure. If patients develop hyperperfusion syndrome, they are treated supportively, while anticoagulants and antiplatelet agents are withheld. The diagnosis can be confirmed with computed tomography, diffusion-weighted magnetic resonance imaging, or transcranial Doppler ultrasound (increase in cerebral blood flow ≥ 100%). The prognosis after cerebral hemorrhage is poor.

After discharge

Peri-incisional hypesthesia

After CEA, patients may complain of numbness of the ear lobe if the greater auricular nerve has been divided or damaged, and they frequently experience diminished sensation in the region of the neck incision because of the interruption of cutaneous cervical nerves. Pain or numbness is rare after common femoral artery puncture for CAS, and occurs due to inadvertent injury to the femoral nerve, or due to a hematoma or seroma compressing adjacent nerves.

Carotid re-stenosis

Recurrent stenosis of ≥ 50% after endarterectomy appears less frequently than after carotid stenting. Fortunately, most re-stenotic lesions are considered less virulent as they seem to carry a lesser risk of stroke when compared with primary atherosclerotic lesions of similar stenotic severity.

Further reading

Bonati LH, Ederle J, McCabe DJ *et al.* Long-term risk of carotid restenosis in patients randomly assigned to endovascular treatment or endarterectomy in the Carotid and Vertebral Artery Transluminal Angioplasty Study (CAVATAS): long-term follow-up of a randomised trial. *Lancet Neurol* 2009; **10**: 908–17.

CREST Investigators. Stenting versus endarterectomy for carotid-artery stenosis. *N Engl J Med* 2010; **363**: 11–23.

Lloyd-Jones D, Adams R, Carnethorn M *et al.* Heart disease and stroke statistics – 2009 update: a report from the American Heart Association Statistic Committee and Stroke Statistics Subcommittee. *Circulation* 2009; **119**: 480–6.

Moulakakis KG, Mylonas SN, Sfyroeras GS, Andrikopoulos V. Hyperperfusion syndrome after carotid revascularization. *J Vasc Surg* 2009; **49**: 1060–8.

Narins CR, Illig KA. Patient selection for carotid stenting versus endarterectomy: a systematic review. *J Vasc Surg* 2006; **44**: 661.

Chapter

82

Abdominal aortic aneurysm repair: open

Naren Gupta

Abdominal aortic aneurysms (AAAs) are dilations of the aorta to a transverse diameter of 3 cm or greater. Although 75% remain asymptomatic, the natural history of AAAs is to grow gradually at the rate of 0.25–0.5 cm a year, with an increasing risk of rupture and death as their transverse diameter increases.

Abdominal aortic aneurysms are predominantly a disease of advanced age, with prevalence from 3–10% among Western populations over the age of 50 years; they are rarely responsible for death below the age of 55 years. Due to the implementation of screening programs and the advent of endovascular repair, annual deaths due to AAAs in the USA have decreased, in spite of the fact that the population aged $\geq$ 50 years increased by over 12 million (20%) in the same time period.

Additional risk factors for AAA include smoking, male sex, atherosclerosis, and a family history of aneurysms. There may be an association with inguinal hernias. Abdominal aortic aneurysms occur less frequently in females, African Americans, and diabetics.

The risk of rupture is closely related to maximal transverse diameter. The annual rupture rate for untreated aneurysms is 0.5–5% for a diameter of 4–4.9 cm, 3–15% for 5–5.9 cm, 10–20% for 6–6.9 cm, 20–40% for 7–7.9 cm, and 30–50% for greater than 8 cm. For patients with aneurysms of the same diameter, rupture risk is greater in females, current smokers, cardiac and renal transplant recipients, and those with hypertension or decreased forced expiratory volume (FEV1).

According to one study, almost three-quarters of patients with a ruptured AAA did not survive long enough to reach the operating room. Of those operated on, the mortality was approximately 50%. This points out the urgency of detecting AAAs early by screening high-risk populations with abdominal ultrasound and repairing aneurysms electively when indicated, either by open or endovascular surgery. Screening high-risk populations by abdominal palpation alone has a mere 15% positive predictive value for identifying AAAs. Abdominal ultrasound screening is a cost-effective way to reduce both short- and long-term aneurysm-related mortality.

Repair is recommended for AAAs with transverse diameters of 5.5 cm or more in patients with at least a 2-year life expectancy, though aneurysms from 5–5.5 cm may be considered for repair on an individual basis in women and in younger, healthy patients who are suitable candidates for endovascular repair. Saccular aneurysms may also be considered for repair at a smaller size.

Ruptured aneurysms should be repaired immediately after a frank discussion with the patient and family about the expected 30–80% perioperative mortality. Patients with known AAAs who are hemodynamically stable but complain of new-onset abdominal or back pain should also be repaired emergently. These stable but symptomatic patients are found by computed tomography to have non-ruptured aneurysms in 50% of cases, contained ruptures in 30%, and some other etiology for abdominal pain in 20%. Non-ruptured but symptomatic aneurysms are considered to be acutely expanding and have a higher operative mortality than elective AAA repair, in part due to the urgent nature of the surgery and suboptimal preoperative work-up.

Lower-extremity ischemia in the presence of an aneurysm may be due to thrombosis of the aneurysm or distal embolization and is an indication for repair. Aneurysms that are tender on palpation or expanding at a rate greater than 0.5 cm over a 6-month interval should also be considered for repair. Rarely, a patient with a known aneurysm will present with a gastrointestinal bleed. This may be a "herald bleed" from a primary aortoenteric fistula due to erosion of the aneurysm into the gastrointestinal mucosa at the third or fourth part of the duodenum. An abdominal computed tomography angiogram (CTA) may diagnose the condition, and urgent surgery is indicated. Rarely, the CTA will reveal an aortocaval fistula in conjunction with the AAA. Such a fistula is usually symptomatic with a hyperdynamic, high-output circulation that rapidly progresses to congestive heart failure and warrants urgent surgery.

Medical Management of the Surgical Patient, ed. Michael F. Lubin, Thomas F. Dodson, and Neil H. Winawer. Published by Cambridge University Press. © Cambridge University Press 2013.

The mean age of American patients undergoing repair is 72 years; nearly 80% are male and 95% are white.

Open or endovascular repair

Open aortic aneurysm repair is the gold standard against which endovascular repair has been measured. A recent large trial conducted at the Veterans Administration hospitals reported perioperative mortality rates of 3% for open and 0.5% for endovascular elective repair. In the USA, the number of AAAs repaired stayed stable at approximately 45,000 per annum from 2001 to 2006, though the number repaired endovascularly doubled and open repairs declined proportionately during that time.

The decision between open and endovascular repair is made after considering the patient's anatomic suitability, comorbidities, and preference. It is important to consider the patient's ability to comply with the lifelong annual radiologic exams that an endovascular repair entails. In this chapter we will outline the management of open surgical repair; Chapter 83 will consider endovascular repair.

Once the diagnosis of an AAA is made, a detailed history and physical exam should be obtained to identify comorbidities and to individualize the risk–benefit ratio for surgery or surveillance with medical management. Ten percent of patients with AAAs also have aneurysms of the common femoral or the popliteal arteries; these locations should be examined along with the pedal pulses.

Prior to elective surgery, patients should be appropriately treated for hypertension, hyperlipidemia, diabetes, and other atherosclerotic risk factors. Aspirin and statins should be started preoperatively if there are no contraindications. Patients on beta-blockers should continue their medication in the perioperative period.

Substance abuse, whether alcohol, tobacco, or illicit drugs, should be identified and managed well before elective AAA repair. Perhaps the most important risk factor modification is cessation of smoking. Moderate exercise does not increase rupture risk and is encouraged.

Open repair presents higher perioperative stress compared with endovascular repair, though it has been argued that patients who are not fit for open repair do not have survival benefit from endovascular repair.

All patients should undergo cardiac risk stratification: patients with moderate to high risk should be referred to a cardiologist for preoperative optimization.

Open repair can be performed through a transperitoneal midline or retroperitoneal left flank approach. In an era when many aneurysms are referred for open repair due to unfavorable anatomy of the aneurysm neck and require a suprarenal clamp, the retroperitoneal approach is receiving renewed attention. The duration of open procedures is typically 3–4 hours with 500–1,000 mL blood loss.

Patients with ruptured AAAs should be transported emergently to the operating room: the practice of permissive hypotension will prevent any delay in induction while maintaining cerebral perfusion. Though most institutions will proceed with open repair, if local expertise and suitable grafts are available, an endovascular approach to repair may be used with good results. In the case of emergent open repair, the abdomen should be prepped and draped prior to induction of anesthesia to allow prompt opening in case the pressure drops due to relaxation of the abdominal wall and loss of vasoconstriction. If there has been a massive resuscitation requirement and abdominal compartment syndrome is a concern, delayed closure or temporary abdominal closure with mesh may be performed.

Usual postoperative course

Expected postoperative hospital stay

The patient should be admitted to an ICU postoperatively, whether extubated or not. An ICU stay of 1–3 days and discharge from hospital in 5–7 days is typical; however, 10% of patients who were ambulatory preoperatively require discharge to a skilled nursing facility, where they stay for an average of 3 months. At 4–6 weeks, a postoperative visit is scheduled and staples are removed. Complete postoperative recovery for the patient takes several weeks and some patients, particularly those of advanced age and/or with significant comorbidities, will report a persistent decrease in functional ability.

Special monitoring required

Continuous electrocardiogram and invasive systemic arterial pressure monitoring is standard due to the marked fluid shifts that occur the first few days after surgery. Pulmonary arterial pressure catheters may be needed in patients with significant cardiac risk. Pulmonary hygiene, urine output, and parameters of coagulation require close management.

Patient positioning and activity

The head of the bed should be maintained at 30°. Respiratory toilet, epidural pain management, and early and frequent ambulation for venous thromboembolism prophylaxis are the cornerstones of early recovery.

Alimentation

The nasogastric tube is discontinued and alimentation started when bowel function returns, normally between the 3rd and 5th postoperative day. Parenteral nutrition may be considered if there is prolonged ileus.

Antibiotic coverage

Antibiotic prophylaxis should not be continued beyond 24 hours after surgery.

Perioperative mortality

Thirty-day mortality after surgery ranges from 1–4% in single-center series to 4–8% in population-based series. Factors that adversely affect outcome include age > 70, creatinine > 1.8, FEV1 < 2.2 L, congestive heart failure, recent myocardial ischemia, female sex, and suprarenal clamp placement.

Perioperative morbidity

Complications occur in 15–30%, including cardiac (15%), pulmonary (10%), renal (10%), DVT (8%), bleeding/wound infection/leg ischemia each approximately 4%, stroke/graft infection/graft thrombosis/ureteral injury each < 1%.

Persistent need for blood transfusion may indicate bleeding from venous injury, splenic injury, or back-bleeding from an undetected lumbar or intercostal artery; it should prompt early re-exploration.

Clinically apparent colonic ischemia (persistent acidosis, leucocytosis, prolonged ileus, fluid sequestration, and bloody bowel movements) occurs in 0.3–3% of elective repairs, and 7–27% of ruptured AAA repair. Sigmoidoscopy can confirm the diagnosis. When limited to the mucosa, it responds to supportive measures like bowel rest, resuscitation, antibiotics, and serial abdominal exams. However, if transmural infarction occurs, it results in 80% mortality.

Postoperative complications

Incisional hernias occur in 10% of transperitoneal repairs; at 2–5 years, 5–6% of patients require reoperation for this. A lateral flank bulge occurs in 10% of retroperitoneal approaches and should be managed conservatively. At 7–15 years, 2–15% of postsurgical patients have experienced graft-related complications, including pseudoaneurysms, graft infections, and limb occlusions. Para-anastomotic aneurysms occur in 1% at 5 years, 6% at 10 years and 20–40% at 15 years. Graft infection occurs in 0.3–1% of patients, and is responsible for 25% of reoperative surgery after open AAA repair. Femoral incisions increase graft infection rate to 3%. Limb occlusions are responsible for 25% of arterial interventions after open AAA repairs, and all such interventions increase the risk of infection.

Long-term survival

Age at the time of repair is the primary determinant of long-term survival. Five-year survival for patients with AAA is 60–70%, compared with 90% for sex- and age-matched patients without AAA. While patients who have undergone AAA repair are successfully protected from aneurysm-related death, the presence of other comorbidities such as cardiac disease, cancer, stroke, pulmonary disease, and renal failure contribute to the decreased survival.

Further reading

Cao P, De Rango P, Verzini F *et al.* Comparison of surveillance versus aortic endografting for small aneurysm repair (CAESAR): results from a randomised trial. *Eur J Vasc Endovasc Surg* 2011; **41**: 13–25.

Chaikof EL, Brewster DC, Dalman RL *et al.* The care of patients with an abdominal aortic aneurysm: the Society for Vascular Surgery practice guidelines. *J Vasc Surg* 2009; **50**: S2–49.

Fillinger, M. Abdominal aortic aneurysms: evaluation and decision making. In Cronenwett JL, Johnston KW, eds. *Rutherford's Vascular Surgery.* Vol. 2. 7th edn. Philadelphia, PA: Saunders Elsevier; 2010, pp. 1928–48.

Lederle FA, Freischlag JA, Kyriakides TC *et al.* Outcomes following endovascular vs open repair of abdominal aortic aneurysm: a randomized trial. *J Am Med Assoc* 2009; **302**: 1535–42.

Malas MB, Freischlag JA. Interpretation of the results of OVER in the context of EVAR trial, DREAM, and the EUROSTAR registry. *Semin Vasc Surg* 2010; **23**: 165–9.

Moll FL, Powell JT, Fraedrich G *et al.* Management of abdominal aortic aneurysms: clinical practice guidelines of the European Society for Vascular Surgery. *Eur J Vasc Endovasc Surg* 2011; **41**: S1–58.

Thompson SG, Ashton HA, Gao L, Scott RA. Screening men for abdominal aortic aneurysm: 10 year mortality and cost effectiveness results from the randomised Multicentre Aneurysm Screening Study. *Br Med J* 2009; **338**: b2307.

Chapter

83

Abdominal aortic aneurysm repair: endovascular

Naren Gupta

Endovascular repair of abdominal aortic aneurysms (EVAR) was introduced in the US market in 1999 and has gained rapid popularity because of decreased perioperative morbidity, shorter length of stay, and rapid recovery compared with open repair. Currently, more than 60% of AAAs are repaired endovascularly. However, there are possible issues of magnetic resonance imaging (MRI) compatibility. While all stent grafts cause image artifacts, the Zenith graft, made of ferro-magnetic stents, is incompatible with MRI. Also, there is increased cost with EVAR when compared with open repair.

The anatomic morphology of the aneurysm and the aorto-iliac system proximal and distal to it is the most important criterion in determining if the patient is a candidate for EVAR.

Anatomic criteria for suitability for EVAR:

- Proximal landing zone (the "neck"): The aortic wall immediately distal to the lowest renal artery and proximal to the aneurysm is the proximal landing zone. The instructions for use (IFUs) for current commercially available grafts specify that the "neck" should be at least 15 mm long; 40% of candidates for EVAR do not meet this criterion.
- Distal landing zone: This is the seal area in the common or external iliac artery where the iliac limbs of the endograft end; it should be at least 10 mm.
- Access vessels: Endovascular devices are inserted into the aorta from the groin, traversing retrograde through the common femoral and iliac arteries. To allow access without rupture, these vessels have to be a minimal diameter that varies according to each device manufacturer and the size of the endograft required.
- Status of critical side branches: The endovascular approach entails occlusion of the inferior mesenteric artery, and may also require the sacrifice of one or more accessory renal or internal iliac arteries. The suitability and configuration of an endovascular approach is thus predicated by the adequacy of collateral supply and the acceptable extent of end-organ ischemia.

Although endovascular repair of abdominal aortic aneurysms can be performed under local anesthesia, the patient needs risk stratification for general anesthesia in case of open conversion. EVAR carries intermediate to high risk of cardiac morbidity (3–7%). Patients should be typed and screened for blood. Screening should be performed for peripheral vascular disease, which can complicate access, and for femoral or popliteal aneurysms. Renal dysfunction may preclude the serial imaging with contrast that is required for EVAR, as will the inability of a patient to participate in regular, lifelong follow-up. Smoking cessation 4–6 weeks prior to surgery and physiotherapy can reduce postoperative morbidity. Statins should be started 1 month preoperatively, and continued postoperatively indefinitely. Unless there are specific contraindications, all patients should be on low-dose aspirin therapy. If the patient receives beta-blockers, these should be continued perioperatively. The patient should drink plenty of fluids the day before surgery.

Unlike the large midline or flank incisions of open surgery, EVAR can be performed through two percutaneous or small transverse groin incisions. There is a 1–2% possibility of failure to complete the initial repair and a similar rate of primary conversion to an open procedure; therefore, the procedure should be performed in a room with operating room standards of sterility. The average operating time is less than 3 hours; the average blood loss is 200 mL with no transfusion requirement. In cases where open exposure of the common femoral arteries has been performed, the groin incisions are closed in layers; the skin is closed with subcuticular absorbable sutures. After percutaneous EVAR, common femoral arteriotomy closure is performed with suture-mediated closure devices. The skin incisions, which are a few millimeters long, can be closed with skin glue alone. The patient is extubated prior to leaving the operating room.

Usual postoperative course
Expected postoperative hospital stay

The EVAR patient goes to a regular ward, where the stay ranges from 1–3 days; 95% of patients are discharged to home. Return to preoperative functional status with percutaneous

Medical Management of the Surgical Patient, ed. Michael F. Lubin, Thomas F. Dodson, and Neil H. Winawer. Published by Cambridge University Press. © Cambridge University Press 2013.

EVAR is achieved within 2 days; patients with groin incisions take less than a week to return to their baseline. Patients undergo a CT angiogram of the abdomen and pelvis one month after the procedure, with follow-up in the clinic immediately thereafter to enable the surgeon to review the images and examine the incision site. Patients need to return for similar consultations after abdominal CT scans at 6 and 12 months after surgery, and then annually lifelong.

Operative mortality

The elective 30-day mortality rate with EVAR is 0.5–1.5%, less than one-third that of open repair.

The mortality and morbidity rate of acute conversion to open surgery (which occurs in 1% of patients) is comparable to that of elective open surgery.

Special monitoring required

Intensive monitoring of vitals does not need to extend past the operation unless specific cardiac or pulmonary risk factors are present. Pedal pulses, groin incisions and urine output should be assessed every 8 hours, and any adverse change investigated. Abdominal pain or tenderness on exam warrants a work-up for mesenteric ischemia. The following morning, a CBC and a Chem-7 should be obtained.

Patient activity and positioning

Following percutaneous EVAR, patients should lie flat in bed without flexing the hips for 2–3 hours: tilting the bed in reverse Trendelenburg may increase comfort during this time. Patients with groin incisions have no restrictions on positioning or ambulation soon after surgery. Oral narcotics or NSAIDs will adequately treat any postoperative pain. If local anesthesia is infiltrated, patients rarely complain of any postoperative pain and can ambulate in a matter of hours after surgery. The Foley catheter should be removed as soon as the patient ambulates.

Alimentation

Patients are encouraged to drink plenty of oral fluids after surgery. If the patient has no complaints and the abdomen and groin exam is benign, regular diet can resume. Intravenous normal saline at 100 mL/hour may be continued for 24 hours after the procedure, especially in patients with renal insufficiency.

Antibiotic coverage

Intravenous cephalosporins are given 10 minutes prior to incision and should be stopped within 24 hours of skin closure.

Postoperative complications
In the hospital

Within the first 30 days, major medical complications occur in 10% of EVAR patients. Endovascular repair has distinct complications that are not associated with open repair; namely, endoleaks, access vessel injuries, and graft migration. Surgical complications, including open conversion to open surgery (rare) or re-intervention, occur in another 10%. These include the 3% who experience a myocardial infarction, stroke, or undergo amputation.

Early rupture

Early ruptures are extremely rare (0.3%) and have been reported only in connection with a single device that is no longer widely used.

Renal complications

Contrast-induced nephropathy occurs 24–72 hours after the procedure and is increased in patients with preexisting renal insufficiency, advanced age, diabetes, and in emergent cases. The risk can be reduced with hydration prior to the procedure, which should be continued postoperatively for 24 hours. Renal failure requiring dialysis occurs in 1% of patients.

Device-related complications

Endoleaks, graft migration, and limb kinking and occlusion are complications related specifically to endovascular repair. Endoleaks result from a failure to completely exclude blood flow from the aneurysm sac after a technically successful deployment of the endograft and its components.

Endoleaks are classified and managed according to their location. Type I describes a leak at the proximal or distal seal zones; it occurs in 5% of endovascular repairs. Due to the risk of aneurysm rupture, Type I leaks must be resolved at the time of operation. If they cannot be treated, then open conversion should be planned. This intervention can be performed as a separate procedure, unless the endograft is deployed in an unstable manner.

Type II describes a retrograde flow from mesenteric, renal or lumbar collaterals into the aneurysm sac. Type II leaks occur in 20% of patients; although intervention used to be performed in as many as half of these cases, currently Type II leaks are followed and managed expectantly. Type III leaks occur between endograft components or through graft fabric and are dealt with like Type I. Lastly, Type IV denotes endotension that causes aneurysm dilation without any evidence of endoleak; this complication is less common with newer, impermeable grafts.

Pelvic ischemia

By virtue of excluding the aneurysm sac from which it arises, the inferior mesenteric artery is excluded in all endovascular repairs. This finding has little adverse effect if collateral supply from the hypogastrics is maintained. In the case of common iliac aneurysms that are treated by embolizing the hypogastric and extending the endograft limbs into the external iliac artery, there is an increased incidence of pelvic ischemia, including: ischemic colitis, buttock claudication, erectile dysfunction and, very rarely, spinal cord ischemia.

Ischemic colitis

Ischemic colitis occurs in less than 2% of patients following elective endovascular repair. Symptoms include low-grade fevers, leucocytosis accompanied by lower quadrant abdominal pain and tenderness with or without a bloody bowel movement. The patient should receive supportive care including resuscitation, broad-spectrum intravenous antibiotics with anaerobic and gram-negative coverage, bowel rest and serial abdominal exams and labs to monitor the response.

Mucosal ischemia will resolve with supportive care alone. Transmural infarction, a rare complication with a 50% mortality rate, is marked by worsening signs and symptoms. Urgent sigmoidoscopic examination and emergent bowel resection are mandatory.

Buttock claudication and erectile dysfunction

With unilateral hypogastric embolization, 30–40% of patients experience buttock claudication; 15% report erectile dysfunction. Although these complications may resolve over time, they are persistent for 12% and 9% of patients, respectively. The reported incidence of persistent severe pelvic ischemic symptoms following bilateral embolization is even greater; this practice has been largely abandoned in favor of a variety of endovascular techniques (e.g., 'snorkeled' or bifurcated iliac limbs) to preserve hypogastric flow.

After discharge

Abdominal aortic aneurysm sac enlargement

An unresolved problem – AAA sac enlargement following EVAR – has recently been reported. In 41% of patients surveyed, the consequences of this enlargement are, as of yet, uncertain.

Long-term radiation exposure

Endovascular repair utilizes preoperative, intraoperative, and postoperative contrast imaging: thus, the patient is exposed to risks associated with contrast media and radiation. Radiation exposure from the initial procedure (12–14 mSv) and the subsequent CT scans (8–20 mSv each) needed for follow-up is cumulative over the patient's lifetime. This exposure can cross the lifetime maximum safe dose threshold limit value (400 mSv) in patients with a long lifespan or a postoperative course complicated by secondary interventions. This information should enter into consideration when choosing between an open or endovascular procedure in young patients.

Late morbidity

The secondary vascular intervention rate is greater for EVAR than for open repair. Indications for secondary interventions after EVAR include endoleak, migration, infection, and limb occlusion. Graft infection is extremely rare, reported in only 0.4% of patients. Long-term results reflect the known inadequacies of early endografts; those devices are no longer in use. New devices continue to improve; however, the long-term results with the newer generation grafts are not known at this time. Current devices have a 16% vascular re-intervention rate and 2% aneurysm rupture risk at 3 years. Endoleaks alone require secondary procedures in 12% of patients at 3 years, although the large majority of these operations are endovascular. Existing long-term data from studies with early-generation devices show that re-intervention rates can be as high as 30% at 8 years.

Late mortality

All-cause mortality at 2 years is 7%, compared with 10% with open repair. This difference largely reflects the early aneurysm-related mortality advantage that EVAR has over open repair. However, this early survival advantage is not maintained beyond 2–4 years. The 3-year survival is 85% for low-to-moderate risk patients after either procedure. Despite concerns about the late aneurysm rupture rate with EVAR, the 6–8 year survival is 55–60%, which is equivalent to that of open repair.

Further reading

Cao P, De Rango P, Verzini F et al. Comparison of surveillance versus aortic endografting for small aneurysm repair (CAESAR): results from a randomised trial. *Eur J Vasc Endovasc Surg* 2011; **41**: 13–25.

Chaikof EL, Brewster DC, Dalman RL et al. The care of patients with an abdominal aortic aneurysm: the Society for Vascular Surgery practice guidelines. *J Vasc Surg* 2009; **50**: S2–49.

Fillinger M. Abdominal aortic aneurysms: evaluation and decision making. In Cronenwett JL, Johnston KW, eds. *Rutherford's Vascular Surgery*. Vol 2. 7th edn. Philadelphia, PA: Saunders Elsevier; 2010, pp. 1928–48.

Lederle FA, Freischlag JA, Kyriakides TC et al. Outcomes following endovascular vs open repair of abdominal aortic aneurysm: a randomized trial. *J Am Med Assoc* 2009; **302**: 1535–42.

Malas MB, Freischlag JA. Interpretation of the results of OVER in the context of EVAR trial, DREAM, and the EUROSTAR registry. *Semin Vasc Surg* 2010; **23**: 165–9.

Moll FL, Powell JT, Fraedrich G *et al.* Management of abdominal aortic aneurysms: clinical practice guidelines of the European Society for Vascular Surgery. *Eur J Vasc Endovasc Surg* 2011; **41**: S1–58.

Schanzer A, Greenberg RK, Hevelone N *et al.* Predictors of abdominal aortic aneurysm sac enlargement after endovascular repair/Clinical Perspective. *Circulation* 2011; **123**: 2848–55.

Thompson SG, Ashton HA, Gao L, Scott RA. Screening men for abdominal aortic aneurysm: 10 year mortality and cost effectiveness results from the randomised Multicentre Aneurysm Screening Study. *Br Med J* 2009; **338**: b2307.

Chapter 84

Aortobifemoral bypass grafting

James G. Reeves and Ravi K. Veeraswamy

Aortobifemoral bypass is performed in patients with atherosclerotic disease that primarily involves the infrarenal aorta and iliac arteries. This condition typically causes predictable, effort-related cramping and burning of the hip and buttock muscles, which is relieved with rest. Vasculogenic impotence (LeRiche syndrome) is also a possible comorbidity for men. On examination, patients with infrarenal aorta and iliac artery involvement have diminished or absent femoral pulses and are frequently younger – 10 years younger on average – than the typical patient with symptomatic femoropopliteal disease.

Preoperative assessment usually includes contrast angiography, which may be performed via a brachial arterial approach if there are no palpable femoral pulses. Alternatively, CTA (computed tomography angiography) and MRA (magnetic resonance angiography) are emerging as anatomically accurate, less invasive alternatives. Because aortobifemoral bypass is a physically stressful operation, an assessment of the patient's overall medical condition is imperative; some evaluation of cardiac function is frequently a part of this preoperative evaluation. If the patient's condition is not suitable for aortobifemoral bypass, other less invasive options are available, including axillary-bifemoral bypass or endoluminal angioplasty and stenting.

Aortobifemoral bypass grafting requires a general anesthetic, a laparotomy incision, and bilateral groin incisions. After the infrarenal aorta is clamped, a prosthetic graft is sewn onto the aorta proximally. The limbs of the graft are then tunneled in a retroperitoneal plane and sewn onto the femoral arteries. The procedure typically takes 2–4 hours and often requires packed red blood cell transfusion or the use of a cell saver autotransfusion system.

Usual postoperative course

Expected postoperative hospital stay

The expected postoperative hospital stay is 7–10 days.

Operative mortality

The operative mortality for aortobifemoral bypass is 1–4%. The most common cause of death in the early postoperative period is myocardial infarction. Along with cardiac events, pulmonary (i.e., atelectasis, pneumonia), and renal complications are the major morbidities associated with the procedure.

Special monitoring required

Postoperatively, the patient typically spends at least the first night in the ICU. During this time, vital signs, hemoglobin, ECG, and urine output are monitored. An epidural analgesia catheter is commonly employed for pain control. Central venous catheters are often employed for volume assessment, with Swan–Ganz catheters reserved for patients with severe cardiac disease.

Patient activity and positioning

The head of the bed is often elevated to improve the patient's pulmonary function. Typically, the patient is allowed to move from the bed to a chair on the first postoperative day, and to walk with assistance on the following day.

Alimentation

Following laparotomy, an ileus is frequently present for 2–5 days. During this period of intestinal inactivity, nasogastric tube decompression may be used at the discretion of the surgeon. Peristalsis is heralded by the return of active bowel sounds, with the passage of flatus as an indication to begin liquids by mouth. The diet is advanced over the next day or two.

Antibiotic coverage

Administration of perioperative antibiotics is imperative for patients receiving prosthetic graft material. The agent of choice is typically a first-generation cephalosporin, with vancomycin or clindamycin reserved for patients with a penicillin allergy. The dosing schedule begins with a preoperative dose prior to

Medical Management of the Surgical Patient, ed. Michael F. Lubin, Thomas F. Dodson, and Neil H. Winawer. Published by Cambridge University Press. © Cambridge University Press 2013.

making the skin incision; routine administration of antibiotics is discontinued within 24 hours, in accordance with Surgical Care Improvement Project (SCIP) guidelines.

Prevention of pulmonary complications

Patients requiring aortobifemoral bypass are frequently active smokers, predisposing them to an increased risk of pulmonary complications. In order to minimize this risk, patients are counseled on the importance of smoking cessation. Despite this, the vast majority of patients will continue to smoke. Pre- as well as postoperative incentive spirometry, bronchodilator treatments, chest physical therapy, and early ambulation are all aimed at minimizing pulmonary complications. Quite possibly the greatest advance in this direction has been the use of epidural analgesia, providing patients with an improved ability to cough and breathe deeply with minimal discomfort.

Prevention of cardiac complications

Preoperative cardiac assessment aimed at diagnosing and treating coronary disease is the key to preventing cardiac complications. If indicated, coronary intervention takes precedence over elective lower extremity revascularization. Perioperative pharmacotherapy frequently consists of nitroglycerin and beta-blockers. ECG is often immediately performed postoperatively and then daily while the patient is in the ICU. When the patient leaves the ICU, cardiac telemetry monitoring can detect ischemic events that are otherwise silent.

Postoperative complications

In the hospital

Cardiac complications

Myocardial infarction is the most frequent cause of death in the early postoperative period. Arrhythmias and heart failure may occur, particularly as the patient experiences the usual postoperative fluid shifts.

Pulmonary complications

Atelectasis is a frequent postoperative finding, with pneumonia seen less commonly. Pulmonary embolus is an infrequent finding, although most patients receive prophylaxis to prevent deep vein thrombosis.

Renal complications

The patient with underlying renal insufficiency is particularly prone to postoperative renal complications. Acute renal failure may have several different etiologies, including intraoperative renal embolization, renal ischemia from suprarenal aortic cross-clamping, hypotension, and significant blood loss that requires large-volume red cell transfusion.

Postoperative bleeding

Bleeding may occur in the immediate postoperative period, but it becomes infrequent after the first postoperative night. The source of bleeding may be from an anastomosis, from the retroperitoneum, from within the peritoneal cavity, or along the tunnel leading to the femoral arteries. Because a large volume of blood can be lost before any significant increase in abdominal size can be detected, the hemoglobin/hematocrit results provide a better assessment of bleeding than does abdominal girth.

Peripheral embolization

Embolization to the lower extremities may occasionally occur as an intraoperative event. Doppler signals at the dorsalis pedis and posterior tibial arteries are noted preoperatively and sites are marked on the feet. Loss of a signal may indicate embolization; further evaluation is mandatory. Microembolization may result in "trash foot" or ischemic changes to the skin with preservation of flow in the vessels at the ankle.

Acute graft occlusion

Graft occlusion in the early postoperative period is an uncommon event. It typically results from a technical problem with an anastomosis, kinking, or extrinsic compression of the graft. This complication requires reoperation, with identification and correction of the problem.

Wound infection

Infection of the abdominal incision is rare, but is more common at the groins where the femoral arteries are exposed. An obese patient with a large panniculus that covers the groins, resulting in an accumulation of excessive moisture, has a heightened risk of wound infection. Attention to hygiene and keeping the groins dry and covered with gauze may help prevent local wound complications.

After discharge

Delayed wound infection

Delayed wound infection is an uncommon complication. It typically occurs in the groins, and is more commonly found in obese patients. Erythema, swelling, discharge, and warmth raise concern for graft infection, and warrant further investigation.

Impotence

Retrograde ejaculation occurs in approximately 20% of male patients as a result of the disruption of sympathetic nerve fibers near the left common iliac artery. Erectile dysfunction is a rare complication of aortobifemoral bypass, but may occur for a variety of reasons.

Graft occlusion

Occlusion of the graft most commonly occurs years after surgery, and involves one of the limbs of the bifurcated graft. Occlusion may result in a recurrence of preoperative symptoms or an acute onset of more severe symptomatology. Intervention consists of thrombolysis, thrombectomy, profundaplasty, femoral–femoral bypass, or a combination of these procedures.

Anastomotic pseudoaneurysm

Discovery of a pulsatile mass in the groin following aortofemoral bypass often signifies an anastomotic pseudoaneurysm. This complication may be due to infection or deterioration of the anastomosis years after graft implantation. Pseudoaneurysms resulting from either etiology require surgical repair.

Aortoenteric fistula

Aortoenteric fistula is an uncommon complication, and most often results from erosion of the proximal aortic suture line into the duodenum. This complication may present with a small "herald" intestinal bleed, followed by massive blood loss. Treatment requires emergent exploration, with repair of the intestinal defect, removal of the infected graft, and restoration of lower extremity perfusion. Aortic reconstruction can be accomplished via extra-anatomical bypass or by reconstruction of the aorta with deep femoral veins, allograft, or antibiotic-soaked prosthetic. A high index of suspicion should be maintained for patients presenting with a GI bleed and a history of aortic graft placement.

Minimally invasive aortoiliac interventions

In addition to bypass, aortoiliac occlusive disease may also be treated by angioplasty with or without stent. The lesions best suited for this modality are focal stenoses or occlusions of the common iliac arteries. Proximal common iliac artery lesions commonly require bilateral iliac stents to prevent narrowing of the contralateral artery with the ipislateral stent placement. Angioplasty and stenting of focal stenoses of the common iliac arteries can provide long-term patency comparable to bypass. Longer lesions, occlusions, and disease involving the external iliac arteries can be treated with angioplasty, although the long-term patency is thereby diminished. Some surgeons believe that these latter lesions are best managed by surgical revascularization.

The prime advantage of angioplasty is that it obviates the morbidity of aortobifemoral bypass. Complications are rare and primarily involve bleeding or pseudoaneurysm formation at the femoral arterial puncture site. The most common long-term problem is restenosis, which typically presents as a return of the preangioplasty symptoms.

Further reading

Burke CR, Henkel PK, Hernandez R *et al.* A contemporary comparison of aortofemoral bypass and aortoiliac stenting in the treatment of aortoiliac occlusive disease. *Ann Vasc Surg* 2010; **24**: 4–13.

Moise MA, Kashyap VS. Treatment of aortoiliac occlusive disease: medical versus endovascular versus surgical therapy. *Curr Treat Options Cardiovasc Med* 2011; **13**: 114–28.

Piazza M, Ricotta JJ 2nd, Bower TC *et al.* Iliac artery stenting combined with open femoral endarterectomy is as effective as open surgical reconstruction for severe iliac and common femoral occlusive disease. *J Vasc Surg* 2011; **54**: 402–11.

Timaran CH, Stevens SL, Freeman MB *et al.* Predictors for adverse outcome after iliac angioplasty and stenting for limb-threatening ischemia. *J Vasc Surg* 2002; **36**: 507–13.

Chapter

Treatment of femoropopliteal disease

Luke P. Brewster and Matthew A. Corriere

Femoropopliteal bypass is a procedure in which an autogenous vein (typically the greater saphenous vein), prosthetic conduit, or a combination of the two is used to improve lower extremity circulation. Femoropopliteal bypass is most commonly performed for symptomatic atherosclerotic disease of the superficial femoral and/or popliteal artery, including intermittent claudication, rest pain, non-healing ischemic ulcers, or gangrene. Patients with mild intermittent claudication symptoms that are not lifestyle-limiting are seldom treated with bypass, as the natural history of this condition infrequently progresses to threaten the limb. However, a failed bypass can significantly worsen ischemic symptoms and may jeopardize the extremity. Patients with asymptomatic or mild lower extremity peripheral arterial disease are therefore managed with exercise therapy and risk factor reduction therapy aimed at lowering the incidence of stroke and myocardial infarction. Therefore, smoking cessation, control of blood pressure (including salt reduction), and dietary modifications are important steps in this effort. Mild intermittent claudication and asymptomatic or mild peripheral artery disease are not benign conditions; however, their presence is not a good predictor of a future need for major amputation.

Less frequent indications for elective femoropopliteal bypass include femoral or popliteal artery aneurysms and non-atherosclerotic occlusive disease such as popliteal entrapment syndrome or cystic adventitial disease.

In addition to a focused history and physical examination, Doppler measurement of the ankle-brachial index (ABI) and associated waveforms is performed as part of the vascular exam. After this assessment, patients scheduled for operation or intervention that requires anatomic identification of the diseased arteries may preoperatively undergo computed tomography angiography (CTA), magnetic resonance angiography or standard catheter arteriography. In the absence of chronic kidney disease, we favor CTA for initial anatomic imaging and usually find it satisfactory for procedural planning. Regardless of the presence or absence of a palpable femoral pulse,

preoperative imaging studies are required to delineate the anatomy and to allow planning for the appropriate operation.

Finally, prior to operative intervention, preoperative risk assessment should be directed toward the status of the cardiac and pulmonary subsystems, since perioperative outcome (morbidity and mortality) is related to the condition of these organ subsystems. Certain patient populations present challenging treatment paradigms. For patients who require coronary artery bypass grafting prior to lower extremity bypass, vein harvest sites need to be chosen carefully. Surgery for patients with bilateral lower extremity disease should be carried out first in the more symptomatic extremity with the best available conduit. Ideally, patients with diabetes, end stage renal disease, gangrene, or infection should not receive prosthetic grafts.

Cilostazol is the only available pharmacologic agent for intermittent claudication that has been approved by the United States Food and Drug Administration. In addition, it has been shown to limit restenosis rates in the coronary and peripheral vasculature. This drug is contraindicated in patients taking monoamine oxidase inhibitors; dosing is adjusted for patients with congestive heart failure. For appropriate patients, risk factor reduction therapy includes smoking cessation, administration of antiplatelet agents (usually aspirin or clopidogrel), perioperative beta blockade, and statin (HMG-CoA reductase inhibitor) therapy. In addition to lowering the risk of adverse cardiovascular events, appropriate risk factor reduction therapy also maximizes bypass patency while lowering risk of disease progression at other anatomic locations.

Femoropopliteal bypass can usually be performed in 2–4 hours under general, spinal, or epidural anesthesia. The operation constitutes a moderate surgical stress, but seldom requires blood transfusion. Factors that may increase the length, complexity, or level of stress to the patient include hostile groins (due to reoperation, infection, or obesity), absence of a femoral pulse (often mandating a simultaneous procedure to improve inflow), previous failed PTA/stent, and diseased distal runoff (such as an isolated popliteal segment). Popliteal entrapment syndrome, popliteal aneurysm, or other

Medical Management of the Surgical Patient, ed. Michael F. Lubin, Thomas F. Dodson, and Neil H. Winawer. Published by Cambridge University Press. © Cambridge University Press 2013.

conditions of non-atherosclerotic etiology may require a less extensive femoral-popliteal bypass.

Drain placement may benefit the obese patient with subsequent difficult wound closure. When drains are used, patients undergoing simultaneous harvest of vein conduit may avoid seroma formation. Heparin anticoagulation, given prior to the clamping of any vessels, is usually allowed to wear off at the conclusion of the procedure, but it can be reversed with protamine to reduce bleeding when no mechanical bleeding is identified. When long-term postoperative anticoagulation is planned, it is usually initiated 24–48 hours following completion of the bypass procedure.

Usual postoperative course

Expected postoperative hospital stay

The expected postoperative hospital stay is 3–6 days.

Operative mortality

Operative mortality is 1–4%.

Special monitoring required

For the first 24 hours, dorsalis pedis and posterior tibial pulses should be evaluated every 2–4 hours by palpation and Doppler assessment. Any change in the exam or symptoms should be promptly evaluated. The wounds are kept dry and covered with a sterile bandage for 48 hours.

Patient activity and positioning

Patients may ambulate with assistance on the first postoperative day. If the patient is in a chair, the leg should be elevated to minimize the edema which is frequently encountered postoperatively.

Alimentation

Food and drink are withheld after midnight prior to surgery. Resumption of the usual diet begins on the first postoperative day.

Antibiotic coverage

A first-generation cephalosporin (or vancomycin if the patient is allergic to penicillin) is administered preoperatively and continued for up to 24 hours. A longer course with a variable antibiotic regimen may be required for patients with open or infected wounds, or may be utilized in patients who require placement of a prosthetic graft.

Postoperative complications

In the hospital

Bleeding

Bleeding, the most common immediate postoperative complication, may arise from the incision, the anastomoses, or from within the tunnel where the conduit is placed. Small hematomas may be observed and will resorb with time. Larger hematomas or suspicion of arterial bleeding should be evaluated in the operating room.

Graft thrombosis

Graft thrombosis in the immediate postoperative period usually indicates a technical problem. Re-exploration, revision of anastomoses, graft thrombectomy, and intraoperative angiography are typically indicated.

Leg edema

Postoperative leg edema is a nearly universal finding, although the severity may vary. The etiology can be multifactorial, and includes reperfusion of the ischemic limb and surgical disruption of venous and lymphatic drainage as the most likely causes. Improvement can be provided by elevation of the limb while in bed. Spontaneous improvement often occurs over a few months following the bypass.

Wound infection

Infection is an uncommon but unsettling problem, particularly when a synthetic conduit has been used. If the synthetic graft material becomes infected, the patient is at an increased risk of death or limb loss. Wound infection overlying an autogenous vein graft is somewhat less critical since this conduit is less likely to become infected. Superficial infections may be treated by opening the wound for drainage of pus, applying dressings or a wound vacuum system to promote healing, and systemic antibiotic therapy.

Deeper infections that involve a synthetic graft or that leave a graft exposed necessitate graft removal and replacement with an autogenous conduit (typically saphenous vein). Exposed autogenous vein may require a sartorius muscle flap to be rotated into position to provide sufficient coverage of the graft. Amputation may ultimately be required in as many as 70% of patients with prosthetic bypass graft infection.

Lymphatic leaks

Lymphatic leaks typically present within the first two postoperative weeks with persistent clear or serous drainage from the wound. When there is established communication to the skin and its flora, we recommend debriding the affected area, identifying and ligating any potential lymphatics, and covering any exposed grafts with a sartorius flap.

After discharge

Vein graft stenosis

Failure of autogenous vein grafts within the first 2 years following bypass is not infrequent (10–35% of patients). During this time period myointimal hyperplasia, which may be due to stenosis within the vein or at the anastomoses, is the most likely cause. Such failure usually presents as a return of preoperative symptoms, which may be worse than the initial presenting symptoms. Prior to failure, failing bypass grafts are usually asymptomatic and may not be detected simply by physical exam or the measurement of ankle pressures. Given the excellent secondary patency results obtained when intervention precedes failure, routine surveillance of the autogenous lower extremity bypass graft is imperative. Prosthetic material behaves differently than saphenous vein grafts. Although anastomotic problems and flow rates within the graft may be accurately determined, routine duplex examination may not have as great an impact on secondary patency in this group.

Graft occlusion

Thrombotic occlusion of a bypass graft may occur suddenly, with an acute onset of symptoms. Such patients may develop a profoundly ischemic limb if the bypass had been performed for limb salvage, or may have a return of their preoperative claudication symptoms. If the patient presents soon after the graft occludes (i.e., within 72 hours), restoration of patency may be obtained by either surgical thrombectomy or catheter-directed thrombolysis. An investigation as to the cause of the occlusion should be made, and the lesion must be treated or the graft revised to prevent recurrent thrombosis.

Percutaneous therapy

Patency and amputation-free survival advantages for primary lower extremity bypass versus percutaneous angioplasty (PTA) have been reported in the recent literature. There is also a suggestion that bypass outcomes are inferior in the setting of a previous PTA. Therefore, proper selection of an initial procedural therapy for patients with peripheral arterial disease remains controversial; however, many patients and clinicians favor primary PTA as the initial intervention, due to the more invasive nature of bypass.

Typically, lower extremity PTA is approached with contralateral femoral artery access, followed by an aortogram with bilateral lower extremity angiography. Wire access across the occlusive lesion is then established, and the patient is systemically anticoagulated. Stenting is reserved for patients whose PTA is technically inadequate due to recoil or residual stenosis, or whose PTA is complicated by dissection. The procedures usually take between 1 and 2 hours, and patients are frequently discharged on the same day.

Further reading

Bradbury AW, Adam DJ, Bell J *et al.* Bypass versus Angioplasty in Severe Ischaemia of the Leg (BASIL) trial: a survival prediction model to facilitate clinical decision making. *J Vasc Surg* 2010; **51**: S52–68.

Bradbury AW, Adam DJ, Bell J *et al.* Bypass versus Angioplasty in Severe Ischaemia of the Leg (BASIL) trial: an intention-to-treat analysis of amputation-free and overall survival in patients randomized to a bypass surgery-first or a balloon angioplasty-first revascularization strategy. *J Vasc Surg* 2010; **51**: S5–17.

Conte MS. Bypass versus Angioplasty in Severe Ischaemia of the Leg (BASIL) and the (hoped for) dawn of evidence-based treatment for advanced limb ischemia. *J Vasc Surg* 2010; **51**: S69–75.

Faries PL, Logerfo FW, Arora S *et al.* A comparative study of alternative conduits for lower extremity revascularization: all-autogenous conduit versus prosthetic grafts. *J Vasc Surg* 2000; **32**: 1080–90.

Gulkarov I, Malik R, Yakubov R *et al.* Early results for below-knee bypasses using Distaflo. *Vasc Endovasc Surg* 2008; **42**: 561–6.

Hugl B, Nevelsteen A, Daenens K *et al.* PEPE II – a multicenter study with an end-point heparin-bonded expanded polytetrafluoroethylene vascular graft for above and below knee bypass surgery: determinants of patency. *J Cardiovasc Surg (Torino)* 2009; **50**: 195–203.

Siani A, Accrocca F, Antonelli R *et al.* Prejudices and realities in the use of 'unsuitable' saphenous vein graft for infrapopliteal revascularization. *G Chir* 2008; **29**: 261–4.

Simosa HF, Malek JY, Schermerhorn ML *et al.* Endoluminal intervention for limb salvage after failed lower extremity bypass graft. *J Vasc Surg* 2009; **49**: 1426–30.

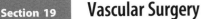

Lower extremity embolectomy

Paul J. Riesenman and Thomas F. Dodson

Acute lower extremity limb ischemia secondary to thromboembolic disease is a common clinical problem with significant associated morbidity and mortality. While embolic sources are primarily cardiogenic in 80–90% of cases, other causes include emboli from proximal atherosclerotic or aneurysmal vessels, paradoxical emboli, and tumors. Additionally, the increase in endovascular techniques has made iatrogenic causes a more commonly appreciated etiology of lower extremity arterial emboli. The majority of embolic material will travel to the lower extremity and lodge near arterial bifurcations, most commonly in the femoral and popliteal arteries.

Patients with thromboembolism of the extremities present with one or more of the six "classic Ps" of limb ischemia: pain, pallor, paresthesia, paralysis, pulselessness, and poikilothermia (cold limb). Since each patient has a critical window before irreversible tissue damage may occur, attempting to determine the duration of symptoms is important. Six hours is commonly considered to be the span before such irreversible damage begins. It cannot be overemphasized that immediate referral to a vascular surgeon is absolutely paramount if a patient presents with acute limb ischemia, as delays in triage or unnecessary imaging can ultimately compromise the potential for limb salvage. Diagnosis can usually be made by history and physical examination, although imaging studies may be necessary to assist with management decisions for some patients.

The algorithm for treating patients with acute thromboembolism can be quite complex, and takes into account the duration and severity of ischemia, presence of preexisting peripheral vascular disease, history of prior vascular surgery, and therapeutic modalities available to the treating surgeon. As a general rule, all patients are immediately anticoagulated with heparin if no contraindications are present. Interventions may include balloon catheter thromboembolectomy, catheter-directed thrombolytic therapy, or percutaneous mechanical thrombectomy. Balloon catheter thromboembolectomy, which was originally described by Fogarty *et al.* in 1962, is performed either through a groin or a medial infrageniculate incision. It is often an effective approach to quickly reestablishing flow to the ischemic extremity. Alternatively, catheter-directed

thrombolytic therapy offers the advantages of a less invasive approach that may facilitate clot breakdown in more distal smaller vessels, which cannot be accessed by balloon thromboembolectomy catheters. The disadvantages with this approach are the potential complications associated with the use of thrombolytic agents, as well as the slower reestablishment of limb perfusion. Finally, several percutaneous mechanical thrombectomy devices that employ different principles to effect thrombus dissolution are commercially available.

Fasciotomy may be performed at the time of the embolectomy procedure if blood flow has been successfully reestablished and there is clinical suspicion of a prolonged severe ischemic period. Alternatively, fasciotomy may be performed in the postoperative period if clinical signs of compartment syndrome develop.

Usual postoperative course
Expected postoperative hospital stay

Following the procedure, patients are in the hospital for approximately 5 days, although this can vary depending upon the patient's condition at presentation, associated comorbidities, and extent of surgery. Although patient recovery time is usually quite short, much of the postoperative hospital stay is spent in ascertaining the etiology of the embolus. Often, hematologists and cardiologists are involved in postoperative care. Transesophageal echocardiography, computed tomography, and angiography are common imaging modalities usually utilized in diagnosing the source of emboli.

Operative mortality

The high hospital mortality rate of 20–30% is a reflection of the underlying disease process and associated comorbidities in this patient population, not necessarily the morbidity of the procedure itself.

Special monitoring required

Patients often recover in the ICU for 24 hours and are placed on telemetry for cardiac monitoring. Frequent monitoring of peripheral pulses is essential as most recurrent thromboses

Medical Management of the Surgical Patient, ed. Michael F. Lubin, Thomas F. Dodson, and Neil H. Winawer. Published by Cambridge University Press. © Cambridge University Press 2013.

occur in the early postoperative period. After revascularization for severe ischemia, an assessment of motor and sensory function is also imperative, with heightened suspicion for compartment syndrome. Measurement of renal function by urine output and serum creatinine determines renal injury that may result from myoglobinuria or contrast-induced nephropathy. Additionally, serum potassium should be closely monitored for elevations resulting from cellular death, acidosis, and impaired renal function.

Patient activity and positioning

Most patients who undergo catheter embolectomy via a single groin incision recover quickly; they are encouraged to ambulate the following day. Patients who undergo an infrageniculate incision and/or have some degree of clinical reperfusion insult to the lower extremity may require assistance with early mobility. For patients who have undergone fasciotomy, function of the affected extremity will be impaired; a more protracted course of physical therapy should be anticipated.

Alimentation

Patients can often resume normal diet the evening of surgery. However, if the potential exists for an early secondary surgical procedure (fasciotomy, amputation), patients should be kept NPO in the early postoperative period.

Antibiotic coverage

Cephalosporin, or an appropriate antibiotic to cover skin flora, is administered immediately prior to the surgical procedure.

Postoperative anticoagulation

Over a period of several days prior to discharge, patients must be converted from intravenous heparin to therapeutic levels of an oral anticoagulant (warfarin). Alternatively, as an outpatient, the patient can be bridged to therapeutic dosage levels with the administration of low-molecular weight heparin. It is necessary to educate patients receiving anticoagulation medications about the risks of warfarin therapy (including possible interactions with certain foods) and the need for lifelong monitoring of prothrombin time.

Postoperative complications

In the hospital

Compartment syndrome

Some degree of leg edema is common following revascularization. When the edema of the revascularized tissue causes elevations in the fascial compartment pressure of the leg, a significant reduction in tissue perfusion pressure can result in ischemia and subsequent muscle necrosis, nerve damage, or thrombosis of the arteries and veins in the affected compartment. The anterior compartment of the lower leg is most frequently involved. Symptoms such as severe leg pain on dorsiflexion of the foot or diminished sensation and paresthesias in the first toe web space are strongly suggestive of anterior compartment syndrome. Early detection is the key to limiting the process; this can be accomplished by frequent clinical assessment of motor and sensory function, or by measurement of compartment pressures. Once compartment syndrome is suspected, immediate decompressive four-compartment fasciotomy must be performed. If the duration of ischemia has been prolonged, some surgeons prefer to perform fasciotomy at the time of initial revascularization. Fasciotomy wounds can usually be closed secondarily after the tissue edema subsides.

Renal failure

Acute renal failure can result either from contrast-induced nephropathy if arteriography was employed, or from myoglobinuria secondary to muscle necrosis. Patients with prolonged ischemia should be monitored closely for acute renal insufficiency and treated aggressively with intravenous hydration. Alkalinization with sodium bicarbonate is essential to diminish precipitation of myoglobin in the renal tubules and prevent further renal tubular injury. Mannitol assists with both diuresis and prevention of reperfusion injury. It should be noted that the urine discoloration associated with myoglobinuria also develops in patients with hemoglobinuria, which is a common side-effect following percutaneous mechanical thrombectomy interventions.

Metabolic acidosis

Progressive, non-resolving metabolic acidosis may indicate that embolectomy and revascularization were not effective. Occasionally, an emergency amputation is the only way to control continued metabolic acidosis and poor tissue perfusion. Hyperkalemia, another concern in cases of severe ischemia, results from cellular breakdown and the release of potassium into the circulation. Maintenance of a brisk urinary output in the postoperative period is an important precaution to maintain renal excretion of elevated extracellular potassium.

Recurrent embolization

When anticoagulation is strictly maintained after the initial procedure, recurrent embolization, while occasionally reported, is relatively uncommon. However, there is heightened suspicion of recurrent embolization for patients who develop worsening symptoms or signs of emboli in other vascular territories.

Hematomas

Hematomas may occur after operation with resumption of heparin therapy. However, they present a minor problem that rarely requires a return to the operating room for evacuation. Some surgeons employ drains to minimize hematoma formation in the groin wound. Patients should be reassured that stable hematomas and ecchymoses will gradually resolve without sequelae.

After discharge

Peripheral nerve deficits

For patients who present with severe ischemia, a peripheral nerve deficit is often the most disabling complication. It can manifest as numbness in the sensory distribution of the affected nerve, loss of motor function, or painful neuropathy. Time and analgesics are the only treatments; in extreme cases, amputation may be required for symptom control.

Pseudoaneurysms

Pseudoaneurysms are a potential complication after any arteriotomy. Indications for treatment are based upon size of the pseudoaneurysm and the associated symptoms.

A pseudoaneurysm typically presents as an expansile mass, thrill, or bruit over the incision site. Duplex ultrasonography or CT scan with contrast confirms the diagnosis. Treatment options include open operation, ultrasound-guided compression, and/or thrombin injection.

Claudication or rest pain

The symptom complex of claudication or rest pain may occur if embolectomy is incomplete or if collateral vessels undergo thrombosis before definitive therapy is achieved. Claudication is usually treated conservatively, whereas rest pain necessitates reevaluation of limb perfusion and an attempt to improve distal blood flow with a surgical bypass or a catheter-based intervention.

Further reading

Fogarty TJ, Cranley JJ, Krause RJ, Strasser ES, Hafner CD. A method for extraction of arterial emboli and thrombi. *Surg Gynecol Obstet* 1963; **116**: 241–4.

Henke PK. Contemporary management of acute limb ischemia: factors associated with amputation and in-hospital mortality. *Semin Vasc Surg* 2009; **22**: 34–40.

O'Connell JB, Quinones-Baldrich WJ. Proper evaluation and management of acute embolic versus thrombotic limb ischemia. *Semin Vasc Surg* 2009; **22**: 10–16.

Rutherford RB. Clinical staging of acute limb ischemia as the basis for choice of revascularization method: when and how to intervene. *Semin Vasc Surg* 2009; **22**: 5–9.

Wissgott C, Kamusella P, Andersen R. Percutaneous mechanical thrombectomy: advantages and limitations. *J Cardiovasc Surg (Torino)* 2011; **52**: 477–84.

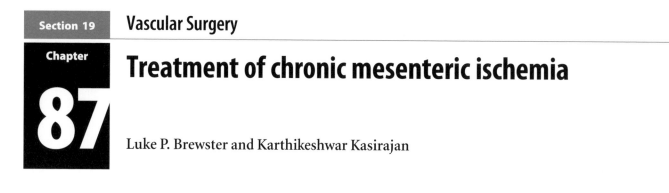

Chapter

87

Treatment of chronic mesenteric ischemia

Luke P. Brewster and Karthikeshwar Kasirajan

Owing to the rich blood supply to the intestines, symptoms of chronic mesenteric ischemia are estimated at 1/100,000 persons. The major vessels supplying the intestines are the celiac artery for the foregut, the superior mesenteric artery for the midgut, and the inferior mesenteric artery for the hindgut. Additionally, the inferior mesenteric artery receives a rich collateral flow from branches of both internal iliac arteries. With chronic mesenteric occlusion, the rich collateral network usually provides adequate collateral flow to the intestines. However, as stenosis or occlusion occurs in two or more of the three major vessels, patients become symptomatic.

The diagnosis of chronic mesenteric ischemia is usually suggested by the presenting symptoms, and it is confirmed by diagnostic tests. Postprandial pain is the most prevalent complaint, which may be accompanied by symptoms of bloating, weight loss, "food fear," nausea, vomiting, diarrhea, and/or constipation. The pain is typically dull and crampy, poorly localized to the midepigastric region or midabdomen, and usually occurs within the first hour after eating. The symptoms are often severe enough to cause the patient to restrict food intake ("food fear"). The weight loss may be so acute as to result in cachexia and prompt a work-up for an underlying neoplasm. The outcome for patients with chronic mesenteric ischemia is dire, with 86% of the patients developing symptoms significant enough to warrant revascularization, or dying from bowel ischemia. Since acute mesenteric ischemia carries a mortality rate that can approach 70%, the timely diagnosis and treatment of patients with chronic mesenteric ischemia is crucial to limiting morbidity and mortality in this patient population.

A non-invasive duplex ultrasound exam of the celiac axis and superior mesenteric artery is often used as the initial screening test; a food bolus may improve the sensitivity of these examinations. The next step is often arteriography (gold standard for diagnosis and planning an operation) with or without angioplasty/stent; or ancillary studies such as computed tomogram or magnetic resonance angiography.

Once the diagnosis has been confirmed, the risks and expected benefits of endovascular or open therapy are aligned with the patient's specific arterial blockages and his/her comorbidities. In general, stenoses that are not overly calcified are well served by angioplasty while total occlusions are best treated with an arterial bypass. Open surgical revascularization has superior long-term patency but has a higher mortality rate and longer hospitalization stay due to associated morbidities. Prior to deciding on an operation, patients should undergo cardiac stress and pulmonary function tests as well as quantification of their malnutrition (albumin, transferrin, pre-albumin levels). Attempted reversal of their catabolic state enterally or parenterally is an important adjunct to their postoperative management. Endovascular therapy does not require these investigations. At the Cleveland Clinic, Kasirajan et al. found technical success of endovascular therapy in ~90% of patients, 30-day mortality of about 10%, 66% freedom of symptoms, and vessel patency of ~75% at 3 years. Given the similarity in outcomes and the lessened morbidity, endovascular therapy should be considered when reasonable, particularly for patients with high operative risk.

Open surgery
Usual postoperative course
Expected postoperative hospital stay
The expected postoperative hospital stay is 8–10 days.

Operative mortality
Operative mortality varies widely, but averages 7% with complications noted in approximately 30% of patients. The most frequent cause of mortality is cardiac disease. Adverse cardiac events are noted in 15% of patients in the postoperative period. Pulmonary, gastrointestinal, and renal complications are the most frequently encountered non-fatal complications. Respiratory failure requiring prolonged

Medical Management of the Surgical Patient, ed. Michael F. Lubin, Thomas F. Dodson, and Neil H. Winawer. Published by Cambridge University Press. © Cambridge University Press 2013.

ventilatory support is noted in 15% of patients, and prolonged ileus or renal failure is observed in 30% and 10% of patients respectively.

Special monitoring required

All patients are placed in the ICU for monitoring and cardiac enzymes are routinely obtained. Liver function tests and amylase are often checked in the early postoperative period. Also, attention is paid to the patient's hemoglobin, lactic acid, and clotting parameters overnight. Abnormalities are corrected aggressively, and untoward trends may require a return to the operating room. Keeping patients euvolemic and preventing prolonged intubation or reintubation limit pulmonary and renal morbidity.

Patient activity and positioning

Patients may be mobilized and out of bed when hemodynamically stable and off the ventilator.

Alimentation

Oral intake is withheld until patient exhibits bowel function.

Antibiotic coverage

Broad-spectrum antibiotic coverage should be extended until there is no longer concern that the intestinal epithelium is threatened.

Postoperative complications
In the hospital

Nasogastric tubes are routinely used to minimize the problems that may result from a prolonged ileus. Early extubation protocols may reduce the risk of pneumonia, and the initiation of total parenteral nutrition may be of benefit in patients with known preoperative nutritional depletion.

Abdominal pain

Abdominal pain may have a variety of causes, among them ileus, bowel ischemia, intestinal edema and pancreatitis. Plain abdominal films and clinical exam should be sufficient to diagnose postoperative ileus. Significant or worsening pain, leukocytosis, elevated lactate, or worsening acidosis may warrant re-exploration to assess for bowel ischemia and exclude acute graft thrombosis. Duplex ultrasound is often not reliable in this situation to exclude graft complications.

After discharge
Recurrent mesenteric ischemia

Restenosis/occlusion of the native artery or bypass graft may result in abdominal angina or acute mesenteric ischemia. Surveillance mesenteric duplex may identify failing bypass grafts and improve assisted patency of these grafts.

Endovascular therapy
Usual postoperative course
Expected postoperative hospital stay

The expected postoperative hospital stay is 1–2 days.

Operative mortality

Mortality occurs in about 5% of patients and complications are seen in about 20%. Mortality is often associated with gastrointestinal complications, especially bowel necrosis, which may be seen in 5–10% of patients. Cardiac and pulmonary events are less frequent. After percutaneous revascularization, the majority of encountered complications are local. Access complications include hematoma, bleeding, pseudoaneurysm, or access vessel thrombosis. Intra-abdominal complications may include vessel rupture, thrombosis, malpositioning of the stent, and distal embolization during angioplasty.

Special monitoring required

Systemic complications are far less frequent with percutaneous revascularization; therefore patients do not need to be monitored in an ICU. However, unlike many other patients who have undergone peripheral angioplasty procedures, percutaneeous revascularization patients should be observed in the hospital overnight with the appropriate attention to volume status and hemodynamic parameters.

Patient activity and positioning

Mobilize progressively as the patient's condition permits.

Alimentation

Oral intake is usually resumed promptly.

Antibiotic coverage

Antibiotics are administered prior to the intervention.

Postoperative complications
In the hospital
Local complications

Careful attention to access techniques should minimize the incidence of access vessel complications. Recent advances in endovascular devices, with smaller device profile and better capacity for tracking around acute angles, have helped eliminate many of the complications reported in the past. In earlier times, the acute downward angle of the mesenteric vessels off the abdominal aorta often required the use of a brachial approach to track the larger and stiffer devices. Historically, this resulted in a higher incidence of brachial complications. Currently, most mesenteric angioplasty procedures may be adequately performed via the femoral approach. Following angioplasty, patients are maintained on aspirin for life. In addition, they are loaded with clopidogrel (Plavix) and continued for 3 months afterwards in order to decrease the incidence of acute stent or vessel thrombosis.

After discharge

Abdominal pain

Elimination of postprandial abdominal pain is one of the primary indicators of the success of the procedure. Similarly, the recurrence of pain may be a reliable indicator of recurrent stenosis.

Nutritional status

Serum albumin and transferrin levels are monitored as a measure of the success of revascularization along with weight gain, which may be apparent within a few weeks after intervention.

Graft or stent restenosis

The treated vessel is routinely monitored for restenosis. Clinical symptoms may not be obvious until the stenosis is critical or results in thrombosis. Hence, we recommend surveillance with non-invasive imaging studies, such as duplex ultrasound, magnetic resonance imaging, or CT angiography. Typically, the bypass graft or stented vessel is assessed at 1 month, every 6 months for 2 years, and then annually for prompt diagnosis and correction of any subclinical restenosis.

Further reading

Cho JS, Carr JA, Jacobsen G et al. Long-term outcome after mesenteric artery reconstruction: a 37-year experience. *J Vasc Surg* 2002; **35**: 453–60.

Gupta PK, Horan SM, Turaga KK, Miller WJ, Pipinos II. Chronic mesenteric ischemia: endovascular versus open revascularization. *J Endovasc Ther* 2010; **17**: 540–9.

Hirsch AT, Haskal ZJ, Hertzer NR et al. ACC/AHA 2005 practice guidelines for the management of patients with peripheral arterial disease (lower extremity, renal, mesenteric, and abdominal aortic): a collaborative report from the American Association for Vascular Surgery/Society for Vascular Surgery, Society for Cardiovascular Angiography and Interventions, Society for Vascular Medicine and Biology, Society of Interventional Radiology, and the ACC/AHA Task Force on Practice Guidelines (Writing Committee to Develop Guidelines for the Management of Patients With Peripheral Arterial Disease): endorsed by the American Association of Cardiovascular and Pulmonary Rehabilitation; National Heart, Lung, and Blood Institute; Society for Vascular Nursing; TransAtlantic Inter-Society Consensus; and Vascular Disease Foundation. *Circulation* 2006; **113**: e463–654.

Kasirajan K, O'Hara PJ, Gray BH et al. Chronic mesenteric ischemia: open surgery versus percutaneous angioplasty and stenting. *J Vasc Surg* 2001; **33**: 63–71.

Kihara TK, Blebea J, Anderson KM, Friedman D, Atnip RG. Risk factors and outcomes following revascularization for chronic mesenteric ischemia. *Ann Vasc Surg* 1999; **13**: 37–44.

Malgor RD, Oderich GS, McKusick MA et al. Results of single- and two-vessel mesenteric artery stents for chronic mesenteric ischemia. *Ann Vasc Surg* 2010; **24**: 1094–101.

Moawad J, McKinsey JF, Wyble CW et al. Current results of surgical therapy for chronic mesenteric ischemia. *Arch Surg* 1997; **132**: 613–18; discussion 618–19.

Mohammed A, Teo NB, Pickford IR, Moss JG. Percutaneous transluminal angioplasty and stenting of coeliac artery stenosis in the treatment of mesenteric angina: a case report and review of therapeutic options. *J R Coll Surg Edinb* 2000; **45**: 403–7.

Oderich GS, Bower TC, Sullivan TM et al. Open versus endovascular revascularization for chronic mesenteric ischemia: risk-stratified outcomes. *J Vasc Surg* 2009; **49**: 1472–9.

Inferior vena cava filters

Jayer Chung and Thomas F. Dodson

The incidence of first-time venous thromboembolic (VTE) events is approximately 70–113 cases per 100,000 people per year. Approximately one-third of these cases are due to pulmonary embolism (PE). Venous thromboembolism will recur in approximately 7% of patients at 6 months, with patients presenting with PE more likely to have recurrent PE. Thirty-day mortality following PE is approximately 12%. While anti-coagulation remains the gold-standard therapy for VTE, patients who have recurrent PE despite adequate anticoagulation, high-risk patients with contraindications to anticoagulation, or patients who have bleeding complications while on anticoagulation therapy meet criteria for inferior vena cava (IVC) filter placement. Inferior vena cava filter placement is contraindicated in patients with complete thrombosis of the IVC, or with an IVC that is otherwise inaccessible by percutaneous means.

Inferior vena cava filters are inserted percutaneously under local anesthesia via the femoral or jugular vein, with fluoroscopic or ultrasound guidance. The procedure usually takes less than 30 minutes, and consists of obtaining central venous access under ultrasound guidance. Venography is performed; fluoroscopic guidance may be used to measure the IVC, locate the renal veins, and identify any possible aberrant anatomy. Procedural morbidity is extremely rare and consists primarily of complications at the insertion site. Long-term complications are more significant and need to be considered when placing filters in young patients. Such complications include device migration, device fracture, caval thrombosis, IVC perforation, and post-thrombotic syndrome.

Multiple devices are currently approved by the Food and Drug Administration for use in pulmonary embolism prevention. Each of these devices possesses its own unique advantages and complication rates, while protecting against PE in over 95% of cases. Our choice for filter placement is the stainless steel Greenfield filter, which has the longest track record of any IVC filter. It boasts the lowest long-term complication rates with a facile over-the-wire delivery system. Its main disadvantage is the requirement of a 12F sheath, the largest of the percutaneous filters. We rarely use the Bird's Nest filter

as deployment can be difficult and high IVC thrombosis rates have been reported; however, it is the filter of choice for an enlarged vena cava. The TrapEase and OptEase have the smallest introducer diameters but suffer from lack of long-term follow-up data. However, an important prospective randomized study recently compared the outcomes between the Greenfield and TrapEase filters. The TrapEase filter had a higher rate of caval thrombosis. Overall, IVC filters are quite successful in preventing recurrent pulmonary embolization, with rates in the range of 2–5% and fatal PE occurring in only 0.3% of cases.

After being successfully used in Europe for years, retrievable filters were introduced into the US marketplace in 2003. These devices may be ideal in patients who require temporary caval interruption before they can be safely anticoagulated, such as multitrauma and pregnant patients or patients undergoing bariatric surgery. Several retrievable filters are currently available: the OptEase (Cordis Endovascular, Warren, NJ) and the Gunther Tulip (Cook Inc., Bloomington, IN) are two of the most frequently used. It is recommended that the OptEase and Gunther Tulip be removed within two weeks of placement. These devices are generally easy to deploy and retrieve, utilize low-profile delivery systems, and should theoretically eliminate the long-term complications of filters such as IVC thrombosis and device migration.

Usual postoperative course
Expected postoperative hospital stay

Depending upon associated medical problems, the patient can be released on the evening of the procedure. In order to minimize bleeding complications, we prefer to have the patient remain flat in bed for 4 hours after manual pressure at the insertion site has been discontinued.

Operative mortality

Death from the procedure itself should approach zero, and has been cited at 0.12%; however, hospital mortality overall is substantial due to medical comorbidities and/or surgical conditions.

Medical Management of the Surgical Patient, ed. Michael F. Lubin, Thomas F. Dodson, and Neil H. Winawer. Published by Cambridge University Press. © Cambridge University Press 2013.

Special monitoring required

None.

Patient activity and positioning

Relates to the patient's condition otherwise, though the patient can often be ambulatory after 4 hours.

Alimentation

Postoperative food intake is permitted as tolerated.

Antibiotic coverage

One dose of antibiotics covering skin flora is administered prior to device insertion.

Anticoagulation

If the patient requires anticoagulation, we prefer to resume heparin 6 hours after the procedure, especially if a large introducer sheath is used.

Radiographs

When jugular venous access is utilized, upright chest radiographs are obtained to ensure that there has been no inadvertent hemothorax or pneumothorax. Otherwise, there is no other radiographic confirmation required.

Postoperative complications

In the hospital

Insertion problems

Procedural morbidity is rare and is usually limited to local complications at the site of device insertion. Hematomas, ecchymosis, and bleeding from the puncture site occur infrequently and are usually controlled by gentle compression at the insertion site. Pneumothoraces and hemothoraces are also rare, and treated with tube thoracostomy as indicated. Air embolism during insertion is also extremely rare, occurring in less than 1% of cases.

Deployment problems

Most serious immediate complications are due to operator error, or to device malfunction. Inadvertent deployment of the device into the iliac veins or suprarenal cava is a minor problem that requires insertion of another device in the correct location. Catheter and wire complications resulting in perforation of the vena cava or right atrium have been reported and require expedient management. Device malfunction resulting in incomplete device expansion or device migration can usually be successfully managed using endovascular techniques.

Other (< 1%)

Infection is extremely rare in terms of the device or insertion site. Rarely seen complications include proximal migration of the filter to the heart or perforation into adjacent vascular or gastrointestinal structures. Other infrequently seen problems such as filter fractures, guide wire entrapment during central line insertion, and arteriovenous fistulas have all been reported. While these complications are rare, awareness of the complications of IVC filter placement is required to prevent undue delays in diagnosis and appropriate treatment.

After discharge

Clinicians must be aware of the long-term complications of permanent IVC filters, especially when considering their use in younger patients. Rates of IVC thrombosis are device-specific, with rates ranging from 0–22%. The Greenfield filter has the lowest rates of IVC thrombosis (0–3%); the Bird's Nest filter has the highest rates of thrombosis (5–21%). Inferior vena cava thrombosis may lead to disabling clinical symptoms such as extensive lower extremity edema, venous ulceration, or phlegmasia cerulea dolens. Recurrent deep venous thrombosis is a highly variable problem (3–46%) after filter placement and probably reflects the underlying disorder rather than a complication of filter placement. When larger sheath sizes were used, venous thrombosis at the entry site was a relatively common occurrence; it now occurs in approximately 2% of cases. Many believe that prevention of fatal PE by IVC filters outweighs the negative effects of any possible delayed large vein thrombotic complications. In all cases of symptomatic venous thrombosis, anticoagulation is the treatment of choice unless otherwise contraindicated.

Further reading

Ingber S, Geerts W. Vena caval filters: current knowledge, uncertainties and practical approaches. *Curr Opin Hematol* 2009; **16**: 402–6.

Kearon C, Kahn SR, Agnelli G *et al.* Antithrombotic therapy for venous thromboembolic disease: American College of Chest Physicians Evidence-Based Clinical Practice Guidelines (8th Edition). *Chest* 2008; **133**: S454–545.

Kinney TB. Update on inferior vena cava filters. *J Vasc Interv Radiol* 2003; **14**: 425–40.

Smoot RL, Koch CA, Heller SF *et al.* Inferior vena cava filters in trauma patients: efficacy, morbidity, and retrievability. *J Trauma* 2010; **68**: 899–903.

Usoh F, Hingorani A, Ascher E *et al.* Prospective randomized study comparing the clinical outcomes between inferior vena cava Greenfield and TrapEase filters. *J Vasc Surg* 2010; **52**: 394–9.

White RH. The epidemiology of venous thromboembolism. *Circulation* 2003; **107**: I-4–I-8.

Chapter

89

Portal shunting procedures

Paul J. Riesenman and Atef A. Salam

Decompressive portosystemic shunts play a significant role in the treatment of patients with portal hypertension and gastroesophageal varices. The main indication for portal shunting procedures is the prevention of recurrent variceal bleeding in patients with cirrhosis and portal hypertension after failure of endoscopic interventions (banding, sclerotherapy). Portal shunting procedures are not indicated for prophylaxis against variceal bleeding in patients who have not yet bled. In these patients, medical management (non-selective beta-blockers) and endoscopic therapies are utilized. The ideal candidates for shunt procedures are Child–Turcotte–Pugh (Child's) class A or B patients who have favorable venous anatomy. The procedures themselves can be divided into two main categories: total shunts and selective distal splenorenal (Warren) shunt.

With total shunts, the entire portal venous blood flow is shunted away from the liver into the systemic venous circulation. This includes end-to-side and side-to-side portacaval shunts, central splenorenal shunts, Marion–Clatworthy mesocaval shunts, interposition mesocaval shunts, and radiologically placed transjugular intrahepatic portosystemic shunts (TIPS). The small graft portacaval interposition shunt is a modification designed to achieve partial rather than total diversion of portal venous flow. If patients who require total shunts are potential candidates for liver transplantation, mesocaval rather than portacaval shunts should be chosen to preclude dissection in the liver hilum, which would complicate subsequent liver transplantation.

With the selective distal splenorenal shunt, the gastroesophageal varices are selectively decompressed by way of the upper stomach through the short gastric veins and the disconnected splenic vein into the left renal vein. The goal of this procedure is to achieve adequate variceal decompression while maintaining enough pressure in the portal and superior mesenteric veins to drive blood through the diseased liver.

Compared with total shunts, the distal splenorenal shunt is associated with a lower incidence of encephalopathy and

hepatic insufficiency, and is therefore used in most patients. Although collateral veins develop over time after this shunting procedure, with progressive diversion of portal blood flow, there is often no parallel progress of encephalopathy. Unlike portacaval shunts, distal splenorenal shunts do not complicate future liver transplantation. In some patients however, adequate splenic or renal veins are not available to make this shunt feasible. Additionally, a selective shunt is not recommended for patients with refractory ascites, and a total shunt should be considered under these circumstances. All surgical portosystemic shunts subject the patient to severe stress and may necessitate multiple perioperative transfusions.

Radiologic shunts (transjugular intrahepatic portosystemic shunts) are often the only option for prevention of variceal rebleeding and refractory ascites in patients with poor liver function (Child's class C) who would not tolerate an abdominal operation and general anesthesia. A TIPS is also employed as rescue therapy for acute variceal bleeding after failure of medical and endoscopic management; in approximately 95% of patients, the variceal bleeding is controlled by use of TIPS. Compared to a surgical shunt, TIPS requires more postoperative interventions to maintain patency. Additionally, TIPS is best employed in cirrhotic patients who are transplant candidates awaiting transplantation. A TIPS functions as a total shunt, and therefore places the patient at risk for portal systemic encephalopathy, a common complication of this procedure.

In this procedure, a connection is created through the hepatic parenchyma between a hepatic vein and a portal vein branch. Access is most commonly obtained to the right or middle hepatic vein using percutaneous guidewire and catheter techniques. A special needle pierces the liver parenchyma between the hepatic vein and, usually, the right branch of the portal vein. The track created is balloon dilated and stented, establishing an intrahepatic portosystemic shunt between these two large veins.

Medical Management of the Surgical Patient, ed. Michael F. Lubin, Thomas F. Dodson, and Neil H. Winawer. Published by Cambridge University Press. © Cambridge University Press 2013.

Liver transplant is the treatment of choice for patients with advanced liver disease (Child's class C). A successful liver transplant eliminates liver failure and variceal hemorrhage, the two main causes of death in cirrhotics. Organ shortage precludes wider application of this modality to include cirrhotics with adequate liver reserve. Therefore, shunts continue to be the preferred treatment when medical management and endoscopic therapy fails to control variceal bleeding in this patient population.

Usual postoperative course

Expected postoperative hospital stay

Without complications, hospital stay is generally 7–10 days.

Operative mortality

Operative mortality varies from 5–30%, depending on the patient's Child's classification and the urgency of the procedure.

Special monitoring required

Intensive care unit observation is necessary for the first 2 or 3 days after surgery. Serial monitoring of all the following is essential: vital signs, intake and output, central venous pressure, body weight, renal function, hematocrit, and liver function.

Patient activity and positioning

Intensive pulmonary care and early ambulation starting on the first postoperative day are important to minimize atelectasis and subsequent pulmonary complications.

Alimentation

Oral intake is allowed when intestinal peristalsis returns, usually the third to fourth postoperative day. Free sodium intake through intravenous fluids and diet should be minimized. Dietary protein is not restricted unless patients have signs of encephalopathy.

Antibiotic coverage

A first- or second-generation cephalosporin is usually administered for 24–48 hours after operation, especially if a prosthetic interposition graft has been implanted.

Reaccumulation of ascites

Ascites is a common occurrence for several days after operation, and it should be monitored by daily weight and abdominal girth measurements. Intravenous colloid solutions coupled with potassium-sparing diuretics (spironolactone 25 mg PO three times daily) should be given to maintain a stable urinary output (30–50 mL/hour). The addition of loop diuretics (furosemide) may be necessary for the management of difficult cases. Diuretic therapy should be closely monitored with serum electrolytes including creatinine.

Postoperative ultrasonography

Shunt patency should be evaluated with duplex ultrasonography.

Postoperative complications

In the hospital

Gastrointestinal bleeding

Recurrence of bleeding after portal shunting can result from postoperative gastritis or peptic ulcer disease. However, variceal bleeding as a result of shunt occlusion must always be considered and angiographic evaluation of the shunt may be required.

Ascites

A mild degree of ascites is a common complication in the early postoperative period. Persistent or massive ascites refractory to medical therapy may require scheduled large-volume paracentesis, or a peritoneovenous shunt. Chylous ascites may occur after a distal splenorenal shunt secondary to disruption of intestinal lymphatics in the vicinity of the superior mesenteric vessels. A peritoneal tap is diagnostic in such cases, and treatment consists of cessation of oral intake and institution of parenteral hyperalimentation.

Hepatic encephalopathy

After total shunt procedures, the incidence of hepatic encephalopathy ranges from 20–60%. The rate is significantly lower after distal splenorenal shunt placement because portal perfusion is maintained, particularly in patients without cirrhosis. Therapy consists of dietary protein restriction and the administration of drugs that alter colonic bacterial flora (lactulose 30 mL PO BID; neomycin 250mg PO QID).

Hepatorenal failure

Serum bilirubin and liver enzyme levels are often mildly elevated during the first postoperative week, but usually decline promptly to preoperative baseline levels if the hepatic reserve is adequate. Progressive deterioration of liver function coupled with hypovolemia secondary to dehydration, postoperative bleeding, or massive ascites can result in hepatorenal syndrome, which is associated with a high mortality once it is established.

Ascitic fluid leakage from the abdominal incision

If ascitic fluid leaks from the abdominal incision, the wound may need to be resutured or reinforced to prevent massive fluid losses and to reduce the risk of peritonitis.

After discharge

Shunt occlusion with recurrent variceal bleeding

Endoscopic interventions or reoperation should be considered if shunt failure is confirmed by angiography.

Progressive hepatic failure

Progressive hepatic failure is the most common cause of late death in patients with cirrhosis who undergo shunt placement.

Ascites reaccumulation

Salt restriction and diuretic administration usually control ascites, but the possibility of shunt failure must be considered.

Chronic alcoholism

Continued alcoholism is generally associated with a poor prognosis for long-term survival.

Further reading

Colombato L. The role of transjugular intrahepatic portosystemic shunt (TIPS) in the management of portal hypertension. *J Clin Gastroenterol* 2007; **41**: S344–51.

Did N, Oberti F, Cales P. Current management of the complications of portal hypertension: variceal bleeding and ascites. *Can Med Assoc J* 2006; **174**: 1433–43.

Garcia-Tsao G, Bosch J. Management of varices and variceal hemorrhage in cirrhosis. *N Engl J Med* 2010; **362**: 823–32.

Henderson JM, Boyd TD, Kutner MH *et al.* Distal splenorenal shunt vs. transjugular intrahepatic portosystemic shunt for variceal bleeding: a randomized trial. *Gastroenterology* 2006; **130**: 1643–57.

Rikkers LF. Portal hypertension: the role of shunting procedures. In Cameron JL, ed. *Current Surgical Therapy*. 9th edn.

Philadelphia, PA: Mosby Elsevier; 2008, pp. 373–80.

Salam A. Distal splenorenal shunts: hemodynamics of total versus selective shunting. In Fischer JE, Bland K, eds. *Mastery of Surgery*. 5th edn. Philadelphia, PA: Lippincott Williams & Wilkins; 2006, pp. 1352–60.

Wolf M, Hirner A. Current state of portosystemic shunt surgery. *Langenbecks Arch Surg* 2003; **388**: 141–9.

Breast reconstruction after mastectomy

Wright A. Jones and Grant W. Carlson

Approximately one woman in eight will develop breast cancer at some point in her life. Among women who undergo mastectectomy, 16–30% will undergo breast reconstruction. Partial and total mastectomies may leave patients with breast defects that produce a tremendous amount of psychological distress. The goal of breast reconstruction is to safely create symmetrical natural-appearing breasts, improving self confidence and relieving the psychological impact of mastectomy or breast conservation therapy. Reconstruction may be performed immediately after mastectomy, or in a delayed fashion months to years after breast removal. Immediate reconstruction allows for several advantages including an additional operation under the same anesthetic, preservation of breast skin by occupying mastectomy space, and placement of an optimally sized structure during single stage procedures. An advantage of delayed reconstruction is that patients have more time to think about reconstructive options; they may postpone reconstruction until after other interventions such as radiation therapy or chemotherapy have been completed.

Breast reconstruction can be divided into two types: autologous tissue reconstruction or implant-expander reconstruction. Several factors are considered to determine the optimal type of reconstruction for each patient including health status, emotional state, cancer stage, and adjuvant therapy. A multidisciplinary approach is essential for the often challenging journey taken by breast cancer patients and their caregivers.

Autologous tissue reconstruction allows the plastic surgeon to create a soft, ptotic breast mound, which tends to match the native contralateral breast in and out of bra support. Various tissue donor sites on the female body can be used for reconstruction, including the abdomen, back, gluteal area, and thigh. However, the transverse rectus abdominus musculocutaneous (TRAM) and latissimus dorsi flaps are most commonly used. The TRAM flap involves dissection of an elliptical pattern of skin and fat below the umbilicus that is tunneled up to the breast defect on either a pedicle (still attached to the rectus muscle and superior epigastric artery) or as a "free" flap (where it is completely detached and then inset into the breast defect

with a microvascular anastomosis of artery and vein using a microscope). Preoperative preparation includes CBC, chemistry profile, PT/PTT, type and screen, pregnancy test, chest X-ray and, if indicated, an ECG. Blood transfusions are usually not needed, though the patient may donate blood preoperatively. The surgery usually lasts 2–4 hours; anesthesia is general, with epidural or PCA pump postoperation for pain control; and primary risk factors are obesity, hypertension, diabetes, history of radiation, and smoking.

Usual TRAM flap postoperative course

Expected postoperative hospital stay

The expected postoperative hospital stay is 3–5 days.

Operative mortality

Operative mortality is very rare (less than 1%).

Special monitoring required

Flap color and warmth are closely followed in the ICU, especially in the first 24–48 hours. With free flaps, monitoring may occur hourly. Also, Doppler probes are often used as an adjunct to assess arterial flow to the free flap within the first 24–72 hours. In addition, assessment of vital signs and Foley catheterization are used to closely monitor fluid status. Other methods of flap monitoring include laser Doppler flowmetry, transcutaneous oxygen tension measurements, and color Doppler ultrasonography.

Patient activity and positioning

The patient is placed in the "beach chair" position for several days postoperatively to reduce tension on abdominal wall closure. Encouraged to be out of bed 24 hours later and ambulating by second day. No heavy lifting or strenuous activity for 6 weeks.

Medical Management of the Surgical Patient, ed. Michael F. Lubin, Thomas F. Dodson, and Neil H. Winawer. Published by Cambridge University Press. © Cambridge University Press 2013.

Alimentation

Ice chips are offered initially, then liquid diet if bowel sounds present on second postoperative day. Typically, regular diet is resumed by the third or fourth day.

Antibiotic coverage

One dose of antibiotics is administered preoperatively, within 30 minutes of incision. Dosage is then continued while in-house and often for several days after discharge while drains are in place. Cephalexin or clindamycin are most commonly used and are intended to cover *Staphylococcus* and *Streptococcus* in the large areas of fascial dissection.

Drains

Drains are placed on bulb suction, and are usually left in place for 4–14 days (in breast, abdomen).

TRAM flap postoperative complications
In the hospital
Flap loss

Total flap loss is rare (less than 1–2%), and partial flap loss only slightly higher. Careful flap monitoring may mitigate some of these losses.

Infection

Infection occurs infrequently: typically, a wound infection or urinary tract infection; less commonly, a pulmonary source.

Hematoma

The large area of surgical dissection creates many potential pockets for hematomas. Drains are intended to prevent hematomas/seromas.

Pulmonary complications

The most serious complication is pulmonary embolus from deep vein thrombosis (less than 1%). Calf sequential compression boots and early ambulation are used as prophylaxis. Also, early post-operation breathing difficulty may be encountered, due to tight fascial closures. Oxygen per nasal cannula is used in the first 24 hours, and incentive spirometry is encouraged. Pneumonia is possible but rare.

After discharge
Abdominal hernia

An abdominal hernia is an infrequent (less than 10%) complication; its occurrence often requires surgical correction. The hernia may be reduced with free flap or perforator flap techniques.

Additional surgery

Two to three months after the initial surgery, a patient may have revision of the reconstructed breast and nipple reconstruction, all in an outpatient setting. Tattoo for areolar recreation is then performed 2 months later.

Implant–expander reconstruction

Implant–expanders offer women a simpler technique for breast reconstruction with less recovery time than a TRAM flap; however, this method requires a permanent prosthesis placed within the tissues of the chest wall. In certain cases, particularly those of thin-skinned individuals or smokers, the latissimus muscle may be transferred from the back to provide additional coverage over the implant. An expander is typically placed in the mastectomy defect at the initial procedure, with an implant exchange months later. Preoperative preparation, anesthesia, blood transfusion issues, and primary risk factors are similar to that of a TRAM flap.

Usual expander reconstruction postoperative course
Expected postoperative hospital stay

The expected postoperative hospital stay is 1–2 days.

Operative mortality

Deaths are rare, and are usually anesthesia related.

Special monitoring required

No special monitoring is required.

Patient activity and positioning

No strenuous activity with the arms is allowed for 3–4 weeks.

Alimentation

Diet is quickly advanced the evening of surgery or the next morning.

Deep vein thrombosis prophylaxis

Deep vein thrombosos (DVT) prophylaxis is based on guidelines set by the American College of Chest Physicians. For moderate-risk patients, 5,000 U of low-dose unfractionated heparin is given BID or less than 3,400 U of low molecular weight heparin (LMWH) is injected once daily. For individuals of higher risk, either 5,000 U of unfractionated heparin is used TID or greater than 3,400 U of LMWH (e.g., enoxaparin 40 mg) is injected subcutaneously. Sequential compression devices are frequently used intraoperatively and postoperatively.

Antibiotic coverage

Prophylaxis with antibiotics (first-generation cephalosporin) is given within 30 minutes of incision and for a few days afterwards.

Expander management

Beginning 1–2 weeks following operation, the expander is slowly inflated in the office over several weeks. In an outpatient procedure the expander is replaced with the final implant, either silicone gel or saline filled.

Drains

Drains are placed on suction, usually left in place for 4–14 days (in breast, abdomen).

Expander reconstruction postoperative complications

In the hospital

Hematoma

The occurrence of hematoma is infrequent. The use of drains is intended to prevent such collections.

After discharge

Implant complications

Implant extrusion through the mastectomy skin flaps, capsular contracture (which can create a hard, painful breast), breast asymmetry, and implant deflation can occur and may require reoperation.

Further reading

Aston SJ, Beasley RW, Thorne CHM. *Grabb and Smith's Plastic Surgery*. Philadelphia, PA: Lippincott-Raven; 2007.

Geerts WH, Pineo GF, Heit JA *et al.* Prevention of venous thromboembolism: the Seventh ACCP Conference on Antithrombotic and Thrombolytic Therapy. *Chest* 2004; **126** (3 Suppl): 338S–400S.

Hartrampf CR, Anton MA, Bried JT. Breast reconstruction with the transverse abdominal island (TRAM) flap. In Georgiade GS, Riefkohl R, Levin LS, eds. *Plastic, Maxillofacial and. Reconstructive. Surgery*. 3rd edn. Baltimore, MD: Williams & Wilkins; 1997.

Jones GE, ed. *Bostwick's Plastic and Reconstructive Breast Surgery*. 3rd edn. Vol II. St. Louis, MO: Quality Medical Publishing; 2010.

Facial rejuvenation

Chapter 91

Kimberly A. Singh and John H. Culbertson

Facial rejuvenation is a broad term that relates to restoring facial structures to a more youthful appearance. Generally, facial rejuvenation is categorized as non-operative or operative.

A thorough preoperative assessment and understanding of patient desires are important in order to optimize outcomes and to create realistic expectations of various treatment modalities. As with any initial patient encounter, a comprehensive history and physical should be performed. Since facial rejuvenation is performed electively, patients with significant comorbidities such as smoking, diabetes, and clinically significant bleeding states should be excluded in most circumstances. A basic psychological assessment that evaluates a patient's motivations for surgery should also be obtained. Adequate time should be allowed for questions and decision making focusing on the patient's specific concerns. Some plastic surgeons also incorporate the use of photographic software that can simulate the effect of specific procedures.

Skin quality is often the first characteristic that is noted on consultation. The general quality of the skin, including elasticity, wrinkles, and actinic damage is assessed.

It is beneficial to divide the face into thirds when examining a patient so as to systematically evaluate the entire face. In the *upper third, or the periorbital zone*, the forehead, brow, eyelids, and upper midface are evaluated. A complete investigation must include brow position, forehead height, glabellar creases, excess skin or wrinkles (crow's feet) in the temporal region and in the upper and lower eyelids, and evaluation of the lateral canthal position and lower lid tone. The *middle third, or perioral zone*, is generally referred to as the lower face; an examination includes the nasolabial folds, the angle of the mouth, the upper and lower lips, chin, nose, and ears. Evaluation of the *lower third of the face, the neck zone*, includes an assessment of the neck with regard to platysmal banding, excess skin, as well as the jawline, submandibular gland, and digastric muscles.

Non-operative facial rejuvenation

Non-operative options for facial rejuvenation include chemo-denervation (Botox), injectable fillers, lasers, and chemical peels. With proper patient selection, all of these modalities can improve facial aesthetics, but patients should be fully informed that the benefits of such therapies are not permanent or long-lasting when compared to operative intervention. Alternatively, these treatments may be combined with surgical rejuvenation to achieve maximal results.

Botulinum toxin

Botulinum toxin is derived from the vacuum-dried exotoxin of *Clostridium botulinum* (types A and B are currently available). It acts by inhibiting acetylcholine release at the neuromuscular junction, thereby inducing partial chemical denervation and reduced muscular activity. Botox is most commonly used to treat the glabellar complex, crow's feet, bunny lines along the nose, perioral wrinkles, a dimpled chin, and platysmal bands. Botox should not be used by patients who have neuromuscular disorders, receive aminoglycoside antibiotics, or are pregnant or lactating. Paralysis typically takes 3–7 days to take effect; patients should be reassessed 2 weeks after the injection. The time between treatments is usually 3–4 months.

The most common adverse event is headache. Complications commonly result from over-treatment or diffusion of toxin into non-targeted neighboring muscles. Over-treatment in the perioral region may result in oral incompetence or speech difficulties. Diffusion to the levator palpebrae muscle of the upper eyelid following corrugator injection may result in eyelid ptosis. This blepharoptosis is transient and can be alleviated by the use of an alpha-adrenergic agonist, which stimulates Mueller's muscle to assist in elevating the eyelid.

Fillers

Soft tissue fillers include autogenous fat, collagen, and hyaluronic acid derivatives, as well as many other synthetic and biologic materials. Each filler has its own characteristics and treatment guidelines.

Complications include discoloration of the overlying skin, edema, contour deformities, and granulomas.

Medical Management of the Surgical Patient, ed. Michael F. Lubin, Thomas F. Dodson, and Neil H. Winawer. Published by Cambridge University Press. © Cambridge University Press 2013.

Lasers

Ablative and non-ablative lasers may be used for facial resurfacing. Lasers work by producing heat, which causes tissue injury and promotes collagen remodeling. The use of the Fitzpatrick classification, which is based on the ability to tan, is helpful to determine which patients may experience pigmentation changes after resurfacing.

Common complications include erythema, pigmentary changes, activation of herpes simplex, hypertrophic scarring, and milia, which are small keratin-filled cysts of the superficial skin. Pretreatment with antiviral medications as well as hydroquinone may lessen the severity of these complications.

Chemical peels

Chemical peels involve the use of exfoliating agents to destroy the epidermis and/or dermis to improve skin turnover. Chemical peels are classified by the depth of injury they cause. The most common peels include trichloroacetic acid (TCA) and phenol/croton oil. The Fitzpatrick classification is also used to optimize patient selection.

Complications include pigmentation changes as well as cardiotoxicity from phenol peels. Pretreatment with tretinoin and hydroquinone for 4–6 weeks improves penetration and helps to prevent hyperpigmentation.

Operative facial rejuvenation

Brow lift

The goals of brow-lift procedures are to optimize the shape and position of the brow and hairline as well as to reduce the appearance of wrinkling of the skin due to age or overexpression. Treatment options vary in the location of the access incision, the extent of release of retaining ligaments, and muscle removal or weakening. Incisions include a direct brow lift, transblepharoplasty browpexy, endoscopic brow lift, coronal, temporal, or pretrichal (hairline) approach. Brow lifts may be accomplished with a subcutaneous, subgaleal, or subperiosteal approach. Muscle weakening of the corrugators supercilii, procerus, and frontalis can be achieved by excision or scoring. Brow fixation can include wires, screws, or sutures when an endoscopic approach is used.

Complications include sensory nerve deficits from injury to the supraorbital or supratrochlear nerves, frontalis paralysis from injury to the frontal branch of the facial nerve, skin necrosis, alopecia, and undercorrection.

Blepharoplasty

Upper blepharoplasty

Upper blepharoplasty should create a well-defined supratarsal fold, remove excess skin, and address fat herniation if present. A thorough preoperative assessment includes evaluation of visual acuity, lacrimal gland ptosis, upper eyelid ptosis, and skin excess. Standard upper blepharoplasty involves marking the upper eyelid crease at the level of the mid-pupillary line, then pinching the excess skin above this to determine the superior extent of resection.

Lower blepharoplasty

Lower blepharoplasty recontours the lower lid through a lateral canthopexy or canthoplasty, and may include fat removal, skin excision, orbicularis suspension, and canthal tightening. Orbicularis oculi ptosis may be addressed by combining lower blepharoplasty with a midface lift. This operation serves to blend the lid–cheek junction to create a smooth transition, thereby addressing festoons, nasojugal folds, and malar fat pad ptosis. Approaches to lower blepharoplasty include subcilliary and transconjunctival pathways.

Postoperative care includes head elevation and ice for the first 48 hours, liberal use of ophthalmic antibiotic ointment, and avoidance of eye make-up or contact lenses for 2 weeks postoperatively. A Frost suture may be used to anchor the lower lid, thereby avoiding ectropion.

Complications include asymmetry, ectropion, dry eye syndrome, lagopthalmos, periorbital hematoma, diplopia, chemosis, and retrobulbar hematoma. Retrobulbar hematoma, which occurs in 0.04% of patients, is the most serious complication following blepharoplasty. It is an ocular emergency because blood behind the globe compromises the blood supply to the optic nerve, and can result in blindness if not addressed within 100 minutes. If retrobulbar hematoma is suspected to have occurred, an emergent lateral canthotomy is performed to relieve the pressure on the globe. Mannitol and acetazolamide are administered, and urgent ophthalmologic consultation should be obtained.

Rhinoplasty

Rhinoplasty is a very challenging procedure that addresses functional airway disorders as well as contour deformities of the nose; it demands a keen understanding of anatomy and applied techniques. Treatment often involves osteotomies to reduce the width of the nasal bones; cartilage manipulation with or without cartilage grafts, altering the underlying nasal architecture; management of the septum; and rasping of dorsal humps. Approaches to rhinoplasty can be open or closed (no external incisions).

Postoperative management includes head of bed elevation; administration of antibiotics, steroids, and nasal spray to prevent congestion; and splinting. Complications can result from contour irregularities and/or airway obstruction due to cartilage overgrowth.

Facelift

Facelift procedures reduce wrinkles, remove excess skin, and reorient facial vectors. There are multiple operative techniques: they involve the removal of the excess skin as well as the removal and/or tightening of the superficial musculoaponeurotic system (SMAS), and the undermining of deeper structures (deep plane facelift). The incisions may be traditional (both in front of and behind the ear), or short scar (minimal access is obtained with incisions mainly in front of the ear).

Complications from facelifts include hematoma (4.2%), superficial skin slough (5% in non-smokers vs 19% in smokers), nerve paresis, and contour irregularities.

Neck lift

The goals of a neck lift are to reduce wrinkling of the skin due to age or over-expression, remove excess skin, and improve the appearance of platysmal bands. Neck rejuvenation can be addressed with liposuction or direct surgical manipulation. It is often combined with a facelift, a choice that depends on the extent of overall facial aging. The platysma is usually addressed with direct excision or tightening. Treatment should result in an improved cervicomental angle, a distinct mandibular angle, and improved contour over the thyroid cartilage and border of the sternocleiodomastoid muscle.

Complications include hematoma, injury to the marginal mandibular or greater auricular nerves, contour deformities, and skin loss. Hematomas occur more in male patients and in patients with elevated high blood pressure preoperatively.

Conclusion

Successful facial rejuvenation involves a keen understanding of facial aging and its effect on the facial structures. An individualized treatment plan that takes into consideration patient goals and thresholds for recovery time and maintenance must be created.

Further reading

Chang S, Pusic A, Rohrich RJ. A systematic review of comparison of efficacy and complication rates among facelift procedures. *Plast Recon Surg* 2011; **127**: 423–33.

Fagian S. Botox for the treatment of dynamic and hyperkinetic facial lines and furrows: adjunctive use in facial aesthetic surgery. *Plast Reconstr Surg* 1999; **103**: 701–13.

Fitzpatrick TB. The validity and practicality of sun-reactive skin types I through VI. *Arch Dermatol* 1988; **124**: 869–71.

Freund RM, Nolan WB. Correlation between brow lift outcomes and aesthetic ideals for eyebrow height and shape in females. *Plast Reconstr Surg* 1996; **97**: 1343–8.

Guerrerosantos J. Neck lift: simplified surgical techniques, refinements, and clinical classification. *Clin Plast Surg* 1983; **10**: 379–404.

Guyuron B. An evidence-based approach to facelift. *Plast Reconstr Surg* 2010; **126**: 2230–3.

Lisman RD, Hyde K, Smith B. Complications of blepharoplasty. *Clin Plast Surg* 1988; **15**: 309–35.

McCord C, Codner MA. *Eyelid and Periorbital Surgery*. St Louis, MO: Quality Medical Publishing; 2008.

Nahai F. *The Art of Aesthetic Surgery: Principles and Techniques*. St Louis, MO: Quality Medical Publishing; 2005.

Chapter 92

Liposuction

Benjamin L. Moosavi and Albert Losken

Liposuction is one of the most popular treatment modalities in aesthetic surgery in the USA. According to the American Society for Aesthetic Plastic Surgery, more than 341,000 liposuction procedures were performed in 2008 and it was ranked second among all invasive cosmetic procedures. Liposuction is used to recontour specific areas of the face and body by removing unwanted deposits of fat. It is best performed on localized areas that do not respond well to diet or exercise, and it is not an alternative to weight loss. The ideal liposuction patient is healthy, exercises, eats a well-balanced diet, has good skin elasticity, desires treatment of minimal-to-moderate localized fat deposits, and is within 20–30% of ideal body weight.

The patient consultation includes evaluation of the patient's goals and realistic expectations. The history is performed to evaluate the patient's suitability for surgical intervention. The physical exam is best performed in front of a mirror to stimulate dialogue and understanding of patient concerns and to reiterate realistic expectations. The exam should detail prior scars, evaluate for hernias, rule out venous insufficiency, and document asymmetry and contour irregularities. It is also important to evaluate skin quality and amount of excess skin. Patients with good skin tone and without excess skin are more likely to have better results. Medical images should be obtained for objective comparison and documentation of postoperative results.

Prior to surgery, preoperative marking is performed in the standing position. This acts as an intraoperative guide and helps confirm with the patient the areas to be addressed during the procedure. The patient is positioned in a way to allow maximum exposure of the areas to be suctioned. Local anesthesia, sedation, or general anesthesia are all options for liposuction procedures.

The procedure involves making small stab incisions for access sites. These access sites are placed in areas that will decrease visibility and avoid neurovascular injury, while still providing the best angle for appropriate contouring, depending on the specific location being addressed. The areas to be suctioned are infiltrated with a solution consisting of crystalloid fluids, lidocaine, and epinephrine. This solution places the tissue under tension, assists in suctioning, and provides local anesthesia and vasoconstriction, which minimizes intraoperative blood loss. After sufficient time to allow the solution to attain its local effects, a cannula is inserted through the access incisions and liposuction is initiated.

Liposuction is performed in the deep fat layer to prevent any surface irregularities. It is repeated in a radial fashion using a "to and fro movement." Large-bore cannulae are used for large-volume fat removal while smaller cannulae are chosen for details and refining contour. Volume measurements (infusion and aspiration) are monitored closely for each location to ensure symmetry. The plastic surgeon determines when the desired amount of lipoaspirate has been suctioned based on volume, contour, and appearance. This is determined by visual exam, palpation of the contour, and the "pinch" test for consistency. Overcorrection is not suggested.

There are numerous liposuction techniques and technologies that vary based on the way the fat cells are broken down. Some of the common techniques include ultrasound, laser, radiofrequency, power-assisted, and suction-assisted liposuction. Each is reported to assist with lysis of fat cells by their respective energy transfer and therefore increase aspirate. Potential benefits over traditional suction-assisted lipectomy include skin-tightening effects from energy transfer into the subdermal tissues and ease of use in areas of increased fibrous tissue.

The access incisions are closed with absorbable sutures or reapproximated and covered with steri-strips or skin glue. Operative time is usually 1–3 hours, depending on the amount of tissue to be removed and number of areas to be suctioned. Liposuction is often performed in conjunction with other procedures.

Usual postoperative course
Expected postoperative hospital stay

Most procedures are performed on an outpatient basis with admission for observation reserved for patients at high risk of volume depletion.

Medical Management of the Surgical Patient, ed. Michael F. Lubin, Thomas F. Dodson, and Neil H. Winawer. Published by Cambridge University Press. © Cambridge University Press 2013.

Operative mortality

According to the American Society of Aesthetic Plastic Surgery, liposuction is considered a safe procedure when done appropriately, with a mortality rate of less than 0.5%. Pulmonary embolism is the most common cause of death in these patients accounting for 25% of fatalities.

Special monitoring required

Vital signs monitoring along with urine output monitoring for higher-volume liposuction procedures are standard with liposuction procedures.

Patient activity and positioning

The patient is allowed to shower after 24–48 hours. Activity is gradually increased according to individual surgeon recommendations; these will depend upon the areas and the amounts suctioned. Compression garments, which reduce swelling and bleeding, are worn continuously over the treated area for 2–6 weeks.

Alimentation

Regular or high-protein diets are allowed immediately after surgery.

Antibiotic coverage

Perioperative antibiotic coverage is usually provided with a single agent.

Postoperative complications

In the hospital

Volume depletion

Volume depletion can result from large-volume liposuction. This is prevented by appropriate intraoperative monitoring and intravenous fluid replacement. Some patients should be admitted for overnight monitoring and fluid replacement.

Pulmonary or fat embolus

Patients are routinely placed in sequential compression devices during the operation. Early postoperative ambulation is encouraged to decrease the risk of these rare complications.

Swelling and bruising

Liquefied fat, injection fluid, and small amounts of blood may leak from the incision sites for about 24 hours. Incision sites should be dressed appropriately. Bruising, swelling, and soreness are expected postoperatively and will resolve over time. Edema resolves in approximately 80% of patients by 4–6 weeks.

After discharge

Hematoma or seroma

Compressive dressings minimize hematoma and seroma formation. Large hematomas or seromas that develop despite compression garments may require evacuation with a large-bore needle.

Wound infection

Perioperative antibiotics are routinely administered with liposuction. If cellulitis occurs, early recognition and oral antibiotics are usually sufficient for treatment.

Loss of sensation/paresthesias

Loss of sensation and/or paresthesias can occur. They usually resolve in a few months.

Cosmetic sequelae

The most common long-term complication is contour irregularity, with 2–10% requiring revision. Rippling or bagginess of the skin may also occur. Skin color changes and skin necrosis are rare, but may occur with aggressive superficial ultrasound or laser-assisted liposuction.

Further reading

Grazer FM, De Jong RH. Fatal outcomes from liposuction: census survey of cosmetic surgeons. *Plast Reconstr Surg* 2000; **105**: 447–8.

Klein JA. The tumescent technique. Anesthesia and modified liposuction technique. *Dermatol Clin* 1990; **8**: 425–37.

Pitanguy I. Evaluation of body contouring surgery today: a 30-year perspective. *Plast Reconstr Surg* 2000; **105**: 1499–514; discussion 1515–16.

Pitman GH, Teimourian B. Suction lipectomy: complications and results by survey. *Plast Reconstr Surg* 1985; **76**: 65–72.

Stephen PJ, Kenkel JM. Updates and advances in liposuction. *Aesth Surg J* 2010; **30**: 83–97.

Teimourian B, Adham MN. A national survey of complications associated with suction lipectomy: what we did then and what we do now. *Plast Reconstr Surg* 2000; **105**: 1881–4.

Facial fractures

J. Nicolas Mclean and John H. Culbertson

Facial fractures are common problems encountered by the plastic surgeon. The increased incidence of patients with facial fractures is related to the frequency of motor vehicle accidents. Management of these fractures requires a team approach, because patients usually present with multiple injuries. Plastic surgeons must be familiar with the best methods of preoperative assessment and imaging to optimally manage the patient with a facial fracture.

Initial management of severe facial fractures and injuries to the face begins with the ABCs of trauma management. The airway is established via either intubation or tracheotomy. High-velocity injuries as well as mandibular injuries have a high rate of airway compromise requiring urgent intervention. Bleeding is controlled with direct pressure, and a secondary survey is performed to evaluate concomitant injuries.

As soon as the patient is stabilized, the initial treatment starts with a clinical examination that focuses on assessment of soft tissue loss if present, occlusion of the mandible, and evaluation of the sensory and motor nerves. In general, patients with facial fractures have limited evaluation of their bony architecture because of the soft tissue swelling, ecchymoses, gross blood, and hematoma. The face and cranium should be palpated to detect bony irregularities, step-offs, and crepitus. Mobility of the midface may be tested preoperatively by grasping the anterior alveolar arch and pulling forward while stabilizing the patient with the other hand. The size and location of the mobile segment may identify which type of Le Fort fracture is present. A thorough nasal and intraoral examination should be completed. The nasal bones are typically quite mobile in Le Fort II fractures, along with the rest of the pyramidal free-floating segment. Intranasal examination may reveal fresh or old blood, septal hematoma, or cerebrospinal fluid rhinorrhea. The intraoral examination should assess occlusion, overall dentition, stability of the alveolar ridge and palate, and soft tissue.

Next, radiographic imaging of the face is obtained to determine the exact fracture patterns. Panorex films of the mandible are sometimes used but a CT scan with fine cuts is the method of choice. Three-dimensional CT scans are highly recommended for the treatment planning of fractures of moderate or greater complexity. Radiographic evaluation is also helpful in determining intracranial injuries, soft tissue loss, and presence of major vascular injury. The patient's C-spine should be evaluated and cleared prior to operative intervention. The goals of the first operation include closure of intracranial injuries, attempted salvage of globe injuries, debridement of foreign material and non-viable tissue, establishment of occlusal relationships in tooth-bearing segments, and bony reconstruction to maintain the soft tissue envelope. Debridement of tissue at the initial operation should be limited to clearly non-viable tissue, with questionable tissue left to declare itself with serial debridements.

Soft-tissue injuries in the form of abrasions, contusions, lacerations, and avulsions are identified and treated primarily. Depending of the severity of these wounds, they can be treated in the emergency department or in the operating room. The definitive treatment of the craniofacial fractures is tailored to specific fracture patterns. Repair of the facial fractures is indicated to restore both appearance and function, particularly in the mandible and orbital floor. In general, it is very important to obtain accurate reduction and stable fixation. Facial fractures can be approached through a variety of incisions. Fixation of unstable fracture segments to stable structures is the objective of definitive surgical treatment of maxillary fractures. This principle, while seemingly simple, becomes more complex in patients with extensive or panfacial fractures.

Upper face fractures

Those fractures include frontal bone, frontal sinus, and orbital fractures. It is very important to evaluate the optic nerve, intercanthal distance, extraocular eye movements, and any possible intracranial component of the fractures. Nasoethmoidal fractures pose a challenge for the reconstructive surgeon due to the complexity and density of the anatomic components of the area. Because of the functional and aesthetic implications of the medial canthus, nasolacrimal system, and intraorbital contents, appropriate and timely treatment is critical to

Medical Management of the Surgical Patient, ed. Michael F. Lubin, Thomas F. Dodson, and Neil H. Winawer. Published by Cambridge University Press. © Cambridge University Press 2013.

avoid unfavorable sequelae. Frontal bone and frontal sinus fractures may extend intracranially and often require a combined approach with neurosurgery.

Midface fractures

Three predominant types are described (Figure 93.1).

Le Fort I fractures may result from the force of injury directed low on the maxillary alveolar rim in a downward direction. The fracture extends from the nasal septum to the lateral pyriform rims, travels horizontally above the teeth apices, crosses below the zygomaticomaxillary junction, and traverses the pterygomaxillary junction to interrupt the pterygoid plates.

Le Fort II fractures may result from a blow to the lower or mid maxilla. Such a fracture has a pyramidal shape and extends from the nasal bridge at or below the nasofrontal suture through the frontal processes of the maxilla, inferolaterally through the lacrimal bones and inferior orbital floor and rim through or near the inferior orbital foramen, and inferiorly through the anterior wall of the maxillary sinus; it then travels under the zygoma, across the pterygomaxillary fissure, and through the pterygoid plates.

Le Fort III fractures, also termed craniofacial dysjunctions, may follow impact to the nasal bridge or upper maxilla. It extends posteriorly through the ethmoid bones and laterally through the orbits below the optic foramen, through the pterygomaxillary suture into the sphenopalatine fossa. This fracture separates facial bones from cranium, causing the face to appear long and flat (i.e., dish face).

Le Fort classification is an oversimplification of maxillary fractures. In most instances, maxillary fractures are a combination of the various Le Fort types. Fracture lines often diverge from the described pathways and may result in mixed-type fractures, unilateral fractures, or other atypical fractures. In addition, in very high-energy blows, maxillary fractures may be associated with fractures to the mandible, cranium, or both.

Mandible fractures

A recent review of the pattern of mandibular fracture presentation at an urban trauma center found that mandible fractures overwhelmingly occur in males and are most often caused by interpersonal altercations. More than one-third of fractures occur in the 25- to 34-year-old age group, and 55% of cases involve illicit drug use. The mandible is the site of injury in approximately 40% of pediatric facial trauma cases, which are most commonly a result of motor vehicle accidents. Fracture location by site includes condylar (36%), body (21%), angle (20%), symphysis (14%), alveolar ridge (3%), ramus (3%), and coronoid fractures (2%). Patients with mandible fractures often have other serious injuries that warrant additional attention, including cervical spine injuries or other facial fractures.

The mechanism of injury can provide valuable information in the examination and treatment of patients with mandibular trauma. For example, motor vehicle accidents tend to result in parasymphyseal fractures. Pediatric fractures usually result after a fall and are frequently condylar fractures, sometimes bilateral.

Usual postoperative course

Expected postoperative hospital stay

Most patients with uncomplicated facial fractures spend 2–5 days in the hospital. Mandible fractures tend to require less time, and upper facial fractures usually require 5–7 days. Patients with multiple trauma should be admitted to the Trauma Service to coordinate care of all injuries.

Operative mortality

It varies with the severity of the fractures, associated injuries, and patients' comorbidities. The mortality rate is as high as 12% in high-impact fractures but is rarely due to maxillofacial injury. The incidence of associated cervical spine injuries has been reported in the 0.2–6% range.

Patient activity

Elevation of the head of the bed at 30° is important to reduce facial edema and pain. The patient is encouraged to ambulate early and resume normal activities.

Alimentation

Patients with mandibular fractures are required to stay on a pureed diet and liquids until healed. Most other patients may stay on a soft mechanical diet. When placed on maxillo-

Figure 93.1 Midface fractures illustrating the Le Fort classification system.

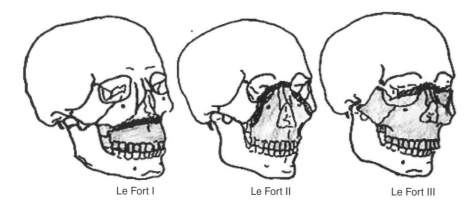

Le Fort I   Le Fort II   Le Fort III

mandibular fixation (i.e., wired shut), the patient must use a straw for oral intake.

Antibiotic coverage

Perioperative antibiotics are used for coverage against both gram-positive and gram-negative organisms and are continued for 2–3 days, depending on the individual case.

Postoperative complications

Patients with maxillo-mandibular fixation are vulnerable to aspiration.

Persistent CSF leaks, meningitis, and abscesses are serious infections that can occur when a CSF leak is present. Observe patients closely for signs and symptoms.

Blindness can occur, usually caused by retrobulbar hematoma.

Malocclusion may result even with the best of care, and orthodontic or surgical intervention may be necessary. Facial deformity, as well, can be expected in some cases that may require revision.

After facial trauma, post-traumatic stress disorder is not uncommon and may require psychiatric intervention.

Further reading

Demetriades D, Chahwan S, Gomez H et al. Initial evaluation and management of gunshot wounds to the face. *J Trauma* 1998; 45: 39–41.

Futran ND, Farwell DG, Smith RB, Johnson PE, Funk GF. Definitive management of severe facial trauma utilizing free tissue transfer. *Otolaryngol Head Neck Surg* 2005; 132: 75–85.

Hollier LH Jr, Sharabi SE, Koshy JC, Stal S. Facial trauma: general principles of management. *J Craniofac Surg* 2010; 21: 1051–3.

Manson P. Facial injuries. In McCarthy JG, ed. *Plastic Surgery*. Vol. 2. Philadelphia, PA: W. B. Saunders; 1990, pp. 979–91.

Ogundare BO, Bonnick A, Bayley N. Pattern of mandibular fractures in an urban

major trauma center. *J Oral Maxillofac Surg* 2003; 61: 713–18.

Sharabi SE, Koshy JC, Thornton JF, Hollier LH Jr. Facial fractures. *Plast Reconstr Surg* 2011; 127: 25e–34e.

Stacey DH, Doyle JF, Mount DL, Snyder MC, Gutowski KA. Management of mandible fractures. *Plast Reconstr Surg* 2006; 117: 48e–60e.

Chapter

94

Flap coverage for pressure ulcers

Neil D. Saunders and Mark D. Walsh

Introduction

For the hospitalized patient, prevention of pressure ulcers requires vigilant surveillance by a dedicated care team. It is estimated that 10–15% of patients who are in the ICU for one week develop a pressure sore. Nursing-home patients have a 10–30% prevalence of pressure ulcers, whereas spinal cord injury patients have a 50–80% lifetime risk. Numerous patient factors, including malnutrition, obesity, smoking, immobility, diabetes, neurologic injury, and hip fractures, are associated with the development of pressure ulcers. Prolonged pressure with resultant tissue ischemia, shear stress, and edema all lead to tissue necrosis. Moisture and infection are factors which may cause additional progression of severity. Pressure ulcers typically occur over bony prominences where pressure and shear stress are the greatest. The most common sites are found over the ischial tuberosities, sacrum, greater trochanters, and heels. Without prompt recognition and treatment, pressure ulcers will progress through stages of increasing tissue damage. Table 94.1 shows the current pressure ulcer staging system, which is based on gross appearance.

Stages I and II will usually resolve with conservative treatment including topical creams, such as silver sulfadiazine, frequent changes in patient position, air fluid beds, protective bandages, and improved nutrition. Few stage III ulcers can be treated effectively with conservative measures and progression

Table 94.1 Pressure ulcer staging, adapted from National Pressure Ulcer Advisory Panel's Updated Staging System, 2007.

Stage	Characteristics
I	Skin intact with non-balancing erythema
II	Partial thickness of dermis lost with open ulcer
III	Full thickness skin loss, subcutaneous fat visible, bone or muscle not visible
IV	Full thickness loss with exposed bone, muscle or tendon

to stage IV generally requires operative intervention. Effective management requires a multidisciplinary team including nurses, dieticians, physical therapists, social workers, and surgeons. Because of the difficulty in treating these wounds and the high rate of recurrence, prevention is of paramount importance. Frequent weight shifts to relieve pressure, proper hygiene, optimal nutrition, and primary education are important measures for prevention.

Operative intervention for established advanced pressure ulcers involves irrigation and debridement to remove devitalized and necrotic tissue, and to decrease bacterial contamination. Removal of infected bone and reduction of bony prominences are necessary for long-term successful reconstruction. Debridement may be followed immediately by reconstruction, but more typically reconstruction is delayed. Repeated debridement may be necessary if significant bacterial contamination is present. Before reconstruction, the patient's nutritional status should be optimized and he/she should be able to successfully complete postoperative rehabilitation. The choice of reconstruction is based on multiple factors including the size of the wound and the location on the patient. Primary closure or split thickness skin grafts may be tried for small and superficial wounds, but are frequently inadequate. The mainstay of pressure ulcer reconstruction is myocutaneous and fasciocutanous flaps. Occasionally, a free flap may need to be employed for large or refractory ulcers.

For sacral wounds, a gluteus maximus myocutaneous flap, or fasciocutaneous flaps based on gluteal artery perforators are the predominant flaps for reconstruction. These are typically designed as large rotational flaps, or as unilateral or bilateral V-Y advancement flaps.

Pressure ulcers over the ischial tuberosities are typically covered first line with gluteal thigh rotation flaps or V–Y hamstring flaps. Since ischial ulcers may frequently reoccur, the rationale for flap selection includes providing adequate soft tissue bulk while preserving tissue for future flap options. Additional flap options include tensor fascia lata flaps or gracilis muscle flaps.

Medical Management of the Surgical Patient, ed. Michael F. Lubin, Thomas F. Dodson, and Neil H. Winawer. Published by Cambridge University Press. © Cambridge University Press 2013.

Trochanteric ulcers can be closed with a tensor fascia lata, inferior gluteus or vastus lateralis muscle flaps. For all flaps, drains are usually left at the donor and recipient sites and non-adherent dressings are placed over the wounds.

Usual postoperative course

Expected postoperative hospital stay

Postoperative recovery is usually not prolonged, but patients will need to be carefully followed for a period of 4–6 weeks.

Operative mortality

Operative mortality is less than 5% and usually is due to patient-specific factors and comorbidities.

Special monitoring required

Frequent flap checks for viability, vascular congestion, or necrosis should be performed by the nursing staff and surgical team. Drain output monitoring and recording can alert the team to postoperative bleeding. Other monitoring is based on the individual patient characteristics.

Patient activity and positioning

Immediate placement on a pressure-distributing mattress is necessary. Patients should also be turned every 2 hours as necessary to prevent formation of additional pressure ulcers. For the first 2–4 weeks, care should be taken not to place focal or prolonged pressure on the operative site. The patient may then begin to put pressure on the area for brief time periods; e.g., 15 minutes 3 times per day, then gradually increasing the amount of time during which pressure is placed on the flap. The flap should be continually assessed for evidence of ischemia or congestion.

Alimentation

Patients should resume their normal diets, tube feeding, or total parenteral nutrition to provide adequate nutrition for wound healing. As part of the multidisciplinary team, the nutrition support services should be involved to ensure that the patient is attaining adequate caloric intake as well as essential amino acids and vitamins needed for wound healing.

Hygiene

Maintaining good wound hygiene is essential. Dressings should be changed daily or more frequently as needed. The suture lines should be covered with a non-adherent permeable gauze such as adaptic or xeroform gauze. On top of this dressing, dry gauze should be placed to allow absorption of moisture from around the wounds. If urinary incontinence is a concern, a Foley catheter should be placed. To prevent fecal soiling postoperatively, fecal diversion should be considered in the preoperative setting. Alternatively, low fiber or constipating bowel regimens may be considered postoperatively to minimize fecal contamination.

Drains

Flap site and donor site drains are utilized to decrease the risk of postoperative flap loss due to hematoma or seroma formation. Low-pressure suction drains allow gentle egress of fluid and maintain contact between the flap and wound bed. Drains at the flap site may be placed for several weeks and can safely be removed when their output is less than 30 mL/day.

Antibiotic coverage

If the patient's wound bed is clean and free of necrosis, perioperative prophylactic antibiotic coverage will be sufficient. If there is necrosis or high bacterial contamination, then antibiotics can be continued for 5–7 days. In cases where osteomyelitis is present, cultures should guide antibiotic coverage; the course of antibiotics can range from 2 weeks to 3 months. Infectious disease consultation should be considered for complex infections.

Postoperative complications

Hematoma

Meticulous hemostasis during the operation is vital as the development of a hematoma postoperatively may lead to flap loss. A large volume of continued drain output may indicate ongoing bleeding, which will require a return to the operating room to find and control the source. If a hematoma develops it should be promptly evacuated in the operating room.

Seroma

As occurs with hematoma formation, seroma formation can also compromise flap viability. To minimize seroma formation, drains placed during the operation should be left in place until their outputs decrease below 30mL/day.

Wound infection

The flap and suture lines should be monitored for signs of infection including erythema and continued drainage. Mild cellulitis can be treated with systemic antibiotics, but purulent drainage will necessitate opening the suture line and allowing the wound to heal by secondary intention.

Suture line dehiscence

Up to 30% of patients will have a portion of their suture line dehisce. If the area is small, it may be allowed to heal by secondary intention using wet-to-dry dressing changes. If the dehiscence is large enough, the patient may need to return to the operating room for revision of the flap and closure of the defect.

Flap loss

Vascular compromise can lead to flap ischemia by loss of inflow from the arterial side or by congestion due to loss of venous outflow. This may lead to partial flap necrosis or loss of the entire flap. If the entire flap appears threatened, the patient will need to return to the operating room for flap revision.

Recurrence

Rates of recurrence are as high as 30–50% at the same site. Recurrences are treated using the same principles and techniques as the treatment of the original pressure sore. Thoughtful flap design frequently allows re-rotation or re-advancement of a preexisting flap. Preventative measures and patient education should be emphasized to decrease recurrence rates. In the postoperative setting, care should be taken to prevent the development of a new ulcer site, and to protect the freshly reconstructed ulcer site.

Further reading

Bass MJ, Phillips LG. Pressure sores. *Curr Probl Surg* 2007; **44**: 101–43.

Black J, Baharestani M, Cuddigan J *et al.*; National Pressure Ulcer Advisory Panel. National Pressure Ulcer Advisory Panel's updated pressure ulcer staging system. *Dermatol Nurs* 2007; **19**: 343–9.

Fulda GJ, Khan SU, Zabel DD. Special issues in plastic and reconstructive surgery. *Crit Care Clin* 2003; **19**: 91–108.

Lefemine V, Enoch S, Boyce DE. Surgical and reconstructive management of pressure ulcers. *Eur J Plast Surg* 2009; **32**: 63–75.

Lemaire V, Boulanger K, Heymans O. Free flaps for pressure sore coverage. *Ann Plast Surg* 2008; **60**(6): 631–4.

Schryvers OI, Stranc MF, Nance PW. Surgical treatment of pressure ulcers: 20-year experience. *Arch Phys Med Rehabil* 2000; **81**(12): 1556–62.

Sørensen JL, Jørgensen B, Gottrup F. Surgical treatment of pressure ulcers. *Am J Surg* 2004; **188**(1A Suppl): 42–51.

Muscle flap coverage of sternal wound infections

Garrett Harper and Albert Losken

The median sternotomy was first described by Julian in 1957 for use in cardiac surgery. A 5% sternal wound infection rate was reported, and the treatment of choice was debridement and open packing. Since that time, management of sternal wounds has changed drastically. Shumacker and Mandelbaum introduced the closed-chest catheter irrigation system in 1963 and reduced mortality from 50 to 20%. The pedicled omental flap was advocated by Lee *et al.* in 1976. A few years later, Jurkiewicz *et al.* revolutionized the treatment algorithm with the introduction of muscle flaps.

Sternal wound infections are divided into superficial (affecting the skin, subcutaneous tissue, and pectoralis fascia only) and deep. It is important to recognize patient risk factors (including, but not limited to): BMI > 30 kg/m^2, diabetes mellitus, urgent operation, sepsis/endocarditis after surgery, smoking history within one year, COPD, renal insufficiency, and history of stroke. The most commonly isolated pathogen is coagulase-negative staphylococcus, followed by *Staphylococcus aureus*, *Propioni*, *Acinetobacter*, *Enterobacter cloacae*, *Escherichia coli*, and *Klebsiella*. There is a subset of patients who never grow bacteria; they are deemed to have non-infectious sternal dehiscence.

Although often a clinical diagnosis, confirmation of infection is done by standard blood work, wound and/or blood cultures, and radiographic studies. Computerized tomography is often the study of choice, with sensitivity and specificity of 93.5% and 81.7% respectively.

Superficial sternal wound infections (SSWI) are treated with intravenous antibiotics and local wound care. Surgical intervention is necessary for deep sternal wound infections (DSWI), and starts with exploration and debridement of all necrotic tissues and removal of foreign materials and exposed cartilage. If the wound then appears clean, muscle or omental transposition is performed, along with placement of closed suction drains in the same setting. Otherwise, serial debridements are performed prior to closure.

There are many different treatment options for sternal wound closure using muscle flaps. The patient's anatomy, wound status, and previous surgeries serve as the reconstructive surgeon's guide to proper flap selection. The most commonly used flaps are the unilateral pectoralis major muscle "turnover" flap, the unipedicled pectoralis major muscle rotation advancement flap, the rectus abdominis muscle flap, bilateral myocutaneous pectoralis major muscle flaps, the latissimus dorsi muscle flap, the omental flap, the microsurgical free flap, and various combinations of all the above.

It should also be noted that some surgeons advocate sternal plating, both as a primary preventive means in high-risk patients and secondarily when used in reconstruction after sternal dehiscence.

Usual postoperative course
Expected postoperative hospital stay

The mainstay of postoperative care continues to include pain control, pulmonary toilet, intravenous antibiotics, nutritional support, and wound monitoring. With the advent of early debridement followed by muscle closure, the average length of hospital stay has been decreased to 12.4 days. Patients are sometimes treated with a prolonged course of intravenous antibiotic therapy, but the bulk of their therapy is received at home with the use of percutaneous intravenous central catheters (PICC lines).

Operative mortality

While the overall mortality in the Emory series was 8.1%, mortality rates have ranged recently from 0–33% depending on many variables. Preexisting end-stage-renal disease, COPD, perioperative MI, and postoperative septicemia or prolonged mechanical ventilation have all been shown to increase mortality rates. Studies have also shown that early referral to plastic surgeons has significantly reduced mortality rates.

Special monitoring required

Patients who are septic, hemodynamically unstable, or undergo a free flap operation require monitoring in the ICU. For most patients, however, standard monitoring on a normal postoperative unit should suffice.

Patient activity and positioning

Patient activity is advanced as tolerated, often with the aid of a physical therapist. Normal poststernotomy precautions are taken with regard to deep breathing and coughing exercises. With most reconstructions, drains are used. Drains are initially placed to continuous wall suction for 24 hours, then converted to bulb suction. Patients with large or pendulous breasts often need support with a bra to minimize tension on the incision.

Alimentation

Diet is advanced as tolerated; enteric feeding is always the preferred route. Diabetic, renal, and American Heart Association diet restrictions should be closely followed for the appropriate patients. Supplementation may be required for those patients with poor preoperative nutritional status. In the event of a laparotomy for omental harvest, appropriate time should be allowed for return of bowel function prior to advancing diet.

Antibiotic coverage

Most patients will have been started preoperatively on broad-spectrum antibiotics. Antibiotics are then tailored according to blood and wound culture results. For patients with sternal osteomyelitis, a prolonged antibiotic regimen of up to 6 weeks or longer may be initiated and a specialist in infectious diseases is often consulted. If there is no bony involvement, a shorter course of antibiotics is often sufficient. Patients should remain on oral antibiotics for as long as drains are in place.

Postoperative complications

In the Emory series, there was an overall complication rate of 18.8%. The most common complications were recurrent wound infections (6.5%), hematoma (6.1%), wound dehiscence (6.1%), re-exploration for wound necrosis (5.9%), partial flap loss (3.8%), and abdominal hernia after rectus abdominis harvest (2.2%). Wound dehiscence occurred most often in the inferior sternum and was more frequent in patients who had COPD, a history of smoking, or large breasts. Hematomas almost always required a re-operation and led to the delay of anticoagulation until 72 hours postoperatively, if medically permissible. Aggressive drain management has also led to a decrease in hematoma and seroma rates.

Further reading

Brandt C, Alvarez J. First-line treatment of deep sternal infection by a plastic surgical approach: superior results compared with conventional cardiac surgical orthodoxy. *Plast Reconstruct Surg* 2002; **109**: 2231–7.

Cabbabe EB, Cabbabe SW. Immediate versus delayed one-stage sternal debridement and pectoralis muscle flap reconstruction of deep sternal wound infections. *Plast Reconstr Surg* 2009; **123**: 1490–4.

Cayci C, Russo M, Cheema F *et al.* Risk analysis of deep sternal wound infections and their long-term survival: a propensity analysis. *Ann Plast Surg* 2008; **61**: 294–301.

Jones G, Jurkiewicz MJ, Bostwick J *et al.* Management of the infected median sternotomy wound with muscle flaps: the Emory 20-year experience. *Ann Surg* 1997; **225**: 766–78.

Patel NV, Woznick AR, Welsh KA *et al.* Predictors of mortality after muscle flap advancement for deep sternal wound infections. *Plast Reconstruct Surg* 2009; **132**: 132–8.

Ridderstolpe L, Gill H, Granfeldt H *et al.* Superficial and deep sternal wound complications: incidence, risk factors, and mortality. *Euro J Cardiothorac Surg* 2001; **20**: 1168–75.

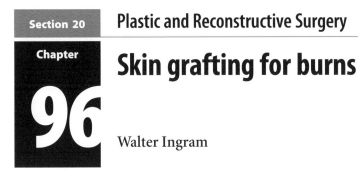

Chapter 96

Skin grafting for burns

Walter Ingram

A burn injury is essentially an injury to the epidermal and dermal layers of the skin. While the epidermis is rapidly and efficiently repaired in humans, the dermis heals poorly if at all. In burns where most of the dermis is not injured (superficial partial thickness burns), the burn heals rapidly with a cosmetically and functionally acceptable scar. In burns where most or all of the dermis is dead (deep partial thickness or full thickness burns), healing is slow (if at all) and the scarring is severe.

Skin grafting for burns consists of repairing the damaged area of skin by harvesting the top layers of an area of uninjured skin. Top layers of undamaged skin are removed with an instrument called a dermatome. This intervention creates an area of exposed dermis called the donor site. The burned skin is debrided by serially slicing off layers of dead dermis until live tissue is reached in a process called tangential excision. The cutting is parallel (tangential) to the surface of the burn. Tissue bleeding and appearance is used as a sign of viability. The harvested skin is attached (using staples, sutures, or glue) to the excised wound bed; it becomes vascularized over the next 3–5 days. The donor site heals by epithelialization from the hair follicles and sweat glands deep in the remaining dermis.

If large areas of burn must be grafted from smaller donor sites, the skin can be meshed (2:1, 3:1) and expanded to cover more area. Meshing the donor skin slows wound coverage and produces a cosmetic and functional result that is inferior to the sheet graft. The best outcome can be obtained by harvesting the full thickness of dermis from the donor site (full thickness skin graft). The donor site for a full thickness graft will not heal and must be sewn closed (thus greatly limiting the size of the available graft).

Attempts have been made to produce an artificial material which, when placed on a wound bed, will function as a template for fibroblasts to produce a normal dermis. The most successful of these dermal templates is Integra®. The dermal template is placed on the wound bed after debridement. Over the next 3 weeks fibroblasts from the patient migrate into the template and secrete collagen and elastin to create a neodermis.

The top silastic layer of the dermal template is then removed and a thin autologous skin graft is applied to the neodermis. The graft grows over the neodermis produced by the dermal template, creating skin.

Usual postoperative course
Patient activity and positioning

The area that received the graft is usually immobilized for about 4–6 days. Then the first (and most painful) dressing is performed. Gentle passive and active range of motion is started with physical or occupational therapy. Daily dressing changes with topical antibiotics are used until the wound completely epithelializes: from several days for sheet grafts and 2:1 meshed grafts to about 14 days for 3:1 and larger meshed skin grafts. In 10 days to 2 weeks, the donor sites spontaneously heal from the skin appendages. The skin on both the donor sites and the new skin grafts is fragile for several months and must be protected from trauma, sunlight, and excessive drying.

Pain management

The skin graft donor sites are often the source of the greatest postoperative pain. Local anesthetics such as marcaine can be infiltrated into the donor sites during the operation, but the mainstay of pain control is postoperative oral and intravenous opioids. The pain usually improves markedly about 48 hours postoperatively.

Postoperative complications
In the hospital
Blood loss

The most common postoperative complications are bleeding and uncontrolled pain. With tangential excision (the most common type of burn excision), tissue bleeding is used as the primary sign of tissue viability. Blood loss during surgery can approach 100 mL for every percentage of body surface area excised. Inadequate intraoperative blood replacement or

Medical Management of the Surgical Patient, ed. Michael F. Lubin, Thomas F. Dodson, and Neil H. Winawer. Published by Cambridge University Press. © Cambridge University Press 2013.

incomplete surgical hemostasis will lead to postoperative hypotension. Since the blood loss is external, postoperative bleeding is easy to localize. The large surface area involved in major burns can lead to underestimation of the blood loss.

Graft failure

Graft failure is one of the most feared complications, leaving the patient with both the same size burn wound and new donor site wounds. Common causes of skin graft failure are:

- Failure to adequately debride the burn wound (the skin graft is placed on tissue that later dies).
- Shearing of the skin graft off its wound bed before it had a chance to adhere.
- Inadequate hemostasis, which leads to hematoma formation under the skin graft.

After discharge

Hypertrophic scarring

At about 14–21 days postoperatively, the skin graft will have completely covered the wound. Daily dressing can be stopped at this point. Usually, the skin graft lacks elasticity and is still tender and erythematous; it often itches. Over the next 6 months the scar undergoes remodeling (also called scar maturation). There is an increase in collagen crosslinking and a decrease in vascularization. Collagenases break down the collagen, which reforms in bundles parallel to the surface of the skin. Wound contraction continues even after the graft has closed the wound. Through this process, the skin graft becomes more supple and stronger. While the meshed pattern of a graft improves with time it rarely disappears completely.

In a subset of patients, hypertrophic scarring develops. Inflammation of the wound persists; the collagen bundles form in whorls instead of parallel to the skin surface; and the scar becomes raised, stiff, and brittle. The scar is often painful and itches. Hypertrophic scarring can occur in isolated areas in a patient with normal scarring or in skin graft donor sites. There is no universal solution to the problem of hypertrophic scarring. The classical remedies are:

- Burn scar compression garments.
- Topical silicone gel sheeting.
- Intralesional steroid injection (usually with triamcinolone).
- Surgical scar revision.

The reduction of scarring and the control of pain in burn patients will be some of the greatest challenges of the twenty-first century for burn surgeons.

Further reading

Brusselaers N, Pirayesh A, Hoeksema H *et al.* Skin replacement in burn wounds. *J Trauma* 2010; **68**: 490–501.

Hawkins H, Pereira C. Pathophysiology of the burn scar. In Herndon DN, eds.

Total Burn Care. 3rd edn. Philadelphia, PA: W. B. Saunders; 2007, pp. 544–59.

Lee JO, Herndon DN. Burns and radiation injury. In Feliciano DV, Mattox KL, Moore EE, eds. *Trauma*. 6th edn.

New York, NY: McGraw-Hill Medical; 2008, pp. 1051–66.

Orgill DP. Excision and skin grafting of thermal burns. *N Engl J Med* 2009; **360**: 893–901.

Abdominal hysterectomy

Cyril O. Spann and Erica C. Dun

Hysterectomy is the most common major gynecologic operation and the second most common major surgical procedure in the USA. More than half a million women undergo hysterectomy each year. It is estimated that by age 65, one third of women will have had their uteri surgically removed. In recent years, alternatives for treating gynecologic disease have decreased the number of hysterectomies performed. Improved systemic hormonal therapies, progestational intrauterine devices, and endometrial ablation techniques have effectively managed menorrhagia without removal of the uterus. Leiomyomas can now be treated with transcervical hysteroscopic resection or uterine artery embolization. In addition, minimally invasive surgery using laparoscopic and laparoscopic-robotic techniques are becoming increasingly common, replacing the traditional abdominal hysterectomy.

Simple total abdominal hysterectomy involves the removal of the uterine corpus and cervix through an abdominal incision. It is performed for a variety of indications including uterine leiomyomas, recurrent dysfunctional uterine bleeding, adenomyosis, chronic pelvic pain, pelvic abscesses, and pelvic organ prolapse. In addition, simple abdominal hysterectomy is performed for three malignant indications: adenocarcinoma of the endometrium, ovarian cancer, and early microinvasive cervical cancer. Preoperative bowel preparation facilitates exposure and reduces trauma to the bowel caused by retraction and packing. Transfusion for simple abdominal hysterectomy is rare, and the operative time is 1 to 2 hours. General anesthesia is usually chosen, although spinal anesthesia can be used.

Usual postoperative course

Expected postoperative hospital stay

The expected postoperative hospital stay is 2–4 days.

Operative mortality

Operative mortality is under 1%.

Surgical wound classification

A Class II/Clean-contaminated surgical wound is an operative wound in which the alimentary, genital, or urinary tracts are entered under controlled conditions and without unusual contamination.

Special monitoring required

No special monitoring is necessary, unless the patient has other medical comorbidities such as heart disease, pulmonary disease, or obstructive sleep apnea.

Patient activity and positioning

Patients are out of bed the day of operation and ambulatory by the next day.

Alimentation

Clear liquids are encouraged on the first postoperative day, with food intake progressing to a regular diet if the patient demonstrates no nausea or vomiting, good bowel sounds, and limited abdominal distension.

Antibiotic coverage

Perioperative intravenous antibiotics aimed at polymicrobial contamination cover gram-negative rods, anaerobes, and gram-positive cocci. The use of prophylactic antibiotics has been shown to significantly reduce postoperative infectious morbidity and decrease the length of hospitalization in women undergoing abdominal hysterectomy. Cefazolin 1 g IV or 2 g IV (for patients with BMI > 35 or weight > 100 kg) is given prior to skin incision. Penicillin-allergic patients can receive clindamycin 600 mg IV plus gentamicin 1.5 mg/kg IV or metronidazole 500 mg IV plus gentamicin 1.5 mg/kg IV. For lengthy procedures, additional intraoperative doses of an antibiotic given at intervals of one or two times the half-life of the drug maintain adequate level throughout the operation. Cefazolin should be redosed after 3 hours of operative time.

Medical Management of the Surgical Patient, ed. Michael F. Lubin, Thomas F. Dodson, and Neil H. Winawer. Published by Cambridge University Press. © Cambridge University Press 2013.

Bacterial vaginosis increases the concentration of pathogenic anaerobic bacteria and increases the risk of post-hysterectomy cuff cellulites. Preoperative treatment and postoperative treatment of bacterial vaginosis with metronidazole for at least 4 days beginning just before surgery significantly reduces vaginal cuff infection.

Catheterization

Indwelling Foley catheter drainage is maintained for patient convenience after surgery and can be removed on the first postoperative day. Urinary retention is seen in 10–15% of patients but can be managed by intermittent self-catheterization.

Vaginal packing

Vaginal packing is not required.

Postoperative complications
In the hospital
Operative injuries

Injuries to the bladder, ureter, and bowel are rare during abdominal hysterectomy, occurring at rates of 1–2%, 0.1–0.5%, and 0.1–1%, respectively. Undiagnosed bladder or ureter injuries result in low urine output, abdominal distension, generalized malaise, and flank or back pain if hydroureter or hydronephrosis is present. A urinoma may form in the abdomen; the contents should be sampled and evaluated for creatinine level. If the creatinine level is similar to that of the urine from the urethra, then a urinary tract injury should be suspected. If the patient has flank or back pain, kidney and ureter imaging should be performed to evaluate the potential for obstruction.

Excessive vaginal bleeding

Intraperitoneal bleeding is associated with tachycardia, low urine output, and low blood pressure. There can be significant loss of blood into the peritoneal cavity before the abdomen becomes significantly distended. Postoperative bleeding predominately occurs from three areas: the infundibulopelvic ligament (when an oophorectomy has been performed), the uterine artery pedicle, and the uterosacral ligament pedicle. If acute blood loss is suspected, an exam under anesthesia should be performed in the operating room and the vaginal cuff sutures removed. The structures of the broad ligament, the uterine artery pedicle, and the uterosacral ligament pedicle can be exposed with long Allis clamps applied to the round ligament and to the uterosacral ligament. Bleeding at these sites can often be secured vaginally. However, if bleeding occurs from vessels higher in the pelvis, such as the ovarian artery and vein located in the infundibulopelvic ligament, the vaginal approach is rarely successful and repeat laparotomy is necessary in order to secure these vessels. The integrity of the ureters is always of concern after bleeding from the pedicles of the uterus is controlled. Indigo carmine dye should be injected intravenously and cystoscopy performed to ensure that the ureters are not obstructed.

Thromboembolic phenomena

The overall risk of a deep vein thrombosis (DVT) after a major gynecologic operation can range between 7 and 45%. Fatal pulmonary embolisms (PEs) are estimated to occur in nearly 1% of women with DVTs. A DVT may be manifested by unexplained fevers and tachycardia. Some patients report swelling and pain in the legs; others do not. Duplex ultrasound evaluation assists in making the diagnosis, but equivocal results may require venography. Postoperative use of sequential compression devices and administration of prophylactic dose unfractionated heparin or low molecular weight heparin decrease the rate of DVTs but have not been found to reduce the rate of PEs.

Dehiscence with or without evisceration

Patients with fascial dehiscence (opening of the fascia along the surgical suture) classically have significant serosanguineous fluid drainage from the incision. In these suspected cases, the patient should be examined to evaluate the integrity of the fascial closure; this may require general anesthesia in the operating room. If a defect is found then the fascia needs to be closed before the bowel eviscerates, or protrudes through the fascial opening and becomes ischemic. The rectus fascia can be resutured with a mass closure technique that uses a No. 1 synthetic delayed-absorbable suture. Dehiscence with evisceration should be managed first by wrapping the intestines in a sterile, moist towel. Once the patient is in the operating room, the incision can be reopened, the intestine replaced in the abdominal cavity, and the wound resutured.

After discharge
Infection

Infection is the most common complication of abdominal hysterectomy. Operative site infections occur in 6.6–24.7% of cases; wound infections in 4–8%; and urinary tract infections in 1.1–5%. The risk of infection increases with longer operative time, major break in sterile technique, obesity, and untreated bacterial vaginosis.

Intestinal obstruction

The location of intestinal obstruction in patients who have undergone gynecologic surgery is almost exclusively in the terminal ileum near the ileocecal junction. Obstruction results predominantly from adhesions to a loop of bowel or from the terminal ileum entering an internal hernia and becoming incarcerated. Therapy with nasogastric tube suction decompression is usually effective. If this method fails, the patient should be taken to the operating room and re-explored in order to relieve the intestinal obstruction.

Vesicovaginal fistula

Vesicovaginal fistulas (VVFs) are uncommon long-term seque-lae of hysterectomy, occurring in 0.1–0.2% of cases. Risk factors for the development of VVFs are large intraoperative cystotomy, tobacco use, larger uterine size, and higher operative blood loss.

Acknowledgment

This chapter is based on material from: Abdominal hyster-ectomy by Hugh W. Randall, which appeared in the 4th edition of *Medical Management of the Surgical Patient.*

Further reading

Antibiotic prophylaxis for gynecologic procedures. *ACOG Practice Bulletin, No. 104*, May 2009. Washington, DC: American College of Obstetricians and Gynecologists.

Dellinger EP, Gross PA, Barrett TL *et al.* Quality standard for antimicrobial prophylaxis in surgical procedures. Infectious Diseases Society of America. *Clin Infect Dis* 1994; **18**: 422–7.

Duong TH, Gellasch TL, Adam RA. Risk factors for the development of vesicovaginal fistula after incidental cystotomy at the time of a benign hysterectomy. *Am J Obstet Gynecol* 2009; **201**: 512e. 1–4.

Farquhar CM, Steiner CA. Hysterectomy rates in the United States, 1990–1997. *Obstet Gynecol* 2002; **99**: 229–34.

Jones HW. Abdominal hysterectomy. In Jones HW, Rock JA, eds. *Te Linde's Operative Gynecology.* 10th edn. Philadelphia, PA: Lippincott, Williams & Wilkins; 2008, pp. 727–43.

Oates-Whitehead RM, D'Angelo A, Mol B. Anticoagulant and aspirin prophylaxis for preventing thromboembolism after major gynaecological surgery. *Cochrane Database Syst Rev* 2003; **4**: CD003679.

Soper DE, Bump RC, Hurt WG. Bacterial vaginosis and trichomoniasis vaginitis are risk factors for cuff cellulitis after abdominal hysterectomy. *Am J Obstet Gynecol* 1990; **163**: 1016–21.

Steed HL, Capstick V, Flood C *et al.* A randomized controlled trial of early versus "traditional" postoperative oral intake after major abdominal gynecologic surgery. *Am J Obstet Gynecol* 2002; **186**: 861–5.

Wingo PA, Huezo CM, Rubin GL *et al.* The mortality risk associated with hysterectomy. *Am J Obstet Gynecol* 1985; **152**: 803–8.

Vaginal hysterectomy

S. Robert Kovac and Gina M. Northington

In the late nineteenth and early twentieth century it was taught that vaginal hysterectomy could not be performed if the uterus was enlarged, but uterine size was never quantified. Other suggested contraindications included a 'narrow vagina' (pubic arch < 90°) and a diminished bituberous diameter (< 8.0 cm). The bituberous diameter represents the distance between the ischial tuberosities (or sitting bones) which are easily palpated when the patient is in the dorsal lithotomy position. Nulliparity and "a uterus that was too high or did not come down" were also considered as contraindications to the vaginal approach, as were "intra-abdominal conditions" such as endometriosis, adhesions, previous pelvic surgery, previous cesarean section, and chronic pelvic pain.

Hysterectomy became the second most common operation performed in the USA in the middle twentieth century, but the complications related to this operation were not re-evaluated until 1982. The Collaborative Review of Sterilization (CREST) from the CDC studied the complications of abdominal and vaginal hysterectomy. For operative indications that could have been performed by either route, abdominal hysterectomy had a complication rate twice that of the vaginal approach.

It was not until the 1950s that gynecologic surgeons began to perform vaginal hysterectomy for conditions other than uterine prolapse and sterilization. As more patients underwent vaginal hysterectomy, many reports of improved outcomes with less invasive technique soon followed.

The early 1990s saw the introduction of laparoscopic-assisted vaginal hysterectomy (LAVH), with the goal to replace abdominal hysterectomy with the use of the laparoscope. The techniques were strikingly different: the more invasive abdominal approach would be replaced by smaller incisions. The first article to employ the term LAVH suggested that the laparoscope could be used for the preoperative evaluation of intra-abdominal anatomy to document the presence or absence of potential disease prior to the selection of a specific route of hysterectomy.

In 2006, the concept of LAVH was modified by laparoscopic surgeons: laparoscopic surgical techniques and instruments could be used to remove the uterus, cervix and/or the fallopian tubes and ovaries through the vagina. Thus, laparoscopic hysterectomy (LH) and LAVH became interchangeable terms; laparoscopic surgeons suggested that all hysterectomies be performed by laparoscopic methods. However, the academic community was slow to adopt the laparoscopic approach, as they felt the case for the use of the laparoscope with hysterectomy had not been adequately presented. The term "traditional hysterectomy," including both abdominal and vaginal hysterectomy, was used in articles that suggested better outcomes for LAVH; however, outcomes comparing the laparoscope to vaginal methods for uterine removal never documented the benefits of the laparoscopic approach over the vaginal approach.

In 2009, the American College of Obstetricans and Gynecologists (ACOG) addressed this controversy in a Committee Opinion, which concluded that ". . . the physician should take into consideration how the procedure may be performed most safely and cost-effectively to fulfill the medical needs of the patient. Most literature supports the opinion that, when feasible, vaginal hysterectomy is the safest and most cost-effective route by which to remove the uterus." In a large population study (n = 5,276) of women undergoing abdominal hysterectomy, vaginal hysterectomy, or laparoscopic hysterectomy, Brummer *et al.* reported that abdominal hysterectomy was associated with a higher rate of wound infection.

Prior to the introduction of laparoscopic hysterectomy, abdominal hysterectomy was performed in more than 65% of cases and vaginal hysterectomy in 35%. The current percentages for the various route of hysterectomy suggest that gynecologic surgeons are performing laparoscopic hysterectomy for cases that previously would have been performed by the vaginal approach.

Not all hysterectomies demand a specific operative approach; some hysterectomies can be performed vaginally, laparoscopically, or abdominally for similar indications. Studies on the outcomes of hysterectomies for similar indications strongly support the vaginal route. The goal of clinical decision making under these conditions would be to select the operative approach that a patient finds desirable; a comparison of the

Medical Management of the Surgical Patient, ed. Michael F. Lubin, Thomas F. Dodson, and Neil H. Winawer. Published by Cambridge University Press. © Cambridge University Press 2013.

outcomes of these alternative surgical approaches and data information should be offered to the patient. A recent Cochrane Review by Nieboer *et al.* of 34 randomized controlled trials including a total of 4,495 women determined that vaginal hysterectomy was associated with a quicker return to normal activities, fewer episodes of febrile morbidity or infections, and a shorter hospital stay. Other recent studies determined that factors associated with conversion from vaginal hysterectomy to abdominal hysterectomy were low parity, previous abdominal surgery, pelvic adhesions, and large uterine weight.

Usual postoperative course

Expected postoperative hospital stay

The expected postoperative hospital stay is 1–2 days, depending on the age and associated medical conditions of the patient.

Operative mortality

Operative mortality is under 1%.

Special monitoring required

Special monitoring is unnecessary.

Patient activity

Patients are usually ambulatory on the day of operation.

Alimentation

Oral intake as desired is permitted on the evening of the day of surgery.

Antibiotic coverage

Intravenous antibiotic coverage for gram-negative rods and gram positive cocci should be administered immediately prior to the induction of anesthesia.

Urinary catheterization

A Foley catheter attached to a sterile bag for continuous bladder drainage may be placed at the start or at the end of a vaginal hysterectomy. Many surgeons prefer to place a urinary catheter at the completion of the operation as this may facilitate anterior dissection of the bladder from the cervix. The urinary catheter is usually removed the following morning.

Vaginal packing

Vaginal packing is often not required.

Postoperative complications

In the hospital

Excessive vaginal bleeding

The most common source of serious bleeding is a uterine artery that has retracted outside the suture ligature; the incidence is approximately one in every 1,000 cases.

This complication can present as vaginal or intraperitoneal bleeding, resulting in tachycardia, low urine output, and low blood pressure. Occlusion of the bleeding artery is best accomplished by interventional radiology. Although it is tempting to open the vaginal cuff if vaginal bleeding appears to be the source, rarely is it possible to identify the source.

Infection

Evaluation of the vaginal pH prior to prepping is the single most important procedure to avoid postoperative infections. If the pH is above 5.5, anaerobic bacteria in the vaginal vault have reached concentrations of 10^6–10^8 above their usual concentrations of 10^3. This elevated concentration is an indicator that the vagina is infected. Therefore, in addition to the prophylactic antibiotics received during surgery, therapeutic antibiotic treatment will be required.

Ureteral injury

The incidence of ureteral injury with vaginal hysterectomy is less than 1%; the rate is 2.2% with abdominal hysterectomy and 7.8% with laparoscopic hysterectomy. Nevertheless, routine cystoscopy with the intravenous injection of indigo carmine dye should be performed after every hysterectomy to determine ureteral patency.

Dyspareunia

There is some suggestion that shortening of the vagina after hysterectomy is associated with postoperative dyspareunia. One observational prospective study has reported that women in the vaginal hysterectomy group were more likely to have shortened vaginal length than women who underwent total abdominal hysterectomy (8.4 + 1.6 cm vs 10.2 + 1.8 cm). In this same study, 20% of women who underwent vaginal hysterectomy reported postoperative dyspareunia compared with 5% in the preoperative group.

To our knowledge, there have been no randomized controlled trials documenting a difference in postoperative sexual function between vaginal hysterectomy and abdominal hysterectomy.

After discharge

Patients are instructed to avoid inserting anything in the vagina until the first postoperative check-up in 4 weeks; slight vaginal bleeding can persist for that period of time. They are allowed to walk as much as they desire, climb stairs, and shower or bathe in the tub. Patients may drive a car as long as they are not taking narcotics. They are instructed to limit lifting anything above 20 pounds. Many patients return to work within 2 weeks if their work does not require heavy lifting.

Further reading

Abdelmonem AM. Vaginal length and incidence of dyspareunia after total abdominal versus vaginal hysterectomy. *Eur J Obstet Gynecol Reprod Biol* 2010; **151**: 190–2.

ACOG Committee Opinion No. 444: Choosing the route of hysterectomy for benign disease. *Obstet Gynecol* 2009; **114**: 1156–8.

Brummer TH, Jalkanen J, Fraser J *et al.* FINHYST, a prospective study of 5279 hysterectomies: complications and their risk factors. *Hum Reprod* 2011; **26**: 1741–51.

Cho HY, Kim HB, Kang SW, Park SH. When do we need to perform laparotomy for benign uterine disease? Factors involved with conversion in vaginal hysterectomy. *J Obstet Gynaecol Res* 2012; **38**; 31–4.

Dicker RC, Greenspan JR, Strauss LT *et al.* Complications of abdominal and vaginal hysterectomy among women of reproductive age in the United States. *Am J Obstet Gynecol* 1982; **144**: 841–8.

Doğanay M, Yildiz Y, Tonguc E *et al.* Abdominal, vaginal and total laparoscopic hysterectomy: perioperative morbidity. *Arch Gynecol Obstet* 2011; **284**: 385–9.

Einarsson JI, Matteson KA, Schulkin J *et al.* Minimally invasive hysterectomies – a survey on attitudes and barriers among practicing gynecologists. *J Minim Invasive Gynecol* 2010; **17**: 167–75.

Guvenal T, Ozsoy AZ, Kilcik MA, Yanik A. The availability of vaginal hysterectomy in benign gynecologic diseases: a prospective, non-randomized trial. *J Obstet Gynaecol Res* 2010; **36**: 832–7.

Kovac SR, Barhan S, Lister M, Bishop M, Das A. Guidelines for the selection the route of hysterectomy: application in a resident clinic population. *Am J Obstet Gynecol* 2002; **187**: 1521–7.

Kovac SR, Cruikshank SH, Retto HF. Laparoscopy-assisted vaginal hysterectomy. *J Gynecol Surg* 1990; **6**: 185–93.

Nieboer TE, Johnson N, Lethaby A *et al.* Surgical approach to hysterectomy for benign gynaecological disease. *Cochrane Database Syst Rev.* 2009; **8**: CD003677.

99

Uterine curettage

Erica C. Dun and Carla P. Roberts

Uterine curettage is the second most frequently performed gynecologic procedure. The primary indications for uterine curettage are both diagnostic and therapeutic:

Polymenorrhea: menstrual cycle interval less than 21 days.

Oligomenorrhea: menstrual cycle interval more than 37 days.

Menorrhagia: excessive or prolonged menstrual bleeding.

Postmenopausal bleeding: uterine bleeding occurring more than 12 months after the last menstrual period in a menopausal woman.

Breakthrough bleeding: intermenstrual bleeding in a menstrual cycle that is the result of exogenous hormones.

Dysfunctional uterine bleeding: any abnormal uterine bleeding in the absence of pregnancy, neoplasm, infection, or uterine lesion.

Other: spontaneous abortion, incomplete abortion, inevitable abortion, fetal demise in utero, septic abortion, termination of pregnancy, dilation and evacuation of gestational trophoblastic neoplasms.

The operation involves dilating the cervix and removing uterine contents and endometrial tissue. The patient is placed on the table in the lithotomy position. The perineum and vagina are cleaned with a povidone-iodine (Betadine) solution. A straight Jacobs (double-tooth) clamp or single-tooth tenaculum is used to grasp and stabilize the cervix. A bimanual exam is performed to confirm the size and position of the uterus and a uterine sound is carefully passed to confirm the length of the uterine cavity and the angulation between the cervical canal and the uterine cavity. Sounding the uterus is contraindicated in the presence of a pregnancy because the increased risk of perforating the soft myometrium. Dilators are subsequently passed through the cervix to achieve the desired cervical canal diameter. After dilation, ureteral stone forceps can be introduced into the uterine cavity to remove endometrial polyps. Curettage is performed with a small serrated curette which can be used to systematically scrape the uterine cavity until a uterine "cry" (vibrations felt as the curette is gently dragged across denuded endometrium) is appreciated. When curettage is performed for the removal of placental tissue, a large, blunt, smooth curette is used to lessen the possibility of perforation and endometrial sclerosis.

It is important that dilation and curettage be performed for the proper indications, as serious complications and even death may result from poor or inappropriate technique. The operative time for the procedure is usually less than 15 minutes. Regional and local anesthesia can be used; however, general anesthesia is more comfortable for the patient, and the procedure is easier to perform with the patient fully relaxed. Transfusion is rarely indicated unless significant preoperative hemorrhage (usually associated with pregnancy) has occurred. Formerly, uterine curettage was believed to be contraindicated in the presence of pelvic infections, pyometra, and septic abortion; however, when indicated and with the use of preoperative antibiotics, dilation and curettage under septic conditions can remove the source of infection (e.g., septic abortion, pyometria) and provide valuable histological information.

Usual postoperative course

Expected postoperative hospital stay

Typically uterine curettage is performed on an outpatient basis. Inpatient hospitalization should be reserved for medical or surgical complications, such as infection, uterine perforation, or hemorrhage.

Operative mortality

Operative mortality is less than 1%.

Special monitoring required

No special monitoring is necessary, unless the patient has other medical comorbidities such as heart disease, pulmonary disease, or obstructive sleep apnea.

Medical Management of the Surgical Patient, ed. Michael F. Lubin, Thomas F. Dodson, and Neil H. Winawer. Published by Cambridge University Press. © Cambridge University Press 2013.

Patient activity and positioning

After recovering from anesthesia, patients are ambulatory on the day of the procedure.

Alimentation

The patient is permitted to resume regular diet as tolerated on the day of surgery.

Antibiotic coverage

Preoperative antibiotic coverage with broad-spectrum antibiotic directed toward polymicrobial contamination of the urogenital tract (gram-negative rods, anaerobes, and gram-positive cocci) is indicated for septic abortions and pyometria. With surgical abortion, antibiotics are recommended for dilation and evacuation: doxycycline 100 mg orally given 1 hour before the procedure and 200 mg orally after the procedure, plus metronidazole 500 mg orally twice daily for 5 days.

Oxytocin

Oxytocin can be administered to patients who undergo abortion to contract the pregnant uterus and prevent hemorrhage.

Postoperative complications

In the hospital

Perforation of the uterus

Most cases of uterine perforation are associated with the use of a sound or cervical dilators and occur in patients with acutely anteflexed or retroflexed uteri. Overnight observation in the hospital is recommended. The two principal dangers of uterine perforation are bleeding and trauma to adjacent abdominal viscera. A lateral perforation may lacerate uterine vessels and cause hemorrhage. When serious damage from perforation is suspected, a diagnostic laparoscopy or laparotomy should be performed so that damage can be assessed and repaired.

Hemorrhage

Bleeding may be obvious or concealed within the peritoneal cavity. Nevertheless, if acute blood loss is suspected or known, immediate abdominal exploration, control of bleeding, and sometimes hysterectomy may be necessary.

Intestinal perforation

Intestinal perforation is a rare complication. It is most often associated with perforation of the uterine fundus during the termination of pregnancy and evacuation of products of conception with a suction curette. Immediate laparotomy should be performed to assess, repair, and resect the injured bowel.

After discharge

Bleeding and fever

If bleeding is copious and sustained, re-exploration of the endometrial cavity is indicated. If fever develops, a culture should be obtained from the endometrial cavity and broad-spectrum antibiotics administered until the culture and sensitivities are identified.

Asherman's syndrome

Asherman's syndrome is a pathologic condition of intrauterine adhesions. It can cause secondary amenorrhea, other menstrual irregularities, infertility, and recurrent abortion. Numerous studies have noted a strong association between puerperal curettage and the formation of synechiae that can partially or completely obliterate the endometrial cavity. A few cases have been reported after uterine tuberculosis, severe endometriosis, myomectomy, and cesarean section. The diagnosis can be confirmed by a hysterosalpingogram and hysteroscopy. Lysis of adhesions can be performed hysteroscopically.

Acknowledgment

This chapter is based on material from: Uterine curettage by Hugh W. Randall, which appeared in the 4th edition of *Medical Management of the Surgical Patient*.

Further reading

Antibiotic prophylaxis for gynecologic procedures. *ACOG Practice Bulletin, No. 104*, May 2009. Washington, DC: American College of Obstetricians and Gynecologists.

Butler WJ, Carnovale DE. Normal and abnormal uterine bleeding. In Jones HW, Rock JA, eds. *Te Linde's Operative Gynecology*. 10th edn. Philadelphia, PA: Lippincott, Williams & Wilkins; 2008, pp. 585–608.

Friedman A, DeFazio J, DeCherney A. Severe obstetric complications after aggressive treatment of Asherman syndrome. *Obstet Gynecol* 1986; **67**: 864–7.

Hefler L, Lemach A, Seebacher V *et al.* The intraoperative complication rate of nonobstetric dilation and curettage. *Obstet Gynecol* 2009; **113**: 1268–71.

Schorge JO, Schaffer JI, Pietz J *et al.* Sharp dilatation and curettage. In Schorge JO, Schaffer JI, Halvorson LM *et al.*, eds. *Williams Gynecology*. New York, NY: McGraw-Hill Companies, Inc.; 2008, pp. 896–900.

Tuncalp O, Gulmezoglu AM, Souza JP. Surgical procedures for evacuating incomplete miscarriage. *Cochrane Database Syst Rev* 2010; **8**: CD001993.

Radical hysterectomy

Leda Gattoc and Sharmila Makhija

Carcinoma of the uterine cervix is the second most common gynecologic malignancy worldwide and the third most common cause of cancer deaths in women all over the world. In 2010, an estimated 12,200 women in the USA were diagnosed with cervical cancer, and 4,210 women died from the disease.

Attempts to treat cervical cancer in the early nineteenth century were deemed largely unsuccessful due to the frequent occurrence of recurrent disease in the vaginal cuff. Surgeons such as Wertheim and Clark postulated that this was likely due to inadequate margin of excision. At the turn of the nineteenth century, these surgeons developed an operation that involved removal of the uterus, along with a wide resection of tissues around the involved cervical tumor.

The primary goal of radical hysterectomy is removal of the cervical tumor with a sufficient surgical margin. This entails removal of the uterus, cervix, superior vaginal margin, and parametrial tissue. Removal of the latter involves extensive dissection of the bladder, ureters, rectum, and lateral pelvic sidewalls.

Cervical cancer is staged clinically. All stages may be treated with a combination of radiotherapy and chemotherapy; however, early-stage cervical cancer may be treated with a radical hysterectomy. While microinvasive disease or stage IA1 can be adequately treated with a vaginal or simple abdominal hysterectomy, radical hysterectomy along with pelvic lymphadenectomy is utilized to treat stages IA2 through IIA. The overall survival of early-stage cervical cancer is similar between radical hysterectomy and radiotherapy. Therefore, patients who are poor surgical candidates due to severe medical illness or morbid obesity are probably best treated with primary radiotherapy.

In addition to treatment of early stage cervical cancer, radical hysterectomy can also be utilized in treatment of centrally recurrent cervical cancer after radiation therapy. Patients with stage II endometrial cancer (primary cancer of the uterus with spread to the cervix) have also been reported to have a significant survival advantage when treated with a radical hysterectomy with lymphadenectomy versus just a simple total hysterectomy with lymphadenectomy.

Patients undergoing surgery must consider the following operative risks: blood transfusion, perioperative infection, thromboembolic disorders, postoperative bladder and bowel dysfunction, fistula formation, nerve injury, and lymphedema. Despite the associated risks, there are potential advantages to radical hysterectomy over primary radiotherapy. Surgery affords the opportunity for ovarian preservation in premenopausal women. Metastatic disease to the ovaries is unusual; removal of the ovaries is not a routine part of the procedure. Radical hysterectomy may inadvertently shorten the remaining vagina but it avoids the fibrotic and stenotic effects caused by radiation therapy. Finally, radical surgery allows for evaluation of nodal metastasis.

Preoperative evaluation of surgical patients should rule out metastatic disease. Bowel prep and availability of type and cross-matched blood should be routine. The estimated blood loss usually ranges from 800–1,500 mL, with one-third to one-half of patients requiring blood transfusion. Operative time can range from 2.5 to 4 hours.

Usual postoperative course

Expected postoperative hospital stay

The expected postoperative hospital stay is typically 3–4 days.

Operative mortality

Improvements in postoperative and critical care medicine including the use of prophylactic antibiotics, thomboprophylaxis, and blood product replacement have reduced the operative morbidity rate for patients undergoing this surgery to 0.6%.

Special monitoring required

Intensive care observation may be necessary for select postoperative patients with certain comorbidities; however, the majority can be monitored on the routine post-surgical ward.

Patient activity and positioning

The routine use of intermittent pneumatic calf compression devices both intra- and postoperatively has decreased the incidence of thromboembolic disease. Postoperative thromboprophylaxis with heparin and calf compression devices should be continued until the patient is fully ambulatory or at the time of hospital discharge. The clinician should be alert to the possibility of thromboembolic events even after patient discharge.

Alimentation

Bowel function usually returns within the first 2–3 postoperative days; diet may be advanced as tolerated.

Antibiotic coverage

A significant reduction in postoperative infectious morbidity and decreased length of hospitalization has been associated with administration of prophylactic antibiotics to women undergoing hysterectomy, as demonstrated in multiple randomized clinical trials and meta-analyses. Preoperative antibiotics should be administered 30 minutes prior to incision. Cephalosporins have emerged as the drugs of choice because of their broad antimicrobial spectrum and low incidence of adverse reactions.

Postoperative complications
In the hospital
Bladder dysfunction

The incidence of postoperative bladder dysfunction after radical hysterectomy has been reported at a rate of 70–85%. Bladder dysfunction results from interruption of the autonomic nerve supply to the bladder, a consequence of anterior, posterior, and lateral dissection of the parametrial tissue and vaginal cuff. Immediate postoperative bladder care usually entails leaving an indwelling catheter to prevent overdistension of the bladder and prolonged dysfunction. Adequate postoperative bladder care will usually restore normal bladder function within 8–12 months.

Urinary fistula formation

Vesicovaginal fistulas and ureterovaginal fistulas have been reported in 0.9–2% of patients after radical hysterectomy. Fistula formation usually presents as a watery uriniferous vaginal discharge within the first 3 weeks following surgery. Diagnosis can be achieved with a simple speculum exam, cystoscopy or a "tampon test" (the bladder is filled with diluted methylene blue solution, then a tampon is inserted into the vagina). Other radiographic studies such as an intravenous pyelogram can rule out a fistula involving the ureter. Prolonged bladder drainage or ureteral stent placement can result in spontaneous closure of a small fistula. To allow for resolution of edema and inflammation, surgical repair, if necessary, is performed after several weeks.

Neural deficits

The majority of nerve injuries sustained during radical hysterectomy are transient. Most patients will regain full sensory and motor function. Nerve injuries can be a consequence of the surgery itself or of the compressive use of retractors. Nerves at risk include: femoral, obturator, sciatic, genitofemoral, ilioinguinal, and lateral femoral cutaneous.

After discharge
Lymphedema

After radical hysterectomy, disruption of the regional efferent lymphatic channels during pelvic lymphadenectomy can result in pelvic pain, lymphocyst formation, lymphedema, and infection. Lymphedema formation usually worsens if a patient undergoes postoperative adjuvant radiotherapy. The condition may be treated with elevation of the involved extremity along with the use of elastic stockings. Placement of retroperitoneal drains can be utilized to prevent lymphocyst formation. Management can include guided percutaneous drainage or laparoscopic surgical resection. Patients with this complication may also develop intermittent lymphangitis, which can be treated with oral antibiotics.

Bowel obstruction

Bowel obstruction is an uncommon complication, although it can occur in patients requiring postoperative adjuvant radiotherapy. It can be managed initially by bowel rest and nasogastric tube decompression. Re-exploration is reserved for those patients who are not helped by conservative treatment.

Further reading

Angioli R, Penalver M, Muzii L et al. Guidelines of how to manage vesicovaginal fistula. *Crit Rev Oncol Hematol* 2003; **48**: 295–304.

Antibiotic prophylaxis for gynecologic procedures. *ACOG Practice Bulletin, No. 104*, May 2009. Washington, DC: American College of Obstetricians and Gynecologists.

Boente MP, Yordan EL Jr, McIntosh DG et al. Prognostic factors and long-term survival in endometrial adenocarcinoma with cervical involvement. *Gynecol Oncol* 1993; **51**: 316–22.

Likic IS, Kadija S, Ladjevic NG et al. Analysis of urologic complications after radical hysterectomy. *Am J Obstet Gynecol* 2008; **199**: 644. e1–3.

Maneo A, Landoni F, Cormio G, Colombo A, Mangioni C. Radical hysterectomy for recurrent or persistent cervical cancer following radiation therapy. *Int J Gynecol Cancer* 1999; **9**: 295–301.

Meigs JV. The Wertheim operation for carcinoma of the cervix. *Am J Obstet Gynecol* 1945; **49**: 542–53.

National Cancer Institute. [December 2010]. Available from: www.cancer.gov/cancertopics/types/cervical

Ware RA, van Nagell JR Jr. Radical hysterectomy with pelvic lymphadenectomy: indications, technique, and complications. *Obstet*

Gynecol Int 2010; Article ID 587610, doi:10.1155/2010/587610.

Wertheim E. The extended abdominal operation for carcinoma uteri (based on 500 operative cases). *Am J Obstet Gynecol* 1912; **66**: 169–232.

Zullo MA, Manci N, Angioli R, Muzii L, Panici PB. Vesical dysfunctions after radical hysterectomy for cervical cancer: a critical review. *Crit Rev Oncol Hematol* 2003; **48**: 287–93.

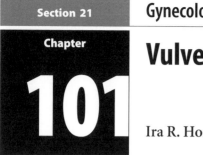

Chapter

101

Vulvectomy

Ira R. Horowitz and Erica C. Dun

Vulvectomy is performed for both preinvasive and malignant conditions of the vulva. This procedure may vary in extent from a skinning procedure performed for multi-centric intra-epithelial neoplasia to a radical vulvectomy combined with bilateral inguinofemoral lymph node dissections for invasive carcinoma. The radical procedure has changed during the past decade; it may range from a hemivulvectomy with unilateral inguinofemoral lymph node dissection to a radical vulvectomy with bilateral inguinofemoral lymph nodes dissection. A three-incision method for radical vulvectomy with bilateral lymph node dissection is preferred over en bloc removal because the multiple incision method has a significantly decreased rate of wound breakdown.

Lateralizing stage T1 lesions that are smaller than 2 cm are treated with a radical hemivulvectomy and ipsilateral lymph node dissection. For larger or midline lesions, attempts are made to perform a radical vulvectomy and bilateral inguino-femoral lymph node dissections through separate incisions (three-incision technique). This approach generally results in fewer postoperative complications (e.g., wound infections) and a shorter hospital stay. The time necessary for this operation is 2–5 hours, and varies according to the extent of resection and reconstruction. Depending on the extent of resection, gracilis or rectus abdominis myocutaneous flaps, Z-plasty full-thickness pedicle flaps, or V–Y advancement flaps may be needed to fill the operative defect. Large defects in the vulva can be reconstructed with split-thickness skin grafts. Closed suction drains are often placed in the operative site to reduce the formation of lymphocysts and to improve wound healing. General, regional, or combination anesthesia can be equally efficacious. Intraoperative transfusions are not routinely required during a radical vulvectomy.

Usual postoperative course
Expected postoperative hospital stay

The duration of hospitalization ranges from 3–21 days, depending on the extent of resection, the required reconstruction, and the rate of wound healing.

Operative mortality

Operative mortality is less than 1%.

Special monitoring required

No special monitoring is required for patients undergoing radical vulvectomy. However, most patients are elderly and may have medical comorbidities, such as heart or pulmonary disease, which necessitate intensive care monitoring.

Patient activity and positioning

Bed rest for 24–48 hours is recommended to allow the myocutaneous flaps or primary closure to begin healing before tension is placed on the suture lines.

Alimentation

Preoperative bowel preparation can decrease the amount of fecal wound soiling in the immediate postoperative period. Although a regular diet would be tolerated on the first post-operative day, clear liquids or a low-residue diet are recommended to further decrease fecal soiling.

Antibiotic coverage

Recent studies report that prophylactic antibiotics do not significantly reduce the number of wound infections or wound breakdowns after radical vulvectomy. Nevertheless, perioperative administration of a first- or second-generation cephalosporin, coupled with postoperative administration of doxycycline, may reduce the incidence of cellulitis in selected patients.

Thromboembolism prophylaxis

To reduce the risk of venous thromboembolisms in women with gynecologic malignancies, the American College of Chest Physicians ACCP (2008) 8th Edition practice guidelines recommend prophylactic doses of unfractionated heparin or low molecular weight heparin, administered either with

Medical Management of the Surgical Patient, ed. Michael F. Lubin, Thomas F. Dodson, and Neil H. Winawer. Published by Cambridge University Press. © Cambridge University Press 2013.

or without the use of perioperative sequential pneumatic compression devices.

Perineal care

Various philosophies exist regarding perineal care in patients undergoing radical vulvectomy. Most surgeons agree, however, that the wound should be kept dry. This may be accomplished with a heat lamp or hair dryer, taking care not to burn the exposed skin.

Postoperative complications

In the hospital

Wound separation and necrosis

The most common complication of radical vulvectomy is wound separation and necrosis, which occurs in about 70–80% of patients. This complication has been significantly reduced by using the three-incision technique. Although the use of myocutaneous flaps and skin grafts can also decrease the incidence of this problem, flaps frequently undergo necrosis at their distal margins. Skin necrosis is treated with aggressive debridement and frequent irrigation. It may take several weeks for complete wound healing to occur. For patients who do experience wound breakdown, no additional skin grafting is necessary; the wound can be allowed to granulate, with satisfactory results.

Wound hematomas and seromas

In a radical vulvectomy, a closed end drain is often placed in the operative site and in the groin if inguinofemoral lymph node dissection is performed. Drain placement can aid in decreasing the collection of fluid, which impedes wound healing.

The saphenous vein may be sacrificed, although some gynecologic oncologists attempt to spare the saphenous vein to decrease postoperative hematomas and leg edema. If small branching arteries and veins from the femoral vessels are not secured in the initial surgery and drains are not effectively emptying the collections, re-exploration may be necessary to evacuate the fluid and achieve hemostasis.

Cellulitis

Cellulitis is the second most common complication of radical vulvectomy. Patients should be treated with a broad-spectrum antibiotic effective against staphylococcal and streptococcal species. Wound cultures should be obtained to identify the predominant species so antibiotics can be appropriately selected. Increasing rates of MRSA infections have been reported in hospitals around the country, especially in patients who have lengthy hospitalizations.

Rupture of femoral vessels

Rupture of femoral vessels is a life-threatening complication. Until patients can be returned to the operating room for repair of the damaged vessel, they should be treated with local compression to control bleeding. Transposition of the sartorius muscle to cover the femoral vessels during the initial operation has almost eliminated this complication. More conservative approaches to node dissection permit a primary closure of the fascia that does not necessitate a sartorius muscle flap to correct the defect.

Femoral neuropathy

The femoral nerve lies lateral to the femoral artery. Femoral nerve injury is rare but can occur during the inguinofemoral dissection. The severing of a few sensory branches results in numbness or paresthesia of the anterior thigh. However, surgical injury of a major portion of the nerve results in significant and permanent difficulty in ambulation.

After discharge

Edema of the lower extremities

Excision or interruption of the regional lymphatics frequently results in chronic lymphedema. Therapy consists of elastic support stockings and limb elevation. In more severe cases, pneumatic compression devices are used.

Lymphangitis and cellulitis

Lymphangitis and cellulitis require aggressive antibiotic coverage.

Vaginal stricture

Cicatricial stenosis around the introitus may result in dyspareunia. The use of vaginal dilators, and, occasionally, surgical correction may be necessary to provide a normal vaginal caliber and to restore the patient's ability to have coitus.

Hernia formation

Inguinal and femoral hernias may develop if care is not exercised in closing the respective fascial planes. Careful closure of the fascia, in addition to the use of a sartorius flap during the initial vulvectomy, further decreases the incidence of this complication.

Incontinence

Urinary or fecal incontinence may occur after resection of the distal urethra or anal sphincter. Attempts should be made to train patients to achieve increased muscle tone. If efforts prove unsuccessful, or if the resection was extensive, additional reconstructive surgery may be warranted.

Further reading

Antibiotic prophylaxis for gynecologic procedures. *ACOG Practice Bulletin, No. 104*, May 2009. Washington, DC: American College of Obstetricians and Gynecologists.

Daly JW, Pomerance AJ. Groin dissection with prevention of tissue loss and postoperative infection. *Obstet Gynecol* 1979; **53**: 395–9.

Duncan A, Horowitz IR, Kalassian K. Postanesthesia and postoperative care. In Jones HW, Rock JA, eds. *Te Linde's Operative Gynecology*. 10th edn. Philadelphia, PA: Lippincott, Williams & Wilkins; 2008, pp. 133–59.

Hacker NF, Leuchter RS, Berek JS *et al.* Radical vulvectomy and bilateral inguinal lymphadenectomy though separate groin incisions. *Obstet Gynecol* 1981; **58**: 574–9.

Hirsh J, Guyatt G, Albers GW, Harrington R, Schunemann HJ. American College of Chest Physicians. Antithrombotic and thrombolytic therapy: American College of Chest Physicians Evidence-Based Clinical Practice Guidelines. 8th edn. *Chest* 2008; **133**: S110–12.

Hoffman MS. Malignancies of the vulva. In Jones HW, Rock JA, eds. *Te Linde's Operative Gynecology*. 10th edn. Philadelphia, PA: Lippincott, Williams & Wilkins; 2008, pp. 1151–207.

Hopkins MP, Reid GC, Morley GW. Radical vulvectomy. The decision for the incision. *Cancer* 1993; **72**: 700–803.

Horowitz IR. Female genital system. In Wood WC, Staley CA, Skandalakis JE, eds. *The Anatomic Basis of Tumor Surgery*. 2nd edn. Berlin: Springer; 2010, pp. 637–80.

Horowitz IR. Surgical conditions of the vulva. In Jones HW, Rock JA, eds. *TeLinde's Operative Gynecology*. 10th edn. Philadelphia, PA: Lippincott, Williams & Wilkins; 2008, pp. 480–507.

Nigriny JF, Wu P, Butler CE. Perineal reconstruction with an extrapelvic vertical rectus abdominis myocutaneous flap. *Int J Gynecol Cancer* 2010; **20**: 1609–12.

Senn B, Mueller MD, Cignacco EL, Eicher M. Period prevalence and risk factors for postoperative short-term wound complications in vulvar cancer: a cross-sectional study. *Int J Gynecol Cancer* 2010; **20**: 646–54.

Stehman FB, Bundy BN, Ball H, Clarke-Pearson DL. Sites of failure and times to failure in carcinoma of the vulva treated conservatively: a Gynecologic Oncology Group study. *Am J Obstet Gynecol* 1996; **174**: 1128–32.

Craniotomy for brain tumor

Kenneth L. Hill, Jr. and Jeffrey J. Olson

Brain tumors have been loosely divided between primary (occurring from the cells native to the CNS) and secondary or metastatic (from spread by direct contiguous contact or hematologic spread). The incidence of primary brain tumors in the USA is roughly 6.4 for every 100,000 people, with the majority comprising the glioblastoma subtype. Metastatic brain tumors occur in 15–20% of all cancer patients with the primary etiology being lung, breast, melanoma, and renal tumors. With the development of new imaging techniques, innovative surgical techniques, and progressive adjunctive therapies, the treatment of brain tumors now involves earlier diagnosis, improved accuracy for surgery, and more medical and radiation options for patients with brain tumors. Despite improved imaging techniques that can better describe the characteristics of brain tumors without tissue evaluation, the role of craniotomy surgery is an important component of both diagnosis and treatment of patients with brain tumors. As opposed to formal craniotomy, stereotactic needle biopsy can be used for those patients with tumor in a deep, functionally important region of the brain and in patients with poor systemic health. Histologic examination of these core needle biopsies is then used to direct therapy. Craniotomy and surgical debulking/excision are especially beneficial in those patients with large lesions that are symptomatic due to size and edema that cause compression of surrounding brain tissue.

Preoperative imaging for brain tumors is technically specific to each individual patient. With expert interpretation, surgical planning can be made with a general understanding of the goal of the procedure. Imaging techniques have progressed to include digital subtraction angiography, MRI, MR spectroscopy and functional MRI, to name a few. These techniques provide valuable information, but are frequently unable to exclude all other non-tumorous lesions like infarction, infection, and multiple sclerosis. Thus a craniotomy or needle biopsy is required to obtain definitive diagnosis.

Many patients with brain tumors also have coexisting systemic medical conditions. Once the decision has been made for surgery, an attempt should be made to optimize the coexisting medical comorbidities. This is typically done with simple

tests to determine any metabolic derangements, cardiac arrhythmias, infectious processes, and pulmonary limitations. If abnormalities are identified through this screening process, consultation with the appropriate service is needed to optimize the patient prior to surgery to decrease his/her surgical morbidity and mortality risk. Patients are also screened for anemia and thrombocytopenia; blood products are ordered as needed, as these may be required during craniotomy surgery.

For many patients, anticonvulsant therapy is used in preoperative treatment. It is indicated in those who present with a convulsive event or in patients whose tumor affects the cortical surface of the brain and will undergo some type of surgical intervention. Though there are guidelines on its use, the length of the course of anticonvulsant therapy postoperatively is based largely on the clinical judgment of the treating physician.

Preoperative corticosteroids are used to decrease swelling associated with vasogenic edema from intracranial tumors as well as to decrease peri-tumoral edema, mass effect, and cerebral edema encountered intraoperatively. The clinical effect is appreciated within the first 1–2 days of treatment.

Once the decision is made to perform a craniotomy, preoperative surgical planning includes image analysis, preparation and use of intra-operative neuronavigation, and surgical decision analysis to create an operative approach that maximizes surgical exposure and access to the tumor with minimal risk to the surrounding brain and patient overall.

In the operative arena, various invasive and non-invasive techniques monitor the patient's cardiovascular, pulmonary, and fluid balance. Prior to the craniotomy portion of the operation, CSF diversion may be required with either ventriculostomy or spinal drain placement to allow for drainage of the fluid during the case.

The craniotomy procedure begins with skin preparation, administration of antibiotics, and the placement of drapes in an aseptic manner. Injection of local anesthetic with epinephrine is then given to help postoperative pain and intraoperative skin bleeding. Epidural hemostasis is critical to the prevention of postoperative epidural hematoma formation.

Medical Management of the Surgical Patient, ed. Michael F. Lubin, Thomas F. Dodson, and Neil H. Winawer. Published by Cambridge University Press. © Cambridge University Press 2013.

A bulging or tense dura mater, a sign of raised intracranial pressure (ICP), is commonly seen during brain tumor surgery. Management of this raised ICP is accomplished with a variety of techniques done simultaneously or in succession. These include elevation of the head to promote venous drainage; confirmation that head position is not restricting the patency of the venous system in the neck; hyperventilation to reduce intracranial blood volume; mannitol or other fast-acting diuretic infusion to decrease cerebral edema; or CSF drainage.

The dura is then incised in a manner that allows for re-approximation at the end of the procedure. Extra-axial tumors are now visible and accessible for removal. Intra-axial tumors that are seen on the cortical surface can be accessed through an incision in the pia and arachnoid overlying the tumor. Identification of safe regions and trajectories for removal of deep intrinsic tumors can be aided by image-guided neuronavigation and intraoperative ultrasonography as well as neuromonitoring with SSEP (somatosensory evoked potential), MEP (motor evoked potential), BAER (brainstem auditory evoked potential), and cortical mapping. These techniques maximize accuracy while helping to preserve highly functional regions of the brain during surgery.

Tumor extirpation is carried out in one of two ways: (1) inside-out method for more interdigitated tumors, or (2) outside-in for those tumors with well-delineated borders. Initial tissue samples are delivered to the pathology department for frozen section analysis. This will provide preliminary results on the type and grade of tumor that will aid the surgical team to individualize the extensiveness of surgical treatment, depending on tumor size and location, age of the patient, and response of the suspected tumor to adjunctive therapies.

When the tumor resection is completed, meticulous hemostasis is obtained and the wound is gently irrigated. The dura mater is then re-approximated and the bone reattached to the skull defect. The soft tissues of the head are closed and a wound dressing is placed as a final means of closure.

Usual postoperative course
Expected postoperative hospital stay
The expected postoperative hospital stay is 1–2 days in the ICU and 1–3 days in a step-down/floor unit.

Operative mortality
Immediate operative mortality is an extremely rare occurrence due to advances in surgical safety and technique, as well as proper anesthesia support. The 30-day mortality for patients with tumors is also rare (less than 5%). Improved short- and long-term outcomes have been demonstrated in institutions with experienced surgeons, dedicated intensive care teams, and collaborations with experienced medical, radiation oncology, and medical oncology teams. Thirty-day mortality is heavily dependent on the medical comorbidities and extent of the patient's systemic tumor, as well as the tumor type, size, and location.

Special monitoring required
The intense monitoring needed by the postoperative craniotomy patient for the first 12–24 hours is provided in the ICU. Early signs of neurologic decompensation (which can be secondary to many different causes) are monitored. Also, the patient receives a higher level of continuous monitoring of cardiac rhythm, blood pressure, volume status, and neurologic function. Expeditious intervention with vasoactive compounds, cardiac supplements, volume resuscitation or other infusions can be facilitated, if necessary. Intracranial pressure monitoring can also be done, and CSF drainage with ventriculostomy or lumbar drainage must be monitored with the assistance of higher-acuity trained nursing staff. Finally, if continuous electroencephalography is desired, more sophisticated technologies as well as skilled staff for the treatment of seizure activity are available.

Patient activity and positioning
Controlled patient activity is desired early postoperatively; early controlled mobilization decreases the incidence of pneumonia, deep venous thrombosis, pulmonary embolism, and hospital-acquired skin breakdown and ulcers. Some limitations to early and aggressive mobilization may be present secondary to the patients' level of consciousness and the presence of a ventricular or lumbar drain. In these patients, as long as there is no contraindication, the head of the bed should be maintained at 30°. Mobilization in the early postoperative period, however, can be accomplished in nearly all patients with the assistance of nursing staff, physical therapists, occupational therapists, and speech therapists.

Alimentation
Nutritional administration is provided as soon as safely possible in the postoperative period. It is initiated with the tolerance of simple clear liquids, and advanced aggressively to a full regular diet as soon as it can be safely tolerated. In surgery for tumors of the brainstem and around the lower cranial nerves (CN IX, X, and XII), formal swallowing evaluation and/or direct visualization of the vocal cords is required prior to the initiation of diet to assess swallowing function and thus prevent aspiration. For those patients who cannot coordinate swallowing function and protect their airway, parenteral or direct gastric feeding is required. It must be stressed that early nutritional support is required for recovery and healing following surgery.

Antibiotic coverage
Antibiotic coverage against gram-positive organisms of the skin flora administered within 30 minutes of skin incision decreases the incidence of wound infection. Continued antibiotics for the 24-hour postoperative period are

surgeon-specific based on the complexity and duration of the case, implantable devices and drains, and quality of skin at skin closure. Antibiotic-impregnated ventriculostomy catheters may decrease the likelihood of developing postoperative infection of this catheter with or without systemic antibiotic prophylactics. Prophylactic systemic antibiotics may be beneficial in cases of continued invasive intracranial or intraspinal monitoring or in patients at risk for infection secondary to suboptimal skin closure, patients who have had previous cranial radiotherapy, or those who are immunosuppressed.

Medications

Few neuromodulating medications need to be considered in the perioperative and postoperative period. Due to cytokine influence on cerebral vasculature causing vasoactive cerebral edema, high-dose corticosteroids may be needed preoperatively as well as in the immediate postoperative period. While the patient is on corticosteroids, the need for GI prophylaxis must be considered. Strict glucose control is advantageous in the treatment of the neurologically injured patient. Cerebral edema is exacerbated by surgical manipulation and this may continue to worsen for the first 3–5 days postoperatively. After this time, steroids are tapered off as tolerated by the patient. Continued corticosteroid therapy may be needed for those patients with continued clinically significant cerebral edema and those who will need to undergo postoperative radiotherapy. The goal once the cerebral edema improves is to discontinue corticosteroid therapy completely, because chronic corticosteroid therapy has many toxicities. Preoperative anticonvulsant therapy is needed only when the patient has a history of seizure activity, and should be continued postoperatively based on the discretion of the treating surgeon. In cases in which cerebral manipulation occurs, a short course of anticonvulsants is used to prevent early postoperative seizure activity that could be devastating to patients who had recently undergone a craniotomy for tumor. The anticonvulsant should be started intravenously while the patient is in the operating room and may need to be continued intravenously postoperatively based on the level of consciousness of the patient. Early transition to an oral agent is recommended. Tight blood pressure control is also needed, especially in the early postoperative period to prevent hematoma formation.

Postoperative complications

In the hospital

In all stages, patient safety must be considered, and special consideration must be paid to all complications. CNS-tumor patients tend to be older and may have other chronic comorbidities including cardiac, pulmonary, renal, or immune dysfunctions. Attempts to mobilize patients early and to remove any unessential indwelling tubes, catheters, and wires will help prevent the development of a host of postoperative complications. While a complete list of possible postoperative medical complications following surgery for a CNS tumor is beyond the scope of this chapter, the following complications are among the most common.

Hemorrhage

Postoperative intracerebral and other types of intracranial hemorrhages can be associated with a number of potential neurologic complications including death. Hemorrhage in this patient population is most likely secondary to bleeding from the tumor bed and can happen immediately or in the early postoperative period. Hypertension either from arousal from anesthesia or from uncontrolled chronic hypertension can also increase the risk of developing postoperative hemorrhages. Aggressive control of blood pressure will help avoid this potential complication. In specific cases, postoperative hematomas may require further intervention with CSF diversion or direct decompression and evacuation. This is determined by the type of hemorrhage and the amount and location of mass effect and dysfunction due to the hemorrhage. Placement of an intracranial parenchymal or ventricular monitor may be necessary to determine the regional or global intracranial pressure on a continuous basis, and to detect early rises in intracranial pressure.

Infection

Prevention of infection of the surgical site, an early risk for increased mortality, requires pre- and perioperative antibiotics. Long-term prophylactic antibiotics are not recommended unless clinically warranted for an individual patient. Infections can occur deep within the cerebral tissue, superficially in the scalp or anywhere in between. These infections can give rise to cerebritis, intracerebral abscess, ventriculitis, subdural empyema, meningitis, epidural abscess, osteomyelitis of the bone flap, subgaleal effusion, cellulitis or infection of implanted hardware/monitoring tools. Signs and symptoms of infection include fever, swelling/pain/erythema/drainage of the wound, headache, mental status changes, and new focal neurologic deficit. Treatment is based on identification of the offending (or likely) organism and antibiotic therapy. Specimens for microbiology analysis may come from superficial wound drainage, but a low threshold should be maintained to utilize surgical methods to obtain samples, debride wounds, and remove devitalized tissue. Techniques used in this circumstance may include needle aspiration or open craniotomy. When there is direct contact between purulent tissue and craniotomy flaps or devascularized tissue, removal of this at-risk tissue may be necessary. In cases where the surgeon believes the infection is less intense, other less aggressive measures should be employed that can preserve the use of the autologous bone. Long-term antibiotics are likely needed for anything more than a simple scalp infection.

Cerebral edema

Postoperative cerebral edema has several possible etiologies. It can be the result of vasogenic edema associated with the tumor itself, the normal physiologic response to direct surgical manipulation of brain tissue, or the interruption of brain arterial or venous supply. In the most severe cases it can cause mass effect on the central gray matter of the brain or the brainstem causing dysfunction and death of these areas. Cerebral edema can be monitored initially by neurologic exam including assessing the degree of swelling of a craniectomy site, if present. In select cases where intracranial pressure monitors are in place, these can be used to detect the early signs of increased cerebral edema. In patients where significant edema is suspected, imaging modalities with CT or MRI will often show worsening edema and mass effect. Treatment options are aimed at decreasing intracranial pressure by decreasing blood flow to the brain and increasing blood return to the heart (hyperventilation, avoidance of hypervolemia, elevation of the head of the bed), osmotic effect to pull excess fluid from the brain (mannitol, hypertonic saline, diuretics) or stabilization of cerebral vasculature and the blood–brain barrier (corticosteroids). Careful consideration is needed when using hyperventilation. Excessive hyperventilation can cause significant vascular constriction which may lead to ischemic events in the brain. When hypertonic saline or diuretics are being used, it is important to prevent excessive dehydration that can lead to impairment of microvascular flow as well as impairment of renal and cardiac function. While these medications are being used, serum osmolality and sodium concentrations are routinely monitored to prevent the previously mentioned complications. When questions about the overall fluid status arise, central venous access is indicated.

Cerebral infarction

Interruption of either the arterial blood supply or venous drainage can cause infarction. Disruption of the arterial supply will impair or destroy the brain tissue in a specific distribution which will impair the function of that region of the brain. It is important to note that damage to even a seemingly small artery of the brain stem can cause a devastating outcome that may even be lethal. In contrast, the venous tributaries can typically drain large amounts of brain tissue. Damage or occlusion of these vessels can also cause an extensive and devastating infarct. Low oxygenation due to hypotension, hypoperfusion, anemia and/or acutely low hematocrit may exacerbate cerebral infarction. Thus careful monitoring and control of these factors before, during, and after surgery are required.

Seizures

Seizure threshold is decreased with irritation of the cerebral cortical surface. This can be from either direct tumor invasion of the cerebral cortex or from iatrogenic effects due to surgical scars obtained by resection of subcortical tumors. Seizures can be detrimental to brain tissue during surgery and in the immediate postoperative phase. Seizures can raise the intracranial pressure, cause temporary hypoxia, or induce hemorrhage in the tumor resection cavity. Anticonvulsant therapy is usually started prior to surgery or during surgery and continued on a scheduled basis afterwards. The choice of agent varies by surgeon. The duration of treatment varies based on the seizure risk of the patient, though it is typically continued for at least 1–2 weeks postoperatively. In those patients with a documented seizure, the anticonvulsant should be continued for at least 6 months postoperatively and tailored to their specific needs thereafter.

Associated fluid and electrolyte imbalances

Brain tumors of, or adjacent to, the hypothalamus and pituitary gland pose specific problems with hormonal secretions. One of the main concerns in these patients is fluid and electrolyte imbalances that can be attributed to abnormal secretion of antidiuretic hormone (ADH) such as SIADH or DI. Other hormonal imbalances may occur, and are treated with the appropriate replacements. Fluid and electrolyte balances deserve special mention here in light of the high-dose corticosteroid therapy in this patient population. Corticosteroids can cause fluid imbalances that lead to third spacing and soft tissue fluid retention. The degree of these effects varies based on each patient and should be carefully monitored and adjusted accordingly.

Cerebrospinal fluid leakage

Diminished absorption of cerebrospinal fluid (CSF) can occur following tumor resection secondary to tumor debris, blood products, or high CSF protein content. It may also occur due to diminished venous outflow, by occlusion or thrombosis of the cerebral venous system. Diminished absorption can manifest as hydrocephalus in the patient with intact CNS coverings, or as a CSF fistula in those without an intact covering. In patients who do not have a watertight dural closure at the time of surgery, CSF will find the path of least resistance and drain through the scalp (CSF fistula), the paranasal sinuses (CSF rhinorrhea), or the mastoid sinuses (CSF otorrhea). Persistent drainage of CSF is a major concern, with the potential of developing lethal meningitis from the persistent leak. Therapy is initiated with non-surgical means, including elevation of the head. Bedside procedures include lumbar drain placement in patients without elevated intracranial pressure, or ventriculostomy drain placement for those with elevated intracranial pressure. In recalcitrant cases, surgical obliteration of the CSF fistula may be required with the use of permanent CSF diversion, often in the form of a ventriculoperitoneal shunt.

After discharge

Each of the above-mentioned complications can also occur following discharge from the hospital. However, delayed hemorrhage, fluid and electrolyte imbalance due to new anatomic changes, and true cerebral infarction are unusual.

Infection

The risk of postoperative wound infection, meningitis and brain abscess is increased in this patient population. This is often secondary to immunocompromise due to the effects of the tumor, chronic corticosteroid therapy, or prior chemotherapy and/or radiation therapy. All these factors can retard wound healing, leaving the wound at risk for contamination, with skin flora being the etiology of the most common organisms. Signs of infection include progressive fever, wound erythema, tenderness and swelling, or any new neurologic deficit that cannot be explained. In patients suspected of having an infection, CT or MRI scans with and without contrast can help identify the extent of the process.

Cerebral edema

Early corticosteroid weaning, as tolerated, should be the goal following tumor resection. This is to help prevent the complications associated with long-term use. In some instances, tapering of corticosteroids is accompanied by neurologic changes ranging from headache and nausea to neurologic deficits and mental status changes. This may be secondary to residual or progressive edema and can be confirmed by cerebral imaging with either a CT or MRI scan. Other possible causes of delayed increase in cerebral edema include tumor recurrence, infectious etiologies, venous occlusion, or impaired venous drainage. In patients with worsening edema secondary to premature taper of corticosteroids, increasing the corticosteroid dose and avoidance of overhydration should quickly reverse symptoms. Close attention needs to be directed to monitoring electrolytes and blood glucose and to treating these abnormalities efficiently, as needed.

Hydrocephalus

As can be seen in the early postoperative course, ventricular enlargement with neurologic changes can develop in a delayed fashion. Hydrocephalus can develop from tumor itself, hemorrhage, broken-down byproducts of tumor or hemorrhage, or from surgical scarring. Signs and symptoms of hydrocephalus range from headache, nausea and vomiting to new neurologic deficits, mental status changes, and obtundation. Treatment includes CSF diversion.

Cerebrospinal fluid leakage

Delayed development of a CSF fistula can occur. The effects of radiation therapy, chemotherapy, and corticosteroid treatment can lead to wound breakdown. If this does occur, particular attention is needed to assure that there is not an associated CNS infection that needs to be treated with temporary CSF diversion and appropriate antibiotics. Active wound or CNS infection is a contraindication to placement of a permanent indwelling diversion catheter. In this situation, temporary diversion can be accomplished. Once the infection is controlled, permanent diversion can be accomplished.

Tumor recurrence

Despite aggressive surgery, radiation, and chemotherapy, all but the completely benign, surgically excised tumors inevitably recur and progress. This is seen most prominently in malignant primary brain tumors. Recurrence itself is not a complication; however, the onset of a new neurologic deficit from recurrence can initially be mistaken as a complication of therapy. Thus it is important to thoroughly investigate neurologic changes with the proper neurologic examinations, laboratory studies, and imaging. Tumor recurrence appears to be most associated with tumor histology (type and grade), patient's age, degree of surgical excision, and performance status at the time of presentation. Once recurrence has been documented, decisions for recovery therapy with reoperation, alternative forms of radiation and new chemotherapy should be made under the counsel of a comprehensive neuro-oncology team composed of neurosurgery, radiation oncology, and medical oncology. In the most devastated patients with irreversible neurologic injury, simple supportive care or hospice may be the most altruistic decision.

Further reading

Berger MS, Hadjipanayis CG. Surgery of intrinsic cerebral tumors. *Neurosurgery* 2007; **61**: S279–304; discussion S304–5.

Kalkanis SN, Kondziolka D, Gaspar LE et al. The role of surgical resection in the management of newly diagnosed brain metastases: a systematic review and evidence-based clinical practice guideline. *J Neurooncol* 2010; **96**: 33–43.

Legriel S, Marijon H, Darmon, M et al. Central neurological complications in critically ill patients with malignancies. *Intensive Care Med* 2010; **36**: 232–40.

Mikkelsen T, Paleologos NA, Robinson PD et al. The role of prophylactic anticonvulsants in the management of brain metastases: a systematic review and evidence-based clinical practice guideline. *J Neurooncol* 2010; **96**: 97–102.

Sawaya R, Hammoud M, Schoppa, D et al. Neurosurgical outcomes in a modern series of 400 craniotomies for treatment of parenchymal tumors. *Neurosurgery* 1998; **42**: 1044–55.

Chapter

103

Intracranial aneurysm surgery

Mark J. Dannenbaum, Sung Bae Lee, C. Michael Cawley, and Daniel L. Barrow

Data on the prevalence of intracranial aneurysms in the general population come from autopsy and from angiography series. A recent review found that the prevalence of intracranial aneurysms for adults without a history of subarachnoid hemorrhage (SAH) is approximately 2%, with a male to female ratio of approximately 1 to 1.3. The same analysis found that the prevalence of aneurysms increases with age, peaking in the 69–79 year age group. Nearly half of all intracranial aneurysms become symptomatic during the patient's lifetime, usually presenting as subarachnoid hemorrhage. In North America, approximately 28,000 cases of aneurysmal SAH occur each year, mostly in adults.

As opposed to fusiform aneurysms, which are encountered in the extracranial peripheral vasculature, intracranial aneurysms are typically saccular in morphology. Intracranial aneurysms possess a well-defined neck and sac distinct from the lumen of the parent vessel and are frequently located at proximal intracranial arterial branching points. Although the pathophysiology of intracranial aneurysms is controversial, they are thought to arise from defects (congenital or acquired) in the muscularis media. Once an aneurysm has developed, conditions such as hypertension and tobacco smoking will likely increase the risk of rupture, leading to SAH. Certain conditions (e.g., autosomal dominant polycystic kidney disease, Ehlers-Danlos syndrome type IV, Alpha-1 Antitrypsin Deficiency (A-1ATD)) are associated with the formation of cerebral aneurysms, presumably from the predisposition for the development of focal weak spots in vessel walls near arterial branch points.

Unruptured aneurysms are believed to bleed at varying rates according to multiple factors, including their diameter at the time of diagnosis. Although evidence suggests that intracranial aneurysms are less likely to bleed if they are less than 7–10 mm, both angiographic and direct intraoperative observational studies have demonstrated that even smaller aneurysms may rupture. About 40–50% of patients die within the first month as a result of the initial hemorrhage and its complications. Of those who survive, approximately 20% succumb to rebleeding in the ensuing 2 weeks (50% in 6 months)

if the aneurysms are not treated, with the highest rate of recurrent hemorrhage (4%) during the first 24 hours after initial rupture.

The most common presentation of intracranial aneurysms is the subarachnoid hemorrhage, which patients will classically describe as the worst headache of their lives. Nuchal rigidity and/or photophobia will often accompany SAH; nausea, vomiting, transient loss of consciousness, and neck stiffness with back pain are often associated conditions. In as many as 50% of cases, there may be a history of minor rupture or symptoms referable to the aneurysm, typically within the 2 weeks prior to the onset of SAH.

Less often, aneurysms may exert mass effect because of their location or size. A common example is an aneurysm of the posterior communicating artery that, by virtue of its intimate relationship with the oculomotor nerve, may expand and compress the latter, resulting in a partial or complete oculomotor nerve deficit. Rarely, a large aneurysm may accumulate thrombus, causing embolization and cerebral ischemia. Another less common although not infrequent presentation includes an ipsilateral optic neuropathy from a large or giant ophthalmic segment aneurysm producing mass effect on the optic nerve. Likewise a cavernous segment internal carotid artery (ICA) aneurysm, when quite large, may produce symptoms of mass effect on cranial nerves traversing the cavernous sinus. An ICA aneurysm can produce occulomotor, trochlear and abducens nerve palsies in addition to retro-orbital pain and facial pain. When medially directed and associated with thinning of the sphenoid bone, cavernous segment ICA aneurysms also may present with massive epistaxis.

After the initial history and physical examination, a noncontrast head CT is obtained to confirm the diagnosis of SAH or intracerebral hematoma. If performed within 48 hours of onset, a high-quality, contemporary, high-resolution CT scan can detect subarachnoid blood in about 95% of cases. When a negative CT scan is obtained but a strong suspicion of SAH exists, lumbar puncture should be performed. Xanthochromia of the cerebrospinal fluid (CSF), a hallmark of SAH, may be detectable within 6 hours after the hemorrhage.

Medical Management of the Surgical Patient, ed. Michael F. Lubin, Thomas F. Dodson, and Neil H. Winawer. Published by Cambridge University Press. © Cambridge University Press 2013.

Although CT angiography is increasingly utilized at many centers, the gold standard remains the four-vessel cerebral angiogram. Catheter-based angiography is the modality of choice to identify the aneurysm thought to be responsible for the hemorrhage and to search for multiple aneurysms, which occur in about 20% of cases.

The two major potential complications of aneurysmal SAH are rebleeding and cerebral arterial vasospasm, both of which are responsible for significant morbidity and mortality.

The incidence of rebleeding is estimated to be 4% in the first 24 hours and 1.5% per day over the next 13 days, although patients with worse neurologic status (graded by Hunt and Hess class; Table 103.1) may rebleed at higher rates. The major supporting argument for early operation in suitable patients is that the risk of rebleeding can be eliminated by prompt and definitive treatment of the aneurysm by either endovascular coiling or clip ligation.

Vasospasm, which usually manifests as mental status changes or a focal neurologic deficit 4–10 days following a subarachnoid hemorrhage, results from delayed arterial narrowing as a consequence of irritation of the outer walls of the cerebral vasculature. It usually becomes clinically apparent during this period of time as cerebral ischemia in 30–40% of patients. Patients with thicker collections and more diffuse patterns of subarachnoid hemorrhage on CT, particularly in the basal cisterns or major cerebral fissures, are at high risk for the development of vasospasm, and should be treated accordingly. Antifibrinolytic agents such as epsilon aminocaproic acid (Amicar), once widely used to reduce the risks of rebleeding, may also increase the risk of ischemic deficits caused by vasospasm. However, these antifibrinolytic agents

Table 103.1 Hunt and Hess Scale for subarachnoid hemorrhage.

Grade	Description
0	Unruptured aneurysm
1	Asymptomatic, mild HA, or nuchal rigidity
2	Cranial nerve palsy, moderate to severe HA, nuchal rigidity
3	Mild focal deficit, lethargy, confusion
4	Stupor, moderate to severe hemiparesis, early decerebrate
5	Rigidity, deep coma, moribund appearance

Add one point for serious systemic disease or severe vasospasm seen on arteriography

HA, headache.

are used selectively in some patients to reduce the risk of re-hemorrhage until definitive aneurysm treatment can be provided.

Vasospasm is treated by the deliberate induction of hypertension and hypervolemic hemodilution in an effort to augment cerebral blood flow and optimize cerebral perfusion. Nimodipine, a selective cerebral calcium channel antagonist, may improve long-term outcomes in patients at risk for vasospasm. This agent is given orally for 3 weeks and used only as a local cerebral vasodilator. Other pressors, if needed, are used to maintain a medically induced hypertension to optimize cerebral perfusion. Vasospasm in the proximal intracranial arteries that is refractory to medical therapy (such as intrathecal nicardipine placed in the patient's external ventricular drain (EVD)) may be treated by catheter-based techniques. These include direct intracranial, intra-arterial infusion of calcium channel blockers. In more extreme cases, transluminal intracranial angioplasty, which involves deploying a balloon in an affected proximal intracranial vessel, is used to mechanically augment flow. Angioplasty, however, should only be performed by an experienced neurointerventionalist. It is contraindicated, and should not be utilized, in patients with a recently ruptured and unsecured aneurysm.

Therapeutic intervention is dictated by the clinical condition of the patient as assessed by the classification of the Hunt and Hess Stroke Scale, which grades the severity of the patient's level of consciousness. If hydrocephalus is present on the admission CT scan and the patient is comatose, judicious blood pressure and intracranial pressure control by external ventricular drainage is done prior to definitive treatment. It must be determined whether poor admission neurological status is secondary to only hydrocephalus, or if it is due to brain injury secondary to elevated intracranial pressure. If the patient is older, has significant medical comorbidities, and presents with a higher Hunt and Hess grade, most practitioners would favor endovascular coil embolization to prevent subsequent aneurysmal rupture.

The timing of aneurysm surgery is controversial, and must be individualized. Patients with large intraparenchymal hematomas causing mass-effect and elevated intracranial pressure are more often considered candidates for craniotomy and clip ligation so that the hematoma can be simultaneously evacuated and, if necessary, hemicraniectomy can be performed to help control refractory elevated intracranial pressure. It has become fairly standard for patients who are not stuporous after initial stabilization (including treatment of hydrocephalus) to have surgical treatment as soon as feasible after SAH. The goal of surgical treatment is to achieve aneurysm obliteration and parent vessel preservation, thereby eliminating the risk of recurrent hemorrhage and allowing for the aggressive treatment of possible cerebral vasospasm. Patients who have poor neurologic function or have presented more than 4 days after the hemorrhage are more often treated by endovascular coil embolization rather than microsurgical clip ligation. This decision is due to a risk of worsening vasospasm that is associated with intracranial vascular manipulation.

During an operative microsurgical clip ligation, administration of mannitol and furosemide, maintenance of mild hyperventilation, and meticulous microsurgical cerebral cisternal dissection are used to relax the brain and minimize retraction injury. Direct surgical exposure of the aneurysm is accomplished by a traumatic dissection of the aneurysm and its parent vessels, after which one or more occlusive clips are placed across the neck or base of the aneurysm.

In the past, hypotensive anesthesia was used to reduce intraluminal pressure during dissection of the aneurysm, thereby decreasing the risk of intraoperative rupture. This technique has been surpassed by a more contemporary strategy of temporary clipping of afferent vessels during critical stages of dissection, carried out under moderate hypertension, mild hypothermia, and pharmacological cerebral protection with barbiturate-induced EEG-burst suppression which is performed by titrating the amount of barbiturate in order to achieve isoelectric intervals interrupted by bursts of 8–12 Hz electrical activity that diminish to 1–4 Hz prior to electrical silence in order to reduce the cerebral metabolic demand during periods of temporary ischemia.

At many centers, an intraoperative angiogram is performed before closure to confirm adequate clip placement and the patency of the parent vessel; otherwise, angiography is performed before patients are discharged from the hospital.

Over the past decade, endovascular therapy has evolved into an alternative treatment for selected aneurysmal SAH patients, particularly for patients with poor medical or neurological conditions. When the angioarchitecture of the aneurysm is favorable, endovascular neurosurgeons can access the lesion and tightly pack thrombogenic materials (usually platinum microcoils) into the aneurysm dome and neck while preserving parent vessel patency. This minimally invasive technique can markedly reduce the rebleeding rate in the acute phase of SAH. Endovascular therapy has some limitations, including uncertain durability and the necessity for long-term follow-up with angiography. Current endovascular techniques are not suitable for all aneurysms, and are dependent on the size, location, angioarchitecture, and presence of an intraluminal thrombus. When there is unfavorable geometry or aneurysm morphology, microsurgical clip ligation (instead of endovascular coiling) is the treatment of choice.

Usual postoperative course
Expected postoperative hospital stay

The usual postoperative hospital stay is at least 2 weeks for patients with SAH, and approximately 3–5 days for patients undergoing surgery for unruptured aneurysms. Patients treated by coil embolization for unruptured intracranial aneurysms are observed overnight in the ICU, and are usually discharged to home the next morning.

Operative morbidity

Morbidity following aneurysm treatment ranges from 1–10%, and is generally related to the patient's preoperative condition, the experience level of the operator and the modality of treatment. While complications may arise from either microsurgical clip ligation or coil embolization, most investigators generally agree that the accepted range for morbidity following the former modality ranges from 5–10%, with a range of 3–5% for the latter. Neurologic morbidity in clip ligation most often is due to perforating vessel injuries, and varies by aneurysm location. Morbidity from coil embolization is most often thromboembolic in nature and is determined by the amount of interface between the coil mass and the parent vessel. There is strong evidence that volume-outcome relationships exist for aneurysm surgery, with a strong correlation between high volume centers and positive outcomes.

Special monitoring required

Intensive care unit observation is necessary. For 48–72 hours, frequent assessment is taken of vital signs, neurologic status, intracranial pressure and intake and output, along with cardiac monitoring. Serial transcranial Doppler studies are conducted along with neurological examination to detect cerebral vasospasm in patients who have presented with SAH. If vasospasm is present, 10–14 days of ICU observation may be required.

Patient activity and positioning

All patients with suspected or documented elevated intracranial pressure should have the head of the bed elevated 30°. Patients may get out of bed and ambulate as soon as possible. The presence of an external ventricular drain does not prohibit the patient from ambulating; however, the drain should be clamped during the period of time the patient is out of bed. If physical therapy is needed, it should commence soon after surgery.

Alimentation

Food intake should be advanced as tolerated. Patients who are unable to eat or who require supplementation may be given nasogastric tube feedings.

Antibiotic coverage

No specific antibiotic coverage is needed in addition to the usual perioperative prophylactic doses. When external ventricular drainage (EVD) is required, frequent CSF surveillance is necessary for early detection of infection. Some EVD systems utilize an antibiotic impregnated design that incorporates antibiotic in the wall of the tubing. These systems may be left in place for long periods of time without the need for antibiotic prophylaxis.

Postoperative complications

In the hospital

Development of a focal neurologic deficit

Complications occur following treatment of intracranial aneurysms, both ruptured and unruptured. With microsurgical clip ligation, injury may be secondary to retraction edema or contusion from frontal and temporal lobe retraction, which may lead to infarction or damaged intracranial vessels or nerves. Focal deficits following coil embolization are usually the result of thromboembolic complications secondary to the interface of the coil mass and the parent artery blood flow. Immediately following either modality of treatment, aggressive investigation for treatable conditions should be conducted. If the patient is unable to follow commands for a prolonged period of time, a non-contrast head CT should be obtained and intracranial pressure should be monitored. Hyperosmolar therapy with mannitol or hypertonic saline administration, mild hyperventilation, and EVD should be used cautiously to treat intracranial hypertension.

Cerebral vasospasm may produce a focal deficit in a delayed fashion (usually, several days following a subarachnoid hemorrhage) as a result of decreased cerebral perfusion; it is detected by serial transcranial Doppler ultrasound. If cerebral vasospasm is suspected, hypervolemic hypertensive hemodilution treatment (triple-H therapy) should be instituted immediately. A formal catheter-based cerebral angiogram or CT angiogram should be obtained to confirm the diagnosis and to evaluate for possible transluminal angioplasty.

Subdural or epidural hematoma

Subdural or epidural hematomas may arise following craniotomy for aneurysm clipping. They are the result of inadequate intraoperative hemostasis or postoperative coagulopathy. In postoperative patients with neurological deterioration, subdural or epidural hematomas should be suspected when there is evidence of worrisome clinical symptoms such as mental status changes, headache, nausea, vomiting, or seizures that may be associated with increased intracranial pressure. A prompt neuroimaging evaluation can provide early detection of these problems. Appropriate surgical evaluation should minimize neurologic damage.

Acute hydrocephalus

Acute hydrocephalus results from the absence of either normal circulation or resorption of CSF by intraventricular or subarachnoid blood. Acute hydocephalus is usually evident preoperatively and should be managed by placement of an external ventricular drain. If the patient cannot be weaned from the EVD by raising the level of the drainage bag over an interval that is determined by the amount of subarachnoid blood, then the device is surgically implanted in a permanent fashion into a ventriculoperitoneal shunt (VPS). About 20% of patients who have early acute hydrocephalus with subsequent ventricular drainage may eventually require CSF drainage via a VPS.

Cardiac problems

In over 50% of cases, a subarachnoid hemorrhage may be associated with cardiac arrhythmia manifested by a wide variety of ECG changes. Occasionally, SAH may produce ECG abnormalities indistinguishable from an acute myocardial infarction ("stunned myocardium"). Most of these cardiac complications resolve spontaneously when the sympathetic surge that follows SAH subsides. Rarely, however, serious cardiac compromise may require invasive cardiac monitoring, inotropic agent use, and the avoidance of hyperdynamic therapy for vasospasm.

Hyponatremia

Hypovolemia and hyponatremia frequently follow SAH as a result of natriuresis and diuresis. Symptoms can include altered mental status or seizures, mimicking delayed cerebral ischemia from vasospasm. Hyponatremia is not routinely attributed to the syndrome of inappropriate antidiuretic hormone (SIADH) as is often the case in patients with central nervous system disorders. Frequently, urinary loss of sodium after SAH is found to contribute to the development of hyponatremia (cerebral salt wasting, CSW). The volume status of the patient is the key factor in differentiating CSW from SIADH since the former is treated with volume repletion, the latter with fluid restriction. In CSW, central venous pressure (CVP) is usually below 6 mmHg and the pulmonary capillary wedge pressure (PCWP) usually less than 8 mmHg, whereas in SIADH these parameters are within normal limits or even slightly elevated. However, routine laboratory values in both conditions may be very similar, with the only difference evident in the patient's volume status. In CSW, the patient is hypovolemic, while in SIADH, the patient is either euvolemic or hypervolemic.

Seizures

Although seizure activity that can be treated with antiepileptic medication is often observed in the acute phase of SAH, it rarely becomes a chronic condition. There is no evidence of benefit from prophylactic use of anticonvulsants. Therefore, medication can be tapered off shortly after recovery if the patient remains seizure-free.

After discharge

Chronic hydrocephalus

Chronic hydrocephalus is typically due to impaired CSF absorption. Acute hydrocephalus occurs in most patients with aneurysmal SAH, but only about 20% develop chronic hydrocephalus requiring a VP shunt. If patients do not reach expected rehabilitation goals or even experience deterioration, efforts should be made to identify the possibility of chronic hydrocephalus or shunt malfunction.

Recurrence

With demonstration of surgical aneurysmal obliteration by appropriate intraoperative or postoperative angiograms, recurrence is extremely rare. Some patients may be predisposed to developing de novo intracranial aneurysms, especially if they have conditions known to be associated with aneurysms, e.g., autosomal dominant polycystic kidney disease, fibromuscular dysplasia, and other connective tissue disorders. For aneurysms occluded with endovascular embolization, serial angiographic and clinical follow-up is essential as recurrence is more common. However, with the advent of newer coiling adjunctive techniques such as stent-assisted coiling and balloon-assisted coil embolization, aneurysmal packing densities are greater and recurrences are becoming less common.

Further reading

Bakker NA, Metzemaekers JDM, Groen RJM, Mooij JJA, Van Dijk JMC. International subarachnoid aneurysm trial 2009: endovascular coiling of ruptured intracranial aneurysms has no significant advantage over neurosurgical clipping. *Neurosurgery* 2010; **66**: 961–2.

Brisman JL, Song JK, Newell DW. Cerebral aneurysms. *N Engl J Med* 2006; **355**: 928–39.

Crowley RW, Medel R, Dumont AS *et al.* Angiographic vasospasm is strongly correlated with cerebral infarction after subarachnoid hemorrhage. *Stroke* 2011; **42**: 919–23.

Dankbaar JW, Rijsdijk M, van der Schaaf IC *et al.* Relationship between vasospasm, cerebral perfusion, and delayed cerebral ischemia after aneurysmal subarachnoid hemorrhage. *Neuroradiology* 2009; **51**: 813–19.

Ferns SP, Sprengers MES, van Rooij WJ *et al.* Coiling of intracranial aneurysms: a systematic review on initial occlusion and reopening and retreatment rates. *Stroke* 2009; **40**: e523–9.

Jun P, Ko NU, English JD *et al.* Endovascular treatment of medically refractory cerebral vasospasm following aneurysmal subarachnoid hemorrhage. *AJNR Am J Neuroradiol* 2010; **31**: 1911–16.

Kim GS, Amato A, James ML *et al.* Continuous and intermittent CSF diversion after subarachnoid hemorrhage: a pilot study. *Neurocrit Care* 2011; **14**: 68–72.

Lefournier V, Krainik A, Gory B *et al.* Perfusion CT to quantify the cerebral vasospasm following subarachnoid hemorrhage. *J Neuroradiol* 2010; **37**: 284–91.

Meyer R, Deem S, Yanez ND *et al.* Current practices of triple-H prophylaxis and therapy in patients with subarachnoid hemorrhage. *Neurocrit Care* 2011; **14**: 24–36.

Molyneux A, Kerr R, Stratton I *et al.* International Subarachnoid Aneurysm Trial (ISAT) of neurosurgical clipping versus endovascular coiling in 2143 patients with ruptured intracranial aneurysms: a randomised trial. *Lancet* 2002; **360**: 1267–74.

Pierot L, Barbe C, Spelle L. Endovascular treatment of very small unruptured aneurysms: rate of procedural complications, clinical outcome, and anatomical results. *Stroke* 2010; **41**: 2855–9.

Raper DMS, Allan R. International subarachnoid trial in the long run: critical evaluation of the long-term follow-up data from the ISAT trial of clipping vs coiling for ruptured intracranial aneurysms. *Neurosurgery* 2010; **66**: 1166–9; discussion 1169.

Taylor CJ, Robertson F, Brealey D *et al.* Outcome in poor grade subarachnoid hemorrhage patients treated with acute endovascular coiling of aneurysms and aggressive intensive care. *Neurocrit Care* 2011; **14**: 341–7.

Wiebers DO, Whisnant JP, Huston J *et al.* Unruptured intracranial aneurysms: natural history, clinical outcome, and risks of surgical and endovascular treatment. *Lancet* 2003; **362**: 103–10.

Winn HR, Richardson AE, O'Brien W, Jane JA. The long-term prognosis in untreated cerebral aneurysms: II. Late morbidity and mortality. *Ann Neurol* 1978; **4**: 418–26.

Yee AH, Burns JD, Wijdicks EFM. Cerebral salt wasting: pathophysiology, diagnosis, and treatment. *Neurosurg Clin N Am* 2010; **21**: 339–52.

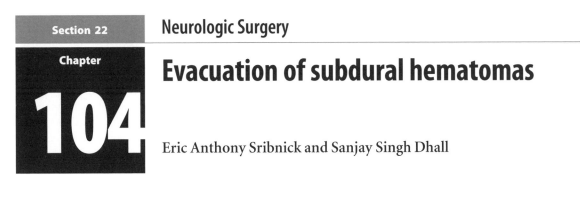

Evacuation of subdural hematomas

Eric Anthony Sribnick and Sanjay Singh Dhall

The meningeal layers covering the brain consist of an outermost layer (the dura mater), a middle layer (the arachnoid membrane), and an inner layer (the pia mater). Between these layers are potential spaces where fluid can collect. Hemorrhage above the dura is called an epidural hematoma. Hemorrhage below the dura is called a subdural hematoma (SDH), and hemorrhage below the arachnoid membrane is called subarachnoid hemorrhage. Bleeding within brain tissue itself is called intraparenchymal hemorrhage, and bleeding into the ventricles is intraventricular hemorrhage. The prognosis and management of these findings are different, so misnomers such as "head bleed" should be avoided when describing an intracranial hemorrhage. Subdural hematomas can grossly be divided into acute, subacute, and chronic. The duration of an acute hematoma is less than 3 days; that of subacute hematoma is from 3–20 days. A chronic hematoma persists for more than 21 days.

Acute subdural hematoma

Historically, the occurrence of acute SDH has been posited to be due to tearing of the bridging veins. This condition can often result from the direct extension of bleeding from a lacerated or contused brain. The most common reported causes of acute SDH are motor vehicle collisions, falls, and assault. This type of injury is seen 3–5 times more often in males than in females; median age is generally in the 40s. As compared with patients with epidural hematoma, patients with acute subdural hematoma are more likely to have associated parenchymal damage and a higher morbidity and mortality. An important category of subdural hematoma patients are those on anticoagulation therapy. Patients taking anti-coagulants are at risk for intracranial hemorrhage following low-impact injuries such as ground level fall or low-velocity motor vehicle collision. Furthermore, in this patient population, SDH often develops spontaneously and without evidence of antecedent trauma.

Preoperative care

Patients with SDH need to be stabilized prior to any neurosurgical procedure. Airway management should be the first priority. Patients requiring intubation should be induced with medications less likely to raise intracerebral pressure (ICP), such as etomidate and vecuronium. Intravenous lidocaine can be given to blunt the transient rise in ICP seen with laryngeal stimulation during intubation. Ventilation should be performed with a goal of normal ventilation. Routine hyperventilation should be avoided as it may lead to decreased cerebral perfusion. Temporary hyperventilation can be used in emergency situations, such as evidence of brain herniation.

Access should include an arterial line and two large-bore venous lines or a central venous line. Basic labs should be obtained, including complete blood count, basic metabolic panel, and coagulation studies. If the patient has a history of antiplatelet therapy, a platelet function assay should be sent. If surgical evacuation seems likely, the patient should be typed and crossed for 2–4 units of packed red blood cells. Patients can be treated with either dilantin or levetiracetam for the first 7 days post-injury to prevent early post-traumatic seizures.

Neurosurgical intervention

Recent surgical guidelines for acute SDH recommend surgical evacuation for hematoma width greater than 10 mm or resultant brain shift greater than 5 mm. Other indications for surgery include an altered neurological exam, acute neurological decline, and increased intracerebral pressure. Additional factors to consider are location of the hematoma, age, and medical comorbidities.

Prior to surgery, prophylactic antibiotics are given (2 g of nafcillin or cefazolin). Surgery for acute SDH generally consists of a craniotomy with incision of the dura and evacuation of the hematoma. Effort is made to find and control the site of bleeding. Once the bleeding has been controlled and the hematoma is removed, the decision is made whether to replace the craniotomy bone flap. If the surgeon notes excessive brain edema after evacuation, the bone flap may be removed altogether and stored either in the patient's abdominal adipose tissue or in a freezer.

One option for asymptomatic, smaller acute SDH is to delay surgery and re-evaluate the patient weeks after the initial presentation. In some cases, the hematoma may resolve; in other cases, the delay allows the clotted blood to break down into liquified hematoma, which can be drained with one or two small burrholes.

Postoperative care

Following evacuation of an acute SDH, the patient will require ICU care with frequent neurological exams. The key tenets for patient management are the prevention of hypoxia, hypotension, and increased intracerebral pressures. Patients should be weaned from the ventilator as soon as possible to avoid complications, but the main goal of therapy should be to keep P_aO_2 above 60 mmHg and oxygen saturation above 90%. Because many of these patients will be neurologically compromised, they may require aggressive pulmonary toilet to avoid pneumonia. For acute SDH patients, the head of bed should be at 30–40° to reduce the risk of pneumonia and to lower ICP.

Deep vein thrombosis (DVT) is a concern in neurologically compromised patients; however, there may be some concern regarding the possible risk of intracranial hemorrhage with the use of perioperative DVT chemoprophylaxis. A recent study showed that, in 287 patients treated with chemoprophylaxis for DVT within 48–72 hours of admission, only 1 patient had hemorrhage expansion while 21 had evidence of DVT. At our institution, all neurotrauma patients wear sequential compression devices. If the hemorrhage is stable on repeat imaging, chemoprophylaxis is started within 48 hours of injury or surgery.

Hypotension should be avoided. There is evidence correlating poorer outcomes with multiple episodes of systolic blood pressures (SBP) below 90 mmHg. Episodes of hypotension may have a greater negative impact than hypoxemia. Fluid resuscitation is the initial treatment for hypotension in the neurotrauma patient.

Hypotonic fluids should be avoided as they can contribute to cerebral edema. Isotonic or hypertonic fluids may be used. If the SBP does not respond to fluid resuscitation, there should be no hesitation in using vasopressors. Permissive hypertension is reasonable, and there are no definitive guidelines for treating elevated blood pressures. At our institution, intravenous calcium channel blockers and beta-blockers are frequently used to maintain a systolic blood pressure less than 160 mmHg. In patients with concomitant hypertension and bradycardia, elevated ICP should be ruled out. Blood pressure is also relevant to brain perfusion, and cerebral perfusion pressure (CPP) should dictate blood pressure goals. The CPP is equal to the mean arterial pressure (MAP) minus the intracerebral pressure (i.e., $CPP = MAP - ICP$). The CPP goal should be 60 mmHg, and CPP less than 50 mmHg may correlate with poorer outcomes.

Patients with severe traumatic brain injury (i.e., Glasgow Coma Scale (GCS) score of 8 or less) require a brain-pressure monitoring device. The use of a ventriculostomy to drain cerebrospinal fluid allows both for monitoring and treatment of elevated ICP. Maintaining ICP at less than 20 mmHg is associated with improved outcome; patients with a subdural hematoma should be treated aggressively to maintain ICP below this threshold. While a comprehensive review of intracerebral pressure management techniques is beyond the scope of this chapter, ICP control begins with simple measures such as raising the head of the bed and straightening the patient's neck to improve venous outflow from the brain. Sedation and hyperosmolar therapies can also be used to control ICP. While there are few current data to support the use of hypothermia, hyperthermia should be avoided. Surface cooling or intravenous cooling catheters can be used to maintain normothermia. For patients with ICP refractory to more conservative measures, paralytics (e.g., vecuronium) and barbituate-induced coma can be used.

To prevent recurrence of the subdural hematoma, sometimes a closed-system drain is left in the subdural space after evacuation. These drains generally remain in place for 24–48 hours and are removed when output is minimal.

The metabolic rate in traumatic brain injury (TBI) patients may be as high as 200% of the normal value; this elevated rate may persist for 30 days post-injury. Because of these findings, every effort should be made to promote enteral nutrition in these patients as soon as possible. Ideally, patients would be meeting their protein-calorie requirements through enteral nutrition, but if this is not possible, then parenteral nutrition should be considered so that all nutritional requirements are met within 7 days of injury. Patients with TBI are known to have an increased incidence of gastrointestinal ulcers ("Cushing's ulcers"). Administration of an H2 blocker or proton pump inhibitor may decrease the incidence of clinically relevant ulcers.

Chronic subdural hematoma

The term chronic subdural hematoma denotes a collection of blood beneath the dura that develops over a longer period of time, giving the brain the length of time needed to accommodate a mass lesion. The brain is displaced by the hematoma. However, the hematoma may become quite large before becoming symptomatic, especially if the patient has cerebral atrophy. Patients with chronic SDH tend to be older. These patients often have a remote history of multiple falls or may present with no definite history of trauma. Chronic SDH likely begins with a smaller acute SDH, which is asymptomatic. The acute blood breaks down, forming pseudo-membranes with neovascularization. These membranes can exude proteinaceous and/or sanguinous fluid. If resorption does not occur, this fluid slowly builds up over time until the brain is displaced to such a degree that symptoms such as headache, altered mental status, or seziure can occur.

Preoperative care

Preoperative management is similar to that of acute SDH. However, when chronic SDH is found incidentally in a largely asymptomatic patient and the lesion causes (exhibits) little radiographic change, monitoring will not need to be as aggressive as that for acute SDH. Any coagulopathy should be treated, and the patient should be placed on seizure prophylaxis.

Neurosurgical intervention

In general, chronic SDH is treated surgically if the patient is symptomatic or if the lesion is large enough to cause significant mass effect or shift. Because chronic SDH is due to entrapped blood that has undergone liquefaction, these lesions can often be managed by saline irrigation through burr holes. If there are loculations within the hematoma, the patient may require more aggressive management, with a larger craniotomy for evacuation. While the choice of intervention is the surgeon's preference, many leave a drain in the subdural space to avoid recurrence.

Postoperative care

Postoperative care for chronic SDH is similar to that of acute SDH. One notable difference is that many clinicians prefer that chronic SDH patients are kept flat in bed for 24–48 hours. Postoperative supine positioning is thought to help the brain to expand back into the subdural space, reducing the risk of hematoma reaccumulation.

Usual postoperative course

The postoperative course can be quite variable, and can depend on the degree of neurological damage and the contribution of any other associated injuries. Prognosis for both acute and chronic SDH correlates with preoperative GCS and age. Patients over 60 have a significantly poorer outcome. The prognosis for chronic SDH tends to be much better than for acute SDH.

Postoperative complications

Recurrence of hematoma

Hematoma recurrence is more common with chronic SDH than with acute SDH. Immediate postoperative scanning is generally done only if a patient has a neurological change, but a head CT is often done several weeks after craniotomy to rule out recurrence.

Seizure

Many clinicians place SDH patients on a 1-week course of prophylactic anti-epileptic medications to avoid early post-traumatic seizures. Later post-traumatic seizures may occur weeks to years after the initial trauma. Post-traumatic seizure should be viewed as a new-onset seizure and treated accordingly.

Infection

A wide range of infections can occur postoperatively, and neurologically debilitated patients are especially at risk. Simple wound infections can occur and may eventually involve deeper tissues if not treated appropriately. Intracerebral abscess or meningitis can occur postoperatively. Subdural empyema, with spread of infection through the hematoma, can also occur and is a neurosurgical emergency. Cortical venous thrombosis can occur if the empyema is left untreated. Any signs of postoperative infection deserve a thorough work-up.

Intracerebral hemorrhage

A postoperative intracerebral hemorrhage can occur spontaneously after SDH, and this complication is thought to be due to local brain hyperemia following removal of the mass lesion. This complication is more common in older patients with chronic SDH.

Hydrocephalus

This can be one cause of postoperative headaches and altered mental status. Hydrocephalus should be considered in any postoperative SDH patient who presents with a declining neurological examination.

Pneumocephalus

A small amount of air underneath the craniotomy site is common postoperatively; if it is thought to be contributing to neurological symptoms, treatment is by administration of 100% F_iO_2 for 24 hours. Simple pneumocephalus should be differentiated from tension pneumocephalus, which may require neurosurgical intervention.

Electrolyte imbalance

Patients with TBI may have a variety of electrolyte disturbances. Hyponatremia may be due to the syndrome of inappropriate antidiuretic hormone (SIADH) hypersecretion or to cerebral salt-wasting syndrome (CSWS). Hypernatremia may occur as a result of central (neurogenic) diabetes insipidus. Post-traumatic clinical changes (e.g., altered mental status, polyuria) should prompt investigation and appropriate treatment.

Further reading

Brain Trauma Foundation. The American Association of Neurological Surgeons. The Joint Section on Neurotrauma and Critical Care. Management and prognosis of severe traumatic brain injury. Part 2: Early indicators of prognosis in severe traumatic brain injury. *J Neurotrauma* 2000; **17**: 559–627.

Bullock MR, Povlishock JT. Guidelines for the management of severe traumatic brain injury. Section XIV: Hyperventilation. *J Neurotrauma* 2007; **24**: S87–90.

Bullock MR, Povlishock JT. Guidelines for the management of severe traumatic brain injury. Section XIII: Antiseizure prophylaxis. *J Neurotrauma* 2007; **24**: S83–6.

Bullock, M.R., Povlishock, J.T. Guidelines for the Management of Severe Traumatic Brain Injury. Section IX: Cerebral Perfusion Thresholds. *J Neurotrauma* 2007; **24**: S59–S64.

Bullock MR, Chesnut R, Ghajar J *et al.* Surgical management of acute subdural hematomas. *Neurosurgery* 2006; **58**: 16–24.

Dudley RR, Aziz I, Bonnici A *et al.* Early venous thromboembolic event prophylaxis in traumatic brain injury with low molecular-weight heparin:

risks and benefits. *J Neurotrauma* 2010; **27**: 2165–72.

Eisenberg HM, Frankowski RF, Contant CF, Marshall LF, Walker MD. High-dose barbiturate control of elevated intracranial pressure in patients with severe head injury. *J Neurosurg* 1988; **69**: 15–23.

Farahvar A, Gerber LM, Chiu YL. Response to intracranial hypertension treatment as a predictor of death in patients with severe traumatic brain injury. *J Neurosurg* 2011; **114**: 1471–8.

Foley N, Marshall S, Pikul J *et al.* Hypermetabolism following moderate to severe traumatic acute brain injury: a systematic review. *J Neurotrauma* 2008; **25**: 1415–31.

Jones PA, Andrews PJD, Midgley S *et al.* Measuring the burden of secondary insults in head-injured patients during intensive care. *J Neurosurg Anesth* 1994; **6**: 4–14.

Manley G, Knudson MM, Morabito D *et al.* Hypotension, hypoxia, and head injury: frequency, duration, and consequences. *Arch Surg* 2001; **136**: 1118–23.

McHugh GS, Engel DC, Butcher I *et al.* Prognostic value of secondary insults in traumatic brain injury: results from the IMPACT Study. *J Neurotrauma* 2007; **24**: 287–93.

Zhang W, Li S, Visocchi M, Wang X, Jiang J. Clinical analysis of hyponatremia in acute craniocerebral injury. *J Emerg Med* 2010; **39**: 151–7.

Chapter

105

Stereotactic procedures

Osama N. Kashlan, David V. LaBorde, and Robert E. Gross

As in all fields of surgery, the current trend in neurosurgery is towards less-invasive procedures and the shorter hospital stays that result from them. Therefore, stereotactic techniques are an indispensable tool for the modern neurosurgeon and have been dramatically improved by the recent revolution in digital image guidance technology. These techniques provide a relatively straightforward, accurate, and safe method to approach intracranial targets that are defined by either anatomical or functional characteristics. Anatomically defined targets include brain tumors and abscesses, as well as other structural lesions. Targeting for anatomical disorders relies entirely on patient-specific anatomy derived from radiographs (e.g., ventriculography, rarely used today) or tomograms (e.g., CT, MRI) for localization. In addition, functional imaging modalities (e.g., fMRI), metabolic imaging modalities (e.g., positron emission tomography (PET)), and MR spectroscopy can be utilized in conjunction with other imaging modalities to help with target planning and visualization. Functionally defined structures include the various nuclei of the basal ganglia and thalamus that are targeted for pain and movement disorders (e.g., Parkinson's disease, essential tremor, and dystonia), as well as other conditions such as obsessive-compulsive disorder. Targeting for functional disorders typically combines computerized imaging with intraoperative electrophysiological mapping for localization, although anatomical techniques can be used alone as well.

Stereotactic brain biopsy – a purely diagnostic tool that does not allow for tumor resection – has been used increasingly during the past decade to aid in the diagnosis and treatment of intracranial lesions. Stereotactic brain biopsy is successful in providing a definitive pathologic diagnosis in 85–98% of patients, with low associated morbidity. Using differing approaches and angles, this procedure is used in characterizing lesions in both non-functional and functional areas of the brain, including the brainstem. Historically, full stereotactic frames have been used but these are increasingly being supplanted by so-called "frameless" techniques. In frame-based procedures, on the day of surgery the patient undergoes a contrast-enhanced imaging study (MRI or CT) following the

attachment to the cranium of the stereotactic base ring and localizer under either local anesthesia and sedation or general anesthesia. General anesthesia is used in uncooperative children, patients with altered mental status, or for patient comfort. In the operating room, a burr hole or twist drill hole is made, through which the biopsy is performed. The procedure is markedly facilitated by the use of neuronavigational computer workstations. Frameless navigational technology – which has diagnostic yield, morbidity and mortality similar to standard frame-based methods – can be significantly less cumbersome. When using frameless technology, typically a reference frame that is tracked must be fixated to the patient's head, usually through a head clamp (and thus is not truly "frameless"). This usually necessitates general anesthesia. Burr hole-mounted guidance tools have also become available. Generally, immediate feedback from an experienced neuropathologist is obtained from the initial specimen prior to the completion of the procedure. Therapeutic measures may also be performed simultaneously, such as aspiration of a cyst or abscess with possible instillation of antibiotics for abscesses or interstitial brachytherapy for specific tumors. The procedure typically lasts less than an hour, after which the patient is transferred to the post-anesthesia care unit. Prior to leaving the unit, a postoperative computerized tomogram (CT) scan is performed in patients who present with new-onset neurological deficits, seizures, or altered consciousness when compared with baseline. Routine postoperative scanning of patients is no longer universally accepted because of visualization of many asymptomatic hemorrhages that might otherwise spontaneously regress.

Deep brain stimulator (DBS) electrode implantation in the basal ganglia and thalamus has supplanted radiofrequency ablation as the therapeutic technique of choice for movement disorders such as Parkinson's disease and tremor (except in some developing regions of the world). These procedures are for symptomatic relief to improve the patient's quality of life, but are not curative. Targeting of the contralateral internal segment of the globus pallidus, subthalamic nucleus, and thalamus has been approved for Parkinson's disease, tremor, and

Medical Management of the Surgical Patient, ed. Michael F. Lubin, Thomas F. Dodson, and Neil H. Winawer. Published by Cambridge University Press. © Cambridge University Press 2013.

dystonia. Overall, deep brain stimulation is a non-destructive and reversible procedure as it produces a functional rather than a structural lesion when compared with ablative procedures such as thalamotomy or pallidotomy. As with brain biopsies, the patient arrives on the day of operation and undergoes a CT or MRI after the stereotactic base ring and localizer are applied; some centers still perform stereotactic ventriculography. Alternatively, imaging can be performed prior to the day of surgery, and co-registered to a stereotactic study on the day of the procedure (although at least one frameless approach involves rapid manufacture of a customized frame which attaches to previously implanted fiducial screws, eliminating the need for day-of-procedure imaging).

The operative procedure is generally done under local anesthesia in the operating room, but in some cases (e.g., dystonia) general anesthesia can be used. A pre-coronal burr hole is performed along a trajectory chosen to avoid veins, sulci, and the ventricle. The initial target is localized by identifying its spatial coordinates in a stereotactic atlas, using indirect references to brain landmarks (anterior and posterior commissures), and/or by direct MR identification. The target is expressed as a set of intraoperative stereotactic coordinates. After opening the dura, electrodes are passed to the initial target to perform intraoperative electrophysiological confirmation while the patient is awake, although not all centers use this technique. Fine adjustments to the initial position are performed as necessary. After this is completed, a DBS lead is implanted. However, even today the target is occasionally ablated using radiofrequency electrocoagulation (e.g., thalamotomy, pallidotomy, subthalamotomy). Stimulation testing for adverse effects and clinical benefits is crucial before and/or after DBS implantation. The overall procedure takes several hours. The pulse generator for the implanted electrode is implanted in the ipsilateral chest wall just below the clavicle, either on the same day or later, along with the extension wire which is tunneled subcutaneously. Postoperatively, the patient is transferred to the post-anesthesia care unit, where a postoperative MRI or CT scan is performed to ensure proper placement of hardware and to rule out intracerebral hemorrhage prior to being transferred to the ward. Similar procedures are being investigated for functional disorders other than Parkinson's disease, such as obsessive-compulsive disorder, depression, and pain.

Stereotactic radiosurgery uses ionizing radiation to eradicate – with minimal exposure to adjacent brain tissue – certain brain tumors, arteriovenous malformations, and a number of functional disorders. Radiating a more select region offers the flexibility to apply stronger doses of radiation to target tissue while at the same time minimizing tissue injury in adjacent regions. Stereotactic radiosurgery can be performed invasively or non-invasively. Invasive radiosurgery follows stereotactic brain biopsy, and typically involves interstitial brachytherapy where radioactive isotopes are placed for a specific amount of time into certain brain tumors. Another investigational form of invasive radiosurgery involves a miniature X-ray generator that is placed stereotactically after biopsy and delivers a single fraction of high-dose irradiation within minutes to small, spherical metastatic brain tumors. Both invasive and non-invasive stereotactic radiosurgery are performed using the frame-based approach described above and under local anesthesia.

Usual postoperative course

Expected postoperative hospital stay

One to 2 days.

Operative mortality

Less than 1%.

Special monitoring required

If the patient is monitored in the post-anesthesia care unit for 1–4 hours with a postoperative scan that was reviewed prior to transfer to the ward, ICU observation is usually unnecessary.

Patient activity and positioning

Initially, the head of the bed is elevated to 30°. Patients may get out of bed as soon as possible. Physical therapy is instituted if required.

Alimentation

A full, regular diet is provided as soon as possible.

Antibiotic coverage

Typically, intravenous antibiotics are given intraoperatively and 24 hours postoperatively.

Medications

Parkinson's disease medications are held after midnight if the pulse generator is to be programmed the following day.

Postoperative radiographic tests

Postoperative brain computed tomographic scan or magnetic resonance image in the post-anesthesia care unit is performed for all patients undergoing stereotactic ablation and deep brain stimulator electrode implantation prior to transfer to the ward. Stereotactic biopsy patients are scanned only if they present with new-onset neurological deficits, seizures, or altered consciousness when compared with baseline.

Postoperative complications

Postoperative complications can become apparent either immediately postoperatively, within hours, or after discharge. According to one study, liver cirrhosis is a risk factor for the occurrence of complications. Medical history of malignancy, diabetes, hypertension, chronic lung diseases, and renal diseases are not considered additional risk factors for the development of complications.

Surgeon preference and hospital resources are the main factors that determine whether frameless or frame-based techniques are used in stereotactic biopsy because both have comparable complication rates. In addition, according to one study, there is no increased incidence of neurological decline in patients whose lesions were in the thalamus, basal ganglia, or deep structures compared with patients whose lesions were in superficial structures. No correlation was found between the number of needle passes made when performing the biopsy and the rate of patient neurologic decline.

In the hospital
Development of a focal neurologic deficit

This complication may be related to hemorrhage, edema, infarction, or accidental passage of needle. The diagnosis is confirmed by an emergent head computed tomographic scan. Hemorrhage is a potentially life-threatening complication, and it usually results from bleeding along the surgical pathway and can lead to formation of an intracranial hematoma. In addition, bleeding may occur into the subarachnoid, ventricular, subdural, epidural, or subgaleal spaces. Selected hematomas or subdural or epidural collections may require surgical evacuation or placement of an external ventricular drainage system. Cerebral edema (swelling of the brain) may result from surgical manipulation of the brain parenchyma, or as an anesthesia complication caused by elevated carbon dioxide due to respiratory depression. Treatment includes hyperventilation, hyperosmolar therapy, furosemide, and possible placement of an intracranial pressure monitoring device or external ventricular drainage system. Cerebral infarction is potentially lethal if the arterial supply to the brain is compromised, placing that particular brain tissue at risk. An extensive infarction may also occur if venous drainage is interrupted or occluded. Care is taken to control blood pressure, volume status, and oxygenation to maintain cerebral perfusion pressure.

Seizure

A seizure that occurs intraoperatively or in the immediate postoperative period may lead to increased intracranial pressure. Thus, antiepileptic medications should be given immediately to stop the seizure, followed by routine maintenance doses for approximately 3–6 months. An emergent head computed tomographic scan should be performed to rule out possible intracranial pathology such as hemorrhage, though seizures can result from intracranial air.

Neuroleptic malignant syndrome

Parkinson's disease patients undergo operations in the "off medication" condition, which can be associated with a typical neuroleptic malignant syndrome. This must be recognized early and is treated with antiparkinsonian medication, fluid resuscitation, and/or dantrolene sodium, as necessary.

Air embolus

Air embolism is a rare, immediate complication that occurs when using a semi-sitting position in certain approaches, such as transcerebellar approach for brainstem lesion biopsy. When this complication becomes a concern in the operating room, the patient is repositioned and an alternative approach is used. Moreover, using a twist drill instead of a drill bit may minimize the risk of an air embolus because of the smaller incision made when using a twist drill.

After discharge
Infection

Infections may be superficial or deep. Skin erosions or cellulitis may be treated with appropriate oral or intravenous antibiotics, but severe infections may also require surgical debridement. Although rare, deep septic contamination may cause such potentially life-threatening complications as meningitis, cerebritis, intracerebral abscess, or subdural or epidural empyema. Treatment includes intravenous antibiotics, surgical debridement for abscesses, and possible hardware removal.

Sterile subcutaneous fluid collections

Postoperative subcutaneous fluid collections from CSF leaks or seromas can occur weeks to months after surgery. Leaks of CSF require surgical repair, and one should be suspicious of hydrocephalus, a known complication of stereotactic procedures. Sterile seromas may be drained by needle aspiration and seldom require surgical intervention.

Other device-related or stimulation-related deep brain stimulation complications

Hardware failure may be due to electrode or extension wire breaks, migration of the electrode, or pulse generator malfunction, all of which can be evaluated and repaired surgically. Adverse effects related to the stimulated target and its vicinity are common and expected. Stimulation of the internal segment of the globus pallidus may induce visual field disturbance, paresthesia, muscle contractions, confusion, and depression; stimulation of the thalamus may provoke paresthesia, muscle cramps, decreased fine motor skills, dysarthria, dizziness, and balance disturbances; and stimulation of the subthalamic nucleus may generate dyskinesia, dysarthria, paresthesia, eyelid-opening apraxia, hemiballismus, confusion, and changes in mental status. In the vast majority of instances, careful adjustments of stimulation parameters and reduction in medications will reverse these side-effects.

Further reading

Air EL, Leach JL, Warnick RE, McPherson CM. Comparing the risks of frameless stereotactic biopsy in eloquent and noneloquent regions of the brain: a retrospective review of 284 cases. *J Neurosurg* 2009; **111**: 820–4.

Chen CC, Hsu PW, Erich Wu TW *et al.* Stereotactic brain biopsy: single center retrospective analysis of complications. *Clin Neurol Neurosurg* 2009; **111**: 835–9.

Chernov MF, Muragaki Y, Ochiai T *et al.* Spectroscopy-supported frame-based image-guided stereotactic biopsy of parenchymal brain lesions: comparative evaluation of diagnostic yield and diagnostic accuracy. *Clin Neurol Neurosurg* 2009; **111**: 527–35.

Dammers R, Haitsma IK, Schouten JW *et al.* Safety and efficacy of frameless and frame-based intracranial biopsy techniques. *Acta Neurochir (Wien)* 2008; **150**: 23–9.

Hariz MI. Complications of deep brain stimulation surgery. *Mov Disord* 2002; **17**: S162–6.

Jain D, Sharma MC, Sarkar C *et al.* Correlation of diagnostic yield of stereotactic brain biopsy with number of biopsy bits and site of the lesion. *Brain Tumor Pathol* 2006; **23**: 71–5.

Kulkarni AV, Guha A, Lozano A, Bernstein M. Incidence of silent hemorrhage and delayed deterioration after stereotactic brain biopsy. *J Neurosurg* 1998; **89**: 31–5.

Pantazis G, Trippel M, Birg W, Ostertag CB, Nikkhah G. Stereotactic interstitial radiosurgery with the Photon Radiosurgery System (PRS) for metastatic brain tumors: a prospective single-center clinical trial. *Int J Radiat Oncol Biol Phys* 2009; **75**: 1392–400.

Perez-Gomez JL, Rodriguez-Alvarez CA, Marhx-Bracho A, Rueda-Franco F. Stereotactic biopsy for brainstem tumors in pediatric patients. *Childs Nerv Syst* 2010; **26**: 29–34.

Umemura A, Jaggi JL, Hurtig HI *et al.* Deep brain stimulation for movement disorders: morbidity and mortality in 109 patients. *J Neurosurg* 2003; **98**: 779–84.

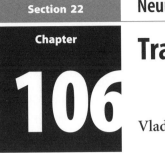

Chapter

106

Transsphenoidal surgery

Vladimir Dadashev and Nelson Oyesiku

Transsphenoidal surgery is the surgical approach of choice in treatment of sellar and parasellar tumors. The pathologies include pituitary adenomas, craniopharyngiomas, meningiomas, Rathke's cysts, chordomas, or, rarely, infectious etiologies and autoimmune disorders. The most common indication for transsphenoidal surgery is a pituitary adenoma that originates from the anterior lobe of a pituitary gland. The anterior lobe secretes prolactin (PRL), adrenocorticotropic hormone (ACTH), growth hormone (GH), thyroid-stimulating hormone (thyrotropin) (TSH), luteinizing hormone (LH), and follicle-stimulating hormone (FSH). Pituitary adenomas can be divided by size into microadenomas (< 1 cm) and macroadenomas (> 1 cm). Pituitary adenomas are also classified as clinically functioning (hyper-secreting, endocrine active) or as non-functioning (no hormone secretion, inactive). Patients can present with symptoms due to mass effect: headaches, visual deficits, cranial nerve neuropathies, and hydrocephalus or endocrine disturbance from hormone hypersecretion or hypopituitarism. The hypersecretory symptoms include amenorrhea-galactorrhea and infertility (hyperprolactinemia); Cushing's disease and hypercortisolism (ACTH); gigantism or acromegaly (GH); and thyrotoxicosis (TSH). Less common presentations of pituitary adenomas occur in association with certain endocrine syndromes (e.g., multiple endocrine neoplasia). In addition to recording the patient history and conducting a physical exam, the diagnostic evaluation for the majority of patients should include obtaining endocrine laboratory and MRI results (especially dynamic pituitary sequences). The main indication for treatment of these tumors is to re-establish normal hormonal secretion and to address the mass effect. The current treatment modalities include transsphenoidal surgical resection, medical management, and radiotherapy.

As our understanding of the physiology and pathophysiology of the hypothalamic-pituitary-end organs (e.g., thyroid, adrenal, gonads) has evolved, medical options have emerged for treatment alternatives for some of the functioning pituitary adenomas, the most common of which are prolactinomas. Currently, prolactinomas are primarily managed medically. The hypothalamic release of dopamine inhibits hypophyseal

prolactin secretion, so dopaminergic-agonists have been developed (i.e., bromocriptine, cabergoline) to suppress prolactin secretion. Approximately 80% of patients with prolactinomas are controlled by medical therapy alone with a resultant normalization of prolactin and significant tumor shrinkage. The treatment is lifelong as agents are tumorstatic; withdrawal of the therapy will lead to tumor re-growth. Another drawback of the dopamine agonist treatment is that it causes tumor scarring and fibrosis, which can make any possible surgery much more difficult. Tumor fibrosis usually occurs in about one year after initiating treatment; therefore, early surgical intervention is preferred if the patient elects to proceed with surgery because of personal preference, management failure, or drug side-effects (headache, dizziness, nausea, postural hypotension).

Similarly, medications have been developed for the treatment of growth hormone (GH) secreting adenomas. Pituitary GH activity is inhibited by hypothalamic somatostatin release; for this reason, somatostatin agonists (i.e., octreotide, lanreotide) are effective in treating patients with acromegaly. Furthermore, a peripheral GH receptor analog (Pegvisomant) that is now available functions by competing for the binding receptor site, leading to decreased IGF-1 secretion. Treatment with somatostatin analogs leads to tumor shrinkage and hormonal normalization in about 50–60% of patients. However, patients on GH receptor analogs must be carefully observed for potential tumor growth, since there is significantly elevated GH activity during treatment (even though IGF-1 levels are suppressed). In cases of incomplete response to medication or cost considerations, many of these patients choose surgical treatment. Medical treatment of GH-secreting adenomas is important as an adjuvant treatment option for incomplete resections or invasive tumors.

There is currently no effective, definitive medical treatment for patients with Cushing's disease, but many agents can be used as adjuvant therapy. Currently, there are three lines of treatment: adrenal glucocorticoid synthesis inhibitors, which inhibit different steps in the metabolic pathway (these agents include ketoconazole, metyrapone, mitotane, and

Medical Management of the Surgical Patient, ed. Michael F. Lubin, Thomas F. Dodson, and Neil H. Winawer. Published by Cambridge University Press. © Cambridge University Press 2013.

aminoglutethimide); a class of glucocorticoid receptor antagonists (e.g., mifepristone); and a class of hypothalamic neuromodulators, which decrease ACTH release (e.g., bromocriptine, octreotide, and cyproheptadine (a serotonin receptor agonist)). All of these agents, especially the steroid synthesis inhibitors, have significant side-effect profiles and are poorly tolerated.

Thyroid-stimulating hormone-secreting adenomas are rare and are usually invasive. Medical treatment is limited. The options include octreotide (a somatostatin analog that downregulates TSH release), anti-thyroid medications, and beta-blockers (for symptom control).

No pharmacologic agents exist for other lesions of the sellar and parasellar region. Steroids are given primarily in the perioperative period in cases when mass effect or vasogenic edema is present.

A transsphenoidal route is the surgical approach of choice in reaching the sellar and parasellar region. There are several variations of the transsphenoidal approach: transseptal (through the septum), sublabial (under the superior lip), or transnasal (through the nostril). The operation can be performed using the microscope or the endoscope (2D or 3D endoscopes are available). Anatomically, the approach leads into the sphenoid sinus, passing through the nasal spaces (or nostrils). The sphenoid sinus is a midline structure right under the anterior skull base. The sella is located in the superior posterior aspect of the sphenoid sinus; it is a recognizable landmark. An arachnoid layer with the surrounding brain cerebrospinal fluid spaces roofs the sella. The optic nerve lies superiorly on either side of the sella. Laterally, on each side of the sella, are the internal carotid arteries. They are essential landmarks and should be carefully identified to avoid injury. An operating microscope or endoscope is required for appropriate visualization, illumination, and magnification. General anesthesia is required and patients are positioned supine with the head in either a 3-point Mayfield fixation or on a horseshoe headrest. Localization can be confirmed with C-arm fluoroscopy or image-guidance (CT or MRI). Lumbar drain placement may be indicated when a CSF leak occurs (for diversion) or when arachnoid manipulation is needed (e.g., to reach suprasellar compartments). The length of surgery is usually 1–3 hours, depending on the pathology treated, the complexity of the lesion, and the extent of the resection. The parasellar and extended or combined approaches usually require more time and dissection, as well as more elaborate skullbase CSF leak reconstructions. If the lesion or the related anatomy is unfavorable for a transsphenoidal approach, transcranial or combined approaches should be considered.

The surgical indication for non-functioning adenomas is a mass effect on the optic pathways with a visual field cut or other compromise on surrounding neural structures. For functioning adenomas, the indication is hormonal over-secretion and mass effect. If a patient presents with hypopituitarism, preoperative hormonal supplementation (especially with levothyroxine and hydrocortisone) and perioperative stress steroids are indicated. About 3–8% of patients with adenomas present with pituitary apoplexy, with abrupt headaches and symptoms from mass effect and endocrine malfunction. The pathogenesis is usually tumor necrosis or hemorrhage with a sudden increase in sellar pressure. These patients usually require urgent surgical attention. Postoperatively, comprehensive hormonal screening is performed; fluid balance is closely monitored and any deficiencies are supplemented. Patients should be carefully examined for signs and symptoms of CSF rhinorrhea.

The goal of surgery for any lesion is gross-total resection or at least significant decompression of neural structures. In functioning adenomas, hormonal normalization is crucial. Long-term data show good microadenoma remission rates for Cushing's disease (up to 70–94%) and acromegaly (70–80%). The tumor control rates are lower for patients with macroadenomas or recurrences.

The role of radiotherapy as an adjunct treatment for sellar and parasellar tumors has grown significantly. Radiotherapy provides an additional modality in treatment. Two primary modes of radiotherapy exist: fractional stereotactic radiotherapy (FSR) and stereotactic radiosurgery (SRS). Fractional stereotactic radiotherapy is usually administered in small fractionated doses (over 4–5 weeks) and is usually administered for invasive large tumors (especially those extending into the cavernous sinus). Fractionation minimizes the risk of radiation-induced injury. Radiosurgery is administered in one dose/session, with the target usually being small residual tumors located away from critical neural structures (optic pathways, hypothalamus). The therapeutic response may take months to years. Radiosurgery for residual functioning tumors has a good outcome, with hormonal normalization seen in 50–66% of patients with Cushing's disease and 20–50% of patients with acromegaly. One side-effect of SRS and FSR radiotherapy is hypopituitarism, which occurs in 13–56% of patients. Newer FSR protocols have been developed that allow for dose fractionation that leads to better tumor control and decreased risk profile. In addition to adenomas, patients with meningiomas and craniopharyngiomas can be controlled with radiation.

Postoperative complications
In the hospital
Hormonal

Diabetes insipidus (DI) can occur as the result of pituitary stalk or posterior lobe injury, and may require medical intervention. Fluid balance is closely monitored and sodium levels are monitored; when appropriate, Pitressin should be administered. Transient DI can occur in up to 10% of patients; if it persists, patients should be transitioned to DDAVP (Desmopressin) supplementation. Also, patients should be evaluated for hypocortisolism; hydocortisone supplementation should be considered if needed.

Cerebrospinal fluid rhinorrhea

The major complications are uncommon ($< 1\%$). Cerebrospinal fluid (CSF) rhinorrhea (up to 5%) can occur and is usually managed by lumbar drain placement. Conditions that persist require surgical intervention.

After discharge

Hormonal imbalances may occur and may require hospitalization and long-term medical supplementation. Delayed CSF leaks may occur months after an operative procedure.

Further reading

Alleyne CH, Barrow DL, Oyesiku NM. Combined transsphenoidal and pterional craniotomy approach to giant pituitary tumors. *Surg Neurol* 2002; **57**: 280–390.

Buchfelder M, Schlaffer S. Surgical treatment of pituitary tumours. *Best Pract Res Clin Endocrinol Metab* 2009; **5**: 677–92.

Gandhi CD, Christiano LD, Eloy JA, Prestigiacomo CJ, Post KD. The historical evolution of transsphenoidal surgery: facilitation by technological advances. *Neurosurgery* 2009; **27**: E8.

Greenberg M. *Handbook of Neurosurgery.* 7th edn. New York, NY: Thieme Medical Publishers; 2010.

Oyesiku NM, Tindall GT. Endocrine-inactive adenomas: surgical results and prognosis. In Landolt AM, Vance ML, Reilly PL, eds. *Pituitary Adenomas.* New York, NY: Churchill-Livingstone; 1996, pp. 377–83.

Oyesiku NM, Tindall GT. Management of hypersecreting pituitary tumors. In Tindall GT, Cooper PR, Barrow DL, eds. *The Practice of Neurosurgery.* Baltimore, MD: Williams & Wilkins; 1996, pp. 1135–52.

Pituitary Surgery. *Neurosurg Clin N Am* 2003; **14**(1): 1–180.

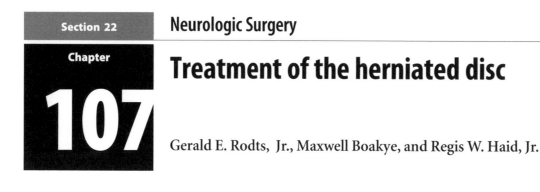

Gerald E. Rodts, Jr., Maxwell Boakye, and Regis W. Haid, Jr.

Herniated discs usually occur in the cervical and lumbar spine. The thoracic spine is relatively non-mobile due to the attached rib cage and therefore is less commonly affected by disc herniations. Herniated discs typically occur in younger patients between ages 30 and 50 years and present primarily with appendicular pain (radicular pain of arm, leg) as well as axial pain (mechanical pain of neck, back). Cervical and thoracic discs may present with myelopathy due to spinal cord compression or radiculopathy from nerve root compression. Sometimes, a combination of myelopathic and radiculopathic symptoms is present. The majority of patients with a disc herniation obtain relief with conservative treatment. Herniated discs are the initial manifestations of the continuum of degenerative disc disease that is later manifested by dehydration of disc material, loss of disc space height, associated facet joint arthropathy, and the development of osteophytes.

Cervical level

Patients with cervical disc herniation typically present with arm and periscapular pain, and often with weakness, numbness, or paresthesias in a nerve root distribution. The majority of patients improve with non-surgical therapeutic options such as cervical collar immobilization rest, non-steroidal anti-inflammatory or corticosteroid medications, traction, and physical therapy. Sometimes epidural steroid injections or foraminal steroid injections are helpful. Typically, patients with troublesome symptoms that do not resolve with these non-surgical measures and that persist beyond 6 weeks–3 months are considered to be candidates for surgery. Patients with significant weakness or sensory loss may opt for surgery sooner.

Central and paramedian cervical disc herniations are treated via an anterior approach. Lateral or foraminal disc herniations can be treated by either an anterior or a posterior cervical approach. Anterior cervical discectomy and fusion is the most common procedure performed for cervical disc herniations. After disc removal, the surrounding vertebral bodies are fused together using a variety of fusion substrates such as autologous iliac crest bone, allograft fibula or iliac crest

or patellar bone, or synthetic fusion implants (also known as "cages") made from materials such as titanium, poly-ether ether ketone (PEEK), ceramic, carbon fiber, etc. Studies have shown that using an allograft alone leads to fusion in approximately 90% of patients. The addition of a cervical plating system increases the fusion rate to 96%. Although adding a plating system raises the cost of the operation, it may allow for faster return to work and can obviate the use of a postoperative collar. Very high rates of fusion associated with the off-label use of bone morphogenetic protein (BMP) have been reported by multiple authors in the peer-reviewed literature. Soft-tissue swelling has been reported in some patients who receive BMP inside a fusion device or bone graft; this adverse condition appears to be dose-related and/or related to the degree of containment of the product within the fusion implant.

Dynamic artificial disc replacements are now available in the USA for single-level disc surgery. These implants appear to work best in patients with soft disc herniations who do not have advanced spondylytic (degenerative) changes such as osteophyte formation, disc space collapse, or facet arthropathy.

Anterior cervical discectomy

Patients are placed supine after general endotracheal intubation has been established. An incision is made that typically extends from the midline to the medial border of the sternocleidomastoid muscle. The medial border of the sternocleidomastoid muscle is identified and the platysma is divided horizontally or vertically to gain access to the loose areolar tissue located medially between the midline strap muscles and lateral to the carotid sheath. The prevertebral fascia is dissected with finger or by blunt sponge or scissor dissection. Radiographs are then taken to confirm the spinal level of interest and the disc is removed with curettes and rongeurs back to the depth of the posterior longitudinal ligament. This ligament is usually removed to allow inspection of the epidural space and dura. Foraminotomies are completed by removal of the medial bone of uncovertebral joints just overlying the nerve root bilaterally. These joints located laterally between two vertebrae can become overgrown with

Medical Management of the Surgical Patient, ed. Michael F. Lubin, Thomas F. Dodson, and Neil H. Winawer. Published by Cambridge University Press. © Cambridge University Press 2013.

osteophytes (bone spurs) causing exiting nerve root compression. A bone graft or synthetic cage is then placed. Plating with screw fixation may be added. If a decision is made to use an autograft, an incision should be made in the anterior iliac crest approximately two fingerbreadths lateral to the anterior superior iliac spine. The dissection is carried to the bone and the graft is removed using a double oscillating saw and bone cutter. The graft site is then closed.

Posterior cervical discectomy and foraminotomy

The posterior cervical discectomy and foraminotomy procedure can be considered for patients with lateral or foraminal disc herniation. Cervical laminoforaminotomy may be performed for patients with foraminal disc herniation and also for patients with cervical spondylosis and foraminal osteophytes or narrowing. Patients with lateral or foraminal soft disc herniations will require removal of the herniated fragment following laminoforaminotomy. Posterior discectomy/foraminotomy is done under general anesthesia with the patient in a prone or sitting position. The head is supported in a Mayfield head clamp. A midline or paramedian incision can be made depending on the surgeon's preference. Standard technique involves opening of the deep fascia and retraction of the paraspinal muscles laterally using a retractor. Dissection is continued until the facet joint and lateral masses are well-visualized. A radiograph or fluoroscopic image is obtained to confirm the cervical level. High-speed drills/Kerrison rongeurs and curettes are used to perform a foraminotomy and to expose the nerve root. Following gentle mobilization of the nerve root, the herniated fragment is then removed by working within the nerve root axilla and/or above the shoulder of the nerve root. This procedure also can be carried out with a less-invasive approach that employs a tubular retractor to bluntly divide the muscle fibers, rather than laterally pulling them off the laminar periosteum. The disc is removed through the tubular retractor using specially designed microinstruments. Many surgeons employ either surgical loupe magnification or the operating microscope.

Usual postoperative course

Expected postoperative hospital stay

The expected postoperative hospital stay is 1–2 days. Some patients are able to leave the same day following either an anterior cervical discectomy and fusion or a posterior laminoforaminotomy with discectomy.

Operative mortality
Rare.

Special monitoring required
None.

Patient activity and positioning
Patients can be out of bed and ambulatory as soon as tolerated. Postoperative X-rays may be desired when grafting and plating are performed (anterior surgery).

Alimentation
Diet is advanced as tolerated.

Antibiotic coverage
Typically for 12–24 hours.

Follow-up
For patients who have undergone anterior cervical discectomy with fusion, follow-up is necessary for 1–2 years to evaluate fusion.

Postoperative complications
In the hospital
Spinal cord or nerve root injury

Spinal cord contusion or nerve root injury may occur during any step of the surgery, including drilling, ligament removal, disc removal or graft/cage placement. The risk of injury can be minimized by careful removal of the disc and posterior longitudinal ligament. In addition, the selected bone graft should be shorter than the depth of the disc space. Graft retropulsion may cause cord injury. Graft migration may be avoided by selecting an appropriate graft size, gently tapping the graft or cage into the disc space, and creating a snug fit.

Vertebral artery injury

Vertebral artery injury may result from aggressive lateral dissection or aggressive foraminotomies, particularly in patients with aberrant vertebral arteries. If an injury occurs, the bleeding should be stopped, an angiogram performed to assess the situation, and a decision made as to whether the artery may need to be occluded endovascularly. Persistent bleeding intraoperatively may require exposure of the vertebral artery proximally and distally to the injury and ligation with suture or vascular clips. The vertebral artery is fragile and difficult to repair. Primary repair has been described but may prove to be a challenge. Patients are often placed on aspirin or anti-platelet therapy postoperatively if the artery has been occluded, dissected, or embolized via endovascular techniques,

Wound hematoma

Soft tissue hematoma formation is a potentially serious complication. Its occurrence is heightened in patients with a history of aspirin use, occult bleeding disorder, or functional platelet disorder. Large symptomatic hematomas may obstruct a patient's trachea and require emergent intubation and surgical evacuation of the clot. The use of a postoperative drain may reduce the risk of postoperative hematoma; not all surgeons agree about its efficacy. Meticulous hemostasis at the time of initial surgical closure is obviously the best preventive measure.

Recurrent laryngeal nerve injury

The complication of recurrent laryngeal nerve injury leads to ipsilateral vocal cord dysfunction or paralysis and usually occurs as a result of retraction or initial dissection. Symptoms include hoarseness, dysphagia or food/fluid aspiration, and vocal cord fatigue. In any patient with previous anterior cervical spine or other neck surgery of any kind (e.g., spine surgery, thyroid surgery, lymph node dissection, etc.), a preoperative assessment of bilateral vocal cord function should be performed to assess the risk of bilateral vocal cord paralysis.

Carotid artery injury

Carotid artery injury is a rare complication that may result from retraction or manipulation, or during dissection for exposure.

Cerebrospinal fluid fistula

A cerebrospinal fluid leak can occur intraoperatively, and should be repaired or treated immediately. The dural rent may be sutured primarily, but this can be difficult due to the limited exposure and field of view in an anterior cervical discectomy procedure. Following a vertebrectomy, primary suturing may be more feasible for a dural tear and spinal fluid leak in the operative field. A cerebrospinal fluid leak can also be treated with the application of a fat or muscle graft or synthetic sealant tissue and fibrin glue with or without postoperative lumbar drainage.

Esophageal or tracheal injury

Esophageal or tracheal injury may be caused by retraction or dissection or from failure to adequately protect the esophagus. If this complication is recognized intraoperatively, the esophagus should be repaired with corresponding consultation of a general or thoracic surgeon to aid in repair. Delayed injuries may manifest as odynophagia, dysphagia, and mediastinitis, and should be evaluated urgently.

Airway compromise

Airway compromise, which may be a result of wound hematoma or laryngeal edema, is more likely to occur in obese patients. This complication should be recognized promptly, and the patient should be reintubated immediately. A CT scan and/or MRI of the patient's cervical spine should be obtained emergently.

After discharge

Discitis, graft infection, osteomyelitis

When infectious complications occur, appropriate radiological studies should be obtained, and the wound should be re-explored. Grafts or cages may be removed and/or replaced. The patient should be treated with 6–12 weeks of intravenous antibiotics. Protracted or new neck pain, night sweats, or early signs of non-union or endplate destruction on radiographic studies should alert the surgeon to a possible surgical site infection. Blood tests such as a C-reactive protein, sedimentation rate, and white blood count with differential are useful in diagnosis and treatment.

Graft extrusion, screw pullout, and plate abnormalities

These abnormalities typically present with dysphagia and require revision of the graft and/or plate. Posterior displacement of grafts or fusion cages may cause acute neurological impairment from spinal cord and/or nerve root compression, and should be corrected immediately.

Pseudoarthrosis

When pseudoarthrosis occurs, there may be a return of symptoms or an increase of symptoms, particularly with neck pain. The graft may need to be revised. In addition, further decompression may be needed due to reactive bone or osteophyte formation. In some cases, a posterior approach with arthrodesis (fusion) is considered to treat an anterior pseudoarthrosis. This is particularly true if the patient has persistent swallowing difficulties or other reasons to avoid another anterior approach.

Donor site infection

Iliac crest graft site infections may require re-exploration, irrigation and debridement followed by 6–12 weeks of intravenous antibiotics. Early or superficial infections may be treated by antibiotics alone.

Thoracic level

Patients with thoracic disc herniations may present with back pain, radicular pain, or myelopathy. Statistically, thoracic herniations are far less common than those in the cervical or lumbar spine due to the more stable nature of the thoracic spine and the attached rib cage. Individuals with thoracic back pain should be treated conservatively, since there is no convincing medical evidence that supports the use of surgery. Patients with radicular pain and intercostal neuralgia may benefit from a trial of intercostal nerve blocks. Since surgical approaches for thoracic disc are fairly major procedures with a potential for blood loss and heightened morbidity, surgery is indicated only in patients with a progressive neurological deficit (myelopathy) or persistent severe thoracic radicular pain. Surgical options include laminectomy, transpedicular, costotransversectomy, lateral extracavitary, and anterolateral transthoracic approaches. Minimally invasive methods using thoracoscopic techniques have also been successfully utilized. Transthoracic, transpleural approaches typically require postoperative chest tube drainage. Fusion is typically not indicated, but may be considered in cases with associated deformity (e.g., kyphosis, scoliosis, listhesis), in cases where significant vertebral body resection is needed, or when a bilateral transpedicular approach has been performed.

Lumbar level

Patients with lumbar disc herniations typically present with buttock and leg pain. Lower lumbar herniations typically present with pain in the distribution of the sciatic nerve (posterior thigh, lower leg below the knee). Upper lumbar herniations may present in the distribution of the femoral nerve (anterior thigh). Weakness and/or paresthesias may also be present in a specific nerve root distribution. The majority of patients without neurological deficit will improve with expectant or non-surgical management. For those patients who present with significant motor or sensory deficit, or especially in those patients with a cauda equina syndrome (bowel and bladder incontinence, perineal sensory loss), urgent surgery is performed. Conservative management in patients without significant neurological deficit includes use of NSAIDs, corticosteroids, narcotics, and muscle-relaxant medication. Several days of bed rest or limited activity is often followed by a course of physical therapy. Epidural steroid injections may be very helpful in reducing the amount of back and leg pain. If a patient initially has incapacitating pain not controlled by IV narcotics, or if a patient has symptoms that persist beyond 6–8 weeks despite the aforementioned non-surgical measures, surgery should be considered.

Treatment involves lumbar discectomy using a thin-bladed retractor or tubular retractor, and is often aided by the use of an operating microscope or by loupe magnification. General anesthesia is preferred, although local sedation with MAC anesthesia or epidural anesthesia is possible. The patient is placed in the prone position and supported on a Wilson frame to create some opening of the interlaminar spaces. Plain radiography or fluoroscopy is performed to determine the appropriate skin incision site for access to the herniated disc. Both "open" or "minimally invasive trans-tubular" discectomies can be performed through a small midline or paramedian incision. The deep fascia is opened in the midline or just off midline, and the paraspinal muscles are either retracted laterally by a flat retractor blade or displaced out radially by a tubular retractor. Repeat imaging is performed to confirm the desired lumbar location. Typically, a small amount of laminar bone is removed laterally from the superior and inferior lumbar levels, and a portion of the medial facet joint is usually removed. A portion of the ligament of flavum is removed and the nerve root is identified and retracted medially. A loose, free fragment can be dissected and mobilized, and then removed. Contained disc herniations can be accessed by incising the posterior longitudinal ligament and/or annulus fibrosis in order to remove the herniated fragment. Excessive curettage of the disc space is not recommended as it has been associated with higher rates of subsequent back pain, disc space collapse, and discitis. Visualization may be enhanced with the operating microscope, surgical loupes or (especially when a smaller tubular retractor is used) rod-lens endoscope.

Theoretically, "minimally invasive," "endoscopic," or "tubular" approaches for the removal of lumbar herniated discs may allow for smaller skin incisions, less muscle trauma and less bone removal; however, a clinical advantage has not been clearly demonstrated.

Usual postoperative course

Expected postoperative hospital stay

The expected postoperative hospital stay is 1–2 days. Many patients can be treated on an outpatient basis (less than 24-hour stay).

Operative mortality

Rare.

Special monitoring required

None.

Patient activity and positioning

Advancement of ambulation as tolerated. No X-rays or brace are needed.

Alimentation

No restriction.

Antibiotic coverage

Typically for 12–24 hours.

Postoperative complications

In the hospital

Hematoma

Hematoma may present with back pain out of proportion to that which is typically expected. A patient may also present with localized weakness, numbness, or even cauda equina syndrome (see above). Prompt surgical re-exploration can be considered, or an imaging study such as MRI, CT, or myelography may first be obtained.

Discitis/wound infection

Wound infections typically present within 2–3 weeks. Disc space infection (discitis) usually presents more sub-acutely and may not present clinically for many weeks or even months. Back pain (especially when supine or resting), malaise, weight loss, and night sweats are classic symptoms that should alert the surgeon to this potential complication. Radiographic work-up to evaluate the disc space and to rule out bony involvement or epidural abscess can include CT or, especially, MRI scans (with and without contrast). Blood cultures should be obtained. Patients without epidural abscesses or significant bone destruction may be treated initially with IV antibiotics alone. For more advanced or resistant infections, the wound and disc space may need surgical exploration by either an anterior or a posterior approach. Wound cultures should be performed, and the patient should be treated for 6–12 weeks with intravenous antibiotics appropriate to the causal organisms. The patient should be followed with serological tests such as erythrocyte sedimentation rate (ESR) and complement reactive protein (CRP). Follow-up radiographic studies are also advised.

Cerebrospinal fluid injury

An intraoperative dural tear should be repaired intraoperatively. Primary suture repair is the optimal method of treatment; adjunctive products can be added such as synthetic dural tissues and fibrin glue or other synthetic sealants. An intrathecal lumbar drain can be placed operatively or postoperatively.

If a spinal fluid leak persists or spontaneously appears postoperatively, the patient will often complain of headaches when upright, which are alleviated by lying flat. Some patients will have clear or blood-tinged fluid draining from the incision. A "target sign" on a dressing is highly suspicious for a CSF leak; fluid can also be sent for laboratory studies to confirm that it is cerebrospinal fluid. Postoperative CSF leaks can be treated with flat bed-rest and lumbar drainage. For persistent leaks, the most effective approach is to re-explore the wound and repair the leak primarily. Meningitis is a rare but potential complication of lumbar CSF leakage.

Nerve root injury

Nerve root injury resulting from surgical manipulation or retraction is uncommon. It can usually be avoided with careful dissection and gentle retraction during disc removal. When operating on foraminal disc herniations, it is important to treat the ganglion as delicately as possible because it is a very sensitive component of any nerve root.

Vascular injury

Blood vessel injury may result from aggressive disc removal, violation of the anterior longitudinal ligament, or overzealous curettage of the anterior disc space with pituitary rongeurs. Some intraoperative vascular injuries may be recognized by a sudden rush of blood into the operative field or by blood that emanates from the disc space. In other cases of vascular injury, no bleeding may be seen; the only signs initially are the development of tachycardia and/or hypotension. Because

bleeding can be concealed in the retroperitoneal space, this complication may also not manifest itself until the onset of anemia and a Grey–Turner sign in the flank area during the early postoperative period. Some patients may present years later with a persistent arteriovenous fistula. When the injury is recognized intraoperatively, emergent vascular or general surgery consultation should be sought. The lumbar wound should be closed rapidly so that the patient can be turned supine for an emergency laparotomy.

Recurrent disc herniations

While uncommon, recurrent disc herniations may occur and will require additional treatment. Repeat discectomy is most often performed. Though there is no Class I or Class II evidence to support fusion, fusion should be considered in patients with radiographically demonstrated instability (scoliosis, spondylolisthesis). Class III medical evidence has demonstrated good results with reoperation that involves discectomy alone as well as with discectomy and fusion.

Arachnoiditis

Arachnoiditis is the clumping and scarring together of the lumbar and sacral nerves as a complication of surgery, prior contrast injection, lumbar punctures, or cerebrospinal fluid leakage. It cannot be treated directly by surgical intervention without significant risk of nerve root injury. Pain medication and other medications such as gabapentin may be useful. In cases of severe, chronic pain due to arachoiditis refractory to medical management, patients may be considered for a percutaneous trial of electrical spinal cord stimulation to ascertain if they would be good candidates for a surgically implanted spinal cord stimulator.

Complications of surgical positioning

Compressive neuropathies of the brachial plexus and of the peroneal and ulnar nerves result from difficulties in surgical positioning. Therefore, special care should be taken to ensure that the patient's elbows have been padded and that there is no excessive pressure on the peroneal nerve (upper lateral knee) during the operative procedure. The upper arms should be adducted no more than 90°, and the elbows flexed no more than 90°.

Further reading

Anand N, Regan JJ. Video-assisted thoracoscopic surgery for thoracic disc disease: classification and outcome study of 100 consecutive cases with a 2-year minimum follow-up period. *Spine* 2002; **27**: 871–9.

Butterman GR. Prospective nonrandomized comparison of an allograft with bone morphogenic protein versus an iliac crest

autograft in anterior cervical discectomy and fusion. *Spine J* 2008; **8**: 426–35.

Moore AJ, Chilton JD, Uttley D. Long-term results of micro-lumbar discectomy. *Br J Neurosurg* 1994; **8**: 319–26.

Mummaneni PV, Rodts GE, Subach BR *et al.* Management of thoracic disc disease. *Contemp Neurosurg* 2002; **23**: 1–8.

Perez-Cruet MJ, Foley KT, Isaacs RE *et al.* Microendoscopic lumbar discectomy:

technical note. *Neurosurgery* 2002; **51**: 129–36.

Righesso O, Falavigna A, Avanzi O. Comparison of open discectomy with microendoscopic discectomy in lumbar disc herniations: results of a randomized controlled trial. *Neurosurgery* 2007; **61**: 545–9.

Rosenthal D, Dickman CA. Thoracoscopic microsurgical excision of herniated thoracic discs. *J Neurosurg* 1998; **89**: 224–35.

Stachniak JB, Diebner JD, Brunk ES, Speed SM. Analysis of prevertebral soft-tissue swelling and dysphagia in multilevel anterior cervical discectomy and fusion with recombinant human bone morphogenetic protein-2 in patients at risk for pseudoarthrosis. *J Neurosurg Spine* 2011; **14**: 244–9.

Stillerman CB, Chen TC, Couldwell WT *et al.* Experience in the surgical management of 82 symptomatic herniated thoracic discs and review of the literature. *J Neurosurg* 1998; **88**: 623–33.

Tumialan LM, Pan J, Rodts GE, Mummaneni PV. The safety and efficacy of anterior cervical discectomy and fusion with polyetheretherketone spacer

and recombinant human bone morphogenetic protein-2: a review of 200 patients. *J Neurosurg Spine* 2008; **8**: 529–35.

Weinstein JN, Lurie JD, Tosteson TD *et al.* Surgical versus nonoperative treatment for lumbar disc herniation: four-year results for the Spine Patient Outcomes Research Trial (SPORT). *Spine* 2008; **33**: 2789–800.

Chapter

108

General considerations in ophthalmic surgery

John F. Payne, G. Baker Hubbard, and Timothy W. Olsen

A vast array of surgical interventions may be performed in the treatment of ocular and periorbital disease. Because of the high technical difficulty, the subspecialist often performs a significant portion of the ophthalmic surgeries. Most procedures in ophthalmology involve microsurgery and are usually limited to the eye and orbit. Thus, typically there is minimal risk to other organs. Ophthalmic surgery offers a high probability of success, with a major positive impact on quality of life. Nevertheless, many patients with eye pathology are elderly, and some have significant systemic illness. Therefore, the risk of elective intervention must be balanced against the expected benefits, and appropriate counseling should be performed prior to surgery. Optimizing the management of medical problems preoperatively can make the surgery safer and minimize patient discomfort.

Anesthesia

The large majority of ophthalmic interventions can be performed under local anesthesia with intravenous sedation. In some cases, even topical anesthetics are sufficient. But there are ophthalmic surgeries that require general anesthesia, such as those that involve significant extraocular manipulation, for which the local anesthetic may not be as effective, or those that may be prolonged, as is often the case in many vitreoretinal and orbital procedures. Some periorbital or facial cosmetic interventions often necessitate general anesthesia as well. General anesthesia is also indicated in younger patients and those who may not be cooperative enough to remain motionless during surgery. In addition, general anesthetics are required in trauma cases with significant ocular laceration, where administration of local anesthetics may raise intraorbital pressure, necessitating subsequent extrusion of intraocular contents. Several choices exist in the route of administration of local ophthalmic anesthesia for intraocular surgery. The most widely used approach is injection of 3–7 mL of a mixture of lidocaine 2% and marcaine 0.75% through a retrobulbar approach using a blunted needle (Atkinson needle). This is often performed with a regional seventh nerve block to paralyze eyelid closure. The risks of local ophthalmic anesthesia are remote, but they may be significant.

They include local damage through retrobulbar hemorrhage, extraocular muscle damage, and penetration of the globe or optic nerve. Systemic exposure to the injected medication through intravascular or subarachnoid injection of the anesthetic has been known to cause hypertension, seizures, apnea, or even death.

Muscular-skeletal problems

Ophthalmic procedures require the patient to be comfortably motionless in a supine position. As many patients in need of eye surgery are elderly, it is not uncommon for them to have associated ailments of the bones and joints, which may interfere with their ability to remain completely supine for any length of time. Similarly, nervous system diseases with involuntary movements or tremors may also be a concern for surgery under local anesthetics. At times, increased use of sedatives and analgesics is enough to make the intervention safe. In some cases, an adjustment in the usual supine position in order to make the patient more comfortable helps. In others, general anesthesia is necessary.

Ventilation under anesthesia

Supplemental oxygen is typically administered throughout all ophthalmic procedures, through either nasal prongs or a mask. Because patients are lying supine with their face covered by surgical drapes, or possibly because of the natural anxiety associated with surgery, it is not uncommon for the patient to have a perception of dyspnea. Ensuring that patients who suffer from true dyspnea or orthopnea are in their best possible ventilatory state is a major factor to be assessed prior to surgery. Elective procedures may need to be postponed until severe chronic obstructive pulmonary disease, respiratory infections, congestive heart failure, or other major medical illnesses are optimally treated. Coughing spasms, which increase venous pressure, may lead to intraocular hemorrhage in an eye that is open to atmospheric pressure, and result in prolapse of intraocular tissues and blindness.

Medical Management of the Surgical Patient, ed. Michael F. Lubin, Thomas F. Dodson, and Neil H. Winawer. Published by Cambridge University Press. © Cambridge University Press 2013.

Patient cooperation

Operations in ophthalmology, when using local anesthesia, rely on the strictest cooperation by the patient. Anxiety, psychological disorders, and psychiatric diseases need to be considered for every patient when deciding between local and general anesthesia. The patient's internist or even family members may have important insight into this information.

Arterial hypertension

Patients with known systemic arterial hypertension should take their oral antihypertensive medications on the morning of surgery with a small amount of water. Not infrequently, chronic hypertensive patients experience acute elevation of their blood pressure during ophthalmic surgery despite good compliance with their medications. This may be a result of the normal stress reaction to surgical intervention, phenylephrine eye drops used for mydriasis, or poor preoperative hypertensive control. In addition to the usual concerns about the systemic effects, an acute increase in blood pressure during eye surgery may cause intraocular hemorrhage. If this occurs in an eye which is open to atmospheric pressure, it may result in blindness. It is important that patients having elective ophthalmic surgery be evaluated for arterial hypertension, and that their therapy is optimized prior to surgical intervention. Patients should be educated to ensure continuation of their daily antihypertensive medications on the day of surgery.

Diabetes mellitus

Patients undergoing ophthalmic procedures often have concomitant diabetes mellitus. It is important, when possible, to try to optimize glycemic control prior to surgery. Patients with non-insulin dependent diabetes are often instructed to continue their oral hypoglycemic medications on the day of surgery. Patients who require insulin are often advised not to use their insulin on the morning of the surgical procedure, and also to reduce or eliminate their insulin use the night prior to surgery. Because the blood sugar control of each patient can be quite variable, it is often beneficial to discuss perioperative management with the patient's internist or endocrinologist.

Blood sugar should be checked prior to surgical intervention in all known diabetic patients to ensure that it is at a safe level. Preoperative hypoglycemia can often be managed with an intravenous dextrose-saline infusion, and mild to moderate hyperglycemia is often treated with a sliding scale of insulin. Patients with severe preoperative hyperglycemia who are undergoing elective ophthalmic surgery should have their surgery rescheduled in order to optimize blood sugar control.

Coagulation

As mentioned earlier, orbital and intraocular hemorrhages pose a serious threat to vision. Normal coagulation makes ophthalmic surgery safer. If medically feasible, patients on chronic anticoagulation and antiplatelet medications should interrupt their therapy in advance to allow for clotting parameters to normalize prior to eye surgery. In most cases, anticoagulant medications can be resumed immediately after the operation. Recent data suggest that some closed-globe vitreoretinal procedures may be safely performed without discontinuing warfarin.

In patients who cannot interrupt anticoagulation for a period of several days, transfusion of fresh frozen plasma and/or platelets immediately prior to surgical intervention is a consideration. Some ophthalmic procedures can be modified enough to avoid the most hemorrhage-prone steps of surgery. For example, scleral buckling surgery can sometimes be executed without trans-scleral drainage, in an effort to avoid an incision through the highly vascular choroid, which is extremely vascular. Additionally, cataract surgery can be performed exclusively through corneal incisions, avoiding ocular structures that are vascular. Retrobulbar anesthesia can be replaced with general anesthesia or, in some instances, substituted for a combination of topical anesthesia and retrobulbar/peribulbar anesthesia using a blunt cannula.

Infection

Intraocular infection, or endophthalmitis, is fortunately a rare event. The onset of acute postoperative endophthalmitis usually occurs within days of the operation. In some instances, onset may be delayed for weeks or months if the causative agent is a slow-growth bacteria or fungus. It often leads to profound visual loss, and if not recognized early enough, even loss of the globe. For most intraocular surgeries, many ophthalmologists inject subconjunctival antibiotics at the end of the procedure, and prescribe prophylactic topical antibiotics during the early postoperative period.

Intraocular infections are typically treated with intravitreal injections of antibiotics, and if severe enough, with vitrectomy as well. Systemic antibiotics, which rarely achieve significant intraocular concentration, are usually not given unless the ocular infection is associated with a systemic infectious origin. Intraocular surgery, and even postoperative endophthalmitis, is very unlikely to cause significant bacteremia or septicemia. It does not require prophylactic systemic antibiotics to prevent endocarditis.

Ophthalmic medications

Dilation of the pupil is usually required prior to intraocular surgery. A combination of a topical sympathomimetic, such as phenylephrine, and a parasympatholytic such as cyclopentolate, atropine or others, is often used. Postoperatively, a topical parasympatholytic is often given to prevent discomfort from spasm of the ciliary body, and a topical steroidal can be used to minimize ocular inflammation. While topical steroid medications have mostly only ocular side-effects, phenylephrine can lead to arrhythmia, arterial hypertension, and tachycardia. Atropine and other parasympatholytic agents can result in headaches, constipation, restlessness, delirium, and urinary retention.

Not infrequently, ophthalmic surgery can cause acute elevation of intraocular pressure in the early postoperative period. Patients typically complain of eye pain, which may be accompanied by a vagal response with nausea, vomiting, and bradycardia. This complication requires administration of anti-glaucoma medications, including beta-blocking agents, such as timolol; topical or systemic carbonic anhydrase inhibitors, such as acetazolamide or dorzolamide; prostaglandin analogs, such as latanoprost; and alpha-2 adrenergics, such as brimonidine. The most common adverse reactions of these topical medications are restricted to the eye surface, causing ocular pruritus, foreign body sensation, and dryness There are occasions when adverse reactions affect other organs. Topical beta-blockers may produce headache, bronchospasm, heart block and exacerbation of congestive heart failure; carbonic anhydrase inhibitors may cause paresthesias, headache, polyuria, and dyspepsia; prostaglandin analogs may result in a rash; and alpha-2 adrenergics may produce somnolence, dry mouth, and hypertension.

Further reading

Dayani PN, Grand MG. Maintenance of warfarin anticoagulation for patients undergoing vitreoretinal surgery. *Arch Ophthalmol* 2006; **124**: 1558–65.

Endophthalmitis Vitrectomy Study Group. Results of the Endophthalmitis Vitrectomy Study Group: a randomized trial of immediate vitrectomy and of intravenous antibiotics for the treatment of postoperative bacterial endophthalmitis. *Arch Ophthalmol* 1995; **113**: 1479–96.

Mason JO 3rd, Gupta SR, Compton CJ *et al*. Comparison of hemorrhagic complications of warfarin and clopidogrel bisulfate in 25-gauge vitrectomy versus a control group. *Ophthalmology* 2011; **118**(3): 543–7.

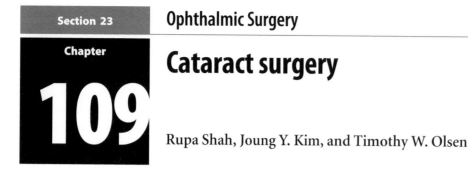

Cataract surgery

Rupa Shah, Joung Y. Kim, and Timothy W. Olsen

Cataracts are characterized by opacity of the crystalline lens of the eye. They represent the primary cause of treatable blindness in the world. Cataracts are generally categorized as congenital or age related; however, they may also result from exposure to drugs, toxins, or radiation; or be the product of various metabolic diseases. Visually significant cataracts are a major public health issue: they are found in 50% of persons 65–74 years of age and 70% of persons 75 years of age or older.

Modern cataract extraction is accompanied by insertion of an intraocular lens (IOL). It is a highly effective and efficient operation that restores visual acuity and contrast sensitivity in patients with visually significant cataracts. Presently, the operation employs a systematic, minimally invasive approach which involves creating a small (2.5–3.5 mm) wound at the edge of the cornea. The incision is carefully created in a beveled manner that minimizes leakage through the wound without sutures. A viscoelastic material is injected into the anterior chamber to protect the cornea and to maintain a working chamber in the eye for instrumentation. Next, a portion of the anterior capsule of the lens is removed to allow access to the lens cortex and nucleus, creating a circular opening in the capsular bag (capsulotomy). An ultrasonic probe (phacoemulsification tip) is then inserted through the anterior chamber and capsulotomy, into the lens. The energy generated at the tip of the probe is used to fragment and remove the cataractous lens nucleus and cortex. The remaining capsule of the lens is left intact (referred to commonly as the capsular "bag"). A custom IOL is selected, with appropriate focusing power to neutralize the refractive error. The measurements are based on the axial length of the eye as well as the corneal curvature. Most lenses are folded and inserted through the incision into the "bag," where the lens can then unfold and rest in the location of the original native lens. After the instruments are removed, the wound is self-sealing and watertight. Occasionally, one or more sutures are required to secure the wound. Despite the highly technical aspects of cataract surgery, experienced surgeons can perform the operation in 30 minutes or less.

Outcomes have steadily improved over the years and the rate of complications has diminished as the procedure has progressed. In the absence of other ocular disease, postoperative visual acuity is often 20/20 or better within 1 week of surgery, with less dependence on the use of glasses for refractive correction. As the risks of the operation are reduced and outcomes have improved, the indications for the intervention have changed. For patients without coexisting ocular disorders, primary current indications for cataract surgery include a symptomatic reduction in visual acuity including reduction in visual function due to glare (i.e., difficulty driving at night), or difficulties with reading. Cataract extraction may also be performed to improve visualization and management of posterior segment disorders. Special care should be taken in eyes with retinal diseases such as diabetic retinopathy, age-related macular degeneration, prior retinal detachments, uveitis, or other retinal disorders.

Cataract extraction is usually performed under local anesthesia with intravenous sedation. Many cataract surgeons now prefer offering topical anesthesia for their cooperative adult patients. The common alternatives include the use of a retrobulbar or peribulbar block that is administered in combination with brief systemic sedation administered by the anesthesia team. Stress to the patient is minimal. Cataract extraction may be possible for even the most debilitated of patients, producing beneficial outcomes.

Usual postoperative course
Expected postoperative hospital stay

With only rare exceptions, the vast majority of cataract extractions are performed on an outpatient basis. The patient must be examined on the first postoperative day by his or her ophthalmologist, usually in an office setting. As a historical footnote, postoperative care for cataract surgery in the mid twentieth century included days to weeks of inactivity with inpatient care. Complete immobilization was achieved by placement of sand-bags on either side of the patient's head!

Operative mortality

In general, operative mortality is solely related to anesthesia or systemic disease.

Special monitoring required

Postoperatively, clinical outpatient exams are usually conducted for the first 2–3 months.

Patient activity and positioning

Routine daily activities may be resumed almost immediately; however, patients must wear protective glasses or a protective shield (especially at night) over the operated eye during the early postoperative period. Eye rubbing must be avoided. After several days, face and hair washing may be performed with eyes closed. Excessively strenuous exercise or heavy lifting should be avoided for approximately 1 week.

Alimentation

Regular preoperative diet may be resumed depending upon the level of operative sedation (usually minimal).

Antibiotic coverage

Topical corticosteroid and antibiotic drops are used 3–4 times daily for 1–3 weeks postoperatively; dosage is adjusted according to the exam. The antibiotic drops are typically discontinued after 1 week. The steroid drops are tapered off over several weeks.

Postoperative complications

In the hospital

Corneal edema

Some swelling of the surrounding structures during the postoperative period is very common and expected. The edema is usually mild and self-limiting. Severe or prolonged edema requires treatment to prevent permanent visual disability. Corneal tissue may be transplanted if severe functional loss of this tissue impairs visual acuity.

Wound dehiscence or wound leak

Wound leaks must be identified and treated promptly to prevent microorganisms from gaining access to the inside of the eye. A test using topical application of fluorescein dye is commonly employed to detect subtle wound leaks. A suture may be needed; this intervention is generally performed using sterile conditions in a minor procedure room with a surgical microscope.

Dislocation of the intraocular lens

Lens dislocation usually results from a defect in the capsule of a native lens that has been left in place to support the implant. Treatment requires reoperation with an alternative form of lens fixation. Lenses may be sewn or fixed to the iris or to the wall of the eye (trans-scleral sutures), or an anterior chamber lens may be inserted.

Residual lens fragments

Fragments of lens left behind after cataract surgery can be highly inflammatory. They often must be removed with a second operation. Vitreoretinal surgeons generally perform these operations at a separate procedure.

Elevated intraocular pressure

Mild pressure elevations are common after cataract extraction and usually respond well to topical pressure-lowering medications. More severe elevations may cause pain, nausea, and vomiting. The response to topical medication is usually adequate to treat this condition and the duration of discomfort is usually limited. Surgical options may be required for severe or prolonged intraocular pressure increases.

After discharge

Infection

Endophthalmitis is a rare but devastating complication of cataract extraction. Treatment involves injection of intraocular antibiotics as well as topical and intravenous antibiotics. When visual acuity is light perception alone or worse, a posterior vitrectomy is indicated.

Retinal detachment

Retinal detachment is a complication of cataract extraction that may occur days, months, or even years after a cataract operation. Standard retinal reattachment surgeries are required to prevent blindness. These procedures include pneumatic retinopexy, laser retinopexy, scleral buckling procedures, or pars plana vitrectomy.

Further reading

Cionni RJ, Snyder ME, Osher RH. Cataract surgery. In Tasman W, Jaeger EA, eds. *Duane's Clinical Ophthalmology*. Vol. 6. Philadelphia, PA: Lippincott, Williams, & Wilkins; 2002.

Devagn U. *Cataract Surgery: A Patient's Guide to Cataract Treatment*. Omaha, NE: Addicus Books; 2009.

Henderson B. *Essentials of Cataract Surgery*. Thorofare, NJ: Slack; 2007.

Yanoff M, Duker J. *Ophthalmology*. 3rd edn. St Louis, MO: Mosby Elsevier; 2009.

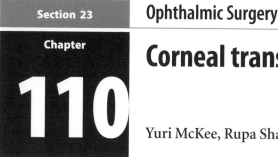

Corneal transplantation

Yuri McKee, Rupa Shah, Joung Y. Kim, and Timothy W. Olsen

Traditional full-thickness corneal transplantation, known as penetrating keratoplasty (PK), was first performed over a century ago and remains the gold standard of corneal transplantation. Penetrating keratoplasty involves replacement of all layers of the central 7–9 mm of the host cornea with allograft tissue, usually derived from eye banks. Donor corneas are harvested from 1–2 weeks prior to transplantation. Tissue or blood typing is not routinely done. The overall optical clarity, integrity of donor tissue, and donor endothelial cell density are evaluated at the eye bank. The tissue is screened for multiple infectious diseases of the donor, a procedure commonly performed for other human allograft tissues.

Surgical technique
Penetrating keratoplasty

Penetrating keratoplasty usually begins with the removal of the diseased central host cornea by use of various forms of trephine. Next, the donor tissue is trephinated from the donor corneal tissue and is usually slightly oversized. The donor tissue is secured in the recipient bed using either interrupted or continuous nylon sutures. When necessary, a cataract extraction may be performed in combination with intraocular lens implantation. Monitored anesthesia care in these cases usually includes brief, intravenous sedation combined with a retrobulbar block. General anesthesia may be required for selected patients unable to be cooperative, such as children or anxious adult patients. Total surgical time is around 30–45 minutes for an experienced surgeon. Corneal graft survival at 1 year is 90% for PK. Indications for PK include haze, ectatic disease, opacities in the cornea, and corneal edema causing decreased vision or pain. In addition, infections, scars, trauma, congenital dystrophies, and corneal decompensation or injury from prior intraocular surgery are also indications.

Lamellar keratoplasty

More recently, attention has shifted from full-thickness PK to partial thickness corneal transplantation, focused on replacing the dysfunctional layers of the cornea, including the stroma or endothelial cells. Endothelial keratoplasty, or EK, has success rates similar to PK for overall graft survival. The EK procedure involves removal of the diseased corneal endothelium from the host through a 3–5 mm incision near the limbus. Next a 7–9 mm lenticule of donor corneal tissue that has donor corneal endothelium, Descemet's membrane, and 100–200 microns of corneal stroma is inserted into the anterior chamber of the recipient. The tissue is positioned to replace the diseased inner surface of the cornea and held in place temporarily with an air bubble injected into the anterior chamber. The corneal wound is typically closed with 2–3 sutures. Eventually the donor lenticule restores a more normal function to the host cornea and the edema resolves. The indication for EK is corneal edema due to corneal endothelial dysfunction. Endothelial keratoplasty has many advantages over PK including the use of a smaller incision, more rapid visual recovery, and less postoperative astigmatism. Final visual acuity after EK may be slightly worse than after PK. An advantage of EK is avoiding the irregular astigmatism that commonly occurs with PK and necessitates the use of a rigid contact lens. Anesthesia is similar to that used in PK.

When corneal disease or opacity is limited to the corneal stroma, a procedure known as deep anterior lamellar keratoplasty (DALK) may be performed. The surgical procedures for DALK are more similar to those for PK than those for EK. However, with DALK, the surgeon performs a meticulous dissection within the corneal stroma, removing the epithelium and deeper diseased tissues, while preserving the host's more normal Descemet's membrane and endothelium. When this delicate dissection proves unsuccessful, a standard PK is performed. While DALK may have a lower rejection and graft failure rate than PK, the technique has not been adopted as quickly as EK, primarily due to the technical difficulty involved with the lamellar dissection.

Usual postoperative course
Expected postoperative hospital stay

These procedures are typically performed in an outpatient surgical setting. Hospital admission is rare and usually associated with systemic complications.

Operative mortality

The operative mortality from these procedures is extremely low. An adverse result is usually due to a complication of underlying disease or general anesthesia.

Special monitoring required

An eye patch and shield are typically placed at the time of surgery and are removed by the surgeon on the first postoperative day. The shield is used to protect the eye during sleep, especially in the first 4 postoperative weeks; the use of eyeglasses or protective eyewear is recommended during waking hours.

Patient activity and positioning

Patients can begin light duties within the first few days after surgery. Heavy exertion is restricted for the first 3–4 postoperative weeks. The patient's head should not go below the waist for the same time period. Swimming should be avoided for 2–3 weeks to minimize the risk for infection. Patients who have undergone EK should remain supine as much as possible for the first 24 hours to aid the air bubble in supporting the graft.

Alimentation

The regular preoperative diet may be resumed following recovery from anesthesia. Diet is advanced cautiously after surgery in order to minimize postoperative nausea and vomiting.

Antibiotic coverage

Topical antibiotics are used prophylactically several times a day for the first 7–10 days after surgery.

Postoperative follow-up

Typical follow-up visits are scheduled on postoperative days 1, 14, and then monthly for the first few months. Sutures may be removed if they become loose or broken, or to minimize astigmatism. Topical corticosteroids are slowly tapered over several months, and may be used indefinitely.

Postoperative complications

In the hospital

Aqueous leaks

Aqueous leaks may develop in the early postoperative period. Small wound leaks are managed with a therapeutic contact lens and topical antibiotics. Larger leaks may require corneal suturing.

Infection

Infection is a rare but serious complication that may occur at any time postoperatively; the area around sutures is the most vulnerable. Intraocular infection in the first 1–2 postoperative weeks represents an urgent and potentially emergent condition (i.e., perforation) that is vision threatening. Especially with long-term topical corticosteroid use, superficial infections of the cornea may present at any time postoperatively and are typically managed with topical antibiotic drops.

Special considerations with endothelial keratoplasty

A small percentage of EK grafts spontaneously dislodge, with resultant corneal edema. In the minor procedure OR, an air bubble may be re-introduced to re-attach the graft. When this is unsuccessful, or if the graft continues to detach, the EK should be repeated.

After discharge

Cataract, glaucoma, and retinal detachment

As with all intraocular surgery, long-term complications may occur, such as glaucoma, cataract formation and retinal detachment. Topical corticosteroid use predisposes to both cataract formation and glaucoma. Intraoperative complications increase the risks of these sequelae.

Graft rejection

Graft rejection most commonly occurs during the first year after surgery. Topical corticosteroids are usually tapered and continued at a low dose for years. Early signs of rejection include ocular redness, sensitivity to light, pain, and decreased vision. A patient experiencing any of these signs or symptoms should seek immediate attention. If the rejection cannot be suppressed, a repeat corneal transplant procedure may be necessary.

Further reading

Brightbill FS. *Corneal Surgery: Theory, Technique, and Tissue.* 4th edn. New York, NY: Mosby Elsevier; 2009.

Krachmer JH, Mannis MJ, Holland EJ. *Cornea: Fundamentals, Diagnosis, and Management.* 3rd edn. New York, NY: Mosby Elsevier; 2011.

Price FW Jr, Price M. *DSEK: What You Need to Know About Endothelial Keratoplasty.* Thorofare, NJ: Slack; 2009.

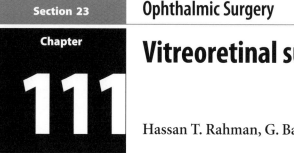

Vitreoretinal surgery

Hassan T. Rahman, G. Baker Hubbard, and Timothy W. Olsen

Vitreoretinal surgical techniques are used to approach disorders of the posterior segment of the eye. Over the past 30 years, great strides have been made in the ability to safely and effectively operate in this segment. The spectrum of disorders menable to operative intervention has broadened significantly with the evolution of advanced, smaller-gauge microsurgical instruments, computer-controlled infusion and aspiration systems, endolaser probes, perfluorocarbon heavy liquid for manipulation of detached retinal tissue, implantable slow-release pharmacological devices, wide-angle optical viewing systems, and long-acting gases and silicone oil for intraocular tamponade. The treatment of intraocular tumors with radioactive episcleral plaques has also become well-characterized and "evidence-based" through large-scale, prospective, randomized clinical trial data. The advent and sophistication of the pars plana approach with microsurgical vitrectomy instrumentation has allowed for the repair of most simple and complex primary and recurrent retinal detachments. The pars plana is the section of the eye located approximately at the junction of the iris and the sclera and is a safe place to insert intraocular instruments without damage to internal structures. However, in certain cases of primary retinal detachment, the most appropriate treatment remains scleral buckling surgery, as has been performed for over 60 years.

Scleral buckling surgery involves the placement of a strip of silicone around the outside of the globe to cause a slight indentation or buckle of the eye wall and support the intraocular retinal breaks and vitreous base. The procedure is effective because the external support helps close the causative retinal tear inside the eye. The retinal tear is repaired by a combination of support from the buckle and the formation of a chorioretinal scar induced by a thermal modality such as cryotherapy (freezing) or laser (heating). The usual procedure for addressing complex retinal detachments with very large or posteriorly located retinal tears, significant retinal scarring, vitreous hemorrhage, or severe cataract formation is to combine scleral buckle surgery with the more advanced intraocular vitrectomy techniques.

A 3-port pars plana vitrectomy is a surgical procedure that involves the insertion of microsurgical instruments into the posterior segment of the eye to extract all or part of the vitreous humor using two ports for instrumentation and a third port for infusion. Intraocular microsurgical instruments that are commonly used include small-gauge forceps, scissors, picks, microcannulae, and endolaser probes. These instruments allow for removal of scar tissue or intraocular foreign bodies, placement of therapeutic laser photocoagulation, and instillation of various long-acting gases or silicone oil for intraocular tamponade, which are often required to repair a detached retina.

In addition to retinal detachment, the list of disorders that may be appropriate for vitreoretinal surgery includes macular hole; epiretinal membranes (also known as macular pucker, fibrosis, surface wrinkling retinopathy, or cellophane maculopathy); subretinal hemorrhage due to macular degeneration and other disorders; proliferative diabetic retinopathy; vitreous hemorrhage; choroidal melanoma and other intraocular tumors; CMV retinitis or other forms of infectious retinitis; retained lens fragments after cataract surgery; dislocated intraocular lens implants; intraocular foreign bodies; and endophthalmitis.

Vitreoretinal surgery is most often performed under local anesthesia with retrobulbar block and intravenous sedation. However, in the setting of reoperation after scleral buckle, adequate local anesthesia may be difficult to achieve and general anesthesia is required. In addition, some operations are of sufficient duration that local anesthesia is less desirable. Low back pain exacerbated by lying flat, claustrophobia, and inability to hold still are relative indications for general anesthesia.

Usual postoperative course
Expected postoperative hospital stay

The vast majority of vitreoretinal procedures are conducted on an outpatient basis. However, select patients with disorders of the posterior segment of the eye also have significant systemic medical conditions. In non-compliant patients, stringent positioning requirements that may affect the outcome of the procedure may require admission to hospital. Monocular patients who have the only eye patched may also require postoperative admission with "blind precautions," as they are functionally blind when their only good eye is patched.

Operative mortality

The operative mortality is very low and generally associated with standard anesthetic risks.

Special monitoring required

Monitoring requirements are based on the underlying disease.

Patient activity and positioning

Strict requirements for head position are common after vitreoretinal operations. Eyes are frequently left with gas or silicone oil filling the posterior segment to provide tamponade after the operation. The tamponade is generally used to help close a retinal tear. Due to the combined properties of buoyancy and surface tension of an intraocular gas or oil bubble, strict head position is needed to provide adequate tamponade of the retinal pathology in the correct location inside the eye. The duration of positioning requirements ranges from 1–14 days or more. Aside from positioning requirements, patients can usually resume normal daily activities within several days of their operation. Eye protection in the form of a shield or protective glasses should be worn for at least several weeks postoperatively.

Alimentation

Regular preoperative diet is usually resumed when the patient recovers from anesthesia.

Postoperative medication

Usual postoperative regimens include a topical corticosteroid, a topical antibiotic, and a topical anticholinergic agent (atropine, cyclopentolate, or scopolamine) to reduce the pain and spasm from the ciliary muscle.

Postoperative complications
Elevated intraocular pressure

Mild pressure elevations are common after vitreoretinal operations and usually respond well to topical pressure-lowering medications. More severe elevations may cause pain, nausea, and vomiting. Even so, response to topical intraocular pressure-lowering medication is usually sufficient, and the duration of elevated pressures is usually brief (days).

Vitreous hemorrhage

Bleeding into the posterior segment after vitrectomy is common, particularly in the setting of proliferative diabetic retinopathy as neovascularization is surgically excised. Most postoperative hemorrhages clear spontaneously but some require reoperation.

Cataract

Cataract formation is inevitable after vitrectomy, but is less rapid in young adults and children. The time to onset of visually significant cataract may be months to many years after the vitrectomy.

Retinal detachment

The rate of postoperative retinal detachment depends on the underlying disease but is generally 1–30%, depending upon the type of surgery being performed. Redetachment is the most common cause for reoperation.

Infection

Endophthalmitis and infected scleral buckle elements are uncommon, yet may become devastating complications with the former resulting in severe visual loss and the latter resulting in minimal morbidity. Treatment of an infected buckle involves removal of buckle elements, while endophthalmitis is treated using injection of intraocular antibiotics and selective use of oral and/or intravenous antibiotics.

Intraocular gas interactions

As noted above, intraocular gas is frequently used after vitreoretinal surgery to provide retinal tamponade. These gas bubbles last from 1–12 weeks before complete reabsorption. *If a patient undergoes another operation during this period, nitrous oxide anesthesia must not be given.* The nitrous gas would diffuse into the intraocular gas bubble, expand, and may cause extreme elevations of intraocular pressure resulting in permanent, severe visual loss. Decompression from atmospheric pressure that may occur during air travel will result in expansion of an intraocular gas bubble with similar results, so air travel, too, must be avoided until the gas bubble resolves.

Further reading

Brinton DA, Wilkinson CP. *Retinal Detachment: Principles and Practice.* New York, NY: Oxford University Press; 2009.

Hart RH, Vote BJ, Borthwick JH, McGeorge AJ, Worsley DR. Loss of vision caused by expansion of intraocular perfluoropropane (C(3)F(8)) gas during nitrous oxide anesthesia. *Am J Ophthalmol* 2002; **134**: 761–3.

Meredith TA. *Atlas of Retinal and Vitreous Surgery.* St. Louis, MO: Mosby; 1999.

Thompson JT. Advantages and limitations of small gauge vitrectomy. *Surv Ophthalmol* 2011; **56**: 162–72.

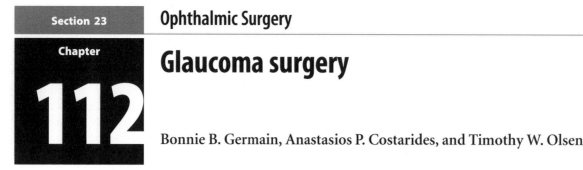

Glaucoma surgery

112

Bonnie B. Germain, Anastasios P. Costarides, and Timothy W. Olsen

Glaucoma is the most common cause of optic neuropathy. Many ocular conditions may lead to the development of glaucomatous nerve damage. In general, therapeutic interventions are directed towards lowering intraocular pressure, a key risk factor for disease progression.

Typically, therapy begins with topical medications, the first and simplest option. These include the prostaglandin analogs, beta adrenergic receptor blockers, carbonic anhydrase inhibitors, alpha adrenergic agonists, and miotics. These agents are used alone or in combination, and are often sufficient to control intraocular pressure. In cases of open-angle glaucoma, laser trabeculoplasty may also be used to lower intraocular pressure. Laser interventions are performed in the clinic either alone or in combination with medical therapy. For cases of angle-closure glaucoma, laser iridotomy may be performed to either treat or prevent pupillary block (iris-lens diaphragm obstruction), an anatomic predisposition that is responsible for the majority of cases. Cyclodestructive surgery (intentional destruction of the ciliary body tissues) is another laser procedure that may be used when other interventions have failed, including incisional surgery. These procedures, which are usually performed in the clinic under local anesthesia, are commonly performed with lasers and, less commonly, cryotherapy.

Incisional intraocular surgery is the treatment of choice when medical and laser procedures have failed to adequately reduce the intraocular pressure to the target level. Trabeculectomy and glaucoma drainage device placement are the most commonly performed intraocular surgical procedures. Both procedures lower intraocular pressure by diverting aqueous fluid from the anterior chamber into the subconjunctival space. Incisional surgeries are performed in the operating room, typically on an outpatient basis with monitored anesthetic care and the use of local anesthesia. Rarely, a patient is admitted to the hospital following incisional surgery, usually due to either systemic complications or when surgery is performed in the patient's only seeing eye.

Ocular complications are usually the result of hypotony (low intraocular pressure). Hypotony may lead to suprachoroidal effusion. A more ominous condition is suprachoroidal

hemorrhage, a complication that may lead to permanent visual loss and even blindness. Endophthalmitis may also occur and result in severe vision loss or blindness. This complication typically becomes symptomatic a few days after surgery; however, it may also be a late complication of the operation.

Usual postoperative course

Expected postoperative stay

Glaucoma surgery usually does not result in hospitalization. Monocular patients may be admitted for brief, overnight observation. A monocular patient who is visually impaired from a suprachoroidal effusion, hemorrhage, or endophthalmitis may also be admitted.

Operative mortality

Mortality in glaucoma surgery is very rare and may be related to systemic complications.

Special monitoring required

Nursing care to help the patient navigate and perform the activities of daily living should be instituted for visually impaired patients. Such precautions are commonly referred to as "blind precautions."

Patient activity and positioning

Activity restrictions are commonly given to patients who have undergone incisional surgery. An eye pad and an eye shield are usually placed over the affected eye for the first postoperative night and removed by the surgeon on the following day. Protective eyewear or eye shields are recommended over the affected eye while the patient is awake. During sleep, an eye shield is used for protection of the surgical site. The Valsalva maneuver increases central venous pressure and predisposes the development of a suprachoroidal effusion or hemorrhage, particularly in a hypotonous eye. Nausea and vomiting, straining at stool, and coughing should be treated

Medical Management of the Surgical Patient, ed. Michael F. Lubin, Thomas F. Dodson, and Neil H. Winawer. Published by Cambridge University Press. © Cambridge University Press 2013.

prophylactically with anti-emetics, stool softeners, and anti-tussives. Patients are instructed to refrain from lifting more than 10 pounds and to maintain a "head above the waist" position at all times for approximately 2 weeks.

Alimentation

Dietary restrictions are unnecessary.

Antibiotic and corticosteroid use

Topical antibiotics and corticosteroids are prescribed following incisional surgery. Topical corticosteroids are tapered over several weeks. For the patient with uveitis, an inflammatory condition of the eye, corticosteroids administered orally or through injection either intravitreally or into the subtenons space may be necessary. The antibiotic regimen is typically discontinued at 5 days in the low-risk patient. Topical cycloplegics are also utilized to manage hypotony. Rarely, intravitreal and intravenous antibiotics are used to treat endophthalmitis.

Postoperative complications

In the hospital

Hypotony

As previously stated, excessive filtration of aqueous humor from the anterior chamber following trabeculectomy or glaucoma drainage device placement may markedly reduce intraocular pressure to a sub-physiologic level. Postoperative hypotony is usually transient, but may also have long-term pathologic consequences. The complication may be accompanied by a shallow or flat anterior chamber, optic disc edema, suprachoroidal effusion or hemorrhage and hypotony maculopathy. Surgical intervention may be required to reverse the manifestations of hypotony and to preserve or maintain vision.

After discharge

Infectious endophthalmitis

Endophthalmitis is an ophthalmic emergency and should be suspected when the postoperative course is complicated by a red, painful eye and vision loss. Blindness may ensue; therefore, rapid and aggressive intervention is necessary. Intravitreal administration of antibiotics or pars plana vitrectomy may be required for management. Infectious endophthalmitis may occur years after a trabeculectomy. During the late postoperative course, breakdown of the surgical filtration site can lead to subsequent bacterial invasion.

Further reading

Chen T. *Surgical Techniques in Ophthalmology: Glaucoma Surgery.* Philadelphia, PA: Saunders; 2007.

Garudadri CS, Rao HL, Senthil S. Three-year follow-up of tube versus trabeculectomy study. *Am J Ophthalmol* 2010; **149**: 685–6.

Shields B. *Shields Textbook of Glaucoma.* Philadelphia, PA: Lippincott Williams & Wilkins; 2011.

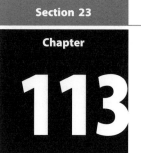

Section 23   Ophthalmic Surgery

Chapter

113 Refractive surgery

Rupa Shah, Yuri McKee, J. Bradley Randleman, and Timothy W. Olsen

Refractive surgery is performed to reduce dependence on glasses or contact lenses. Refractive surgical techniques reshape the cornea using incisions, heat, various forms of laser, or implantation of intraocular lenses to decrease myopia (nearsightedness), astigmatism, or hyperopia (farsightedness). The excimer laser is currently the technology of choice for keratorefractive surgeons. The laser can reshape the cornea by ablating the anterior corneal surface in procedures such as photorefractive keratectomy (PRK), and more commonly in laser-assisted *in situ* keratomileusis (LASIK). In LASIK, the surgeon performs corneal stromal ablation using the excimer laser directed to the corneal tissue under a thin lamellar flap. This flap is created by either a microkeratome or a laser.

In order to select the best candidates for refractive surgery, a thorough preoperative history, assessment, and complete eye exam is required. Parameters such as corneal topography, central corneal thickness, degree of refractive error, ocular surface health and patient expectations are all carefully considered in order to determine whether the individual is a good refractive surgical candidate, as well as for selecting the most appropriate procedure. Absolute contraindications to laser vision correction include diagnoses of keratoconus or ectatic corneal dystrophies. Relative systemic contraindications include poorly controlled rheumatoid arthritis and diabetes, pregnancy, and AIDS.

Refractive surgery is carried out under topical anesthesia as an outpatient procedure performed in a laser suite. LASIK or PRK usually lasts about 15 minutes; the patient experiences minimal discomfort. Both eyes may be operated upon on the same day. In LASIK, a thin corneal flap is created and then lifted to allow the laser to reshape the cornea. The laser is programmed with the patient's refractive error. After the refractive error is corrected, the corneal flap is realigned. In PRK, only the epithelium of the cornea is removed; the laser is then used to correct the patient's refractive error. A bandage contact lens is applied after the procedure and removed after 3–4 days.

Usual postoperative course

The patients are operated upon as outpatients. The operations are performed in a laser suite or in the physician's office.

Special monitoring required

The patient's eyes are not patched, although sunglasses may be helpful when there is sensitivity to light. Discomfort is minimal postoperatively for LASIK. Following PRK, patients typically experience more discomfort for 2–3 days, while the epithelium of the cornea is healing. These patients may be treated conservatively with topical non-steroidal anti-inflammatory agents during the first 3 days following surgery.

Patient activity and positioning

After LASIK surgery, most patients will be able to see well enough on the first postoperative day to return to regular activity. With PRK, healing time is more variable, and may take up to 3–4 weeks. To minimize the risk of postoperative infection, patients are instructed not to rub the eye during the first few days following surgery and to avoid swimming for several weeks.

Antibiotic coverage

The patient is instructed to instill topical antibiotics and steroids for the first week following LASIK. Corticosteroids are to be continued longer following PRK, and are used to modulate the healing response. Dry eye symptoms are common during the first few months, and patients are instructed to use artificial tears as needed.

Postoperative follow-up

Follow-up examinations include the first day after surgery and a second visit at 1–2 weeks postoperatively. After PRK, the patient will return 3–4 days postoperatively to remove the bandage contact lens. Subsequent follow-up visits are generally at 3 months, 6 months, and 1 year. Up to 2–3 months after surgery, there may be small fluctuations in refraction or in visual acuity. Some patients may require enhancement surgery (further laser vision correction) if the refractive result is not achieved.

Medical Management of the Surgical Patient, ed. Michael F. Lubin, Thomas F. Dodson, and Neil H. Winawer. Published by Cambridge University Press. © Cambridge University Press 2013.

Postoperative complications

Dry eye

Laser vision correction may induce or exacerbate dry eye symptoms. For the vast majority of patients who have undergone refractive surgery, dry eye symptoms are at most mild and/or transient, lacking significant morbidity. For most symptomatic patients, dry eye symptoms resolve within 6 months. Dry eye symptoms are treated with lubricating eye drops, punctal (lacrimal) plugs, or prescription eye drops.

LASIK flap complications

A multitude of rare complications can occur involving the flap created in LASIK. These include a free flap, a perforated flap, a dislocated flap, striae within the flap, or debris in the flap interface. These complications are treated conservatively and usually resolve without serious permanent visual sequelae.

Halos and glare

Patients may experience halos and glare at night; these sequelae diminish with time. With recent improvements in laser technology, such side-effects have been reduced. These side-effects, which are thought to be related to preoperative scotopic pupillary diameter, are reported to occur in 3–40% of patients.

Infection

Topical antibiotics are used to minimize the risk of corneal infection. This problem can occur at any time following refractive surgery, and can lead to loss of vision.

Decentered laser ablation, irregular corneal surface

While there is a small risk of complications that would lead to an aberrant corneal refractive surface, many such outcomes may be improved with subsequent laser ablation.

Corneal ectasia

Following LASIK or PRK, an acceleration of corneal ectasia may occur in patients with preexisting corneal conditions such as forme fruste keratoconus or ectatic corneal dystrophies. Therefore, laser vision correction is not currently advised for patients with these comorbidities.

Further reading

Alió y Sanz J, Azar D. *Management of Complications in Refractive Surgery*. Berlin: Springer-Verlag; 2008.

Azar D, Gatinel D, Hoang-Xuan T. *Refractive Surgery*. 2nd edn.

New York, NY: Mosby Elsevier; 2007.

Buratto L, Brint S. *LASIK: Surgical Techniques and Complications*. Thorofare, NJ: Slack Inc.; 2000.

Krachmer J, Mannis M, Holland E. *Cornea*. 3rd edn. New York, NY: Mosby Elsevier; 2010.

Vinciguerra P, Camesasca F. *Refractive Surface Ablation*. Thorofare, NJ; Slack Inc.; 2007.

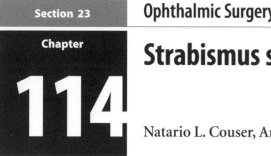

Extraocular muscle surgery is performed to correct strabismus. Strabismus includes any horizontal, vertical, or torsional misalignment of the eyes and can affect either children or adults. The disease can be categorized as congenital, acquired, restrictive, or paralytic. The goal of surgery is to restore the eyes to their normal anatomical position and to maximize the potential for binocularity. Other indications include eliminating diplopia, relieving mechanical restriction or restoring normal head position. In cases of nystagmus, surgery has the potential to improve vision. Either individual or multiple extraocular muscles may be operated upon during surgery; bilateral procedures are common. In selective cases, adjustable suture surgery may be performed.

Strabismus surgery is most commonly performed under general anesthesia. However, in selected cases, local anesthesia may be preferred. Topical anesthesia may be used for standard "muscle weakening" procedures for surgical patients who are good candidates for conscious sedation. Retrobulbar or peribulbar anesthesia may be useful for strabismus correction if strabismus correction surgery is only being performed in one eye under monitored anesthesia.

Usual postoperative course
Expected postoperative hospital stay

Most strabismus surgery is performed on an outpatient basis. Hospitalization is uncommon.

Operative mortality

The mortality rate associated with strabismus surgery is exceedingly low and generally due to complications of anesthesia. The incidence of malignant hyperthermia may be slightly higher in children undergoing strabismus surgery since strabismus can be an early sign of an undiagnosed congenital myopathy.

Special monitoring required

No special monitoring is required.

Patient activity and positioning

For the first 2 weeks after surgery, patients are advised to avoid swimming and other activities that may introduce foreign material or debris into their eyes. Young children should be carefully supervised during the postoperative period and discouraged from eye-rubbing behavior. Eye patches are usually not necessary.

Alimentation

Oral intake should be resumed gradually, since nausea and vomiting are common after strabismus surgery, especially in children.

Antibiotic coverage

Topical antibiotic or antibiotic/steroid combination drops are commonly prescribed after surgery.

Postoperative complications
In the hospital
Perforation of the sclera

Intraoperatively, a suture needle may perforate the sclera and injure either the choroid or even the neurosensory retina. The needle track may also provide an access for infections to enter the globe. Needle perforation may also lead to vitreous hemorrhage or retinal detachment. Usually, perforation leads to the formation of a chorioretinal scar. In general, observation with periodic fundus examination is recommended. Only rarely is further treatment needed, although some advocate laser treatment around the perforation site at the time of injury.

Slipped or lost muscle

A "slipped muscle" occurs when the muscle is severed and retracts within its capsule. A "lost muscle" occurs when a muscle is completely detached from the sclera and retracts into the sheath of the muscle toward the orbital apex. Such a muscle may be difficult to retrieve. Patients who present with an abrupt change in their ocular alignment, limited duction of

Medical Management of the Surgical Patient, ed. Michael F. Lubin, Thomas F. Dodson, and Neil H. Winawer. Published by Cambridge University Press. © Cambridge University Press 2013.

the muscle, or acute diplopia following strabismus surgery should be considered candidates for surgical exploration.

Diplopia

Transient diplopia is common after strabismus surgery. However, persistent diplopia is less common. When diplopia persists after surgery, additional surgery, prism glasses, or occlusion may be required. Reoperations are occasionally necessary as in the case of a "slipped" or "lost" muscle.

Anterior segment ischemia

Anterior segment ischemia is an uncommon complication that results from insufficient blood flow to the anterior segment of the eye. The ciliary arteries supply anterior segment circulation to the eye; transection occurs during most strabismus surgery. The likelihood of ocular ischemia increases when surgery is performed on three or more muscles in one eye, leaving fewer arteries to supply the anterior segment. Older patients who have compromised circulation may be adversely affected even after surgery on one or two muscles. The signs and symptoms of the anterior segment ischemic syndrome include decreased vision, ocular pain, and anterior chamber inflammation with signs of vascular incompetence (i.e., cell and flare on slit lamp examination). Operating on as few muscles as possible may prevent this complication; supportive treatment includes frequent administration of topical or systemic corticosteroids. Most cases resolve through the eventual development of collateral circulation; in its absence, end-stage disease (hypotony and/or phthisis bulbi) may occur.

After discharge
Infections

Although they are uncommon, periocular infections may occur; most at risk are children with poor hygiene or those who introduce foreign material through eye rubbing. Infectious complications usually occur between 1 and 5 days postoperatively. Pain, edema, and eyelid erythema are common signs and symptoms of infectious complications. Mild cases are usually treated with oral antibiotics; more severe cases may necessitate hospitalization and intravenous antibiotic administration. Endophthalmitis is rare following strabismus surgery, but may occur even without scleral perforation.

Conjunctival inclusion cysts or foreign-body granuloma

The conjunctival epithelial edges may be incidentally buried during closure of surgical incisions; a translucent cystic vesicle that becomes visible several days to years following surgery is thus created. Foreign-body granulomas may develop as a result of an allergic reaction to suture material, creating a tender, elevated, and hyperemic nodule that is visible at suture sites. The nodule remains visible from several weeks to months after surgery. Topical corticosteroids may be used; surgical excision is occasionally required in persistent cases.

Changes in eyelid position

Widening or narrowing of the palpebral fissures may occur following surgery on the vertical rectus muscles. In general, recessions of vertical muscles are associated with lid fissure widening; resections are associated with narrowing of the palpebral fissures. In addition, changes in lid position may result from stress on the orbicularis oculi muscle from eyelid speculum placement or from altered tone of a yoke, agonist, or antagonist muscle.

Unsatisfactory postoperative alignment

Multiple operations may be necessary to achieve the desired alignment; candidates should be appropriately counseled preoperatively. Before a reoperation is undertaken, patients should be observed for 4–6 weeks or until alignment is stable. An adjustable suture technique may be implemented with patients under conscious sedation. Under the direction of the cooperative patient, the surgeon is able to adjust the position of the muscles in the early postoperative period to help achieve the final desired outcome.

Further reading

Coats DK. Strabismus surgery complications. *Int Ophthalmol Clin* 2010; **50**: 125–35.

Coats DK, Olitsky SE. *Strabismus Surgery and its Complications*. Berlin: Springer-Verlag; 2007.

Kushner BJ. The efficacy of strabismus surgery in adults: a review for primary care physicians. *Postgrad Med J* 2011; **87**: 269–73.

Simon JW, Aaby AA, Drack AV *et al.* Pediatric ophthalmology and strabismus. *Am Acad Ophthalmol*

BCSC 2006; Section **6**: 173–93.

Lambert SR, Hutchinson AK. Strabismus surgery. In Spaeth GL, Danesh-Meyer H, Goldberg I, Kampik A, eds *Ophthalmic Surgery: Principles and Practice*. 4th edn. Philadelphia, PA: Saunders; 2011

Chapter

Enucleation, evisceration, and exenteration

Jill R. Wells, G. Baker Hubbard, and Timothy W. Olsen

Removal of an eye or the contents of an orbit may be indicated when the eye is affected by neoplasia or a severe infectious process, or when an end-stage ocular disease in a blind eye causes pain. These ophthalmic interventions are usually classified as:

1. Enucleation: the removal of the entire globe, including the sclera, intraocular contents, and the cornea. The stump of the optic nerve as well as the extraocular muscles are left behind.
2. Evisceration: the removal of intraocular contents including the lens, uvea, retina, vitreous humor, and in some cases the cornea. Only the sclera and extraocular muscles remain intact.
3. Exenteration: the removal of the globe and all of the orbital contents. This procedure may include removal of selective sections of orbital bone.

Following enucleations and eviscerations, an orbital implant is used to replace the globe and restore the lost orbital volume. The implant or sphere serves to maintain the structure of the orbit and to provide motility to the overlying prosthesis. For children, it additionally serves to maintain more normal growth of the surrounding orbital bones. In cases of exenteration, an osseointegrated prosthesis may be attached within the orbit, secured with metal support elements or magnets that are attached to bone.

Enucleation is the most frequently performed surgical approach, especially when there is a need to remove intraocular lesions such as tumors or blind painful eyes. When ocular disease results in an eye being classified as totally blind or NLP ("no light perception": incapable of perceiving the brightest light), a chance for visual recovery is highly unlikely. One exception would be that of an immediately post-traumatic eye that is filled with blood. When an eye has severe, end-stage pathology and has progressed to an eye that is painful and cosmetically unacceptable, enucleation may be recommended. Such a procedure is widely accepted. For example, after severe ocular trauma, the recommendation may be to remove the blind eye within 2 weeks after trauma. Some

believe that electing to perform this surgery will reduce the incidence of sympathetic ophthalmia. This rare complication results from the exposure of uveal tissue, which leads to an immune-mediated attack of the contralateral healthy eye. Other indications for enucleation include infectious endophthalmitis, end-stage glaucoma, and malignant intraocular tumors. Retinoblastoma and choroidal melanoma are relatively common intraocular tumors that may require enucleation.

Evisceration is an alternative to enucleation. Some believe that evisceration may lead to improved prosthesis motility. Evisceration should be considered only if the presence of an intraocular malignancy has been excluded. When there is no view of the posterior pole, an ultrasound or other definitive imaging modality must be performed to exclude the presence of an intraocular malignancy.

Exenteration is rarely recommended. It should be considered for the following scenarios: destructive tumors extending into the orbit from the sinuses, face, eyelids, and conjunctiva; intraocular malignancies that have extended from the globe to the orbit; and severe infectious processes such as mucormycosis in a diabetic patient.

In most cases, these procedures are performed under general anesthesia. Adequate local anesthesia may be difficult in cases of severe infectious globe disease; these cases may require general anesthesia. Additionally, the psychological effects of removal of the eye related to loss of function may be diminished by the use of general anesthesia. Patients prefer not to be "aware" of the loss while a surgery is being performed. This effect is not present when a restorative procedure for vision is being performed under local monitored anesthesia care.

Usual postoperative course
Expected postoperative hospital stay

Although there may not be a need to stay overnight in hospital after the surgery, it is not unusual to admit pediatric patients or even adults that may require additional pain control or hematologic management.

Medical Management of the Surgical Patient, ed. Michael F. Lubin, Thomas F. Dodson, and Neil H. Winawer. Published by Cambridge University Press. © Cambridge University Press 2013.

Operative mortality

Intraoperative mortality is very low and generally associated with general anesthesia. In the case of exenteration, postoperative mortality can occur if the ophthalmic disease progresses to involve other critical intracranial structures such as the cerebral vasculature or cavernous sinus.

Special monitoring required

Monitoring requirements may be necessary for underlying systemic diseases. Typically, special monitoring is not required other than the standard postoperative ophthalmologic examinations. The orbit is commonly secured with a postoperative pressure dressing that is removed within the following 24 hours. A plastic conformer that maintains the tissues within the eyelids is positioned in the conjunctival cul-de-sac to prevent contraction of the fornix. The conformer is generally left in place until a more sophisticated prosthesis can be placed.

Patient activity and positioning

The usual recommendation is minimal physical activity for a few days postoperatively. At one week, most patients may return to their usual activities.

Alimentation

Dietary restrictions are individualized. Usually, regular preoperative diet is resumed as patient recovers from anesthesia.

Postoperative medications

Postoperative medications are also individualized, and often include topical antibiotic ointment plus systemic medications for pain and nausea. When infection is the surgical indication for enucleation or evisceration, systemic antibiotics may be recommended.

Psychological support

Patients may feel that removal of an eye represents a major loss. The loss of vision, followed by the loss of an eye, may become an afflictive emotional event; the physical loss may be very distressing. The treating physician should be sensitive to the potential adverse psychological impact on the individual, and recommend psychological consultation and support as indicated.

Fitting an external prosthesis

Six to 8 weeks following an uncomplicated postoperative period, patients are referred to a professional ocularist. The ocularist creates and molds an external prosthesis that fits into the healed tissues of the orbit with attention to size and color. The prosthesis is artistically created, matching the size and coloration of the contralateral eye. Through education about periodic removal, cleaning, maintenance, and reinsertion of the orbit, patients are trained to care for their external prostheses.

Medical follow-up

The patient's internist may assist with the postoperative course when indicated. For example, when an eye is removed due to infectious endophthalmitis of unknown and possibly endogenous etiology, a systemic evaluation to find the nidus of infection is critical.

A systemic metastatic work-up is indicated with a neoplasm that is metastatic to the eye.

When the indication for enucleation was a primary intraocular malignant neoplasm, most physicians suggest regular intervals of surveillance for metastatic disease. All monocular patients should also wear protective polycarbonate glasses.

Postoperative complications

Orbital and periorbital edema

Immediately postoperatively, edema and even hemorrhage is common. Edema of the remaining periocular tissue may occur long-term. In general, either edema or mild hemorrhage tends to resolve spontaneously. The customary pressure patch is meant to minimize these problems. Long-term edema may require a re-assessment of the implant or may prompt an investigation for recurrent orbital disease.

Sympathetic ophthalmia

Of the three operations discussed, evisceration is associated with the greatest risk of sympathetic ophthalmia. This condition is theorized to follow evisceration in instances where remnants of uveal tissue, attached to the sclera of the involved eye, sensitize the immune system. Manifestations of sympathetic ophthalmia are treated with aggressive systemic immunosuppression.

Exposure and extrusion of implant

The implanted orbital prosthesis may extrude through the periocular soft tissues, either early postoperatively, or even as a late complication. Exposed implants may cause an orbital infection; they should be re-covered with a scleral patch graft or autogenous tissue graft. In cases of extrusion, a second operation is necessary to replace the implant.

Contraction of fornices

The fornices may contract following surgery, resulting in improper fitting of the prosthesis. To minimize this complication, as much as possible of the conjunctiva should be preserved during surgery. To prevent foreshortening of the fornices, the patient also should have a conformer in place immediately postoperatively. The conformer remains until a permanent prosthesis is in place.

Further reading

Dortzbach RK, Woog JJ. Choice of procedure: enucleation, evisceration, or prosthetic fitting over globes. *Ophthalmology* 1985: **92**: 1249–55.

Kersten RC, Codere F, Dailey RA *et al*. Orbit, eyelids, and lacrimal system: the anophthalmic socket. *Am Acad*

Ophthalmol BCSC 2006–2007; Section **7**: 119–29.

Nerad JA, Kersten R, Neuhans R *et al*. Orbit, eyelids and lacrimal system. *Am Acad Ophthalmol BCSC* 1996; Section **7**: 116–17.

Nunery WR, Hetzler K. Enucleation. In Hornblass, A., ed. *Oculoplastic, Orbital, and Reconstructive Surgery*. Vol **2**.

Baltimore, MD: Williams & Wilkins; 1990, pp. 1200–20.

Raflo TG. Enucleation and evisceration. In Tasman W, Jaeger EA, eds. *Duane's Ophthalmology*. Vol. **5**. Philadelphia, PA: Lippincott Williams & Wilkins; 2000.

Soares JP, Franca VP. Evisceration and enucleation. *Sem Ophthalmol* 2010; **25**: 94–7.

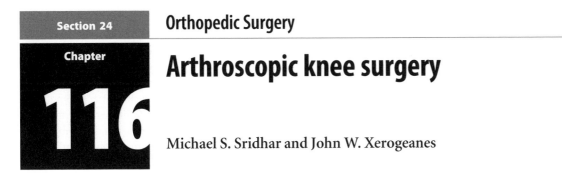

Arthroscopic knee surgery

Michael S. Sridhar and John W. Xerogeanes

Arthroscopy is the most performed procedure in orthopedics, with the knee being the most common site of surgical treatment. Advances in surgical technique and technology have led to increasing indications for knee arthroscopy. The advantages of arthroscopic surgery include the ability to function in an outpatient surgical setting, limited incisions and resultant improved cosmesis, and lowered risks for perioperative complications such as infection, substantial blood loss, and thromboembolic disease. Image capture systems and the ability to take still photographs and videos intraoperatively provide illustrations of specific pathology and procedures carried out, thereby fortifying the medical record and enhancing postoperative communication with the patient. The benefits carry over to the postoperative period in the form of lower requirements for analgesia and earlier initiation of rehabilitation protocols.

While the utility of knee arthroscopy has primarily been observed in its ability to administer therapeutic maneuvers, the arthroscope remains the gold standard as a powerful diagnostic tool. The process of preoperative counseling with the patient and obtaining informed consent is paramount, as the treatment plan can be modified based on arthroscopic findings. Surgeries performed most regularly include partial meniscectomy, meniscal repair, and anterior cruciate ligament (ACL) reconstruction. The arthroscope is also utilized for complex isolated or multiligamentous reconstructions including posterior cruciate ligament (PCL) and medial collateral ligament (MCL) work, meniscal transplantation, articular cartilage restoration, the irrigation and debridement of a pyoarthrosis, and osseous injuries such as low-energy tibial plateau fractures. A requisite for the arthroscopic management of intra-articular soft-tissue derangements is motion, as preoperative knee motion is the best predictor of postoperative motion. An exception is a locked knee joint secondary to a large bucket-handle meniscal tear.

Patients with meniscal pathology will often recall a specific twisting or squatting injury, describing a sharp pain on the medial or lateral side of their knee, occasionally radiating posteriorly. Mechanical symptoms such as clicking, catching, or locking are highly suggestive of a flap tear to either meniscus

that is physically impairing knee motion. On exam, patients have tenderness along the respective joint line, positive Thessaly and McMurray's tests, and localized pain with hyperflexion and/or hyperextension of the knee. Exam findings are often confirmed by a high-resolution MRI, but it should be mentioned that plain radiographs should always be the first imaging modality ordered in the setting of knee trauma to evaluate for fracture, dislocation, and/or osteoarthritis. Modern MRIs are capable of visualizing the articular surface, allowing for refined decision-making and counseling of patients with regard to their expected outcome. The decision to perform a meniscal repair or partial meniscectomy is made at the time of surgery.

Patients with injuries to the ACL usually report a twisting injury to the knee, with or without contact. They experience immediate or early swelling and pain, and usually have a sensation of subjective "looseness" or instability with rotatory movements that often correlates with objective laxity. Upon examination, the patient typically has an effusion, sometimes significant enough to warrant aspiration for pain relief and improvement in motion, the downside being the potential avenue for infection. With an acute, complete tear, patients usually have positive Lachman's (most sensitive), anterior drawer, and pivot shift tests. Briefly described, a Lachman's test is done with the knee in 30° of flexion and an anterior shift is applied to the tibia with one hand while the femur is held in place with the other hand. The contralateral, unaffected knee should always be examined first to have a frame of reference with which to compare the injured extremity. MRI is highly sensitive and specific for visualizing ACL rupture. Most tears involve a complete disruption of the tendinous substance. Avulsion injuries occur and are typically diagnosed in children.

An ACL tear, in and of itself, is not an indication for reconstruction. The decision for surgery should be individualized, as low-demand patients do not require an ACL for activities of daily living and reconstruction is usually contraindicated in the setting of concomitant arthrosis. Lifestyle modification to avoid certain sports and knee positions can allow for reasonable outcomes in some patients. For more active patients who are uninterested in lifestyle modification and will commit to

Medical Management of the Surgical Patient, ed. Michael F. Lubin, Thomas F. Dodson, and Neil H. Winawer. Published by Cambridge University Press. © Cambridge University Press 2013.

vigorous rehabilitation postoperatively, ACL reconstruction is a reasonable option. Preoperative counseling is vital, as the rehabilitation required to have a successful reconstruction is time-consuming and strenuous.

Medial and lateral collateral ligament (LCL) and PCL injuries can occur in isolation or in a multiligamentous knee (i.e., knee dislocation). The MCL is intra-articular and along with ACL and medial meniscus tears, is historically reported as a component of the "terrible triad" knee injury. Suspicion for an MCL or LCL tear should be raised when the mechanism of injury includes a non-physiologic valgus or varus stress respectively. Patients often report "buckling" or "giving way" of the knee, and the clinical exam often reveals laxity with valgus stress for an MCL tear and varus stress for an LCL tear. Typically, collateral ligament injuries heal via scar tissue without surgical intervention with a period of knee immobilization in the coronal plane. It is essential to have stable collaterals prior to cruciate ligament reconstruction. The mechanism involved in a PCL tear is a posteriorly directed force on the tibia. Exam findings include a positive posterior drawer, quadriceps active test, and posterior sag test. These injuries are typically treated conservatively unless in the setting of a multiligamentous knee or in a high-demand patient such as an elite athlete. Magnetic resonance imaging is a valuable tool in the diagnosis and management of these injuries.

Articular cartilage injuries, including osteochondritis dissecans and osteonecrosis, pose a particular challenge to the treating orthopedic surgeon due to the limited healing potential of this tissue type. Chondral defects can result from trauma or degeneration and if left untreated can lead to significant functional deterioration, debilitating joint pain, and degenerative arthritis. Modern techniques of cartilage transplantation and bone marrow stimulation techniques (microfracture) have provided much-needed tools for dealing with these conditions. These advanced techniques must be administered under stringent indications and should be avoided in patients with an elevated body mass index, those older than 40–50 years, and in the setting of preexisting, primary osteoarthritis, inflammatory arthropathy, or limb malalignment. Such injuries may be difficult to glean from the history and physical examination and are often determined on MRI. Failure of conservative management may necessitate surgical intervention.

Meniscus

Knowledge regarding the importance of the meniscal fibrocartilage and its shock-absorbing and joint-stabilizing properties has gone through significant evolution. Once thought to be vestigial tissue, menisci were routinely excised in the form of a total meniscectomy when injured. During diagnostic arthroscopy, a characterization of the meniscal tear can be made in multiple planes and correlated with the MRI findings. Various tear patterns may occur through the anterior horn, body, and posterior horn. Repair should only be carried out in young, active patients and those without degenerative changes. If the

tear is not amenable to repair, the torn meniscus may be removed with a combination of a mechanical shaver and meniscal biters under direct visualization through the arthroscope. Isolated meniscectomies are performed under MAC (minimum alveolar concentration) and local anesthesia without antibiotic prophylaxis or a pneumatic tourniquet. Routine, degenerative meniscal tears can take as little as 10 minutes with minimal blood loss, and patients are discharged from an ambulatory surgery center fully weightbearing. With meniscal repair, the procedure may take longer, a tourniquet may be used, and preoperative antibiotic prophylaxis is administered given the need for suture placement. The repair is done arthroscopically, sometimes with an accessory incision either posteromedially or posterolaterally for passage of suture needles. Meniscal repairs are also done in an ambulatory setting, immediate knee motion is allowed, and weightbearing is protected for 4–6 weeks.

Although many meniscal tears are repairable, not all are salvageable. Meniscal transplantation has been developed for a certain subset of younger, active patients without preexisting, advanced arthritis who have undergone a prior, total meniscectomy and who would stand to benefit from a decrease in pain with daily activities, restoration of the load-bearing capacity of the transplanted meniscus, and protection of the subjacent articular surface. Much research is currently being devoted to the improvement of this technique and the encouragement of host cellular repopulation of the transplanted tissue and organization of the collagen matrix to match the native meniscus's ability to withstand the many forces applied to an athletic knee.

Anterior cruciate ligament

The poor performance of primary repair of ACL tears has led to the development of techniques for arthroscopically assisted ACL reconstruction. The three most popular graft choices are autograft bone-patellar tendon-bone (BPTB), autograft hamstrings (HS), and allograft. While there is some dependence on surgeon preference and familiarity, the pros and cons are as follows. Allograft tissue eliminates donor-site morbidity and patients often enjoy a less painful procedure and quicker rehabilitation, making it an attractive option for adult patients and recreational athletes. The major concern with allograft tissue lies in its potential for antigenicity, disease transmission, and slower biologic incorporation. Modern techniques of sterilization have made the risk of disease transmission remarkably low with only a handful of case reports in the literature.

Bone-patellar tendon-bone grafts require a harvesting of the middle third of the native patellar tendon. These grafts are extremely stout, are easily secured with bioabsorbable screws in the tibial and femoral tunnels, and benefit from bone-to-bone integration. Complications arise in the form of patellar fractures, patellar tendon rupture, and persistent anterior knee pain.

Hamstring autografts are relatively simpler to harvest by using a small incision over the hamstring insertion at the pes anserinus on the proximal tibia. Concern lies in the less reliable anatomy of the hamstring tendons, potentially less durable soft-tissue fixation, reliance on tendon-to-bone healing, postoperative sensory disturbances through the distal, cutaneous branches of the saphenous nerve, and the sacrificing of a potential dynamic stabilizer of the knee joint.

Once the graft is selected, the arthroscope is used to determine where the graft will be placed with the hope of recreating the anatomic footprint of the ACL on the tibial and femoral sides. Any remnant of the torn ACL is typically removed except in the setting of an intact, singular bundle. The graft is secured on both sides with a variety of fixation devices depending on the graft choice and preference of the surgeon.

Anterior cruciate ligament reconstruction typically requires less than an hour for an allograft and about an hour for an autograft. Preoperative antibiotics, in the form of a first-generation cephalosporin or clindamycin in penicillin-allergic patients, are administered and a tourniquet is used. The procedure is usually performed under general anesthesia with a laryngeal mask airway (LMA), blood loss is minimal, and patients are discharged home shortly after their procedure with motion encouraged and weightbearing restricted for about a week.

Cartilage

A discrete cartilage defect, similar to a meniscal tear, can be the source of debilitating pain and can lead to the development of osteoarthritis. Newer techniques and the modification of older techniques have shown some success in the treatment of these lesions. Bone marrow stimulation or microfracture employs an arthroscopic awl to perforate the subchondral bone, delivering a blood clot with multipotent mesenchymal stem cells to the defect in the hope of differentiation into fibrochondrocytes capable of establishing a fibrocartilaginous repair of the lesion. With involvement of the femoral side, weightbearing is restricted for 6 weeks, while involvement of the patellofemoral joint allows for immediate weightbearing. Most surgeons typically treat their patients with continuous passive motion postoperatively to enhance cartilage nourishment. Other, newer procedures involve whole-tissue transplantation, typically done via a mini-arthrotomy. One option is autologous osteochondral mosaicplasty, sometimes referred to as OATS (osteoarticular transfer system). This involves the harvest of multiple, small cylindrical osteochondral plugs from the less weightbearing periphery of the articular surface of the femoral condyle and transfer to create a congruent and durable resurfaced area in the defect. Another option is osteochondral allograft transplantation, which involves articular resurfacing with a fresh cadaver graft of hyaline cartilage and its underlying subchondral bone. Lastly, there is the option of autologous chondrocyte implantation (ACI), a two-staged procedure requiring an initial chondrocyte harvest and subsequent re-implantation of the approximately 12 million cultured chondrocytes (Carticel, Genzyme Tissue Repair, Cambridge, MA)

into a full-thickness chondral defect. With these more involved cartilage restoration techniques, weightbearing is usually protected for at least 6 weeks and up to 3 months if a realignment osteotomy is simultaneously performed.

Osteoarthritis

The effectiveness of arthroscopy for degenerative joint disease of the knee is controversial. The results of these procedures are unpredictable at best. However, it is believed that there is a subset of patients with primary knee osteoarthritis in whom arthroscopy may be beneficial, namely those with mechanical symptoms of locking, catching, or clicking that are the result of degenerative meniscal tear or an osteoarticular loose body.

Usual postoperative course
Antibiotic coverage

Preoperative broad-spectrum prophylaxis will have been administered and is extended for 24 hours if the patient is admitted. Much recent attention has deservedly been focused on community-acquired methicillin-resistant *Staphylococcus aureus* (MRSA) and its implication in postsurgical infections. Patients with a prior MRSA wound or deep infection receive a preoperative dose of vancomycin. Some high-risk centers are moving towards preoperative screenings for asymptomatic MRSA carriers via nasal swabs. If positive, we recommend the prophylactic use of mupirocin nasal ointment and/or chlorhexidine soap bath/showers.

Pain management

It is customary to inject a local anesthetic into the arthroscopy portal sites and incisions to cause preemptive desensitization of nociceptors. Many surgeons also inject a local anesthetic to distend the joint preoperatively and for pain control postoperatively. Postoperative pain ranges from minimal after arthroscopic partial meniscectomy to moderate after ACL reconstruction. We typically also administer an intra-articular dose of Toradol for its anti-inflammatory properties. Narcotic analgesics may be required for several days, and we often prescribe a course of Naprosyn to control postoperative inflammation in patients without contraindications to non-steroidals.

Rehabilitation

With an ACL reconstruction, it takes 9–12 months before full return to sports. In the early postoperative period, knee motion is key, especially the pursuit of knee extension comparable to the unaffected knee. Immediately after surgery, range of motion exercises and light strengthening exercises are begun. More aggressive strengthening may begin when the reconstruction has been afforded the time to heal. This is slowly combined with functional activities and then sport-specific activities, finally ending with return to competition on a gradual basis. Patients undergoing a partial meniscectomy do not require extensive rehabilitation and may return to full activity when their strength and motion are optimized and their swelling and pain are minimal.

Postoperative complications

Hemarthrosis

Hemarthrosis may occur in approximately 1% of cases and is more common after release of the lateral patellofemoral retinaculum due to disruption of the superior lateral geniculate artery.

Thromboembolic disease

Several factors have been associated with a greater risk for patients, including age over 40 years, prolonged surgical and/ or tourniquet time, and having a history of thromboembolic disease. Thrombi distal to the popliteal circulation do not require systemic anticoagulation. Intraoperatively, the well leg receives a pneumatic compression sleeve.

Infection

While a rare occurrence, infections can be a devastating complication, especially in the setting of cruciate reconstruction or tissue transplant. They require arthroscopic lavage and debridement, may require graft resection, and usually up to 6 weeks of intravenous antibiotics. After extended antibiosis, an arthrocentesis is performed and if the synovial fluid is clear of infection, a graft may be reimplanted.

Neurovascular injury

Nerve injuries are typically due to direct injury intraoperatively (transection or traction-induced), postoperative compartment syndrome, external compression due to improper patient positioning and ineffective padding, or compression underneath the tourniquet. Most direct injuries are seen with lateral, inside-out meniscal repairs where the suture needle may perforate the popliteal neurovascular bundle or the common peroneal nerve as it courses around the fibular neck.

Compartment syndrome

Compartment syndrome may be caused by fluid extravasation into the thigh or calf via rupture of the suprapatellar pouch or the semimembranosus bursa respectively. The syndrome can also occur in the well leg if it is left in an extreme position, wrapped too tightly in an attempt to secure the limb, or insufficiently padded.

Tourniquet-related injury

Complications associated with prolonged tourniquet use include the self-limited post-tourniquet syndrome, compartment syndrome, direct vascular injury, compressive neuropraxia, soft-tissue damage, and myonephropathic-metabolic syndrome resulting from the systemic return of toxic metabolites after deflation of the tourniquet. Symptoms of the latter include metabolic acidosis, hyperkalemia, myoglobinemia, myoglobinuria, and renal failure.

After discharge

Delayed problems generally relate to inadequately controlled pain, residual instability, or graft rerupture or meniscal retear and may require additional treatment.

Further reading

Allum R. Complications of arthroscopy of the knee. *J Bone Joint Surg* 2002; **84B**: 937–45.

ElAttrache NS, Harner CD, Mirzayan R, Sekiya JK, eds. Anterior cruciate ligament reconstruction: general considerations. In *Surgical Techniques in Sports Medicine*. Philadelphia, PA: Lippincott Williams & Wilkins; 2007, pp. 309–18.

Bedi A, Feeley B, Williams RJ III. Current concepts review. Management of articular cartilage defects of the knee. *J Bone Joint Surg* 2010; **92A**: 994–1009.

Carey JL, Dunn WR, Dahm DL, Zeger SL, Spindler KP. A systematic review of anterior cruciate ligament reconstruction with autograft compared with allograft. *J Bone Joint Surg* 2009; **91**: 2242–50.

Carey JL, Huffman GR, Parekh SG, Sennett BJ. Outcomes of anterior cruciate ligament injuries to running backs and wide receivers in the National Football League. *Am J Sports Med* 2006; **34**: 1911–17.

Cerynik DL, Lewullis GE, Joves BC, Palmer MP, Tom JA. Outcomes of microfracture in professional basketball players. *Knee Surg Sports Traumatol Arthrosc* 2009; **17**: 1135–9.

Grontvedt T, Engebretsen L, Benum P et al. A prospective, randomized study of three operations for acute rupture of the anterior cruciate ligament: five year follow-up of one hundred and thirty-one patients. *J Bone Joint Surg* 1996; **78A**: 159–68.

Moseley JB, O'Malley K, Petersen NJ et al. A controlled trial of arthroscopic surgery for osteoarthritis of the knee. *N Engl J Med* 2002; **347**: 81–8.

Nelson JD, Hogan MV, Miller MD. What's new in sports medicine. *J Bone Joint Surg* 2010; **92A**: 250–63.

Taylor DC, DeBerardino TM, Nelson BJ et al. Patellar tendon versus hamstring tendon autografts for anterior cruciate ligament reconstruction: a randomized controlled trial using similar femoral and tibial fixation methods. *Am J Sports Med* 2009; **37**: 1946–57.

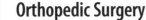

Chapter

117

Total knee replacement

Greg Erens and Thomas Bradbury

Total knee replacement is indicated for end-stage degeneration of the knee joint with loss of articular (joint surface) cartilage. The most common reasons for this operation are osteoarthritis (idiopathic or post-traumatic) and inflammatory arthritis (rheumatoid, psoriatic, etc.). Total knee replacement is typically considered once all other conservative modalities (oral medications, intra-articular injections, physical therapy, weight loss, etc.) have failed to relieve the pain and dysfunction associated with knee degeneration.

The natural knee joint consists of three compartments: lateral, medial, and patellofemoral. A total knee replacement is designed to resurface the damaged articular surfaces of these compartments. Both the femoral and tibial components are typically made from metal. A high-density plastic (polyethylene) insert is placed between the metal components to serve as the artificial cartilage of the joint. Highly crosslinked polyethylene may be utilized as a more wear-resistant bearing surface; however, long-term results with this type of plastic are not yet available. Most total knee replacements also resurface the patella with an all-polyethylene component. Fixation of the metal components to the bone is typically done with bone cement, but some designs allow for fixation by bony ingrowth into porous metal surfaces applied to the surface of the implant, which is placed against the bone. By removing all damaged surfaces of the knee, pain can be alleviated and function restored.

The procedure is commonly performed through a midline skin incision over the anterior aspect of the knee. The joint capsule is typically entered medially along the border of the patella. Standard approaches extend into the quadriceps mechanism. Some minimally invasive approaches that do not extend into the quadriceps can be utilized, but complications from poor visualization and component position have been described. The patella may or may not be everted for exposure of the joint. Once it is exposed, sizing and cutting guides direct the preparation of the distal femur and proximal tibia. Careful attention is given to the alignment of the components and the balancing of the knee ligaments. The operation usually takes less than 2 hours, though complicated total knee replacements can take longer.

Special attention to pain management is recommended. Many different techniques have been described. General, spinal, epidural, and/or regional anesthesia may be used. Often, multimodal therapies are combined to help with perioperative pain control. A tourniquet is typically used on the upper thigh to limit intraoperative blood loss and improve cement fixation of the components. Postoperative bleeding may occasionally require a transfusion, although the trigger for transfusion is variable among physicians. Most transfusions are recommended for patients with symptomatic anemia not responding to intravenous (IV) fluids. There has been a trend away from autologous blood donation. Statistics show that over 50% of autologous units are not transfused and that the cost of autologous donation may be significant.

Unicompartmental (partial) knee replacement has gained some popularity, and involves replacement of either the medial or lateral compartment only. By replacing only the damaged compartment, there is less overall surgical trauma which may translate into an easier recovery and more natural knee function. Some reported results demonstrate nearly equivalent results to total knee replacement, with failure typically occurring due to wearing out of the opposite compartment.

Usual postoperative course

Expected postoperative hospital stay

The expected postoperative hospital stay is 2–4 days.

Operative mortality

Operative mortality is less than 1%.

Special monitoring required

Neurovascular checking of the extremity should be performed during the early postoperative period to rule out neural or vascular injuries, which are rare. Monitoring for clinical signs of deep vein thrombosis (DVT) should be conducted during the remainder of the hospital stay.

Medical Management of the Surgical Patient, ed. Michael F. Lubin, Thomas F. Dodson, and Neil H. Winawer. Published by Cambridge University Press. © Cambridge University Press 2013.

Patient activity and positioning

Early mobilization is encouraged following total knee replacement. Physical therapy is critical to the success of the surgery. It is initiated in the hospital and is often continued for a total of 3 months postoperatively. Weightbearing (as tolerated) is started within the first 24 hours after surgery. Often, a walker or crutches are required to help with balance and proper gait. The patient may be weaned from an assistive device once pain, strength, and balance allow. Many patients are able to get out of bed, walk in the hall, and even negotiate stairs independently prior to discharge. For patients who experience delays in achieving these goals, a short stay in a rehabilitation facility may be recommended.

Alimentation

Diet is typically advanced as tolerated. Patients are transitioned to oral pain medication as part of a multimodal regimen. Postoperative ileus is rare.

Antibiotic coverage

Appropriately timed and selected prophylactic antibiotics are part of the current set of hospital-based Joint Commission core measures, and are a critical component to help prevent periprosthetic infection. Administration of a first-generation cephalosporin within 1 hour prior to incision is recommended. For patients with penicillin or cephalosporin allergy, vancomycin is given within 2 hours prior to incision. Antibiotics are discontinued within 24 hours postoperatively. No additional benefit has been demonstrated beyond 24 hours.

Postoperative complications

In the hospital

Fever

Postoperative fever is quite common following total knee replacement. Low grade temperatures less than 38.5 °C (101.3 °F) may be seen for up to 3 days postoperatively. Infectious work-up in these patients is usually negative unless other clinical findings are apparent. Fevers occurring after postoperative day 3 and above 39.0 °C (102.2 °F) have a higher rate of positive findings.

Thromboembolism

Without prophylaxis, DVT occurs in 50–80% of patients following total knee replacement. Prophylactic measures such as early mobilization, sequential compression devices, epidural anesthesia and pharmacologic prophylaxis (aspirin, low molecular weight heparin (LMWH), or warfarin) reduce the incidence to 30–40%. While warfarin is still used by many orthopedists for DVT prophylaxis after knee replacement, at our institution we typically use LMWH (Lovenox). Without prophylaxis, symptomatic pulmonary embolism occurs in 2–7% of patients; fatal pulmonary embolism has been reported in 0.2–0.7% of patients. There continues to be debate regarding the best pharmacologic agent. Each one has its own risks and benefits, and the choice can be tailored to the patient and their individual risk. Prophylaxis is started with 24 hours of surgery and may be continued for up to 2–4 weeks postoperatively. Use of a pharmacologic agent must be weighed against the possibility of bleeding complications.

Bleeding

Minimal blood loss typically occurs during a total knee replacement because of the common use of a tourniquet. However, bleeding does occur following deflation of the tourniquet. Meticulous attention to hemostasis is recommended to prevent hematoma formation. Coagulopathy or medications may heighten the risk of bleeding. Coagulopathies should be corrected preoperatively, and medications such as warfarin, Plavix and NSAIDs should be withheld for 5–7 days before the operation. Drains can be utilized, but recent studies have not demonstrated improved results.

Hematomas may result in increased postoperative pain and stiffness. In addition, a hematoma can lead to prolonged drainage. If persistent drainage occurs for more than 5–7 days despite immobilization and local wound care, operative intervention may be recommended. A higher risk of infection has been associated with this scenario.

Neurovascular injury

Nerve injury during total knee replacement is quite rare. The most common injury is injury to the peroneal nerve. This typically presents as a "foot drop" and decreased sensation in the peroneal distribution of the foot. This nerve injury is usually associated with a preoperative flexion contracture and a valgus (knock-kneed) deformity. If peroneal palsy is detected postoperatively, the surgical bandage should be loosened and the knee flexed. An ankle–foot orthosis (AFO) may be required to help with gait. Resolution is variable, with best results in patients with early recovery of function.

Vascular injury is even more uncommon. It is usually detected once the tourniquet is released or by neurovascular exam immediately postoperatively. Prompt attention is critical, and timely vascular surgery consultation is recommended.

After discharge

Extensor mechanism problems

The extensor mechanism consists of the quadriceps tendon, the patella, and the patellar tendon. This mechanism is critical to the function of the knee to maintain stance and to allow gait. A tear of the quadriceps or patellar tendon or a fracture of the patella may lead to disruption of the extensor mechanism. Inability to extend the knee, particularly after a fall or trauma, should prompt an evaluation of extensor integrity. If disruption is noted with evidence of an extensor lag, surgical intervention is often required.

Infection

Infection following primary total knee replacement has an incidence of approximately 1%. This is a very serious complication and needs urgent attention. Obesity, diabetes, and immunosuppression increase the risk of periprosthetic infection. The diagnosis of infection early in the immediate postoperative period is difficult. Common signs of infection are masked by the swelling, pain, and hyperemia around the surgical incision associated with a normal postoperative recovery. Persistent fever > 38.5 °C or drainage from the incision occurring for longer than 7 days after surgery warrants further investigation. Serum C-reactive protein and erythrocyte sedimentation rate are often used to aid in the diagnosis of infection postoperatively. In the uncomplicated total knee replacement, the C-reactive protein peaks by postoperative day 3 but can remain elevated for up to 6 months after surgery. An increasing C-reactive protein rate after postoperative day 3 is suggestive of infection. Confirmation of infection is typically obtained from a knee aspirate analysis of cell count, gram stain, and culture. It is imperative that antibiotics are withheld until the diagnosis is confirmed and the treating orthopedist has been notified. Antibiotic administration will temporarily improve the clinical picture but will not eradicate deep infection. The delay in diagnosis may result in a delay in surgical intervention. Early infection can often be successfully managed with surgical irrigation and debridement with polyethylene liner exchange, followed by a course of intravenous antibiotics. If the infection is believed to be more chronic in nature (longer than 1 month), then removal of all components, with irrigation, debridement, and insertion of an antibiotic spacer, may be required. Prolonged administration of IV antibiotics (6–8 weeks) is often needed. A reimplantation should only be considered once the infection has been eradicated. Infections that persist despite aggressive therapy may require chronic suppressive antibiotics or even amputation.

Late hematogenous seeding of a total knee replacement is a rare complication. However, routine antibiotic prophylaxis prior to any invasive procedure that may cause bacteremia (dental procedures, colonoscopy, etc.) is recommended for 2 years postoperatively. See Table 117.1 for a list of patients who should receive antibiotic prophylaxis for life prior to invasive procedures.

Stiffness

Decreased range of motion in the early postoperative period, usually related to pain and swelling, should be expected. Range of motion will typically improve steadily over the first 6–8 weeks as pain and swelling subside. Physical therapy is also critical to help this process. However, some patients may not

Table 117.1 Patients at potential increased risk of hematogenous total joint infection

Immunocompromised/immunosuppressed patients
Inflammatory arthropathies (e.g., rheumatoid arthritis, systemic lupus erythematosus)
Drug-induced immunosuppression
Radiation-induced immunosuppression
Patients with comorbidities (e.g., diabetes, obesity, HIV, smoking)
Previous prosthetic joint infections
Malnourishment
Hemophilia
HIV infection
Insulin-dependent (Type 1) diabetes
Malignancy
Megaprostheses. A megaprosthesis is a prosthesis used for limb salvage when extensive bone loss is present or when a large amount of bone is removed (e.g., tumor surgery). The prosthesis uses metal to replace the absent bone.

progress as expected. Inability to achieve 90° flexion within 4–6 weeks may require intervention (manipulation) under anesthesia. Beyond 3 months, manipulation may not provide significant benefit and stiffness may become permanent. Skillful surgical technique, avoidance of postoperative hematoma, and patient education can usually prevent problems with stiffness.

Polyethylene wear and loosening

The most common long-term problem following total knee replacement is wear of the prosthesis. Over time, the polyethylene bearing surface experiences wear and microscopic wear particles are released into the joint. These wear particles can lead to an inflammatory response causing destruction of bone around the prosthesis. This is called osteolysis. If enough bone is lost, fracture or implant loosening can occur. This often presents as pain, typically with weightbearing activities. Revision surgery for total knee replacement is often required in this scenario. With improved polyethylenes now available, we can hope to delay or arrest the occurrence of prosthetic wear, loosening, and failure.

Further reading

AAOS Information Statement 1033. *Antibiotic Prophylaxis for Bacteremia in Patients with Joint Replacements.* 2009. http://www.aaos.org/about/papers/advistmt/1033.asp.

Ayers DC, Dennis DA, Johanson NA, Pelligrini VD. Common complications of total knee arthroplasty. *J Bone Joint Surg Am* 1997; **79**: 278–311.

Bozic KJ, Kurtz SM, Lau E *et al.* The epidemiology of revision total knee arthroplasty in the United States. *Clin Orthop Relat Res* 2010; **468**: 45–51.

Hirsh J, Guyatt G, Albers GW *et al.* Antithrombotic and Thrombolytic Therapy. American College of Chest Physicians Evidence-Based Clinical Practice Guidelines (8th Edition). *Chest* 2008; **133**; 110S–12S.

Moyad TF, Thornhill T, Estok D. Evaluation and management of the infected total hip and knee. *Orthopedics* 2008; **31**(6): 581–8.

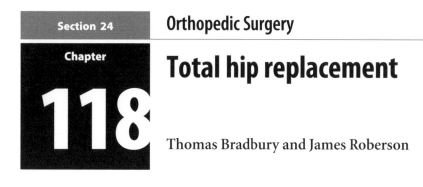

Chapter

118

Total hip replacement

Thomas Bradbury and James Roberson

The hip joint is a constrained ball and socket joint capable of withstanding repeated forces in excess of ten times body weight. The articulating surfaces of the femoral head (the ball) and the acetabulum (the socket) are covered with articular cartilage which allows smooth and painless motion. Pain, stiffness, and declining function due to cartilage and bone damage in the hip joint are the primary indications for total hip arthroplasty. Most commonly, these symptoms are the result of osteoarthritis, but can also occur with inflammatory arthritis (e.g., rheumatoid arthritis), bone death (e.g., avascular necrosis) or the sequelae of traumatic injury (e.g., previous fracture). It is now recognized that most cases of hip osteo-arthritis are a result of subtle variations in the shape of the femoral head and/or acetabulum. These variations result in hip impingement (abnormal contact forces across the joint that eventually result in destruction of articular cartilage).

When the symptoms of hip arthritis are no longer responsive to conservative measures including medication and reduction in hip joint force (e.g., weight loss or use of a cane), total hip arthroplasty may produce dramatic improvements in pain management, function, and quality of life. The operation is performed through an incision over the outside of the hip. The joint is exposed and an osteotomy (bone cut) in the femoral neck allows removal of the femoral head from the acetabulum. The acetabulum is prepared to accept a hemispherical metal socket. A hemispherical socket liner is then snapped into the socket. The hollow canal of the femur bone is prepared to accept a metal stem. A ball that perfectly matches the shape and size of the liner of the socket is attached to the top of the stem. The soft tissues around the hip are then repaired and protected while they heal.

The materials used for stem and socket are most commonly metal alloys (titanium). The liner is mostly commonly made of hardened plastic (high molecular weight polyethylene) but can also be manufactured from metal or ceramic. Polished chrome cobalt is the most commonly used material for the ball although ceramics are also used. These combinations of modular prosthetic components then serve as the ball and socket of the joint. Both the acetabular socket and femoral stem are most commonly initially attached to bone using a "press–fit" or "interference fit" between the bone and implant. Those terms indicate a precise contouring of bone with instruments to allow an exact and tight fit of the prosthetic device within the confines of the socket and shaft of the femur. The outer surface of the socket and stem are coated with a porous metal surface which allows for bone growth into the prosthesis and biologic fixation. Biologic fixation by bone ingrowth to the implant has proven highly successful and durable. Thus, bone cement is less commonly used for fixation of the component in total hip replacement than in the past.

The typical surgery time for total hip replacement is 2 hours or less, although more complicated operations such as revision of a failed replacement may require much more time. Depending on surgeon and patient preference, general, spinal, or epidural anesthesia can be used. Anticipated blood loss for uncomplicated cases is usually 250–500 mL. Postoperative blood transfusion may be required; hematocrit and hemoglobin should be monitored during the first couple of days after surgery. Because of cost, complexity, and questionable efficacy, autologous donation of blood prior to surgery has fallen out of favor.

Usual postoperative course
Expected postoperative hospital stay

The expected postoperative hospital stay is 1–3 nights for uncomplicated cases.

Operative mortality

Operative mortality is significantly less than 1%.

Special monitoring required

Neurovascular examination of the extremity should be performed in the early postoperative period. Monitoring for clinical signs of deep vein thrombosis (DVT) must continue during the subsequent hospital stay, and duplex scanning is useful to rule out DVT if symptoms arise. Spiral CT is the

Medical Management of the Surgical Patient, ed. Michael F. Lubin, Thomas F. Dodson, and Neil H. Winawer. Published by Cambridge University Press. © Cambridge University Press 2013.

best imaging study to rule out pulmonary embolus. Because of fluid shifts in the first couple of days following surgery, the patient should be carefully monitored for possible orthostatic hypotension when first mobilizing and beginning physical therapy.

Patient activity and positioning

The patient is mobilized and encouraged to walk either on the day of surgery or the first postoperative day. Generally, patients are allowed to weight bear as tolerated with a walker or crutches unless otherwise specified by the surgeon. Patients should be able to get out of bed independently, walk in the hall, and maneuver a few stairs prior to leaving the hospital. If the patient is having difficulty achieving these goals in a timely manner, a short stay at a rehabilitation hospital is encouraged. Most patients use either a walker or crutches for 2–4 weeks, followed by use of a cane for 2–4 weeks. The duration of weightbearing activity can be incrementally increased as discomfort subsides. Postoperative pain subsides relatively quickly.

Alimentation

Typically, patients take clear liquids on the day of operation; diet can be advanced as tolerated. Occasionally, postoperative ileus occurs, delaying oral intake. Pain medications may also contribute to nausea, which may be alleviated by anti-emetics.

Antibiotic coverage

Administration of prophylactic antibiotics immediately prior to the start of total hip arthroplasty has been shown to decrease the postoperative infection rate. A first-generation cephalosporin is the drug of choice in most cases but vancomycin or clindamycin are used in patients who are allergic to penicillin or cephalosporins. Antibiotics should not be continued longer than 24 hours after surgery.

Postoperative complications

In the hospital

Fever

Slight to moderate elevations in temperature are commonly observed following hip replacement surgery. This may be related to a subclinical marrow embolus that does not cause changes in the chest radiograph. Embarking on an investigation for infection during this period is expensive and invariably negative if no other clinical findings are apparent.

Thromboembolism

When preventive measures have not been used, a high percentage of patients undergoing total hip arthroplasty have been found to have DVTs on routine venograms. This incidence can be reduced by administration of low molecular weight heparin, aspirin, or warfarin; use of sequential compression stockings; early mobility; or combinations of the above. Fortunately a high percentage of thrombi occurring after hip replacement are asymptomatic and located at, or below, the popliteal vein. Symptomatic pulmonary emboli occur in about 1% of patients; fatal pulmonary emboli occur in 0.1–0.2% of cases.

Multiple regimens have been proven to decrease the incidence of thrombosis. The type of prophylaxis used should be weighed against the risk of bleeding complications in the initial postoperative period. Postoperative bleeding and hematoma are usually prevented by meticulous hemostasis prior to wound closure. The medications used for prophylaxis of DVT and pulmonary embolism increase the risk of bleeding. In addition, when a pulmonary embolus is suspected in the early postoperative period, proof of the embolus with a spiral chest CT or ventilation–perfusion scan (VQ scan) is highly recommended prior to full anticoagulation. Pulmonary emboli are less likely to occur in the first few days following the procedure; full anticoagulation within 48–72 hours following total hip replacement greatly increases the risk of hematoma and its subsequent morbidity.

After discharge
Dislocation

Dislocation occurs when the hip is placed in extremes of flexion or extension. Historically, this complication has been noted in about 2% of prosthetic hips in the first year; the incidence increases to 7% by 25 years. Closed reduction under conscious sedation or general anesthesia is usually successful, but recurrent dislocations may require reoperation and revision of the components.

The incidence of dislocation has significantly decreased over the last 10 years as material and design improvements have allowed the use of larger-diameter femoral heads with increased intrinsic stability. Anatomic repair of the joint capsule at the completion of the procedure has also been shown to decrease the rate of dislocation. The rate of dislocation with these changes is generally less than 1%. Despite these improvements, dislocation is the most common reason for reoperation within the first year following surgery.

Infection

Infection is a significant but relatively uncommon complication. The incidence should be approximately 1% or less. Early diagnosis, although difficult, is imperative. A persistent fever higher than 38.5 °C, or drainage from the surgical incision for longer than 2 weeks after the operation, are suggestive of infection. Antibiotic administration will mask but not cure a deep infection after total hip arthroplasty. Under all circumstances, antibiotic administration should be withheld until the diagnosis is confirmed and the treating orthopedic surgeon has been notified. Early diagnosis of infection (i.e., within 2–3 weeks) greatly improves the success rate for surgical debridement of the wound. If the infection has persisted for longer than 4 weeks, there is little chance for eradication of the infection unless the metal components are removed and intravenous antibiotics are administered for 6 weeks. The components should in most cases not be re-implanted until resolution of the infection is confirmed.

Infections from hematogenous seeding of the prosthetic joint may occur either in the perioperative period or later. After total hip replacement, routine antibiotic administration prior to routine dental cleaning is recommended only within the first 2 years after surgery or for immunosuppressed patients. It is important to ensure that any existing bacterial infections such as dental abscess, pneumonia, urinary tract infection, etc. are promptly evaluated and treated for all patients with hip replacements.

Prosthetic wear and loosening

Improvements in the wear properties of the materials used for the articulating surfaces have drastically decreased the incidence of wear-related failure and the need for reoperation. Wear in the socket liner generates small particles that can elicit a biologic response causing destruction (osteolysis) of bone supporting the implants. The resulting bone loss may then lead to loosening of components. Loosening of the components may cause pain and destruction of the surrounding bone. In such cases, radiographs often show lucent lines around the prosthesis. For various reasons, about 1% of hip replacements require revision operations each year. Revision procedures are technically more difficult and are associated with increased operative time, blood loss, and complications compared with first time or primary hip replacement operations.

Further reading

Berry DJ, von Knoch M, Schleck CD, Harmsen WS. Effect of femoral head diameter and operative approach on risk of dislocation after primary total hip arthroplasty. *J Bone Joint Surg Am* 2005; **87**: 2456–63.

Colwell CW Jr, Froimson MI, Mont MA *et al*. Thrombosis prevention after total hip arthroplasty: a prospective, randomized trial comparing a mobile compression device with low-molecular-weight heparin. *J Bone Joint Surg Am* 2010; **92**: 527–35.

Dorr LD, Gendelman V, Maheshwari AV *et al*. Multimodal thromboprophylaxis for total hip and knee arthroplasty based on risk assessment. *J Bone Joint Surg Am* 2007; **89**: 2648–54.

Matar WY, Jafari SM, Restrepo C *et al*. Preventing infection in total joint arthroplasty. *J Bone Joint Surg Am* 2010; **92**: S36–46.

Pedersen AB, Sorensen HT, Mehnert F, Overgaard S, Johnsen SP. Risk factors for venous thromboembolism in patients undergoing total hip replacement and receiving routine thromboprophylaxis. *J Bone Joint Surg Am* 2010; **92**: 2156–64.

Chapter

119

Fractures of the femoral shaft

William M. Reisman

The femur is the largest bone in the body and has a large soft tissue muscle mass surrounding it. The femoral shaft includes the region 5 cm below the lesser trochanter and 9 cm above the knee joint, and is termed the diaphysis. The estimated incidence of fractures of the femoral shaft in the USA is around one fracture per 10,000 persons per year. There is a bimodal age distribution of femur fractures with one peak in the 20s and one peak in the 60s.

Most femur fractures tend to occur secondary to high-energy trauma such as motor vehicle accidents, pedestrians struck by vehicles, falls from a height, or gunshots. The force required to fracture a femur may also cause a multitude of other associated injuries, most commonly to the head and chest. Therefore, a thorough and complete evaluation by a systematic protocol is warranted followed by any needed resuscitation. High-energy femoral shaft fractures may lose up to 1–3 units of blood into the thigh musculature causing hemodynamic instability, so close monitoring is indicated.

A femur fracture from a ground-level fall should be investigated for the underlying cause. Low-energy femur fractures usually have some pathologic process that has allowed the diaphysis of the femur to weaken and fracture. Common etiologies include osteoporosis, metastatic disease, or primary neoplasm. Several recent case reports have suggested a link between long-term bisphosphonate use and proximal femur fractures. While a review of three bisphosphonate study groups showed no significant increase in low-energy fractures among the drug users, the Federal Drug Administration has issued a warning due to the concern and suspicion that there may be a link. A delay of surgical stabilization may be indicated if the pathology would change the treatment plan.

Non-operative management of femoral shaft fractures with traction is of historical value. The advent of intramedullary nailing by Kuntscher revolutionized the stabilization of femur fractures by allowing early mobilization and decreasing the non-operative complications. Advances in design have allowed for union rates to be reported as high as 97–100%. Additional definitive management options include external fixation and plate fixation when patient factors such as age,

body size, or soft tissue defects dictate a deviation from intramedullary nailing.

While the timing of stabilization of femur fractures remains controversial, most agree intramedullary nailing of stable patients within 24 hours decreases pulmonary dysfunction such as fat emboli, acute respiratory distress syndrome, and pneumonia by allowing early mobilization. However, a multiply injured patient may warrant delay in order to avoid a second insult to their pulmonary injury. This remains a controversial topic.

Usual postoperative course

Expected postoperative hospital stay

Patients with a femoral shaft fracture usually stay in the hospital for 2–4 days but may stay longer depending on the presence of other associated injuries.

Operative mortality

The overall mortality with unilateral femur fractures is reported to be relatively low at 1.5%. However, the rate of mortality for bilateral femur fractures is significantly higher at 5.6%, but has been reported to be as high as 26%. Mortality of the patient is closely associated with concomitant injuries and those with bilateral fractures are more likely to also have head, thoracic, and abdominal pathology.

Special monitoring required

Prior to and following surgical stabilization the patient's neurologic, cardiovascular, and pulmonary status should be closely monitored. Quick recognition of fat emboli syndrome, acute respiratory distress syndrome, compartment syndrome, or pulmonary embolus is imperative in the treatment algorithm. In addition, the patient's hematocrit level as well as urine output should be used to monitor their need for further resuscitation.

Medical Management of the Surgical Patient, ed. Michael F. Lubin, Thomas F. Dodson, and Neil H. Winawer. Published by Cambridge University Press. © Cambridge University Press 2013.

Patient activity and positioning

After stabilization of the fracture, the typical patient is up on postoperative day 1 with physical therapy. The weightbearing status is dependent on fracture fixation, intramedullary nail size, number of interlocking screws, and associated injuries. Early mobilization and range of motion of the affected leg are encouraged to decrease postoperative complications.

Alimentation

In the absence of concomitant injuries, the patient's diet is advanced as tolerated. Multiply injured patients may require supplementation to meet the metabolic demands in order to ensure proper mineralization during fracture healing.

Antibiotic coverage

For closed femur fractures, a first-generation cephalosporin administered preoperatively within one hour of the surgical incision and continued for no more than 24 hours is the standard of care. Open fractures require urgent debridement as well as immediate administration of antibiotics to prevent infection. For Grades I and II open fractures, a first-generation cephalosporin as well as the appropriate tetanus prophylaxis are given immediately upon arrival at the treating facility. For Grade III open fractures, an aminoglycoside is added. For fractures that are grossly contaminated, the addition of penicillin is recommended. These antibiotics are continued until surgical debridement and then for 24 hours after stabilization.

Clinical and radiographic evaluation

Daily wound evaluation while in the hospital is recommended. After discharge the patient should return for a wound check and suture/staple removal between 14 and 21 days. The patient is encouraged to work on range of motion and strengthening during the recovery process. Anteroposterior and lateral view radiographs are typically obtained at the 6-week and 12-week points following surgery to follow the progression of healing. The patient should be seen at a minimum of every 6 weeks thereafter until clinical and radiographic union is achieved.

Postoperative complications

In the hospital

Fat embolism syndrome

Fracture of the femur as well as instrumentation of the intramedullary canal for nail insertion can cause the embolization of fat and marrow contents into the circulatory system. The signs and symptoms typically develop within 12–48 hours after a femur fracture or stabilization of the femur fracture. The diagnosis of the fat embolism syndrome is primarily a clinical diagnosis based on pulmonary dysfunction secondary to hypoxemia and tachypnea. Forty percent of patients with fat embolism syndrome will develop axillary and subconjunctival petechiae, while 70% will have alterations in mental status. The rate of mortality is reported to be between 10% and 20%. The treatment for fat embolism syndrome is supportive therapy with supplemental oxygen or mechanical ventilation for respiratory failure in order to maximize the patient's pulmonary and cardiac output.

Thromboembolism and pulmonary embolus

Patients with femur fractures are at high risk for a deep vein thrombosis (DVT). Early mobilization along with pneumatic compression devices and drugs such as heparin, warfarin, or low molecular weight heparin, are used to help prevent the development of a DVT. Deep vein thromboses can lead to fatal pulmonary embolism (PE) which manifests as tachypnea, tachycardia, pleuritic chest pain, and mental status changes. Immediate diagnosis and treatment is needed for a favorable outcome. Diagnostic tests include chest X-ray, ECG, and arterial blood gas. Pulmonary angiography is the gold-standard imaging study; however, a spiral CT scan is often more readily available. A ventilation-perfusion scan can also be used in the diagnosis of a PE. The treatment can consist of supportive care, anticoagulation therapy, and the use of thrombolytics.

Acute respiratory distress syndrome (ARDS)

Respiratory failure and pulmonary edema are the hallmarks of ARDS. The orthopedic literature has debated over the past one-and-a-half decades whether early stabilization of femur fractures has an effect on the development of ARDS. It is generally accepted that intramedullary nailing produces measurable transient effects on the pulmonary system, but whether that effect changes the clinical course in the development of ARDS is still controversial. Signs and symptoms include tachypnea, tachycardia, and hypoxemia. Treatment consists of mechanical ventilation support with high PEEP.

Compartment syndrome

Acute compartment syndrome occurs when the swelling secondary to trauma causes the pressure in the fibro-osseous compartment to exceed the perfusion pressure, thereby diminishing blood flow to the tissue leading to ischemia and irreversible damage. While compartment syndrome of the femur is rare, one must remain vigilant in the examination of patients with femur fractures. The diagnosis remains a clinical diagnosis with pain out of proportion to the injury and pain with passive stretch of the muscles as the main indicators. The patient may also have paresthesias, pallor, and/or pulselessness, but these are late findings. Emergent surgical fasciotomy is the treatment.

Nerve paresis

Nerve injury is uncommon with femur fractures because of the large soft-tissue envelope around the femur. However, if excessive traction is used with a fracture table where the leg is pulled distally against a peroneal post, nerve palsies can occur to the pudendal, sciatic, femoral, and obturator nerves.

After discharge

Infection

Infections with intramedullary nailing are rare. In the event of acute infection, immediate irrigation and debridement with long-term parenteral antibiotics are indicated. The goal is to eradicate the infection and preserve the hardware. If the infection becomes chronic, debridement with antibiotic suppression of the infection until the fracture is healed is recommended. Once the fracture is healed, removal of the implant may be necessary.

Non-union and delayed union

Cases of non-union and delayed union of the femur are extremely infrequent. When they do occur, the diagnosis is based on the patient's clinical symptoms as well as the failure of progression on radiographic evaluation. Treatment algorithms consist of: dynamization of the nail by removing any static interlocking screws, thus allowing compression; exchange nailing; repair of the non-union by compression plating; or applying bone graft to the fracture site. Medical optimization includes a complete work-up for nutritional deficiencies such as vitamin D and calcium along with the cessation of smoking and the use of any anti-inflammatories.

Further reading

Black D, Kelly M, Genant H *et al.* Bisphosphonates and fractures of the subtrochanteric or diaphyseal femur. *N Engl J Med* 2010; **362**: 1761–71.

Brumback RJ, Virkus WW. Intramedullary nailing of the femur: reamed versus nonreamed. *J Am Acad Orthop Surg* 2000; **8**: 83–90.

Copeland CE, Mitchell KA, Brumback RJ, Gens DR, Burgess AR. Mortality in patients with bilateral femur fractures. *J Orthop Trauma* 1998; **12**: 315–19.

Fabian TC, Hoots AV, Stanford DS, Patterson CR, Mangiante EC. Fat embolism syndrome: prospective evaluation in 92 fracture patients. *Crit Care Med* 1990; **18**: 42–6.

Kuntscher G, Rinne HH (trans): *Practice of Intramedullary Nailing.* Springfield, IL: Charles C Thomas; 1967.

Nork SE, Agel J, Russell GV *et al.* Mortality after reamed intramedullary nailing of bilateral femur fractures. *Clin Orthop Relat Res* 2003; **415**: 272–8.

Pape HC, Auf'm'Kolk M, Paffrath T *et al.* Primary intramedullary femur fixation in multiple trauma patients with associated lung contusion: a cause of posttraumatic ARDS? *J Trauma* 1993; **34**: 540–8.

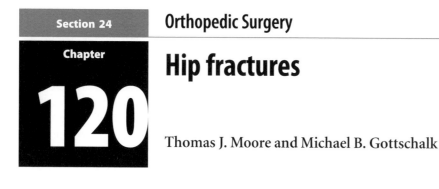

Hip fractures

Thomas J. Moore and Michael B. Gottschalk

The treatment of hip fractures is the prototype for the orthopedic management of geriatric patients. Because of the demographics of the USA (increasing age of the population), the incidence of hip fractures will increase in the next few decades, with the yearly incidence increasing to 500,000 in 2040 from 250,000 in 1990. Prevention of hip fractures is becoming increasingly important due to significant morbidity and mortality associated with a hip fracture. Modalities that have been shown to decrease the incidence of geriatric hip fractures include analysis of conditions that predispose to falls, prevention, and treatment of bone fragility, and, possibly, the use of hip protectors. Therefore, especially in patients who already have sustained a hip fracture, reviewing the patient's medications to identify those that may interfere with cognition and balance (e.g., diazepams), evaluating eyesight (poor vision may predispose to a fall), and diagnosing and treating osteoporosis may decrease the risk of subsequent hip fractures.

Classification of hip fractures

It is not the purpose of this chapter to discuss the complete classification of hip fractures and subsequent treatment; however, it is useful to describe hip fractures and the goal of surgical treatment. Femoral neck fractures occur mostly in elderly patients; displaced fractures often are treated with arthroplasty to avoid the known complications of non-union and avascular necrosis and to allow for immediate ambulation. Intertrochanteric hip fractures are almost always treated with internal fixation. This intervention provides a high union rate; with newer implants, unrestricted weightbearing is usually allowed. The goal of treatment of all geriatric hip fractures is a rapid return to the pre-injury ambulatory status, as this has been shown to decrease the morbidity of hip fractures.

Timing of surgery

The optimal timing for surgical intervention for hip fractures is not well defined. In general, hip fracture patients should be treated urgently, but a short delay in surgery to correct minor comorbidities (metabolic abnormalities) does not increase

mortality. In a large retrospective study of hip fracture patients by Moran *et al.*, a delay in operation of 4 days in patients without significant comorbidities did not increase the 30-day mortality. However, hip fracture patients with significant comorbidities such as pneumonia and an operative delay of greater than 4 days had a 30-day mortality rate 2.5 times greater than that of the patients treated within 4 days. Therefore, it may be important to have internal medicine input for medical comorbidities for preoperative orthopedic patients. When compared with hip fracture patients, similar orthopedic patients (e.g., arthroplasty patients) treated by internal medicine hospitalists had shorter hospital stays. However, there was no decrease in mortality in comparison with patients managed solely by orthopedists.

Preoperative evaluation of hip fracture patients

The goal of preoperative evaluation of elective surgery patients is to determine any clinical situation that, if corrected, will decrease perioperative morbidity and mortality. The goal of preoperative evaluation in emergent surgery is to determine the risk–benefit of the proposed surgery in comparison to non-operative treatment. The American Society of Anesthesiologists (ASA) has attempted to correlate preoperative testing and subsequent adverse postoperative events. A meta-analysis of the literature found few high-level evidence-based studies on this topic, and the current ASA recommendations are based largely on clinical experience. Despite the lack of such studies documenting positive outcomes of preoperative testing or perioperative medical management in hip fracture patients, preoperative testing and perioperative medical management are indicated.

Preoperative cardiac assessment

Predictably, patients with coronary artery disease (CAD) have a higher than average incidence of perioperative cardiac complications than non-cardiac patients undergoing non-cardiac surgery. The estimated incidence of cardiac complications following non-cardiac surgery in all patients is between

Medical Management of the Surgical Patient, ed. Michael F. Lubin, Thomas F. Dodson, and Neil H. Winawer. Published by Cambridge University Press. © Cambridge University Press 2013.

0.03% and 1.5%. A prospective study by Ashton *et al.* of men over the age of 40 undergoing non-cardiac surgery had an incidence of 4.1% of postoperative myocardial infarction in patients with known CAD, and no myocardial infarctions (MI) in patients without known preexisting cardiac disease. Certain other medical conditions are known to increase cardiac events in the perioperative period: an MI within 6 months of the proposed procedure, emergency surgery, history of congestive heart failure, and a non-sinus cardiac rhythm. In addition, specific surgical procedures have varying adverse cardiac events, with orthopedic procedures in the intermediate range.

Hip fractures in geriatric patients are classified as urgent rather than elective or emergent. There are significant negative sequelae for prolonged bed rest in geriatric patients; operative stabilization and subsequent mobilization decreases the morbidity following hip fractures. Basic preoperative cardiac assessment in the geriatric hip fracture patient is available in all hospitals, and should consist of 12-lead ECG, which will demonstrate acute ischemia, arrhythmias, or remote MI. In postmenopausal women, other ECG abnormalities have been associated with postoperative cardiac events, such as first and second degree AV block, left ventricular hypertrophy without ST-T wave elevation or frequent atrial or ventricular premature beats. In general, other preoperative cardiac evaluations in geriatric hip fracture patients should emphasize conditions that can be corrected or modulated to decrease perioperative morbidity. Correction of metabolic abnormalities (electrolyte abnormalities), intraoperative monitoring of hemodynamic status (including central line placement to monitor fluid status), and postoperative medications to decrease cardiac workload (beta-blockers) may decrease cardiac complications in geriatric patients with hip fractures.

Coagulation and transfusion requirements

Patients with hip fractures may have preexisting coagulopathy, and a risk of resultant excessive intraoperative bleeding. A history of prolonged bleeding following minor surgery, a family history of excessive bleeding, and the presence of significant hepatic disease or a known coagulation factor deficiency indicates the possibility of coagulopathy. Standard coagulation profiles should be obtained for these patients. In addition, aspirin and other over-the-counter medications can inhibit platelet adhesion, and result in excessive intraoperative bleeding. Several conditions are associated with a hypercoagulable state, such as certain malignancies, nephrotic syndrome, and multiple traumas. Estrogen use may also be associated with a hypercoagulable state. In addition, there are several known inherited conditions that result in a hypercoagulable state (deficiencies of Protein S or Protein C, Antithrombin III, or the presence of Factor V Lieden or other factors).

Patients with a proximal femur fracture are at high risk for deep venous thrombosis (DVT) and, in turn, pulmonary embolus (PE). Hip fracture patients who do not receive prophylactic DVT treatment incur fatal PEs up to 7% of the time. Patients who undergo total hip replacement without prophylaxis have a reported symptomatic PE rate of 20%. This complication is secondary to long periods of immobilization preoperatively and postoperatively, traumatic release of thrombogenic factors, and possible intimal damage to veins during surgery. Prior to surgery, patients should receive both mechanical (sequential compression devices) and pharmacologic DVT prophylaxis. Examples of preoperative and postoperative pharmacotherapy include warfarin, subcutaneous heparin, and low molecular weight heparin (LMWH). Pharmacotherapy should be held at midnight prior to surgery to avoid surgical bleeding complications. Patients on chronic anticoagulation should have an INR of 1.5 or below prior to proceeding to surgery. Low molecular weight heparin has been proven to be safe and more efficacious than other modalities secondary to its pharmacokinetic profile.

The treatment of anemia, either chronic or acute from the hip fracture, has evolved in the past several years. The concept of 30/10 as a preoperative criterion for surgery (30% hematocrit and 10 g hemoglobin) originated in the 1940s with little physiologic evidence. Currently, preoperative blood transfusion in hip fracture patients should take into account the cardiopulmonary status of the patient.

Usual postoperative course
Expected postoperative hospital stay
Routine hospital stay generally ranges from 2–5 days.

Patient activity and positioning
The goal of treatment of all geriatric hip fractures is a rapid return to the pre-injury ambulatory status, as this has been shown to decrease the morbidity of hip fractures. Failure to return to pre-injury ambulatory status is associated with age, pre-fracture ambulation, American Academy of Anesthesia (ASA) operative risk, and fracture type (9). With the advent of new-generation implants, most hip fracture patients, including those with internal fixation and arthroplasty, are allowed to weight bear to tolerance.

Assistive devices, such as a walker, are routinely used within the immediate postoperative time frame to aid ambulation and prevent subsequent falls. After several weeks and the return of muscle strength, the walker can usually be transitioned to a cane to be used in the opposite hand as the operative side. Patients who do well postoperatively can expect to walk with a cane at 3 months. At 6 months, no assistive device is normally needed (unless used prior to surgery). At 1 year, the patient should be back to baseline function and normal activities.

Most patients with significant comorbidities, poor pre-injury function, or inability to weight bear to tolerance require referral to a sub-acute rehabilitation facility. Patients who do not require a referral to a rehabilitation facility may benefit from home healthcare physical therapy and occupational therapy. The number of visits provided is normally dependent on insurance status and social circumstances (i.e., family help at home). Postoperative orthopedic follow-up is normally scheduled at 2 weeks, 6 weeks, 3 months, and 1 year.

Operative mortality

Despite improvements in medical management, implants, and surgical technique, there is a continued increased mortality in the perioperative period following a hip fracture, as well as a decreased overall life expectancy. The mortality in the immediate postoperative period is 5%, and the mortality rate in the first year following a hip fracture is between 20% and 25%. Risk factors for mortality following a hip fracture include an ASA physical classification of 3 (severe systemic disease) or 4 (severe systemic disease that is a constant threat to life); poor nutrition; age greater than 85 years; and lack of independent ambulation prior to the hip fracture.

Special monitoring required

Postoperatively, further cardiac testing and cardiac intervention should be done in those patients with preoperative cardiac abnormalities. Following hip fracture surgery, patients with an identified hypercoagulable state should be monitored and prophylactically treated for thromboembolic disease.

Administration of LMWH does not need monitoring; it may be initiated as soon as 24 hours postoperatively to avoid immediate post-surgical bleeding complications. The dose should be adjusted for obese patients and those with impaired renal function. Patients unable to ambulate in the early postoperative period should continue DVT prophylaxis for 4–6 weeks.

Antibiotic coverage

In general, antibiotic prophylaxis should be given within an hour of the surgical incision and be terminated 24 hours postoperatively. Cefazolin or cefuroxime is the preferred prophylactic antibiotic for elective orthopedic procedures involving an implant. In hospitals with a high incidence of methicillin-resistant *Staphylococcus aureus* surgical site infections, vancomycin antibiotic prophylaxis can be considered.

Further reading

Ashton CM, Petersen NJ, Wray NP *et al.* The incidence of perioperative myocardial infarction in men undergoing noncardiac surgery. *Ann Intern Med* 1993; **118**: 504–10.

Boersma E, Kertai MD, Schouten O *et al.* Perioperative cardiovascular mortality in noncardiac surgery: validation of the Lee cardiac risk index. *Am J Med* 2005; **118**: 1134–41.

Butler M, Forte M, Siddharth J, Swiontkowski M, Kane R. Evidence summary: systematic review of surgical treatments for geriatric hip fractures.

J Bone Joint Surg Am 2011; **93**: 1104–15.

Decker R, Foley J, Moore T. Perioperative management of patients with cardiac disease. *J Am Acad Orthop Surg* 2010; **18**: 267–77.

Goldman L, Caldera DL, Nussbaum SR *et al.* Multifactorial index of cardiac risk in noncardiac surgical procedures. *N Engl J Med* 1977; **297**: 845–50.

Huddleston JM, Long KH, Naessens JM *et al.* Medical and surgical comanagement after elective hip and knee arthoplasty: a randomized, controlled trial. *Ann Intern Med* 2004; **141**: 28–38.

Lindskog DM, Baumgaertner MR. Unstable intertrochanteric hip fractures in the elderly. *J Am Acad Orthop Surg* 2004; **12**: 179–90.

Moore TJ. Perioperative medical management. In Fischgrund JS, ed. *Orthopedic Knowledge Update 9.* Rosemont, IL: The American Academy of Orthopaedic Surgeons; 2007, pp. 105–14.

Moran CG, Wenn RT, Sikand M, Taylor AM. Early mortality after hip fracture: is delay before surgery important? *J Bone Joint Surg Am* 2005; **87**: 483–9.

Lumbar spine surgery

Dheera Ananthakrishnan and John G. Heller

Lumbar surgery in adults can be divided into three general levels of complexity and associated morbidity. The first, an operation to treat herniated lumbar nucleus pulposus, is relatively straightforward from a medical management perspective. The second, an operation for multilevel lumbar stenosis, is usually more involved and tends to be performed for older patients with more comorbidities. The most complicated surgeries are fusion surgeries, which may be carried out with a posterior or anterior approach, or with both approaches.

Patients with a lumbar disc herniation present with radiculopathy in a dermatomal pattern, and may exhibit motor weakness or reflex changes which correspond to the anatomic level of neural compression. The patient is typically a young adult in good health. Axial back pain is not a predominant symptom of this condition and is generally unimproved with a discectomy. If the symptoms produced by lumbar disc herniation fail to respond to appropriate non-operative therapy, laminotomy and discectomy are indicated. Patients are placed either prone or in the knee–chest position on a specially designed operating table; the latter position affords decompression of the abdominal cavity and the epidural veins. The procedure is performed with either loupe magnification or use of the surgical microscope through a posterior midline incision measuring 2.5–5 cm. The operative level is confirmed radiographically to prevent harm to an otherwise normal intervertebral disc. Blood loss is minimal and the total anesthetic time is usually 1–2 hours. A subset of these patients will present with acutely worsening neurologic dysfunction with or without cauda equina syndrome. In these cases, the herniated nuclear fragment is so large that it causes ischemia of the nerve roots. Although unusual, this situation is a true surgical emergency and requires prompt clinical diagnosis to give the patient the best chance of neurologic recovery.

Operative treatment of lumbar spinal stenosis requires a laminectomy with or without foraminotomies. The term laminectomy refers to the removal of one or more spinous processes and their associated laminae, traditionally for the purpose of decompressing the cauda equina or lumbar nerve roots. Such exposure of the spinal canal allows the removal of facet joint osteophytes and thickened ligamentum flavum (foraminotomy), which may contribute to neural compression. The typical patient with spinal stenosis is older than the herniated disc patient and complains of leg pain, heaviness, numbness and/or tingling in one or both lower extremities. The symptoms may be difficult to discern from claudication, in that they increase in intensity with weight-bearing activity and are relieved by sitting or supine rest. While axial back pain is not a primary feature of spinal stenosis, a fusion procedure may be added to the laminectomy in selected cases when pain is clinically significant. Fusion is also indicated in conjunction with a laminectomy when instability is present on the preoperative X-rays (e.g., with degenerative spondylolisthesis or degenerative scoliosis). Compared with laminotomy and discectomy, laminectomy takes longer to perform, requires a larger incision, and engenders more blood loss (usually less than 500 mL). As stenosis patients are usually older, they often have more coexisting medical conditions and greater operative risk factors than discectomy patients. Their preoperative medical clearance and perioperative medical care must take into account these incremental risks.

Under certain circumstances, fusion of a lumbar motion segment (a motion segment comprises two adjacent vertebral bodies, the intervertebral disc between them, the facet joint created by their articular processes, and associated soft tissues) may be required, which can be done by itself or in concert with either of the decompressive procedures described above. If lumbar instability exists before operation or is created during a laminotomy or laminectomy, fusion is performed. Posterolateral (intertransverse) fusion requires a far more extensive posterior muscle dissection. Bleeding from the branches of the lumbar segmental vessels can be copious, with blood loss increasing with each additional level fused. During the harvest of autologous bone graft, significant blood loss from the posterior iliac crest also occurs. Intraoperative red blood cell salvage is a common adjunct to reduce transfusion exposure. Laminectomy and fusion procedures generally require 3.5–5 hours. If segmental pedicle screw fixation is used as an adjunct to the fusion procedure, operative times may

Medical Management of the Surgical Patient, ed. Michael F. Lubin, Thomas F. Dodson, and Neil H. Winawer. Published by Cambridge University Press. © Cambridge University Press 2013.

increase by 1–2 additional hours. While the use of screw fixation increases the risk of certain technical complications and the volume of blood loss, it also improves the likelihood of achieving a successful fusion. With the recent advances in spinal instrumentation and the biotechnology of bone graft substitutes, an anterior lumbar fusion procedure may be a viable substitute for some posterior fusion operations, resulting in less blood loss and faster recovery.

Fusion of lumbar motion segments can also be performed via an anterior procedure, which can employ either a transabdominal or a retroperitoneal approach. The operation may be performed with autologous iliac crest bone, allograft bone, or a bone graft substitute. Any of the available techniques can be performed in conjunction with various forms of spinal instrumentation systems. A single-level fusion can generally be completed in 1.5–3 hours. The advantages of this approach are easier recoveries, generally less postoperative pain, and avoidance of lumbar muscle dissection. With the single-level fusion, the foraminotomy is accomplished indirectly by restoring height to the intervertebral space and the neural foramen. One disadvantage is that decompression of spinal stenosis as a result of facet osteophytes and ligamentum flavum cannot be addressed with this technique. There are additional considerations unique to transabdominal or retroperitoneal surgery. They include inadvertent visceral injury, prolonged ileus, intra-abdominal adhesions, vascular injury, deep venous thrombosis, and retrograde ejaculation.

Minimally invasive surgery

The last 10 years have been witness to an increase in minimally invasive surgery in many specialties; spinal surgery is no exception. For posterior operations, both the use of smaller incisions during tubal dilation of paraspinal musculature and the use of microscopes for decompression and percutaneous instrumentation have become more and more common. Anterior lumbar surgeries via a direct lateral transpsoas approach have also become prevalent. All of the above operations can be performed with less tissue trauma and a reduction in blood loss. Nevertheless, the learning curve for surgeons is often steep; there are lengthened initial operative times, as well as a great reliance on fluoroscopy. Also, it must be kept in mind that even though the incisions for minimally invasive operations may be small, the tissue trauma beneath the skin is often equivalent to that of open procedures. The goals of using minimally invasive techniques are to decrease pain, limit blood loss, and shorten hospital stays; some studies have reported modest advances in the last two criteria.

Preoperative evaluation

Among the key medical points to consider before surgical intervention is the patient's ability to tolerate a prone procedure. The risks of large fluid shifts during fusion procedures and/or prolonged postoperative intubation raise respiratory considerations and a possible need for ICU care postoperatively. Prior to surgery, patients with medical issues such as diabetes, coronary artery disease, and hypertension should have a definite perioperative plan outlined by the medical and anesthesia teams. Diabetes and obesity are known to increase the risks of infections and other perioperative complications after lumbar spine surgery; these issues should be discussed with patients prior to surgery. For elective procedures, weight loss can be a prerequisite.

Many patients undergoing preoperative evaluation for spine surgery have a long history of chronic narcotic use, which can complicate anesthesia selection and postoperative pain management. Therefore, non-judgmental identification of patients who are addicted to alcohol or other drugs is of paramount importance in providing appropriate perioperative care.

Usual postoperative course
Expected postoperative hospital stay

Many lumbar discectomies are performed on an outpatient basis, although it is not unusual to expect a stay of 1 postoperative hospital day. The inpatient stay generally increases in proportion to the magnitude of the surgical dissection: 2–4 days for a laminectomy and 4–6 days for a posterior fusion procedure. Unless the operation is prolonged by an ileus, anterior lumbar interbody fusion techniques generally allow for shorter hospital stays (2–4 days). Medical comorbidities may impact the duration of hospitalization and may also necessitate acute inpatient rehabilitation.

Operative mortality

Mortality for all lumbar surgical procedures in the postoperative period is under 1%, although it increases in proportion to the magnitude of the procedure and the preoperative medical status of the patient.

Special monitoring required

Frequent neurologic evaluation should be performed during the first 24–48 hours after the operation. Any significant change should be reported at once; appropriate and prompt investigation must be pursued in the event of objective change. Bleeding into the paraspinal tissues continues for 2–3 days, especially after posterior fusion procedures. The hematocrit decreases after surgery in proportion to the magnitude of the procedure, generally reaching its nadir by postoperative day 3. Platelet counts and coagulation studies should be monitored after large volumes of blood have been lost. For anterior lumbar procedures, pedal pulses should be checked pre- and postoperatively since manipulation of the aorta, vena cava, and iliac vessels is occasionally needed for surgical exposure. Additionally, postoperative ileus may be more common for anterior procedures; consideration should be given to the use of nasogastric suction and the withholding of oral intake until the ileus resolves. Fevers below 38.5 °C are the rule more than the exception following fusion procedures; however, persistent fever or elevated temperatures should be investigated thoroughly.

Patient activity and positioning

Following lumbar surgical procedures, ambulation usually begins on the first postoperative day. Patients should receive preoperative instruction regarding isometric trunk and lower extremity exercises, body mechanics, and bending and lifting restrictions. A lumbar support may be worn for comfort after laminotomy and laminectomy but is not required. The need for rigid bracing after fusion varies according to the specifics of the procedure and the preference of the surgeon. The routine use of instrumentation for a fusion adjunct has greatly decreased the need for rigid bracing and immobilization after these surgeries. Unrestricted activity can be expected within 6–12 weeks after laminotomy and laminectomy and within 4–6 months after a fusion procedure.

Alimentation

Identifiable nutritional deficiencies should be corrected prior to operation, especially in patients undergoing elective fusion. After the procedure, food intake is advanced as tolerated. Patients undergoing fusion may have a significant adynamic ileus. If oral feeding is delayed more than 3 days, parenteral support should be contemplated.

Antibiotic coverage

Prophylaxis with a first-generation cephalosporin is the standard of care for spinal surgery. Additional doses are given during surgery (based on the duration of the procedure and the magnitude of blood loss) and for 24 hours afterwards. Antibiotics with a broader spectrum of activity may be used in patients who are immunocompromised hosts, who have colonized urinary tracts, or who have required prolonged preoperative hospitalization.

Deep venous thrombosis

Prophylaxis to guard against deep venous thrombosis (DVT) is recommended. Thigh-high elastic hose should be used in combination with sequential pneumatic compression stockings throughout the operative procedure, and until the patient achieves independence with ambulation. The use of low molecular weight heparin can result in an increased risk of bleeding complications (e.g., a hematoma that may require repeat surgical intervention); therefore, it should be administered with caution. If a patient is at particularly high risk for DVT, a vena cava filter should be placed prior to surgery. Circumstances which warrant consideration of a filter include a history of DVT or pulmonary emboli, hypercoagulable states (e.g., protein S deficiency), morbid obesity, anticipation of prolonged immobility or bed rest, paraplegia or quadriplegia, and combined anterior/posterior spinal procedures. The literature does not support the routine use of anticoagulation in elective lumbar spinal surgery, although anticoagulation is often recommended for trauma patients.

Blood transfusion

Lumbar discectomies and straightforward laminectomies rarely require transfusions. Intraoperative red cell salvage and reinfusion is often practiced during posterior fusion procedures. The need for transfusion must be weighed against the patient's general medical condition, degree of anemia symptoms, and their wishes regarding blood product use.

Cigarette smoking

Tobacco interferes with bone graft and wound healing. Fusion potential may be maximized by preoperative cessation of all tobacco and nicotine products. Nicotine patches and analogous products are contraindicated when fusion is included in the procedure. Surgeons will often avoid fusion procedures in nicotine users, with the exception of urgent cases such as trauma, myelopathy, or tumors.

Medications

Medications that impair platelet function should be discontinued 2–4 weeks before operation to minimize intraoperative bleeding, especially when a fusion is planned. Oral narcotics may be appropriate as an alternative analgesic during the preoperative period. Non-steroidal anti-inflammatory drugs should not be used for at least 3 months after fusion procedures because they have been shown to inhibit the fusion process.

Postoperative complications
In the hospital
Hematoma

Subcutaneous hematomas or seromas occur most commonly when the iliac crest is exposed through the same midline incision. Such collections are best prevented through careful wound closure and drainage of the wound, as determined by the operating surgeon at the time of closure. Surgical evacuation is seldom required. Epidural hematomas usually present within 2–4 days as a cause of severe back or leg pain with progressive neurologic deficit. Emergent surgical exploration and decompression is required.

Infection

The incidence of infection varies from 0.5–5%, depending on the complexity of the operation and the status of the patient. Diagnosis can be delayed since the appearance of the wound is often deceptively normal. Treatment is by surgical debridement, closure over drains, and administration of parenteral antibiotics. Treatment with antibiotics alone or with antibiotics in combination with local wound care is contraindicated, especially for patients receiving bone grafts and/or spinal instrumentation.

Cerebrospinal fluid leakage

A dural tear should be surgically repaired when it is identified. If primary repair or patching of the dura is not possible, a closed subarachnoid drain should be used to divert the cerebrospinal fluid. Strict supine bed rest may be necessary for up to 48 hours after a dural repair. The wound dressing should be inspected for cerebrospinal fluid and patients should be observed for signs of meningitis. Prophylactic antibiotic coverage may be extended during the period that a subarachnoid drain is in place, but the agent chosen should have good blood–brain barrier penetration.

Persistent/recurrent radicular pain or neurologic deficit

Complications of continued or recurrent pain or neurological deficit are not uncommon. These may result from inadequate decompression, recurrent herniated disc, persistent foraminal stenosis, radiculitis or chronic radiculopathy in the face of adequate decompression. Malposition of hooks or pedicle screws may also cause such symptoms after an instrumented fusion. If sufficient symptoms or signs persist, myelography with computed tomography or magnetic resonance scanning is recommended to clarify such issues in the immediate postoperative period. Generally speaking, it is both wiser and easier to address identifiable problems early in the postoperative course.

Bowel or bladder dysfunction

Injury to the sacral nerve roots which results in neurogenic bowel or bladder dysfunction is rare. More often, especially in older patients, an underlying degree of dysfunction caused by high-grade stenosis and bladder or prostate problems becomes more pronounced under the influence of bed rest, bladder catheterization, and various medications. An intermittent catheterization program should be instituted as soon as possible to minimize the risk of urinary tract infection. Urologic consultation is advised if the symptoms do not resolve rapidly once patients are ambulatory. The possibility of postoperative retrograde ejaculation (which occurs in 1–3% of males undergoing anterior interbody fusions) should be discussed with the patient preoperatively, especially in regards to family planning. If the dysfunction persists, urologic consultation may be beneficial.

Vision loss

Vision loss after spinal surgery is an extremely rare but devastating consequence. The etiology is not clearly defined, but it is thought to be related to optic nerve ischemia. Vision loss tends to occur after operations of long duration (usually in the prone position), and in patients with large fluid shifts. It is important to discuss this complication with patients scheduled to undergo lengthy and complex spinal reconstructions, in much the same manner as paralysis and death are discussed. Pressure on the globe of the eye should be minimized, and hypotension and anemia must be adequately controlled. Educating the nursing staff about potential vision loss after spinal surgery, and the need for monitoring the patient's vision and visual fields, is of paramount importance.

After discharge

Recurrent radicular pain

If radicular pain recurs after hospital discharge, each of the possible causes mentioned above should be re-evaluated. In addition, postlaminectomy instability or fatigue fracture of the pars interarticularis can cause similar symptoms.

Back pain

The quantity and duration of local wound pain is proportional to the magnitude of the procedure performed. Incisional pain should be managed with analgesics as needed for a reasonable period. Debilitating post-discectomy back pain may occur in 15% of patients and can be treated by lumbar fusion if warranted. Intervertebral discitis or deep wound infection should also be considered, especially if the pain persists at night and is associated with diaphoresis and/or low-grade fevers. The external appearance of an infected wound may be deceptively normal, but the sedimentation rate and C-reactive protein levels of the patient are often consistently elevated and should be monitored. Recurrent or new back pain may also be related to post-laminectomy instability or failed fusion.

Pseudarthrosis

The incidence of failed fusion varies with the number and location of the dissected segments, use of instrumentation, and the type of bone graft used. Pain is usually activity related. The diagnosis of pseudarthrosis is made with appropriate radiographic studies, bearing in mind that plain radiographs are commonly misleading.

Instrumentation failure

Broken or loose implants are a hallmark of pseudarthrosis. Surgical repair of the non-union is recommended if the symptoms are sufficiently severe.

Wound infection

The diagnosis of a postoperative spinal wound infection is frequently delayed. Increasing back pain in association with malaise, sweats, chills, and an elevated erythrocyte sedimentation rate and C-reactive protein strongly suggest the presence of wound infection. Treatment is surgical, followed by administration of parenteral antibiotics.

Psychosocial dysfunction

For many patients who have undergone back surgery, re-entry into the workplace requires a coordinated effort by patient, doctor, therapists, employer, and others. Patients must be strongly motivated in order to help themselves resume a normal lifestyle.

Further reading

Browne JA, Cook C, Pietrobon R, Bethel MA, Richardson WJ. Diabetes and early postoperative outcomes following lumbar fusion. *Spine* 2007; **32**: 2214–19.

Cheng JS, Arnold PM, Anderson PA, Fischer D, Dettori JR. Anticoagulation risk in spine surgery. *Spine* 2007; **35** (9 Suppl) : S117–24.

Glassman SD, Alegre G, Carreon L, Dimar JR, Johnson JR. Perioperative complications of lumbar instrumentation and fusion in patients with diabetes mellitus. *Spine J* 2003; **3**: 496–501.

Park P, Upadhyaya C, Garton HJ, Foley KT. The impact of minimally invasive spine surgery on perioperative complications in overweight or obese patients. *Neurosurgery* 2008; **62**: 693–9.

Petrozza PH. Major spine surgery. *Anesthesiology Clin North Am* 2002; **20**: 405–15.

Rodgers WB, Gerber EJ, Patterson J. Intraoperative and early postoperative complications in extreme lateral interbody fusion: an analysis of 600 cases. *Spine* 2011; **36**: 26–32.

Rodriguez-Vela J, Lobo-Escolar A, Joven-Aliaga E *et al*. Perioperative and short-term advantages of mini-open approach for lumbar spinal fusion. *European Spine J* 2009; **18**: 1194–201.

Spivak JM. Degenerative lumbar spinal stenosis. *J Bone Joint Surg Am* 1998; **80**: 1053–66.

Surgery for adult spinal deformity (scoliosis or kyphosis)

John M. Rhee and William C. Horton

The most common indications for surgery in adults with scoliosis or kyphosis are debilitating pain from the deformity or associated spinal stenosis with neurological symptoms. Other indications include documented progression of deformity or instability that hinders erect posture. Although surgery may be considered in the adolescent with spinal deformity to prevent long-term development of restrictive lung disease or cor pulmonale (which may occur in patients with scoliosis > 90–100°), adult deformity correction surgery is rarely if ever indicated to improve established cardiopulmonary impairment. In fact, spinal deformity surgery in the adult may actually lead to long-term deterioration of pulmonary function, particularly if the chest is entered during the approach.

Because of the potential for major physiologic insult, an extensive preoperative medical work-up should be conducted when indicated in the patient considering surgery for spinal deformity correction. The combination of careful preoperative screening, risk stratification, and medical optimization in consultation with medical specialists is paramount to successful outcomes. Depending on the magnitude of associated comorbidities, the surgical procedure may need to be appropriately curtailed to address the underlying medical conditions. Therefore, complete correction of the deformity may not be achieved. However, because adequate correction of deformity (in particular, deformity in the sagittal plane) has been shown to be associated with significantly better outcomes, the majority of operations for spinal deformity should be designed to achieve, at a minimum, the restoration of spinal balance in both the coronal and sagittal planes.

The surgeon can choose the operative approach (posterior, anterior, or combined). In severe, rigid deformities, an osteotomy may be required. Osteotomies involve correction of deformity by removing wedges of bone from the vertebral column. Although there are several types of osteotomies, they generally require prolonged operative times and are associated with greater blood loss as well as significant potential neurologic risk. The principal goals of surgery are decompression of symptomatic neural structures, correction of major spinal imbalance, and stabilization of deformity with fusion and

instrumentation. Depending on the magnitude of surgery, operations can last 4–14 hours, and blood loss may range from 500 to 5,000 mL or more, involving multiple transfusions and significant fluid shifts. If the procedure is expected to last longer than 12 hours, it may be divided into anterior or posterior stages performed on different days during the same hospitalization. General endotracheal anesthesia is used. Neurologic monitoring with somatosensory and motor-evoked potentials is used routinely during deformity correction surgery.

Usual postoperative course
Expected postoperative hospital stay

Depending on the severity of surgery, postoperative hospital stay ranges from 3–7 days; most patients are fully independent at the time of discharge. If the anterior and posterior portions need to be staged and separated by several days, then the hospital course will be longer. Patients who undergo thoracotomy for anterior thoracic fusion will require a chest tube until the output is serous and less than 25–50 mL per shift, which typically occurs on postoperative day 3 or 4. Patients undergoing prolonged surgery and/or experiencing large blood loss often require postoperative stays in the ICU. Common ICU issues include postoperative intubation until airway edema subsides, and monitoring for coagulopathy and neurologic changes. Spinal deformity patients occasionally need inpatient rehabilitation prior to their ultimate discharge home.

Operative mortality

The operative mortality rate ranges from under 1% in uncomplicated cases to 6–8% in patients with severe comorbidities.

Special monitoring required

In most cases, central venous access is necessary to manage volume resuscitation both intra- and postoperatively. Spinal deformity surgery can place major metabolic and nutritional demands on the patient; therefore, dedicated central venous

Medical Management of the Surgical Patient, ed. Michael F. Lubin, Thomas F. Dodson, and Neil H. Winawer. Published by Cambridge University Press. © Cambridge University Press 2013.

access for postoperative hyperalimentation is of benefit for patients who have staged surgery or who are likely to experience prolonged ileus. An arterial line may also be used intraoperatively for hemodynamic monitoring (especially since hypotensive anesthesia may be employed to minimize blood loss), and also for the monitoring of arterial blood gases.

Spinal deformity patients often undergo prolonged surgery with resultant large volume shifts, facial and airway edema from prone positioning, or the need for a transthoracic approach with resultant surgical trauma to the lung and chest. For all of the above reasons, postoperative intubation is common. However, patients are rapidly weaned as conditions permit, and tracheostomy is rarely required.

Patient activity and positioning

Early mobilization aids in the recovery of the deformity patient; it helps to prevent thromboembolic, pulmonary, and decubitus complications. Initially, patients are 'logrolled' frequently (every 2–3 hours) while in bed and encouraged to spend time in the lateral position to prevent pressure sores to the extremities and to any posterior incision. The head of the bed may be raised 30–45°. Aggressive pulmonary toilet, which ideally includes deep breathing, coughing, and incentive spirometry for every patient, may initially be limited by pain. Physical therapy (mainly for mobilization and gait training) is prescribed in the hospital starting on postoperative day 1.

Patients who have received implants are usually stable for mobilization. Patients having severe osteoporosis, a staged initial procedure without internal fixation, or corrective osteotomies may have a relatively unstable spine; mobilization in these cases should be discussed on an individualized basis. In rare circumstances, early mobilization may be contraindicated. The patient who has sustained an intraoperative cerebrospinal fluid leak may need to lie with the head of their bed flat for 24–72 hours. This positioning will allow the dural repair to seal without excessive hydrostatic pressure. Although bracing may be necessary for some patients, improvements in spinal fixation implants have greatly decreased its use.

Alimentation

Postoperative ileus is common for 1–4 days, especially in patients undergoing anterior lumbar spine surgery. Postoperative narcotics and lack of mobilization contribute to intestinal ileus. Oral feedings should be delayed until the ileus clears and the patient passes flatus; however, judicious consumption of ice chips is generally well tolerated. Because of the severe metabolic demands placed on the postsurgical deformity patient, nutritional supplementation is mandatory. Proper nutrition is critical for healing and for avoiding wound and infectious complications. Although oral supplementation is instituted as soon as possible, hyperalimentation should be

used if the period of ileus is expected to be prolonged. For patients undergoing staged deformity surgery, hyperalimentation is recommended until oral feedings are tolerated.

Antibiotic coverage

An intravenous cephalosporin or vancomycin is administered for 24 hours.

Pain management

Severe pain is common for 1–5 days following surgery. A patient-controlled analgesia pump (PCA) is commonly used. As ileus resolves, there is a transition to oral medications. Toradol and non-steroidal anti-inflammatory drugs (NSAIDS) are avoided due to deleterious effects on platelets and on fusion formation.

Blood loss

The fusion procedure can expose raw cancellous bone surface; therefore, postoperative blood loss is common. Even with aggressive intraoperative resuscitation with blood products, postoperative coagulopathies can develop from transfusions, hypocalcemia, and factor/ platelet consumption. The INR, PT, PTT, and platelet count may need to be followed for 2–3 days after surgery or until stabilization occurs. Postoperative bleeding is monitored by suction drain output and serial hematocrits; it usually decreases to less than 30 mL per shift by 72 hours after surgery. Coagulation defects must be aggressively reversed while active bleeding is occurring. Postoperative anemia should be anticipated and corrected as medically necessary.

Thromboembolism prophylaxis

Some form of prophylaxis for thromboembolism is necessary. However, early anticoagulation is risky, due to both expected ongoing bleeding from decorticated cancellous bone in the fusion area and to the potential for epidural hematoma. Therefore, elastic stockings, pneumatic compression hose, frequent turning, early leg motion, and mobilization (as conditions allow) are prescribed instead.

Postoperative complications
In the hospital
Spinal cord and nerve root injury

Injury to the spinal cord and/or nerve root is a serious potential problem in all patients undergoing major deformity correction surgery. Late neurologic changes can arise 1–3 days postoperatively. Therefore, detailed and well-documented serial neurologic examinations (motor, sensory, reflexes, and rectal) are the keystone of postoperative monitoring. All new complaints of postoperative numbness, weakness, clonus, perianal anesthesia, or incontinence should be rapidly evaluated. Any signs of acute spinal cord dysfunction should prompt consideration of high-dose steroids (methylprednisolone); aggressive correction of any significant anemia, hypoxia, or hypotension; and urgent diagnostic work-up of the spine.

Wound infection

Progressive and increasing incisional pain with drainage suggests possible infection. If infection is suspected but not obvious, aspiration of the hematoma (with meticulous sterile technique) may be helpful. Surgical incision and drainage should proceed promptly if infection is likely present. However, it is rare for surgical wound infections to present until about 2 weeks postoperatively.

Pulmonary insufficiency

Incentive spirometry and pulmonary therapy should be given prophylactically. Poor ventilation caused by "self-splinting" due to pain is especially common after thoracotomy, thoracoplasty, or an anterior approach to the spine. If a patient has preexisting pulmonary compromise, or if the procedure is associated with surgical trauma to the chest cavity, supplemental chest physical therapy or intermittent positive pressure breathing (IPPB) treatments (administered every 4–6 hours via a bronchodilator, e.g., albuterol nebulizer) may be very useful. Pneumonia, pulmonary embolus, and pulmonary edema may be causes of postoperative pulmonary insufficiency. However, the possibility of pneumothorax must also be considered for patients who have undergone a transthoracic approach or placement of a central line. Appropriate physical examinations, serial chest radiographs, pulse oximetry, and arterial blood gas determinations may be performed.

Myocardial infarction

Patients are at risk of coronary complications from major spinal deformity surgery, as they would be with any other surgery of similar magnitude. Prolonged prone surgical positioning, with pads pressing on the sternum and ribs, can cause local chest pain or costochondritis that can be confused with a cardiac etiology. If a patient sustains a myocardial infarction, the standard treatment measures should be considered. However, decision making regarding the use of thrombolytics and anticoagulants must proceed with awareness of the potential for severe surgical site bleeding and the risk of paralysis from epidural hematoma.

Pulmonary embolism

If an embolism occurs, standard therapeutic intervention is necessary. Generally anticoagulants should be strictly avoided for at least 48–72 hours postoperatively due to the potential of extensive bone bleeding and the risk of epidural hematoma. These concerns are present when a decompression or osteotomy has been performed. If the risk of thrombosis is unusually high, placement of a caval filter should be considered, or anticoagulants can be administered (with great caution).

Bladder atony

Postoperative bladder atony is common in patients undergoing decompression, due to a combination of narcotic administration and immobilization with neurologic manipulation. In general, Foley catheters should be removed 2–4 days postoperatively when the patient is more mobile and can more comfortably void. Removing the catheter too soon introduces the risk of a later reinsertion if the patient develops urinary retention with narcotic use, or with an inability to sit or stand to void. There is also a possibility of infection with prolonged catheterization, which should be avoided. Intermittent sterile catheterization can be performed as needed, but the residual volumes should be kept low in order to prevent a cycle of bladder stretching and atony.

Intestinal atony

The high doses of narcotics frequently required for pain control exacerbate the atony induced from surgery, anesthesia, and immobilization. Oral intake is restricted until peristalsis is established. A nasogastric tube may occasionally be necessary to treat persistent ileus.

Anemia secondary to blood loss

Postoperative hematocrit levels are used to monitor for anemia related to blood loss, and replacement packed red blood cells (PRBC) should be given as necessary with close attention to orthostatic symptoms and signs.

After discharge

Bone graft pain

Currently, iliac crest bone graft harvest is not always performed due to the availability of alternatives such as bone morphogenetic protein. However, this procedure may be necessary in some situations. Donor site pain from the harvest of autologous bone is common but gradually dissipates over 1–3 months. Increasing pain at the graft site should raise the suspicion of infection.

Skin ulceration under a brace or cast (pressure and/or friction)

Patients must be closely monitored for the possibility of a poorly fitting brace or cast, especially if they are very thin or if their deformity is severe. Cast revision or brace modification should be done immediately if skin irritation occurs.

Wound infection

Many wound infections manifest at 2–4 weeks postoperatively. Progressive and increasing (rather than decreasing) incisional pain suggests possible infection. Fevers, chills, and drainage may not be present, but all symptoms must be aggressively evaluated. An elevated white blood count may or may not be present. The sedimentation rate and C-reactive protein should be checked in those with suspected infection; either or both may be artificially high due to the postoperative state. In general, the sedimentation rate may take up to 7 weeks to normalize postoperatively, whereas the C-reactive protein usually normalizes more quickly (as early as 2–3 weeks postoperatively). Surgical management is recommended for the majority of postoperative infections, except for the most benign superficial infections.

Implant failure

Internal fixation devices occasionally loosen or break. Problems may occur in the early postoperative period (1–3 months) if bone density is poor, or later (6–12 months) if the fusion fails to heal. There may be an associated new pain or possible deformity; radiographic examination is necessary for diagnosis. Revision is usually performed unless the fusion is found to be solid.

Pseudarthrosis

Pseudarthrosis (failure of a fusion to heal solidly), can occur for any number of reasons related to the mechanical environment (e.g., poor bone quality, inadequate fixation of the spine, technical surgical factors), patient non-compliance (e.g., smoking or using NSAIDS during the early postoperative period), or the biological milieu (e.g., malnourishment, immunocompromise, inadequate bone graft, or multiple prior operations with scar). Smoking, in particular, has negative effects on the healing of fusions; many spinal surgeons will not perform elective fusions on smokers. Pseudarthrosis usually manifests as increasing pain at the site of non-union. Implant breakage and/or loosening are commonly associated findings, and progression of deformity may also be seen. The diagnosis is not always evident on plain radiographs alone: thin-cut computed tomography and bone scans may be necessary. Revision surgery is usually required and may necessitate anterior, posterior, or combined approaches.

Acknowledgment

The author wishes to acknowledge the contributions of Dr. Thomas E. Whitesides, Jr. to this chapter.

Further reading

Ali RM, Boachie-Adjei O, Rawlins BA. Functional and radiographic outcomes after surgery for adult scoliosis using third-generation instrumentation techniques. *Spine* 2003; **28**: 1163–9.

Polly DW, Kuklo TR. Perioperative blood and blood product management for spinal deformity surgery. In DeWald RL, ed. *Spinal Deformities: The Comprehensive Text*. New York, NY: Thieme; 2003.

Sansur CA, Smith JS, Coe JD *et al.* Scoliosis research society morbidity and mortality of adult scoliosis surgery. *Spine* 2011; **36**: E593–7.

Suk SI, Chung ER, Lee SM *et al.* Posterior vertebral column resection in fixed lumbosacral deformity. *Spine* 2005; **30**: E703–10.

Cervical spine surgery

Samuel M. Davis, Gerald E. Rodts, Jr., and John G. Heller

Cervical spine disorders that require surgical intervention can include degenerative disorders causing radiculopathy or myelopathy, trauma, tumors, and infections. Radiculopathy can present as parasthesias or weakness in a specific root level(s). Myelopathy is a condition caused by spinal cord compression; once manifest clinically, the only treatment for this process is surgery to prevent further neurologic decline. Tumors or infections can present in the cervical spine as radiculopathy, myelopathy, or pain due to instability or pathologic fracture.

The cervical spine can be accessed via anterior or posterior approaches; a combined anterior–posterior approach (360° approach) may be utilized when necessary. The choice of approach is largely dependent upon location of the pathology, history of previous surgery, body habitus, and patient comorbidities. The anterior approach allows exposure of the spine by mobilization of the trachea and esophagus to exploit the interval between these structures and the carotid sheath. The anterior approach allows performance of anterior cervical discectomy and fusion (ACDF) as well as vertebral corpectomy.

Anterior cervical discectomy and fusion involves removing the pathologic disc material and then replacing this void with a spacer fashioned from autograft bone, allograft bone, or synthetic devices. This procedure is employed primarily in treating radiculopathy and multilevel (< 3 levels) cervical spondylitic myelopathy. Anterior cervical discectomy and fusion can also be used in the treatment of certain fractures (e.g., unstable facet fractures or floating lateral mass fractures) and for infections.

Vertebral corpectomy involves removing the vertebral body itself, with the two lateral walls and their adjoining transverse foramen (which house the vertebral arteries) as the only remaining structures. This procedure allows for unparalleled decompression of the cervical spinal cord, and can be employed to treat calcified herniated discs, multilevel cervical spondylytic myelopathy, ossification of the posterior longitudinal ligament (OPLL), fractures, tumors, and infection.

Posterior cervical procedures (laminoforaminotomy, laminoplasty, laminectomy with fusion) can also be employed to treat the conditions mentioned above. Laminoforaminotomy (also known as "key-hole" foraminotomy) involves removal of a portion of the lamina as well as a portion of the medial facet joint to decompress the nerve root of interest. It is quite useful for treating radiculopathy in those patients with amendable pathology (e.g., a herniated disc fragment in the foramen). The nerve root is decompressed and pain relieved, while avoiding a fusion.

Laminoplasty is used to treat multilevel cervical spondylitic myelopathy without fusing multiple cervical vertebrae. This procedure involves creation of a hinge on one side of the cervical lamina while performing a complete cut through the lamina on the other side. The lamina is then opened like a book to effect expansion of the spinal canal and decompression of the spinal cord. The "door" or opened lamina is then held open with use of small metallic plates, bone, or suture.

Laminectomy involves the complete removal of the lamina from the vertebral body. Often, it is combined with posterior instrumentation and arthrodesis to restore stability to the spine after removing the posterior elements. Laminectomy allows decompression of the spinal cord and is commonly used to treat multilevel myelopathy. Foraminotomy can be used in addition to this procedure for further nerve root decompression.

Prior to surgery, cervical spine surgery patients should receive a thorough history and physical exam performed by their primary-care physician in addition to the spine specialist to discover issues that may pose a threat to the patient's well-being while attempting to provide anesthetic or surgical care. The incorporation of other healthcare specialists (e.g., pulmonologist, cardiologist, gastroenterologist) should be sought as necessary.

Many patients receive anticoagulants for various reasons. The risk of intraoperative and postoperative bleeding necessitates that these drugs be discontinued far enough preoperatively to allow for normal clotting function. The timing of both cessation and reinstitution of these medications should be agreed upon by the surgeon and the patient's physician to

Medical Management of the Surgical Patient, ed. Michael F. Lubin, Thomas F. Dodson, and Neil H. Winawer. Published by Cambridge University Press. © Cambridge University Press 2013.

reduce the risk of postoperative complications such as hematoma formation, stroke, and even death.

A small subset of patients, particularly those with rheumatoid arthritis and basilar invagination, may require preoperative cervical traction to aid in reestablishing more normal spinal alignment and surgical planning. This may require hospitalization up to a week in advance of the planned surgery. Cervical traction is routinely placed in the ICU where close attention can be paid to the patient's neurologic as well as cardiopulmonary status. The patient should be mentally prepared for immobilization during this period of time.

Patients who are dependent on maintenance dosages of steroids will require "stress doses" of corticosteroids during surgery as well as perioperatively. They should be weaned down to their pre-surgery dose once the risk of an adrenal crisis has passed.

Patients with significant spinal cord malfunction may benefit from administration of dexamethasone while awaiting surgical treatment. For patients with infections, the treating team must weigh the potential for immunosuppression. The drug is weaned as rapidly as possible postoperatively to avoid adrenal and immune suppression.

For the last two decades there has been a tendency to administer very high-dose methylprednisolone to acute spinal cord injury patients immediately after injury. Though this treatment option has largely been abandoned, the pattern of behavior lingers due to a lack of awareness outside the spine surgery community. Meaningful neurologic benefit is not experienced by patients treated with high-dose methylprednisolone, while significant complications do occur. Patients with myelopathy are routinely given 10 mg of dexamethasone intraoperatively to attenuate any swelling that may occur during the procedure.

Intraoperatively, mean arterial pressure (MAP) is maintained at 90 mmHg or at/above the baseline MAP, whichever is greater. This requires adequate control of hypertension preoperatively as a precipitous drop in the blood pressure, which can occur with induction, places the spinal cord at further risk due to ischemic insult. Mechanical prophylaxis for deep venous thrombosis is begun intraoperatively.

Usual postoperative care

Expected postoperative hospital stay

The vast majority of patients undergoing a single level ACDF can expect to be discharged on postoperative day 1 after postoperative X-rays are made and reviewed. Longer hospital stays may be required for more extensive anterior decompression procedures. After laminoplasty and laminectomy with fusion, patients can expect a 3–4 day hospital stay.

Operative mortality

Operative mortality is less than 1% (anterior, posterior, or combined).

Postoperative patient activity

Healthy, younger patients with an ACDF are allowed out of bed on the day of surgery, ambulating as tolerated. They are generally asked to refrain from strenuous upper body activities for up to 12 weeks. Non-impact aerobic activity is encouraged to maintain general fitness while their fusion heals. Laminoplasty patients are encouraged to begin active neck range of motion as soon as possible after having the procedure. Successful outcome depends in part on maintaining flexibility within the spine after having this procedure. After a laminectomy with fusion, patients can expect to lose $\sim 50\%$ of the range of motion present preoperatively, in all directions. This may be larger depending on the number of levels fused within the cervical spine.

Elderly patients with significant cervical myelopathy are likely to have preoperative mobility impairment and multiple medical comorbidities, and to have undergone more extensive and prolonged surgeries. Therefore, they are mobilized as conditions permit under the supervision of qualified physical and occupational therapists. This subgroup of patients may need inpatient rehabilitation services before resuming activities of daily living.

Alimentation

Virtually every patient will experience some level of discomfort in swallowing after having anterior cervical surgery due in part to retractors placed to adequately visualize the spinal column. For this reason, they are started on a liquid diet that is advanced as tolerated. Patients at high risk for dysphagia, aspiration and/or inability to manage secretions should be kept NPO until cough and gag reflexes are assessed. Some patients may require evaluation by a speech therapist for swallowing evaluation and dietary recommendations. To assist in postoperative healing, enteral or parenteral supplementation may be required. Rarely, prolonged postoperative dysphagia may require the insertion of a gastrostomy tube.

Antibiotic coverage

A first-generation cephalosporin is given preoperatively and re-dosed every 4 hours if needed during the procedure. Postoperatively, antibiotics are continued for 24 hours only.

Postoperative pain control

Generally speaking, patients undergoing posterior cervical procedures will have greater pain medicine requirements than anterior procedure patients. Opiates are the mainstay of postoperative analgesia. Patient-controlled analgesia (PCA) pumps are commonly used for pain control after surgery until the patient can tolerate adequate oral medication. Patients on a chronic preoperative narcotic regimen will typically require an increased dosage to achieve pain relief. For these patients, the anesthesiologist plays a vital role in adjusting the PCA dose level by adding a basal rate or instituting multimodal drug therapy (which may require additional ICU monitoring).

Patients undergoing fusion operations are generally advised to avoid non-steroidal anti-inflammatory drugs (NSAIDs), as they may impede bone graft healing. However, patients whose procedures do not require fusions to heal (e.g., laminoplasty, laminoforaminotomy, or artificial cervical disc replacement) may benefit substantially from NSAIDs such as Toradol, substantially reducing opiate requirements.

Special equipment

Collars are not necessary for patients undergoing a single level ACDF. Patients undergoing more extensive anterior decompression procedures or laminectomy with fusion may require a postoperative cervical orthosis for 6–12 weeks, since bone graft healing will require at least 3–6 months. No brace is needed following laminoplasty.

Postoperative complications

In the hospital

Deep venous thrombosis

Deep venous thrombosis and subsequent emboli can have devastating permanent effects. Mechanical prophylaxis continues postoperatively in the form of sequential compression devices maintained on the legs at all times while the patient is not actively ambulating. For patients at higher risk of developing thrombi, retrievable intravenous filters can be placed. Chemical prophylaxis is not routinely administered due to the increased risk of epidural hemorrhage in the acute postoperative period. Should the patient develop a thrombus that requires treatment during the early postoperative period, heparin should be titrated slowly to the therapeutic range.

Airway compromise

Potential complications following cervical surgery include obstructive hematoma, re-intubation, dysphagia, hoarseness, dysphonia, recurrent laryngeal nerve injury, esophageal perforation, and respiratory failure due to obstruction of the airway. Airway compromise after anterior cervical surgery is rare, but risk factors include severe myelopathy, prolonged surgical time, and multilevel surgical procedures.

Re-intubation after anterior cervical surgery can be technically demanding due to retropharyngeal swelling and limited neck mobility. Maintenance of the endotracheal tube should be considered for those patients with significant swelling due to prolonged prone positioning, as this may indicate increased risk of postoperative airway compromise. Emery et al. reported on seven patients requiring re-intubation after anterior cervical surgery, and found patients had massive laryngeal and hypopharyngeal edema. They recommended maintaining the endotracheal tube for 24–72 hours postoperatively in those patients who had anterior cervical corpectomy and fusion. The authors tend to keep patients intubated overnight when anterior procedures exceed 4 hours in duration, especially if they end later in the day. They are extubated based on standard parameters, and when qualified personnel are present if re-intubation is required.

Retropharyngeal hematoma

Though rare, an expanding retropharyngeal hematoma can be life-threatening and its presence requires prompt evaluation and treatment. This phenomenon can occur at any point in the first 24–36 hours after surgery, but occurs most commonly immediately after the surgery and often presents in the post-anesthesia care unit. Patients complain of increasing difficulty breathing, a feeling of impending doom, or extreme pressure in the neck area. Examination may reveal use of accessory respiratory muscles, stridor, or an expanding mass in the surgical area or tracheal deviation. Early recognition of this problem is critical, and emergent evacuation is paramount, be it in the postanesthesia care unit or the operating room.

Dysphagia

Dysphagia tends to peak on postoperative days 3–5 and then slowly gets better. A small percentage (12%) of patients can have symptoms > 6 months. Patients are encouraged to eat a mechanically soft diet and avoid large food boluses.

After discharge

Laryngeal nerve dysfunction

Hoarseness associated with laryngeal nerve dysfunction due to prolonged intubation and elevated cuff pressures has been reported in up to 51% of patients after anterior cervical surgery. Frank vocal fold paralysis occurs in < 5% of cases and can result in hoarseness, aspiration, dysphagia, and even airway compromise. Superior laryngeal nerve dysfunction can also occur, leading to aspiration and difficulty with singing while maintaining a normal speaking voice.

Further reading

Bracken MB, Shepard MJ, Holford TR et al. Methylprednisolone or tirilazad mesylate administration after acute spinal cord injury: 1-year follow up. Results of the third National Acute Spinal Cord Injury randomized controlled trial. *J Neurosurg* 1998; **89**: 699–706.

Coleman WP, Benzel D, Cahill DW et al. A critical appraisal of the reporting of the National Acute Spinal Cord Injury Studies (II and III) of methylprednisolone in acute spinal cord injury. *J Spinal Disord* 2000; **13**: 185–99.

Daniels AH, Riew KD, Yoo JU et al. Adverse events associated with anterior cervical spine surgery. *J Am Acad Orthop Surg* 2008; **16**: 729–38.

Emery SE, Smith MD, Bohlman HH. Upper-airway obstruction after multilevel cervical corpectomy for myelopathy. *J Bone Joint Surg Am* 1991; **73**: 544–51.

Matz PG, Holly LT, Mummaneni PV et al. Anterior cervical surgery for the treatment of cervical degenerative myelopathy. *J Neurosurg Spine* 2009; **11**: 170–3.

Rihn JA, Kane J, Albert TJ *et al.* What is the incidence and severity of dysphagia after anterior cervical surgery? *Clin Orthop Relat Res* 2011; **469**: 658–65.

Ryken TC, Heary RF, Matz PG *et al.* Cervical laminectomy for the treatment of cervical degenerative myelopathy. *J Neurosurg Spine* 2009; **11**: 142–9.

Sagi HC, Beutler W, Carroll E, Connolly PJ. Airway complications associated with surgery on the anterior cervical spine. *Spine* 2002; **27**: 949–53.

Woods BI, Hohl J, Lee J *et al.* Laminoplasty versus laminectomy and fusion for multilevel cervical spondylotic myelopathy. *Clin Orthop Relat Res* 2011; **469**: 688–95.

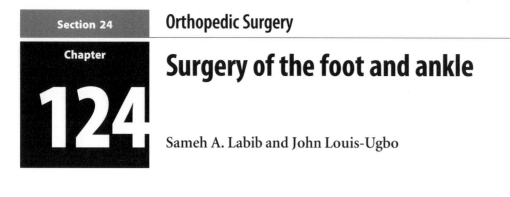

Surgery of the foot and ankle

Sameh A. Labib and John Louis-Ugbo

The foot and its related anatomical structures are specialized for weight-bearing and support, balance, shock absorption, and propulsion and direction. The foot has very complex bony, ligamentous, and musculotendinous units that enable it to function both as a flexible structure that conforms to uneven surfaces and as a fairly rigid and strong platform able to provide push-off and spring during various activities. During ambulation, the foot may have to support repetitive loads equal to eight times body weight.

Except in fracture care, surgery of the foot and ankle is often considered as a last option when more conservative measures fail to alleviate symptoms. Surgeries of the foot and ankle include bunion surgery and lesser toe surgery, deformity correction, fracture fixation, arthrodesis (fusion of joint spaces) for inflammatory processes, and surgical reconstruction that involves invasive manipulation of musculoskeletal structures to treat deformities. After foot surgery, it is important to allow enough time for bony and soft tissue healing in order to attain normal function. Orthotics, physical therapy, NSAIDs, and a change of shoes are useful modalities that complement surgical intervention, and in most cases will be required for optimal recovery.

General rules for operating on the foot

- Special monitoring required: Neurovascular monitoring is required in the immediate postoperative period. Tight casts or bandage should be recognized and corrected.
- Patient activity and positioning: Foot rest and elevation is encouraged to minimize postoperative pain and swelling. Ice packs may be applied. Patients are usually non-weight bearing on the operated foot. Crutches or walker are provided and patients are encouraged to ambulate early.
- Alimentation: No change in diet is needed following foot surgery except for post-anesthetic nausea or vomiting.
- Prophylactic antibiotics: First-generation cephalosporins are routinely given before tourniquet use and for 24 hours post-surgery. Appropriate substitutes are given to patients with known allergic reactions.

- Deep venous thrombosis (DVT) prophylaxis: This is indicated only in high-risk patients during hospital stay, and discontinued with resumed ambulation.

Surgery of the diabetic foot

Complications affecting the feet are major sources of mortality and morbidity among the diabetic population. Patients usually present with non-healing foot ulcers and superficial or deep infections, and will require immediate antibiotic treatment. Management and prognosis depends on the extent of the infection, vascular and sensory status of the extremity, and foot deformity. Interdisciplinary collaboration between medical subspecialists, nurses, physical therapists and social workers is needed to provide effective treatment.

Patients with a surgical abscess in the foot will require debridement and culture-specific antibiotic treatment. The basis of antibiotic therapy should be culture of a tissue specimen obtained at the time of surgical debridement, because swab cultures of the lesions in such cases are notoriously unreliable. The wound should be converted to a clean wound that can heal by secondary intention, with the use of modern adjuncts to wound healing. Both percutaneous lengthening of the Achilles tendon and recession of the gastrocnemius muscle have been shown to be effective in healing forefoot ulcers by creating a motor balance between the overpowering equinus-producing plantar flexors in the ankle and the neuropathically weakened dorsiflexors of the foot and ankle.

Exostectomy or correction of neuropathic (Charcot) deformity may be required when the wound in the foot cannot be accommodated with pressure-dissipating orthoses.

Amputations may be necessary if the infection cannot be controlled with conservative treatment or if the foot remaining after adequate debridement is judged to be inadequate for ambulation.

Hospital course and postoperative rehabilitation

Hospital stay is dictated by the severity of the infection and the associated medical problems. Broad-spectrum antibiotics should be started after appropriate deep tissue cultures are

Medical Management of the Surgical Patient, ed. Michael F. Lubin, Thomas F. Dodson, and Neil H. Winawer. Published by Cambridge University Press. © Cambridge University Press 2013.

obtained. In the presence of osteomyelitis, surgical debridement is followed by 6 weeks of appropriate antibiotics.

Postoperative activity

Rest and non-weight bearing splints or casts are important adjuncts to medical and surgical treatment. Once infection is brought under control, a well-padded total contact cast is applied to relieve local pressure on healing tissues; this has been the most successful method to heal chronic foot ulcers.

Discharge plan

Dressing and cast change is done weekly to follow up healing and ensure complete resolution of infection and ulcer healing.

Recurrence

Diabetic patients are at high risk for recurrence of ulceration or infection. Diabetic foot care should be done daily, and patients should be prescribed appropriate shoes and inserts to prevent recurrent ulceration.

Foot fusion

Degenerative and inflammatory arthritis are common causes of foot pain and deformity. Often, anti-inflammatory medications, orthoses, and shoe modification can provide relief for these disabling conditions. Elective surgical procedures are offered to those patients who fail conservative treatment. Fusion of various foot joints has been the mainstay of treatment for correcting advanced arthritis.

Hospital course and postoperative rehabilitation

Patients are admitted on the day of surgery. Fusion surgery is usually done through a longitudinal incision made directly over the involved joint. Transverse and plantar incisions are usually avoided in the foot. Internal fixation and supplemental autologous or allograft bone are routinely used to improve fusion rate. After surgery, patient is placed in a below-the-knee non-walking cast or splint. Drains may be used and are usually removed within 48 hours. Prophylactic antibiotics are given for 24 hours or until drains are discontinued.

Discharge plan

Patients are discharged in a below-the-knee cast and should remain non-weightbearing with crutches or a walker for 6 weeks. Dressing changes and suture removal is done at 10–14 days post-surgery.

Foot trauma and fracture treatment

Foot trauma is commonly missed, and delayed diagnosis has been recognized in the multiply injured patient. That often leads to long-term foot pain and deformity that could have been avoided. It is imperative that the treating physician look for and help manage foot trauma. Trauma can involve the forefoot, midfoot, hindfoot, and ankle. Management goals in the care of foot and ankle trauma include appropriate care of the soft-tissue envelope, temporary immobilization of the fractures, urgent treatment of open wounds and factures, use of broad-spectrum antibiotics for open wounds, and surgical stabilization of fractures to allow for optimal recovery.

Hospital course and postoperative rehabilitation

Most patients will require cast treatment and non-weightbearing restrictions following surgery.

Discharge plans

Continue non-weightbearing for 6 weeks. Foot elevation, icing, and rest are necessary for recovery. Deep vein thrombosis prophylaxis is often not required for most foot and ankle trauma.

Foot and ankle amputations

Foot and ankle amputations are commonly performed due to chronic infection, neoplasm, congenital deformity, mangled foot trauma and, more commonly, for diabetic foot complications. Important perioperative considerations include the number of comorbidities the patient has, and the tissue viability and functional status of the residual limb. Amputation of the foot and the ankle requires a multidisciplinary approach involving the surgeon, endocrinologist or internist, prosthetist, and physical therapist, among others.

Preoperatively, a complete history and physical examination should be obtained. The presence of systemic disease as well as medication or tobacco use that could potentially impede the healing process should be identified. Palpation of distal pulses is a critical component of the physical assessment; a palpable popliteal pulse with an absent dorsalis pedis pulse or posterior tibial pulse may indicate significant vascular disease that is not amenable to bypass. The patient's nutritional status is also of prognostic value with regard to wound healing and, therefore, should be evaluated preoperatively.

The goal of amputation is to optimize patient mobility and independence. Studies have shown that energy demand for walking is associated with the level of amputation. A functional residual limb, no matter what the amputation level, requires a stable weightbearing surface with smooth loading contours and balanced, unopposed motor control around the limb; therefore, the functional status of the residual limb is an important consideration when determining the level of amputation. Any change in the length and relative relationship of the columns of the foot will alter the normal biomechanics.

Postoperatively, to obtain good outcomes, wound care is very important, as well as the cessation of smoking; in a diabetic patient, control of blood sugar must be meticulous. Prosthetic care is also needed in the postoperative period.

Complications of foot and ankle surgery
Postoperative complications in foot and ankle surgery

Unfortunately, complications after foot/ankle surgery do occur, and must be dealt with from time to time. Many of these complications and postoperative problems are minor, and may be no more than a superficial wound infection or dehiscence, excessive swelling, or delayed healing. Occasionally, complications could lead to complex deformity, infection, non-union or contracture. Postoperative wound infection may require an aggressive debridement; otherwise one could be faced months later with a deep infection or osteomyelitis that necessitates more extensive soft-tissue coverage. The same occurs with a non-union or a delayed union of an arthrodesis, which could easily be salvaged with revision at an early stage. As time progresses, avascular necrosis, bone resorption and increasing deformity occur, making subsequent salvage extremely complicated.

However, when faced with a postoperative complication, how rapidly do you reassure the patient, and appraise the situation openly and honestly? It is essential to acknowledge to the patient as well as to oneself that a course of treatment may not be proceeding as planned. There is nothing worse than coasting along, hoping for the best in a situation that gradually turns into disaster. It is not easy to face up to and treat complications following surgery. However, early recognition, frank discussion with the patient, and appropriate intervention are essential.

Acute foot compartment syndrome

Acute foot compartment syndrome can occur as a result of severe local trauma or may be associated with multiple skeletal injuries from high-energy trauma situations. Commonly patients present with progressive foot pain, numbness in toes, and decreased motion. Occasionally, patients with foot injuries such as calcaneal fractures will present with tense tissue bulging, skin blisters, and paralysis. Compartmental pressures are often elevated and this is often missed in the acute trauma setting. Pain alone is not sufficient for diagnosis; however, increased pain on passive dorsiflexion of metatarsophalangeal joints is diagnostic, and poor capillary refill and absent pulses are late findings.

Surgical decompression including immediate and complete fasciotomy of the nine compartments of the foot is the appropriate treatment for a suspected compartment syndrome of the foot. Two parallel dorsal incisions along the lengths of the second and fourth metatarsals and a medial approach are commonly sufficient to decompress the foot compartments.

Further reading

Bonutti PM, Bell GR. Compartment syndrome of the foot. *J Bone Joint Surg* 1986; **68**(A): 1449.

Brodsky JW. The diabetic foot. In Coughlin MJ, Mann RA, Saltzman CL, eds. *Surgery of the Foot and Ankle*. 8th edn. Philadelphia, PA: Mosby Elsevier; 2007, pp. 1281–369.

Coughlin MJ, Mann RA, Saltzman CL, eds. *Surgery of the Foot and Ankle*. 8th edn. Philadelphia, PA: Mosby Elsevier, 2007.

Fakhouri AJ, Manoli A. Acute foot compartment syndromes. *J Orthop Trauma* 1992; **6**: 223–8.

Myerson MS. Management of compartment syndromes of the foot. *Clin Orthop* 1991; **271**: 239–48.

Ng VY, Berlet GC. Evolving techniques in foot and ankle amputation. *J Am Acad Orthop Surg* 2010; **18**(4): 223–35.

Pell RF, Myerson MS, Schon LC. Clinical outcome after primary triple arthrodesis. *J Bone Joint Surg Am* 2000; **82**: 47–57.

Philbin TM, Berlet GC, Lee TH. Lower-extremity amputations in association with diabetes mellitus. *Foot Ankle Clin* 2006; **11**: 791–804.

Pinzur MS, Slovenaki MP, Trepman E *et al.* Diabetes Committee of American Orthopaedic Foot and Ankle Society. Guidelines for diabetic foot care: recommendations endorsed by the Diabetes Committee of the American Orthopaedic Foot and Ankle Society. *Foot Ankle Int* 2005; **26**: 113–19.

Chapter

125

Lower extremity amputations

James C. Black, Shervin V. Oskouei, Alonzo T. Sexton, and Lamar L. Fleming

Lower extremity amputations are performed for tumors, trauma, peripheral vascular disease, infection, or congenital deformity. The goal of treatment is to return the patient to a functional level allowing pain-free ambulation, which is best achieved through a multidisciplinary approach involving physician, physical therapist, and prosthetic team. Due to the psychological aspects of care, it is important to involve the patient in the decision-making process. This will help the patient to understand the intervention and (hopefully) to concur with the medical staff regarding the importance and necessity of performing the amputation, as well as postoperative expectations.

The vast majority of amputations are performed for vascular disease and infection resulting from diabetic neuropathy; the most common level is a below-knee amputation. The more proximal the amputation, the greater the metabolic cost of walking. Studies have shown that walking speed is decreased and oxygen consumption is increased with more proximal amputations.

Preoperative consideration of several important factors will directly affect the patient's ability to successfully recover from the amputation. The goal of surgery is to leave enough viable tissue that will heal and allow for prosthetic fitting. A serum albumin level below 3.5 g/dL indicates a malnourished patient and an absolute lymphocyte count below 1,500/mm^3 is a sign of immune deficiency; these values should be corrected prior to any elective amputation. Some advocate the optimization of serum glucose levels in patients with diabetes, but this treatment choice is not entirely clear. To maximize the health and nourishment of the patient, an internist and nutritionist should be included in the treatment team.

An essential step in gauging post-amputation healing potential is preoperative assessment of the vascular status of the lower extremity. Standard Doppler ultrasound measurements of arterial pressure may be falsely elevated in patients with diabetes and peripheral vascular disease; measurements of toe pressures are more accurate. The gold standard is to determine the transcutaneous partial pressure of oxygen, which reflects the oxygen-delivering capacity of the vascular

system. Values greater than 40 mmHg correlate with acceptable wound healing rates; values less than 20 mmHg suggest poor healing potential. Consultation with a vascular surgeon is indicated if the vascular status of the limb is in question.

Lower extremity amputations are performed under general anesthesia or regional (spinal or epidural) block. The duration of operation ranges from 45 minutes for a transmetatarsal amputation, 1 hour for a below-knee amputation, and as long as 2 hours or more for a hip disarticulation. The magnitude of the surgical stress is directly related to the level of amputation. When a tourniquet is used for amputations distal to the knee, blood loss is usually minimal; in more proximal amputations, 2–4 units of packed red blood cells may be required.

Usual postoperative course

Expected postoperative hospital stay

The expected postoperative hospital stay is usually 3–5 days.

Operative mortality

The operative mortality depends on the indication for amputation, level of amputation, age, and general medical condition. Mortality rates range from 0.5% for young, healthy patients undergoing amputation for trauma to 20% for elderly patients undergoing above-knee amputation for vascular insufficiency.

Special monitoring required

Pain control, deep vein thrombosis prophylaxis, and pulmonary hygiene are important for all amputations. A well-padded splint or cast should be used postoperatively to facilitate wound healing, prevent flexion contractures, and reduce stump edema. Postoperatively, immediate attention should be directed to the placement of casts. Pressure on the stump by the cast may lead to severe patient discomfort, creating a need for splitting of the cast. Drains are often used to prevent postoperative hematoma and may be removed once the output measures less than 30 mL per 8 hour shift.

Medical Management of the Surgical Patient, ed. Michael F. Lubin, Thomas F. Dodson, and Neil H. Winawer. Published by Cambridge University Press. © Cambridge University Press 2013.

Patient activity and positioning

Patients are mobilized out of bed on the first postoperative day. Physical therapy – including quadriceps, abductor, and hip extension strengthening exercises – is begun on the second day. The cast or rigid dressing is changed 5–7 days after operation, both to allow inspection of the wound and to ensure proper cast fitting after the early postoperative edema has subsided. Skin sutures are removed at approximately 2 weeks and the cast is changed again at 3–4 weeks. A temporary prosthesis can be fitted to the limb when the incision has healed. Touch-down weightbearing with the use of crutches or a walker is then increased over the next month to weightbearing as tolerated. When the stump size has not changed for 6 weeks, a permanent prosthesis may be fitted. Young patients with well-vascularized stumps may be candidates for early fitting of their prosthesis and immediate weightbearing.

Alimentation

Because trauma or infection increases energy requirements 30–50% above basal values, patients should undergo at least baseline nutritional assessments, including serum albumin, prealbumin, and total lymphocyte counts. Nutritional supplementation should be provided as necessary.

Antibiotic coverage

Prophylactic antibiotics (usually first-generation cephalosporin) are administered at the initiation of the surgical procedure and continued for 24 hours postoperatively. For patients with infections, cultures should be obtained and broad-spectrum antibiotics should be utilized until the cultures and sensitivities return. Antibiotics can then be tailored to the identified organisms.

Postoperative complications

In the hospital

Wound necrosis

Insufficient arterial circulation, excessive local pressure, hematoma formation, or skin closure under tension account for most cases of wound necrosis. Small areas of necrosis often heal by secondary intention with local wound care and dressing changes. Vacuum-assisted wound closure devices can be very beneficial. Flap revision or more proximal amputation may become necessary for the treatment of larger areas of necrosis, especially in patients with poor vascularity.

Joint contracture

Joint contracture is best prevented by proper positioning, extension splinting or casting, and early physical therapy. Knee flexion contractures greater than 15° and hip flexion contractures greater than 25° make conventional prosthetic fitting difficult.

Wound infection

The risk of infection increases in patients with vascular insufficiency, diabetes, or previous distal infection. Wound debridement, irrigation, and appropriate antibiotic coverage are the standard treatment, although revision of the amputation to a more proximal level is sometimes necessary.

Pulmonary embolism

Deep vein thrombosis and thromboembolism are potential threats to partially immobilized patients undergoing lower extremity surgery. Prophylaxis with subcutaneous heparin or low molecular weight heparin should be initiated on postoperative day 1.

After discharge

Stump edema

Postoperative edema may impede wound healing and make prosthetic fitting difficult. The edema should be treated with compressive dressings. Edema developing after stump maturation is typically due to a poorly fitted prosthesis.

Phantom sensation

Phantom sensation is defined as non-painful awareness of the amputated limb. This sensation lasts a variable amount of time and may be permanent in some patients. It is a normal phenomenon and treatment is unnecessary.

Phantom pain

Phantom pain is experienced as a burning, painful sensation in the amputated part. It occurs in 2–10% of adults who have undergone amputation and is most frequently observed in patients with pain in the limb prior to surgery. Organic causes such as neuroma, compartment syndrome, and infection should be ruled out. Phantom pain may be diminished by prosthetic use, physical therapy, compression, and transcutaneous nerve stimulation. There is controversy over the effectiveness of other treatments, such as epidural injections, regional neural blockade, beta-blockers, and gabapentin.

Residual limb pain

Residual limb pain in the stump most often resolves in 2–3 weeks with the healing of the incision.

Skin problems

Abrasion of the skin from excessive local pressure or blisters due to friction between the skin and the prosthesis may be managed by providing local skin care and temporarily discontinuing use of the prosthesis. Areas of local pressure should be treated by redistributing the pressure over a larger area of the skin through modification of the prosthetic socket liner.

Psychosocial issues

Potential psychosocial issues should be considered preoperatively as well as after discharge. Studies have shown that young children adapt well to amputations, while adolescents are particularly sensitive to peer acceptance or rejection and may require more assistance. The elderly may be at greater risk than other groups with regard to development of psychiatric disturbances such as depression. Cognitive therapy and psychological support should be utilized to address issues that may arise with limb loss.

Further reading

Bodily KC, Burgess EM. Contralateral limb and patient survival after leg amputation. *Am J Surg* 1983; **146**: 280–2.

Canale ST, Beaty JH. *Campbell's Operative Orthopaedics*. Vol. 1. 11th edn. Philadelphia, PA: Mosby Elsevier; 2008, pp. 561–75.

Eneroth M, Persson BM. Risk factors for failed healing in amputation for vascular disease: a prospective, consecutive study of 177 cases. *Acta Orthop Scand* 1993; **62**: 369–72.

Knetsche RP, Leopold SS, Brage ME. Inpatient management of lower extremity amputations. *Foot Ankle Clin* 2001; **6**: 229–41.

Tintle SM, Keeling JJ, Shawen SB, Forsberg JA, Potter BK. Traumatic and trauma-related amputations. Part I: general principles and lower extremity amputations. *J Bone Joint Surg Am* 2010; **92**: 2852–68.

Volpicelli LJ, Chambers RB, Wagner FW Jr. Ambulation levels of bilateral lower extremity amputees: analysis of one hundred and three cases. *J Bone Joint Surg Am* 1983; **65**: 559–605.

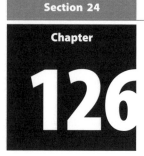

Surgical procedures for rheumatoid arthritis

Michael S. Sridhar and Gary R. McGillivary

Rheumatoid arthritis (RA) is a chronic, systemic, inflammatory disorder that affects nearly 1% of the adult population, with women being affected earlier and more often than men. The disease typically strikes between the third and sixth decades of life, but children and the elderly can be affected as well.

Despite markedly improved and more aggressive medical management, rheumatoid arthritis continues to be, for many, a progressive disease that ultimately leads to significant joint destruction, severe disability, a lower quality of life, and a shorter life expectancy.

Patients with RA typically present with complaints of overall fatigue, morning stiffness that may improve throughout the day, joint swelling, and pain. Patients have serology positive for rheumatoid factor (Anti-IgG IgM antibodies) and antibodies to cyclic citrullinated peptides (CCP) in addition to plain radiographic findings including subchondral bony erosions, periarticular osteopenia, and soft-tissue edema. Synovial hypertrophy precedes joint destruction and can be diagnosed on ultrasound or MRI. Anti-CCP antibodies can be present and detected months to years before the autoimmune attack on the articular surfaces. These antibodies are positive in 50–60% of individuals with RA; antibodies may be present in otherwise seronegative patients (negative serology for rheumatoid factor). Clinical RA will develop in 95–98% of patients with a positive anti-CCP antibody screen. Early diagnosis is paramount as any delay can often lead to irreversible joint destruction and the resultant morbidity.

Rheumatoid arthritis is an autoimmune disorder with a multifactorial etiology including a presumed genetic predisposition. The synovial destruction is theorized to be caused by CD4+ T-cells attacking synovial antigens lining cartilaginous surfaces and the subchondral bone. This initiates an inflammatory cascade, including the elaboration of degradative enzymes and the production of antibodies by monoclonal B-cells.

Early in the disease process, medical management prescribed by a rheumatologist can be effective in stalling disease progression. Patients are typically started on disease-modifying anti-rheumatic drugs (DMARDs), such as methotrexate alone or in combination with biological response modifiers (BRMs)

such as Infliximab, Etanercept, Adalimumab (anti-TNF-alpha antibodies), or Anakinra (IL-1 receptor agonist). Caution is still appropriate with the use of these drugs as their long-term safety and efficacy have not been proven and they may cause complications including infection, hypersensitivity, and possibly lymphoma. Once a patient is in remission, non-steroidals may be relied upon. Glucocorticoids are still used to control acute flares, although they carry the risk of osteoporosis and hyperglycemia and should be used with caution in diabetics.

In a 2004 study from the UK that included more than 1,000 patients, the investigators found that 11% underwent small or large joint surgery within 5 years of disease presentation despite aggressive medical management that included DMARDs. Poor prognostic factors leading to a surgical outcome included a high erythrocyte sedimentation rate and low hemoglobin. The major and intermediate surgical patients had worse functional grades at 5 years when compared with non-operative patients, but conclusions are difficult to draw because preoperatively their functional scores were worse, indicating the advancement of their disease necessitating surgery.

The primary indication for almost all surgical procedures remains pain relief, with improvement in cosmesis, functional improvement, reduction in joint laxity, and prevention of deformity being lesser goals. In general, in the upper extremity, the proximal deformity should be corrected first, i.e., the shoulder and elbow before the wrist and hand. The goal of lower extremity surgery is improvement in mobilization and in the upper extremity to position the hand in space. Common operative procedures are as follows.

Arthroplasty

Arthroplasty procedures are effective at relieving pain because they replace the entire articular surface and subchondral bone and they also preserve motion. Joint replacements are routinely performed at the hip, knee, ankle, shoulder, elbow, wrist, metacarpophalangeal joints (MCP), and less often the proximal interphalangeal joints (PIP). In the upper extremity, interpositional arthroplasty is an option as well. This is a

Medical Management of the Surgical Patient, ed. Michael F. Lubin, Thomas F. Dodson, and Neil H. Winawer. Published by Cambridge University Press. © Cambridge University Press 2013.

technique where synthetic allograft tissue, or autologous tissue (i.e., fat, fascia, or tendon) is placed in between two articulating surfaces.

Older patients with RA who sustain intracapsular hip fractures should undergo a total hip arthroplasty (replacing the femoral head and acetabulum) as opposed to a hemiarthroplasty (addressing only the femur). The former procedure is preferable because older patients are predisposed to synovitis and articular destruction, even if there is no striking evidence of arthritic changes across the acetabulum. This same principle applies to the knee and shoulder: a diagnosis of RA is a contraindication to a unicompartmental knee replacement and a shoulder hemiarthroplasty, respectively. Of note in the knee, the posterior cruciate ligament should always be sacrificed and a posterior-stabilized prosthesis should be used. Similar to the hip, intra-articular fractures at the distal humerus in elderly patients with RA may be best treated with a total elbow arthroplasty. In general, arthroplasty at the MCP joint has better outcomes than at the PIP joint, and a relative contraindication to a PIP arthroplasty is a preexisting MCP arthroplasty at the same digit.

Rheumatologists and orthopedists often disagree with regard to the role of implant arthroplasty in the hand in patients with RA. A recent study by Chung *et al.* investigated the outcomes in two cohorts of patients with RA. One cohort was managed with silicone MCP joint arthroplasties; the other cohort was managed medically. The patients in the surgical treatment group began with a more severe impairment of hand function, but after one year the two groups had achieved similar function. The patients in the surgical treatment group had improved significantly, whereas the outcomes for the patients in the medical treatment group were unchanged. The authors concluded that implant arthroplasty does improve hand function, at least in the short term, and is a good option for patients with poor hand function, for whom medical therapy alone has been ineffective.

Despite the groundbreaking advancements in biomaterials and surgical technique, joint replacements do not last forever. Orthopedists must maintain stringent criteria related to age, compliance with postoperative recommendations, and overall medical health when recommending arthroplasty procedures to their patients. The outcomes of arthroplasty at the ankle and the upper extremity are not yet as favorable as those at the hip and knee. Patients undergoing arthroplasty at the upper extremity often have permanent activity restrictions including light lifting, sometimes no more than a gallon of milk.

Arthrodesis

Joint fusion remains an excellent salvage procedure in some areas, such as the wrist, PIP joints, ankle, spine, and selected others in certain clinical situations. It is reliable at relieving pain but does so at the expense of motion. It should be noted though that often patients already have significantly compromised motion and do not sacrifice much more with a joint fusion. Surgeons must be meticulous with respect to the position of the joint at fusion to maximize function and take full advantage of the compensatory capacity of neighboring joints. Bilateral disease is not a contraindication. For example, patients with bilateral wrist fusions are able to perform activities of daily living with minimal hindrance and their function is not adversely affected.

Soft-tissue procedures

In the hand and wrist, synovectomy, tenosynovectomy, carpal tunnel release, tendon transfers, tendon repair, reconstruction/arthrodesis procedures to address swan neck and boutonnière deformities, and resection of symptomatic rheumatoid nodules all have roles in certain patients. These occasionally are prophylactic and may help alter the course of the disease. Synovectomy is an option early in the disease course before radiographic evidence of significant joint destruction. A prerequisite includes supple passive range of motion.

Surgical considerations

Consultation with internists should be routine to optimize the preoperative medical conditions of patients undergoing general or epidural/spinal anesthesia for significant arthroplasty procedures. In general, surgical stress is related to the magnitude of the specific procedure. On occasion, multiple procedures may be carried out at one time if they are not too substantial. For more significant interventions, such as revision arthroplasty, isolated procedures tend to be the standard approach. Most primary procedures, alone or in combination, do not require more than 2–3 hours of anesthesia. Complicated operations (e.g., revisions at the shoulder, hip, or knee) may demand more time.

Procedures on the distal portions of the extremities (below the shoulder and hip) are generally done with tourniquet control, with blood loss typically being minimal. Although shoulder surgery is done without tourniquet control, the amount of bleeding is usually not excessive and transfusion is fairly uncommon. If arthroplasty at the shoulder is carried out in the beach-chair position, the operative team and patient need to be aware of the risks, albeit small, of blindness and a cerebrovascular accident secondary to cerebral hypoperfusion. Hip and knee arthroplasties involve the most blood loss and sometimes a blood transfusion is required. In certain situations where excessive blood loss is expected (i.e., a complex revision arthroplasty), intraoperative blood salvage, commonly known as a "cell saver" machine, can be used to recycle and intraoperatively transfuse the patient's blood. Stimulants of the hematopoietic system, such as erythropoietin, are also being utilized more commonly in some patients. Closed-suction drainage is sometimes used in the spine and at the hip and knee but carries the increased risk of a transfusion requirement postoperatively and theoretically can serve as a portal for infection.

Many RA patients have significant disease and potential instability of their cervical spines. In addition to a routine history and physical examination, cervical spine films and even preoperative consultation with a spine surgeon and anesthesiologist may be necessary to prevent a serious untoward outcome related to positioning of the head and neck.

The staging and timing of surgical procedures are primarily dependent upon patient needs and wants, which basically means that the most symptomatic joints are usually treated first. However, if there is no clear indication from the patient, lower extremity procedures are probably best done before upper extremity corrections, thus avoiding the problem of crutch-weight bearing down on reconstructed upper extremity joints. In the lower extremity, foot and ankle problems are preferentially addressed either operatively or non-operatively (i.e., orthoses, therapy) ahead of more proximal joints to provide a stable weightbearing base during rehabilitation. The sequencing of hip and knee arthroplasty can vary depending on the degree of joint morbidity involved at each level. If there is a choice, the hip should be done before the knee as it is easier to rehabilitate a hip with a poorly functioning, symptomatic knee than vice versa. Currently, simultaneous bilateral hip or knee arthroplasties can be done, albeit at the risk of increased perioperative cardiopulmonary complications, blood loss, thromboembolic disease, and infection. Patients must be chosen carefully, and if problems arise during or at the end of the first procedure, one should not hesitate to forego the contralateral side. In the setting of simultaneous hip arthroplasties, the approach is usually anterior because the patient does not have to be repositioned to address the other side.

Usual postoperative course
Expected postoperative hospital stay
Even in patients with RA, the hospital stay can be as brief as overnight for distal extremity procedures. For hip, knee, and spine procedures the stay is typically longer, possibly a few days in the uneventful scenario.

Operative mortality
Operative mortality should be less than 0.3%.

Special monitoring required
Occasionally, spine surgery will require somatosensory and possibly motor evoked potentials intraoperatively. Beyond that, monitoring is dictated by the general condition of the patient.

Patient activity and positioning
Both patient activity and positioning will vary a great deal, based on the previous level of function, general health, and conditioning, the specific surgical procedure, and the

intraoperative problems encountered (e.g., poor bone quality). Most patients will need physical or occupational therapy. It seems that hips and elbows require less intensive therapy than other joints. Patients undergoing hip arthroplasty very often need to use abduction pillows when in bed and, if undergoing a posterior approach for hip arthroplasty, should observe posterior hip precautions (avoiding the combination of hip flexion and internal rotation) for several months to avoid dislocation. These patients may require other aids such as an elevated toilet seat. The use of continuous passive motion machines for knees, elbows, and shoulders has been advocated by some but remains unproven and controversial. Following hand and wrist surgery, prolonged use of special splinting techniques and regular occupational therapy may be necessary.

Alimentation
No special dietary requirements are recommended.

Antibiotic coverage
For all patients who have received implants, antibiotic prophylaxis is recommended. A first-generation cephalosporin (or clindamycin for the penicillin-allergic patient) is standard. The initial dose is given preoperatively in the operating room, followed by two doses postoperatively for a total of 24 hours of coverage. Lately, more attention has been devoted to methicillin-resistant *Staphylococcus aureus* (MRSA). For asymptomatic carriage, patients in centers are now more routinely screened by nasopharyngeal swabbing. Patients positive for MRSA are treated with mupirocin ointment and/or chlorhexidine baths/showers. Vancomycin should be considered for perioperative use for patients with a prior infection or for those undergoing a procedure at an at-risk center.

Corticosteroid therapy
Patients who have been on long-term steroids will need stress doses of intravenous corticosteroid perioperatively, due to suppression of their adrenocortical axis. Typically, 100 mg of hydrocortisone is given in the operating room and then tapered over a few days.

Postoperative complications
In the hospital
Neurovascular injury
Orthopedic surgeries carry the risk of neurovascular injury. Meticulous technique and a thorough knowledge of the surrounding anatomy are crucial to avoiding such complications.

Tourniquet-related injury
Microvascular injury occurs in muscle after ischemia of greater than 2 hours. Prolonged tourniquet use can lead to the self-limited complication of post-tourniquet syndrome.

After release of the tourniquet, increased vascular permeability leads to interstitial and intracellular edema. Post-tourniquet syndrome is characterized by edema, stiffness, pallor, weakness without paralysis, and subjective numbness without objective anesthesia. Other tourniquet-related complications include compartment syndrome, direct vascular injury, compressive neuropraxia, soft-tissue damage, and myonephropathic-metabolic syndrome resulting from the systemic return of toxic metabolites after deflation of the tourniquet. Symptoms of the latter include metabolic acidosis, hyperkalemia, myoglobinemia, myoglobinuria, and renal failure.

Infection

Wound infection typically does not present until approximately 5 days after surgery. For this patient population, there is a greater risk of infection due to immunosuppression related to their disease and to many of the medications they take. Irrigation and debridement, coupled with a course of antibiotics, is warranted for acute infection. The patients' state of relative immunosuppression predisposes them to contracting atypical infections. As an example, there is a suppurative mycobacterial species that causes particularly difficult-to-treat hand infections; treatment requires serial debridements and a protracted course of antibiotics. There are few data related to the role of withholding immunomodulatory agents in the setting of arthroplasty surgery to avoid infection. Anecdotally, some surgeons will recommend suspension of a DMARD or BRM (sometimes, for up to a month after surgery) while others are comfortable continuing their use to reduce flares at other joints.

Acute adrenal insufficiency

Despite perioperative corticosteroid supplementation, acute adrenal insufficiency may still occur; it needs to be considered in the gravely ill patient with hypotension, nausea, vomiting, weakness, and hyperthermia. The associated hyponatremia, hyperkalemia, and low hematocrit mandate aggressive and urgent treatment with glucocorticoid replacement.

Delayed wound healing

Both the rheumatoid condition and many of its medical treatments lead to an impaired ability to heal wounds. Skin, soft tissues, and bone are all affected. Skin sutures may be left in place for prolonged periods.

Periprosthetic fracture

Patients with RA may have poor bone quality. Periprosthetic fractures may occur intraoperatively during arthroplasty. These fractures often need to be addressed with supplemental fixation, a different prosthesis, and/or weightbearing precautions.

After discharge
Thromboembolic disease

Patients undergoing total hip and knee arthroplasty are at an increased risk for the development of venous thromboembolic disease; these patients require prophylaxis. The selection of an agent and duration of treatment involves balancing the efficacy and safety of a drug, and often needs to be individualized for specific patients and institutions. Potential agents include low-molecular-weight heparin, warfarin, aspirin, and fondaparinux. The use of pneumatic compression boots is also helpful.

Synovitis

Synovitis is typically associated with silicone implants in the hand. Newer designs use different materials; these include pyrolytic carbon, which is less deleterious to the remaining synovium.

Postoperative fractures

Osteoporosis is such a severe problem in patients with rheumatoid arthritis that postoperative fractures around an implant or elsewhere are not uncommon. To ensure that patients with osteoporosis have adequate calcium and vitamin D intake and receive evaluation for potential bisphosphonate therapy, they should be followed by an internist or endocrinologist in consultation with an orthopedist.

Late infection

Occasionally, an artificial joint may become infected well after the immediate postoperative period. This is often due to seeding from another source, since these patients are at increased risk due to chronic immunosuppression. In the setting of a late, deep infection, patients may require resection arthroplasty and, possibly, antibiotic cement spacer placement (in the larger joints). Once the infection has cleared, the decision to choose reimplantation instead of fusion should be based on patient history, examination, possible joint aspiration, and decreasing inflammatory markers. For at least 2 years after their surgery, patients who have undergone major joint arthroplasty should receive a course of broad-spectrum antibiotics prior to any dental procedure. Patients who are immunocompromised or who have a history of a periprosthetic joint infection should be considered for lifetime prophylaxis.

Loosening of prosthesis and wear

All total joint arthroplasties may fail over time, with the most frequent cause being loosening secondary to wear or loss of fixation. Failure tends to occur at roughly the same rate for all artificial joints, about 1–2% per year. The patient usually complains that the joint has once again become painful.

Instability

Due to component malposition, incompetent soft tissues, implant loosening, advanced disease, or trauma, patients can experience unstable joints and even dislocation. For example, dislocation of a hip prosthesis requires urgent reduction and possible revision.

Disease progression

Since nothing that is done either medically or surgically will cure this disease, its progression may ultimately affect the long-term outcome of any surgical procedure.

Further reading

Amadio PC. What's new in hand surgery. *J Bone Joint Surg Am* 2010; **92**: 783–9.

Chung KC, Burns PB, Wilgis EF *et al.* A multi-center clinical trial in rheumatoid arthritis comparing silicone metacarpophalangeal joint arthroplasty with medical treatment. *J Hand Surg Am* 2009; **34**: 815–23.

Cohen RG, Forrest CJ, Benjamin JB. Safety and efficacy of bilateral total knee arthroplasty. *J Arthroplasty* 1997; **12**: 497–502.

Dodds SD, Brugel-Sanchez V, Swigart CR. Rheumatoid arthritis of the hand – soft tissue reconstruction. In Trumble TE, Budoff JE, eds. *Hand Surgery Update IV*. Rosemont, IL: American Society for Surgery of the Hand; 2007.

Green DP, ed. *Operative Hand Surgery.* 2nd edn. New York, NY: Churchill Livingstone; 1988.

Hollander JL, ed. *Arthritis and Allied Conditions.* 8th edn. Philadelphia, PA: Lea & Febiger; 1972.

James D, Young A, Kulinskaya E *et al.* Orthopaedic intervention in early rheumatoid arthritis. Occurrence and predictive factors in an inception cohort of 1064 patients followed for 5 years. *Rheumatology (Oxford)* 2004; **43**: 369–76.

Lieberman JR, Hsu WK. Current concepts review: prevention of venous thromboembolic disease after total hip and knee arthroplasty. *J Bone Joint Surg Am* 2005; **87**: 2097–112.

Little KJ, Stern PJ. Rheumatoid arthritis – skeletal reconstruction. In Trumble TE, Budoff JE, eds. *Hand Surgery Update IV*. Rosemont, IL: American Society for Surgery of the Hand; 2007.

Millender LH, Sledge CB. Symposium on rheumatoid arthritis. (Foreword) *Orthop Clin North Am* 1975; **6**: 601–2.

O'Dell JR. Therapeutic strategies for rheumatoid arthritis. *N Engl J Med* 2004; **350**: 2591–602.

Papp SR, Athwal GS, Pichora DR. The rheumatoid wrist. *J Am Acad Orthop Surg* 2006; **14**: 65–77.

Parker MJ, Roberts CP, Hay D. Closed suction drainage for hip and knee arthroplasty. *J Bone Joint Surg Am* 2004; **86**: 1146–52.

Chapter

127

Otologic surgery

Adrienne M. Laury and Douglas E. Mattox

Otologic surgery encompasses a wide variety of surgical procedures with the main goals being elimination of chronic or acute ear infections and/or restoration of hearing. The various types of otologic procedures can best be divided based on the anatomic location of the disease or impairment. Working from lateral to medial, the external auditory canal (EAC) is the first landmark which can be subject to injury; this is followed by the tympanic membrane, then the middle ear space, and finally the inner ear.

1. External Auditory Canal – EAC stenosis is an infrequent but challenging problem often found as a result of previous surgery or as an idiopathic phenomenon in the immunocompromised patient. A stenotic canal prevents adequate evaluation of the tympanic membrane; cerumen impacted deep to the stenosis often creates hearing impairment as well. A *canaloplasty*, which involves remodeling the EAC to widen its lumen, is the surgery of choice for this problem.

2. Tympanic membrane – Perforation of the tympanic membrane is a relatively common finding and can often be dealt with asymptomatically for decades in certain patients. However, a majority of patients will suffer either persistent ear drainage or hearing loss as a result of a perforation. Subsequently, a *tympanoplasty* can be performed. A tympanoplasty uses autologous tissue, either temporalis fascia or perichondrium, as a graft to replace the injured tympanic membrane.

3. Middle ear space – A cholesteatoma is a benign but destructive and expanding growth of keratinizing squamous epithelium, which can fill the middle ear space and cause hearing loss and ear drainage. While this is the most common mass found in the middle ear, other etiologies such as a glomus tumor or even malignant carcinomas can be identified here. A *mastoidectomy* is the surgery of choice for removal of these tumors, especially if they extend into the mastoid bone. A *canal-wall up mastoidectomy* keeps the EAC intact and allows the mastoid to drain through the middle ear in the usual fashion, while a *canal-wall down mastoidectomy*

(used for more severe disease) exteriorizes the mastoid cavity through an enlarged EAC.

4. The ossicles are also present in the middle ear space and can likewise be implicated as a cause of hearing loss. Ossicular bone overgrowth (otosclerosis), bone erosion from cholesteatoma, or ossicular dislocation secondary to trauma can all cause malfunction of the normal hearing process. Reconstructive surgery for hearing – *ossicular prosthesis placement* and *stapedectomy* – can be used to remove and replace the injured or malfunctioning ossicles.

5. Inner ear – A malfunctioning cochlea can often result from an infection, trauma, or genetic insult. *Cochlear implantation* has been a revolutionary solution, which allows previously deaf patients an opportunity to regain auditory function.

While otologic procedures are numerous and extremely varied in their techniques and desired outcomes, the operations themselves are relatively similar in their intraoperative and postoperative courses. Most otologic procedures are performed under general anesthesia. Often a cranial nerve monitor will be employed due to the surgical proximity of this nerve to CN VII (facial nerve). Consequently, muscle relaxants are often avoided in order to accurately monitor for facial nerve stimulation.

Usual postoperative course

Expected immediate postoperative course

Most otologic surgery is performed as an outpatient procedure, or an outpatient procedure with 23-hour observation. Patients are typically discharged with analgesics and, usually, antibiotic otic drops. Major postoperative issues include nausea and vomiting from manipulation of the vestibular system. Hearing can also be worse temporarily due to the presence of packing in the EAC.

Operative mortality

The operative mortality equals the anesthetic risk.

Special monitoring

The surgical field is in close proximity to the facial nerve; muscle relaxants are avoided so that facial activity may be monitored intraoperatively. Epinephrine is used as a vasoconstrictor agent; therefore, cardiac monitoring is required.

Patient activity and diet

The patient may resume normal daily activity within a few days of surgery. Heavy physical exercise, lifting, air travel and nose blowing are avoided for 4 weeks to prevent intracranial pressure differences which might displace a new graft. Patients have no dietary restrictions after otologic surgery.

Wound care

During surgery, the ear canal is usually packed with dissolvable sponge material that will remain for 1–2 weeks after surgery. This packing must be kept dry except for the application of antibiotic eardrops. The incision behind the ear should also not be submerged under water for at least the first 2 weeks postoperatively.

Antibiotic coverage

A single dose of preoperative antibiotics is used in all cases. Postoperative oral antibiotics may be continued if a prosthesis is left in the middle ear space. Antibiotic eardrops are used to soften the ear canal packing and make its removal easier.

Postoperative complications

Major complications of otologic surgery are neurologic and intracranial in nature and very rare. Minor complications include vertigo/nausea, canal stenosis, or recurrent disease.

Major complications
Facial paralysis

Facial paralysis is a rare but life-altering complication of otologic surgery. The facial nerve traverses both the middle ear and the mastoid. The bony covering over the nerve may be naturally dehiscent or eroded by disease, exposing the nerve to intraoperative injury. If facial weakness is noted, its initial timing and severity should be noted using the House–Brackmann scale (Table 127.1).

Subsequently, if any unexpected facial paresis or paralysis is identified, the operative site should be re-explored, and the nerve should be decompressed, repaired, or grafted according to the extent of the injury.

Cerebrospinal fluid leak

Cerebrospinal fluid leak can also be a rare but critical complication. The lifetime risk of meningitis with a persistent CSF leak can be as high as 19%. Cerebrospinal fluid leaks can occur during otologic surgery due to the fact that the roof of the

Table 127.1 House–Brackmann scale of facial weakness.

Grade	Definition
I	Normal symmetrical function
II	Slight weakness but complete eye closure with minimal effort
III	Obvious weakness but complete eye closure with maximal effort
IV	Incomplete eye closure and asymmetry of mouth with maximal effort
V	Motion barely perceptible
VI	No movement, loss of tone, no synkinesis

mastoid also plays a role as the floor of the middle cranial fossa. Removal of that excessive bone can lead to a temporal lobe encephalocele and penetration of the dura produces an intraoperative cerebrospinal fluid leak. A CSF leak should be repaired immediately when recognized. Lumbar drainage is not routinely used for small leaks, but it may be helpful in large defects.

Minor complications
Inner ear irritation

Excessive nausea, vomiting, vertigo and/or hearing loss all suggest irritation of the labyrinth (inner ear) during the procedure. The surgical procedure should be carefully reviewed and the ear possibly re-explored if these symptoms are unexpected. The administration of intravenous fluids and antiemetic drugs may be needed.

Stenosis

Stenosis of the external canal is an infrequent complication that may need reoperation if the canal or mastoid cavity cannot be examined and cleaned.

Recurrent disease

Despite a perfect surgical procedure, recurrent disease and the need for repeat procedures is a relatively common complication. Poor Eustachian tube function is the root cause of chronic ear disease. If antibiotics, decreased inflammation, and surgical correction are unsuccessful in restoring Eustachian tube function the ear may develop recurrent perforation, retraction, or cholesteatoma. Continued monitoring is critical to detect recurrent disease at an early stage. Some surgeons routinely perform "second look" operations approximately 6 months after removal of cholesteatoma to thoroughly re-examine for recurrent disease.

Prognosis

Although it is difficult to compare otologic procedures due to their variations in operative goals, the overall success rate in eradicating disease or restoring hearing is relatively high.

For the first few weeks postoperatively, a moderate amount of blood-tinged or brownish otorrhea can be expected as the EAC packing dissolves. However, over the long term, few permanent sequelae exist, except for those who have undergone a canal-wall down mastoidectomy.

Since the ear canal and the mastoid are one continuous skin-lined space, the natural self-cleaning mechanisms of the ear are often disturbed for these patients. Therefore, lifelong semi-annual or annual follow-up for routine cleaning with suction and operative microscope may be required. More recently, one specific prognostic factor has been identified which appears to directly relate to both the incidence of otologic pathology and the success of subsequent surgery. Smoking was found to be directly related to more severe chronic ear disease, more extensive surgical procedures, and worse surgical outcomes.

Further reading

Cummings CW, Flint PW, Harker LA *et al. Cummings Otolaryngology: Head and Neck Surgery.* Philadelphia, PA: Elsevier-Mosby; 2005.

Daudia A, Biswas D, Jones NS. Risk of meningitis with cerebrospinal fluid rhinorrhea. *Ann Otol Rhinol Laryngol* 2007; **116**: 902–5.

Glasscock ME, Gulya AJ, Shambaugh G. *Glasscock–Shambaugh Surgery of the Ear.* 5th edn. Philadelphia, PA: BC Decker; 2002.

House JW, Brackmann DE. Facial nerve grading system. *Otolaryngol Head Neck Surg* 1985; **93**: 146–7.

Kaylie DM, Bennett ML, Davis B, Jackson CG. Effects of smoking on otologic surgery outcomes. *Laryngoscope* 2009; **119**: 1384–90.

Myers EN. *Operative Otolaryngology: Head and Neck Surgery.* Philadelphia, PA: Saunders; 2008.

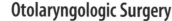

Chapter

128

Tympanotomy tubes

N. Wendell Todd and Katherine L. Hayes

The placement of tympanotomy or pressure equalization tubes is the most common minor ambulatory procedure performed in the USA. Most often done in children, it is also needed in some adults. In appropriately selected patients the procedure can be straightforward and extremely beneficial, but these patients should be monitored to identify complications.

The normal middle ear is an air-filled space which functions to transmit sound from the outside world to the inner ear (Figure 128.1). Basic functions of its mucosal lining are the production of a small amount of mucus and the absorption of air from the middle ear space. In a physiologically normal state, the Eustachian tube functions to open with swallowing and yawning to allow for adequate ventilation and mucociliary clearance of the middle air space. About 1 mL per 24 hours is the usual amount of air which must be transported through each Eustachian tube to maintain near-atmospheric pressure in the middle ear.

It follows then that any disruption of the normal function of the Eustachian tube can offset the pressure balance within the middle ear and create problems. Abnormal sub-atmospheric middle ear pressure occurs if there is failure of the Eustachian tube to transmit sufficient air; if there is undue loss of air from the middle ear through the Eustachian tube during sniffing; or if there is a special circumstantial need (e.g., descent portion of aircraft travel, descent in a submarine, diving, or during hyperbaric therapy) for greatly increased gas transport through the Eustachian tube. Such abnormal sub-atmospheric middle ear pressure may lead to otitis media, and can create scarring or negatively affect hearing. When the Eustachian tube is dysfunctional, placement of a trans-tympanic tube serves to restore adequate drainage and ventilation of the middle ear space.

The procedure itself involves placement of a tympanotomy tube through a full-thickness incision of the tympanic membrane. The incision is usually placed anteriorly to avoid the posterior-superior ossicular chain and the posterior-inferior round window membrane. Because the tympanic membrane is exquisitely sensitive to pain, a brief general anesthetic is usually used for a pediatric patient. Local anesthetic is often adequate for an adult.

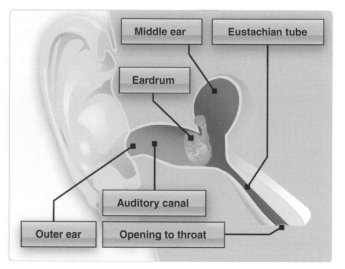

Figure 128.1 The Eustachian tube allows air pressure to equalize between the nasopharynx and the middle ear.

Surgical tympanotomy tube insertion violates a surgical principle of treating inflammation: the introduction of foreign material typically worsens inflammation and infection. During tympanotomy tube insertion, a foreign body is placed into a region which is already inflamed! Nevertheless, at the tympanic membrane, modern medical-grade materials are usually tolerated, even if bathed in pus.

Myringotomy without tube insertion is sometimes performed, but usually affords only a few days of an open tympanic membrane. Even if the tympanic membrane is opened with a laser procedure, spontaneous healing with closure of the opening usually occurs in 1–2 weeks. As a result, a tube is placed to allow for longer-lasting trans-tympanic ventilation.

Usual postoperative course

Expected postoperative hospital stay

Tympanotomy tube placement is performed as an outpatient procedure.

Medical Management of the Surgical Patient, ed. Michael F. Lubin, Thomas F. Dodson, and Neil H. Winawer. Published by Cambridge University Press. © Cambridge University Press 2013.

Operative mortality

The operative mortality is essentially the anesthesia-related risks, unless the practitioner encounters a dehiscent carotid artery or jugular vein (i.e., dehiscence of cortical bone that normally separates the vessel from the middle ear space).

Special monitoring required

None.

Patient activity and positioning

Patients resume normal levels of non-aquatic activity and normal diet once the effects of anesthesia have subsided.

Alimentation

Patients resume normal diet once the effects of anesthesia have subsided.

Antibiotic coverage

Topical and/or systemic antibiotics are prescribed as needed, based on findings at the time of tympanotomy tube placement.

Postoperative complications

Hearing is typically improved after normal atmospheric pressure has been reestablished in the middle ear. Common postsurgical complaints are ear fullness and itchiness for a couple of days. These complaints are, respectively, attributable to alteration of pressure in the middle ear and disturbance of the epithelium of the tympanic membrane and external ear canal. Note that aural fullness is a symptom of abnormal middle ear pressure, whether that pressure is above or below atmospheric.

If a preoperative conductive hearing impairment is not relieved despite relief of middle ear fluid, then the ear has some sort of problem with vibration of the ossicles or with the round window or tympanic membrane. The decision to resume use of a hearing aid in an operated ear is determined by surgeon preference and patient preference.

Otorrhea

Liquid drainage from an ear with a tympanotomy tube is disturbingly common, especially in children. Persistent or recurrent otorrhea occurs in 3–38% of patients.

Most otorrhea is mucoid, purulent, or some combination thereof and typically correlates with recent water contamination or an upper respiratory infection. Such tympanotomy tube otorrhea usually responds promptly to topical otic drops (quinolone 4–6 gtt twice a day for about 5 days) without the need for systemic antibiotics. However, if otorrhea persists despite topical treatment, culture-directed antibiotics should be administered. The ideal culture specimen is obtained under direct microscopic visualization, after removal of potentially contaminating debris from the external ear canal. If tympanotomy tube otorrhea nevertheless persists on systemic antibiotics, the tube must be removed, since it is the presumed nidus of persistent infection.

Bloody otorrhea can also be seen, and is alarming to patients and families. However, it is often of the order of a few drops and is rarely clinically significant. Mechanical trauma to the ear canal (e.g., Q-tip, fingernail) is often the cause. Sometimes bleeding occurs when the tympanotomy tube wobbles in the tympanic membrane; this happens with head banging, or with migration or extrusion of the tube from the tympanic membrane. In addition, bleeding can occur from "granulation tissue" at the tympanotomy tube (Figure 128.2). Regardless, topical quinolone drops typically calm the problem.

A rare but more disconcerting form of otorrhea is clear watery fluid which worsens with coughing, sneezing, or head-hanging posture. Such otorrhea is cerebrospinal fluid until determined otherwise. This is a serious finding which places the patient at risk for retrograde travel of bacteria and resultant meningitis. Cerebrospinal fluid otorrhea should be promptly diagnosed and addressed.

Water precautions

The amount of liquid that gets into the middle ear is a function of the pressure pushing the liquid in, the viscosity of the liquid, and the compliance of the Eustachian tube in relieving positive middle ear pressure. A child with comparatively healthy Eustachian tubes and repeated otitis media that fully resolves between bouts is at minimal risk for water-induced tympanotomy tube infection from surface-swimming in a chemically treated swimming pool. However, exposure to contaminated water (e.g., ear under-water in bathtub) should be strictly avoided.

In general, the ear should be kept free of shampoo and water to prevent transmission of microbes that could prompt acute infection. Earplugs and custom swim molds are helpful in preventing such contamination, but nothing is consistently waterproof. Active evaporization of water inside the ear canal, e.g., use of a blow dryer (warm air setting), is often advised.

Monitoring

The ear should be checked every few months to monitor for satisfactory ventilation of the middle ear, hearing, foreign body reaction, infection, extrusion of the tube, and cholesteatoma. Over time, tympanotomy tubes migrate laterally from the tympanic membrane into the external ear canal. Retention time of a tympanotomy tube in the tympanic membrane is related to size of the flange medial to the tympanic membrane and incorporation of a locking feature (e.g., clothes-pin type connection to the manubrium of the malleus; shaft-style tube placed in a bony trough "under" the annulus of the tympanic membrane). Interestingly, data suggest a genetic mechanism of retention time. Persistent tubes may have to be removed if they are no longer useful.

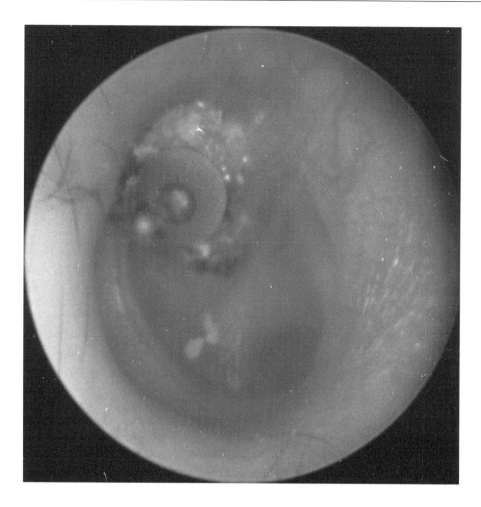

Figure 128.2 Granulation tissue in lumen of extruded Pope style tympanotomy tube. Crusted debris surrounds the grommet. Left ear: top of patient's head is up in this image.

Reinsertion

A myringotomy tube establishes a surgical trans-tympanic membrane ventilation route into the middle ear space in lieu of natural ventilation via the Eustachian tube. If the underlying pathology of the Eustachian tube has resolved (usually occurring concomitant with growth in stature by the child), the patient will have satisfactory trans-Eustachian middle ear function after extrusion of the myringotomy tube. However, if Eustachian tube function remains poor, tubes may need to be reinserted. In an attempt to improve Eustachian tube function, reinsertion of tubes in children is often combined with adenoidectomy. For refractory cases, semi-permanent or permanent tubes may be used for long-term ventilation. In children, the overall rate of continuing Eustachian dysfunction which requires another set of tympanotomy tubes is about 19%.

Residual perforation

About 1–2% of tympanotomy tube patients will have a persistent perforation after extrusion or removal of the tube. In many cases this is fortunate, as it obviates the necessity of reinsertion of a new tube. Otologists sometimes term such an opening through the tympanic membrane "nature's myringotomy." In other cases, when Eustachian function has improved and the physiologic advantage of a perforation is no longer necessary, the perforation may be closed surgically with tympanoplasty.

Cholesteatoma

A cholesteatoma (more aptly termed a keratoma) is a histologically benign cyst of keratinizing squamous epithelium in the middle ear or mastoid. A cholesteatoma usually forms in ears with chronic inflammation; rarely, its development is directly related to keratinizing epithemium (skin) growing into the middle ear space adjacent to a myringotomy tube. In either event, surgical removal of the cholesteatoma is required. If excision is not performed, the growth of the cholesteatoma leads to infection and/or erosion into important structures (e.g., a middle ear ossicle, the facial nerve with resultant paralysis, or the inner ear or brain).

Nasopharyngeal carcinoma

A rare but serious cause of middle ear effusion is impaired middle ear drainage due to obstruction of the Eustachian apparatus by a mass within the nasopharynx. Middle ear effusion, especially if unilateral, should prompt direct visualization of the nasopharynx and Eustachian orifice. Because

Eustachian tube function is almost always symmetrical, unilateral pathology should alert the provider to the possibility of more serious conditions such as nasopharyngeal carcinoma.

Atlantoaxial rotatory subluxation

Too much neck rotation (60° is usually tolerable), recent upper respiratory infection, and comorbidities such as Down syndrome (or any syndrome associated with spinal instability) may contribute to atlantoaxial rotatory subluxation, a rare though serious complication. Patient symptoms include a twisted and stiff neck, and pain that worsens with movement. Examination findings include torticollis: the head is rotated in one direction but tilted in the opposite direction (the so-called "cock-robin posture").

Flying

Trans-tympanic ventilation with a tympanotomy tube precludes a middle ear problem of recompression: air pressure differences are equalized through the tube. Thus, there is no device-related contraindication to flying immediately after tube placement. For individuals who fly frequently, recurring otalgia from pressure changes during aircraft flights is a rare but legitimate indication for the insertion of tympanotomy tubes.

Further reading

Azadarmaki R, Gaughan JP, Isaacson G. Failed tube extrusion is not a random event in children or their siblings. *Laryngoscope* 2008; **118**: 1248–52.

Behar PM, Todd NW. Management of the draining pressure equalization tube. In Pensak M, ed. *Controversies in Otolaryngology*. New York, NY: Thieme; 2001, pp. 196–202.

Kim B, Iwata K, Sugimoto K *et al.* Significance of prevention and early treatment of a postoperative twisted neck: atlantoaxial rotatory subluxation after head and neck surgery. *J Anesth* 2010; **24**: 598–602.

Todd NW. What your colleagues think of tympanostomy tubes – 28 years later. *Laryngoscope* 1999; **109**: 1028–32.

Heslop A, Lildholdt T, Gammelgaard N, Ovesen T. Topical ciprofloxacin is superior to topical saline and systemic antibiotics in the treatment of tympanostomy tube otorrhea in children: the results of a randomized clinical trial. *Laryngoscope* 2010; **120**: 2516–20.

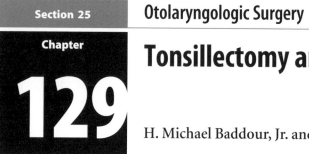

Section 25
Otolaryngologic Surgery

Chapter
129

Tonsillectomy and adenoidectomy

H. Michael Baddour, Jr. and Melissa M. Statham

The palatine tonsils, pharyngeal tonsils (adenoids) and lingual tonsils together comprise a ringed, lymphoid tissue complex within the naso- and oropharynx known as Waldeyer's ring. This structure is known to be involved in inducing secretory immunity and regulating secretory immunoglobulin production. Both the adenoids and the tonsils are subject to infection. They can be potential contributors to upper airway obstruction due to hypertrophy. The number of adenotonsillectomies has been decreasing over the last 60 years. Historically, recurrent tonsillitis was the most common indication for adenotonsillectomy. Though this remains an indication for surgical intervention, airway obstruction secondary to adenotonsillar hypertrophy is currently the most common indication. Manifestations of such obstruction fall within the spectrum of sleep-disordered breathing ranging from primary snoring (PS) to upper-airway resistance syndrome (UARS) to obstructive sleep apnea syndrome (OSAS).

Depending on the extent of adenotonsillar hypertrophy, obstructive symptoms can include loud snoring, chronic mouth breathing, hyponasal speech, frequent night-time awakenings, enuresis, parasomnias, daytime somnolence, poor school performance, dysphagia, failure to thrive, and witnessed apneic episodes. On physical exam, adenotonsillar visualization should be performed as well as a speech evaluation to assess for the presence of hyponasality secondary to nasal obstruction. In addition, craniofacial structures should be noted to assess for the stigmata of adenoid facies associated with chronic mouth breathing. The need for preoperative polysomnographic testing to diagnose OSAS should be based primarily on the history and physical examination. Patients with adenotonsillar hypertrophy, clinical stigmata of OSAS, and a history of loud snoring with witnessed obstructive apneic events may be considered for polysomnographic testing. However, this may not always be necessary before proceeding with surgery, and such symptomatology should warrant overnight hospital observation. If the physical examination is inconsistent with the patient's history, preoperative testing should be performed. In addition, polysomnographic testing should be strongly considered for patients with high perioperative risks, including children less

than 3 years of age; obese patients; patients with craniofacial anomalies, neuromuscular, or neurologic disease; and patients with other medical conditions (e.g., bleeding diatheses, sickle cell disease, or substantial pulmonary disease) that may complicate postoperative management. The apnea–hypopnea index (AHI), peak end-tidal CO_2 and severity of oxygen desaturation are useful data recorded during testing. Based on polysomnography, an AHI of $\geq$ two events per hour with a clinical history consistent with sleep-disordered breathing is appropriate evidence to proceed with adenotonsillectomy.

Though the aforementioned information pertains to adenotonsillar disease of childhood, tonsillectomy is still performed in adults with OSAS undergoing uvulopalatopharyngoplasty (UPPP). Tonsillectomy is also performed when tonsillar neoplasia is suspected or in the setting of recurrent or chronic tonsillitis. Adenoidal tissue physiologically atrophies during pubertal growth; therefore, prominent adenoidal tissue in adults should raise concern for occult neoplasia or HIV infection.

Preoperatively, patients should have a thorough history and physical examination performed to recognize specific high-risk patients as previously mentioned. General anesthesia is used for the procedure. For pediatric patients undergoing adenotonsillectomy, intraoperative corticosteroids should be administered as this has been shown to improve recovery in this population. Multiple surgical techniques are currently used, and the indications for use of techniques vary among centers. It is noteworthy that no one particular technique has been proven definitively to be superior.

Usual postoperative course
Expected postoperative hospital stay

The following are the AAO-HNS indications for 23-hour inpatient monitoring: age younger than 3 years; evidence of obstructive sleep disorder; systemic disorders that put the patient at increased perioperative risk; poor socioeconomic status or other confounders that would limit the patient's ability to return quickly to the hospital; other medical problems

Medical Management of the Surgical Patient, ed. Michael F. Lubin, Thomas F. Dodson, and Neil H. Winawer. Published by Cambridge University Press. © Cambridge University Press 2013.

(substantial heart disease, bleeding disorder, pulmonary disease, mental retardation, Down syndrome, craniofacial disorder, cerebral palsy, morbid obesity); and procedures undertaken to treat a peritonsillar abscess. Patients without a history of the above indicators who demonstrate adequate fluid intake can be observed for 4–6 hours postoperatively, and may be discharged the same day.

Operative mortality

The mortality rate for adenotonsillectomy is one per 16,000 to one per 35,000, usually related to anesthetic complications or excessive bleeding.

Special monitoring required

For those patients with an increased chance of postoperative respiratory complications (e.g., severe OSAS, less than 3 years of age, neurological impairment), continuous pulse oximetry should be used. Intensive care monitoring may be needed, depending on patient factors.

Patient activity and positioning

Light activities are recommended for approximately 7–10 days. When in bed, patients are encouraged to elevate the head of the bed to 30° to reduce postoperative swelling.

Alimentation

Beginning the day of surgery, patients are encouraged to drink ample amounts of liquids. Liquids are encouraged as dehydration can worsen postoperative pharyngeal pain and can also lead to desiccation of the tonsillar eschar, which can result in bleeding. Patients should avoid foods that may abrade the pharynx, and can progress to a soft diet as tolerated.

Antibiotic administration

Antibiotics have been found to reduce pain, fever, and halitosis related to tonsillectomy. In addition to perioperative prophylactic antibiotics, patients are placed postoperatively on a 7-day course of an antibiotic to which oropharyngeal flora are susceptible.

Analgesia considerations

Pain can be severe following tonsillectomy and is generally better tolerated by children than adults. Adequate analgesia can usually be achieved with narcotics, such as elixir preparations of acetaminophen combined with codeine or hydrocodone. Non-steroidal anti-inflammatory medication, specifically ketorolac, should be avoided postoperatively as it has been shown to increase bleeding.

Anti-emetic considerations

Nausea and vomiting commonly occur in the postoperative period due to remaining circulating anesthesics and narcotic analgesics. Ondansetron should be considered for first-line anti-emetic coverage. Given its adverse event profile, promethazine should generally be avoided in children less than 6 years of age.

Postoperative complications
Acute and perioperative
Hemorrhage

Postoperative hemorrhage is the most common serious complication related to adenotonsillectomy. The rate of postoperative hemorrhage varies in reports, but remains below 2%. Bleeding can occur primarily (within 24 hours) or have a delayed presentation (after 24 hours). Presentation may vary from epistaxis, hemoptysis, or hematemesis from swallowed blood. For immediate postoperative bleeding, bedside cautery may be considered. However, patients with continued or severe bleeding should return to the operating room for definitive treatment. Delayed postoperative bleeding usually manifests between the fifth and seventh postoperative day. Management of these patients may require return to the operating room as well.

Dehydration

Though patients are encouraged to begin an oral liquid diet immediately postoperatively, many suffer from dehydration secondary to refusal to drink, poorly controlled pain and/or intractable nausea and vomiting. Patients should be maintained on intravenous hydration until they demonstrate adequate oral intake. Narcotics and anti-emetics should also be used as needed to promote oral intake.

Airway obstruction and pulmonary edema

Postoperative airway obstruction can occur after adenotonsillectomy, especially in children under 3 years of age. Obstruction usually results from edema of the nasopharynx, palate or pharyngeal mucosa, and requires the temporary placement of a nasopharyngeal airway and corticosteroid administration. Post-obstructive pulmonary edema (POPE) can also occur after surgical relief of substantial chronic upper airway obstruction, necessitating the use of diuresis, intensive care monitoring, and, potentially, mechanical ventilation.

Velopharyngeal insufficiency

Transient mild velopharyngeal insufficiency (VPI), may occur following adenoidectomy. This condition (defined by hypernasal resonance and/or nasopharyngeal regurgitation) may persist for days to weeks following adenoidectomy, but usually resolves spontaneously. Patients at risk for VPI after adenoidectomy include those with a history of bifid uvula, repaired cleft palate, occult submucous cleft palate, or palatal hypotonia. In these particular patients, adenoidectomy should be carefully considered and only superior adenoidectomy should be performed. All patients with persistent VPI postoperatively should be referred to a speech pathologist for evaluation.

Nasopharyngeal stenosis

Nasopharyngeal stenosis (NPS) is an exceedingly rare complication of adenotonsillectomy. Most cases of NPS are caused by excessive cauterization during adenotonsillectomy with extensive mucosal destruction of opposing mucosa in the nasopharynx (e.g., superior palate injury during adenotonsillectomy). Patients may present with nasal obstruction with mouth breathing, persistent or worsened snoring, rhinorrhea, hyponasality, dysphagia and otalgia. Management of this condition is difficult and requires surgical intervention for correction. Often, repeat procedures are required to obtain an optimal result.

Atlantoaxial subluxation (Grisel's syndrome)

This rare postoperative complication of adenotonsillectomy results from decalcification of the atlas and laxity of the anterior transverse ligament resulting in non-traumatic subluxation of the atlantoaxial joint. Adjacent tissue inflammation from infection or surgical trauma is theorized as an etiology. Patients will present postoperatively with persistent neck pain, limited neck motility, and torticollis. Urgent CT and MRI imaging is warranted to detect bony and/or ligamentous injuries. Early neurosurgical consultation is advised if radiographic abnormalities and/or atypical physical exam results are found. Depending on the degree of injury, cervical stabilization may be achieved with a cervical collar or may require more invasive treatments such as cervical traction. Systemic antibiotics as well as non-steroidal anti-inflammatory medications should be given to all patients with suspected Grisel's syndrome. Patients with Down syndrome have a heightened susceptibility to subluxation of the atlantoaxial joint due to possible bony deformities of the cervical spine and ligamentous laxity. Particular caution to avoid excessive head movements and neck extension should be taken with at-risk patients during adenotonsillectomy.

Further reading

Afman CE, Welge JA, Steward DL. Steroids for post-tonsillectomy pain reduction: meta-analysis of randomized controlled trials. *Otolaryngol Head Neck Surg* 2006; **134**: 181–6.

Bailey BJ, Johnson JT, Newlands ST, eds. *Head and Neck Surgery – Otolaryngology*. 4th edn. Philadelphia, PA: Lippincott Williams & Wilkins; 2006.

Brown OE, Cunningham MJ. Tonsillectomy and adenoidectomy inpatient guidelines: recommendations of the AAO-HNS Pediatric Otolaryngology Committee. *AAO-HNS Bull* 1996; **15**: 1–4.

Cummings C, ed. *Cummings Otolaryngology – Head and Neck Surgery*. 4th edn. Philadelphia, PA: Mosby Elsevier; 2005.

Darrow D, Siemens C. Indications for tonsillectomy and adenoidectomy. *Laryngoscope* 2002; **112**: 6–10.

DelGaudio, J. Tonsillectomy and adenoidectomy. In Lubin MF, ed. *Medical Management of the Surgical Patient*. 4th edn. Cambridge: Cambridge University Press; 2006, pp. 753–4.

Friedman M. *Sleep Apnea and Snoring: Surgical and Non-surgical Therapy*. Philadelphia, PA: Saunders; 2009.

Johnson LB, Elluru RG, Myer CM 3rd. Complications of adenotonsillectomy. *Laryngoscope* 2002; **112**: 35–6.

Statham M, Myer C. Complications of adenotonsillectomy. *Curr Opin Otolaryngol Head Neck Surg* 2010; **18**: 539–43.

Statham MM, Elluru RG, Buncher R, Kalra M. Adenotonsillectomy for obstructive sleep apnea syndrome in young children: prevalence of pulmonary complications. *Arch Otolaryngol Head Neck Surg* 2006; **132**: 476–80.

Telian SA, Handler SD, Fleisher GR *et al.* The effect of antibiotic therapy on recovery after tonsillectomy in children. A controlled study. *Arch Otolaryngol Head Neck Surg* 1986; **112**: 610–15.

Chapter

130

Surgery for obstructive sleep apnea

Eric E. Berg and John M. DelGaudio

Obstructive sleep apnea (OSA) is a serious and chronic condition affecting as many as 15–20 million American adults. Resulting sleep deprivation has been linked to motor vehicle and workplace accidents. The incidence of OSA is increasing with the obesity epidemic, and it is increasingly recognized as a mediator of cardiovascular disease including atrial fibrillation, stroke, myocardial infarction, and sudden cardiac death. The importance of appropriate diagnosis and timely treatment thus cannot be overstated.

Obstructive sleep apnea manifests by repeated episodes of apnea or hypopnea during sleep. During deeper levels of sleep, especially that characterized by rapid eye movement (REM), there is loss of the normal tone of the pharyngeal and tongue muscles that keep the pharynx open, resulting in collapse of the oropharyngeal and nasopharyngeal airway. In the majority of the population this decrease in airway diameter is clinically insignificant. However, in OSA patients the varied degree of airway obstruction can have clinical consequences. Narrowing of the airway causes increased velocity of inspiratory airflow in the pharynx, causing decreased intraluminal pressure, further tissue collapse, and increased airway obstruction (Bernoulli's principle). In instances of complete airway obstruction, the patient will experience apnea, a cessation of breathing for at least 10 seconds. Incomplete obstruction may result in hypopnea, a reduction in airflow with associated oxygen desaturation, which is more common. Each apnea or hypopnea episode continues until the patient awakens to a more shallow level of sleep, which results in a recovery of pharyngeal muscle tone and recovery of airway integrity. The more frequent the apnea and hypopnea, the more fragmented the sleep, which results in greater sleep deprivation due to the lack of adequate REM activity.

Continuous positive airway pressure (CPAP) remains the most efficacious treatment when used appropriately, decreasing both apneas and cardiovascular morbidity. Unfortunately, these effects are most significant only when CPAP is used on a regular basis. Reported long-term compliance rates, defined as ≥ 4 hours use per night for > 70% of days, range from 40–80% of prescribed patients. Only in these patients, who have failed

CPAP treatment or have proven unable to tolerate it, should surgical intervention be considered. In such cases, the continued morbidity associated with OSA makes effective alternative interventions a necessity.

Weight loss, though difficult for most patients to achieve and maintain, can lead to significant improvement in OSA. Mechanical devices that aim to alter upper airway anatomy are of varied efficacy. Multiple surgical procedures are used, the most definitive of which is tracheotomy. As obstructive sleep apnea is a multilevel phenomenon, these procedures address multiple levels of potential obstruction such as the nasal cavity, palate, and tongue base.

Nasal cavity surgery aims to open the nasal airway. Septoplasty corrects obstruction caused by septal deviation from the midline and is performed by resecting the deviated portion of septal cartilage and bone via an intranasal, mucosa-preserving incision. Inferior turbinate reduction can be achieved via a number of techniques, and aims to decrease the size of hypertrophic laterally based turbinate tissue. While correcting nasal cavity obstruction may assist with adherence to CPAP, meaningful surgical control of sleep apnea is achieved primarily through intervention in the oropharynx and/or the hypopharynx.

In the evaluation of oropharyngeal and hypopharyngeal obstruction, defined patterns of obstruction exist based upon retropalatal and hypopharyngeal obstruction. Uvulopalatopharyngoplasty (UPPP) is a procedure designed to address retropalatal obstruction. Uvulopalatopharyngoplasty involves removing redundant tissue from the posterior aspect of the soft palate including the uvula and lateral pharyngeal mucosa (or tonsils if present), thereby enlarging the oropharyngeal and nasopharyngeal airway, and limiting collapse during deeper levels of sleep. While highly effective for snoring alone, the overall success rate for treating OSA is roughly 40%, though it is felt to be more efficacious in mild OSA and in cases of isolated retropalatal obstruction.

The multilevel nature of airway obstruction in OSA is a significant contributor to this low surgical efficacy, so UPPP is often combined with other site-specific procedures for better

Medical Management of the Surgical Patient, ed. Michael F. Lubin, Thomas F. Dodson, and Neil H. Winawer. Published by Cambridge University Press. © Cambridge University Press 2013.

results. To better address the hypopharynx and tongue base, a number of procedures have been described. Procedures such as midline glossectomy and tongue radiofrequency ablation aim to decrease the size of the obstructing tongue base via either direct resection or scarring after introduction of an inflammatory stimulus, respectively. They do not alter the anatomic position of the tongue base. Tongue base and hyoid suspension, the most established of these procedures, differs in that it does alter the anatomic position of the tongue base. Through a variety of techniques, the tongue base and hyoid bone are essentially anchored anteriorly, limiting posterior collapse and airway obstruction. Such a multi-level approach improves surgical efficacy, with success rates of 60–75% in many reviews.

This multi-level approach to surgery for obstructive sleep apnea has been condensed into a well-defined surgical protocol by Riley and Powell. Phase I treatment involves site-specific intervention with UPPP for oropharyngeal obstruction; tongue base and hyoid suspension for hypopharyngeal obstruction; and UPPP and tongue base and hyoid suspension for multi-level obstruction. Overall success rates, as stated above, range from 40–75% dependent upon disease severity. Patients who fail Phase I surgery are offered Phase II orthognathic surgery, consisting of more aggressive skeletal surgery with maxillo-mandibular advancement via bilateral sagittal split mandibular ramus osteotomies and Le Fort I maxillary osteotomy. While significantly more invasive, Phase II surgery offers success rates as high as 95%.

Usual postoperative course
Expected postoperative hospital stay

The anticipated hospital stay is highly dependent on the operation(s) performed. Nasal surgery alone is generally performed on an outpatient basis. When UPPP is performed alone, patients usually stay overnight and are discharged the next day after demonstrating the ability to take fluids orally. Phase I hypopharyngeal surgery, namely genioglossus advancement and hyoid myotomy, generally results in a longer 2–3 day hospital stay while adequate analgesia is achieved and tolerance of oral liquids proven. Phase II surgery with skeletal intervention will generally result in a 2–3-day hospital stay as well.

Operative mortality

Operative mortality is rare.

Special monitoring required

Intensive care unit observation may be prudent for patients with severe OSA; it should include continuous postoperative pulse oximetry because postobstructive pulmonary edema and decreased respiratory drive may occur in rare cases. Continuous postoperative pulse oximetry in patients with mild to moderate severity OSA is advocated by some, but generally not required.

Patient activity and positioning

Postoperatively, the head of the patient's bed should be elevated approximately 30–45° to help with edema. Ambulation should be initiated as early as possible. Strenuous activities should be avoided for 2 weeks in order to minimize the risk of bleeding.

Alimentation

Patients receive a liquid diet the day of operation and are advanced to a soft diet on the first postoperative day. Severe throat pain is common after UPPP and hypopharyngeal surgery and narcotic analgesia is almost universally required to make oral intake tolerable. As the patient heals and his or her pain decreases, the diet can be advanced as tolerated.

Perioperative antibiotic coverage

Intravenous ampicillin or cefazolin is administered preoperatively and for 24 hours postoperatively with clindamycin substituted in penicillin-allergic patients. Patients are continued on oral antibiotics in liquid form for 7 days.

Analgesia

Postoperative pain is severe and can severely compromise the patient's oral intake. Intravenous narcotics are often required initially, and adequate pain control using oral medication alone must be ensured prior to discharge. Oral narcotics, usually oxycodone in liquid form, are generally necessary for up to 2 weeks postoperatively.

Postoperative complications
In the hospital
Bleeding

Postoperative bleeding can occur in the immediate postoperative period. Minor mucosal bleeding can be observed, since this will usually resolve spontaneously. More significant bleeding requires return to the operating room for control. If tonsillectomy has been performed, bleeding can occur up to 10–14 days after surgery as eschar sloughs from the wound bed.

Velopharyngeal insufficiency (VPI)

Due to involuntary splinting of the palate in an attempt to reduce pain, nasopharyngeal reflux of liquids and a hypernasal voice are common in the immediate postoperative period. As pain diminishes, so will the condition.

Post-obstructive pulmonary edema

Chronic upper airway obstruction is believed to produce a modest level of positive end expiratory pressure (PEEP) and increase end expiratory lung volumes. Relief of the obstruction removes the PEEP and returns lung volumes to normal, but interstitial fluid transudation and pulmonary edema may result.

Septal hematoma

If septoplasty is performed as part of the management of OSA, a septal hematoma can form in the immediate postoperative period, and this will require drainage to prevent septal necrosis.

After discharge

Velopharyngeal insufficiency (VPI)

Permanent velopharyngeal insufficiency is rare but can occur if excessive resection of the soft palate is performed. With over-resection of the palate, there is insufficient palatal tissue to contact the posterior pharyngeal wall and adequately seal the nasopharynx during phonation and swallowing, leading to a hypernasal voice and nasal reflux of food and liquids when swallowing. This is a difficult problem to remedy.

Nasopharyngeal stenosis

During healing, nasopharyngeal stenosis can occur with posterior contraction of the palate and tonsillar fold, resulting in nasal obstruction, a hyponasal voice, and resumption of sleep apnea symptoms. Conservative resection of the posterior tonsillar pillars and avoiding injury to the posterior pharyngeal wall reduce the likelihood of this complication.

Dehydration

Patients who are not tolerating adequate fluids by mouth are maintained on intravenous fluid while in the hospital, however dehydration may occur in a patient who is prematurely discharged.

Septal perforation

If septoplasty is performed as part of the management of OSA, septal perforation may develop and result in altered nasal airflow, chronic nasal crusting, and whistling.

Lip and palate numbness

If Phase II skeletal surgery is required, nerve swelling or injury may result in temporary or permanent lower lip or palate numbness.

Bony non-union

When Phase II skeletal surgery is performed, failure of the bone segments to heal in proper position may occur if intra-operative fixation is inadequate.

Further reading

Epstein LJ, Kristo D, Strollo PJ *et al.* Clinical guideline for the evaluation, management, and long-term care of obstructive sleep apnea in adults. *J Clin Sleep Med* 2009; **5**: 263–76.

Franklin KA, Anttila H, Axelsson S *et al.* Effects and side-effects of surgery for snoring and obstructive sleep apnea – a systematic review. *Sleep* 2009; **32**: 27–36.

Fujita S, Conway W, Zorick F, Roth T. Surgical correction of anatomic abnormalities in obstructive sleep apnea syndrome: uvulopalatopharyngoplasty. *Otolaryngol Head Neck Surg* 1981; **89**: 923–34.

Kakkar RK, Berry RB. Positive airway pressure treatment for obstructive sleep apnea. *Chest* 2007; **132**: 1057–72.

Lin HC, Friedman M, Chang HW *et al.* The efficacy of multilevel surgery of the upper airway in adults with obstructive sleep apnea/hypopnea syndrome. *Laryngoscope* 2008; **118**: 902–8.

Lopez-Jimenez F, Sert Kuniyoshi FH, Gami A *et al.* Obstructive sleep apnea: implications for cardiac and vascular disease. *Chest* 2008; **133**: 793–804.

Mickelson SA, Hakim I. Is postoperative intensive care monitoring necessary after uvulopalatopharyngoplasty? *Otolaryngol Head Neck Surg* 1998; **119**: 352–6.

Riley RW, Powell NB, Guilleminault C *et al.* Obstructive sleep apnea surgery: risk management and complications. *Otolaryngol Head Neck Surg* 1997; **117**: 648–52.

Riley RW, Powell NB, Kasey KL *et al.* Surgery and obstructive sleep apnea: long-term clinical outcomes. *Otolaryngol – Head Neck Surg* 2000; **122**: 415–21.

Schendel SA, Powell NB. Surgical orthognathic management of sleep apnea. *J Craniofacial Surg* 2007; **18**(4): 902–11.

Sher AE, Schechtman KB, Piccirillo JF. The efficacy of surgical modifications of the upper airway in adults with obstructive sleep apnea syndrome. *Sleep* 1996; **19**: 156–77.

Young T, Palta M, Dempsey J *et al.* The occurrence of sleep-disordered breathing among middle-aged adults. *N Engl J Med* 1993; **328**: 1230–5.

Endoscopic sinus surgery: indications, prognosis, and surgical complications

Adrienne M. Laury, Sarah K. Wise, and Giri Venkatraman

Rhinosinusitis is a very common and often debilitating disease affecting approximately 1 in 10 people. Billions of dollars are spent annually on medical and surgical treatments for rhinosinusitis. Rhinosinusitis is defined as the inflammation of the mucosa of the paranasal sinuses and the nasal cavity. Various etiologies of sinusitis have been identified, including environmental (e.g., pollution/allergies, viral upper respiratory tract infections (URIs)), systemic (e.g., diabetes, HIV), and host issues (e.g., autoimmune diseases, cystic fibrosis). Regardless of the inciting event, the mucosal inflammation leads to obstruction of the paranasal sinus ostia, stasis of secretions, and often, superimposed bacterial infections. The causative organisms in the acute setting are usually *Streptococcus pneumoniae*, *Hemophilus influenzae* and *Moraxella catarrhalis*. The diagnosis of sinusitis requires at least two major symptoms including:

1. Facial pain/pressure.
2. Nasal congestion or obstruction.
3. Nasal discharge or purulence.
4. Anosmia or hyposmia.
5. Clinical finding of purulence in nasal cavity.

Or one major symptom and two minor:

1. Headache.
2. Fever.
3. Halitosis.
4. Dental pain.
5. Ear pain, pressure, or fullness.

Accurate diagnosis is often quite difficult since viral URIs and allergic rhinitis may present with similar symptoms. This may lead to inappropriate usage of antibiotics in the acute setting. However, with the increased availability of sinus CT scans, radiographic evidence of sinus opacification has become a major criterion in the diagnosis of chronic rhinosinusitis (CRS). Sinus CT scans are also used in the preoperative evaluation of paranasal sinus anatomy.

Rhinosinusitis is a medical disease and initially should be treated as such. Treatment typically involves the use of antibiotics, mucolytic agents, decongestants and systemic steroids for a minimum of 2 weeks. Adjuvant therapies such as nasal saline irrigations and topical nasal steroids provide symptomatic relief but have not been shown to expedite bacterial clearance. Most cases of acute sinusitis will resolve completely. However, the inflammation persists in certain subsets of patients, leading to chronic symptoms or recurrent episodes of acute sinusitis, and, occasionally, to the development of inflammatory sinonasal polyps. Endoscopic sinus surgery (ESS) is usually reserved for patients with persistent inflammation, infection, or anatomical obstruction of the paranasal sinus ostia.

Endoscopic sinus surgery is currently the procedure of choice for surgical management of CRS. Endoscopic sinus surgery involves the use of an endoscope for visualization of the paranasal sinuses and specially designed endoscopic instruments to widen the natural sinus ostia, resect inflammatory tissue, and clear anatomic defects that interfere in normal mucociliary clearance. Studies have shown that mucociliary clearance in the paranasal sinuses is always directed toward the natural ostium of the respective sinus. A major advantage of ESS over open sinus procedures is our ability to visually identify diseased mucosa or polyps, remove them, and accurately identify the various sinus ostia. The ostia are then widened, thus maintaining and augmenting the native mucociliary flow patterns.

In addition to surgery for CRS, ESS is also employed for correction of a variety of other disease processes. Sinus surgery is used for the treatment of allergic fungal sinusitis; invasive fungal sinusitis; excision of benign and malignant tumors of the nose, sinuses, and skull base; repair of CSF leaks and encephaloceles; and drainage of intraorbital abscesses. More recently, ESS has developed a role in neurosurgical pituitary resections, by providing a direct pathway, through the resection of sinus cells, to the pituitary sella.

Image guidance systems have also become an important supplement in complex or repeat ESS. These systems allow for improved localization and identification of critical structures within the paranasal sinuses through the use of a preoperative

CT scan which is anatomically synchronized with the patient intraoperatively. This anatomic synchronization is performed in the operating room via the use of fiducial markers or surface-matching registration to the patient's facial features. With line-of-sight or electromagnetic technology, the surgical instruments can be tracked to the preoperative image. Image guidance systems have improved our ability to perform more complex and extensive skull-based resections.

Usual postoperative course

Expected immediate postoperative course

Usually ESS is an outpatient procedure. Patients are typically discharged with analgesics, antibiotics, and nasal saline irrigations. Exceptions are patients with severe reactive lower airway disease or other medical conditions that would necessitate an overnight hospital stay. The major postoperative issues include postoperative nausea or vomiting (mostly from blood in the pharynx which may be swallowed). Postoperative pain is fairly mild and easily controlled with mild narcotic analgesics.

Operative mortality

Currently, operative mortality after ESS is almost non-existent.

Special monitoring

No special monitoring is typically required beyond standard general anesthesia monitoring devices, except in cases where patients have CRS in association with severe asthma, where the respiratory status needs monitoring.

Patient activity and diet

To reduce the likelihood of nasal bleeding due to raised intra-abdominal/intrathoracic pressure, patients are advised to not lift items heavier than 10 lb. This is especially important after endoscopic repairs of CSF leaks or encephaloceles. In these cases, a mild laxative is also prescribed to avoid straining. Patients are also advised to refrain from sneezing, drinking through a straw, or nasal manipulations. Patients have no dietary restrictions after ESS.

Postoperative course

Postoperative management after ESS is probably as important as the surgery itself. A regimen of aggressive nasal saline irrigations is started postoperative day 1 to minimize blood clots and collection of mucus and crusts, as well as to begin dissolving any temporary nasal packing. These irrigations should be performed multiple times a day and may result in mild, discolored drainage. Patients must also undergo routine debridements in the office as early as 1 week postoperatively. Debridement expedites mucosal healing and, more importantly, minimizes scar formation. Aberrant scarring leading to

obstruction of the sinus ostia is probably the most common reason for revision surgery.

Postoperative complications

Major complications of ESS are ophthalmologic and intracranial and have a rate of occurrence of 0.85%. Minor complications include bleeding and scar formation; these complications occur in approximately 7% of cases.

Ophthalmic complications

Ophthalmic complications include the possibility of blindness. Most complications occur when the lamina papyracea (orbital lamina) or anterior ethmoid artery is violated and there is bleeding into the orbit, leading to increased intraorbital pressures and optic nerve damage. Immediate recognition is paramount, followed by steps to reduce intraorbital pressures – steroids, mannitol and a lateral canthotomy with cantholysis, which also helps to drain blood and clots. Occasionally, the optic nerve itself is injured, especially in the setting of sphenoid sinusitis.

Cerebrospinal fluid leak

The most common intracranial complication is a cerebrospinal fluid (CSF) leak. This usually occurs at or near the cribriform area where the skull base is very thin; a CSF leak also may occur in the region of the sphenoid sinus. Management involves early recognition of the leak (difficult in the acute setting due to the fact that blood-tinged CSF is difficult to differentiate from blood-tinged mucus) and immediate patching with a mucosal graft. Postoperatively, these patients are admitted and observed for at least 24 hours to rule out meningitis and/or a pneumocephalus. At times, the implementation of a lumbar drain can be useful in decreasing intracranial pressure and improving the integrity of the patch. Very rarely, more significant violations of the skull base occur, with injuries to the subfrontal or olfactory areas.

Bleeding

Bleeding is usually minimal and controlled with topical oxymetazoline or neosynephrine. More major bleeding may require postoperative nasal packing. Occasionally, major arteries supplying the nose such as the sphenopalatine or anterior ethmoid arteries are injured, which may require open approaches or the use of electrocautery for proximal control. These complications, fortunately, are quite rare since these vessels course through bony canals.

Scar formation

Scar formation is probably the most common complication and requires diligent, aggressive postoperative surveillance and lysis of the adhesions in the office.

Prognosis

Although it is difficult to compare results from ESS due to the variety of disease states, patients with chronic rhinosinusitis have been found to have significant improvement in quality of life following sinus surgery. Studies have shown significant symptom reduction or complete resolution over the first 17 months postoperatively for approximately 80–90% of ESS patients. Furthermore, 70% of patients reported an improvement in their overall quality of life following surgery. Additionally, anosmia, when identified preoperatively, has been found to be remarkably improved with the intervention of ESS. Overall, ESS, when used appropriately, can significantly alter a number of intranasal and skull-based disease states, and it often has a direct impact on a patient's ability to function daily.

Further reading

Cummings CW, Flint PW, Harker LA *et al.* *Cummings: Otolaryngology Head and Neck Surgery*. Philadelphia, PA: Mosby Elsevier; 2005.

Glicklich R, Metson R. The health impact of chronic sinusitis in patients seeking otolaryngologic care. *Otolaryngol Head Neck Surg* 1995; **113**: 104–9.

Levine HL. Functional endoscopic sinus surgery: evaluation, surgery, and follow-up of 250 patients. *Laryngoscope* 1990; **100**: 79–84.

Litvack JR, Mace J, Smith TL. Does olfactory function improve after endoscopic sinus surgery? *Otolaryngol Head Neck Surg* 2009; **140**: 312–19.

May M, Levine H, Mester S, Schaitkin B. Complications of endoscopic sinus surgery: analysis of 2108 patients – incidence and prevention. *Laryngoscope* 1994; **104**: 1080–3.

Ray N, Baraniuk J, Thamer M. Healthcare expenditures for sinusitis in 1996: contributions of asthma, rhinitis and other airway disorders. *J Allergy Clin Immunol* 1999; **103**: 408–14.

Smith TL, Litvack JR, Hwang PH *et al.* Determinants of outcome of sinus surgery: a multi-institutional prospective cohort study. *Otolaryngol Head Neck Surg* 2010; **142**: 55–63.

Williamson IG, Rumsby K, Benge S *et al.* Antibiotics and topical nasal steroid for treatment of acute maxillary sinusitis: a randomized controlled trial. *J Am Med Assoc* 2007; **298**: 2487–96.

Chapter

132

Aesthetic facial plastic surgery

Seth A. Yellin and H. Michael Baddour, Jr.

Facial plastic surgery is conceptually divided into aesthetic and reconstructive disciplines. Indications for aesthetic surgery include the sequelae of facial aging: rhytidosis, facial and cervical skin laxity and redundancy, brow ptosis, dermatochalasis and generalized periorbital aging, and cervical fat excess. Additional indications include refinement of nasal, ear, or chin deformities as well as cheekbone and lip enhancement. Reconstructive procedures are indicated for correction of nasal airway obstruction, deformities following facial trauma or cancer resection, and birth defects. Surgical interventions vary in complexity and duration based on the indications and goals of the procedure. Regardless of the indication, facial plastic surgery is most often an elective procedure done to improve the patient's quality of life. Knowledge of relevant complications and sequelae is essential to enlighten the patient so that an informed decision can be made. Realistic expectations including surgical limitations should be thoroughly addressed with each patient preoperatively to avoid postoperative psychological distress and dissatisfaction.

The choice of anesthetic techniques for these procedures is evenly divided between general anesthesia and a combination of local anesthesia with intravenous sedation. Patient preference, surgical expertise, and expected procedure duration should all be considered in the choice of anesthesia. Blood loss from facial plastic and reconstructive procedures is usually minimal and cases requiring transfusions are the rare exception.

Usual postoperative course
Expected postoperative hospital stay

Most patients undergo operations on an outpatient basis. The remainder of patients can usually be discharged from the hospital after overnight observation.

Operative mortality

The operative mortality rate for an aesthetic procedure is less than 1%. Most of these procedures are performed in an elective setting on patients with few coexisting medical conditions.

In cases of complex reconstructive procedures on patients with multiple medical problems, the mortality rates rise proportionally.

Special monitoring required

No special monitoring is necessary.

Patient activity and positioning

Patients are permitted to ambulate on the evening of the procedure. They are advised to avoid straining, bending over, heavy lifting, or vigorous nose blowing when nasal procedures are performed. When in bed, patients are recommended to have their head elevated 30° and to place ice on the affected areas. Ice should be maintained for 48 hours intermittently while awake to reduce postoperative ecchymoses and edema.

Alimentation

A regular diet is permitted as tolerated.

Antibiotic administration

Perioperative prophylactic antibiotics are routinely used. The antibiotics selected should have adequate gram-positive coverage for most routine facial plastic surgery procedures as well as anaerobic coverage when the oral cavity is violated. Further antibiotic selection is determined by the patient's allergy profile.

Postoperative complications
Nasal surgery

Rhinoplasty and septoplasty are common nasal procedures, which involve reshaping of the nose and straightening of the septum, respectively. Each may be performed for a cosmetic and/or functional reason; regardless of the indication, a variety of complications can arise postoperatively following either procedure. Bleeding is the most common complication. Minor postoperative bleeding is normal and usually ceases spontaneously. Profuse bleeding may require the use of topical vasocontrictors and/or nasal packing and occasionally

Medical Management of the Surgical Patient, ed. Michael F. Lubin, Thomas F. Dodson, and Neil H. Winawer. Published by Cambridge University Press. © Cambridge University Press 2013.

surgical ligation. Septal hematoma is another dreaded complication, most commonly following septoplasty. This requires urgent incision and drainage to prevent septal perforation, septal abscess and possible permanent deformity. Infection is a rare occurrence with a reported incidence of less than 2%. This is usually related to local wound infection; however, systemic disease (e.g., toxic shock syndrome) can occur as a result of lack of appropriate antibiotic coverage with nasal packing. Following osteotomy, some facial and periorbital ecchymoses is to be expected. A thorough ocular evaluation should be performed to rule out orbital hemorrhage and/or nerve entrapment. Lacrimal duct injury can also occur secondary to osteotomy, requiring fistulization of the lacrimal sac into the nasal cavity for repair. With such close proximity to the skull base, CSF rhinorrhea can be a complication of nasal surgery, though this is rare. Depending on the size and location of the defect, this may be treated conservatively or may require surgical intervention. Undesirable cosmetic results requiring surgical correction occur with an incidence of 5–10% depending on whether the nasal surgery is a primary or secondary procedure. Finally, for any nasal procedure the patient needs to be reassured that nasal obstruction, olfactory limitation, and postoperative swelling will likely improve with time.

Facelift surgery

Facelift surgery, or rhytidectomy, is performed to correct the stigmata of the aging face and neck, specifically, skin redundancy, platysmal bands, and the redistribution of cervicofacial fat. Rhytidectomy undermines, repositions, and contours these superficial and deep soft tissues to restore youthful facial tone and appearance. Complications related to rhytidectomy include hematoma formation, nerve injury, flap skin necrosis and hairline/earlobe deformities. Hematoma is the most common complication of facelift surgery with a higher predominance in men than women. The risk of occurrence has been shown to be associated with the use of NSAIDs, systolic hypertension, postoperative retching or coughing, and poor intraoperative coagulation. Patients with major hematomas will usually present within the first 12 hours with worsening pain, swelling, and duskiness of the facial flap. Treatment involves surgical evacuation for major hematomas to avoid skin flap necrosis and infection. Nerve injury is another complication of rhytidectomy with branches of the facial nerve and the great auricular nerve at most risk. Transient or permanent muscle paralysis and/or numbness can occur depending on the mechanism of injury; treatment varies accordingly. Skin flap necrosis occurs most commonly with long, thin flaps and in patients who smoke. Treatment of skin flap necrosis depends on the degree of soft tissue injury and can result in some degree of depigmentation and scarring. Cosmetic complications include hairline and earlobe deformities, which are related to incision design, soft tissue realignment, and excess tension with closure.

Eyelid surgery

Eyelid surgery, or blepharoplasty, is performed to correct drooping lids and puffiness under the eyes that naturally occur with age. In addition to obvious poor cosmetic appeal, the weakened periorbital tissues themselves can cause visual impairment. The procedure involves removal of periorbital fat and skin and reinforcement of the surrounding muscles. Postoperative bleeding occurs most commonly with periorbital adipose removal. Both periorbital and orbital hematomas can develop and should be monitored closely. Hemorrhagic retrobulbar extension can occur and patients may present with decreased visual acuity, proptosis, ocular pain, ophthalmoplegia, and progressive chemosis. Urgent ophthalmologic consultation and orbital decompression are the mainstays of treatment. Untreated, retrobulbar hemorrhage can lead to the most feared potential complication of blepharoplasty, blindness. In addition to hemorrhage, both cosmetic and functional problems can follow blepharoplasty, related mostly to the extent of tissue removal and realignment. Cosmetic deformities include lid malposition, asymmetry, and contour irregularity. One functional problem related to extensive tissue removal is the inability to fully close the eye, termed lagophthalmos. This causes a dry eye sensation and increases the risk of corneal abrasion. This can often be treated conservatively with artificial tears, lubricating ointments and taping the eyelid during sleep. Permanent complications from overly aggressive tissue removal include eyelid retraction, ectropion and epiphora, all of which often require surgical correction. Postoperative lid swelling is common and can cause apparent ptosis of the upper lid. This is a self-limiting condition; however, true ptosis can occur secondary to levator muscle injury. This complication requires surgical correction. Wound healing can be complicated by dehiscence, milia at or around the suture line, and hypertrophic scarring. Ocular injury can also occur, including corneal abrasion, globe puncture, and extraocular muscle injury. These problems should be evaluated by an ophthalmologist.

Skin resurfacing

Skin resurfacing is performed to reduce the appearance of fine to medium depth lines and wrinkles, scarring and areas of skin dyschromia. Resurfacing techniques include chemical peeling, dermabrasion and laser resurfacing. Chemical peels involve the application of a caustic solution to the skin to destroy superficial skin layers. Dermabrasion utilizes a diamond fraise or high-speed rotary metal brushes to achieve mechanical desquamation. Laser resurfacing uses a CO_2 laser beam to vaporize the skin. Regardless of the technique used, similar complications can occur following skin resurfacing. Expected sequelae include skin erythema and photosensitivity often lasting several months following the procedure. Bacterial infection and herpes simplex outbreaks can occur within several days following resurfacing and should be aggressively treated with standard antibiotics and antiviral medications. Undesirable hyperpigmentation can be reduced with skin lighteners, steroid creams, and sun avoidance. Hypopigmentation can also occur and may be improved with micropigmentation. Hypertrophic scarring is a disastrous outcome of resurfacing that should be avoided if proper technique is followed; its occurrence indicates that the depth of resurfacing was too extensive, injuring the deeper dermal layers of skin. In general, skin resurfacing should not be routinely performed on dark-skinned individuals. There is a significantly higher incidence of dyschromia in this population, which precludes predictable recovery.

Further reading

Becker FF, Castellano RD. Safety of face-lifts in the older patient. *Arch Facial Plast Surg* 2004; **6**: 311–14.

Cummings CW, Flint PW, Harker LA, Haughey BH *et al.*, eds. *Cummings Otolaryngology – Head and Neck Surgery*. 4th edn. Philadelphia, PA: Mosby Elsevier; 2005.

Demas PN, Bridenstine JB. Diagnosis and treatment of postoperative complications after skin resurfacing. *J Oral Maxillofac Surg* 1999; **57**: 837–41.

Fulton JE. Dermabrasion, chemabrasion, and laserabrasion: historical perspectives, modern dermabrasion techniques, and future trends. *Dermatol Surg* 1996; **22**: 619–28.

Grover R, Jones BM, Waterhouse N. The prevention of hematoma following rhytidectomy: a review of 1078 consecutive facelifts. *Br J Plast Surg* 2001; **54**: 481–6.

Lelli GJ, Lisman RD. Blepharoplasty complications. *Plast Reconstruct Surg* 2010; **125**: 1007–17.

McCollough EG. *Nasal Plastic Surgery*. Philadelphia, PA: WB Saunders; 1994.

Nauman HH, Jahrsdoerfer RA, eds. *Head and Neck Surgery*. 2nd edn. New York, NY: Thieme; 1996.

Papel ID, Frodel JL, Holt GR *et al.*, eds. *Facial Plastic and Reconstructive Surgery*. 3rd edn. St. Louis, MO: Mosby Elsevier; 2009.

Teichgraeber JF. Nasal surgery complications. *Plast Reconstr Surg* 1990; **85**: 527–31.

Chapter

133

Surgical treatment of head and neck cancer

William J. Grist

Head and neck cancer comprises about 3–6% of all cancers in the USA. Despite the relatively small numbers, it can have great effects on appearance and affects important functions of daily living, such as speech and swallowing. For the purposes of this discussion, only the oral cavity, pharynx, larynx, and the neck will be covered.

The treatment of head and neck cancer is best undertaken by a multidisciplinary team of physicians and others, including head and neck surgeons, oral surgeons, medical oncologists, radiation oncologists, and diagnostic radiologists. Other important members of the team include speech and swallowing therapists, nurses and nurse practitioners, dieticians, social workers, and physician assistants. The team usually meets regularly to discuss the patients who have been seen recently or to discuss follow-up and status of patients after treatment. The multidisciplinary approach provides the patient with a comprehensive plan developed from many different perspectives. The treatment of a patient with head and neck cancer is frequently demanding, regardless of the method; careful attention to detail and to the subtleties of treatment is necessary to optimize the outcome.

Depending on the location of the tumor and its size and extent, most patients will be treated with radiation alone or with radiation and concomitant chemotherapy.

For the patient, the head and neck surgeon is usually the initial contact with the multidisciplinary team. In many cases the patient has already been diagnosed with cancer; in other cases, a diagnosis is suspected but not yet formally confirmed by tissue examination. A tissue diagnosis is necessary for treatment to be given.

All patients need a complete head and neck exam by a head and neck surgeon. This is performed both to assess the primary tumor and to look for a second primary tumor (which occurs 5–10% of the time). If a biopsy has not been performed, it can often be done at the time of the initial visit.

Most patients with head and neck cancers are smokers and many are drinkers. These patients can have what is known as "field cancerization" or multifocal disease. An examination of the larynx and hypopharynx (at a minimum) is necessary for

assessment. Many evaluations will need to be carried out with fiberoptic laryngoscopy in order to optimally visualize the larynx and hypopharynx.

Many patients will also have had difficulty with swallowing due to odynaphagia; they will be nutritionally compromised. Most will require a feeding gastrostomy, particularly if they are going to receive chemoradiation.

Although modern endoscopic equipment can provide an excellent view of the tumor in many cases, it is often necessary to take the patient to the operating room for direct laryngoscopy. This medical procedure will more accurately determine the size and extent of the tumor; it can also determine the site of the primary tumor, since the tumor nidus is not always obvious. Tonsillectomy may be necessary if the primary site has not been identified. Usually esophagoscopy is also performed to look for second (synchronous) primary tumors of the esophagus. This is also an excellent opportunity to place a feeding gastrostomy tube if one is needed.

In addition, if the patient is going to receive radiation therapy, a dental consult is necessary. This appointment should include a dental cleaning and a discussion of strategies to avoid dental decay caused by xerostomia. If the patient's teeth are found to be in poor condition, dental extraction may be necessary before medical treatment to avoid dental complications after radiation is completed.

Radiographic imaging of the neck is necessary to fully evaluate the primary tumor and the neck. Chest CT or PET scanning may also be performed to look for a second primary tumor in patients with large tumors. Computerized tomography scanning of the neck with contrast is the most commonly used imaging modality. In addition, MRI scanning can be used to provide information not obtained by CT. It may be possible to use MRI when the patient's renal function cannot permit CT with IV contrast. Positron emission tomography scanning with FDG is also used frequently to look for distant spread of disease or for second primary tumor.

Patients will benefit from being evaluated by a speech and swallowing therapist and a dietician regardless of whether

---

Medical Management of the Surgical Patient, ed. Michael F. Lubin, Thomas F. Dodson, and Neil H. Winawer. Published by Cambridge University Press. © Cambridge University Press 2013.

they will receive surgical or non-surgical treatment. A speech therapist will educate laryngectomy patients about the many differences in their lives after laryngectomy and assist them as they begin to use an electrolarynx. To help the patient and the patient's family cope with any socioeconomic problems that may be encountered, a social worker may be needed as well.

Usual postoperative course

The usual postoperative course of patients requiring reconstructive surgery will be covered in the chapter on head and neck reconstruction.

Expected postoperative hospital stay

Patients who have small oral cavity lesions excised will either be discharged after the operation, or stay overnight for observation. Depending on factors such as pain level, nausea, and the ability to eat, some patients will need to be converted to inpatient status.

Patient activity and positioning

Patients who have large oral cavity lesions and/or have undergone neck dissections are usually ambulatory by the first postoperative day. Patients who undergo neck dissection are very functional after surgery. They have postoperative pain but are ambulatory.

Alimentation

For oral cavity tumors, the excision site of the primary tumor will likely be painful. A nasogastric (NG) feeding tube should be placed if it is expected that the patient will be unable to eat. Patients who have larger lesions and/or have undergone neck dissections may not be able to take nourishment orally and must rely on enteral alimentation. Patients undergoing surgery for very large tumors will be NPO after surgery and will probably also receive a tracheotomy. Following laryngectomy, patients are kept NPO for a week and rely on their feeding tube for nutrition. Patients who undergo neck dissection can resume oral alimentation if they were eating preoperatively.

Antibiotics

Antibiotics are given perioperatively to all patients who have oral or laryngeal surgery. Depending on the choice of the antibiotic, one dose is administered preoperatively and two or three doses postoperatively. Cefazolin or clindamycin is administered depending on penicillin allergy. Unless there is wound contamination from orocutaneous or pharyngocutaneous fistulization, postoperative head and neck wound infections are rare.

Blood transfusion

Blood loss from most head and neck procedures is usually low and blood transfusions are rarely necessary.

Drains

Patients who undergo neck dissection usually have a closed drain in the neck, which is removed when the amount that accumulates has decreased to less than 30 mL in 24 hours.

Postoperative complications
Infection

Small or moderate-sized oral cavity lesions heal without complication. Larger lesions (particularly those of the floor of the mouth) can potentially communicate with a neck dissection and then fistulize and contaminate the neck wound. The neck incision may need to be opened and the wound packed with gauze, which must be changed at least daily. It is the responsibility of the surgeon to inspect the wound and make a determination if such treatment is needed.

Wound breakdown and postoperative fistulization is rare but must be anticipated after laryngectomy. Fever lasting more than 1–2 days after surgery is considered to be the sign of a fistula until proven otherwise. Inspection of the wound and the secretions accumulating in the drain may aid with recognition of this problem. Antibiotics in this setting are not helpful. The wound must be opened and treated locally with packing daily or more often.

Neck dissection without surgery of the primary site rarely becomes infected.

Hematoma

Hematoma formation can occur following neck dissection, as with any surgical wound. This rare complication usually necessitates that the patient be taken back to the operating room for wound exploration, evacuation of the hematoma, and cautery or ligation of the bleeding vessel.

Chyle leak

The thoracic duct can be injured during neck dissection, especially when operating on the left side. Chyle leak can occur postoperatively when the patient begins to eat and there is a flow of chyle through the injured duct. The most effective solution for a leakage of chyle is to return to the operating room. However, if the leak is small, removal of the drain and placement of a pressure dressing will sometimes work. Total parenteral nutrition is occasionally necessary.

Shoulder dysfunction

Injury to the spinal accessory nerve during neck dissection is usually temporary but not rare. Early movement of the arm prevents shoulder fixation at the glenohumeral joint. Physical therapy should be started early after surgery and continued after discharge from the hospital.

Airway obstruction

Mucous plugging after laryngectomy can lead to airway obstruction. Laryngectomy patients no longer breathe through the nose and mouth; therefore, they require humidity in inspired air. If humidification is not applied, these patients may develop a plug in the trachea below the laryngectomy tube. Suctioning is usually not helpful in cases of obstruction. The plug needs to be removed with a forceps or hemostat; sometimes the patient can blow the plug out, akin to expelling a cork from a popgun. Patients need to be taught how to remove mucous plugs on their own; in any case, all of their caregivers should be able to perform this task as well.

After discharge

Patients may need additional time for healing, for pain to decrease, and for swelling to subside. It is common for them to feel depressed and anxious after surgery. For those patients who undergo neck dissections, continued physical therapy for the shoulder and the neck are recommended.

Laryngectomy patients are usually visited by a volunteer who has undergone the same surgery. This individual can answer many of the patients' questions, and can demonstrate by example that life goes on productively after laryngectomy. Laryngectomy patients should continue to practice speaking using their electrolarynx.

For those patients who will receive postoperative radiation or chemoradiation, the window of opportunity is approximately 6 weeks from surgery. This gives the patient enough time to heal while any remaining tumor is still microscopic in size.

Further reading

Close L, Shah J, Larson D, eds. *Essentials of Head and Neck Oncology*. New York, NY: Thieme Medical Publishers; 1998.

DSouza G, Kreimer AR, Viscidi R *et al.* Case-control study of human papilloma virus and oropharyngeal cancer. *N Engl J Med* 2007; **356**: 1944–56.

Jemal A, Siegel R, Ward E *et al.* Cancer statistics, 2006. *Cancer* 2006; **56**: 106–30.

Pazdur R, Wagman LD, Camphausen KA, Hoskins WJ, eds. *Cancer Management: A Multidisciplinary Approach: Medical, Surgical & Radiation Oncology*. 13th edn. London: UBM Medica; 2010.

Srinivasan A, Mohan S, Mukherji SK. Biologic imaging of head and neck cancer: the present and the future. *AJNR Am J Neuroradiol* 2012; **33**: 586–94.

Chapter

134

Reconstruction after cancer ablation

Candice C. Colby and J. Trad Wadsworth

Reconstruction of head and neck defects following cancer ablation presents a difficult challenge to the reconstructive surgeon. The upper aerodigestive system serves multiple important functions such as speech, swallowing, respiration, and protection of the airway that reconstruction must attempt to preserve in both form and function. During surgery, the normal anatomy of this system is disrupted and can impair all of these functions. The goal of reconstruction is to recreate the normal anatomy as best as possible in order to maintain function and decrease morbidity following cancer ablation, while taking into consideration aesthetics, body image and quality of life of the patient.

Multiple techniques for reconstruction are available. These include primary closure, skin grafting, local-regional flaps, pedicled fasciocutaneous or myocutaneous flaps, and free tissue transfer flaps. Each type of flap has a vascular pedicle supplying the tissue; a free tissue transfer will require microvascular anastamosis of this pedicle to local recipient vessels. Patients must be rigorously evaluated preoperatively to define the lesion and the anticipated defect, as well as to determine the best options for reconstruction. The reconstructive surgeon must have multiple options available prior to initiating cancer resection, as the final defect often cannot be determined until the lesion has been removed and all margins are free of cancer.

Free tissue transfer has multiple advantages over more traditional loco-regional flaps. These include versatility, simultaneous flap and resection harvest, possible dental rehabilitation, and improved function and cosmesis. Following cancer ablation, common defects that are best reconstructed using free tissue transfer include composite or three layer defects of the oral cavity, near or total pharyngoesophageal defects, and extensive skull or skull base defects. Although multiple donor sites are available for free tissue transfer, there are a few that are utilized most commonly for head and neck reconstruction: radial forearm fasciocutaneous, fibula osteocutaneous, rectus abdominis muscular or myocutaneous flap, and jejunum flaps for reconstruction of tubular defects such as the pharynx or cervical esophagus. Neck dissection may also be necessary to perform cervical lymphadenectomy

for cancer removal and to identify vessels for microvascular anastamosis, depending on the location of the defect.

Usual postoperative course
Expected postoperative hospital stay

Patients generally stay in the hospital for 7–10 days, depending on the extent of their operation and/or comorbidities. Patients who undergo free tissue transfer reconstruction often stay in the ICU for 3 days prior to transferring to the general medical ward, and may require a longer length of stay overall secondary to the extent of the operation. Some hospitals may have specialty Head & Neck Surgery units that take these patients immediately postoperatively in lieu of an ICU placement.

Operative mortality

Operative mortality is less than 2% overall depending on the patient's comorbidities.

Special monitoring required

Free tissue transfer reconstruction requires additional monitoring in the ICU, most commonly for the initial 72-hour postoperative period. Multiple monitoring techniques have been used; these are dependent on the reconstructive surgeon. No monitoring technique has been shown to be superior to any other in outcomes. The authors' "flap checks" are performed every 6 hours by the Otolaryngology team during this time period to ensure viability of transferred tissue. The flap check (carried out under halogen lighting) consists of pricking the tissue paddle (skin paddle) with a 25-gauge needle, then watching for immediate bright red blood return. Patients undergoing extensive operations or with significant comorbidities may also require care in the ICU.

Patient activity and positioning

Most patients undergoing reconstruction typically require tracheostomy placement and airway management. Care should be taken to avoid stretching, compressing, or applying pressure

Medical Management of the Surgical Patient, ed. Michael F. Lubin, Thomas F. Dodson, and Neil H. Winawer. Published by Cambridge University Press. © Cambridge University Press 2013.

to the tissue flap vascular pedicle. For all patients, the head of the bed should be elevated to 30–45° to decrease risk of edema and ventilator-associated pneumonia.

Patients with a free tissue transfer may need to be sedated to maintain a stable head position (typically the neutral position) for 72 hours postoperatively. This head position helps to maintain the position and patency of the delicate arterial and venous anastamoses of the vascular pedicle. Often this positioning will require the patient to be maintained on mechanical ventilation while sedated. Pillows or propping up of the head are avoided to maintain neutral position and to protect the pedicle. Postoperatively, hypo- or hypervolemia, hypotension, and hypothermia should be avoided. Patients usually receive some sort of anticoagulation postoperatively during this 72-hour period. No form of anticoagulation has been shown to be superior in outcomes. The authors' patients receive aspirin starting on postoperative day 1, along with standard deep vein thrombosis and pulmonary embolism (DVT/PE) prophylaxis.

Suction drains in the neck and/or chest should be placed on continuous wall suction while the patient is in the ICU. Once the patient is on the general medical ward, the drains can be placed onto bulb suction, provided that the output is decreasing. The drains are then removed once the output has decreased to less than 30 mL in 24 hours. Patients are encouraged to ambulate as soon as possible.

Venous thromboembolism prophylaxis

Patients who have undergone major head and neck ablative and reconstructive procedures of over 8 hours duration should be considered to be at high risk for VTE, in the same way that major trauma or abdominal surgery patients are considered to be in need of DVT/PE prophylaxis. Sequential compression devices are commonly used both intraoperatively and postoperatively, and subcutaneous heparin or other adjuncts are administered, until the patient is ambulatory.

Alimentation

Most patients who undergo reconstruction after cancer ablation will not be able to obtain nutrition by mouth in the immediate postoperative period. The patient may have suture lines within the oral cavity or pharynx; NPO status is necessary to prevent oro- or pharyngocutaneous fistula formation. The exception is any operation performed on the neck or face without distortion of pharyngeal tissues; these patients may also have a significant degree of dysphagia secondary to edema and other perioperative issues that distort normal anatomy. For patients who are NPO, a small flexible nasogastric Dobhoff feeding tube is placed intraoperatively to allow for nutrition during this period. If long-term tube feeding is anticipated, a percutaneous gastrostomy tube is placed at the time of the original operation or in the postoperative period. Tube alimentation typically is initiated on postoperative day 1 at a slow continuous rate; it is progressively increased until the goal level (determined by the patient's estimated caloric needs) is reached. Reconstruction, like other lengthy operations, can cause a significant catabolic trend; attention to nutritional support is essential.

Any suture line placed in the oral cavity or pharynx typically requires 5–10 days to heal completely. Patients who have a history of radiation therapy treatment in the surgical area may take slightly longer to heal, since radiation causes decreased vascularity and, potentially, delayed wound healing in the affected tissues.

For patients with pharyngeal reconstruction, a barium swallow is performed prior to the initiation of clear liquids to ensure adequacy of healing and absence of fistula.

Antibiotic coverage

Except for sterile interventions in the neck or soft tissue, where there is no contact with the aerodigestive tract, the majority of head and neck operations are performed in a clean contaminated field. Perioperative antibiotics that cover the polymicrobial aerodigestive flora (including anaerobes) are administered immediately prior to the procedure and during the 48-hour postoperative period. Patients with drains in place often continue antibiotic coverage until these are removed, as drains can serve as a nidus for infection and a portal of entry into the sterile wound. No good data exist showing the superiority of one antibiotic regimen over another or of the timing of withdrawal of antibiotics.

Management of the airway

Patients undergoing extensive cancer ablation and reconstruction typically require tracheostomy as a precautionary measure to secure the airway. Postoperative edema of the pharynx and airway can cause compromise; typically this subsides within days. The tracheostomy tube must be sutured in place to secure the airway.

Patients undergoing free tissue transfer are sedated to maintain a stable head position; during this period of sedation, the patient will most often be maintained on mechanical ventilation. Tracheostomy provides a more secure airway than an oral endotracheal tube during this tenuous 72-hour postoperative period, when the vascular pedicle is most vulnerable. To prevent injury to the vascular pedicle, no ties should be placed around the neck until after the first tracheostomy tube change.

Frequent suctioning of secretions is essential after a tracheostomy is performed, since the airway is newly exposed to irritants that have not first passed through the nasal and oral filters. Humidification is also essential to decrease scabbing, bleeding, and drying of secretions – all of which can cause significant airway obstruction.

Wound care

If a free tissue transfer is performed using tissue from the arm or leg, a splint dressing is placed on the donor site wound intraoperatively; this dressing is removed on postoperative days 5–7. Once removed, a soft dressing is placed with a splint over the wound. Skin graft sites are covered with Xeroform dressing intraoperatively, and are slowly removed starting postoperative day 7.

Analgesia

Patients with free tissue transfer will usually be sedated for 72 hours postoperatively, and may require mechanical ventilation for at least 24 hours after the operation. Intravenous narcotics are typically required for the first 48–72 hours. Oral narcotics, such as oxycodone derivatives, can be given in liquid form through a feeding tube.

Speech therapy/physical therapy/occupational therapy

Following cancer ablation, and even with extensive reconstruction, patients can have significant speech and swallowing impairments secondary to distortion of normal anatomy and/or impairment of cranial nerves. It is optimal to obtain a speech and swallowing consultation within the immediate postoperative period to assist with identification of speech and swallowing difficulties. Rehabilitation with an experienced team of speech pathologists should begin as soon as possible.

Physical therapy is essential to assist with weightbearing exercises of the leg for patients receiving free tissue transfer with fibula reconstruction. Therapy is also extremely important to prevent deconditioning and long-term dysfunction. Occasionally, shoulder pain and/or weakness can occur following neck dissection because the spinal accessory nerve is routinely dissected and traced in order to perform cervical lymphadenectomy. As a result of this dissection, patients can develop a neuropraxia that may benefit from physical therapy.

Management of comorbidities

Consultations are obtained by the critical care team when performing free tissue transfers, and coordinated management is often necessary following other major operations, or for patients with significant preexisting comorbidities. Once the patient is on the general medical ward, a hospitalist medicine service may be consulted to assist with complex medical issues.

Postoperative complications

In the hospital

Vascular compromise of free tissue transfer

Vascular compromise is a rare complication, occurring in approximately 4% of cases; over half of these are salvageable upon re-exploration. If compromise occurs, it is almost always within the first 72 hours. The most common cause is thrombosis of the venous anastamosis. Early signs include vascular congestion, increased flap turgor, and increased capillary refill with brisk return of dark red blood when the flap is pricked with a needle. Compromise of the arterial pedicle results in a pale, cool flap, with the absence of capillary refill upon examination. If flap compromise is suspected, an immediate return to the operating room for re-exploration is necessary, as time is of the essence. After approximately 6 hours of ischemia, most fasciocutaneous flaps are not salvageable; this time is significantly less for muscular or enteric (jejunum, gastric/omental) flaps.

Bleeding

Extensive care is taken intraoperatively to control any bleeding. However, bleeding can occur postoperatively following any surgical procedure. Large vessels are encountered routinely during surgery of the head and neck but are not typically the source for postoperative bleeding. Most often, the sources of a postoperative bleed or hematoma are small superficial veins that were retracted during the operation, and which become exposed once tension is relieved.

Speech and swallowing impairment

Patients may have continued speech and swallowing impairments secondary to distortion of normal anatomy and cranial neuropathies. It is optimal to obtain a speech and swallowing consult in the immediate postoperative period and to continue rehabilitation throughout the hospital stay. Patients may also require home therapy sessions to continue this rehabilitation.

Airway obstruction

When adequate care has been taken intraoperatively to secure the airway with tracheostomy placement, airway obstruction rarely occurs. Tracheostomy tube obstruction can occur in the presence of dried secretions, extensive mucus plugging, or bleeding from the airway or from around the tracheostomy site proper. Humidification and proper tracheostomy care will help to prevent airway obstruction.

Infection

Fortunately, postoperative infections are relatively uncommon, given that the majority of head and neck operations are clean contaminated cases. Any infectious fluid collection that is present in a post-surgical wound must be opened and drained. Antibiotics are used to cover polymicrobial aerodigestive flora, including anaerobic coverage.

Fistula

A fistula is an abnormal connection or communication between two organs or spaces that should not connect. Postoperative fistulas commonly occur between the oral cavity or oropharynx and the neck (orocutaneous fistula), especially if extensive loss of native tissue occurs. During a laryngectomy, a pharyngotomy is created; occasionally, the repair suture line can break down and develop a passageway to the neck (pharyngocutaneous fistula).

Close observation with conscientious wound care and packing are usually sufficient to allow the wound to heal and close. Rarely, more aggressive reconstruction may be required to close the defect.

Chylous fistula

Chylous fistula is an infrequent complication that can occur following neck dissection secondary to an injury of the thoracic duct or surrounding lymphatics. Management consists of close observation, diet management, and pressure dressing. Only rarely does this complication require re-exploration and/or surgical repair.

After discharge

Wound care

Typically, no special wound care is required once the patient leaves the hospital. If an infection or fistula has occurred, local wound care with packing or dressing changes may be required. Patient care is usually performed with the aid of a home healthcare nurse.

Tumor recurrence

Vigilant postoperative surveillance, including frequent otolaryngologic exams and radiologic examinations, is required to identify and treat local or distant tumor recurrence.

Further reading

Chien W, Varvares MA, Hadlock T, Cheney M, Deschler DG. Effects of aspirin and low-dose heparin in head and neck reconstruction using microvascular free flaps. *Laryngoscope* 2005; **115**: 973–6.

Farwell DG, Reilly DF, Weymuller EA Jr *et al.* Predictors of perioperative complications in head and neck patients. *Arch Otolaryngol Head Neck Surg* 2002; **128**: 505–11.

Futran ND, Wadsworth JT, Villaret D, Farwell DG. Midface reconstruction with the fibula free flap. *Arch Otolaryngol Head Neck Surg* 2002; **128**: 161–6.

Luu Q, Farwell DG. Advances in free flap monitoring: have we gone too far? *Curr Opin Otolaryngol Head Neck Surg* 2009; **17**: 267–9.

Momoh AO, Yu P, Skoracki RJ *et al.* A prospective cohort study of fibula free flap donor site morbidity in 157 consecutive patients. *Plast Reconstr Surg* 2011; **128**: 714.

Smeele LE, Irish JC, Gullane PJ *et al.* A retrospective comparison of the morbidity and cost of different reconstructive strategies in oral and oropharyngeal carcinoma. *Laryngoscope* 1999; **109**: 800–4.

Tsue TT, Desyatnikova SS, Deleyiannis FW *et al.* Comparison of cost and function in reconstruction of the posterior oral cavity and oropharynx. Free vs pedicled soft tissue transfer. *Arch Otolaryngol Head Neck Surg* 1997; **123**: 731–7.

Wadsworth JT, Futran N, Eubanks TR. Laparoscopic harvest of the jejunal free flap for reconstruction of hypopharyngeal and cervical esophageal defects. *Arch Otolaryngol Head Neck Surg* 2002; **128**: 1384–7.

Wei FC, Jain V, Celik N *et al.* Have we found an ideal soft-tissue flap? An experience with 672 anterolateral thigh flaps. *Plast Reconstr Surg* 2002; **109**: 2219–26; discussion 2227–30.

Chapter 135

Surgical management of thyroid malignancies

Amy Y. Chen

In 2010, thyroid cancer was estimated to affect 44,670 individuals in the USA, according to data provided by the American Cancer Society; in the same year, 1,690 affected individuals died. The risk of developing thyroid cancer is approximately 1 in 286 or 0.35%. The risk of dying of thyroid cancer is even lower, approximately 1 in 2,500 or 0.04%. Differentiated thyroid cancer incidence is increasing annually at 3–5% per year. This increase is predominantly seen among the smallest thyroid cancers (those less than 2 cm); however, increases have been reported among the largest thyroid cancers as well. The reason for this increase is thought to be mainly due to increased diagnostic scrutiny and imaging for non-thyroid related ailments. However, the rise in incidence rates among the larger thyroid tumors suggests that other mechanisms may be at work.

Differentiated thyroid cancer comprises 90% of all thyroid cancers, and thus the discussion in this chapter will focus on these cancers. These cancers are pathologically defined as papillary and follicular thyroid cancer. The remaining 10% of thyroid cancers include medullary, anaplastic, poorly differentiated thyroid carcinoma, and lymphoma. Papillary thyroid cancers have a strong predilection to produce lymph node metastases. Follicular thyroid cancer tends to metastasize by hematogenous spread. Radiation exposure is the single highest risk factor in the development of thyroid cancer; however, more research has identified other molecular changes such as in the bRAF protein that leads to thyroid carcinogenesis. Approximately 45% of papillary thyroid cancers exhibit mutations of the bRAF protein. Research into the molecular changes necessary for development of differentiated thyroid cancer is ongoing.

Surgical management

The preferred first treatment for differentiated thyroid cancer is surgical resection of the thyroid gland. Pathology should be verified prior to obtaining consent from the patient for thyroidectomy. Recent efforts have been made to clarify fine needle aspiration findings and to standardize them.

Total thyroidectomy is preferred over subtotal thyroidectomy for surgical management of thyroid cancer. A recent study reported that disease-free survival was better for patients who had undergone total thyroidectomy for papillary thyroid cancers greater than 1 cm.

Management of the central compartment portion of the neck is controversial. American Thyroid Association (ATA) guidelines recommend central compartment neck dissection (CCND) for thyroid cancers measuring T3 or T4. Some authors report increased complications such as hypocalcemia and vocal cord dysfunction after CCND. However, others report that the complication rate is not higher, especially in the hands of experienced surgeons. A subsequent paper also reported on the inverse relationship between volume of a surgeon's practice and complication rates: high-volume surgeons had decreased odds for recurrent laryngeal nerve injury and hypocalcemia.

Lateral compartment neck dissections are recommended only for patients with pathologically proven lymph nodes in the lateral neck. These surgeries are accomplished in a comprehensive fashion rather than by "node plucking."

A preoperative work-up for thyroid cancer patients should include thyroid function testing. For women of childbearing age, a pregnancy test should be considered. For any patients who are hyperthyroid prior to surgery, an endocrinology consult preoperatively may be very helpful to avoid anesthetic complications from the hyperthyroid state. Examination of vocal cord function is also important. Otolaryngologists and head and neck surgeons routinely examine the larynx either by mirror laryngoscopy or by flexible fiberoptic nasopharyngolaryngoscopy. Prior to surgery, it is very important to document whether each vocal cord is functioning normally. During surgery, visual monitoring of the recurrent laryngeal nerve can be enhanced by intraoperative neural monitoring (IONM), which is usually obtained via a specially adapted endotracheal tube. Recently, standards for the optimal execution of IONM have been described, including standard procedures for placement and testing, the appropriate use of muscle relaxants, monitoring, and efforts to decrease false

Medical Management of the Surgical Patient, ed. Michael F. Lubin, Thomas F. Dodson, and Neil H. Winawer. Published by Cambridge University Press. © Cambridge University Press 2013.

negatives. However, the efficacy of IONM in decreasing recurrent laryngeal nerve injury has not been established.

Ultrasound of the thyroid and neck is recommended prior to surgery. This should ideally be done by a skilled technologist and radiologist who are accustomed to evaluating thyroid cancer and its related lymph nodes metastases. Ultrasonographic features such as a presence of microcalcifications or an absence of the fatty hilum are more common among lymph nodes that are positive for thyroid cancer. The sensitivity and specificity for predicting central compartment disease were reported as 30% and 86.8%, respectively; for the lateral neck, sensitivity and specificity were 93.8% and 80.0%.

Traditional surgical resection is an open thyroidectomy. Most commonly a transverse incision is made, measuring 3–6 cm over the thyroid gland. Once the superior and inferior skin flaps are elevated, dissection of the superior thyroid pedicle begins, taking care to preserve the superior laryngeal nerve which runs medial to the pedicle. The superior parathyroid gland should also be preserved. Next, the lateral aspect of the gland is carefully dissected, and the gland reflected medially to identify the recurrent laryngeal nerve prior to clamping and ligating the inferior thyroid artery. The recurrent laryngeal nerve runs most often just medial and inferior to the inferior thyroid artery. On the right, the recurrent laryngeal nerve travels in a more oblique path in the neck. In contrast, the left recurrent laryngeal nerve travels in a more vertical fashion in the neck. Once the nerve is identified and protected, the inferior thyroid vein and inferior thyroid artery are then identified, clamped, and ligated. The artery is ligated as close to the thyroid gland as possible to preserve the vascular structure to the inferior parathyroid gland.

Another option is to remove the parathyroid gland and to reimplant it in the sternocleidomastoid muscle. Some surgeons prefer this approach, especially if there is a risk of a re-operation in the central compartment. The gland is then carefully dissected off the anterior wall of the trachea. The surgeon takes great care in removing thyroid tissue so that little native thyroid tissue remains. Any residual thyroid tissue that remains may adversely impact the patient's ability to respond to radioiodine ablation. The procedure is then duplicated on the contralateral side and the thyroid gland is then removed.

Central compartment neck dissection (CCND) is performed by dissecting the recurrent laryngeal nerve and removing all soft tissue medial to the nerve and overlying the trachea. The superior limit of dissection should be the hyoid bone and the inferior extent should be several tracheal rings below the cricoid cartilage.

Lateral compartment neck dissection is performed by first skeletonizing the sternocleidomastoid muscle. Dissection is then carried down to identify the spinal accessory nerve. The spinal accessory nerve is then dissected superior to its intersection with the internal jugular vein. The superficial layer of the deep cervical fascia is then incised, taking care to preserve the cervical rootlets. Dissection is then carried medially to the internal jugular vein. Inferiorly, the surgeon should include fascia and lymphatics inferior to the omohyoid muscle. If dissection is extensive in the left inferior neck, he/she should ensure that the thoracic duct is adequately ligated to avert formation of a chyle leak. Usually, an induced Valsalva maneuver of 20 cm H_2O can be performed by anesthesia to ensure adequate ligation of the duct. Another option is to infuse cream through the orogastric tube and observe whether or not chyle leaks from the thoracic duct. A drain is commonly used prior to closure.

Newer modalities of thyroid surgery include endoscopic approaches and trans-axillary robotic approaches. The benefits of these procedures are a smaller neck incision (endoscopic) or no cervical incision (robotic). However, these two techniques are not as feasible for large thyroid masses or if a total thyroidectomy is attempted.

Usual postoperative course

Thyroid hormone replacement is begun on postoperative day 1. Endocrinologists are a vital part of the team in the postoperative period.

Postoperative complications

Postoperative complications can include bleeding, seroma, chyle leak, hypocalcemia, and recurrent laryngeal nerve injury.

Hematoma and seroma

A hematoma can form when the patient is emerging from anesthesia. This can be a fatal complication if not acted upon promptly. The most effective treatment for a neck hematoma is to evacuate the hematoma, ideally in the operating room. However, if this is not feasible, the incision can be opened at the bedside prior to going to the operating room. A hematoma can compress the airway and cause death; therefore, recognizing and treating a neck hematoma is of utmost importance.

A seroma is a collection of serosanguinous fluid from the operative site. A drain that is placed at the time of surgery most often controls this complication.

Chyle leaks

Chyle leaks are not common after thyroid surgery; however, if a left neck dissection is performed in addition, then one must be able to recognize a chyle leak. The drain fluid will turn milky white once the patient resumes a normal diet. Management of chyle leaks is usually conservative with a low-fat diet. Only on rare occasions is ligation of the thoracic duct necessary to control the chyle leak. Replacement of electrolytes and fluids is the mainstay of chyle leak management.

Hypocalcemia

Hypocalcemia can occur when a total thyroidectomy is performed. Oftentimes, it is the result of devascularization of the parathyroid glands. Calcium replacement as well as Rocaltrol administration is often used to prevent any adverse effects, such as tetany, due to hypocalcemia. Early symptoms of hypocalcemia include perioral numbness and tingling.

Recurrent laryngeal nerve injury

A unilateral recurrent laryngeal nerve injury can result in dysphonia or hoarseness. Watchful waiting is recommended for the first 6 months. If after 6 months, the unilateral vocal cord palsy is present, a thyroplasty can be considered to medialize the vocal cord and improve voice quality. Bilateral recurrent laryngeal nerve injury can result in complete airway obstruction. A tracheotomy is usually necessary to manage this complication. An arytenoidectomy can be performed later in order to allow the patient to be decannulated.

Conclusion

Thyroid malignancies are increasing in frequency in the USA. One possible explanation is an increase in the use of diagnostic imaging. Surgery remains the mainstay of treatment of thyroid cancer. Treating the cervical lymphatics is also an important and vital aspect of thyroid cancer treatment. In addition to traditional open surgery, minimally invasive surgery such as endoscopic thyroidectomy and robotic-assisted thyroidectomy is being increasingly explored. Risks of surgery include hematoma, recurrent laryngeal nerve injury, and hypocalcemia. High-volume surgeons appear to have lower odds of these complications.

Further reading

Cibas ES, Ali SZ. The Bethesda system for reporting thyroid cytopathology. *Am J Clin Pathol* 2009; **132**: 658–65.

Cooper DS, Doherty GM, Haugen BR *et al.* Revised American Thyroid Association management guidelines for patients with thyroid nodules and differentiated thyroid cancer. *Thyroid* 2009; **19**: 1167–214.

Franco AT, Malaguarnera R, Refetoff S *et al.* Thyrotrophin receptor signaling dependence of Braf-induced thyroid tumor initiation in mice. *Proc Natl Acad Sci USA* 2011; **108**: 1615–20.

Gourin CG, Tufano RP, Forastiere AA *et al.* Volume-based trends in thyroid surgery. *Arch Otolaryngol Head Neck Surg* 2010; **136**: 1191–8.

Hwang HS, Orloff LA. Efficacy of preoperative neck ultrasound in the detection of cervical lymph node metastasis from thyroid cancer. *Laryngoscope* 2011; **121**: 487–91.

Randolph GW, Dralle H, Abdullah H *et al.* Electrophysiologic recurrent laryngeal nerve monitoring during thyroid and parathyroid surgery: international standards guideline statement. *Laryngoscope* 2011; **121** (Suppl 1): S1–16.

Seybt MW, Terris DJ. Minimally invasive thyroid and parathyroid surgery: where are we now and where are we going? *Otolaryngol Clin North Am* 2010; **43**: 375–80, ix.

Shen WT, Ogawa L, Ruan D *et al.* Central neck lymph node dissection for papillary thyroid cancer: comparison of complication and recurrence rates in 295 initial dissections and reoperations. *Arch Surg* 2010; **145**: 272–5.

Shindo M, Stern A. Total thyroidectomy with and without selective central compartment dissection: a comparison of complication rates. *Arch Otolaryngol Head Neck Surg* 2010; **136**: 584–7.

Terris DJ, Stack BC Jr. Current technology in thyroid surgery. *J Otorhinolaryngol Relat Spec* 2008; **70**: 305–12.

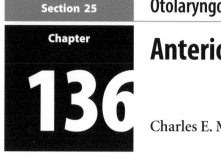

136

Anterior cranial base surgery

Charles E. Moore

Anterior cranial base surgery has been greatly enhanced with new advances in diagnostic and surgical techniques. These new advances incorporate a comprehensive, multidisciplinary approach to the removal of anterior skull-base lesions. Approaching the anterior cranial base from anterior and below has gained increasing popularity. The principal advantage is the minimal amount of frontal lobe retraction. In addition, this approach eliminates the need for facial incisions and therefore eliminates facial scarring. It also allows for the preservation of smell, depending on the location of the lesion, in contradistinction to more traditional techniques that often ensure anosmia. With the advent of improved endoscopic equipment and surgical techniques, endoscopic approaches have gained increased popularity in certain surgical cases as a different approach when compared with open surgical techniques.

Imaging plays an important role in the surgical and reconstructive planning of craniofacial tumors. It allows for assessment of the extent of the disease process and determination of the operability of the lesion. If the lesion is operable, the extent of the disease will also determine whether the surgical procedure is best done through an endoscopic or open approach. This chapter will focus on the open approach. The imaging modalities commonly employed include axial and coronal two-dimensional, three-dimensional, and interactive three-dimensional CT imaging, MR imaging, and angiography.

The use of the subcranial approach, an open approach, in anterior cranial base surgery allows intracranial access extending along the posterior planum sphenoidal, anterior clinoid, and tuberculum sellae. The lateral aspect of the exposure is determined by the type and extent of craniotomy that is performed. Extra-cranial exposure extends to the foramen magnum. After tumor extirpation, closure is routinely accomplished with a pericranial flap. A tracheotomy is rarely necessary if nasal trumpets are placed to divert air away from the skullbase closure.

All anterior cranial base procedures are performed under general anesthesia. The operative time may range from 3–10 hours depending on the extent of the disease process. Blood transfusion may be required depending on the tumor pathology. The approach to the brain is sterile via a craniotomy; the subcranial approach from below is semi-sterile since the sinuses are exposed.

Usual postoperative course

Expected postoperative hospital stay

The expected overall hospital stay is 5 days. The overall hospital stay is determined primarily by the neurological status, and the ability to tolerate removal of a cerebrospinal fluid (CSF) monitoring device.

Operative mortality

Operative mortality is 1% or less.

Special monitoring required

A lumbar drain or ventriculostomy is routinely placed intra-operatively to monitor and adjust CSF pressure.

Patient activity and positioning

Each patient is observed initially in an ICU setting. The neurological status is closely monitored. The patient may remain intubated for 24 hours. This may be extended based upon the neurological status. A lumbar drain or ventriculostomy, along with nasal trumpets, are in place for approximately 5 days.

Alimentation

Patients are not allowed to have any oral intake if they have ventilatory support. Otherwise, a liquid diet is initiated and progressed to a regular diet as the patient is able to tolerate the oral intake.

Medical Management of the Surgical Patient, ed. Michael F. Lubin, Thomas F. Dodson, and Neil H. Winawer. Published by Cambridge University Press. © Cambridge University Press 2013.

Antibiotic coverage

Antibiotics are administered intraoperatively and continued until the lumbar drain or ventriculostomy is removed. The antibiotic chosen should have good central nervous system penetration.

Humidity

Irrigation of the nasal trumpets is performed while they are in place in order to prevent their occlusion.

Analgesia

Pain is routinely controlled with morphine or meperidine. Patients are introduced to an oral pain medication such as Tylenol with codeine prior to their discharge in order to provide pain relief.

Postoperative complications

In the hospital

Excessive pneumocephalus

A certain degree of pneumocephalus is expected as a result of performing a craniotomy. If a continued air leak occurs through the surgical closure, this may lead to obtundation or herniation. The lumbar drain or ventriculostomy in conjunction with the nasal trumpets will usually provide adequate time for the surgical closure to seal. In rare cases, the closure does not seal and a tracheostomy should be performed to divert air from traversing the surgical closure.

Cerebrospinal fluid leak

The chance for a CSF leak increases in direct proportion to the increase in size of the defect and therefore the size of the reconstructed surgical site. Uncommonly, a lumbar drain or ventriculostomy is inadequate to prevent a CSF leak in the standard period of time. In most cases, continued use of one of these devices will eventually result in resolution of the leak in the immediate postoperative period.

Cerebral edema

Surgical manipulation of the brain or as a characteristic of the tumor itself may lead to swelling of the brain. This can be monitored by imaging studies and managed by hyperventilation, steroids, mannitol, and furosemide.

Seizures

Tumors that involve the cortex or surgical manipulation of the cortex can lead to seizures. Anticonvulsants are given routinely in an effort to avoid seizure development. The duration of the anticonvulsant therapy is often dependent on the location and pathology of the mass.

Low-pressure headache

A protracted headache may occur from the loss or removal of CSF. Most cases will resolve as the CSF pressure equilibrates. A blood patch may prove helpful in low-pressure headaches that are prolonged.

After discharge

Delayed cerebrospinal fluid leak

A CSF leak after discharge may present as CSF rhinorrhea. In the later postoperative period, elevation of the head of the bed and CSF drainage, either by spinal taps or by a continuous device, often will treat the problem. If leakage is persistent, an additional surgical procedure is needed to repair the leak.

Crusting

Severe nasal cavity crusting is common, resulting in nasal obstruction and potential superimposed bacterial infection. This can be avoided when the patient strictly adheres to a nasal irrigation regimen.

Diplopia

Diplopia is a transient complication from mobilization of the orbital contents, in particular the trochlea. In severe cases, an eye patch may be used intermittently until the diplopia resolves.

Further reading

Browne JD, Mims JW. Preservation of olfaction in anterior skull base surgery. *Laryngoscope* 2000; **110**: 1317–22.

Darrouzet V. Subcranial approach to tumors of the anterior cranial base. *Otolaryngol Head Neck Surg* 2000; **122**: 466–7.

Fliss DM, Zucker G, Cohen A *et al.* Early outcome and complications of the extended subcranial approach to the anterior skull base. *Laryngoscope* 1999; **109**: 153–60.

Moore CE, Marentette L. Subcranial approach to tumors of the anterior cranial base. *Otolaryngol Head Neck Surg* 2000; **122**: 466–7.

Moore CE, Olson JJ. *Skull Base Surgery: Basic Techniques*. San Diego, CA: Plural Publishing; 2010.

Moore CE, Ross DA, Marentette LJ. Subcranial approach to tumors of the anterior cranial base: analysis of current and traditional surgical techniques. *Otolaryngol Head Neck Surg* 1999; **120**: 387–90.

Pinsolle J. Subcranial approach. *Arch Otolaryngol Head Neck Surg* 1994; **120**: 676–7.

Raveh J, Turk JB, Ladrach K *et al.* Extended anterior subcranial approach for skull base tumors: long-term results. *J Neurosurg* 1995; **82**: 1002–10.

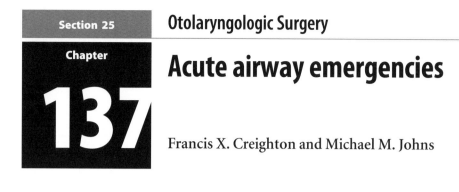

Chapter

137

Acute airway emergencies

Francis X. Creighton and Michael M. Johns

Acute airway distress is a medical emergency that requires immediate treatment to limit morbidity and mortality. Airway distress arises from any process in the larynx, trachea, or bronchi that obstructs pulmonary ventilation. A wide variety of pathologic processes can result in airway distress. Management of patients experiencing acute airway distress depends greatly on the severity of distress as well as the specific etiology, but restoring adequate ventilation to the pulmonary system is the goal of all treatments. Oxygen administration, intubation, cricothyrotomy, and tracheotomy are all treatment options for patients in acute airway distress.

Differential diagnosis

Since the treatment of acute airway distress can depend greatly on the etiology of the problem, it is important to know the clinical presentation of different causes of airway distress. Interpreting both patients' presenting signs and symptoms in conjunction with physical examination, laryngoscopy when appropriate, and ancillary testing is essential to determine the etiology of obstruction and proper management. Causes of acute airway obstruction include infections, immunologic reactions, trauma, and foreign body obstruction.

Infection
Epiglottitis/supraglottitis

Supraglottitis and epiglottitis are often used interchangeably, both indicating inflammation of the glottis and surrounding structures. Epiglottitis typically refers to a pediatric patient while supraglottitis refers to an adult. For epiglottitis the classic signs and symptoms are a child with stridor, drooling, and muffled voice. Many patients will lean forward when sitting to aid in breathing. A left shifted and elevated white blood cell count is also often present. The causative agent is classically *Haemophilus influenzae* type B (Hib), but with widespread vaccination the percentage of cases caused by streptococcal infection is increasing. Supraglottitis in adults

follows a different course and its classical presenting symptoms are fever, sore throat with odynophagia and anterior neck tenderness. An elevated white blood cell count is also common. While Hib is the most common etiologic agent in epiglottitis, no definitive etiologic agent is identified in a majority of cases. The thumb print sign (thickening of the glottis on lateral radiography) can be seen in both supraglottitis and epiglottitis but is not required for diagnosis. Definitive diagnosis for both diseases is made by direct visualization of swelling of the glottis by flexible laryngoscopy.

Pediatric patients with epiglottitis and signs of airway obstruction should be brought to the operating room by the surgeon and anesthesiologist for immediate laryngoscopy, bronchoscopy, and intubation by an experienced airway specialist. Medical treatment follows with antibiotic coverage of Hib and streptococcus. If intubation is unsuccessful or unattainable due to swelling or anatomically difficult airway, surgical tracheotomy should be performed. Cricothyroidotomy should not be attempted in a patient under the age of 12. Throughout this process, all efforts should be made to not disturb the patient and to make the patient comfortable, because crying or anxiety can worsen the airway distress.

Adult supraglottitis less often leads to complete airway obstruction. Patients with obvious signs of severe distress such as stridor, dyspnea, or cyanosis should immediately be intubated or scheduled for tracheotomy, but proper airway management of milder cases may consist of ICU monitoring, corticosteroids, and antibiotics.

Ludwig's angina

Ludwig's angina is a rapidly progressing cellulitis of the sublingual and submandibular spaces that often causes elevation and protrusion of the tongue and edema of the anterior neck that can cause airway obstruction. Ludwig's angina commonly arises from dental infections and the typical etiologic agents are staphylococcus, streptococcus, and bacteroides. Classic presenting signs and symptoms include prominent and painful neck swelling, dysphagia, dysphonia, odynophagia, and a woody, edematous sublingual region.

Medical Management of the Surgical Patient, ed. Michael F. Lubin, Thomas F. Dodson, and Neil H. Winawer. Published by Cambridge University Press. © Cambridge University Press 2013.

Treatment involves prompt antibiotic therapy, classically ampicillin/sublactam and metronidazole. Airway management is imperative and patients with signs of respiratory distress should be intubated and scheduled for surgical access of the airway. Cricothyrotomy is the intervention of choice in acute airway collapse. If the patient's respiratory status allows, surgical tracheotomy is preferred rather than cricothyrotomy because of its associated complications.

Immunologic reactions

Immunologic causes of acute airway distress result from angioedema. When angioedema causes swelling of the structures surrounding the airway it often leads to acute airway distress. Patients classically present with localized, non-pitting, painless edema of the face and neck. The three main types of angioedema are allergic, hereditary, and drug-induced.

Allergic angioedema

Allergic angioedema is in response to a specific allergen such as foods, contrast media and Hymenoptera stings. Allergic angioedema is often accompanied by superficial skin changes such as urticaria.

Hereditary angioedema

Hereditary angioedema has multiple subtypes but is classically due to a deficiency or defect in C1 esterase, an enzyme that inhibits the complement system and, subsequently, the release of vasoactive substances such as bradykinin. The Type I subset involves mutations that result in decreased production of C1 esterase, while the Type II variant involves production of defective C1 esterase. Diagnosis can be confirmed by measuring serum levels of C1 esterase blood levels.

Drug-induced angioedema

Finally, drug-induced angioedema is a type IV sensitivity reaction. Drug-induced angioedema is most often associated with ACE-inhibitors. ACE-inhibitors block the ability of angiotensin-converting enzymes to degrade bradykinin, leading to angioedema. This reaction is more common in African American patients.

Obtaining a pertinent history if possible is important to determine the etiology and allow for removal of any offending agents. Patients with suspected angioedema should be treated with epinephrine 0.1–0.5 mg subcutaneously or intramuscularly. This can be repeated every 5–10 minutes to avoid airway compromise. Antihistamines and steroids should also be administered. This treatment regimen has greatest efficacy in allergic and drug-induced angioedema but is minimally effective in hereditary angioedema. In emergent situations it is rarely possible to immediately discriminate between these different etiologies. Therefore treatment with epinephrine, steroids, and antihistamines should be initiated for all patients presenting with angioedema and signs of airway distress.

Patients with known history of hereditary angioedema can be treated with synthetic or blood-derived C1 esterase, also known as C1-INH, if available; otherwise fresh frozen plasma can be used as a substitute treatment.

Trauma

Laryngeal trauma is a relatively rare presentation that can result in acute airway distress. It can result from both penetrating and blunt injuries. Penetrating trauma is typically from stab or gunshot wounds, while blunt trauma is often caused by steering wheels in motor vehicle accidents. Patients can present with a wide variety of symptoms but dysphonia, hemoptysis, odynophagia, and loss of normal anatomical landmarks are common. Stridor is also a classic symptom and can provide information as to the location of the trauma. Inspiratory stridor is seen in extrathoracic trauma, while expiratory stridor is seen in intrathoracic injury. Continuous stridor often is indicative of injury at the level of the glottis or subglottis. It is important to note that many patients with laryngeal trauma will be asymptomatic. CT scan and direct visualization of the airway with laryngoscopy are the best methods for diagnosis of laryngeal trauma. Patients presenting with acute airway distress following laryngeal trauma should, if possible, undergo tracheotomy or cricothyrotomy at the bedside or in OR because intubation risks further damage to the airway. To decrease the chances of long-term deficits in phonation and airway patency, it is important to have a high degree of clinical suspicion and to avoid delay of treatment in cases of laryngeal trauma. Significant laryngeal injury with mucosal disruption and cartilage exposure requires open surgical repair within 48 hours.

Foreign body obstruction

Commonly referred to as choking, partial or complete airway obstruction caused by aerodigestive foreign bodies is a medical emergency. Emergent obstruction typically occurs with foreign bodies lodged in the larynx or trachea, while those lodged in the bronchi or esophagus follow a more sub-acute course. Pediatric patients, especially those 1- to 3-years old, are at greatest risk. Pediatric patients are at risk secondary to their lack of molars, immature closure of the glottis, and propensity to place objects in their mouth. Greater public awareness of the hazards of choking has decreased the mortality of this condition, but despite these efforts approximately 150 children per year die secondary to asphyxiation. The most important factor in decreasing mortality and morbidity associated with choking is to rapidly recognize the patient with airway obstruction. The signs and symptoms of foreign body obstruction often mimic those of other airway disorders, which delays diagnosis. To ensure prompt diagnosis, a high level of suspicion for foreign body ingestion should be maintained in any patient presenting with respiratory distress. For patients presenting with complete obstruction the most common presenting sign is the patient performing the internationally recognized sign for choking by placing both hands around their neck. Breathlessness is also seen, but gagging, wheezing, and coughing are not present in complete obstruction. For patients with partial obstruction, initial symptoms are often acute onset choking, gagging and cough. These signs will often subside once the object has become lodged and these reflexes diminish. Further symptoms and signs depend on the location of the obstruction.

Laryngeal partial obstruction is typically associated with hoarseness and stridor. These symptoms often mimic those of croup in the pediatric patient; therefore in patients with suspected croup, it is important to consider the potential presence of foreign bodies. Tracheal obstruction presents similarly to laryngeal obstruction, but without hoarseness. Furthermore a palpable thud as well as an audible slap can often be heard as the object comes into contact with the trachea. Both laryngeal and tracheal foreign bodies resulting in initial partial obstruction can result in edema, ultimately leading to complete obstruction. Obstruction in the bronchi, which is the most common location of foreign body obstruction, often results in coughing and wheezing heard on chest auscultation and unilateral decreased breath sounds.

Initial treatment depends on whether partial or complete obstruction is present. For complete obstruction, the Heimlich maneuver should be initiated in an attempt to dislodge the obstruction in a conscious adult patient. For unconscious patients and children over the age of 1 year, abdominal thrusts with the patient in the supine position should be used. In infants, back thrusts or chest compressions can be used. If efforts to dislodge the obstruction are unsuccessful, immediate access to the airway should be obtained via surgical cricothyrotomy. In children, and when an individual trained in surgical cricothyrotomy is not available, percutaneous cricothyrotomy is the treatment of choice. Partial obstruction should be treated conservatively and laryngoscopy should be used to try to visualize and remove the foreign body. Unlike treatment for patients with complete obstruction, the Heimlich maneuver and other efforts to dislodge the obstruction should not be initiated because they have the potential to convert the partial obstruction to a complete obstruction.

Surgical management

Surgical treatment options for acute airway distress aim to restore ventilation and maintain adequate blood oxygen levels. Initial treatment for any patient in respiratory distress with decreasing oxygen saturation is oxygen administration. Oxygen administration through a nasal cannula or non-rebreather should be attempted and heliox, if available, can also be used as an adjuvant therapy. Heliox is a mixture of oxygen and helium which generates less airway resistance than normal air, thereby reducing the patient's overall work of breathing. If oxygen administration fails to revert decreasing oxygen saturation, bag mask ventilation should be initiated.

Worsening respiratory status indicates that intubation should be attempted. Although subacute airway compromise can be managed with fiberoptic intubation, it should generally be avoided in trauma or neoplastic obstruction. Awake tracheotomy or cricothyrotomy is the preferred approach to airway management.

If intubation cannot be obtained secondary to edema or difficult airway, or if an intubated patient is expected to have prolonged or progressive obstruction, invasive measures to access the airway are indicated. Options to access the airway include tracheotomy and cricothyrotomy. Tracheotomy is performed to establish an airway in patients with existing or impending airway obstruction. In an emergency situation, mask ventilation or endotracheal intubation is done to gain control of the airway, followed by tracheotomy under more controlled circumstances. For patients who cannot be ventilated or intubated, cricothyrotomy is preferable since tracheotomy is a difficult emergency procedure.

Tracheotomy

Tracheotomy is typically performed in the operating room after an airway has been secured by intubation, but can be performed at the bedside with local anesthesia. A horizontal incision is made typically two fingerbreadths above the sternal notch. Dissection is performed down through the subcutaneous tissue until the trachea is exposed. Any overlying veins are ligated and tied off, and the thyroid isthmus, if encountered, is divided or reflected. Stay sutures are placed in the second or third tracheal ring. A vertical incision is then made through the trachea. A tracheal dilator expands the incision and finally a tracheostomy tube is placed in the airway and secured. Usually, fiberoptic bronchoscopy is performed simultaneously through the existing endotracheal tube to ensure proper placement of the dilators and the tube. Regardless of the technique, the end result should be the same: a dependable, stable airway in the lower neck. Tracheotomy in children should always be performed in the operating room, where anesthesia, monitoring, adequate light, suction, and assistance are available. Following the placement of a tracheotomy, adequate measures must be taken to ensure that accidental displacement doesn't occur. Until a tract has formed, a displaced tracheotomy tube can be difficult and dangerous to replace.

Cricothyrotomy

Cricothyrotomy, performed through the cricothyroid membrane located between the larynx and the cricoid cartilage, involves a higher anatomic level than that of tracheotomy. The highly vascular thyroid gland is avoided and airway access can be established in seconds, making cricothyrotomy a more favorable emergent procedure than tracheotomy. Following emergency cricothyrotomy, tracheotomy is then done to reposition the tube in a more suitable location in the trachea so that injury to the cricoid cartilage can be avoided and subglottic stenosis will not develop.

There are two techniques to perform a cricothyrotomy: one surgical and one percutaneous. For a surgical cricothyrotomy, the cricothyroid membrane is palpated inferior to the laryngeal prominence and superior to the cricoid cartilage. A vertical incision is made through the skin and subcutaneous tissue. A horizontal incision is then made through the cricothyroid membrane. An endotracheal or tracheotomy tube is then inserted and secured. Surgical cricothyrotomy should not be performed in children under the age of 12. For percutaneous cricothyrotomy a 12- or 14-gauge-needled catheter attached to a syringe is inserted through the skin overlying the cricothyroid membrane. The needle is advanced while pulling back on the syringe until air is aspirated, confirming positioning in the trachea. The catheter is then advanced off of the needle and a wire can be threaded through the catheter to guide an endotracheal tube or dilator into the trachea. Increasingly larger dilators can be passed over the wire until a tracheotomy tube can be placed.

In most cases patients are initially fitted with a cuffed tracheotomy tube. The balloon cuff helps to keep blood out of the trachea and can usually be deflated 24 hours after the procedure unless the patient is being mechanically ventilated. Traction sutures should be placed in the trachea, and the tracheotomy tube should be sewn to the skin of the patient. In addition, a security strap should be placed around the patient's neck. The retaining sutures are usually removed 3–5 days after the procedure.

Postoperative course
Expected postoperative hospital stay
Usually depends on the underlying reason for the acute airway distress.

Operative mortality
The operative mortality rate for tracheotomy is < 1% for elective procedures and 10–50% for emergency procedures.

Special monitoring required
Patients with acute airway distress who are not treated surgically should be closely monitored for worsening airway distress by assessing work of breathing, blood gases through a radial artery A-line, or by using pulse oximetry. A low threshold should exist to proceed with surgical access of the airway.

If possible, all patients with a new tracheotomy should be monitored closely in the ICU for bleeding from the tracheotomy site and for security of the tube to avoid displacement from the trachea. Tracheal suctioning should be performed as needed and continuous pulse oximetry is required. A chest radiograph is not routine except in children, but should be considered for patients whose hemoglobin–oxygen saturations are low.

Patient activity and positioning
Activity and positioning depend greatly upon the etiology of airway distress.

Patients who require surgical access of the airway should have their head elevated, and a high-humidity collar is essential for the first few days. Ambulation is dependent on the patient's overall status and on the underlying condition responsible for the tracheotomy. If the patient is being ventilated, the cuff pressure should be kept just above the pressure at which air leak occurs during inspiration. Mucosal capillary perfusion pressure is approximately 25 cm H_2O; cuff pressures above this level can potentially damage the tracheal mucosa. If the cuff or the cuff valve begins leaking, the tube will need replacing. Otherwise, there is no need to automatically change a tracheotomy tube when it is functioning properly.

If a patient is alert and does not require mechanical ventilation, the original cuffed tracheotomy tube can often be changed to a non-cuffed tube on the third day (after a tract has formed around it). Following placement, the patient may be able to phonate by occluding the tube. In some cases, the tube can be fitted with a one-way valve that allows the patient to speak without digital occlusion.

When a tracheotomy is no longer needed, it can be removed and the tract is allowed to close. While most tracts close spontaneously, there are cases in which a persistent tracheocutaneous fistula requires surgical closure.

Alimentation
Alimentation depends on the etiology of airway distress.

For patients requiring surgical access of the airway, oral intake may be resumed after operation if the oral cavity and gastrointestinal tract are normal and if the patient's mental status permits. However, due to tethering of the trachea by the tube, the larynx fails to rise normally during swallowing and aspiration is common. Similarly, if gastroesophageal reflux above the upper esophageal sphincter occurs, the patient may aspirate even if oral intake is not allowed.

Antibiotic coverage
Antibiotic coverage depends on the etiology of airway distress.

A patient with infectious causes of airway distress should have antibiotics covering the common microorganisms responsible for his or her condition. Patients with epi/supraglottitis should be covered with antibiotics directed toward *Haemophilus* and *Streptococcus* species. Patients with Ludwig's angina should be covered for *Staphylococcus*, *Streptococcus*, and *Bacteroides* species.

For patients undergoing tracheotomy in the operating room, perioperative antibiotics should be given using a first-generation cephalosporin or, if the patient is penicillin allergic, clindamycin.

Postoperative complications of tracheotomy

In the hospital

Displacement of the tube

Coughing is often vigorous during the first few hours and can displace the tube unless it is well secured.

Bleeding

The most common site is from the thyroid gland and can usually be controlled with surgical gauze or oxidized cellulose packed around the tube.

Infection

Wound infection is uncommon, but aspiration may cause tracheal secretions to increase and to become more purulent.

Obstruction

Thick, tenacious secretions can be difficult to clear. Irrigation with 3–5 mL of sterile saline solution, and use of humidified air or oxygen delivered by tracheotomy collar are helpful. Suctioning should be performed as needed.

Pulmonary edema

Acute relief of airway obstruction can cause post-obstructive pulmonary edema, which is recognized by frothy abundant secretions and hemoglobin-oxygen desaturation. Positive pressure ventilation is often necessary and diuretics may be helpful.

Pneumothorax

Pneumothorax occurs in 25% of infant tracheotomies because of the high reflection of the pleura into the root of the neck. Chest auscultation and postoperative chest radiographs should identify the condition.

Cervical or mediastinal emphysema

Pneumothorax should be considered. No treatment is necessary unless pneumothorax is present.

After discharge

For successful care at home, patient education in care and maintenance of the tracheotomy is crucial. Patients should be instructed on cleaning the tube and the tracheotomy site, as well as what to do if the tube becomes obstructed or displaced. Home health services can provide home nursing or respiratory therapy care, which allows continued reinforcement of tracheotomy care principles while also relieving much patient anxiety.

A home humidifier can help keep secretions moist. A suction machine can also be useful, but requires additional patient and caregiver instruction. Deep suctioning of the trachea is uncomfortable and unnecessary if the patient has a good cough.

If the conditions responsible for tracheotomy are no longer present or the patient has improved, the tracheotomy can be removed. Decannulation should be performed only after careful consideration of the patient's pulmonary mechanics and airway patency.

Further reading

Al-Qudah M, Shetty S, Alomari M, Alqdah M. Acute adult supraglottitis: current management and treatment. *South Med J* 2010; **103**(8): 800–4.

Hwang SY, Yeak SC. Management dilemmas in laryngeal trauma. *J Laryngol Otol* 2004; **118**(5): 325–8.

Rosbe Kristina W. Foreign bodies. In Lalwani AK, ed. *Current Diagnosis & Treatment in Otolaryngology – Head & Neck Surgery*. 2nd edn. New York, NY: McGraw-Hill Medical; 2007.

Shockley WW. Ludwig angina: a review of current airway management.

Arch Otolaryngol Head Neck Surg 1999; **125**(5): 600.

Temiño VM, Peebles RS Jr. The spectrum and treatment of angioedema. *Am J Med* 2008; **121**(4): 282–6.

Management of upper urinary tract calculi

John G. Pattaras

The term "Endourology" has been adopted for the minimally invasive endoscopic surgery of upper urinary calculus disease. Since the introduction of shock wave lithotripsy, this modality has become the most common form of stone therapy, allowing an almost completely hands-off treatment for radio-opaque calculi. Due to the technological advances of endourologic procedures such as ureteroscopy and percutaneous nephrolithotomy (PCNL), the incidence of open kidney stone surgery is almost non-existent. Due to the popularity of the daVinci robot (Intuitive, CA), traditional open calculus surgeries are being performed robotically for stones that would otherwise require several endoscopic procedures. It is important to note that as advanced as surgical intervention has evolved for nephrolithiasis, medical management and prevention of complicated urolithiasis still fall short of the ideal.

Nephrolithiasis affects as much as 12% of the population in industrialized nations. Urolithiasis patients will agree that the sensation of stone passage is perhaps the most painful and intense experience of their lives, surpassing even childbirth. Urolithiasis may present as hematuria (ranging from asymptomatic microscopic hematuria to painful gross hematuria), abdominal/flank/back pain, urinary tract infection, renal failure, or as an incidental radiologic finding.

Decompression of the acutely obstructed system with either cystoscopic stenting or percutaneous nephrostomy drainage is emergently mandatory for patients with a solitary kidney, infected obstruction, immunocompromised state (e.g., diabetes, AIDS, transplant), history of renal insufficiency, and worsening renal function.

Work-up of the potential nephrolithiasis patient should include at a minimum the following: general history, prior history of personal/family nephrolithiasis, physical examination, urine analysis (and culture for any hematuria, pyuria, fevers, or elevated WBC count) and radiologic examination if clinically warranted. The "gold standard" of radiologic examination for stone disease is a non-contrast helical computerized tomography (CT) scan of the abdomen/pelvis rather than the traditional intravenous urogram (IVU). The distinct advantages of the CT over the IVU are the ability to visualize other abdominal pathology and the absence of intravenous contrast. Unfortunately, the indiscriminate use of CT imaging has led to concern about excessive radiation exposure. A combination of ultrasonography and plain X-ray abdominal/pelvic imaging, however, can be beneficial when following the known stone patient.

Open surgical management of renal and ureteral calculi still has a place in modern-day urology, but it is limited to less than 1% of stone therapy. Our experience with robotic stone surgery has been limited but successful in relatively complicated cases, including patients with coagulopathy. American Urological Association practice guidelines were established for ureteral and staghorn renal calculi and should be referred to for procedural options, with the important variables being stone size, location, and clinical status.

Shock wave lithotripsy (SWL) is the most common treatment for renal calculi. This non-invasive management relies on focused sound energy to fragment calculi. Absolute contraindications to SWL include pregnancy, active complicated urinary tract infection, uncontrollable hypertension, and irreversible coagulopathy. Ureteroscopy can be performed using semi-rigid scopes for lower ureteral calculi (below iliac vessels). For upper ureteral or renal stones, flexible ureteroscopes as small as 7F ($\sim$2.5 mm) can be introduced for basket extraction or laser lithotripsy. Ureteroscopy is more invasive than SWL, but the direct visual lithotripsy has a higher success rate. Ureteroscopy is indicated for almost any calculus under 1.5 cm, calculi which have failed SWL or high-risk patients (coagulopathy, arrhythmias, pregnancy).

Percutaneous nephrolithotomy is indicated for stone burden greater than 1.5–2 cm, lower pole stones that have failed SWL, and infectious or staghorn calculi. Percutaneous nephrolithotomy involves placing a percutaneous nephrostomy tract(s), dilating the tract (24–30F), and using a rigid or flexible scope for lithotripsy. Second-look procedures are performed through an established tract when excessive stone burden or complicated staghorn calculi cannot be managed in a single setting. Laparoscopic ureterolithotomy or pyelolithotomy have been described, but these procedures are more

Medical Management of the Surgical Patient, ed. Michael F. Lubin, Thomas F. Dodson, and Neil H. Winawer. Published by Cambridge University Press. © Cambridge University Press 2013.

invasive than endoscopy and are therefore performed less frequently. Ultrasonography or non-contrast CT in a patient with suspected complications generally can delineate the problem. Interventional or surgical correction of the obstruction – especially in medically frail or infected patients – should be accomplished in a timely fashion.

Usual postoperative course
Expected postoperative hospital stay

Ureteroscopy and shock wave lithotripsy are routinely performed as outpatient procedures. Medical comorbidities including sleep apnea, morbid obesity, bacteremia or chronic infections can require admission for observation or postoperative care. Percutaneous nephrolithotomy and robotic/laparoscopic procedures usually require 2–4 days of hospitalization.

Operative mortality

The overall operative mortality for stone procedures is 0.01–1% for more invasive procedures such as percutaneous nephrolithotomy. The operative mortality for ureteroscopy is less than 1% and, in the author's experience, this outcome usually involves a high-risk patient.

Special monitoring required

General anesthesia monitoring for ureteroscopy, robotic/laparoscopic and percutaneous nephrolithotomy is standard. Shock-wave lithotripsy can be performed under intravenous sedation, but still requires continuous electrocardiography monitoring because of the possibility of shock-induced arrhythmias. Percutaneous nephrolithotomy requires diligent electrolyte monitoring (even more so than ureteroscopy procedures) to assess the absorption of intraoperative irrigating fluids. A postoperative chest X-ray is necessary for nephrostomy placement above the 10th rib, or if a pneumo- or hydrothorax is suspected.

Patient activity and positioning

Patient position differs by procedure. Shock-wave lithotripsy is usually performed in the supine position for most stones and prone for mid-ureteral calculi. Ureteroscopy is performed in dorsal lithotomy but can be accomplished in split-leg prone as well. Percutaneous nephrolithotomy is commonly accomplished in the prone position and second-look procedures in lateral decubitus position. Immediate ambulation is normal for outpatient procedures.

Alimentation

Oral food intake is immediate in most cases in the absence of ileus, nausea, or vomiting.

Antibiotic coverage

For shock-wave lithotripsy, patients should have a negative urine culture, and therefore they do not routinely require antibiotics. However, most patients receive a single dose just prior to the procedure for prophylaxis. For ureteroscopy and percutaneous nephrolithotomy procedures, irrigation fluid and drains increase chances of complicated urinary infection; therefore, all patients should receive preoperative intravenous antibiotics at least 30 minutes to one hour prior to the procedure. Medically complicated and infected-stone patients should be admitted for 24–48 hours prior to surgery for intravenous antibiotics, which should be continued orally for a course of 7 days. Fevers are common after PCNL procedures and are not always infectious in source.

Drains

For shock-wave lithotripsy procedures performed for stones greater than 1.5 cm or for solitary kidneys, internal double-J ureteral stents should be placed. Internal indwelling stents are commonly placed for ureteroscopy procedures and are the surgeon's preference for percutaneous nephrolithotomy. Stents are left indwelling for 3–7 days for uncomplicated procedures but remain longer if complications such as ureteral perforations or stricture disease are encountered. Ureteral stents can be removed as a simple outpatient procedure in the urologist's office. Stents with an attached string that exits the urethra can be self-removed by the patient. A single dose of oral urinary-specific antibiotic should be administered at the time of removal. Percutaneous nephrolithotomy requires that the establishment of a nephrostomy tract for infectious stones occurs at least 24 hours prior to a definitive procedure. This allows time for adequate drainage of the affected kidney, and may disclose a worsening infection that would otherwise not present until after surgery. Otherwise, nephrostomy tubes can be placed intraoperatively by the experienced surgeon or radiologist. Postoperatively, the tubes are left to straight drainage for 24–48 hours, capped if the patient experiences no obstructive symptoms, and removed if significant hematuria has resolved and all stone burden has been removed.

Postoperative complications
In the hospital
Fever

Fever is common after percutaneous surgery, especially with infected stones. Patients should be kept on appropriate antibiotics until they become afebrile. Fevers may occur from release of bacteria from lithotripsy, renal trauma, or pulmonary atelectasis. Clinical assessment is mandatory for prolonged fever and should include chest X-ray, blood, and urine cultures.

Gross hematuria

Gross hematuria is commonly seen during and after shockwave lithotripsy and should clear within 24 hours after the procedure. Because of their more invasive nature, percutaneous nephrolithotomy procedures may produce gross hematuria for days before resolving; recurrent bleeding may also start as long as 2 weeks post-surgery. Ureteroscopy usually produces the least amount of hematuria in routine cases because of the lack of incision and the focal nature of stone basketing or intracorporeal lithotripsy. Hemorrhage and hematomas also may occur, especially in patients with undiagnosed coagulopathies, undisclosed blood thinner (ASA) usage, and uncontrolled hypertension. Arterial-venous malformation should be ruled out for patients with a persistent gross hematuria necessitating transfusion. Should the patient become clinically unstable, super-selective embolization may be performed at the time of angiography.

Renal/ureteral obstruction

Stone fragments or ureteral edema may cause transient yet substantial obstruction resulting in pain, nausea, and infection in the unstented patient. *Steinstrasse* (German for street of stone) is the term urologists use to describe a ureteral obstruction from a lead fragment followed by smaller fragments or a stone. Stenting, nephrostomy tube placement, or ureteroscopy with lead fragment lithotripsy are treatment options for *steinstrasse*.

Pneumothorax

The pleura may be punctured during percutaneous nephrolithotomy access (typically, above the 11th rib), leading to a pneumothorax, hydrothorax (from irrigation during the procedure), or hemothorax. Chest X-rays are typically ordered postoperatively for complicated cases, and they should be obtained for persistent fevers, respiratory compromise, or chest pain. Percutaneous drainage should be performed if the patient is symptomatic from the blood or fluid in the pleural cavity.

Pain

Pain can arise from a multitude of sources.

After discharge

Urinoma

Perforation of the collecting system or ureter may occur during instrumentation. Nephrosto-ureterogram, which is usually performed at the conclusion of a percutaneous nephrolithotomy procedure, may not identify a small tear with urinary extravasation. Complicated ureteroscopy with laser perforation or difficult stone extraction may also cause a ureteral tear. A CT scan or ultrasound may identify free fluid in the retroperitoneum, which suggests the diagnosis.

Subcapsular hematoma

Subcapsular hematomas are seen in 0.1–0.3% of shock-wave lithotripsy procedures. They are usually self-limiting complications, but may cause pain and discomfort. A close follow-up post shock-wave lithotripsy CT scan or ultrasound should be obtained and blood-pressure monitoring should be performed. A resultant Page kidney (a compressed kidney decreasing renal blood and resulting in hypertension) may occur. The trauma and pressure of the hematoma causes capsular distension and parenchymal compression. If uncontrollable hypertension occurs with this complication, nephrectomy will be necessary.

Organ damage

There are a few scattered reports about damage to surrounding organs (pancreas, spleen, and liver contusions) from the shockwave path during SWL. Colonic perforation may occur during percutaneous tube placement, especially in patients with previous colonic or gastric bypass surgery.

Late-onset hypertension and diabetes

Delayed hypertension after shock wave lithotripsy has been reported, but has not been substantiated at the present time. Delayed diabetes secondary to SWL has been reported in a large Mayo Clinic retrospective study. However, several other studies have questioned this finding; it is considered controversial as well.

Further reading

Collado SA, Huget PJ, Monreal GF *et al.* Renal hematoma as a complication of extracorporeal shockwave lithotripsy. *Scand J Urol Nephrol* 1999; **33**: 171–5.

Hemal AK, Nayyar R, Gupta NP *et al.* Experience with robotic assisted laparoscopic surgery in upper tract urolithiasis. *Can J Urol* 2010; **17**: 5299–305.

Kraft K, Pattaras JG. Medical management of urolithiasis. *AUA Update Series* 2007; **26** (Lesson 36): 353–64.

Preminger GH, Assimos DG, Lingeman JE *et al.* AUA guideline on management of staghorn calculi: diagnosis and treatment recommendations. *J Urol* 2005; **173**: 1991–2000.

Preminger GH, Tiselius HG, Assimos DG *et al.* 2007 guideline for the management of ureteral calculi. *J Urol* 2007; **178**: 2418–34.

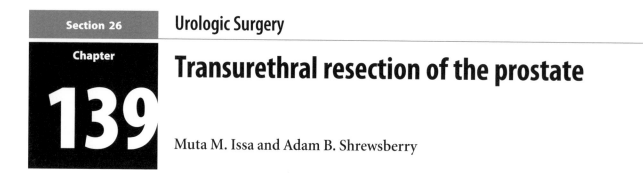

Chapter 139

Transurethral resection of the prostate

Muta M. Issa and Adam B. Shrewsberry

Transurethral resection of the prostate (TURP), developed in the 1920s, remains the gold standard surgical treatment for benign prostatic hyperplasia (BPH) throughout the world. Over the years, the procedure has undergone significant modifications that improved its efficacy and safety. The most significant recent improvement is bipolar TURP. Conventional monopolar TURP employs hypo-osmolar fluids for irrigation during the procedure. As a result, patients are at risk of developing perioperative dilutional hyponatremia and TUR syndrome, which is a severe form of serum electrolyte and osmolar derangement. Since the new bipolar TURP system utilizes normal saline for irrigation, these risks and complications are completely eliminated. Bipolar TURP thus allows for safer resection.

Indications for transurethral resection of the prostate

Transurethral resection of the prostate is the treatment of choice in patients with moderate to severe BPH symptoms and significant compromise to their quality of life who:

- Are unable to tolerate or do not respond to other forms of management (e.g., watchful waiting, medical therapy and/or minimally invasive thermal therapy).
- Are experiencing urinary retention thought to be secondary to BPH.
- Have recurrent urinary infection secondary to BPH.
- Have bladder stones secondary to BPH.
- Have renal failure secondary to BPH.
- Have recurrent bleeding (gross hematuria) secondary to BPH.

Spinal or general anesthesia can be used for the procedure; spinal anesthesia administration is the preferred method since it permits closer intraoperative monitoring of the patient and allows for easier postoperative recovery. The patient is placed in the dorso-lithotomy position. The urologist uses a specially designed cystoscopic instrument (resectoscope) to perform the procedure under direct vision. The resectoscope has an energy-active (radiofrequency) metal loop that is used to resect the obstructing prostatic tissue into small chips (0.5–1 g). The tissue fragments are then evacuated out of the bladder. Hemostasis is secured by coagulating all bleeding vessels on the resected surface of the prostate. A three-way Foley catheter is then inserted into the bladder and placed on traction by taping it stretched onto the patient's thigh. This traction enables the Foley balloon to tamponade the vessels at the resected surface. To prevent clot formation during the initial postoperative period, continuous bladder irrigation is instituted by running normal saline through the Foley; the solution will circulate inside the bladder before draining out. Once the urine clears, the Foley traction and the continuous bladder irrigation are discontinued. Prior to discharge, the Foley is removed and the patient is given a voiding trial. Most patients (> 90%) will void spontaneously. However, some patients may require a prolonged period of Foley catheterization.

All prostatic chips resected during TURP are sent for pathological examination. The pathologist will confirm the diagnosis of BPH. There is often an inconsequential degree of inflammatory changes in the specimen (prostatitis). In approximately 10% of patients, prostate cancer is incidentally found in the specimen. Depending on the percentage of tissue affected by cancer and its histological grade (Gleason grade), the diagnosis is then referred to as either stage T1a or T1b prostate cancer.

Usual postoperative course
Expected postoperative hospital stay

Hospitalization ranges from 1–2 days depending on the size of the prostate, the extent of resection, and the overall health status of the patient.

Operative mortality

Over the past 50 years, there has been a gradual reduction in operative mortality due to improvement in instrumentation and technique of TURP as well as advances in anesthesia; the mortality rate has dropped from 5% (1930s) to 0.2% (1980s).

In 1995, the Veterans Affairs Cooperative Study Group on Transurethral Resection of the Prostate reported similar mortality rates between TURP and watchful waiting.

Special monitoring required

Urinary output and degree of hematuria should be observed as long as the catheter remains in place.

Patient activity and positioning

The resected "raw" prostatic fossa usually takes 4–8 weeks to heal completely. During this period, patients are required to refrain from excessive physical activities, straining, heavy lifting, and sports since such activities may precipitate delayed bleeding. For the same reason, it is not unusual for patients to experience gross hematuria after a bowel movement or physical activity such as walking. In addition, patients should be warned about the possibility of a clot or "scab" being expelled in the urine during this recovery period. It is unusual for the patient's voiding symptoms to resolve immediately after TURP. Improvement in voiding will take a few weeks. Patients with advanced bladder outlet obstruction often have significantly dysfunctional bladders. Therefore, it may take a few months for bladder function to normalize and for improvement in voiding symptoms to become apparent.

Alimentation

To avoid constipation, patients should be placed on oral hydration, a fiber-rich diet, and stool softeners.

Antibiotic coverage

Broad-spectrum prophylactic antibiotics are given perioperatively.

Bladder function

Many years of urinary obstruction will cause the bladder muscle to hypertrophy because the urine is "pushed out" through a narrowed channel. Following TURP and relief of the obstruction, the bladder continues to function abnormally for a few weeks until readjustment. During this period, patients are warned of continued symptoms of frequency, urgency, and nocturia.

Postoperative complications

In the hospital

Bleeding

Generally, an average of 10 mL of blood is lost for every gram of prostate tissue resected. However, this may be variable, with less bleeding emanating from those prostates referred to as "dry glands" (2–5 mL per resected gram of tissue), and more bleeding from those prostates referred to as "wet glands" (15 mL per resected gram of tissue). The frequency of blood transfusion is significantly lower with bipolar-TURP (0–0.8%) compared with monopolar-TURP (2.0–5.4%).

Prostatic capsular perforation

Prostatic capsular perforation, which occurs in less than 5% of procedures, may be associated with urine extravasation outside the prostate into the pelvis. In the majority of cases, this can be managed conservatively by Foley catheter drainage for an extended period. Occasionally, extensive extravasation may necessitate placement of a suprapubic drain for a few days.

Transurethral resection syndrome

Transurethral resection (TUR) syndrome is considered to be a historical adverse event. It occurs only with the old monopolar TURP system, which allows hypotonic irrigation fluid to be absorbed, leading to hyponatremia. In a small percentage of patients (1–2%), the hyponatremia can be sufficiently excessive to cause TUR syndrome. This syndrome is characterized by mental confusion, nausea, vomiting, hypertension, slow heart rate, and visual disturbances (related to the glycine content of the irrigation fluid). The risk is increased when the prostate gland is larger than 35 g and resection time exceeds 90 min. Early recognition of the syndrome is important: upon discovery, the procedure should be terminated and a diuretic given. Occasionally, hypertonic saline is infused to counteract the blood dilution. This adverse event is eliminated with the use of newer bipolar-TURP systems.

Urinary retention

The Foley catheter may be blocked by a residual prostate chip or a blood clot that has developed in the bladder, causing urinary retention. Clot retention is infrequent (2–3%), and is treated by irrigation of the Foley to evacuate the clot.

Urinary infection

Prior to the TURP, every effort should be made to ensure that the patient has sterile urine and that any active infection has been adequately treated. Prophylactic antibiotics are recommended to reduce the possibility of dissemination of an unrecognized urinary infection, but patients may develop signs of infection despite these precautions. Infection is usually successfully treated with antibiotics.

After discharge

Urinary incontinence

True urinary stress incontinence (which occurs in less than 1% of TURP patients) results from damage to the external urinary sphincter during the procedure, rendering it weak and incapable of retaining urine. The risk increases in patients with previous TURPs, significant prostate cancer, or severely damaged bladders. True permanent "stress-type" urinary incontinence should be distinguished from the more common transient "urge-type" urinary incontinence; the latter is self-limiting, resolving when healing is complete.

Erectile dysfunction (impotence)

Because the nerves for erection are situated between the prostate and the rectum, there is a theoretical risk of nerve damage from the heat generated by the resecting loop during the procedure. Traditionally, patients were informed about a 10% risk of erectile dysfunction; however, this figure was not supported by pre- and postoperative validated questionnaires. More recent literature shows no significant change in erectile function as assessed with a validated questionnaire 6 months post-TURP.

Retrograde ejaculation

Retrograde ejaculation (RGE) is a backward flow of the ejaculatory fluid (semen) into the bladder instead of the normal forward propulsion through the urethra. Retrograde ejaculation is a direct result of the anatomical debulking of the prostate, with resultant bladder neck incompetency. Retrograde ejaculation is common after TURP (70–90%). While most patients are unconcerned by this complication, in some, especially the young, it may be considered undesirable. In these individuals, a more conservative resection should be performed to minimize the risk of developing RGE.

Bladder neck contracture

Obstruction from scar formation at the bladder neck may occur in 7%. After confirming the diagnosis by cystoscopy, the contracture is treated by transurethral incision of the bladder neck (TUIBN).

Urethral strictures

Instrumentation during TURP causes a certain amount of trauma to the urethra. In the majority of cases the urethra heals without sequelae. However, in a small percentage of patients (1.8–10%), scar formation develops and causes urethral strictures of the lumen. The frequency of this adverse event is related to the size of the resection. It occurs in 1.8% and 3.8% following < 70 g TURP and 70–150 g TURP, respectively. The treatment to reestablish patency is either dilation or transurethral incision.

Regrowth benign prostatic hyperplasia

Since the peripheral rim of the prostate is left in place after TURP, there is a potential risk for the residual tissue to grow in the years following the operation. During the initial 10 years following operation, the risk for this growth to become symptomatic is 20%. A number of patients may require a second TURP after 15–20 years.

Transurethral incision of the prostate

Transurethral incision of the prostate is an efficacious surgical therapy for BPH. Transurethral incision of the prostate (TUIP) consists of establishing incisions (usually two) along the obstructing prostate to release the obstruction. It only works on relatively small BPH glands (< 20 g), but TUIP is a simpler

and safer technique and carries less risk of urinary incontinence, impotence, and retrograde ejaculation.

Alternative surgical procedures

Over the last two decades, the urology community has witnessed a procedure-frenzy era with the birth and demise of many new BPH surgical treatments, each claiming to be "the" treatment. This charged environment created much confusion and frustration among patients, urologists, and third-party payers. The touted benefits of these alternative procedures have tended to be exaggerated, and surgical realities have been overlooked.

Modifications of monopolar-transurethral resection of the prostate

Modifications of the standard monopolar TURP procedure include transurethral electrovaporization of the prostate (TUEVP), in which the obstructing prostate is vaporized with a specially designed roller-ball device. Significantly higher radiofrequency energy than with the standard monopolar TURP procedure is utilized during TUEVP to produce the very high temperatures required for evaporization. Another modification is transurethral vaporesection of the prostate (TUVRP), which modifies the configuration of the standard TURP loop component to allow a combination of resection and vaporization of tissue. The theoretical objective of all of these modified procedures is to decrease blood loss and fluid absorption during the procedure. For the most part, bipolar-TURP has outperformed all monopolar TURP modifications.

Minimally invasive thermal therapies

The last 20 years have seen the emergence (and disappearance) of various forms of minimally invasive thermal therapies. These include transurethral needle ablation (TUNA), transurethral microwave thermotherapy (TUMT), high intensity focus ultrasound (HIFU) thermal therapy, and interstitial laser thermal therapy (ILTT). These modalities utilize various forms of energy (e.g., laser, radiofrequency (RF), microwave, and ultrasound) to achieve the desired effect. Irrespective of the type of energy used, the final common objective is to achieve sufficient therapeutic intraprostatic temperatures to reduce obstructing tissue, usually in the range of 80–110 °C.

The advantages these minimally invasive thermal therapies offer include the option of an outpatient procedure in a clinic setting or cystoscopy suite and the possibility of local anesthesia with sedation in place of spinal or general anesthesia. Patients can resume work and regular daily activities within a few days. The newer procedures offer greater safety, and complication rates for conditions such as bleeding, impotence, retrograde ejaculation, and urinary incontinence tend to be lower than standard surgical procedures. The efficacy of minimally invasive thermal procedures in the treatment of BPH is not as great as that of standard surgical procedures. While the adoption of these newer methods by the urological community continues to face challenges due to high cost, inconsistent reimbursement, limited patient selection, lower treatment efficacy, and unknown long-term durability, we believe that these therapies have an important place in the armamentarium of BPH surgical treatment.

Laser therapy

Laser TURP attempts to achieve a TURP-like resection through various types of laser energies and techniques. These include Holmium Laser Ablation of the Prostate (HoLAP), Holmium Laser Enucleation of the Prostate (HoLEP), Holmium Laser Resection of the Prostate (HoLRP), Potassium-Titanyl-Phosphate Photovaporization of the Prostate (PVP) and Thulium:YAG Laser. The choice between laser therapy and bipolar TURP is primarily driven by the surgeon's preference and the availability of the system.

In our experience, the optimal surgical procedure is bipolar-TURP, which allows for hemostatic tissue resection in a normal saline medium. With the use of this newer system, perioperative and short-term complication rates have become negligible.

Further reading

Issa MM, Marshall FF. *Contemporary Diagnosis and Management of Diseases of the Prostate*. 3rd edn. Newtown, PA: Handbooks in Healthcare; 2005, pp. 103–12.

Issa MM. Technological advances in transurethral resection of the prostate – bipolar *versus* monopolar TURP. *J Endourol* 2008; **8**: 1587–95.

Issa MM, Young MR, Bullock AR, Bouet R, Petros JA. Dilutional hyponatremia in TURP syndrome – a historical event in the 21st century. *Urology* 2004; **64**: 298–301.

McVary KT, Roehrborn CG, Avins AL *et al. American Urological Association Guideline: Management of Benign Prostatic Hyperplasia*. Linthicum, MD: American Urological Association, 2010. www.auanet.org/content/guidelines-and-quality-care/clinical-guidelines/main-reports/bph-management/authors.pdf.

Wasson JH, Reda DJ, Bruskewitz RC *et al.* A comparison of transurethral surgery with watchful waiting for moderate symptoms of benign prostatic hyperplasia. The Veterans Affairs Cooperation Study Group of Transurethral Resection of the Prostate. *N Engl J Med* 1995; **332**: 75–9.

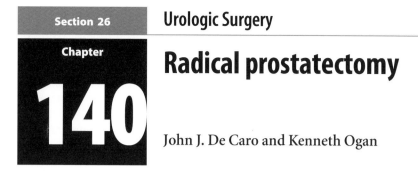

Chapter

140

Radical prostatectomy

John J. De Caro and Kenneth Ogan

Radical prostatectomy is typically offered to patients with clinically localized prostate cancer (stage T1 to T3 disease) with a life expectancy > 10 years. The operation involves total removal of the prostate, seminal vesicles and ampullae of vas deferens. Radical prostatectomy may be performed using perineal, retropubic, or laparoscopic approaches. The three goals ("trifecta") common to all approaches are: oncologic control, urinary continence, and preserved erectile function. While key differences in technique influence optimum patient selection and expected perioperative morbidity, level I evidence is lacking comparing available surgical approaches with regard to outcomes. A comparison with other treatment options for clinically localized prostate cancer (e.g. "watchful waiting" and radiation therapy) is beyond the scope of this chapter.

All surgical approaches can be effectively combined with nerve-sparing techniques whereby one or both neurovascular bundles alongside the prostate are spared to preserve erectile function and urinary continence. However, nerve-sparing should not be performed at the expense of oncologic control. Staging pelvic lymphadenectomy, once routinely combined with radical prostatectomy, is now more selectively performed based on nomograms that allow predictions of disease stage and pelvic lymph node involvement based on prostate specific antigen (PSA), clinical stage, and Gleason pathologic score. Unlike other approaches, the perineal approach does not permit lymphadenectomy, however it can be combined with laparoscopic lymphadenectomy. Lymphadenectomy risks pelvic lymphocele formation; however, this does not commonly require further intervention.

The robot-assisted laparoscopic prostatectomy (RALP) combines the minimal-invasiveness of laparoscopy with a three-dimensional view of the operative field and control of robotic instruments that mimic the dexterity of human hands. The RALP has rapidly become the most popular approach to laparoscopic radical prostatectomy in the USA. A pure laparoscopic approach has become uncommon. Those who are cautious about the rapid shift to this new technology highlight potential increased healthcare costs and the absence of level I evidence demonstrating a clear long-term benefit to the patient. Patient selection considerations include morbid obesity, large prostate size and prior abdominal/pelvic surgery, prostate surgery, pelvic irradiation, or neoadjuvant chemotherapy. Virtually all reported experiences with RALP are with the daVinci Surgical System (Intuitive Surgical, Inc., Sunnyvale, CA), a master-slave system consisting of a remote-surgeon console in control of a surgical robot with camera and working arms. A RALP is typically performed through five 8–12 mm incisions with the patient positioned supine in steep Trendelenberg with legs in low lithotomy or spread apart. A key feature of RALP versus other approaches is transperitoneal access to the prostate, however a comparable extraperitoneal approach has also been described.

The radical retropubic prostatectomy (RRP) remains the gold standard for surgical treatment of clinically localized prostate cancer with proven long-term oncologic control, high rates of urinary continence and the ability to perform nerve-sparing techniques to preserve erectile function. Patient selection is similar to other techniques. However, compared with RALP the open approach may be more suitable for those with a large prostate size, a history of abdominal/pelvic surgery, pelvic irradiation, or neoadjuvant chemotherapy. An RRP, with the patient supine, is performed through a relatively small (8–10 cm) lower abdominal incision that avoids cutting of rectus muscles while permitting entry into the preperitoneal space. Aside from the reduced blood loss, the current data suggest that RALP is no better than RRP with regard to long-term outcomes.

The radical perineal prostatectomy (RPP) is seldom performed today, but it offers cost-effective proven long-term oncologic control and excellent urinary continence with newer techniques permitting nerve-sparing for improved erectile function. Individuals unable to tolerate exaggerated lithotomy position are not candidates; however, RPP may be more suitable for those considered poor candidates for RALP or RRP, such as those with morbid obesity and extensive prior abdominal/pelvic surgery. An RPP is performed through a small curvilinear perineal incision between the scrotum and anus.

Laparoscopic approaches must be performed under general anesthesia, while RRP and RPP may be performed under either

Medical Management of the Surgical Patient, ed. Michael F. Lubin, Thomas F. Dodson, and Neil H. Winawer. Published by Cambridge University Press. © Cambridge University Press 2013.

regional or general anesthesia. A RALP typically takes longer than RRP and RPP, with operative times of 5–6 hours for less experienced surgeons and < 3 hours for more experienced surgeons.

Usual postoperative course

Expected postoperative hospital stay

Following robot-assisted laparoscopic prostatectomy, patients typically are discharged postoperative day 1 compared with 1–2 days following radical perineal prostatectomy and 2–3 days following radical retropubic prostatectomy. Studies consistently support a shorter length of stay following RALP versus RRP.

Estimated blood loss and transfusion rates

The RALP and RPP appear to have decreased blood loss compared with RRP. The pneumoperitoneum in RALP is believed to limit blood loss and contribute to low transfusion rates (0–17%). Decreased blood loss during RPP is attributed to reflecting the dorsal venous complex (a common source of bleeding) instead of transecting it during apical prostatic dissection as required during other approaches. In a recent comparison, transfusion rates following laparoscopic, retropubic, and perineal approaches were 2.7%, 20.8%, and 7.2%, respectively.

Operative mortality

With judicious patient selection operative mortality is rare for all approaches (< 1%).

Special monitoring required

Patients are observed for postoperative hematuria. Surgical drain output is monitored for evidence of urine leakage or bleeding.

Patient activity

Patients generally rest overnight, then ambulate postoperative day 1.

Alimentation

Patients generally progress as tolerated to a regular diet.

Pain control

Low pain scores have been reported for all approaches; however, there are data to suggest lower narcotic use for RALP and RPP compared with RRP.

Antibiotic coverage

Perioperative prophylactic antibiotics are administered for 24 hours.

Deep venous thrombosis prophylaxis

Thromboembolic events are uncommon. Sequential compression devices are applied in the operating room, and postoperative chemical prophylaxis, e.g., low molecular weight heparin, is recommended.

Drains

A Foley catheter is typically in place for 10–14 days following RRP and RPP versus 7–10 days following RALP. A surgical drain is placed and removed when there is minimal output, generally prior to discharge. Drain fluid can be checked for creatinine levels with high levels indicating an anastomotic urine leak.

Postoperative complications

In the hospital

In-hospital complications such as ileus, wound infection, venothromboembolic events, rectal injury and anastomotic urinary leak are rare. In a recent review, overall complication rates were similar between RALP (3–17%) and RRP (6–27%) with a trend toward fewer complications following RALP. Rectal injury appears to have a slightly higher occurrence during RPP (1–11%) as do transient neuropraxia unique to positioning in RPP (typically < 2%).

After discharge

Rectourethral fistula

Rectourethral fistula is an uncommon event that occurs following an unrecognized rectal injury, reported in 0–5.3% of published case series. More contemporary surgical series report an even lower incidence (< 1%). The majority present within 7 days of surgery, and necessitate operative repair.

Deep venous thrombosis and pulmonary embolism

Lymphoceles may cause impeded venous flow from the lower extremity, leading to deep venous thrombosis (DVT). While lymphocele rates vary, they have been shown to be higher following extended lymphadenectomy. Subsequent rates of DVT and pulmonary embolism are less than 1% in recent series.

Incontinence

Urinary incontinence is common during the first few months following surgery, however, most men will recover continence (78–98%) depending upon the definition of continence used and upon patient age with older men more likely to be incontinent. Nerve-sparing techniques are believed to improve rates of urinary incontinence. Recent data suggest a trend toward more rapid return to continence and higher rates of continence for RALP.

Impotence

Post-prostatectomy erectile dysfunction is common with 20–90% of men affected, depending on baseline sexual function, patient age, comorbidities (e.g., diabetes and hypertension), and use of nerve-sparing techniques. The RALP has not demonstrated a clear benefit to RRP. Potency tends to improve with time. Best results are reached beyond 12 months of follow-up. As with continence, there is a trend toward more rapid return of erectile function following RALP compared with RRP.

Bladder neck contracture

Bladder neck contracture typically occurs 4 months postoperatively with similar but variable rates when comparing approaches (ranging from 0–16% for retropubic and laparoscopic approaches).

Further reading

Berryhill R Jr, Jhaveri J, Yadav R *et al.* Robotic prostatectomy: a review of outcomes compared with laparoscopic and open approaches. *Urology* 2008; **72**: 15–23.

Cadeddu JA, Gautam G, Shalhav AL. Robotic prostatectomy. *J Urol* 2010; **183**: 858–61.

Ficarra V, Novara G, Artibani W *et al.* Retropubic, laparoscopic, and robot-assisted radical prostatectomy: a systematic review and cumulative analysis of comparative studies. *Eur Urol* 2009; **55**: 1037–63.

Finkelstein J, Eckersberger E, Sadri H *et al.* Open versus laparoscopic versus robot-assisted laparoscopic prostatectomy: the European and US experience. *Rev Urol* 2010; **12**: 35–43.

Janoff DM, Parra RO. Contemporary appraisal of radical perineal prostatectomy. *J Urol* 2005; **173**: 1863–70.

Prasad SM, Gu X, Lavelle R, Lipsitz SR, Hu JC. Comparative effectiveness of perineal versus retropubic and minimally invasive radical prostatectomy. *J Urol* 2011; **185**: 111–15.

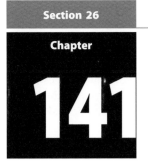

Nephrectomy

John G. Pattaras

Nephrectomy is a common urologic procedure indicated for malignancy, certain benign conditions of the kidney and renal transplantation. Simple, radical, partial and donor nephrectomies and nephroureterectomy all have common surgical steps but have unique complications. Renal tumor ablative interventions are the more commonplace attempts to limit patient morbidity.

Simple nephrectomy is indicated for benign but not trivial conditions. Indications include non-functioning kidneys causing pain (usually from congenital obstruction or urolithiasis), reno-vascular disease causing uncontrollable hypertension, benign symptomatic tumors (angiomyolipomas), trauma, or treatment of infectious diseases (xanthogranulomatous pyelonephritis, chronic or emphysematous pyelonephritis, and tuberculosis). During simple nephrectomy, the kidney is removed within Gerota's fascia along with a small amount of ureter. Nephrectomy for inflammatory conditions can be the most exacting of procedures; medical comorbidities add to the challenge of patient management.

Donor nephrectomy is a simple nephrectomy in which a healthy kidney (usually the left because of increased vein length) is removed and transplanted as an allograft in a controlled scheduled situation. These donor patients are all healthy and have had extensive preoperative evaluations. Transplant nephrectomy is a simple nephrectomy in which the renal allograft is removed, usually because of rejection complications.

Radical nephrectomy involves the removal of all structures within Gerota's fascia, which includes the adrenal, kidney, and peri-renal tissue. Adrenal-sparing radical nephrectomy, especially for lower pole tumors, has become commonplace because of the low incidence of ipsilateral adrenal invasion or metastases. Most renal tumors are found incidentally by CT or MRI, or during the process of hematuria screening. Upwards of 95% of enhancing renal masses are malignant; therefore, needle biopsy or pathologic proof before surgery is not routinely obtained.

Complicated radical nephrectomy includes renal tumor thrombus extension into the renal vein, vena cava, or even the right atrium. Large renal masses invading surrounding organs such as the liver, spleen, colon, pancreas, duodenum, or diaphragm are also surgical challenges as well. These difficult cases are managed in various fashions, which can even include thoracoabdominal surgery or cardiopulmonary bypass for tumor thrombus extension into the right atrium. In advanced tertiary centers, the majority of radical nephrectomies are often accomplished laparoscopically and, more recently, robotically.

Alternatively, upper tract urothelial carcinoma, which differs in surgical and chemotherapeutic management, can be encountered. The entire urothelial lining from the renal pelvis to the urinary bladder should be excised in continuity. Nephroureterectomy involves removing the kidney (sparing the adrenal if not involved) and the entire ureter down to and including the ureteral orifice in the bladder.

Nephron-sparing surgery is the present-day goal for the urologic oncologist. Presently, smaller (less than 4 cm), bilateral tumors or tumors in patients with borderline renal function may require only partial nephrectomy, with fairly equivalent oncologic results. There is growing evidence that, in experienced hands, even larger tumors can be excised, as long as half of the renal parenchyma and renal hilum are preserved. Depending on tumor location and size, the surgical approach may include renal hypothermia, vascular control and temporary occlusion, or renal cortical occlusion. Reconstruction of the renal parenchyma, collecting system, ureter, or major vasculature are all possibilities.

Most minimally invasive laparoscopic partial nephrectomies are now being performed robotically. The versatility of the robot in respect to improving three-dimensional visualization and instrument control has been demonstrated by successful outcomes for partial nephrectomy with minimal morbidity. Presently, in our institution, more than 80% of renal tumors are treated with nephron-sparing surgery; robotic-assisted partial nephrectomy is our main approach. Renal tumor ablation therapy with cryosurgery or radiofrequency techniques is the most recent treatment for small masses. It has growing mid- and long-term successful follow-up, but is still mostly considered an option for high-risk surgical candidates. For certain patients, it has proven to be a viable and efficacious option over nephrectomy or partial nephrectomy. Long-term studies to prove oncologic success are ongoing.

Nephrectomy is almost always performed under general anesthesia. Incisional placement varies by surgeon preference/experience, patient body habitus, and surgical goals. If feasible, extraperitoneal approaches are favored, but transperitoneal surgery is common for advanced tumors or difficult infectious cases. Laparoscopic nephrectomy, first performed in 1991, is now a standard approach even for larger tumors (upwards of 14 cm) and for cytoreductive goals prior to chemotherapy. Laparoscopic nephrectomy can be performed transperitoneally (more common) and retroperitoneally. The obvious advantages of the former choice include less pain, quicker recovery, and better cosmesis. High anesthetic risk patients are also candidates for laparoscopy and have been shown to have equivalent surgical outcomes, decreased hospitalization, and decreased convalescence when compared with similar open nephrectomy patients.

Transfusion rates for nephrectomy also vary with regard to surgical approach. In general, the overall rate is low. Simple nephrectomy for xanthogranulomatous or emphysematous pyelonephritis can be more difficult than most radical nephrectomies, requiring a higher rate of transfusion. Radical nephrectomy with tumor thrombus, advanced partial nephrectomy, or extensive dissections all increase the possibility of blood transfusion.

Usual postoperative course

Expected postoperative hospital stay

For simple or uncomplicated radical nephrectomy, a hospital course of 3–5 days is expected. Laparoscopic nephrectomy usually decreases hospital stays to as short as 1 day for simple retroperitoneal nephrectomies to an average of 3 days for radical cases. Medical comorbidities greatly influence hospital stay, which can extend to 7 days, even for laparoscopic cases.

Operative mortality

Operative mortality is generally low: less than 1% for simple uncomplicated nephrectomy to as high as 5% for higher-risk patients with advanced disease, tumor thrombus above the liver, or present metastatic disease, extensive dissection, or preexisting medical comorbidities.

Special monitoring required

Intraoperative monitoring of general anesthesia may include arterial lines, central venous pressures, and special attention to urine output. Laparoscopic and robotic surgical patients commonly have decreased intraoperative urine output, which increases with cessation of pneumoperitoneum. The goal is to properly hydrate the patient before pneumo-insufflation, especially in nephron-sparing cases, to decrease postoperative renal acute tubular necrosis. Postoperative urine output and daily chemistries should be closely followed. Transient elevations in creatinine and BUN are common.

Patient activity and positioning

Patients are usually encouraged to ambulate within 24 hours of the procedure unless extensive reconstructive or vascular surgery prohibits activity. Patient position depends on the surgical approach. The most common positioning is modified or full lateral decubitus position for subcostal or flank approaches. Laparoscopic and robotic approaches are almost exclusively flank positioning except for cases where a bilateral nephrectomy is performed. Supine positioning is necessary for midline or chevron incisions.

Alimentation

Open surgery will usually result in a short ileus, which resolves in 24–48 hours but may take days. Laparoscopic surgery usually decreases postoperative ileus; with pure retroperitoneal approaches, patients are fed the same day. High-protein diets should be avoided short term for nephron-sparing patients and long term for patients undergoing complete nephrectomies because of potential hyperfiltration injury to the kidney.

Antibiotic coverage

Antibiotics are usually used for short-term prophylaxis and stopped after 24 hours. Exceptions include simple nephrectomies for complicated pyelonephritis, infected stone surgery, or opening the gastrointestinal tract. Broad-spectrum antibiotic use should then be continued until the patient is clinically deemed to be stable. Doses should be adjusted to renal function.

Diaphragmatic/pleural injury

Entry into the chest cavity is a common and well-known complication of nephrectomy. Disruptions in the pleura or diaphragm discovered intraoperatively can be managed by a small chest tube or diaphragmatic closure during deep inspiration. Postoperative chest X-rays should be followed until signs of pneumothorax have resolved.

Drains

Drains are not routinely placed for radical nephrectomies. Surgical drains are placed for patients with infections, partial nephrectomy with entry into the collecting system, and nephroureterectomy requiring partial cystectomy.

Drain fluid should be measured and checked for creatinine levels that exceed serum levels, an indication of urinary extravasation.

Laboratory values

After nephrectomy, a transient rise in serum BUN and creatinine may occur. Pancreatic or hepatic involvement may cause brief rises in amylase and liver function tests, respectively. Preoperative anemia may be seen with large tumors, paraneoplastic syndromes, or renal insufficiency.

Analgesia

Pain control varies in relation to surgical approach. Thoracoabdominal or flank approaches may require epidural placement. Laparoscopic approaches may require minimal parenteral analgesia, quickly switched to oral medication. Non-steroidal anti-inflammatory medication should be avoided in the immediate postoperative period and should be limited lifelong secondary to nephrotoxic effects.

Postoperative complications

In the hospital

Ileus

Short-term ileus may occur from any surgical approach and should resolve. Nasogastric decompression and bowel rest are usually curative. A prolonged ileus should be evaluated by CT with oral contrast to rule out herniation or volvulus.

Wound infection

Wound infection is an uncommon complication, even in patients with renal infections. Obesity and malnutrition are predisposing factors. Local wound care and drainage may be necessary.

Pneumothorax

Postoperative chest X-ray in the recovery room may reveal a pneumothorax. This complication can be managed conservatively by observation for a small asymptomatic pneumothorax. For larger or symptomatic pneumothoraces, chest tube placement, oxygen supplementation, and positive pressure inspiration will all aid in healing.

Urinary leak/extravasation

The increasing use of nephron-sparing surgery, particularly partial nephrectomy, is not without cost. There is a 10–15% incidence of post-operative bleeding or urinary extravasation when the renal collecting system is entered. Meticulous surgical technique and experience decreases the incidence, but intraoperative drain placement is usually standard to monitor for this possibility.

Deep venous thrombosis and pulmonary emboli

Deep venous thrombosis and resultant pulmonary emboli are serious complications, usually resulting from extensive dissection of the vena cava or iliac veins. Prevention starts with placement of sequential compression stockings in the operating room prior to anesthesia induction. In addition, subcutaneous heparin (5,000 units BID or TID) can be administered (with clinical judgment) to hemodynamically stable patients.

Bowel injury

Bowel injury is a rare and potentially life-threatening complication somewhat unique to laparoscopy. It may occur as a consequence of unrecognized thermal injury. The classic peritoneal symptoms are absent. Nausea/vomiting, trocar pain, fever, and leukopenia are signs that should be immediately investigated by CT. Exploration or CT drainage with conservative management are emergent issues.

After discharge

Flank/abdominal hernia or weakness

Abdominal wall herniation or weakness in the flank is more common in obese, elderly, or malnourished patients. Disruption of the fascial closure is a cause of hernias. Herniations may occur at larger trocar sites even when fascial closure is performed. Surgical intervention is necessary for incarceration or symptomatic hernias. Flank weakness results from a denervation of the musculature secondary to incision of the intercostal and subcostal nerve branches. Weakness may not be correctable, but vigorous physical therapy may help.

Renal insufficiency/failure

Renal insufficiency may occur and be transient, stable, or progressive after nephrectomy. If possible, the contralateral kidney should be evaluated preoperatively; evaluation results may influence the surgical decision of total nephrectomy versus nephron-sparing surgery.

Delayed bleed/arteriovenous malformation

Partial nephrectomy may lead to a delayed vascular complication in the form of gross hematuria or flank hematoma. Significant unexplained anemia should be evaluated by angiography to rule out active tumor bed bleeding or the formation of an arteriovenous malformation. Treatment is typically super-selective embolization after conservative management has failed.

Further reading

Beemster PW, Barwari K, Mamoulakis C *et al.* Laparoscopic renal cryoablation using ultrathin 17-gauge cryoprobes: mid-term oncological and functional results. *BJU Int* 2011; **108**: 577–82.

Bishoff JT, Allaf ME, Kirkels W *et al.* Laparoscopic bowel injury: Incidence and clinical presentation. *J Urol* 1999; **161**: 887–90.

Haber GP, Lee MC, Crouzet S, Kamoi K, Gill IS. Tumor in solitary kidney: laparoscopic partial nephrectomy vs laparoscopic cryoablation. *BJU Int* 2012; **109**: 118–24.

Hsiao W, Pattaras JG. Not so "simple" laparoscopic nephrectomy: outcomes and complications of a 7-year experience. *J Endourol* 2008: **22**: 2285–90.

Petros F, Sukumar S, Haber GP *et al.* Multi-institutional analysis of robotic partial nephrectomy for renal tumors > 4 cm vs. ≤ 4 cm in 445 consecutive patients. *J Endourol* 2012; **26**: 642–6.

142

Cystectomy and urinary diversion

Peter T. Nieh

Cystectomy is most often performed for bladder cancer, either superficially invasive disease that has failed to respond to topical chemotherapy, or more aggressive disease that has invaded into the muscular layer of the bladder. In males, the procedure will usually include removal of the prostate, thus the term cystoprostatectomy is used. In women, the traditional radical cystectomy would include hysterectomy, oophorectomy, and removal of the anterior vaginal wall, which would also be referred to as anterior pelvic exenteration. More recently, there has been a trend towards preservation of the anterior vaginal wall.

When dealing with bladder cancer, pelvic lymphadenectomy has a therapeutic role, showing improved survival when more lymph nodes are removed. Thus, a more extensive dissection to include the common iliac nodal tissue has become routine. With such extended dissections in the pelvis/retroperitoneum, there is more risk for lymph leak, bleeding, and fluid losses in the early postoperative period.

Other indications for cystectomy include neurogenic bladder, pyocystis from defunctionalized bladder, salvage cystoprostatectomy for radiation therapy failure for prostate cancer, radiation cystitis, and refractory interstitial cystitis.

Once the bladder has been removed, the reconstruction of the urinary tract is performed. The ideal bladder replacement would fill and empty without leakage, would protect the kidneys from reflux or obstruction, would have no metabolic or nutritional consequences, would not require an appliance or instrumentation, and would have low risk of infection or stones. There have been numerous types of urinary diversions, each with advantages and unique disadvantages, but none have attained that ideal. There are several options for permanent urinary diversion.

The ileal loop or conduit, which was popularized by Bricker in 1950, uses a short 15–20 cm segment of the distal ileum to continuously transport urine to the skin surface through a stoma, where an external appliance collects the urine. The ureters are anastomosed separately to the proximal end of the ileal segment in a refluxing fashion. Factors that contributed to the widespread use of this technique were the

generous length of small bowel available, even after pelvic radiation; the reliable vascular arcades of the small bowel mesentery; ease of construction; fewer metabolic complications compared with the use of the sigmoid colon as a conduit (ureterosigmoidostomy); and improved urinary drainage with the use of silicone stents.

Continent, or catheterizable, reservoirs permit urine to collect in a bowel reservoir, and are drained by intermittent catheterization through a small, often recessed, skin stoma. This type of diversion may be used when the urethra has been removed for disease beyond the bladder neck or involving the urethra, or is unsuitable for an orthotopic neobladder, such as following radiation therapy. Continent reservoirs are created using lengthy (50–75 cm) segments of small bowel only, combination of small and large bowel (ileocecal, ileocolonic), and, rarely, a wedge of stomach. These segments are then detubularized to diminish intra-reservoir pressures, and re-shaped into spherical reservoirs. The ureters are anastomosed to the reservoir, relying on either an isoperistaltic ileal segment or "chimney," intussuscepted nipple, or tunneled reimplant into the tenia of large bowel to prevent reflux. The catheterizable stoma may be created from appendix or tailored small bowel, using a tunneled implant into the reservoir. These reservoirs take several months to expand to a volume permitting catheterization at 6-hour intervals. Younger patients who wish to avoid an external appliance are the best candidates for this approach. Selected patients for this technique must be highly motivated and well informed of the more rigorous rehabilitation than that of ileal loop diversion.

Continent orthotopic neobladder avoids an external appliance and stoma, and is feasible when the urethra has been preserved. In this form of diversion, the detubularized bowel reservoir is placed in the pelvis and attached to the native urethra, making the external sphincter responsible for continence. Similar to post radical retropubic prostatectomy vesicourethral anastomosis, this procedure was originally used only in males, though the indications have now been extended to females. In this procedure, preservation of the distal two-thirds of the urethra is required for excellent continence. Patients

Medical Management of the Surgical Patient, ed. Michael F. Lubin, Thomas F. Dodson, and Neil H. Winawer. Published by Cambridge University Press. © Cambridge University Press 2013.

void by abdominal straining, have a less forceful stream, and sometimes may need self-catheterization to empty completely. The rehabilitation period during which the reservoir gradually increases in capacity is more prolonged than for ileal loop surgery, taking up to several months before achieving 6-hour intervals between voiding. While daytime continence is excellent, most patients will need to awaken at night to empty or risk nocturnal incontinence. This occurs because the small bowel mucosa will permit free water to equilibrate with the more concentrated urine excreted by the kidneys at night, increasing urine volume despite dehydration. An important caveat about continent reservoirs, whether orthotopic or catheterizable, is to avoid them in patients with impaired renal function (Cr > 2.0), for they are more likely to have significant metabolic problems from the large absorptive surface.

The combination of cystectomy, pelvic lymphadenectomy, and urinary diversion is an extensive major surgical procedure, taking 5–8 hours to perform depending on the type of urinary diversion. Since 2003, the standard management of muscle-invasive bladder cancer now includes chemotherapy prior to surgery (neoadjuvant), so these patients may have some nutritional issues, limited exercise tolerance, and anemia. Because most of these patients were smokers, pulmonary and coronary disease is common. The medical oncologist has a critical role in handling the various toxicities of chemotherapy in these individuals with multiple medical comorbidities to get them ready for major surgery.

For small bowel urinary diversion, full mechanical bowel preparation is no longer required. A clear liquid diet starting the day before surgery ensures minimal small bowel content and volume contraction problems in elderly patients. We still use standard oral and perioperative parenteral antibiotics with or without full mechanical bowel preparation. Most patients are admitted the day of surgery. However, those more debilitated patients with bowel dysfunction, including fragile diabetics or those with a neurogenic bladder such as myelomeningocele patients, require inpatient bowel preparation with cleansing enemas, and may require intravenous fluids to prevent volume contraction due to the preparation. Venous thrombosis prophylaxis with lower extremity venous compression devices and mini-dose heparin is employed. Arterial and central venous monitoring is routine, since significant fluid shifts from extensive pelvic dissection require aggressive crystalloid resuscitation. Even with use of cell saver, blood replacement may be necessary as baseline anemia is common after neoadjuvant chemotherapy.

Usual postoperative course
Expected postoperative hospital stay
The expected postoperative hospital stay is 6–10 days.

Perioperative mortality
Perioperative mortality is approximately 3%.

Special monitoring required
Many bladder cancer patients have a smoking history with compromised pulmonary function; therefore, monitoring of blood gases during weaning from assisted ventilation is necessary. Since many patients also have coronary disease, the hematocrit should be maintained above 30. Urine output should exceed 60 mL/hour. Patients have significant fluid losses, which will typically begin to mobilize around the third postoperative day.

Patient activity and positioning
Early mobilization from bed on postoperative day 1 and ambulation on postoperative day 2 is recommended for prevention of deep venous thrombosis. Pain pumps for infusing local anesthesia for several days around the incision will decrease narcotic requirement and facilitate early ambulation.

Alimentation
Use of postoperative nasogastric tube drainage is the surgeon's preference. This author prefers to remove the tube in the recovery room, because tube-induced posterior pharyngeal discomfort causes many patients to perform air-swallowing, with resultant increase in gaseous distension (which is not well-evacuated by the tube) and more prolonged ileus. Patients are permitted to moisten their lips and oral cavity with swabs, and gum chewing is encouraged, but they are not allowed oral intake until bowel activity returns. Stimulation of lower gut function with Dulcolax suppositories begins on the second postoperative day. Bowel function usually returns around the third or fourth postoperative day, when clear liquid diet is started. The diet is advanced to regular as tolerated.

Antibiotic coverage
Preexisting urinary infections are treated beginning a few days before surgery. Perioperative broad-spectrum antibiotic coverage for prophylaxis is routine, beginning just before the operation, and continued for 1 day afterwards. To minimize problems with *C. difficile* colitis, prolonged courses of broad-spectrum antibiotics should be avoided. A low-dose uroselective antibiotic such as nitrofurantoin may be used until catheters are removed.

Postoperative complications
In the hospital
Most of the early postoperative complications do not require surgical intervention.

Ileus
In any procedure where the bowel is manipulated, there is risk for delayed return of bowel activity. Prolonged ileus occurs in 2.4% of cases. For patients with abdominal distension, nausea,

and vomiting, placement of a nasogastric tube may be necessary for relief. Persistent ileus may prompt evaluation with CT scan to ascertain contributing causes for the ileus, such as urinary leak, small or large bowel leak, obstructed ureteral stent, or infected lymphocele.

Stomal ischemia

When the mesentery is released to deliver adequate length of bowel through the fascia to create a protruding stoma, the distal end of the bowel used for creating the stoma may have its blood supply compromised. The mucosa may appear edematous and dusky for the first 48 hours, but maneuver may still result in a healthy stoma. If it becomes darker, however, there may be compromised perfusion of the entire bowel segment requiring surgical intervention. This problem can be avoided in obese patients by using a loop-end Turnbull stoma; the terminal segment of the stoma is brought to the skin surface with the mesentery intact, and the stoma is created by everting the bowel through a transverse opening in the bowel.

Infarcted urinary diversion

This catastrophic complication may be recognized at surgery when the vascular pedicle to the bowel segment is damaged by excessive traction, compression, or surgical injury. The entire bowel segment becomes dark, the pulse cannot be palpated in the mesenteric pedicle, and intraoperative Doppler examination confirms the lack of perfusion. Delayed infarction may occur following hemorrhage into the mesenteric pedicle. Surgical resection and revision are required.

Urinary leak

The use of ureteral stents and drainage catheters has minimized urinary leaks. Whenever there is persistent drainage from suction or Penrose drain, analysis of the fluid for creatinine should quickly determine whether the leak is urine or lymph. Irrigation of catheters or stents to eliminate mucus occlusion might be required. Most urine leaks will resolve with conservative management.

Oliguria or anuria

Inadequate fluid resuscitation accounts for most low urine output situations, but mucus or blood clot obstruction must be evaluated to prevent over-distension of the reservoir in the early postoperative period. Careful and regular irrigation of catheters should be performed. Edema of the ileal loop stoma may obstruct drainage; insertion of a small catheter into the loop should relieve this blockage.

Bleeding

Most oozing stops once the abdominal cavity is closed, and coagulation abnormalities are corrected. Ongoing bleeding through drains or from the vaginal wound may require re-exploration if no medically correctable bleeding problems

exist and the patient demonstrates ongoing transfusion requirement.

Deep venous thrombosis and pulmonary embolus

There is an increased risk of deep venous thrombosis (DVT) with any major pelvic surgery, particularly with extended pelvic lymphadenectomy, where there is dissection around the iliac veins, and malignant involvement. If clinical signs of DVT or pulmonary embolism occur, either full anticoagulation or inferior vena cava filter placement should be considered in the postoperative period, depending on bleeding risk in the postoperative period.

Obturator nerve injury

While rare, obturator nerve injury may occur during the pelvic lymphadenectomy or with excessive traction from a deep retractor blade. If possible, the injury should be repaired when recognized at surgery. Patients with this complication may have difficulties with leg adduction, ambulation, and possibly driving.

Urosepsis

Perioperative antibiotics should cover most urinary tract organisms, but colonization may lead to active infection during prolonged hospital stays. Judicious antibiotic use, central venous pressure monitoring, and volume resuscitation are routine. In addition, a CT scan or ultrasound should be performed to identify upper tract obstruction from a poorly positioned or obstructed stent, or to locate any fluid collection in the abdomen or pelvis (possible infected lymphocele, urinoma, mucus collection, or hematoma), which would require percutaneous drainage.

Mucus production

In the early postoperative period with continent reservoirs, mucus may occlude the catheters or stents. Regular and rigorous irrigation with 50 mL volumes of saline or bicarbonate solution will prevent such mucus plugs from causing leakage. As the reservoir expands, the increased urinary volume tends to diminish this problem.

After discharge

Incontinence

Urinary incontinence is common in the early months after continent reservoir creation, since the reservoir has relatively high intraluminal pressures from high wall tension with small reservoir diameters (LaPlace's Law). The wall tension and intraluminal pressure drop as the pouch gradually distends, permitting improved continence.

Difficult catheterization

In the older reservoirs, the cutaneous stoma was created with a wide lumen with redundancy of the suprafascial portion of the stoma, resulting in buckling of the catheter. Use of the appendix or tailoring of the stoma over a smaller catheter improves this problem.

Stomal stenosis

Stomal stenosis is typically caused by chronic scarring; it is occasionally accelerated by urine-induced skin irritation. Stomal narrowing occurs in about 20% of ileal loop patients. When urinary infection or hydronephrosis occurs, surgical correction is needed.

Nocturnal incontinence

While most patients achieve daytime continence, nocturnal control is more difficult. Contributing factors are surgical injury to distal sphincter complex; pelvic nerve damage affecting reflex recruitment from bladder distension that normally increases to maintain sphincter tone; increased intrapouch pressures at capacity despite detubularization; and the absence of the usual diurnal variation in urine volume, with more free water being drawn passively into the pouch lumen through the reservoir wall to equilibrate the osmolarity of the more concentrated urine. The ileum is slower to achieve osmotic equilibrium than the jejunum, but more rapid than colon or stomach. Patients may need to awaken to catheterize or void to prevent over-distension and incontinence.

Metabolic or nutritional disorders

Each bowel segment used in the urinary tract has different metabolic consequences. The stomach may cause a hyponatremic, hypochloremic metabolic alkalosis, which may be useful in patients with preexisting metabolic acidosis. The jejunum may cause a hyponatremic, hypochloremic, hyperkalemic metabolic acidosis, while the ileum and colon are associated with hyperchloremic metabolic acidosis, since chloride is exchanged for bicarbonate. These metabolic abnormalities are related to the amount of bowel used, and rarely occur in patients with normal renal function. Previous concerns that chronic acidosis from ileal diversion would result in bone loss have not been substantiated.

The use of lengthy segments of ileum (up to 75 cm) for continent reservoirs is rarely (< 1%) associated with intractable diarrhea or malabsorption. However, loss of more than 50 cm of terminal ileum may result in vitamin B_{12} malabsorption, increasing the risk of megaloblastic anemia or irreversible neurologic symptoms. As the liver stores of vitamin B_{12} last approximately 3 years, it is recommended that vitamin B_{12} levels be monitored beginning from 1 to 5 years after surgery in patients who required more than 50 cm of terminal ileum to be used as a conduit. Replacement therapy for vitamin B_{12} is 100 µg intramuscularly every month.

Urinary tract infection

With the freely refluxing ileal loop, bacteria introduced into the stoma can ascend into the upper tracts. Thus, any stomal stenosis or appliance difficulties might predispose to pyelonephritis. Chronic infections may result in renal deterioration; therefore, prompt stomal revision or conversion to a non-refluxing system is required.

Bacteriuria is common in intermittently catheterized continent reservoirs because of bacterial adherence on the extensive mucosal surface provided by the villi. While urine cultures are often positive, most patients are asymptomatic. When these patients develop symptomatic infection ("pouchitis"), they tend to experience more local discomfort, having the sense of pouch fullness despite recent catheterization, sudden onset of urinary incontinence from the stoma or the urethra, fever, abdominal pain in the region of the stoma, low back pain, nausea, and increased mucus drainage with cloudy, strong-odored urine. While the initial picture may resemble pyelonephritis, these patients generally respond more rapidly to antibiotic treatment. By maintaining self-catheterization to drain the reservoir regularly and proper antibiotic selection, excellent tissue and urinary antibiotic levels are achieved, which are enhanced by the active reabsorption of antibiotic through the permeable pouch wall.

Calculus formation

Stone formation occurs in association with exposed staples, hair, or other foreign bodies introduced with self-catheterization, mucus, and chronic urinary infection. Most stones will be detected incidentally, but the remainder may present with symptomatic urinary tract infections or new-onset urinary incontinence. Most of these stones are struvite or infection-related, and can become quite sizable, causing obstruction and upper tract infections. The smaller stones may be fragmented by extracorporeal shock wave lithotripsy or endoscopic lithotripsy. They may be removed via standard endoscopic instruments through the older wide-caliber stomas. For patients with tailored or tunneled stomas, for whom repeated instrumentation would endanger the continence mechanism, stones are removed by the percutaneous route. Generous irrigation is necessary to remove all fragments, particularly the primary nidus (staple or foreign body) of the stone. However, the larger calculi may require open surgical removal.

Urinary stasis with mucus production and bacteriuria contribute to stone problems. Daily irrigation of any catheterized reservoir is advisable to prevent mucus accumulation and stone formation.

Metabolic factors also contribute to stones in continent reservoirs. Such patients tend to have increased urinary excretion of calcium, phosphate, and magnesium. Many will have metabolic acidosis, which further promotes hypercalciuria and hypocitraturia. Thus, a complete metabolic evaluation with 24-hour urine collections is recommended for recurrent stone formers. Treatment with oral citrates may be necessary.

Pouch distension

An overdistended pouch may occur with any type of continent urinary reservoir if the regular catheterizations are not performed on schedule. Rupture of a continent reservoir is extremely rare, but augmented bladders in children for neurogenic bladder are more susceptible to spontaneous rupture. Patients experience severe cramping abdominal pain with nausea and even vomiting from the distended small bowel of the reservoir, which produces a tense lower abdomen around the stoma. The entry into the reservoir may become acutely angulated with distension, making passage of the relatively flimsy smaller catheters difficult. When the pouch is distended to this degree, catheters, scopes, and most guidewires usually fail to negotiate the angulation. Using ultrasound guidance, if available, and a spinal needle with local anesthesia to drain a small volume of urine from the pouch will often decrease the pouch pressure sufficiently to straighten out the catheterizable stoma so that regular catheterization may be resumed.

Parastomal hernia

A parastomal hernia may occur where the mesenteric portion of the stoma is most difficult to secure to the abdominal wall fascia, and thus vulnerable to herniation. Most herniations are asymptomatic bulges, but some may affect adherence of the appliance or may become symptomatic. Either of these last situations requires parastomal hernia repair. With tapered or tailored catheterizable stomas, the smaller fascial defect has a significantly reduced risk for hernia.

Hydronephrosis

Hydronephrosis may occur from reflux, obstruction from a stenotic stoma or afferent nipple, stricture at the ureterointestinal anastomosis, or recurrent cancer. Most patients are asymptomatic, while the remainder present with urinary tract infections. Urine cytology should be ordered; if recurrent disease is present, surgical resection is necessary. For benign obstruction, endoscopic dilation or incision and stenting of the obstruction has limited success, as ischemia is often the underlying problem. Surgical revision is required for durable relief.

Cancer at ureterointestinal anastamosis

Cancer of the bowel has been reported to occur in patients 15–20 years following ureterosigmoidostomy diversions. Periodic endoscopic monitoring of the reservoir is recommended, particularly if gross hematuria is present.

Further reading

Bricker EM. Symposiums on clinical surgery: bladder substitution after pelvic evisceration. *Surg Clin North Am* 1950: **30**: 1511–21.

Gore JL, Yu HY, Setodji C *et al.* Urologic Diseases in America Project: urinary diversion and morbidity after radical cystectomy for bladder cancer. *Cancer* 2010; **116**: 331–9.

McDougal WS. Metabolic complications of urinary intestinal diversion. *J Urol* 1992; **147**: 1199–208.

Pruthi RS, Nielsen M, Smith A *et al.* Fast track program in patients undergoing radical cystectomy: results in 362 consecutive patients. *J Am Coll Surg* 2010; **210**: 93–9.

Shimko MS, Tollefson MK, Umbreit EC *et al.* Long-term complications of conduit urinary diversion. *J Urol* 2011; **185**: 562–7.

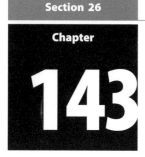

Female stress urinary incontinence surgery

Niall T. M. Galloway

It is estimated that more than 20 million American women have moderate or severe stress urinary incontinence. Despite the negative impact on quality of life, many patients are slow to complain and fail to seek medical care – a typical patient will suffer symptoms for more than 7 years before talking to a physician. For the elderly, problems of incontinence often weigh heavily towards institutional care.

There are many causes for stress urinary incontinence, and surgery is not always needed to resolve it.

Current practice guidelines clearly promote non-surgical therapies first, and pelvic floor muscle exercises are often effective, notably when combined with fluid regulation, diet, and bowel management, because bladder control is always better when the lower bowel is empty. Surgery should be reserved for those who have failed these methods, and have severe or moderate incontinence that can be demonstrated on examination.

Pelvic support anatomy varies widely from patient to patient: some pelvic floors are versatile and balanced; others are asymmetrical and incomplete, causing problems of bladder control, pelvic organ prolapse, and bowel dysfunction. Bladder, bowel, and vaginal prolapse problems may occur in the same patient, and other female family members are likely to be similarly afflicted. Acquired diseases with a role in promoting stress urinary incontinence include diabetes, lumbar or cervical disc disease, and spinal stenosis, as well as a history of pelvic floor insults such as vaginal delivery, hysterectomy, and other pelvic surgery. Surgical procedures in the abdomen or retroperitoneum may also disturb bladder function, and a history of radiation therapy or peripheral neuropathy may compromise surgical treatments.

On abdominal examination, one looks for evidence of abdominal distension, surgical scars, and hernias. Two-point discrimination should be tested in the perianal and postanal dermatomes; muscle tone and grip of the circumvaginal and anal sphincter muscles should be noted on the right and left. Examination of the perineum should be done when the bladder is full and with the patient in the standing as well as supine position. One should use both a bivalve (Graves') speculum to examine the vaginal vault and a Sim's speculum to examine the anterior and posterior vaginal walls.

All patients should be asked to keep a bladder diary of every voided volume and the time of the void; a standard graduated measuring "hat" that fits in the commode will assist in making these recordings. Patients are instructed to maintain their usual practices during the recording period so that the fluid intake will reflect their usual pattern. The resulting chart provides critical information about the largest voided volume (functional bladder capacity), the pattern of voiding throughout the day and night, and the total output in 24 hours. Total 24-hour urine volume should be on the order of 1.5–2 liters for the average adult, but it is not unusual to find that patients with urinary frequency and incontinence may have daily voided volumes in excess of 6–8 liters a day. If there is no organic cause, moderation of fluid intake can readily improve or eliminate their troublesome urinary symptoms.

Almost every patient without organic causes is offered non-surgical treatment. The treatment plan must be tailored to the needs of the individual patient and every effort made to initially address the most troublesome symptom. Preliminary strategies might include fluid restriction, bowel management, and review of prescription and non-prescription medications; timed or prompted voiding might also be considered. It is often effective to team the patient with a continence nurse for coaching and personal support. If the symptoms are moderate or severe and the patient has pelvic support defects or detachments that could be corrected, one should proceed with urodynamics to assess bladder and urethral function prior to surgical correction.

Surgery for stress urinary incontinence is elective, and it is rarely appropriate to accept a patient for surgery who is in less than optimal condition. Initial evaluation should include clinical history, physical examination, post-void residual, and urinalysis; also assessment of gait, the lumbosacral spine, lower extremities, and the feet.

The feet will mirror the pelvic floor because they share the same sacral nerve roots (feet: S2 and 3 immediately adjacent to the pelvic floor; sphincters: S3, 4, and 5). If the feet and toes are

Medical Management of the Surgical Patient, ed. Michael F. Lubin, Thomas F. Dodson, and Neil H. Winawer. Published by Cambridge University Press. © Cambridge University Press 2013.

not fully formed and versatile, the pelvic floor will not be, either. If the cause of incontinence is one or more anatomical defects, correction of those defects is likely to resolve the problem because surgical procedures for stress incontinence change the anatomy. However, if there are other causes, such as neurological deficits, the incontinence is likely to persist in spite of surgery.

Responsibility for care of the female pelvis is divided among several specialists: urologists, gynecologists, and colorectal surgeons. In the prevailing climate, it is not uncommon for these competing factions to treat only one part of the problem and to ignore other correctable pelvic support defects. Lack of an integrated care plan may result in incomplete treatment and imperfect outcomes that will often demand further surgical revisions.

It is estimated that more than 200,000 surgical procedures are done in the USA each year for the treatment of stress urinary incontinence. Since there is no standard operation to treat it, many approaches are used, all of which have their own risks and benefits. Gynecologists favor vaginal repairs, and the current vogue is to introduce a compensatory abnormality by placement of a mesh sling in an effort to support the anterior vaginal wall and urethra. Surgeons have adopted these procedures because they are minimally invasive, and simple and quick to perform in an outpatient setting. The marketing of surgical mesh products has been aggressive and directed to both patients and the medical community, resulting in a stampede for surgical care. The early claims for these treatments and the short recovery times were favorable, but adverse outcomes have led to the withdrawal of some mesh products and the FDA has issued warnings about the use of mesh in vaginal surgery.

Outcomes are best when surgery restores normal nulliparous pelvic support anatomy without mesh. Vaginal prolapse and urethral hypermobility occur because the vagina is no longer attached as it should be within the pelvis. The vaginal apex should be in continuity with the utero-sacral ligaments, and the anterior vaginal wall should be attached to the pelvic side wall along the arcus to the ischial spines. When there is a bulge, there is always a defect or detachment of pelvic support anatomy, but the bulge is often not at the point of detachment. The surgeon should identify all defects and detachments in a particular case, repair the defects, and restore the attachments, just as she would repair a hernia.

Preparation of the patient should include a general medical assessment and consideration of comorbidities and risk factors. Patients may be taking hormone replacement therapy, which should be withheld 1 week prior to surgery to reduce the risk of deep venous thrombosis and pulmonary embolism.

Usual postoperative course
Expected postoperative hospital stay
Hospital stay should be 1–3 days.

Operative mortality
Not greater than 0.1%.

Special monitoring required
A urinary catheter may be used in the first 24 hours to maintain bladder drainage and to monitor urinary output.

Patient activity and positioning
The patient is positioned in a modified dorsal lithotomy position for surgery. Serial compression is applied to the legs as prophylaxis against deep venous thrombosis.

Alimentation
A fluid diet is prescribed for 2 days prior to operation, and use of an enema is recommended the day before and the morning of surgery, but full bowel prep is not indicated. With the first passage of flatus following surgery, food intake is permitted as tolerated.

Antibiotic coverage
A preoperative antibiotic (single dose fluoroquinolone 1 hour before operation) is appropriate. Urinalysis should be repeated 1 week preoperatively, and a urine culture is appropriate if the urinalysis suggests possible infection. Urinary tract infection should be resolved or thoroughly treated before elective surgery.

Instrumentation
Cystoscopy is appropriate for all patients.

Urodynamic studies
Urodynamic studies involve measurement of pressure within the bladder, urethra, and abdomen during bladder filling, as well as provocative maneuvers to provoke leakage and mimic patient symptoms. Primary surgical correction may be done without urodynamics if the clinical features and findings are clear, but for secondary procedures and when features are not typical, pressure studies are recommended to confirm the clinical diagnosis and to guide the surgical plan.

Postoperative complications
In the hospital
Bleeding
Typically, intraoperative blood loss is minimal, but bleeding disorders or inappropriate medications might pose a risk. Patients should avoid aspirin and non-steroidal anti-inflammatory medications for 5 days prior to operation. Wound hematoma and vaginal bleeding are uncommon.

Abdominal distension

This is generally due to inertia of the large bowel rather than paralytic ileus. Minimal use of opiates, anticholinergic medications, and epidural analgesia may limit bowel problems.

Early voiding difficulty and incomplete bladder emptying

These are to be expected for most patients when the catheter is removed on the first postoperative day. Pain and local swelling might impair voiding function at first. Some surgeons leave a suprapubic catheter in place for a few days and remove it after a successful voiding trial; others prefer to teach clean intermittent catheterization to empty the bladder after voiding efforts in order to measure the residual volumes. Bladder function is usually better when bowel function has resumed. Catheterization is usually continued until the bladder is emptying well (residuals consistently less than 100 mL).

After discharge
Wound problems

These are uncommon, but late hematoma or wound infection may occur. Worsening pain at the operative site together with feeling of malaise and fever suggest infection, and local signs of swelling, redness, tenderness, and discharge confirm the clinical suspicion. It may be necessary to open the wound to allow for optimal drainage and to encourage healing by secondary intention. Antibiotics are indicated and are based on wound cultures.

Urinary tract infection

Increased frequency and bladder pain might suggest urinary infection. It is appropriate to use a daily antimicrobial such as nitrofurantoin as a prophylactic against infection for the patient who is learning to manage clean catheterization.

Urinary frequency, urgency, and nocturia

These symptoms suggest incomplete emptying or a small bladder capacity. Pelvic hematoma can form a capsule around the urinary bladder, reducing the space that is necessary to permit effective bladder filling and causing a tendency to frequency and urgency until the hematoma resolves. At times, a similar pattern of urinary symptoms can be provoked by constipation and bowel inertia.

Deep venous thrombosis

Special measures should be used to minimize the possibility in high-risk patients. Early ambulation in the hospital and sustained daily walking exercise after discharge are to be encouraged.

Postoperative anemia

Since signs of anemia are sought and treated effectively before surgery, and the operative blood loss is typically small, this is a rare problem, but postoperative treatment with iron supplements may be indicated.

Further reading

Albo ME, Richter HE, Brubaker L et al. Burch colposuspension versus fascial sling to reduce urinary stress incontinence. *N Engl J Med* 2007; **356**: 2143–55.

FDA Safety Communication: UPDATE on Serious Complications Associated with Transvaginal Placement of Surgical Mesh for Pelvic Organ Prolapse, July 13, 2011. Available at: www.fda.gov/MedicalDevices/Safety/AlertsandNotices/ucm262435.htm.

Swift SE. The distribution of pelvic organ support in a population of female subjects seen for routine gynecologic health care. *Am J Obstet Gynecol* 2000; **183**: 277–85.

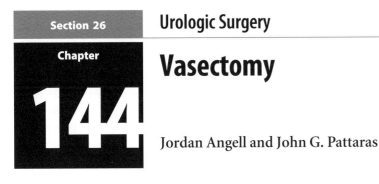

Vasectomy

Chapter

144

Jordan Angell and John G. Pattaras

Vasectomy is an extremely common, cost-effective, and permanent form of contraception dating back to the late 1800s. Presently, in the USA, approximately 500,000 vasectomies are performed annually. An approximated 11% of the USA population uses vasectomy as their means of contraception, making it the most commonly performed urologic procedure in the USA.

In comparison with other methods, vasectomy has been estimated to produce a 5-year saving of nearly $14,000. Contraception saves the USA $19 billion a year in medical costs. The three most cost-effective forms of contraception when comparing all types are the copper-T IUD, vasectomy, and the LNG-20 IUS.

Couples often come to a personal decision on contraception, and therefore must choose from various options. Urologists can educate patients regarding vasectomy as a safe, cost-effective, permanent form of contraception.

The initial office visit of a patient seeking a vasectomy should begin with a complete history/physical and specific questions regarding the patient's reasons for seeking a vasectomy. Questions to the patient should include: if discussion about vasectomy has occurred with the partner; how many children they have, and if they know anyone else who has had a vasectomy. Other pertinent questions should include family history of bleeding disorders, patient use of antiplatelet or anticoagulant medications, and any past history of surgery/trauma to the testis or inguinal canal (i.e., hernia). The exam, while complete, should focus on palpation of both vasa deferentia. The feasibility of performing the vasectomy procedure is based on the patient's anatomy. Complications to be discussed include epididymitis, recanalization, chronic orchialgia, and anti-sperm antibodies.

Surgical treatment

Vasectomy is performed in two different ways: scalpel and no-scalpel techniques. Both function to ligate the left and right vas deferens, so that no sperm is found subsequently in the semen on ejaculation.

A "scalpel" vasectomy involves making either a very small midline scrotal incision or two very small hemi-scrotal incisions, dissecting down to the vasa deferentia, and ligating them. The argument for two incision vasectomy is a lessened chance of ligating the same vas deferens twice; however, two (albeit small) incisions are made.

A "no scalpel" vasectomy employs the same techniques. However, it entails the use of a special fine instrument so that the vas deferens can be grasped through the skin. The vas is dissected and ligated though tiny puncture sites, a procedure requiring neither a knife incision nor closure sutures. Surgeon preference will include removing a portion of the vas (5–10 mm), cauterization, clip placement, and/or absorbable suture ligation prior to delivering the ends back through the wound.

There is no "gold standard": each technique has equal outcomes. Both are outpatient procedures and are usually carried out with administration of some anxiolytic medication and local injectable anesthesia (lidocaine ± bupivicaine). For patients with significant obesity, extreme anxiety, or a stated treatment preference, general anesthesia may be required.

Usual postoperative course

Expected postoperative course

Patients are told they will be sore after the local anesthesia wears off. Patients are advised to stay off their feet for 24 hours following surgery, and then to "just relax" for 2–3 days. Most men will need 2–3 days off from work. They should postpone showering until the next day, and wear scrotal support for a week in the form of boxer briefs or supportive underwear. Patients are asked to avoid strenuous physical activity for at least 1 week. We ask patients to refrain from any activity involving a saddle, such as riding a bicycle, for an additional week.

Operative mortality

There are no data regarding operative mortality except in cases of significant comorbidity.

Medical Management of the Surgical Patient, ed. Michael F. Lubin, Thomas F. Dodson, and Neil H. Winawer. Published by Cambridge University Press. © Cambridge University Press 2013.

Special monitoring required

None.

Patient positioning

Patients are supine for individual dual incisions or in lithotomy position for a midline scrotal single incision.

Alimentation

Oral food intake is immediate, even for operations performed under general anesthesia.

Antibiotic coverage

There is no consensus concerning prophylaxis, but a negative urine analysis should be documented. Our preference is to have the patient start a 5-day course of doxycycline hyclate orally prior to the procedure; this regimen has been shown to limit postoperative epididymitis.

Drains

None.

Postoperative complications

The most common early complications for the procedure are hematoma, infection, and scrotal edema, which occur in about 2–4% of patients. These complications seem to be decreased in the no-scalpel vasectomy population.

Post-vasectomy pain syndrome

Patients may have some postoperative orchialgia, which is usually short-lived. The incidence of true chronic pain, however, has been cited to be less than 5%. Patients with persistent or worsening pain beyond a week should be evaluated immediately for bacterial epididymitis. We typically administer urinary specific antibiotics to these patients, and consider non-steroidal anti-inflammatory medication or Medrol dose pack in severe cases.

Sperm granulomas

Sperm granulomas are spherical collections of extravasated sperm that are found along the cut edges of the vasa deferentia or epididymis in vasectomized men. A local immune response causes sperm granulomas to be palpated as a marble-like mass. The occurrence of this complication should be expected in 4–60% of patients. About half of vasectomized patients are inconvenienced by the granuloma. Sperm granulomas can be locally painful with certain movements, on palpation, and during sexual activity.

Recanalization

An extremely small number of patients (less than 1%) will have recanalization of the vas deferens, which may allow sperm back into the ejaculate. Patients should be counseled to have postoperative semen analyses.

After discharge
Vasectomy failure

All patients will need two semen analyses to be declared sterile; these tests should be obtained at 3 and 6 months after vasectomy. Most surgeons will ask the patient to ejaculate at least 20 times prior to the analysis. Some patients will have an analysis that shows rare, non-motile sperm. Some urologists go ahead and declare these patients sterile; however, a discussion about the remote possibility of conception should occur. If motile sperm are noted at 6 months after the procedure, it should be recognized that the operation was not successful.

Multiple studies have shown that vasectomy has a greater than 99% success rate, with less than a 1% chance of failure or continued fertility. A large survey of 586 urologists showed 1 pregnancy per 1,000 vasectomies, 50% of which occurred immediately post-vasectomy. A prospective study from the US Collaborative Review of Sterilization reported the cumulative probability of failure of vasectomy at 9.4/1,000 procedures at 1 year after vasectomy, and 11.3/1,000 at years 2, 3, and 5.

Further reading

Deneux-Tharaux C, Kahn E, Nazerali H, Sokal DC. Pregnancy rates after vasectomy: a survey of US urologists. *Contraception* 2004; **69**: 401–6.

Sandlow JI, Winfield HN, Goldstein M. Surgery of the scrotum and seminal vesicles. In Wein AJ, ed. *Campbell's Urology*. 9th edn. Philadelphia, PA: Elsevier; 2007, pp. 1089–127.

Stein DG. Vasectomy. In Graham SD, Keane TE, eds. *Glenn's Urologic Surgery*. 7th edn. Philadelphia, PA: Wolters Kluwer/ Lippincott Williams & Wilkins; 2010, pp. 372–8.

Trussell J, Lalla AM, Doan QV *et al.* Cost effectiveness of contraceptives in the United States. *Contraception* 2009; **79**: 5–14.

Trussell J, Leveque JA, Koenig JD *et al.* The economic value of contraception: a comparison of 15 methods. *Am J Public Health* 1995; **85**: 494–503.

Chapter

145

Inflatable penile prosthesis

S. Mohammad A. Jafri and Chad M. W. Ritenour

In 1998, the introduction of sildenafil allowed erectile dysfunction to gain public recognition and acknowledgment among men. Subsequently, more and more patients have become comfortable in seeking treatment for this condition. Once erectile dysfunction becomes refractory to medical measures, motivated patients may consider undergoing surgical placement of an inflatable penile prosthesis (IPP). Since its introduction in 1973, the IPP has undergone many revisions and improvements. These changes have allowed for easier surgical insertion, decreased complications, and patient and partner satisfaction rates consistently greater than 90%.

The inflatable penile prosthesis typically comes in two forms: two-piece and three-piece. The difference between the two is that the latter contains a fluid reservoir within the pelvis, which is typically placed below the rectus abdominis fascia. A manually operated internal pump allows for the movement of fluid between the reservoir and cylinders to create an erect penile state. The reservoir within the three-piece IPP allows for greater changes in penile size when compared with the two-piece model, which relies on the movement of much smaller amounts of fluid from the base of the cylinders to the distal ends. In both cases, the penile cylinders are placed within the paired corpora cavernosa, and the pump is located within the base of the scrotum. There are two surgical approaches for placing the implant: infrapubic and penoscrotal. It is currently estimated that ~85% of IPPs are placed penoscrotally, with an occasional abdominal counter-incision for placement of the reservoir. The principle of the IPP is that a patient can squeeze the scrotal pump to allow fluid to fill the penile cylinders, creating tumescence for successful coitus. At the conclusion of intercourse, the release mechanism on the pump is pushed and fluid exits the cylinders, allowing for detumescence. While the basic principles of the device are similar, the specific components depend on the manufacturer of the prosthesis.

After insertion, the cylinders may be left inflated for a short period to provide for better hemostasis. A urethral catheter may be placed at the time of surgery and also left in place for a short interval. Because there can be significant discomfort (often lasting several weeks) in the scrotal area in the initial perioperative period, patients are given a prescription for oral narcotics when they are discharged from the hospital. On a daily basis, patients are instructed to "milk" the scrotal pump towards the base of the scrotum; this will allow the pump to settle into a more dependent and easily accessible position during the healing process. Additionally, patients are advised to wear close-fitting underwear, with the penis pointing cephalad: this will facilitate normal upward deflection of the erect penis. After a period of approximately 6 weeks, patients are trained to cycle the device at least daily to help stretch the newly formed pseudocapsule around the penile cylinders, as well as to practice operating the prosthesis. When inflation can be performed without discomfort, the patient may begin to use the prosthesis for intercourse.

Usual postoperative course

Expected postoperative hospital stay

Hospital stay will last 1 day.

Operative mortality

Operative mortality is very rare.

Special monitoring required

Surgery is performed via general or spinal anesthesia.

Patient activity and position

During surgery, patients may be placed either in the frog-leg, lithotomy, or supine position. Postoperatively, they are allowed to ambulate as desired.

Alimentation

Patients are kept NPO the midnight before surgery. No bowel preparation is required. After surgery, a general diet is restarted.

Antibiotic coverage

Broad-spectrum antibiotics providing both gram-positive and negative coverage should be administered before the incision, and continued for 24 hours after surgery. Examples include

Medical Management of the Surgical Patient, ed. Michael F. Lubin, Thomas F. Dodson, and Neil H. Winawer. Published by Cambridge University Press. © Cambridge University Press 2013.

vancomycin, aminoglycosides, cephalosporins, fluoroquinolones, or ticarcillin-clavulanate. Many surgeons will continue oral antibiotic coverage for up to 1 week after discharge.

Postoperative complications
Infection

Postoperative infection is a feared complication of any prosthetic surgery. With increased understanding of implantation and prosthesis design, the risk of infection has decreased over the years. Careful patient preparation at the time of surgery, including shaving just prior to incision, broad-spectrum perioperative intravenous antibiotics, and a meticulous skin preparation are paramount in reducing this complication. Avoidance of wound infection is especially important given that *Staphylococcus epidermidis* is the most common organism found in infected penile prostheses. Additionally, changes in prosthetic design, specifically the use of antimicrobial-impregnated materials, have lessened the risk of infection. Currently, for virgin placement of an IPP, the risk of infection is 1–3%; however, this risk increases up to 7–18% for revision surgery. Another important risk factor for IPP revision occurs in patients with diabetes. However, recent advances in the device (e.g., an antibiotic-impregnated coating) have helped to lessen this risk to around 1.5%.

Infection of the prosthesis does not typically lead to significant illness. However, serious systemic infections, although rare, can occur. Unfortunately, a prosthetic infection necessitates complete removal of the device. Infections can be defined as early (within a few weeks of implantation) or late (months–years after implantation). Early infections commonly present with erythema, edema, and/or purulent drainage. Late infections may only manifest with persistent or recurrent penile pain. The diagnosis of an infection is made clinically; radiographic assessment does not aid in management. Treatment is with appropriate antibiotics and surgical explantation of all components or, depending on the clinical scenario, washout of the infected spaces and replacement (salvage) with a new device.

Penile cylinder complications

Perforation is an intraoperative event that occurs typically while the corpus cavernosum is being dilated for the eventual placement of the penile cylinders. If urethral injury occurs, the procedure is abandoned and a urethral catheter is left in place for 7–10 days; implantation is performed at a later date. Early implant infections may be related to missed urethral perforations.

Erosion of the cylinders is a postoperative event that can occur along the glans, penile shaft, or scrotum. This complication will typically occur secondary to an infection, or in patients with poor sensation, which can allow pressure on the device components to proceed unheeded. If erosion leads to exposure of the device, all or part of it should be removed. In the case of erosion of a solitary cylinder through the glans and/or meatus, the cylinder should be removed expeditiously. Prompt intervention will avoid the spread of bacteria to the rest of the prosthesis and the potential of a devastating perineal soft-tissue infection. Despite removal of the exposed cylinder, many men are able to achieve coitus with just one cylinder in place. Additionally, after healing, the cylinder may be replaced at a later date as well. The risk of erosion is less with a three-piece IPP; however, this complication may still occur.

Reservoir complications

With the three-piece IPP, a fluid-filled reservoir is placed in the pelvis. Placement is usually below the rectus abdominis fascia, so that the device is non-palpable for the patient. Complications associated with the reservoir include auto-inflation, erosion into surrounding structures, and deep venous thrombosis from iliac compression. Newer-generation IPPs have valves that have significantly reduced the risk of auto-inflation of the penile cylinders from 11% to 1.3%. Case reports have demonstrated that the reservoir can potentially erode into the bladder and/or bowel. Similarly, the reservoir may compress adjacent vasculature, resulting in venous thromboembolism.

Further reading

Bettocchi C, Palumbo F, Spilotros M et al. Patient and partner satisfaction after AMS inflatable penile prosthesis implant. *J Sex Med* 2010; 7: 304–9.

Eldefrawy A, Kava BR. An unusual complication during inflatable penile prosthesis implantation. *Urology* 2010; 76: 847.

Govier FE, Gibbons RP, Correa RJ et al. Mechanical reliability, surgical complications and patient and partner satisfaction of the modern three-piece inflatable penile prosthesis. *Urology* 1998; 52: 282–6.

Leach GE, Shapiro CE, Hadley R et al. Erosion of the inflatable penile prosthesis reservoir into the bladder and bowel. *J Urol* 1988; 131: 367–8.

Mulcahy JJ. Long-term experience with salvage of infected penile implants. *J Urol* 2000; 163: 481–2.

Mulcahy JJ, Carson CC. Long-term infection rates in diabetic patients with antibiotic-impregnated versus nonimpregnated inflatable penile prostheses: 7-year outcomes. *Eur Urol* 2011; 60: 167–72.

Scott FB, Bradley WE, Timm GW. Management of erectile impotence: use of implantable inflatable prosthesis. *Urology* 1973; 2: 80–2.

Wilson SK, Henry GD, Delk JR et al. Mentor Alpha 1 penile prosthesis with reservoir lock-out valve: prevention of auto-inflation with improved capability for ectopic reservoir placement. *J Urol* 2002; 168: 1475–8.

Wilson SK, Delk JR Jr, Salem EA et al. Long-term survival of inflatable penile prostheses: single surgical group experience with 2,384 first-time implants spanning two decades. *J Sex Med* 2007; 4: 1074–9.

Index